MW01174874

Aviation Medicine

Aviation Medicine

Second Edition

Edited by

Air Commodore John Ernsting,
OBE, BSc, PhD, MB, BS, MRCP, MFOM, FRAeS
Royal Air Force Consultant Adviser in Aviation Medicine

Air Vice-Marshal Peter King,
CB, OBE, FRCS(Ed), MFOM, DLO, (RAF Rtd)
Consultant Otolaryngologist, King Edward VII Hospital, Midhurst

Butterworths
London Boston Singapore Sydney Toronto Wellington

All rights reserved. No part of this publication may be reproduced or transmitted in any form or by any means, including photocopying and recording, without the written permission of the copyright holder, application for which should be addressed to the Publishers. Such written permission must also be obtained before any part of this publication is stored in a retrieval system of any nature.

This book is sold subject to the Standard Conditions of Sale of Net Books and may not be resold in the UK below the net price given by the Publishers in their current price list.

First edition published by Tri-Med Books Ltd, 1978
Second edition published by Butterworths, 1988

© **Butterworths & Co (Publishers) Ltd, 1988**

British Library Cataloguing in Publication Data

Ernsting, J.
    Aviation medicine.—2nd ed.
    1. Aviation medicine   2. Space medicine
    I. Title   II. King, Peter
    616.9′8021   RC1062

    ISBN 0-407-01470-5

Library of Congress Cataloging-in-Publication Data

Aviation medicine.

    Includes bibliographies and index.
    1. Aviation medicine.   I. Ernsting, John.   II. King,
P. F.   [DNLM: 1. Aerospace Medicine. WD 700 A957]
RC1062.A95   1988   616.9′80213   87-38209
ISBN 0-407-01470-5

Phototypeset by Scribe Design, Gillingham, Kent
Printed and bound in England at the University Press, Cambridge

Foreword to the first edition

Aviation Medicine, a branch of occupational medicine, developed from the need to adapt man to the hostile environment of the air. At first it was a minor branch of medicine, confined to a small group of mainly military doctors with a preponderantly physiological interest. With the spread of a mass market in air travel, it has become a subject about which no doctor, whatever his specialty, can afford to be ignorant.

The present textbook, written by those concerned with the Farnborough course for the Diploma in Aviation Medicine, brings together all the information which previously existed in a variety of sources – textbooks, journals, papers, records – and the unrecorded experience of those who have spent their lives in aviation medicine research or practice. It is in two volumes in order that the physiological principles may be studied side by side with an occupational or clinical problem – and vice versa. I consider that it is a considerable achievement which will be invaluable to all doctors who have any professional contact with aviation: and an authoritative source-book for the aviation industry, which, more than any other, has to pay heed to the physiological and psychological limitations of man.

Air Marshal Sir Geoffrey Dhenin,
KBE, AFC, GM, QHP, MA, MD, FFCM, FRAeS
Director-General of Royal Air Force Medical Services
(1974–1978)

Preface to the second edition

The unavailability of the first edition of *Aviation Medicine* in 1986 indicated the need either to reprint the book in its original form or to carry out a complete revision and publish a second edition. Consultations with colleagues suggested that the latter was the better course to follow, having regard to the major changes in the past 10 years in aviation physiology and psychology and in clinical aviation medicine. With the demise of Tri-Med Books Limited, the original publishers, Butterworths were approached and they welcomed the opportunity to publish the second edition.

Like the first edition, this book is intended to provide a basic reference textbook for those engaged in the practice of aviation medicine or of occupational medicine when it relates to aviation. It is believed that it will also prove of interest to others in the wider field of aviation. It remains the standard text for those studying for the examination for the Diploma in Aviation Medicine of the Royal College of Physicians of London. While the authorship of the book is wholly British, the ideas expressed and the practices described are the distillate of work carried out by researchers and practitioners worldwide. It is for this reason and for the universality of aviation that this textbook is suitable for reference on a world-wide basis.

Sadly, since the publication of the first edition several of the original authors have died. These are Air-Vice Marshal C.R. Griffin (1979), Air Commodore I.W.H.R. Cran (1978), Air Commodore I.A. McIntosh (1978) and Air Commodore T.J.G. Price (1979). Each of these clinicians made a noteworthy contribution to the specialty and to the first edition, and this is commemorated in this volume. Others have retired, and this alone has necessitated a wide re-selection of authors. Those who have retired include Mr J. Bailey, Mr A.F. Barnes, Mr R.O. Belton, Mr J.G. Boulding,

Squadron Leader R.C. Humphrey, Mr O. Graham-Jones, Dr A.S. Peffers and Dr J.G. Taylor. The Editor-in-Chief, Air Marshal Sir Geoffrey Dhenin, and the editor of Volume 2 of the first edition, Group Captain T.C.D. Whiteside, have retired but continue in medical practice as have several of the original authors including Air Vice-Marshals Sir Ralph Jackson, H.B. Kelly and P.J. O'Connor. Finally, the following have left the practice of the speciality but are still active in other fields: Dr M.H. Harrison, Dr P. Marcus, Dr J.M. Rolfe, Squadron Leader C.A.P.D. Saxton, Wing Commander G.R. Sharp and Dr J.L. Waddell. Wing Commander Sharp made a noteworthy contribution to the first edition, being sole author of 11 chapters and joint author of a further four as well as joint editor of Volume 1.

A major change has been made in presentation in the second edition. All parts of the book have been bound into one volume for greater ease of cross-reference and handling. Hopefully, this new format will find favour.

Three major changes in the contents of the book have been introduced in this edition. First, the section on Aviation Psychology has been completely rewritten; second, Group Captain Nicholson's chapter on Irregular Work and Rest has been expanded into two chapters and moved to the clinical section; third, a whole new section deals with the important topics of Accident Investigation and Aviation Pathology. Group Captain Cullen, whilst withdrawing from authorship, continued to make a valuable contribution to this section. Other changes in the second edition include the radical rewriting of most of the chapters on the clinical aspects of aviation medicine. This is to accommodate the many changes that had occurred in clinical practice, the increasing importance of certain aspects of the specialty and to provide a wider text of information for clinicians.

Finally, all the chapters on aviation physiology have been revised either by the original authors or new authors, all of whom except one are members of the staff of the RAF Institute of Aviation Medicine.

The references have been expanded to include key papers and further reading for those wishing to pursue the literature on specific aspects of the subject.

Systéme Internationale (SI) Units have been employed throughout the text but the convention of specifying aircraft altitude in feet and aircraft speed in knots has been retained. Furthermore, respired gas tensions and blood pressure values have been expressed primarily in millimetres of mercury. The Appendix on Units of Measurement has been expanded to include the derivation of relevant SI units and tables for conversions between SI and other commonly used units.

We wish to express our appreciation to successive Directors General of the Royal Air Force Medical Services and Air Vice-Marshal P. Howard OBE, QHP, Commandant, Royal Air Force Institute of Aviation Medicine for continued encouragement and support; to Dr Geoffrey Bennett, Chief Medical Officer of the Civil Aviation Authority, for his help in planning the layout and in the selection of authors; and finally to Dr Frank Preston, Director of Medical and Safety Services, British Airways, for advice on the practical aspects of aviation medicine related to commercial flying.

Our thanks are also due to Ms Sue Deeley of Butterworths for continued help during the production of this book and to Mr Alan Taman for his valuable contribution to the final product. As in all works of this nature, the secretaries of the editors and authors have borne a heavy burden, and we are grateful to them.

J. Ernsting
P.F. King

Preface to the first edition

Volume 1—Physiology and human factors

The environment of flight is essentially unnatural to man and one which imposes considerable demands on him. For the successful practice of civil and military aviation medicine it is necessary to have an understanding of those aspects of physiology and psychology which deal with the human response to the stresses of flight and to be familiar with with principles of protecting man against the hostile environment of flight. This volume provides the fundamentals of these aspects of aviation medicine in a comprehensive yet easily assimilated form.

When Air Vice-Marshal H.L. Roxburgh CBE QHS, Commandant of the Royal Air Force Institute of Aviation Medicine from 1967 to 1973, originally conceived the idea of a textbook of aviation medicine he believed that the uniformity of style and presentation of single authorship would be of advantage in a work of this type. Accordingly, the formidable task of writing such a textbook was undertaken by Wing Commander D.I. Fryer OBE, then a Consultant in Aviation Medicine at the Institute. With little more than a few chapters written in draft form, the preparation of the textbook was halted by Wing Commander Fryer's untimely and tragic death. Following the loss of such a wealth of personal experience and an inimitable literary style, it was decided that this textbook should be of multiple authorship and consist of two companion volumes, one dealing with the physiological and psychological aspects and the other with the occupational and clinical aspects of aviation medicine.

This volume has been prepared by members of staff of the Royal Air Force Institute of Aviation Medicine. An attempt has been made to maintain a style normally associated with single authorship and the aims of the textbook have been maintained as close as possible to those originally conceived. In general, the structure of the text for each major environmental stress, such as changes of pressure (Part I), long and short duration acceleration (Part II) and extremes of temperature (Part III) follows the same arrangement. This includes an introductory resumé of the relevant normal functions and performance, the manner in which these are affected by the stress, the limits of human tolerance and finally the applied physiology and psychology of the methods used to minimize impairment of performance in flight due to the stress. By its three-dimensional nature, flight may engender unusual inputs to the central nervous system which can grossly impair performance. The fourth part of this volume is devoted, therefore, to the special senses of sight, hearing and spatial disorientation. Since irregular rest and work frequently arise in both civil and military aircraft operations, the effects of these on performance and the manner in which resulting impairment can be reduced is the subject of a separate chapter in this part of the text. A significant part of the volume is devoted to the basic concepts and methods of psychology as applied to aviation. This emphasis is necessary because of the importance of an understanding of human behaviour in maintaining safety and efficiency in flight.

Written primarily for physicians and biological scientists involved in aviation matters and those in the field of industrial medicine, the text of this volume assumes that the reader has a basic knowledge of human physiology to the standard taught to medical students. It contains the basic and applied physiology and psychology required by physicians studying for the Diploma in Aviation Medicine of the Royal College of Physicians (London) and Royal College of Surgeons (England). This and its companion volume will also serve as a concise source of information for the aircraft industry generally, its engineers, designers, component manufacturers and operators for whom a knowledge of aviation meicine topics which arise within their own specialized fields is essential.

We wish to express our appreciation of the general advice and guidance given by Group Captain P. Howard OBE, Commandant, Royal Air Force Institute of Aviation Medicine, the specialist advice given by Wing Commander D.H. Glaister and D.C. Reader, the assistance provided by the Drawing Office, Photographic and Typing Sections of the Institute and the excellent secretarial support by Miss L. Couzens.

G.R. Sharp
J. Ernsting
(Editors, Volume 1)

Volume 2—Health and clinical aspects

Aviation Medicine is one aspect of occupational medicine and, as such, before applying medical knowledge to its special problems, the doctor must first understand the environment and its interaction with the man, whether professional aviator or a passenger who may be well or unwell.

Since man is not naturally adapted to it, the flight environment is particularly demanding. Usually, adaptation to the environment takes place through physiological mechanisms which are concerned with maintaining what Claude Bernard called the stable 'milieu interieur', but in aviation, the environment may change so quickly that these adaptive mechanisms may compensate too slowly or even inappropriately. It is therefore essential for the good practice of aviation medicine, that the doctor should be familiar with the physiological and psychological effects of this particular environment upon the individual. The reader who requires that insight into the specialty would therefore be well advised to study this volume in conjunction with its companion volume *Aviation Medicine—Physiology and Human Factors*.

As regards the professional aviator, it is necessary to select individuals who are most suited to an occupation which requires physiological aids of one sort or another; to train them in the use of these aids; to keep them under surveillance while they follow the occupation; and to relate any pathological or psychological changes in them, temporary or permanent, to the demands of the occupation. On the other hand, those who enter the environment temporarily as passengers, being usually unselected, are bound to present the widest spectrum of age and health and, though their exposure to the environment may be short, it may well be critical.

In the following chapters, the authors have been mainly concerned with the professional aviator but they have also included both clinical and epidemiological information which, taken with a good scientific basis, will equip the reader with the means to promote the health of all those connected with aviation, whether they be aircrew or passengers.

Inevitably the topics have tended to be considered on the basis of UK civil and military practice, but throughout, an attempt has been made to play down the more parochial questions and to bring into focus, principles which, if sufficiently broad, should avoid any shade of chauvinism. With a multi-author book, the degree of detail and the styles are bound to vary. The Editorial Board have therefore tried to achieve a degree of uniformity in the presentation whilst interfering as little as possible with the styles of the individual contributors.

Of the clinical chapters, it will be obvious that ophthalmology, otorhinolaryngology and neuropsychiatry are much fuller in their treatment of the subject. This has been largely planned, since the Editors considered that these three areas were perhaps those in which the non-specialist may find the biggest gap between his clinical practice, and the searching examination required of an individual on whose physical and mental fitness under stress, depend the lives of hundreds of passengers.

T.C.D. Whiteside
(Editor, Volume 2)

Contributors

J R Allan, MB, BS, MFOM
Principal Medical Officer Research, Royal Air
Force Institute of Aviation Medicine, Farnborough,
Hants GU14 6SZ

E Anthony, MD, FRCPsych, DCH, *Group Captain,*
Royal Air Force Consultant Adviser in Psychiatry,
Central Medical Establishment, Royal Air Force
Kelvin House, Cleveland Street, London W1P 6AU

D J Anton, MSc, MB, BS, DAvMed, MFOM, *Wing
Commander*
Royal Air Force Consultant in Aviation Medicine,
Royal Air Force Institute of Aviation Medicine,
Farnborough, Hants GU14 6SZ

M Bagshaw, MB, BCh, MRCS, LRCP, DAvMed, AFOM,
FRAeS, *Squadron Leader (RAF Rtd)*
Lately Senior Medical Officer Pilot, Royal Air
Force Institute of Aviation Medicine, Farnborough,
Hants GU14 6SZ

A J C Balfour, CBE, MA, MB, BChir, FRCPath, DCP,
DTM&H, MRAeS, *Group Captain*
Royal Air Force Adviser in Aviation Pathology and
Consultant in Pathology and Tropical Medicine,
Royal Air Force Institute of Pathology and Tropical
Medicine, Halton, Aylesbury, Bucks HP22 5PG

A J Benson, BSc, MSc, MB, ChB, FRAeS
Senior Medical Officer Research, Royal Air Force
Institute of Aviation Medicine, Farnborough, Hants
GU14 6SZ

D H Brennan, MA, LMSSA, DO, AFOM
Medical Officer Research, Royal Air Force Institute
of Aviation Medicine, Farnborough, Hants GU14
6SZ

J W Chappelow, BSc
Senior Psychologist, Royal Air Force Institute of
Aviation Medicine, Farnborough, Hants GU14 6SZ

Muriel A Churchill, BSc, PhD
Psychologist, Royal Air Force Institute of Aviation
Medicine, Farnborough, Hants GU14 6SZ

J K Cloherty, MB, BCh, DO, FRCS, *Group Captain*
Royal Air Force Consultant Adviser in
Ophthalmology, Central Medical Establishment,
Royal Air Force Kelvin House, Cleveland Street,
London W1P 6AU

J N C Cooke, CB, OBE, MD, BS, FRCP, FRCP(Edin),
MFOM, MRCS, *Air Vice-Marshal (RAF Rtd)*
Consultant Physician to the Civil Aviation
Authority, CAA House, 45–59 Kingsway, London
WC2B 6TE

J Ernsting, OBE, BSc, PhD, MB, BS, MRCP, MFOM, FRAeS,
Air Commodore
Royal Air Force Consultant Adviser in Aviation
Medicine, Royal Air Force Institute of Aviation
Medicine, Farnborough, Hants GU14 6SZ

E W Farmer, BSc, PhD
Senior Psychologist, Royal Air Force Institute of
Aviation Medicine, Farnborough, Hants GU14 6SZ

G A Faux, MRCS, LRCP
Principal Medical Officer, Health Control Unit,
Heathrow Airport (London), Hounslow, Middlesex

D H Glaister, BSc, PhD, MB, BS, *Group Captain*
Royal Air Force Consultant in Aviation Medicine,
Royal Air Force Institute of Aviation Medicine,
Farnborough, Hants GU14 6SZ. Also Whittingham

Professor of Aviation Medicine, Royal College of Physicians, London

R G Green, BSc
Principal Psychologist, Royal Air Force Institute of Aviation Medicine, Farnborough, Hants GU14 6SZ

R L Green, MB, ChB, DAvMed, MFOM
Principal Medical Officer, British Airways Medical Service, Heathrow Airport (London), Hounslow, Middlesex

R M Harding, BSc, PhD, MB, BS, DAvMed, MRAeS, FBIS
Royal Air Force Consultant in Aviation Medicine, Royal Air Force Institute of Aviation Medicine, Farnborough, Hants GU14 6SZ

T C Harris, SDA
Harris Associates Ltd, Crab Hill Farm, South Nutfield, Redhill, Surrey

I R Hill, MA, MD, BChir, LDS, MRAeS, *Wing Commander*
Royal Air Force Senior Specialist in Pathology, Royal Air Force Institute of Pathology and Tropical Medicine, Halton, Aylesbury, Bucks HP22 5PG

J A C Hopkirk, MB, FRCP, *Wing Commander (RAF Rtd)*
Royal Air Force Civilian Consultant in Chest Diseases, Royal Air Force Chest Unit, King Edward VII Hospital, Midhurst, West Sussex

D H Hull, MA, MB BChir, FRCP *Air Commodore*
Royal Air Force Consultant Adviser in Medicine, Central Medical Establishment, Royal Air Force Kelvin House, Cleveland Street, London W1P 6AU

P J Jerram, AIMLS, MRSH
Principal Hygiene Adviser, British Airways, Heathrow Airport, Hounslow, Middlesex

G E Joss, MRCVS
Veterinary Adviser to International Aviation Transport Association, 10 Park Lane East, Reigate, Surrey

C T Kirkpatrick, BSc, MB, BCh, BAO, MD
Medical Officer Research, Royal Air Force Institute of Aviation Medicine, Farnborough, Hants GU14 6SZ

P F King, CB, OBE, FRCS(Ed), MFOM, DLO, MRAeS, *Air Vice-Marshal (RAF Rtd)*
Consultant Otolaryngologist, King Edward VII Hospital, Midhurst, West Sussex. Lately the Senior Consultant Royal Air Force, Royal Air Force Consultant Adviser in Otorhinolaryngology and Whittingham Professor in Aviation Medicine, Royal College of Physicians, London

A J F Macmillan, BSc, MB, ChB, MFOM
Senior Medical Officer Research, Royal Air Force Institute of Aviation Medicine, Farnborough, Hants GU14 6SZ

Margaret M MacPherson, MB, ChB, DA
Airport Medical Officer, Health Control Unit, Heathrow Airport (London), Hounslow, Middlesex

R T G Merry, MB, MRCPsych, FRCP, *Wing Commander*
Royal Air Force Consultant and Adviser in Neurology, Princess Alexandra Hospital, Royal Air Force Wroughton, Nr Swindon, Wilts SN4 0QJ

Sandra Mooney, MB, ChB, MFOM, DAvMed
British Airways Medical Service, Heathrow Airport (London), Hounslow, Middlesex

A N Nicholson, OBE, DSc, FRCP(Ed), FRCPath, *Group Captain*
Royal Air Force Consultant in Aviation Medicine, Royal Air Force Institute of Aviation Medicine, Farnborough, Hants GU14 6SZ

A J Palmer, BSc, CEng, MRAeS
Principal Engineer, Mechanical and Safety Systems, British Airways, Heathrow Airport (London), Hounslow, Middlesex

F S Preston, OBE, VRD, MB, ChB, DA, FFOM, FRAeS
Consultant Physician to British Heart Foundation. Lately Director Medical Services, British Airways Medical Services, Speedbird House, Heathrow Airport (London), Hounslow, Middlesex

D J Rainford, MBE, MB, BS, FRCP, *Wing Commander*
Royal Air Force Consultant and Adviser in Renal Disease, Princess Mary's Royal Air Force Hospital, Halton, Aylesbury, Bucks HP22 5PG

C C G Rawll, MB, ChB, MFOM, DTPH, CIH
Principal Medical Officer (Ground), British Airways Medical Services, Speedbird House, Heathrow Airport (London), Hounslow, Middlesex

G M Rood, MSc, PhD, CEng, MI Mech E, MRAeS
Principal Scientific Officer, Flight Systems Department, Royal Aircraft Establishment, Farnborough, Hants GU14 6TD

P J Sowood, MA, BM, BCh, DAvMed, *Squadron Leader*
Royal Air Force Specialist in Aviation Medicine, Royal Air Force Institute of Aviation Medicine, Farnborough, Hants GU14 6SZ

J M Stewart, MB, ChB, DTM&H
Senior Medical Officer (Immunizations), British Airways, British Airways Medical Service, 75 Regents Street, London

J R R Stott, MA, MB, BChir, MRCP, DCH, DIC, DAvMed
Medical Officer Research, Royal Air Force Institute
of Aviation Medicine, Farnborough, Hants GU14
6SZ

D W Trump, MB, ChB, DAvMed
Senior Medical Officer, Civil Aviation Authority
(London), 45–59 Kingsway, London WC2B 6TE

J C D Turner, MB, BS, MRCS, LRCP, DAvMed, AFOM,
MRAeS, *Surgeon Commander*
Royal Navy Senior Specialist in Occupational
Medicine, Royal Air Force Institute of Aviation
Medicine, Farnborough, Hants GU14 6SZ

H J K Vieyra, MBE, MCh Orth, MB, BS, FRCS, FRCS(Ed),
Air Commodore
Royal Air Force Consultant Adviser in Orthopaedic
Surgery, Central Medical Establishment, Royal Air
Force Kelvin House, Cleveland Street, London
W1P 6AU

Contents

Part I – The Pressure Environment

3   1   The Earth's Atmosphere   R.M. Harding

13   2   The Effects of Pressure Change   G.R. Sharp, revised by A.J.F. Macmillan

19   3   Decompression Sickness   A.J.F. Macmillan

27   4   Respiratory Physiology   J. Ernsting

45   5   Hypoxia and Hyperventilation   J. Ernsting and G.R. Sharp, revised by R.M. Harding

60   6   Prevention of Hypoxia   G.R. Sharp and J. Ernsting, revised by A.J.F. Macmillan

72   7   Oxygen Equipment and Pressure Clothing   R.M. Harding

112   8   The Pressure Cabin   A.J.F. Macmillan

127   9   Toxic Gases and Vapours in Flight   G.R. Sharp, revised by D.J. Anton

Part II – Biodynamics

139   10   The Effects of Long Duration Acceleration   D.H. Glaister

159   11   Protection Against Long Duration Acceleration   D.H. Glaister

166   12   Crash Dynamics and Restraint Systems   D.J. Anton

174   13   Head Injury and Protection   D.H. Glaister

185   14   Vibration   J.R.R. Stott

200   15   Escape from Aircraft   D.J. Anton

Part III – Thermal Stress and Survival

219   16   The Thermal Environment and Human Heat Exchange   J.R. Allan

235   17   Thermal Physiology   C.T. Kirkpatrick

247   18   Thermal Protection   J.R. Allan

261   19   Survival   P.J. Sowood and J.R. Allan

Part IV – The Special Senses

277   20   Spatial Disorientation – General aspects   A.J. Benson

297   21   Spatial Disorientation – Common illusions   A.J. Benson

318   22   Motion Sickness   A.J. Benson

339 23 Vision in Flight   D.H. Brennan

353 24 Noise and Communication   G.M. Rood

Part V – Aviation Psychology

385   Introduction to Aviation Psychology   R.G. Green

391 25 Perception   R.G. Green

402 26 Cognitive Processes   E.W. Farmer

414 27 Individual Differences   E.W. Farmer

423 28 Selection and Training   J.W. Chappelow and M. Churchill

435 29 Stress and Workload   E.W. Farmer

445 30 Ergonomics   R.G. Green and E.W. Farmer

458 31 Social Psychology   R.G. Green

Part VI – Special Types of Flight

471 32 Medical Aspects of Special Types of Flight   R.M. Harding (with contributions by J.C.D. Turner and M. Bagshaw)

Part VII – Commercial Aviation and Health

493 33 Commercial Aviation and Health – General Aspects   F.S. Preston

497 34 Health and Safety Aspects of Aircraft Design   A.J. Palmer

501 35 Medical Standards for Civilian Aircrew   D.W. Trump

Part VIII – Health and Hygiene

517 36 International Health Regulations   G.A. Faux and M.M. MacPherson

527 37 Epidemiological and Immunological Problems in International Travel   J.M. Stewart

534 38 Airline Hygiene   P.J. Jerram

542 39 Health of Airline Ground Staff   C.C.G. Rawll

551 40 Carriage of Invalid Passengers by Civil Airlines   R.L. Green and S.E. Mooney

558 41 Airfreight – Health and Safety in the Air Transport of Animals   G.E. Joss and T. Harris

Part IX – Clinical Aspects of Aviation Medicine

565 42 Sleep and Wakefulness: Clinical Considerations   A.N. Nicholson

576 43 Aircrew and their Sleep   A.N. Nicholson

585 44 Cardiovascular Diseases   J.N.C. Cooke

597 45 Respiratory Diseases   .J.A.C. Hopkirk

604 46 Renal Disease   D.J. Rainford

609 47 Other Important Medical Conditions   D.H. Hull

619 48 Psychiatry   E. Anthony

644 49 Neurology   R.T.G. Merry

649 50 Otorhinolaryngology   P.F. King

666 51 Ophthalmological Conditions and the Examination of the Eye   J. Cloherty

688 52 Orthopaedics   H.J.K. Vieyra and D.J. Anton

Part X – Accident Investigation

697   53   Accident Investigation and its Management   A.J.C. Balfour

703   54   Aviation Pathology   A.J.C. Balfour

710   55   Dental Identification   I.R. Hill

715   **Appendix – Units of Measurement**   R.M. Harding

725   **Index**

Part I

The Pressure Environment

1

The Earth's atmosphere

R.M. Harding

Introduction

This chapter is concerned with the nature of our atmosphere: its physics, its composition, and its structure. It is also concerned with those aspects of applied atmospherics that are of direct relevance to aviation in general and aviation medicine in particular. Thus the chapter includes a brief description of International Standard Atmospheres, and ends with a discussion of the elementary gas laws and conditions of measurement with especial emphasis on the implications that these have for human physiology.

The biosphere is that part of the universe in which life can be sustained without artificial support. At present, this comprises the Earth's land and sea masses, the lithosphere and hydrosphere respectively, and the enveloping mass of air, the atmosphere, above them. This gaseous atmosphere is essential to life on our planet: it supplies the oxygen required for the release of biological energy, it forms a barrier which protects life from the harmful effects of incident cosmic radiation, and it provides a temperature environment at the Earth's surface which is compatible with life. Man has evolved in the gaseous environment maintained by the atmosphere at the surface of the Earth, and ascent into the upper layers of the atmosphere produces the gross physiological disturbances that are described in succeeding chapters.

Physics of the atmosphere

Density and pressure

The atmosphere extends from the surface of the Earth to a distance determined by two opposing factors: thermal radiation from the Sun and the gravitational attraction exerted by the Earth. Thermal solar radiation tends to expand gases in the outer atmosphere into the surrounding vacuum of space, whilst the Earth's gravitational attraction tends to contract the gases back towards its surface. Thus the density (that is, mass per unit volume) of the atmosphere, and hence the pressure (that is, force (i.e. mass) per unit area) exerted by it, falls progressively with ascent from the surface of the Earth towards space. Because gas is compressible, density and pressure both fall in an approximately exponential manner with vertical distance (altitude) from the Earth's surface, although small departures from a true exponential decline are caused by variations in temperature at different altitudes.

The pressure exerted at sea level by the weight of the atmosphere is 14.7 lb/in^2 (101.3 kPa), and this *atmospheric pressure* will support a column of mercury (Hg) in an evacuated tube to a height of 760 mm. The atmospheric pressure at sea level can therefore be expressed as 760 mm Hg. As *Figure 1.1* shows, this pressure is halved to 380 mm Hg at an altitude of 18 000 feet, and reduced to one quarter (190 mm Hg) at an altitude of 33 700 feet. At 100 000 feet, the atmospheric pressure is one-hundredth of that at sea level.

At an altitude of about 262 000 feet (50 miles, 80 km) (the von Karman Line), collisions between molecules within the atmosphere (that is, the physical nature of pressure) become so infrequent that aerodynamic forces are no longer effective and manoeuvrability of craft must be achieved by rockets or reaction jets powered by internally carried fuel. At even greater altitudes, the density of the atmosphere is so low that particles within it travel considerable distances without colliding with each other at all. Some of the lighter particles with

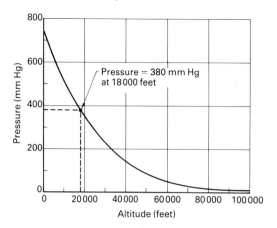

Figure 1.1 The exponential relationship between the pressure exerted by the atmosphere and altitude.

high velocities escape from the Earth's gravitational attraction and move out into space. The altitude at which this occurs can be regarded as the upper limit of the atmosphere and is the beginning of true space. The escape level is about 435 miles (700 km) above the surface of the Earth, and the transitional zone above it, where the atmosphere thins out into the complete vacuum of space, is termed the exosphere (*see* below). Even at this altitude, the influence of Earth's gravitational attraction is considerable, and it is not until an altitude of 1700 miles (2735 km) is reached that it has fallen to half its sea level value.

Temperature

The temperature of the atmosphere varies markedly with altitude (*Figure 1.2*). Furthermore, for any given altitude, there are considerable geographical and temporal differences in temperature. Clearly, both the Earth and its atmosphere are warmed by the Sun, but there are several different mechanisms in this process. Whilst some solar radiation is reflected away into space by the outermost layers of the atmosphere, and some is absorbed in the upper layers, the bulk of the infra-red radiation from the Sun penetrates the atmosphere and reaches the Earth's surface. The warm ground then heats the air immediately above it, partly by conduction but mainly by radiation, again in the infra-red spectrum but at different frequencies (wavelengths). This radiation is absorbed by carbon dioxide and water vapour in the lower atmosphere and, in turn, these lower layers re-radiate part of the infra-red energy. Some returns to the surface of the Earth to be radiated yet again, whilst the remainder passes up to be absorbed in the higher layers of the atmosphere.

The overall effect of these processes is that the Earth's surface is rather warmer than it would be if it received heat direct from the Sun in the absence of the atmospheric blanket: the so-called 'greenhouse effect'.

Heating the surface of the Earth in this manner creates convection currents in the lower layers of the atmosphere, and these play a key role in the circulation patterns of weather and climate. The temperature of the lower layers, heated primarily by infra-red radiation from the Earth's surface, normally falls progressively as altitude increases (although temperature inversions do occur at low altitudes and are, for example, the reason why fog does not disperse). This fall in temperature is, however, halted and reversed above about 60 000 feet at the equator (42 000 feet at the poles) by the heat produced in the ozonosphere (*see* below), and the consequent inversion inhibits convection so that weather is a phenomenon that is present only at lower altitudes. Above the ozonosphere there is another region in which cooling predominates, while further still from the surface of the Earth, above an altitude of about 50 miles, the temperature rises yet again. Despite this progressive increase in temperature, the rise has no thermal significance since the density of the particles is so low. In this region, however, the combination of the very low density of the air and the intense ultraviolet radiation means that virtually all gases are present as charged atoms and there is a relatively high concentration of free electrons. The layers of charged particles form the ionosphere, the structure of which varies with the input to it of energy from the Sun, and which is markedly affected by the 11-year cycle of solar flare activity. The ionosphere acts as a reflector for the long-wavelength electromagnetic radiation which is used for radio communication between distant points on the Earth's surface.

Ionizing radiation

The Earth is continuously bombarded from space by high-energy sub-atomic primary particles consisting of protons (about 79%), alpha particles (helium nuclei) (20%) and nuclei of heavier atoms (heavy primaries) (1%). This particulate material originates either from the Sun (solar cosmic radiation) or from other stars (galactic cosmic radiation), and enters the atmosphere travelling at high velocity; in some cases approaching that of light. As the ionizing radiation enters the upper regions of the atmosphere the primary particles collide with atoms within it at altitudes between 60 000 and 120 000 feet to produce a secondary radiation of protons, electrons, neutrons, mesons and gamma rays. Such secondary radiation has considerably less energy than does its precursor but is capable of intense ionization. Secondary rays penetrate the lower regions of the atmosphere but, although some reach the surface of the Earth, their ionizing power diminishes rapidly at altitudes below 50 000 feet as further collisions occur with atmospheric molecules. At sea level, the ionizing effect of cosmic radiation is only about one-seventieth of that encountered at an altitude of 70 000 feet. The implications of ionizing radiation upon the occupants of supersonic transport aircraft and manned spacecraft are discussed in Chapter 32.

Composition of the atmosphere

The composition of the atmosphere is remarkably constant between sea level and an altitude of about 300 000 feet. Air is a mixture of nitrogen, oxygen and argon, together with traces of carbon dioxide and certain rare gases such as neon and helium. *Table 1.1* lists the percentage by volume constituents of dry air.

Table 1.1 The composition of the atmosphere

Gas	Concentration in dry air (% by volume)
Nitrogen	78.09
Oxygen	20.95
Argon	0.93
Carbon dioxide	0.03
Neon	1.82×10^{-3}
Helium	5.24×10^{-4}
Krypton	1.14×10^{-4}
Hydrogen	5.00×10^{-5}
Xenon	8.70×10^{-6}

The composition of air close to the surface of the Earth is sometimes modified slightly from that listed in the table by the products of human activity, such as factory effluent and engine exhausts, or by natural phenomena, such as volcanoes and geysers. There may be significant increases in the concentration of carbon dioxide in the air near such activity, as well as measurable levels of toxic contaminants such as carbon monoxide and methane. The lower regions of the atmosphere, up to an altitude of about 30 000 feet, may also contain significant quantities of water vapour. The concentration of water within a given mass of air depends largely upon its location (that is, whether it is or has recently been located over an area of water) and upon the air temperature. The higher the temperature of the mass of air, the greater will be its capacity for water vapour. Despite this, for most practical purposes, dry air may be regarded as a mixture consisting of 21% oxygen and 79% nitrogen.

Ozone

Ozone (O_3), the triatomic form of oxygen, is another important constituent of the atmosphere and is present in significant concentrations at altitudes between 40 000 feet and 140 000 feet. It is a blue, unstable gas formed by the irradiation of molecular oxygen in the upper atmosphere by short-wavelength (200 nm) ultraviolet light from the Sun. The ultraviolet radiation is absorbed and the oxygen molecules are split into free atoms which then either recombine with each other, to reform molecular oxygen, or combine with other oxygen molecules to form ozone. The amount of ozone formed at a given altitude thus depends upon the concentration of oxygen molecules and the intensity of ultraviolet radiation. Above about 350 000 feet, ultraviolet radiation is so intense that all molecular oxygen is dissociated into oxygen atoms; whilst below that altitude, molecular oxygen is more abundant and the ultraviolet radiation less intense so that conditions for ozone production are created. Consequently, the concentration of ozone increases progressively as altitude is reduced below about 140 000 feet to reach a maximum level of approximately 10.0 parts per million by volume (ppmv) by 100 000 feet (*see Figure 1.2*). Below this altitude,

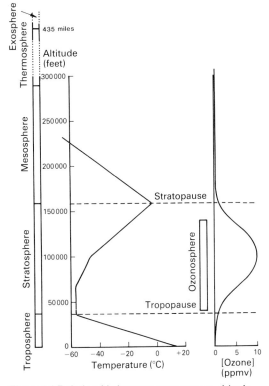

Figure 1.2 Relationship between temperature, altitude, and the layers of the atmosphere (including the ozonosphere).

ultraviolet radiation is much less intense, as a consequence of atmospheric absorption, and oxygen molecules are more numerous, and so the concentration of ozone falls progressively to a value of less than 1.0 ppmv at altitudes below 40 000 feet, and to about 0.03 ppmv at sea level. Furthermore, at these lower altitudes, ozone is dissociated to molecular oxygen by longer wavelength (210–300 nm) ultraviolet light.

The formation and destruction of ozone in the atmosphere is of great physical and biological importance. The absorption of ultraviolet light, of wavelengths between 200 and 300 nm, associated with these processes in the upper parts of the atmosphere greatly reduces the intensity of this biologically harmful radiation reaching the surface of the Earth. In addition, the continuous destruction of ozone in the same regions is associated with the release of heat, and this exothermic reaction is largely responsible for the progressive rise in temperature that occurs during ascent from about 70 000 feet to 160 000 feet.

Ozone itself is a highly toxic gas, exerting its clinical effects primarily upon the respiratory tract. Acute exposure to concentrations of 0.6–0.8 ppmv for 2 hours is sufficient to reduce vital capacity and forced expiratory volume, and to cause a fall in diffusing capacity for carbon monoxide, presumably as a consequence of alveolar oedema. Exposure to just 1.0 ppmv is sufficient to cause lung irritation, while 10.0 ppmv can cause fatal pulmonary oedema. In addition, ozone has been shown to impair night vision in man, and exposure of human cell cultures to ozone induces chromatid breakages similar to those produced by X-rays. The potentially serious implications of supersonic travel within the ozone layer are considered in Chapter 32.

Structure of the atmosphere

It is convenient to consider the atmosphere as comprising a number of concentric shells, each with its own characteristics. One of the most valuable and widely used approaches is that based upon the thermal features of each region. The successive layers of the atmosphere from the surface of the Earth outwards are: the troposphere, the stratosphere, the mesosphere, the thermosphere and the exosphere. The outer edge of each 'sphere' is termed a 'pause'; thus, for example, the edge of the troposphere is the tropopause and the edge of the stratosphere is the stratopause.

The original form of this description was produced before variations of temperature and pressure in the upper atmosphere had been measured directly. Thus, as originally defined, the air temperature within the troposphere fell linearly with increasing altitude to the tropopause where it became a constant value ($-56.5°C$), and remained so throughout the stratosphere. As data on the physical characteristics of the upper atmosphere became available, it was apparent that there were large changes of temperature within the stratosphere, especially in its upper region, and several sub-divisions of that layer are now recognized. *Figure 1.2* depicts the relationship of temperature and altitude to these various regions. It must be noted, however, that the divisions of the atmosphere are somewhat arbitrary, and that the extent of a given sphere will vary markedly with latitude and season.

The troposphere

The troposphere is characterized by a relatively constant rate of fall of temperature with increasing altitude, the presence of water vapour, and the presence of large-scale air turbulence (weather). The fall of temperature with altitude is termed the temperature lapse-rate and depends largely upon local conditions. The mean lapse-rate in still air is about 2°C per 1000 feet. The decline in temperature ceases at the tropopause, the altitude of which varies with latitude and time of year. Since the intensity of solar energy received at the surface of the Earth is greater at the equator than at the poles, the air at the equator is hotter and consequently rises further than the air at the poles. Thus the altitude of the tropopause varies from approximately 58 000 feet at the equator to approximately 26 000 feet at the poles. The temperature gradient seen in the troposphere therefore ranges from an average 15°C at sea level to about $-83°C$ over the equator and to about $-53°C$ over the poles. It is this gradient that is partly responsible for weather phenomena; phenomena confined to the troposphere.

The stratosphere

As originally defined, the stratosphere was characterized by a fairly uniform temperature and an almost complete absence of water vapour. It extends from the tropopause to an altitude of about 158 000 feet (30 miles, 50 km). It is now known that the temperature is only constant in the lower part of the stratosphere, termed the isothermal layer, and that temperature increases with altitude from about 90 000 feet to reach a maximum of $-3°C$ at the stratopause. The increase in temperature is produced by the heat liberated by the dissociation of ozone in this region, which is consequently termed the ozonosphere and which extends from an altitude of about 40 000 feet to 140 000 feet.

The mesosphere

The mesosphere, or middle region, is characterized by a rapid decline in temperature, from the $-3°C$ of its base at the stratopause, to about $-113°C$ at an altitude of 290 000 feet (55 miles, 85 km).

The thermosphere

The thermosphere is the uppermost region of the atmosphere and is characterized by a continuous increase in temperature to values that are dependent upon the activity of the Sun. Temperatures can exceed 1500°C during days of maximum solar activity but may fall to 227°C during nights of solar calm. In air of such low density, however, temperature has no thermal significance for the air itself; but does of course for any body within it, hence the nature of Icarus' demise. The upper limit of the thermosphere lies at an altitude of about 435 miles (700 km); that is, at the extreme edge of the atmosphere. Since most of the particles within this layer are charged, it is also known as the ionosphere.

The exosphere

Within the exosphere, which is the start of true space, collisions between particles are so rare as to be considered not to occur at all, and gas atoms may be regarded as having free-space trajectories. The concept of temperature no longer has the customary meaning, although if it did the exosphere would be an isothermal layer which extended into deep space.

Standard atmospheres

The need to standardize the description of the relationship between barometric pressure and altitude has been recognized ever since pressure-measuring instruments were introduced to indicate the altitude of a balloon or aircraft above the ground. Such a standard can be used as the basis for calibration of flight instruments, and to allow accurate comparisons to be made between the performance of various aircraft and aircraft systems. The first internationally accepted standard atmosphere was prepared by the International Committee on Air Navigation (ICAN) in 1924, and this used simple laws to define the relationship between pressure and altitude. Over the following years, a number of different standards were prepared and adopted both nationally and internationally: for example, the United States (US) Standard, the

Wright Air Development Centre (WADC) Standard, the Air Research and Development Centre (ARDC) Standard, and the International Civil Aviation Organization (ICAO) Standard. These standards, which differ one from another in the temperature–altitude convention employed in their construction, are very similar (and indeed identical in their most recent versions) for altitudes up to 65 000 feet. The most commonly used standard atmospheres are the US (1962) and ICAO (1964) constructions, and these are identical from mean sea level to an altitude of 100 000 feet.

The ICAO Standard Atmosphere (1964)

The widely used 1964 ICAO Standard Atmosphere closely represents the pressure and temperature characteristics of the real atmosphere at the temperate latitude of 45°North. The relationship between pressure and altitude defined by this standard, and listed in an abbreviated form at *Table 1.2*, is based upon the following 'ideal' assumptions:

1. The air is dry, devoid of dust, and has a stated composition (that given in *Table 1.1*).
2. The atmospheric pressure at mean sea level is 760 mm Hg.
3. The atmospheric density at mean sea level is 1.225 kg/m^3.
4. The relative molecular mass of air at mean sea level is 28.9644.
5. Acceleration due to gravity is 9.80665 m/s^2, and is constant.
6. The temperature–altitude profile is:
   (a) Temperature at mean sea level = +15°C.
   (b) Mean temperature lapse rate = +1.98°C per 1000 feet from sea level to 36 089 feet.
   (c) Height of tropopause = 36 089 feet.
   (d) Temperature of the isothermal layer of the stratosphere, from 36 089 to 65 616 feet = $-56.5°C$.
   (e) Temperature rises progressively above 65 616 feet to $-46°C$ at 100 00 feet.

It must be emphasized that a given standard atmosphere merely defines the variation of *pressure* with altitude for a given relationship between *temperature* and altitude. As described above, however, there are in reality considerable variations in the temperature profile both with season of the year and with latitude. *Table 1.3* illustrates this by comparing the ICAO standard with measured maximum and minimum temperatures at various altitudes. Such deviations will clearly change the relationships defined by the standard.

These temperature variations are of practical importance both to the physiologist and to the aeronautical engineer. Thus the physiological disturbances induced by exposure to low pressure in a

Table 1.2 The ICAO (1964) International Standard Atmosphere

Altitude ft	Altitude m	Pressure mm Hg	Pressure lb/in²	Temperature °C
0	0	760	14.70	+15.0
1 000	305	733	14.17	+13.0
2 000	610	706	13.67	+11.0
3 000	914	681	13.17	+ 9.1
4 000	1 219	656	12.69	+ 7.1
5 000	1 525	632	12.23	+ 5.1
6 000	1 829	609	11.78	+ 3.1
7 000	2 134	586	11.34	+ 1.1
8 000	2 438	565	10.92	− 0.9
9 000	2 743	543	10.50	− 2.8
10 000	3 048	523	10.11	− 4.8
11 000	3 353	503	9.72	− 6.8
12 000	3 658	483	9.35	− 8.8
13 000	3 962	465	8.98	−10.8
14 000	4 267	447	8.63	−12.7
15 000	4 572	429	8.29	−14.7
16 000	4 879	412	7.97	−16.7
17 000	5 182	395	7.64	−18.7
18 000	5 486	380	7.34	−20.7
19 000	5 791	364	7.04	−22.6
20 000	6 096	349	6.75	−24.6
21 000	6 401	335	6.48	−26.6
22 000	6 706	321	6.21	−28.6
23 000	7 010	307	5.95	−30.6
24 000	7 315	294	5.70	−32.6
25 000	7 620	282	5.45	−34.5
26 000	7 925	270	5.22	−36.5
27 000	8 230	258	4.99	−38.5
28 000	8 534	247	4.78	−40.5
29 000	8 839	236	4.57	−42.5
30 000	9 144	226	4.36	−44.4
31 000	9 449	215	4.17	−46.4
32 000	9 754	206	3.98	−48.4
33 000	10 058	196	3.80	−50.6
34 000	10 363	187	3.63	−52.4
35 000	10 668	179	3.46	−54.2
36 000	10 973	170	3.30	−56.3
37 000	11 278	162	3.14	−56.5
38 000	11 582	155	3.00	−56.5
39 000	11 887	147	2.95	−56.5
40 000	12 192	141	2.72	56.5
41 000	12 497	134	2.59	−56.5
42 000	12 802	128	2.47	−56.5
43 000	13 107	122	2.36	−56.5
44 000	13 411	116	2.24	−56.5
45 000	13 716	111	2.14	−56.5
46 000	14 021	106	2.04	−56.5
47 000	14 326	101	1.95	−56.5
48 000	14 630	96.0	1.85	−56.5
49 000	14 935	91.5	1.77	−56.5
50 000	15 240	87.3	1.68	−56.5
51 000	15 545	83.2	1.61	−56.5
52 000	15 850	79.3	1.53	−56.5
53 000	16 155	75.6	1.46	−56.5
54 000	16 459	72.1	1.39	−56.5
55 000	16 764	68.8	1.32	−56.5
56 000	17 069	65.5	1.27	−56.5
57 000	17 374	62.4	1.21	−56.5
58 000	17 679	59.5	1.15	−56.5
59 000	17 983	56.8	1.10	−56.5
60 000	18 288	54.1	1.04	−56.5
65 000	19 812	42.3	0.828	−56.5
70 000	21 336	33.3	0.644	−55.2
75 000	22 860	26.2	0.507	−53.6
80 000	24 384	20.7	0.401	−52.1
85 000	25 908	16.4	0.317	−50.6
90 000	27 432	13.0	0.251	−49.1
95 000	28 956	10.3	0.199	−47.5
100 000	30 480	8.2	0.158	−46.0

Table 1.3 World-wide maximum and minimum recorded air temperatures at various altitudes (frequency of occurrence of 10 days in any one year)

Altitude (ft)	ICAO (1964) Standard	Temperature (°C) Maximum recorded	Temperature (°C) Minimum recorded
0	+15.0	+50	−26
10 000	− 4.8	+16	−34
20 000	−24.6	− 3	−48
30 000	−44.4	−21	−62
40 000	−56.5	−40	−68
50 000	−56.5	−40	−78
60 000	−56.5	−40	−86
80 000	−52.1	−40	−86
100 000	−46.0	−30	−90

hypobaric chamber are determined by the pressure altitude tables uncorrected for temperature, whilst the aerodynamic behaviour imparted to an airframe during its passage through the air is determined by the density altitude. Density altitude is the pressure altitude corrected for the difference between the observed temperature and the temperature adopted by the standard atmosphere, and may therefore be regarded as a 'real' or 'true' altitude.

The gas laws and conditions of measurement

The physical laws that govern the behaviour of gases in both gaseous mixtures and in liquid media have an important bearing on the understanding of mechanisms whereby changes in altitude affect human physiology. The laws of particular relevance are those that describe changes in the volume of a gas in response to changes in pressure (Boyle's law) and to changes in temperature (Charles's law), the behaviour of gases reacting together (Gay-Lussac's law), the behaviour of the individual components making up a mixture of gases (Dalton's law), and the behaviour of gases in solution (Henry's law and the laws of gaseous diffusion).

Other concepts that are of importance include those of absolute and gauge pressures, and the complexities surrounding conditions of measurement.

The gas laws

Boyle's law

Boyle's law states that, at a constant temperature, the volume of a given mass of gas is inversely proportional to the pressure to which it is subjected. Expressed mathematically, therefore:

$$\frac{P_1}{P_2} = \frac{V_2}{V_1}$$

Where P_1 is the initial pressure, P_2 is the final pressure, V_1 is the initial volume, and V_2 is the final volume.

It should be noted that the pressure here is expressed in absolute terms and not as a differential (gauge) pressure (*see* below). The law is modified by the presence of water vapour and so, since the gases in body cavities may be regarded as being saturated with water vapour at a constant (body) temperature, the equation becomes, for physiological purposes:

$$\frac{P_1 - P_{H_2O}}{P_2 - P_{H_2O}} = \frac{V_2}{V_1}$$

Where P_{H_2O} is water vapour pressure at body temperature. Since body temperature is constant so too is P_{H_2O}.

Charles's law

Charles's law states that the volume of a given mass of gas at constant pressure is directly proportional to its absolute temperature. The absolute temperature of a gas, which is measured in degrees Kelvin, is obtained by adding 273 to its Celsius temperature since absolute zero is −273°C. [At absolute zero, molecular motion ceases and theoretically gases then have no volume.] Charles's law may be expressed mathematically thus:

$$\frac{V_1}{V_2} = \frac{T_1}{T_2} = \frac{(t_1 + 273)}{(t_2 + 273)}$$

Where V_1 is the initial volume, V_2 is the final volume, T_1 is the initial absolute temperature (and is itself the sum of the initial temperature t_1 in °C plus 273), and T_2 is the final absolute temperature (and is itself the sum of the final temperature t_2 in °C plus 273).

Gay-Lussac's laws

Gay-Lussac's law of thermal expansion is similar to Charles's law and states that, at constant pressure,

all gases expand by the same amount for the same increase in temperature. Gay-Lussac's law of gaseous volumes states that when gases combine chemically, the volumes of the reacting gases and gaseous products are in simple proportion if measured at the same temperature and pressure.

Dalton's law

Dalton's law of partial pressures states that the pressure exerted by a mixture of gases is equal to the sum of the pressures that each would exert if it alone occupied the space filled by the mixture. The pressure that a single component of a gas mixture would exert if it alone occupied the total space filled by the mixture is termed the partial pressure of the component. The law may be expressed mathematically thus:

$$P_t = P_1 + P_2 + P_3 \ldots P_n$$

Where P_t is the total pressure of the mixture, and P_1, P_2, P_3 ... P_n are the partial pressures of each component.

The partial pressure of any gas in a mixture is given by the relationship:

$$P_x = F_x \times P_t$$

Where P_x is the partial pressure of gas x, F_x is the fractional concentration of gas x in the mixture, and P_t is the total pressure of the gas mixture.

Thus, for example, the partial pressure of oxygen (Po_2) in the dry atmosphere at mean sea level pressure is:

$$Po_2 = \frac{20.95}{100} \times 760 = 159.2 \, \text{mm Hg}$$

Henry's law

Henry's law states that the mass of gas absorbed by a given mass of liquid, with which it does not combine chemically, is directly proportional to the partial pressure of the gas above the liquid at a given temperature. At equilibrium, the partial pressure of the gas in the liquid phase will be the same as that of the gas directly above the liquid. The absolute amount of gas dissolved at equilibrium is determined by the solubility of the gas in the liquid as well as by its partial pressure. Thus if the partial pressure of a gas in a liquid is reduced, then the amount of that gas that can be held in solution will be reduced in proportion. This behaviour underlies the basis of bubble formation (leading to decompression sickness) in body fluids on exposure to low environmental pressures.

Laws of gaseous diffusion

Diffusion is the process whereby molecules in

different solutions move from regions of higher to those of lower concentration, or the molecules of one gas intermingle with those of another. Several precepts govern the rate of diffusion of a single gas through a liquid or gaseous mixture. Thus the rate of diffusion is proportional to the difference between the pressures of the gas at the two points, it is inversely proportional to the square root of its molecular weight (Graham's law), and, in a liquid, it is proportional to the solubility of the gas within the liquid such that the more soluble the gas the faster its diffusion.

Diffusion of a gas through a tissue medium, such as the alveolar membrane, is described by Fick's law, which states that the rate of gas transfer is proportional to the tissue area and the difference between the gas partial pressures on the two sides, and inversely proportional to the tissue thickness. It is also proportional to a diffusion constant described by Graham's law. Fick's law can be expressed mathematically, thus:

$$\dot{V}_{gas} \propto \frac{A}{T} \cdot D \cdot (P_1 - P_2)$$

and $D \propto \dfrac{Sol}{\sqrt{MW}}$

Where $\dot{V}_{gas}$ is the rate at which gas is transferred, A is the surface area of the tissue and T its thickness; $(P_1 - P_2)$ is the difference in gas partial pressure across the tissue; D is the diffusion constant, Sol is the solubility of the gas, and MW its molecular weight.

Conditions of measurement

Measurement of pressure

Pressure may be defined as perpendicular force per unit area. A column of liquid or gas will therefore exert a pressure which is proportional to the height of the column, the density of the material within it, and the acceleration due to gravity. Accordingly, *atmospheric pressure* is a reflection of the force imparted by the mass of a column of air which, at sea level, will exert a pressure on the Earth's surface of $1 \, kg/cm^2$ ($14.7 \, lb/in^2$, $760 \, mm \, Hg$, 1 atmosphere, 1 bar). Aeronautical engineers, however, routinely further describe pressures in terms of either *absolute* (abs) or *gauge* (g) values, and it is important to appreciate the difference between these two expressions.

The *absolute pressure* of a gas or (confined) liquid is the total pressure it exerts, and includes the effect of atmospheric pressure. Thus an absolute pressure of zero corresponds to a complete vacuum (as is found in deep space). Pressure measuring devices, such as a pneumatic tyre pressure gauge, however,

respond to the pressure present in excess of any atmospheric component. So, for example, a tyre pressure gauge may indicate a pressure of $30 \, lb/in^2$ within a tyre, and this is termed the *gauge pressure*, but the absolute pressure exerted by the air within the tyre must include the atmospheric component and thus at sea level will be $44.7 \, lb/in^2$. The gauge reading given by such an instrument is therefore the *difference* between two pressures; and so the instrument will register zero whenever the pressure applied to the measuring point equals that of its surroundings. The total or absolute pressure is the algebraic sum of the gauge and the atmospheric pressures. That is:

Absolute pressure = gauge pressure + atmospheric pressure

Pressures less than atmospheric will produce negative gauge pressures and these correspond to partial vacuums. An absolute pressure, however, cannot be less than zero.

In physiology, the distinction between absolute and gauge pressures is important. In the case of a diver, for example, where a man is already under a pressure of 1 atmosphere at sea level (1 bar) before descending, a dive to a depth of $30 \, m$ will produce a gauge reading of 3 bar (3 atmospheres), but the absolute pressure will be 4 bar.

In aviation physiology, this concept is of particular relevance when considering cabin pressurization schedules (*see* Chapter 8). The absolute pressure within the cabin of an aircraft equals the sum of the atmospheric pressure at its external surface (measured by static probe) and the *cabin differential pressure*. And the cabin differential pressure is the difference between the absolute pressure within the aircraft and that of the atmosphere outside it. Thus:

Cabin differential pressure = internal cabin pressure (abs) − atmospheric pressure (abs)

and so

Cabin absolute pressure = cabin differential pressure + atmospheric pressure (abs)

As an example, the atmospheric pressure surrounding an aircraft flying at 25000 feet is $282 \, mm \, Hg$ ($5.45 \, lb/in^2$ abs) and if the cabin differential pressure is $236 \, mm \, Hg$ ($4.55 \, lb/in^2$ g) then the absolute pressure within the cabin will be the sum of these; that is, $518 \, mm \, Hg$ ($10.0 \, lb/in^2$ abs) and the cabin altitude will be just over 10000 feet.

Measurement of gas volumes

In physiology and medicine, the gas laws will have their greatest influence in the study of respiratory behaviour. The brief description of the laws governing the behaviour of gases implies that changes in temperature and pressure will have profound effects on the numerical values of any variables studied. It is therefore vital to a clear appreciation of this subject that relationships between the various conditions of measurement are understood.

It is generally accepted that body temperature, including that of the lungs, is constant and that water vapour when present, as in the lungs, is at its saturation pressure. The values commonly used are a temperature of 37°C and the saturated water vapour pressure at that temperature, which is 47 mm Hg. The gas in the lungs under these conditions is stated to be at *body temperature and pressure, saturated* with water vapour; and is abbreviated to BTPS. BTPS conditions are those regarded as most appropriate for *respiratory* studies (cf. metabolic – *see* below).

Under most circumstances, however, ambient air is at a lower temperature than gas in the lungs and, furthermore, contains less water vapour. This is not only because atmospheric air is not usually saturated with water vapour but also because, *ipso facto*, at a lower temperature the saturated water vapour pressure is lower. If measurements are made under these conditions, they are said to be at *ambient temperature and pressure* (ATP). If, however, as is usual in the laboratory, respiratory measurements are made via a water spirometer, gas in the circuit is regarded as saturated with water vapour and the conditions of measurement are the familiar *ambient temperature and pressure saturated with water vapour* (ATPS).

Ambient air is heated and humidified as it passes through the upper respiratory tract, and it consequently expands in accordance with Gay-Lussac's law of thermal expansion and by virtue of water molecules evaporating within the airway. The physiological importance of this is that the volume of gas inspired (as measured by a spirometer or similar device) is less than the volume of gas taking part in respiratory exchange. The shortfall may be of the order of 10% in temperate climates, and for the precision required by respiratory physiologists a correction from ATPS to BTPS is therefore necessary. The correction may be expressed mathematically, thus:

$$V_{BTPS} = V_{ATPS} \cdot \frac{273 + 37}{273 + t_a} \cdot \frac{P_B - P_{H_2O}}{P_B - 47}$$

Where 273 is the melting point of ice in K, 37 is body temperature in °C, t_a is ambient temperature in °C, P_B is barometric pressure in mm Hg. P_{H_2O} is saturated water vapour pressure at t_a, and 47 is the saturated water vapour pressure at body temperature.

The first fraction in this equation is the term describing expansion due to heat, while the second fraction is the term describing the volume increase as a consequence of added water vapour. The product is therefore the factor by which the ATPS volume must be multiplied to give the lung volume at BTPS.

When dealing with *metabolic* physiology, however, different requirements exist. In this case, it is the *number* of molecules of oxygen used and carbon dioxide produced which are of interest and not the *volume* which they happen to be occupying at the time of measurement. It is essential, therefore, to express oxygen and carbon dioxide volumes under the precisely defined standard or normal conditions; that is, at *standard temperature and pressure, dry* (STPD). Standard temperature is 273 K (0°C) and standard pressure is 760 mm Hg. When defined in this way, the number of molecules contained within the STPD volume can be calculated readily since, under STPD conditions, gases comply with Avogadro's law; that is, 1 gram-mole of a gas will have a volume of 22.4 l (STPD).

Just as BTPS conditions can be derived from ATPS measurements, corrections for STPD conditions can be applied mathematically, thus:

$$V_{STPS} = V_{ATPB} \cdot \frac{273}{273 + t_a} \cdot \frac{P_B - P_{H_2O}}{760}$$

Where 273 is the melting point of ice in K, t_a is ambient temperature in °C, P_B is barometric pressure in mm Hg, P_{H_2O} is saturated water vapour pressure at t_a, and 760 is standard pressure.

Finally, in the context of breathing system definition (*see* Chapter 7), two further conditions of measurement are encountered that are of particular use to life support engineers. Thus system specifications may often quote gas volumes under *atmospheric temperature and pressure, dry* (ATPD) conditions; while consumption figures are quoted under *normal temperature and pressure* (NTP) conditions. In the United Kingdom, temperature and pressure under ATPD conditions are considered to be +15°C and the absolute pressure of gas within the site under study (for example, within a mask delivery hose). Similarly, the temperature and pressure under NTP conditions are +15°C and 760 mm Hg absolute respectively.

The need to express quantities of gas under NTP conditions is a reflection of the expansile behaviour of gases on exposure to low environmental pressures; that is, once at altitude, the *volume flow* of a gas is not the same as its *mass flow*, the difference increasing with altitude. As an example, a mass flow of 4.0 litres (NTP)/min will provide a volume flow of about 8.0 litres (ATPD)/min at an altitude of 18 000 feet, where atmospheric pressure is half its sea level value and expansion has occurred roughly in accordance with Boyle's law. In fact, the volume flow of a gas is never the same as its mass flow, even at sea level; although the magnitude of the difference increases with altitude. This has particular relevance for respiratory physiology at altitude, since respiration is a volume flow phenomenon, and this aspect is dealt with further in Chapter 4.

Further reading

BILLINGS, C.E. (1973). Atmosphere. In *Bioastronautics Data Book*, edited by J.F. Parker and V.R. West. 2nd edn. Washington, DC: NASA SP-3006

DEJOURS, P. (1966). *Respiration*, pp. 10–19. New York: Oxford University Press

Her Majesty's Stationery Office (1971). *Handbook of Aviation Meteorology*. London: HMSO

International Civil Aviation Organization (1964). *Manual of the ICAO Standard Atmosphere*, 2nd edn. Montreal: ICAO

2

The effects of pressure change

G.R. Sharp, revised by A.J.F. Macmillan

Introduction

The body contains a number of gas-filled cavities which communicate with varying degrees of ease with the external environment. During changes of environmental pressure, for example, on ascent or descent in an aircraft or on sudden loss of cabin pressurization, the pressure of the gas within these cavities must attain equilibrium with that of the surrounding environment or the individual will suffer adverse effects.

The behaviour of the gas within a cavity during pressure change and the ultimate effect on the body if equilibration of the pressure of the gas with that of the surrounding atmosphere fails, depends to some extent on whether the cavity is *semi-closed* or *closed*. The gas-containing cavities of the lungs, middle ears and paranasal sinuses are typical examples of the semi-closed; the gastro-intestinal tract provides an example of the closed type of cavity. This chapter describes the important gas-filled cavities of the body, the mechanisms that allow pressure equilibration during changing environmental pressure and the problems that can arise when gas equilibration does not occur.

Mechanism of gas expansion

The gas contained within distensible body cavities is influenced by changes in the pressure outside the body: so that, as atmospheric pressure decreases (during ascent or on loss of cabin pressure), the volume of the gas increases. During descent, the process is reversed and the volume of the gas within cavities decreases.

Apart from any consequence of physical restraint affecting the gas, the degree of expansion of

contained gas during change of atmospheric pressure might be expected to follow Boyle's law; that is, the volume of a gas varies inversely with its absolute pressure. However, since the walls of all body cavities are always moist, the gases contained within them are normally saturated with water vapour. If the volume of a gas is increased by a reduction of pressure, the partial pressure of the water vapour will tend to fall: but the very rapid evaporation of water from the lining film maintains full saturation under virtually all conditions. The partial pressure exerted by the water vapour is determined solely by the temperature. It is normally 47 mm Hg (at a temperature of 37°C). The relative gas expansion, that is, the ratio of final to initial volume of a given quantity of gas in a body cavity, is expressed by the relationship:

$$\text{Relative gas expansion} = \frac{(P_c - 47)}{(P_f - 47)}$$

where P_c = initial pressure of gas in cavity expressed in mm Hg and P_f = final pressure of gas in cavity expressed in mm Hg.

Thus, for a given pressure ratio, the greater the altitude the greater the gas expansion, until at 63 000 feet (19 000 m) the gas expansion is theoretically infinite – atmospheric pressure at that altitude being 47 mm Hg. In practice, however, the gases enclosed within unventilated body cavities cannot expand completely freely, since an increasing resistance is offered by the surrounding tissue as it stretches, and this causes a local rise in internal pressure. Thus the process tends to be self-limiting and infinite gas expansion does not occur, even during prolonged exposure to atmospheric pressures less than 47 mm Hg.

When there is unrestricted communication between a gas-filled cavity and the outside atmosphere, gas expansion occurs with little difficulty and no discomfort. If, however, the pressure of the gas in the cavity fails to equilibrate with the outside environmental pressure there may be considerable discomfort, frank pain, or damage to tissues or organs of the body which may well incapacitate the individual. The various sites where gases can be trapped and pressure fail to equalize will be discussed individually in terms of the behaviour of semi-closed and closed cavities.

Effects of changes of pressure on semi-closed cavities

The middle ear

The cavity of the middle ear is separated from the outer ear by the tympanic membrane (*Figure 2.1*). It communicates with the nasopharynx and hence the atmosphere by way of the Eustachian tube, the proximal two-thirds of which has soft walls which are normally collapsed. During ascent to altitude, the gas in the middle-ear cavity expands and the expanding gas escapes along the Eustachian tube into the nasopharynx, so that pressure remains equal on both sides of the tympanic membrane. Since the anatomical structure of the pharyngeal portion of the Eustachian tube is such that it acts as a 'one-way' valve, expanding air can escape easily to the atmosphere, and it is very unusual for passive venting of the middle ear to present difficulties during decompression. This intermittent passive ventilation of the middle ear during ascent may be appreciated as a 'popping' sensation as air escapes from the mouth of the Eustachian tube into the pharynx. On ascent, the Eustachian tube opens and gas escapes from the middle ear into the nasopharynx approximately once every 500–1000 feet.

During descent, gas from the nasopharynx must enter the middle ear in order to maintain equilibrium between the atmospheric pressure outside and the gas pressure in the middle ear. In most individuals, the one-way valve mechanism of the Eustachian tube prevents the passive flow of gas back into the middle-ear cavity. The resultant relative increase of pressure on the outside of the tympanic membrane pushes the membrane into the middle-ear cavity. As descent continues, the membrane is pushed further into the middle-ear cavity unless gas enters it through the Eustachian tube. This distortion leads to a sensation of fullness in the ear and a decrease in hearing acuity. If descent continues further without equalization of pressure between the atmosphere and the middle ear, the

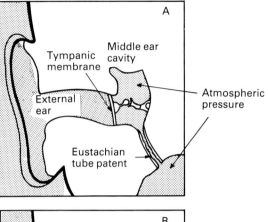

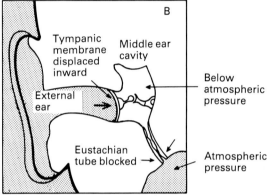

Figure 2.1 Diagram of external and middle ear (*a*) at a constant altitude with a patent Eustachian tube, and (*b*) during descent with an occluded Eustachian tube. Whilst the Eustachian tube is patent the pressure in the middle-ear cavity equals that in the nasopharynx which in turn is equal to that of the atmosphere. If, however, the Eustachian tube is occluded during descent (*b*) the pressure in the middle-ear cavity is less than that in the nasopharynx and the atmospheric pressure and the pressure difference across the tympanic membrane displaces it into the middle-ear cavity.

differential pressure across the ear drum causes pain. In certain susceptible individuals, a rapid change of pressure in the middle-ear cavity may also affect the organs of balance in the inner ear and so cause vertigo.

In order to equalize the pressure across the tympanic membrane during descent and thus prevent the development of otic barotrauma, it is usually necessary to perform some active manoeuvre to open the Eustachian tubes. Although there are several simple manoeuvres such as swallowing, yawning and jaw movements which may open the tube, these are not effective in about half the aircrew population. These individuals have to raise the pressure in the nasopharynx in order to force gas into the middle ear cavities. This rise in pressure is usually achieved by performing either a

Valsalva or Frenzel manoeuvre. The Valsalva manoeuvre is carried out by attempting a forced expiration with the lips closed and the nostrils occluded by compressing the nose. This manoeuvre is used commonly in flight, but the raised intra-thoracic pressure generated during the procedure may, under certain circumstances, impair cardiovascular function.

The Frenzel manoeuvre raises the pressure locally in the nasopharynx. It is performed by closing the glottis and the lips while occluding the nostrils and simultaneously contracting the muscles of the floor of the mouth and pharynx. These co-ordinated actions are similar to those employed when 'blowing one's nose' or stifling a sneeze and have to be learnt. The Frenzel manoeuvre has the advantages of opening the Eustachian tube at lower nasopharyngeal pressures and being capable of performance during any phase of respiration.

Mention must also be made of the Toynbee manoeuvre which consists of swallowing while the nostrils are pinched. This action also opens the Eustachian tubes at ground level but does so by generation of a reduced pressure in the nasopharynx. It is therefore useful for checking the patency of the tubes but is not recommended as a procedure for use during descent.

The frequency with which trained aircrew perform one or other of these 'ear clearing' manoeuvres varies considerably, from once every 1000 feet to once every 4000 feet or more. There is, however, a limit to the pressure rise that can be created within the nasopharynx, and the Eustachian tube may become 'locked' closed when the differential pressure between the middle ear and the environment exceeds 90–120 mm Hg.

Upper respiratory tract infection causes congestion and oedema of the mucosal lining of the Eustachian tube, particularly where it opens into the nasopharynx. This congestion may restrict the passage of gas into the middle-ear cavity during descent. The tympanic membrane will then be driven into the middle ear causing deafness and pain. If descent is continued, the grossly distorted membrane may rupture, with immediate relief of the pain. The changes in the tympanic membrane and middle ear produced by failure of adequate ventilation of the latter during descent is termed otic barotrauma. The condition commonly arises in association with upper respiratory tract infections but may be caused by too rapid descent or inadequate knowledge of the correct procedures for ventilating the middle ear.

The paranasal sinuses

The paranasal sinuses are cavities located in the bones of the face and skull. The frontal sinuses communicate with the nose by a relatively long duct whilst each of the other sinuses is connected to the nose by a hole in its wall. During ascent and descent, the expanding and contracting gas contained within a sinus is thus free to communicate with the gas in the nose, and a pressure difference does not develop between the gas in the sinus and the external atmosphere. If, however, the mucous membrane lining the passage connecting a paranasal sinus to the nose becomes inflamed and oedematous, the normal passive ventilation of the sinus cavity may be obstructed, particularly during descent. Such a failure causes severe pain in the cheeks, forehead or deep in the head, often accompanied by watering of the eyes. Auto-inflation of the sinus cavity is not achieved easily during this condition, even by manoeuvres in which the pressure in the mouth and nose is raised above that of the environment. Nasal decongestants may help to re-establish auto-ventilation of the sinus cavity but the airman may have to limit the aircraft's rate of descent. Damage to the mucosal lining may occur with subsequent haemorrhage into the sinus cavity. This condition of acute sinus barotrauma frequently recurs and may eventually require surgical treatment.

The lungs

The large volume of gas in the alveoli, the relatively narrow passages that connect the alveoli to the external environment, and the susceptibility of the lung tissue to damage when it is overstretched, combine to make the lungs a vulnerable part of the body during a very rapid reduction of environmental pressure such as occurs in sudden loss of cabin pressure. Although no serious injuries have been reported so far in human decompression with open airways, studies on experimental animals have shown that fast decompressions over large pressure ranges can cause structural damage to pulmonary tissue with haemorrhagic, emphysematous and atelectatic changes in various lobes of the lung. The ability of the human lung to withstand and adapt to sudden changes in pressure is the limiting factor in the rate or range of decompression that can be tolerated, and strict attention is paid to this factor in the design of pressurized cabins.

The decompression rate of the lungs is limited by the flow resistance offered by the pulmonary and upper airways. Thus any environmental decompression that is faster than the maximum decompression rate of the lungs will result in a transient positive differential pressure between the gas within the lungs and the surrounding cabin environment. The faster the decompression rate of the cabin the greater will be the transient pressure difference. The magnitude and duration of the difference between the pressure of the gas in the lungs and that of the cabin environment during a rapid decompression depend on the following factors:

1. The rate of decompression of the cabin in relation to the simultaneous rate of decompression of the lungs.
2. The total change of cabin pressure during the decompression.
3. The volume of gas in the lungs at the beginning of the decompression.
4. The ability of the lungs and thorax to expand within normal limits during decompression.

The normal expansion of the lungs and chest wall, and the flow of gas from the lungs through the airways to the environment will reduce considerably the pressure within the lungs during a rapid decompression.

A simple model which illustrates the dynamic relationships between the pressure in the lungs and that in the cabin during a rapid decompression is depicted in *Figure 2.2*. The model represents the situation in which the lungs and chest wall behave as a rigid container. The ratio of the volume of the lungs to the area of the opening from the lungs to the cabin environment (the area of an orifice equivalent to the airways) is greater in this model than the ratio of the volume of the cabin to the area of the defect in the cabin wall. Curve I shows the behaviour of the pressure in the cabin as it decompresses through the defect; while Curve II depicts the time course of the pressure changes in the lungs. Curve III is the difference between Curves I and II and represents the pressure difference between the gas in the lungs and that in the cabin – the transthoracic pressure. This pressure difference builds up rapidly to a peak and then declines gradually as the lungs progressively decompress.

Lung damage in rapid decompression is caused by stretching of the lung tissue beyond its elastic limit. As the gas within the lungs expands, the chest wall and diaphragm are displaced outwards. If the expansion of the gas within the lungs can be taken up without the final lung volume exceeding the normal total lung volume, no damage will occur. If, however, the lung expansion induced exceeds the normal total lung volume, the lung tissue will be overstretched. Eventually it will tear and blood vessels will be severed. The transthoracic pressure difference required to tear the lungs when the chest and abdominal muscles are relaxed is of the order of 80–100 mm Hg. When lung tissue tears, air passes along tissue planes into the mediastinum, and even up into the neck, to produce surgical emphysema; whilst gas entering torn blood vessels passes into the systemic circulation (generalized gas embolism).

The worst case is when the gas within the lung cannot escape during the fall of environmental

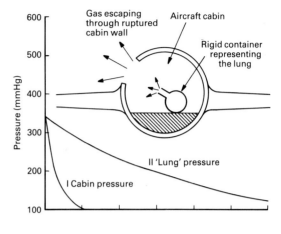

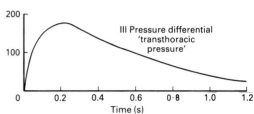

Figure 2.2 Simple model to demonstrate effects of a rapid decompression of the cabin of an aircraft flying at high altitude (at approximately 47 000 feet) upon the pressure difference between the gas within the lung and the gas surrounding the body (the transthoracic pressure differential). The lung is represented by a rigid container with a relatively narrow opening into the cabin. On rupture of the cabin wall the pressure in the cabin (Curve I) falls to that of the environment in about 0.2 seconds. The rate at which gas escapes from the 'lung', and hence the rate at which lung pressure (Curve I) falls, is much slower than the rate of decompression of the cabin so that there is a transient but large pressure difference between the lung and cabin gas (Curve III).

pressure. The free flow of expanding gas to the atmosphere may be prevented by closure of the glottis such as occurs during breath-holding, swallowing and straining, or by the characteristics of any breathing equipment being used at the time. Thus the compensated outlet valve fitted in a typical pressure demand oronasal mask may well be held shut throughout and immediately after a rapid decompression. The range of decompression that is safe (i.e. the transthoracic pressure after the decompression does not exceed 50 mm Hg when no gas can escape from the lungs) can be calculated if the initial volume of gas in the lungs is known. Typical limiting conditions are presented in *Table 2.1*. When the gas within the lungs is free to escape, it is difficult to predict whether the individual circumstances – the initial and final altitudes, the ratio of the volume of the cabin to the effective area

Table 2.1 Safe limits to rapid decompression without venting of the lungs

Initial altitude (ft)	Initial lung volume (fraction of total lung capacity)	Maximum 'safe' final altitude (ft)
8000	0.25*	44000
	0.50†	29700
	0.75	20000
	1.00‡	13000
25000	0.25*	61000
	0.50†	46500
	0.75	37500
	1.00‡	31500

*Minimum lung volume (residual volume).
†Resting end expiratory lung volume (functional residual capacity).
‡Maximum lung volume (total lung capacity).

of the orifice through which it is being decompressed – will produce a transthoracic pressure difference of the order of 80 mm Hg and hence cause lung damage. Most of the available information has been obtained by animal experimentation, although there is some information with regard to 'safe' decompression for man. The limiting conditions of the initial-to-final pressure ratio and the cabin volume-to-orifice area ratio beyond which lung damage is likely to occur in man are presented in *Figure 2.3*.

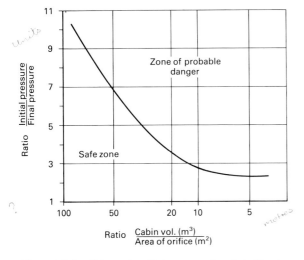

Figure 2.3 Conditions of rapid decompression that will not cause lung damage (safe zone) and in which lung damage may occur (zone of probable danger). The range and speed of decompression are expressed in terms of the ratio of the pressure in the cabin before the decompression (initial pressure) to the pressure in the cabin after the decompression (final pressure) and the ratio of the volume of the cabin (in cubic metres) to the area of the orifice (in square metres) through which the cabin is decompressed. It is assumed that the glottis is open and that there is no external obstruction to the flow of gas from the lungs.

Whilst it is reasonably certain that conditions of decompression that lie to the left of the curve are 'safe' provided that the glottis is open and there is no external obstruction to the flow of gas from the lungs, decompression under conditions that lie to the right of the curve may or may not cause lung damage. In practice, lung damage due to decompression either in an aircraft or in a decompression chamber is a very rare event.

Effects of changes of pressure on closed cavities

The alimentary canal

In normal, healthy individuals the stomach and intestines contain a quantity of gas, the volume of which varies between 0 and 400 ml, with an average value of 100 ml. This gas is derived from swallowed air, from the action of bacteria within the gut, and from exchange with the gases in the tissues and blood.

During ascent, the gas contained within the stomach expands and usually escapes up the oesophagus and out through the mouth. Gas bubbles within the large bowel coalesce to form large bubbles which are vented out of the anus. Certain individuals, usually inexperienced aircrew, have difficulty in venting gas from the mouth and anus even with low rates of ascent. At very high rates of ascent and during rapid decompression this difficulty increases, and even experienced aircrew have some difficulty in expelling gas from the alimentary tract as quickly as it expands. In these cases, the individual may develop symptoms which vary from mild upper or lower abdominal discomfort to, in exceptional cases, very severe pain. In some sensitive individuals, the abdominal pain caused by the expanding gas may cause vasovagal syncope. Expansion of the gas in the gastrointestinal tract has never produced visceral damage.

The problem of gas expansion in the alimentary tract may be aggravated if the individual is suffering from mild intestinal infection or has eaten a large quantity of foodstuffs known to be gas forming (peas, beans, cauliflower, cabbage, high roughage foods, or carbonated drinks). With experience, aircrew learn which foodstuffs cause excessive gas formation and adjust their diets accordingly. The incidence of abdominal discomfort or pain in healthy aircrew who are frequently exposed to high altitude is negligible when the maximum altitude does not exceed 25000 feet. Even when such individuals are decompressed to altitudes above 40000 feet the incidence of abdominal pain on short-duration exposures is only 2–3%.

Question of units   F(y) cannot equal F(x)
unless units are same on both sides?

The teeth

Expansion of gas in the teeth during ascent to
altitude may cause severe toothache – aerodontalgia. The source of gas in the teeth may be air
trapped between the tooth substance and a deep
cavity filling – particularly in unlined cavities.
Modern dental filling materials have reduced the
incidence of trapped gas in dental fillings and
aerodontalgia from this source is now rare. Aerodontalgia may, however, be experienced by aircrew
with unhealthy teeth where, for example, gas of
putrefaction gathers in a small bubble at the apex of
a tooth in the condition of chronic or acute apical
abscess.

Further reading

ARMSTRONG, H.G. and HEIM, J.W. (1937) The effect of flight
in the middle ear. *Journal of the American Medical
Association*, **109**, 417–421

FRENZEL, H. (1950) *Otorhinolaryngology in German
Aviation Medicine, World War II*, Vol. 2, p. 20.
Washington, DC: Government Printing Office

GILLIES, J.A. (1965) *A Text Book of Aviation Physiology*,
1st edn. Chapters 5–7. Oxford: Pergamon Press

JONES, G.M. (1957) *Current Problems Associated with
Disorientation in Man-Controlled Flight*. Flying Person-
nel Research Committee, Report No. 1021. London:
Air Ministry

KING, P.F. (1979) The Eustachian tube and its significance
in flight. *Journal of Laryngology and Otology*, **93**,
659–678

PEARLMAN, H.B. (1967) Normal tubal function. *Archives of
Otolaryngology (Chicago)*, **86**, 632

3

Decompression sickness

A.J.F. Macmillan

Introduction

The preceding chapter has dealt with the effects of lowered barometric pressure on the gas-containing cavities of the body. Later chapters deal with disturbances produced by the reduction in the partial pressure of oxygen which occurs on ascent. There remains, however, another group of effects produced by exposure to low pressure which are known collectively as decompression sickness. Since the manifestations of decompression sickness are so variable and the underlying mechanism is not well understood, this condition is usually identified by exclusion. Thus decompression sickness is the group of effects produced by exposure to altitude which are not due to expansion of trapped or enclosed gas or to the lowered partial pressure of oxygen.

Although the clinical syndrome of decompression sickness was recognized in divers and compressed-air workers as caisson disease in the 1850s, the first clear description of the condition arising in men exposed to subatmospheric pressures was not made until 1930. Indeed, the production of the condition by exposure to altitude did not gain general recognition until the end of the third decade. Although decompression sickness is the most generally accepted term, other terminology is sometimes used to describe the condition. These include: 'bends' (often the commonest symptom-pain in or around the joint of a limb), dysbarism, aeropathy and aeroembolism.

There are distinct differences between compressed-air and sub-atmospheric decompression sickness, although they share the same colloquial nomenclature for the common manifestations. Classically, the main manifestations are limb pain (the 'bends'), respiratory disturbances (the 'chokes'), skin irritation (the 'creeps'), various disturbances of the central nervous system (the 'staggers') and cardiovascular collapse (syncope). These symptoms of sub-atmospheric decompression sickness virtually always subside or disappear during descent to ground level. Rarely, however, recovery does not occur after recompression to ground level, and in some cases the severity of the symptoms may increase, accompanied by a generalized deterioration in the individual's condition (post-descent collapse).

The cause of decompression sickness

Although the details of the processes underlying some of the manifestations of altitude decompression sickness remain unknown, the basic mechanism is undoubtedly the supersaturation of the tissues with nitrogen. Thus the syndrome does not occur if the nitrogen normally dissolved in the body tissues and fluids is removed by breathing 100% oxygen before exposure to altitude. The tissues and body fluids of a man breathing air at ground level contain dissolved nitrogen, which exerts a partial pressure approximately equal to that of the nitrogen in the inspired air. The quantity of nitrogen contained in the body in this manner is approximately 1 litre (NTP). As the partial pressure of nitrogen in the inspired air falls with ascent to altitude, nitrogen is carried by the blood from the tissues to the lungs where it leaves the body in the expired gas. Since the solubility of nitrogen in blood is relatively low, and some tissues contain large amounts of nitrogen, the rate of fall of the absolute pressure of the body tissues associated with the ascent to altitude is greater than the rate of fall of the partial pressure of nitrogen in the tissues. These tissues, therefore,

19

become supersaturated with nitrogen. Under certain circumstances, this supersaturation gives rise to the formation of bubbles of gas, the main constituent of which is initially nitrogen, in specific tissues of the body. This supersaturation concept identifies a critical component in the formation of bubbles of gas as the ratio of the tension of the inert gas in the tissues to ambient pressure (supersaturation ratio). Thus gas exchange is the governing mechanism in the formation of the bubbles and these bubbles subsequently grow in size by the diffusion of nitrogen and other gases such as oxygen and carbon dioxide into them from surrounding tissues. It is virtually certain that the occurrence of decompression sickness is due to this bubble formation in the tissues. Bubbles that form at one site may be carried by the circulation to another organ, where their presence disturbs the function of the part. Although there has been no unequivocal demonstration that bubbles are formed in the tissues under conditions in which altitude decompression sickness occurs in man, there are reports of Doppler (ultra-sound) identified intravascular bubbles developing during exposure to reduced atmospheric pressure. A causal relationship between these Doppler intravenous bubbles and the development of symptoms has yet to be established.

The driving pressure for bubble formation in a fluid is the difference between the partial pressure of the gas dissolved in the fluid and the absolute hydrostatic pressure. The greater the partial pressures of the gas and the lower the absolute hydrostatic pressure, the greater is the tendency for bubble formation. The increase in the partial pressure of nitrogen produced in a tissue by a given decompression depends on the solubility and the rate of diffusion of the gas in the tissue and the local blood flow. Thus the rise of the partial pressure of nitrogen—and hence the magnitude of the pressure causing bubble formation—is greater in a tissue with a high lipid content, with its high solubility for nitrogen and low blood flow. Bubbles will not form in a fluid, however, even when the driving pressure is large unless suitable nuclei are present. Nuclei for bubble formation consist of microscopic masses of gases attached to irregularities on the walls of a cavity, such as a blood or lymph vessel, or small particles suspended in the fluid. The distribution of such gas nuclei may account for the sites at which the disturbances occur in decompression sickness. It is very probable, also, that bubbles have to grow to a certain critical size before the deformation which they produce is sufficient to cause symptoms or a disturbance of function. This hypothesis fits the observation that the rate of production of symptoms of decompression sickness is very low immediately after ascent, and that it increases to reach a peak in 20–60 minutes. The manner in which the bubbles formed by supersaturation of the tissues with

nitrogen produce the various manifestations of decompression sickness are considered in association with the descriptions of each of the main symptoms of the syndrome given in the next section of this chapter.

Presentation of decompression sickness

Decompression sickness may arise either in flight or during exposure to reduced atmospheric pressure in an hypobaric chamber. There is considerable evidence for the existence of an altitude threshold at approximately 18000 feet, although under certain circumstances, for example where decompression closely follows hyperbaric exposure in self-contained underwater breathing apparatus (scuba diving), the condition may occur at a much lower altitude. The incidence of decompression sickness at altitudes between 18000 feet and 25000 feet is low. However, the proportion of individuals who develop decompression sickness increases greatly with altitude above 25000 feet.

Clinical manifestations

The clinical manifestations of the condition are extremely varied. The relative incidences of symptoms and signs during 2-hour exposures to 28000 and 37000 feet are presented in *Table 3.1*. The clinical manifestations of decompression sickness are as follows.

Table 3.1 Relative incidence of symptoms of altitude decompression sickness

Symptom	Incidence (%)	
	28000 ft for 2 hr	37000 ft for 2 hr
Joint and limb pains	73.9	56.5
Respiratory disturbances	4.5	6.5
Skin disturbances	7.0	1.6
Visual disturbances	2.0	4.8
Neurological disturbances	1.0	0
Collapse	9.0	25.8
Miscellaneous	2.5	4.8

Joint and limb pains

Often referred to as 'bends', pain in a joint or a limb is the commonest severe symptom of decompression sickness (*Table 3.1*). When it occurs, the pain is usually ill localized and deep seated. Mild aches will often develop into severe or agonizing pain if altitude is maintained or increased; and, ultimately, if no corrective actions are carried out, the individual may collapse. Less frequently, the pain disappears without becoming severe. More than one site may be involved, and, in descending order of frequency, the commonly affected parts are as follows: knee, shoulder, elbow, wrist or hand, ankle or foot and, rarely, the hip. The pain starts as a mild ache which develops into a severe pain that spreads up and down the affected limb. Mild pain often encourages the subject to move or rub the aching part, but this action tends to increase rather than alleviate the pain. Local pressure by means of a tight bandage, a pneumatic cuff or immersion of the limb in fluid generally relieves the pain. Symptoms virtually always disappear during descent, although residual stiffness and even mild aches may persist for some time.

Although bubbles may be radiologically demonstrated in the synovial spaces of an affected joint, in tendon sheaths and even in fascial planes, bends pain may be present in the absence of radiological changes and, conversely, bubbles may be seen in the absence of symptoms. A pain that closely resembles that of bends can be produced by the local injection of small quantities of physiological saline into the muscles and ligaments around a joint. It is probable, therefore, that bends is due to the formation of extravascular bubbles in these tissues.

Skin disturbances

Itching, tingling ('creeps') and formication often occur at altitude (*Table 3.1*) and are usually transient. They are of little significance, and only rarely do these symptoms progress to more serious manifestations. In rare cases, the itching may be severe and accompanied by a marked hyperaesthesia. Occasionally, localized skin rashes, mottling and urticaria are observed, often in association with other symptoms and signs. Thus, chokes is commonly accompanied by mottling of the skin over the chest; bluish-red patches of variable size appear, and itch intensely. Discomfort associated with mottling may persist for 2–3 days.

The more severe skin manifestations of decompression sickness are probably due to embolism by gas bubbles carried in the blood to the skin from other tissues of the body.

Respiratory disturbances

Respiratory disturbances (chokes), which are a serious manifestation of decompression sickness, occur relatively infrequently (*Table 3.1*). The first symptom is almost invariably a sense of constriction around the lower chest, often with a tight feeling in the epigastrium. An attempt to take a deep breath causes an inspiratory 'snatch' which limits inspiration, and soreness develops beneath the sternum. There is frequently a general feeling of malaise and, as the condition develops, any attempt to take a deep breath causes coughing, which frequently becomes paroxysmal. If the exposure to altitude is maintained, chokes almost invariably progresses to collapse. The symptoms of chokes may persist for several hours after descent and may be precipitated during this period by tobacco smoke or a deep inspiration.

Chokes is probably part of the reflex response to irritation of the pulmonary tissues caused by the occlusion of pulmonary arterioles and capillaries by gas bubbles carried to the lungs from the peripheral tissues by the circulating blood. Thus the clinical picture produced by the intravenous injection of air in man often resembles chokes.

Neurological disturbances

Neurological disturbances ('staggers') are rare in aviation decompression sickness (*Table 3.1*). Paralysis, paraesthesia, anaesthesia and fits may be present in a wide variety of clinical pictures. No disturbance of smell, taste or hearing and only one case of permanent paralysis have been reported. The focal disturbances of function in the central nervous system are most probably the result of gas-bubble embolism.

Visual disturbances

The most commonly noted effects are blurring of vision, scotomata, 'fortification' patterns and hemianopia. These often occur in conjunction with other symptoms such as headache and are comparable with the visual symptoms of migraine. It is not known whether these symptoms are primarily vascular or neurological, but again they are probably the result of gas embolism.

Collapse

A small but significant proportion of cases of decompression sickness present with a general feeling of malaise, anxiety and diminished consciousness (*Table 3.1*). This syndrome may occur either in the absence of any other manifestations of decompression sickness (primary collapse) or in association with the bends, the chokes or central nervous system disorder (secondary collapse). Typically, the individual becomes restless and pale and his hands and face are cold and clammy with sweat. At this stage he generally feels hot and cold alternately. It is followed by impairment of consciousness. The radial pulse is virtually absent and there is usually bradycardia. Finally, the subject loses consciousness and he may or may not jactitate. Descent is usually followed by a rapid recovery. Vomiting is quite common and most cases develop a frontal headache.

Post-decompression collapse

The vast majority of individuals with decompression sickness recover either immediately or very shortly after descent to ground level. In a few instances, however, the symptoms may persist after return to ground level and, in a small number of cases, the symptoms and signs may become worse after descent. Post-decompression collapse occurs in 1 in 2500 exposures to altitudes greater than 30 000 feet. It virtually never follows an altitude exposure in which no symptom of decompression sickness occurred. Also, post-decompression collapse has never been reported when the only symptoms at altitude were mild bends at a single site or mild skin effects.

The clinical picture is variable. There may be an interval of several hours between the descent to ground level and the appearance of symptoms. Typically, the patient becomes anxious, develops a frontal headache, and feels sick. He has facial pallor and cold, sweaty extremities. There is nearly always peripheral cyanosis. General or focal signs of neurological involvement, such as weakness of the limbs, apraxia, scotomata and convulsions may occur. Mottling of the skin across the chest and shoulders is commonly very marked. The arterial blood pressure is generally well maintained until late in the development of the illness. Finally, in the worse cases, coma supervenes. Recovery can occur at any stage, although in the past it has been very rare once coma has developed. To date there have been 18 deaths due to decompression sickness reported in the world literature. A very consistent, early finding in all cases of severe post-decompression collapse is an increase in the blood haematocrit. Typically the haematocrit rises to 55–65+ There is often also a polymorphonuclear leucocytosis, and the patient may have a high fever.

The collapses seen in decompression sickness appear to be caused by air emboli scattered throughout the body by way of the systemic arterial tree. The main pathological changes found in the fatal cases—effusions in serous cavities, congested and oedematous lungs and marked haemoconcentration—indicate a massive loss of blood plasma to the extravascular compartment. These changes are most probably triggered by bubbles, in both the pulmonary and systemic arteries, obstructing capillary flow throughout the body. It is suggested that these bubbles arise in fat and pass, together with fat emboli, into the venous side of the circulation to produce a large-scale pulmonary gaseous embolism. The bubbles gain access to the systemic arterial tree through capillaries and shunts in the lungs. The delay of the onset of collapse until after return to ground level may be due to the descent reducing the size of many bubbles to that which allows them to traverse the lungs.

Incidence of decompression sickness

The factors that influence the incidence of decompression sickness can be considered under two main headings: general and personal.

General factors

Altitude

The altitude threshold for decompression sickness is 18 000 feet. Above this altitude (*Figure 3.1*) the incidence increases with altitude although the condition occurs only very rarely below 20 000 feet and rarely below 25 000 feet.

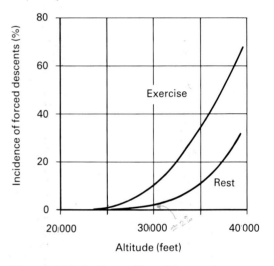

Figure 3.1 The incidence of forced descents due to decompression sickness during 2-hour exposures to various altitudes of subjects either seated at rest or carrying out moderate exercise.

Base altitude

Exposure to breathing air at pressures greater than 1 atmosphere during the 24 hours prior to flight increases the susceptibility to decompression sickness, since the amount of nitrogen present in the tissues may be increased and bubbles may have been formed in the tissues asymptomatically. This effect may be avoided by not undertaking ascents to altitude for at least 12 hours after exposure to a pressure of up to 2 bar abs (10 m of sea water) and at least 24 hours when the pressure to which the individual has been exposed exceeds 2 bar abs.

Rate of ascent

Within the range normally encountered in aviation, the rate of decompression *per se* has no significant effect on the incidence of decompression sickness.

Duration of exposure

Decompression sickness does not occur immediately on exposure to altitude (*Figure 3.2*). It is very rare for a case to occur before at least 5 minutes have passed at altitude. The rate of occurrence increases to reach a maximum at between 20 and 60 minutes exposure to altitude. The occurrence of new cases then falls, so that the total incidence approaches a plateau value which may or may not be 100% of those exposed.

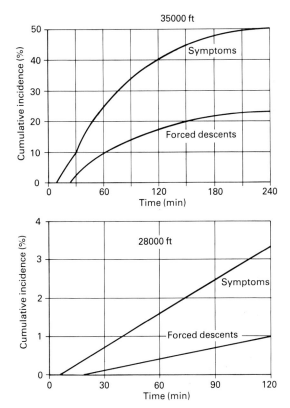

Figure 3.2 Time course of the development of symptoms and of forced descents due to decompression sickness in normal seated subjects exposed to simulated altitudes of 35 000 feet for 4 hours (upper graph) and 28 000 feet for 2 hours (lower graph).

Re-exposure

Re-exposure to altitude immediately after the first exposure greatly increases the susceptibility to decompression sickness. The longer the interval between the two exposures the less the increase in susceptibility but even when the interval is 24 hours, this effect is still apparent. The interval between two exposures must be increased to 48 hours to avoid an increase in susceptibility.

Exercise

Exercise at altitude greatly increases the susceptibility to decompression sickness (*see Figure 3.1*). It raises the incidence of symptoms at a given altitude and lowers the altitude at which symptoms appear. The effect of heavy exercise is roughly equivalent to an increase in the altitude of exposure of 5 000 feet.

Temperature

A low environmental temperature slightly increases the incidence of decompression sickness.

Hypoxia

The presence of hypoxia increases the incidence and severity of decompression sickness.

Personal factors

There is a true individual susceptibility to decompression sickness. Thus on repeated exposures to the same altitude an individual who developed decompression sickness on the first exposure is much more likely to develop the condition on a second exposure than an individual who did not have symptoms of decompression sickness on the first.

Age

Susceptibility to decompression sickness increases with age. Thus, there is a nine-fold increase in the liability to develop symptoms during a 2-hour exposure to 28 000 feet between the ages of 17–20 and 27–29 years.

Body build

The incidence of decompression sickness is greater in obese individuals. A reduction of the weight of an obese individual who has experienced serious symptoms of decompression sickness does not, however, usually reduce his susceptibility to the condition.

Injury

There is some evidence to suggest that recent joint or limb injury increases the local incidence of 'bends' pain.

General health

The after-effects of alcohol ingestion and the presence of infection both increase the susceptibility to decompression sickness.

Management of cases of decompression sickness

Differential diagnosis

It may be necessary to make a retrospective diagnosis when an individual has developed symptoms in flight and has either recovered or collapsed on descent. The differential diagnosis of decompression sickness includes the following:

1. Intercurrent illness—Myocardial ischaemia; spontaneous pneumothorax; limb pains due to cramp or injury; septicaemia.
2. Flight stresses—Pressure vertigo (at low altitude); abdominal distension; hypoxia; motion sickness (nausea and retching); acceleration atelectasis.
3. Psychological stresses—Anxiety; claustrophobia; anxiety-induced hyperventilation.

A careful history and clinical examination should allow most of these conditions to be excluded; but, in difficult cases, the haematocrit value is a useful diagnostic aid (a high value initially, for example 45% or over, or a significant increase in the haematocrit value over half an hour is highly suggestive of decompression sickness). The presence of pyrexia and leucocytosis are valuable but not specific confirmatory features.

Further observation and assessment of cases

The vast majority of cases of decompression sickness recover if rapid descent is carried out to low altitude (below 10000 feet). If the affected individual is suffering from severe bends, chokes, neurological disturbances or collapse he should, where possible, be laid flat and given 100% oxygen to breathe.

An individual who has had to make an emergency descent because of symptoms of decompression sickness should be examined medically as soon as possible. If, at this time, the symptoms have disappeared or shown marked improvement, he should be observed for at least 4 hours, and a close watch kept for any deterioration in his condition. The symptoms suggesting deterioration include frontal headache, nausea, visual disturbances, anxiety and sweating. The signs of deterioration include haemoconcentration, pyrexia, peripheral vascular failure, peripheral cyanosis, a weak, distal arterial pulse in the presence of a normal or near normal blood pressure; and neurological disturbances. If symptoms fail to improve within the first hour after

return to ground level, or new symptoms or signs appear within the first few hours, active treatment must be instituted.

Treatment of decompression sickness

The primary treatment of decompression sickness arising at altitude is recompression to ground level as rapidly as possible.

The effects of bubbles in tissues and body fluids can be decreased by overcompression—that is, exposure to a pressure greater than 1 atmosphere—and removal of nitrogen by the administration of 100% oxygen. Breathing 100% oxygen will also tend to relieve the tissue hypoxia produced by the reduction of local blood flow. Thus in practice, the treatment of choice in decompression sickness is compression of the patient in a hyperbaric chamber to a pressure of 2.8 bar abs (equivalent to the pressure at 18 m of sea water) with intermittent oxygen breathing.

The actual management of a case of serious decompression sickness must depend on geographical situation and availability of a suitable hyperbaric chamber. Therefore, the order of preference of available treatment is as follows:

1. Immediate hyperbaric compression with or without intermittent oxygen breathing.
2. Where no chamber facility exists, institution of treatment for circulatory collapse and early transfer to a hyperbaric chamber where this facility is available at a reasonable time or distance (less than 6 hours travel time). Surface transport is preferable: flight to a suitable chamber should be at an altitude below 1000 feet if possible and not higher than 3000 feet.
3. Full supportive treatment for circulatory collapse where there is no possibility of transfer within a reasonable time to a hyperbaric chamber.

Supportive treatment for circulatory collapse

The supportive treatment does not differ significantly from those methods already proven for circulatory collapse of different aetiology. The aim is to support the circulation and maintain the blood pressure by expanding the plasma volume. To this end, small molecular size dextran or plasma should be administered intravenously, and this may be supplemented by glucose/saline solution. In a seriously ill patient with hypotension which does not respond promptly to other measures, high doses of steroids should be given intravenously, e.g. hydrocortisone 500 mg over a few minutes. Throughout the treatment, the patient should be given 100% oxygen. Pleural effusions have been found in most fatal cases and, where the presence of a sizeable effusion is detected, fluid should be withdrawn to improve pulmonary expansion. If electrolyte imbalance or acidosis occurs, it should be corrected. Morphine should not be given because of the danger of respiratory depression.

Compression therapy

The patient, breathing 100% oxygen, should be compressed rapidly to 2.8 bar abs. If this procedure produces a marked improvement in his condition within 10 minutes then the exposure to 2.8 bar abs should be maintained for a further 30–60 minutes, with short periods of air breathing to reduce the possibility of oxygen toxicity. If the improvement is maintained, he is brought slowly to the surface with the intermittent administration of oxygen. If there is not a marked improvement after 10 minutes of oxygen breathing at 2.8 bar abs, or if deterioration occurs at any time during the treatment, oxygen breathing is discontinued and the patient is compressed immediately to 6 bar.

The subsequent decompression depends on the clinical state of the patient and is carried out according to standard diving therapeutic tables. It may be necessary to carry out supportive therapy during the overpressure treatment (for example, to administer fluids intravenously to restore the circulating blood volume). The need for this form of treatment is decided on clinical signs and the results of serial measurement of the hematocrit and blood electrolyte concentrations.

Disposal of cases

After recovery from decompression sickness, the patient should not be allowed to fly at a cabin altitude of 18 000 feet or above in an aircraft or be exposed to reduced atmospheric pressure in a decompression chamber until specialist medical opinion has been sought. It may well be necessary, when the symptoms have been severe, to recommend that he should never again be exposed to a pressure altitude in excess of 18 000 feet. In fatal cases of sub-atmospheric decompression sickness, or in deaths suggestive of decompression sickness occurring within 48 hours of exposure to altitude, the body should be conserved for autopsy.

Sequelae of decompression sickness

A striking feature of sub-atmospheric decompression sickness is the rapid and complete recovery which occurs in the vast majority of cases and the absence of permanent sequelae. However, it has been known since the beginning of the twentieth century that a significant proportion of compressed-air workers develop bone lesions later in life. Typically, these lesions comprise areas of aseptic or ischaemic necrosis in the head and neck of the femur, the head of the humerus and, less commonly, the lower end of the femur and the upper end of the tibia. Infarcts also occur in the medulla of the femur, the humerus and the tibia. These lesions are symptomless, unless and until a joint surface is involved. Thus the true incidence of this condition can best be determined by radiological surveys of the femur, the humerus and the tibia.

In spite of several radiological surveys of groups of individuals who have been exposed repeatedly to altitudes above 25 000 feet, only four unequivocal cases of aseptic bone necrosis due to altitude exposure have been reported in the literature. Two of these individuals had repeatedly suffered severe bends pain during flights at cabin altitudes above 30 000 feet. The lesions presented with pain and limitation of movement of the affected joint (shoulder, hip or knee). The bone lesions produced by exposure to high altitude are almost certainly due to intravascular bubbles.

Prevention of decompression sickness

Decompression sickness may be prevented by limiting the reduction of environmental pressure and/or the duration of the exposure to low pressure, or by eliminating nitrogen from the tissues and body fluids prior to the exposure to altitude.

Ideally, since the threshold for the occurrence of decompression sickness is 18 000 feet, aircrew and passengers should not be exposed to altitudes greater than this height. In practice, however, especially in military aircraft, the reduction of aircraft operating performance imposed by such a limitation may be unacceptable. The possible harmful effects of the rapid decompression of the pressure cabin led in the past to the selection of a maximum cabin altitude of 25 000 feet, as an acceptable compromise between the need to reduce the incidence of hypoxia and decompression sickness on the one hand, and to avoid a high cabin pressure differential on the other. If, however, a cabin altitude of 25 000 feet is maintained for several hours, decompression sickness may occur with sufficient frequency to be of practical importance. Since subsequent experience has shown that the incidence and harmful effects of rapid decompression of low differential pressure cabins had been overestimated, the best practical compromise now is that the maximum cabin altitude should not exceed 22 000 feet. The need to avoid exposures to pressures greater than 1 atmosphere absolute in the

12–24 hour period before a flight has already been mentioned.

The removal of the nitrogen which is normally dissolved in the tissues and body fluids is accomplished by breathing 100% oxygen before exposure to reduced pressure, a procedure termed 'pre-oxygenation' or 'denitrogenation'. The removal of nitrogen from the tissues, especially those that contain a high concentration of lipid and those with a low blood flow, takes an appreciable time. The protection afforded against decompression sickness is related to the amount of nitrogen removed from the tissues, and hence to the time for which 100% oxygen is breathed. This in turn depends on the altitude and the duration of the intended exposure. Thus pre-oxygenation for 30 minutes will ensure that an individual will not develop decompression sickness during a short-duration exposure to an altitude of 48 000 feet in which the time for which he is at altitudes above 25 000 feet does not exceed 10 minutes. On the other hand, pre-oxygenation must be carried out at ground level for 3 hours in order to prevent decompression sickness occurring during a subsequent exposure to an altitude of 40 000 feet for 3 hours. This method of prevention is widely used in the training of aircrew in the use of personal oxygen equipment and pressure clothing. It is present policy for aircrew who are undergoing such training in hypobaric chambers to breathe 100% oxygen for 30–60 minutes (depending on the nature of the subsequent exposure) before they are exposed to altitudes in excess of 25 000 feet. Pre-oxygenation can also be used to protect experimental subjects who are to be exposed to high altitudes in hypobaric chambers, and aircrew flying to high altitudes in unpressurized aircraft. It is, however, a time-consuming and complicated procedure which is not practical in many operational situations.

Finally, since there is a wide variability in individual susceptibility to decompression sickness, the relatively unsusceptible may be selected by testing in a hypobaric chamber. This technique was widely used during and immediately after World War II to avoid decompression sickness in aviation. Such testing is uncommon today. However, in certain circumstances, such as the use of unpressurized training aircraft at high altitudes, selection tests are still used to eliminate those aircrew who have a high susceptibility to decompression sickness. Experience has shown that the most successful approach to the design of such tests is to simulate, in a hypobaric chamber, exposure to the most severe cabin altitude/time profile to which the aircrew will be exposed during flight. In order to reduce the occurrence of serious cases of decompression sickness in selection testing to an absolute minimum, it is essential that the tests should be carried out by experienced medical officers and that full facilities, including a 6-atmosphere absolute hypobaric chamber, should be immediately available for the treatment of any case that may arise.

Further reading

BUCKLES, R.G. (1968) The physics of bubble formation and growth. Symposium on Undersea Aerospace Medicine, 39th Meeting. *Aerospace Medicine*, **39**, 1062–1069

FRYER, D.I. (1969) *Sub-Atmospheric Decompression Sickness in Man*. AGARD-ograph (NATO) No 129

MACMILLAN, A.J.F. (1970) *The Management of Sub-Atmospheric Decompression Sickness*. IAM Report No 489 (Revised 1983). London: Ministry of Defence.

OLSON, R.M., KRUTZ, R.W. and DIXON, G.A. (1986) Validity of ultra-sonic monitoring at altitude for bends protection. *Aviation, Space and Environmental Medicine*, **57**, 511

RAYMAN, R.B. (1983) Decompression sickness: USAF experience 1970–80. *Aviation, Space and Environmental Medicine*, **54**, 258–260

4

Respiratory physiology

J. Ernsting

Introduction

A clear understanding of the physiological disturbances induced by lack of oxygen rests on a knowledge of the processes whereby oxygen and carbon dioxide are exchanged between the tissues and the environment. It is convenient to consider respiration as occurring in a series of steps as follows:

1. Consumption of oxygen and production of carbon dioxide by the tissues.
2. Exchange of gases between blood and the tissues.
3. Carriage of gases by the blood between the tissues and the lungs.
4. Exchange of gases between the blood in the lungs and the environment.

The processes underlying the exchange of gases between the blood and the environment is called external respiration: the carriage of gases to and from the tissues and the gas exchange in the tissues constitute internal respiration.

Tissue respiration

Cellular metabolism

The immediate source of energy for virtually all biological processes is the chemical energy held in the special energy-rich bonds of adenosine triphosphate (ATP). In living material, hydrolysis of the terminal energy-rich phosphate bond of ATP with the formation of adenosine diphosphate (ADP) and a phosphate radical is intimately associated with the performance of work. The work associated with the hydrolysis of ATP to ADP may be mechanical

(contraction of a muscle), chemical synthesis (formation of protein and fat), electrical (passage of a nerve impulse), osmotic (the formation of urine), or simply the liberation of heat. The amount of ATP in the cellular cytoplasm is relatively small. Although most cells contain reserve stores of energy-rich bonds in the phosphate bond of creatine phosphate, which can in the short term regenerate ATP from ADP, new energy-rich bonds must be generated eventually in order to restore the resting levels of ATP and creatine phosphate.

Energy-rich bonds are generated by the disruption of the chemical bonds of complex molecules, such as glucose and fatty acid, by oxidation (*Figure 4.1*). This process in the presence of oxygen (aerobic catabolism) results eventually in the oxidation of the complex molecules to carbon dioxide and water and the formation of large numbers of energy-rich phosphate bonds. Thus one molecule of glucose, when completely oxidized, yields 38 molecules of ATP. The breakdown of glucose can, however, proceed part way in the absence of oxygen (anaerobic metabolism), the process ceasing at the 3-carbon-atom molecule pyruvic acid, which is transformed to lactic acid, allowing more glucose to be broken down to pyruvic acid. This anaerobic process is, however, much less efficient than the complete oxidation of glucose. The breakdown of glucose to lactic acid yields only 2 molecules of ATP per molecule of glucose. Furthermore, the accumulation of lactic acid eventually limits the activity of the working tissues, although it is completely oxidized by heart muscle and synthesized to glycogen in the liver.

The complete oxidation of the 2- and 3-carbon-atom compounds produced by the breakdown of glucose, fats and proteins occurs in the mitochondria of the cytoplasm. Here, in a series of complex

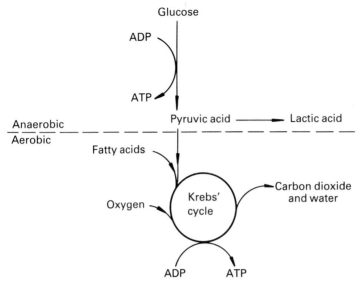

Figure 4.1 The major steps in the breakdown of glucose and fatty acids to carbon dioxide (and water) and the generation of energy-rich phosphate bonds of adenosine triphosphate (ATP). The initial steps in the breakdown of glucose to pyruvic acid can proceed in the absence of oxygen (anaerobic) when lactic acid is formed. In the presence of oxygen, however, the pyruvic acid is oxidized to carbon dioxide and water by a complex series of reactions catalysed by numerous enzymes (the Krebs' cycle). The energy-rich phosphate bonds generated in this manner are captured in the terminal phosphate bond of ATP which is formed from adenosine diphosphate (ADP).

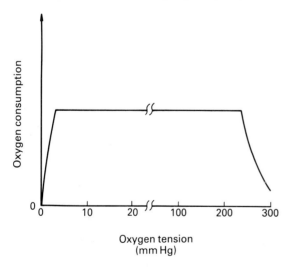

Figure 4.2 The relationship between the rate of oxidative phosphorylation expressed as rate of consumption of oxygen and the local oxygen tension at the surface of the mitochondria. Over a very wide range of oxygen tensions the rate of oxygen uptake is independent of the oxygen tension. Only at oxygen tensions below 0.5–3.0 mm Hg (0.07–0.4 kPa) is the oxidative rate of phosphorylation limited by the supply of oxygen. The fall in rate of oxygen consumption at high oxygen tensions is due to disruption of enzymes by the high oxygen tension (oxygen toxicity).

reactions known as the Kreb's cycle, these compounds are oxidized to carbon dioxide and water, with the generation of many molecules of ATP. This process is termed oxidative phosphorylation. The final step of the chain, oxidation with the formation of water, is catalysed by the enzyme cytochrome oxidase. Oxidative phosphorylation requires a certain minimum molecular concentration i.e. partial pressure (tension) of oxygen (*Figure 4.2*). Above this critical value, however, the rate of oxidation is independent of the local oxygen tension, although of course it is affected by many other factors such as the availability of substrate, the activity of the tissue, etc. The value of this critical oxygen tension required at the mitochondria varies with the type of cell but typically lies within the range 0.5–3.0 mm Hg (0.07–0.4 kPa). Thus if aerobic metabolism is not to be limited by the available oxygen supply, the oxygen transport system must maintain the oxygen tension at the mitochondria greater than 0.5–3 mm Hg (0.07–0.4 kPa). It may be seen from *Figure 4.2* that the rate of oxygen consumption of the mitochondria falls at very high oxygen tensions. This phenomenon, which is due to disruption of some of the enzymes of the Krebs' cycle, is one of the mechanisms involved in oxygen poisoning. Between these two limits, the rate of consumption of oxygen by the mitochondria is independent of the local oxygen tension. The primary determinant of the rate of oxygen consumption is the demand for energy-rich phosphate bonds, that is, the activity of the tissue.

More than 90% of the oxygen consumed by the tissues is involved in the generation of energy-rich bonds by oxidative phosphorylation under the influence of the enzyme cytochrome oxidase. Most of the remaining consumption of oxygen also involves the removal of hydrogen from complex molecules such as amino acids and amines. The activities of many of the enzymes controlling these oxidations vary with the oxygen concentration at oxygen tensions considerably greater than 100 mm Hg (13.3 kPa). Finally, a very small proportion (about 1%) of the oxygen consumed by the tissues is involved in reactions in which oxygen is incorporated into complex organic molecules, a process known as oxygenation. They include the reactions responsible for the production and destruction of biogenic amines and steroid hormones. The activity of the enzymes (oxygenases) controlling these reactions is affected by relatively high tensions. The rates of certain oxygenations are significantly reduced by a fall of oxygen tension from 100 to 60 mm Hg (13.3 to 8.0 kPa). Thus while the consumption of oxygen by the tissues to generate the energy-rich bonds of ATP is virtually unaffected by a reduction of the local oxygen tension to as low as 3 mm Hg (0.4 kPa) changes of cellular oxygen tension in the range 5–100 mm Hg (0.68–13.3 kPa) may have very significant effects on the rates of certain oxygenation reactions.

The major products of the complete oxidation of foodstuffs are carbon dioxide, ammonia and water. The rate at which carbon dioxide is produced is closely related to the rate at which oxygen is consumed. The ratio of the volume of carbon dioxide produced to the volume of oxygen consumed per unit time by the tissues is termed the respiratory quotient (RQ). This ratio varies with the nature of the foodstuff being oxidized. The oxidation of carbohydrates (sugars) gives a RQ of 1.0; that of fat or protein about 0.7. The RQ of an individual on a normal mixed diet lies in the range 0.80–0.85.

In contrast to the rapid, gross effects when the oxygen supply is cut off, a rise in the molecular concentration of carbon dioxide of itself does not disrupt tissue function. Throughout the body, however, carbon dioxide is in equilibrium with hydrogen ions and bicarbonate ions according to the equation:

$$CO_2 + H_2O \rightleftharpoons H_2CO_3 \rightleftharpoons H^+ + HCO_3^-$$

A rise of the concentration of carbon dioxide will, therefore, result in an increase in the concentration of hydrogen ions. This increase of acidity is much less well tolerated by the tissues than the causative rise of carbon dioxide concentration.

Tissue oxygen requirements

The rate of oxygen consumption varies with the tissue and its activity, for example, the oxygen consumption of cerebral tissue is 3.5 ml/min/100 g whilst that of skeletal muscle varies from 0.2 ml/min/100 g at rest to 11 ml/min/100 g during hard work. The partition of the total oxygen consumption of a resting man between the major organs of the body is summarized in *Table 4.1*. At rest, the brain, which is

Table 4.1 Partition of oxygen consumption in a normal subject (70 kg body weight) at rest

Organ/region	Oxygen consumption	
	ml (STPD)/min	% Total
Brain	47	18
Heart	28	11
Kidney	18	7
Splanchnic region	62	25
Skeletal muscle	75	30
Skin	5	2
Other organs	15	6
Total	250	100

Note: The oxygen consumed by the respiratory muscles which is included in the figure for skeletal muscles amounts to 5 ml/min or 2% of the total.

2% of the body weight, consumes almost one-fifth of the total oxygen uptake and, even at rest, skeletal muscle, which is 40% of the body weight, uses nearly one-third of the total oxygen supply. In moderate exercise, sufficient to increase the total oxygen consumption to twice that at rest (that is, 500 ml/min), the oxygen uptake of skeletal muscle rises to about 300 ml/min, 60% of the total oxygen consumption.

The total oxygen consumption of an individual at rest in a thermally neutral environment is proportional to the surface area of the body. The basal metabolic oxygen consumption varies slightly from one individual to another and falls progressively with age. The average basal oxygen consumption of normal young men amounts to 1.33 l (STPD)/min/m^2 of body surface. A man weighing 70 kg who is 1.8 m tall (body surface area = 1.9 m^2) has a basal oxygen consumption of 253 ml (STPD)/min. Although extremes of environmental temperature and changes of deep body temperature affect total oxygen consumption to a limited extent, by far the most important determinant of oxygen consumption is the level of physical activity. Typical values of the total oxygen consumption for various activities are presented in *Table 4.2*.

Table 4.2 Total oxygen consumption during various activities for average sized young men

Activity	Total oxygen consumption (l(STPD)/min)
Sleep	0.24
Lying fully relaxed	0.24
Lying moderately relaxed	0.28
Sitting at rest	0.34
Standing relaxed	0.36
Walking (5 km/h)	0.85
Running (10 km/h)	2.80
Flying an aircraft	
DC3 level flight	0.34
Light aircraft in rough air	0.54
Taxiing DC3	0.58
Aerobatics	0.65
Air combat manoeuvring	1.00

+ Basal O₂ consumption DECREASES with age.

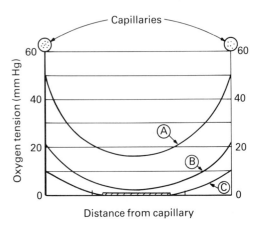

Figure 4.3 A cross-section of a simple model of the distribution of tissue oxygen tension in which symmetrically arranged parallel capillaries carry blood in one direction through a tissue with uniform oxygen consumption. The solid curves (A, B and C) depict the magnitude of the oxygen tension with distance from a capillary. The tension falls to a minimum at a point mid-way between the two capillaries. When the oxygen tension in the capillary blood is high (curve A) the oxygen tension everywhere in the tissue exceeds 15 mm Hg (2.0 kPa). When the capillary oxygen tension is reduced to about 20 mm Hg (2.7 kPa) (curve B) the oxygen tension in the tissue mid-way between the capillaries falls to about 2 mm Hg (0.27 kPa) whereas when the capillary oxygen tension falls to about 10 mm Hg (1.33 kPa) the oxygen tension of a significant part of the tissue is zero.

Blood–tissue gas exchange

The oxygen required for oxidation is brought to a tissue by the blood flowing through its capillaries. This flow of blood also removes the carbon dioxide produced by respiration in the tissue. The exchange of oxygen and carbon dioxide between the blood in the capillaries and the cells of a tissue occurs by simple physical diffusion. The molecules of each gas move through the blood, the capillary wall and the cells of the tissue down the concentration gradient in accordance with Fick's law of diffusion. The latter states that the rate of diffusion of a gas between two points in a fluid is proportional to the difference of the concentrations (partial pressures) of the gas at the two points and inversely proportional to the distance between them. The rate of diffusion is also proportional to the solubility of the gas in the fluid and inversely proportional to the square root of the molecular weight of the gas. Since the solubility of carbon dioxide in tissue is much greater than that of oxygen, carbon dioxide diffuses about 20 times more rapidly than oxygen. The transfer of carbon dioxide to the blood is, therefore, much less of a problem than the delivery of oxygen from the blood in the capillaries to the mitochondria of the tissues.

The consumption of oxygen by the cells causes the partial pressure tension of oxygen to fall progressively with distance from the blood in the capillary (*Figure 4.3*). As the distance from the capillary increases beyond a certain point, the oxygen supply ceases to come from that capillary and is provided by another neighbouring capillary. There are, therefore, points within a tissue where the oxygen tension is a minimum. The value of this minimum oxygen tension is determined by the oxygen tension in the capillary blood, the tissue oxygen consumption and the intercapillary distance. A lowering of the oxygen tension in the blood, a rise in oxygen

consumption or an increase in the distance between capillaries all reduce the minimum oxygen tension. The condition of the local oxygen supply becomes critical when the minimum oxygen tension falls to a level at which it limits the rate of oxidative phosphorylation, that is, a value of 1–3 mm Hg (0.13–0.4 kPa) (*Figure 4.3*, curve B). If the minimum oxygen tension is reduced further, then the tissue in that region turns to anaerobic metabolism with the formation of lactic acid (*Figure 4.3*, curve C). Such regions are termed lethal areas or corners. The fall of oxygen tension in the blood as it flows through the capillary bed is determined by the oxygen content of the arterial blood, the rate at which oxygen is removed by the tissue, the blood flow and the relationship between oxygen tension and oxygen content in the blood. The reduction of the oxygen content of the blood is related simply to the blood flow and oxygen consumption by the tissue as follows (the Fick principle):

Arteriovenous blood oxygen content difference =
$$\frac{\text{Rate of oxygen consumption}}{\text{Blood flow}}$$

The fall of oxygen content from the arterial blood to any given point in the capillary is therefore proportional to the rate at which oxygen passes from that length of the bed into the tissue and inversely proportional to the blood flow. The manner in which oxygen tension falls along the capillary is determined by the sigmoid relationship between oxygen content and tension of blood, which is defined by the oxygen haemoglobin dissociation curve (*see* Carriage of Gases by the Blood).

There are two important mechanisms whereby the oxygen tension in potential lethal corners can be raised when the oxygen consumption of a tissue increases: an increase in the flow of blood through the capillaries, which reduces the fall of oxygen tension along the length of the capillary bed; and the opening up of additional capillaries which reduces the maximum distance over which oxygen has to diffuse and thus reduces the fall of oxygen tension from the capillary to potential lethal corners. Both of these mechanisms operate in most tissues even at rest. Thus the capillary bed is normally in a dynamic state with new capillaries opening up as the local tissue oxygen tension falls to a low level and other capillaries closing down. These changes in the capillaries are almost certainly mediated locally—a fall of oxygen tension, a rise of carbon dioxide tension and an increase in acidity, which usually occur together, all cause the opening up of previously closed capillaries and dilatation of capillaries are almost certainly mediated locally—a evidence that the changes in tissue oxygen and carbon dioxide tension associated with local hypoxia can cause dilatation of the arterioles feeding that particular capillary bed and thus increase blood flow. The magnitude of the changes of blood flow and capillarity that can occur in response to an increase in activity and hence in the demand for oxygen and removal of carbon dioxide varies from one tissue to another. The number of open capillaries in muscle during maximum exercise is 100–200 times greater than that at rest. There is at the same time a 20-fold increase in the blood flow. In many regions of the brain, most of the capillary bed is open even at rest, and there is only a 2- to 4-fold increase in the number of open capillaries during intense activity or in the face of a threat of tissue hypoxia.

The supply of oxygen to a tissue is virtually always more critical than the removal of carbon dioxide since (1) accumulation of carbon dioxide causes much less disruption of tissue function than hypoxia; (2) carbon dioxide requires only one-twentieth of the partial pressure difference needed for oxygen to diffuse at the same rate; and (3) the tissue storage capacity for carbon dioxide (which is stored by conversion to bicarbonate ion) is much greater than for oxygen. In most circumstances, the adjustments of the blood flow through, and the capillarity of, a

tissue are set by the demand for oxygen. Paradoxically, in certain circumstances lowering of the tension of carbon dioxide in the arterial blood, which increases the removal of carbon dioxide from the tissues, induces hypoxia. A reduction of the arterial carbon dioxide tension causes intense vasoconstriction of the cerebral arterioles, so that a halving of the normal carbon dioxide tension reduces the blood flow through the brain by half. Thus although hyperventilation on air increases slightly the oxygen tension of the arterial blood it induces hypoxia in brain tissue.

When the oxygen tension in the lethal corners of a tissue is inadequate to maintain oxidative phosphorylation, energy-rich phosphate bonds can only be generated by anaerobic metabolism, with the formation of lactic acid. This situation occurs at the beginning of even light muscular exercise, since it takes time for the blood flow to the working tissue to increase to the required level. Once the blood flow has increased to raise the oxygen tension throughout the tissue, the formation of lactic acid ceases. With very high levels of exercise, the increase in the demand for oxygen cannot be met by the circulation and lactic acid formation continues until the muscles can no longer contract.

Carriage of gases by the blood

Oxygen

Oxygen is carried in the blood in physical solution and in chemical combination. The concentration of dissolved oxygen varies directly with the tension of this gas in accordance with Henry's law. The concentration of oxygen dissolved at an oxygen tension of 100 mm Hg (13.3 kPa) is 0.3 ml/100 ml blood, which is about 1.5% of the concentration of oxygen in chemical combination with haemoglobin (*Figure 4.4*). Even when the arterial oxygen tension is raised to about 650 mm Hg (86.6 kPa) by breathing 100% oxygen at one atmosphere, the quantity of oxygen in physical solution (1.95 ml/100 ml blood) is only about 40% of that removed from the blood by the tissues.

Oxygen undergoes an easily reversible combination with haemoglobin to form oxyhaemoglobin. Haemoglobin is a conjugated protein composed of haeme, an iron-porphyrin compound, and globin, a protein consisting of four polypeptide chains. Each haemoglobin molecule contains four iron atoms which are in the ferrous state. The haemoglobin is contained in the red cells, and the normal concentration of haemoglobin is 15 g/100 ml blood. The maximum amount of oxygen which can combine with one gramme of haemoglobin is 1.39 ml; so that the total amount of oxygen which can be carried in

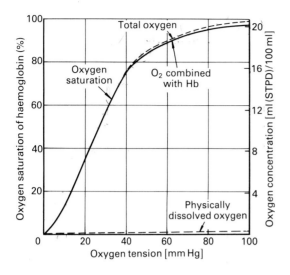

Figure 4.4 The oxygen dissociation curve of blood. The relationship for normal blood (haemoglobin concentration = 15 g/100 ml) at pH = 7.4, P_{CO_2} = 40 mm Hg (5.3 kPa) and 37°C between oxygen tension and oxygen concentration (broken curve) and oxygen saturated (solid line). The concentration of physically dissolved and chemically combined oxygen are shown separately.

combination with haemoglobin in normal blood (the *oxygen capacity* of the blood) is 1.39 × 15 = 20.8 ml/100 ml blood. The quantity of oxygen present in the blood in combination with haemoglobin is frequently expressed as the *oxygen saturation* of haemoglobin which is given by the relationship:

$$\text{Oxygen saturation} = \frac{\text{Concentration of } O_2 \text{ combined with Hb}}{\text{Oxygen capacity of blood}} \times 100\%$$

The relationship between the oxygen saturation of haemoglobin and the oxygen tension is described by the oxygen dissociation curve, which is sigmoid in shape (*Figure 4.4*). The oxygen saturation of the haemoglobin of blood (at pH 7.4, P_{CO_2} = 40 mm Hg (5.3 kPa) and 37°C) is about 97.5% at an oxygen tension of 100 mm Hg (13.3 kPa). For practical purposes it can be assumed that the haemoglobin is fully saturated with oxygen at oxygen tensions greater than 200 mm Hg (26.6 kPa). At low oxygen tensions, below about 50 mm Hg (6.7 kPa), the oxygen saturation increases rapidly with tension, whereas at higher oxygen tension the curve is much flatter. Thus a 10 mm Hg (1.3 kPa) change of oxygen tension from 90 to 100 mm Hg (12.0 to 13.3 kPa) increases the saturation by only 1% whereas a similar change of oxygen tension from 35 to 45 mm Hg (4.7 to 6.0 kPa) increases the saturation

by 14%. The haemoglobin is half saturated with oxygen (P_{50}) at an oxygen tension of about 26 mm Hg (3.5 kPa).

The shape of the oxygen dissociation curve of blood is of great physiological significance. The flat upper portion of the curve means that moderate variations of the alveolar oxygen tension about the normal value (103 mm Hg (13.7 kPa)) produced by breathing air at one atmosphere have relatively small effects on the concentration of oxygen in the arterial blood. Furthermore, the steep part of the curve between oxygen tensions of 40 and 55 mm Hg (5.3 and 7.3 kPa) ensures that, during the passage of the blood through the pulmonary capillaries, the oxygen tension does not rise until much of the oxygen has been transferred to the blood. Thus a high oxygen tension gradient aiding diffusion of oxygen into the blood is maintained over much of the time for which transfer of oxygen is taking place. The steep portion of the curve at lower oxygen tensions greatly aids the unloading of oxygen from the blood in the tissues. The loss of a large amount of oxygen results in only a relatively small fall in the oxygen tension in the blood, which is an important factor in maintaining the oxygen tension in the tissue cells. Finally, the steep part of the oxygen dissociation curve tends to maintain the tension at which oxygen is delivered to the tissues when the arterial oxygen tension is lowered in hypoxia.

The shape of the oxygen dissociation curve is unaffected by the concentration of haemoglobin in the blood. It is, however, affected by pH, carbon dioxide tension, temperature and the concentration of 2,3-diphosphoglycerate (2,3-DPG) in the red cells. A fall in pH, a rise of carbon dioxide tension and a rise of temperature all shift the curve to the right. All these changes, which occur in working

Table 4.3 Oxygen content of arterial and mixed venous blood of man at rest (haemoglobin concentration = 15 g/100 ml)

	Arterial blood	Mixed venous blood
Oxygen tension (mm Hg)	95.00	42.00
(kPa)	12.7	5.6
Oxygen concentration (ml/100 ml)		
Physically dissolved	0.29	0.13
Combined with haemoglobin	20.23	15.37
Total	20.52	15.50
Oxygen saturation (%)	97.00	74.00
Arteriovenous difference (ml/100 ml)		
Physically dissolved		0.16
Combined with haemoglobin		4.86
Total		5.02

tissue, increase the amount of oxygen given up by the blood at a given oxygen tension, thus favouring oxygen delivery in the tissues. Most of the effect of carbon dioxide (the Bohr effect) can be attributed to associated changes of pH within the red cell. The Bohr effect also operates in the pulmonary capillary blood, so that the affinity of haemoglobin for oxygen increases; that is, the oxygen dissociation curve moves to the left as carbon dioxide diffuses out of the blood into the alveolar gas. The Bohr effect accounts for about 10% of the total oxygen uptake in the pulmonary capillaries.

The total concentration of oxygen in the blood is the sum of that in physical solution and that carried in combination with haemoglobin (*Figure 4.4*). Typical values for the concentrations of oxygen in the arterial and mixed venous blood of a normal individual at rest are given in *Table 4.3*.

The difference between the concentrations of oxygen $[O_2]$ in the arterial and mixed venous blood is related to the total oxygen consumption and the cardiac output by Fick's equation:

$$[O_2] \text{ arterial} - [O_2] \text{ venous} =$$

$$\frac{\text{Oxygen consumption}}{\text{Cardiac output}}$$

Thus a man seated at rest with a total oxygen consumption of 250 ml (SPTD)/min and a cardiac output of 5 l/min has an arteriovenous oxygen concentration difference of 5 ml/100 ml blood. Although the cardiac output increases in exercise, the increase is inadequate to meet the rise in the oxygen consumption of the tissues; so that the arteriovenous oxygen difference is also increased. Thus in exercise sufficient to raise the oxygen consumption to 1.0 l (SPTD)/min, the cardiac output averages 10 l/min; so that the arteriovenous oxygen difference is 10 ml/100 ml blood. Since the concentration of oxygen in the arterial blood is virtually unchanged by slight and moderate exercise, the increased arteriovenous oxygen difference results in a reduction of the oxygen concentration in the mixed venous blood. The venous oxygen concentration falls from about 15.5 ml/100 ml at rest to 10.5 ml/100 ml in exercise, with an oxygen uptake of 1.0 l (SPTD)/ min. The corresponding oxygen saturations of the mixed venous blood are 74% and 50%.

Carbon dioxide

Carbon dioxide is carried in the blood in three forms: in physical solution, as bicarbonate and in combination with protein. As with oxygen, the concentration of dissolved carbon dioxide is proportional to the tension of the gas, but carbon dioxide is some twenty times as soluble as oxygen. Thus the concentration of dissolved carbon dioxide in blood at a tension of 40 mm Hg (5.3 kPa) is 2.6 ml (SPTD)/100 ml. Bicarbonate is formed by the dissociation of carbonic acid which is produced by the hydration of carbon dioxide:

$$CO_2 + H_2O \rightleftharpoons H_2CO_3 \rightleftharpoons H^+ + HCO_3^-$$
carbonic anhydrase

The hydration of carbon dioxide to carbonic acid proceeds very slowly in the plasma, but the enzyme carbonic anhydrate in the red cells catalyses the reaction; so that significant formation of carbonic acid occurs only within the red cell. The subsequent dissociation into bicarbonate and hydrogen ions is very rapid. The bicarbonate ions formed from dissolved carbon dioxide pass back into the plasma, whilst the hydrogen ions are buffered by the proteins within the red cell. An important buffer is haemoglobin. Reduced haemoglobin is a more effective buffer than oxyhaemoglobin, so that the deoxygenation of the blood which occurs in the tissue capillaries favours the formation of bicarbonate and hence the uptake of carbon dioxide. Conversely, oxygenation of blood in the lungs favours the conversion of bicarbonate to carbon dioxide. The concentration of carbon dioxide carried as bicarbonate in arterial blood at a carbon dioxide tension of 40 mm Hg (5.3 kPa) about 44 ml (SPTD)/100 ml, which is approximately 90% of the total carbon dioxide concentration. The remaining 5% of the total carbon dioxide is carried as carbamino compounds with the amine groups of proteins, especially the globin of haemoglobin:

$$HbNH_2 + CO_2 \rightleftharpoons HbNHCOOH \rightleftharpoons HbNHCOO^- + H^+$$

This type of reaction occurs rapidly; and since oxyhaemoglobin binds less carbon dioxide as carbamino compound than reduced haemoglobin, it favours uptake of carbon dioxide in the tissues and the reverse process in the pulmonary capillaries.

The carbon dioxide dissociation curve of whole blood (*Figure 4.5*) is much more linear over the physiologically significant range than the oxygen dissociation curve (*Figure 4.4*). Since the oxygen saturation of haemoglobin affects both the bicarbonate concentration and the concentration of carbamino haemoglobin, the oxygen saturation affects the carbon dioxide dissociation curve (*Figure 4.5*). *In vivo*, the oxygen saturation of the blood falls as the carbon dioxide tension rises; so that the 'physiological' dissociation curve is of the form depicted by the broken line in *Figure 4.5*. Typical values for the concentrations of carbon dioxide in the arterial and venous bloods of a normal individual at rest are given in *Table 4.4*. Although 90% of the carbon dioxide content of blood is in the form of bicarbonate, only just half of the arteriovenous carbon dioxide concentration difference is accounted for by the change in bicarbonate concentration. A third of the arteriovenous carbon dioxide difference is due to changes in the concentrations of carbamino compounds.

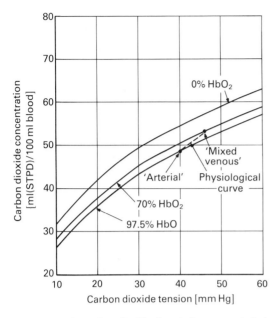

Figure 4.5 The carbon dioxide dissociation curve of whole blood at oxyhaemoglobin saturations of 0% (fully reduced), 70% (mixed venous blood at rest) and 97.5% (arterial blood breathing air at rest). The broken line depicts the relationship (the 'physiological curve') between carbon dioxide tension and carbon dioxide concentration which is followed as blood takes up carbon dioxide in the tissues and gives it up in the pulmonary capillaries.

Table 4.4 Carbon dioxide content of arterial blood and mixed venous blood of man at rest

	Arterial blood	Mixed venous blood
Carbon dioxide tension:		
(mm Hg)	40.0	46.0
(kPa)	5.3	6.1
Carbon dioxide concentration (ml/100 ml):		
Physically dissolved	2.6	3.0
As bicarbonates	43.8	46.4
As carbamino compound	2.6	3.9
Total	49.0	53.3
Arteriovenous difference		
Physically dissolved		0.4
As bicarbonate		2.6
As carbamino compound		1.3
Total		4.3

Gas exchange in the lung

Functional anatomy

The primary function of the lung is the exchange of oxygen and carbon dioxide between the venous blood and the air. It also has other important functions, such as filtering toxic materials, for example, blood thrombi from the circulation, metabolism of certain biologically active agents such as vasoconstrictor agents, serotonin, bradykinin and histamine and substances such as heparin which are involved in blood clotting. It also acts as a reservoir of blood.

The structure of the lung is such that air and blood are brought into intimate contact in some 300 million air sacs or alveoli, each of which is approximately 0.3 mm in diameter. Gases are exchanged across the alveolar capillary membrane. The vast number of alveoli gives the membrane a total area of 50–100 m². The membrane is also very thin, its thickness averaging 0.5 μm. Both the very large area and the thinness of the alveolar capillary membrane serve to minimize the resistance to gas diffusion between the blood and gas phases (*see* Fick's law of diffusion).

The arrangement of the lung, which may be regarded as a collection of some 300 million interconnected bubbles, is inherently unstable. The forces normally generated by surface tension at the air–wall interface in bubbles of this size are relatively large. The surface tension forces tend to cause collapse of the smaller alveoli (the force generated by surface tension being inversely proportional to the radius of the bubbles): but some of the cells lining the alveoli secrete a material (surfactant) which profoundly lowers the surface tension of the alveolar lining fluid. The surfactant (which contains dipalmitoyl lecithin) greatly reduces the tendency of small alveoli to empty into larger ones and hence promotes the stability of the lung structure. It also decreases the stiffness of the lung, reducing the effort required to ventilate it, and reduces the forces tending to draw fluid from the blood into the alveoli.

Functionally, the respiratory passages can be divided into two regions, the conducting airways and the respiratory zone. The upper conducting airways comprise the nose, the mouth, the pharynx, the trachea and the main, lobar, segmental and terminal bronchi (these comprise the first 16 generations of branches of the respiratory tree). The latter are the smallest airways without alveoli. The conducting airways carry inspired air down to the gas-exchanging regions of the lungs. The gas within the conducting airways cannot exchange with the blood and it constitutes the anatomical dead space. It has a volume of about 150 ml. The terminal bronchioles divide into respiratory bronchioles, which have alveoli attached to their walls. The final division of the airways constitutes the alveolar ducts, which are lined completely with alveoli. These lower parts of the airways, which comprise the remaining seven generations of the respiratory tree, are termed the transitory and respiratory zones of the lung, since the gas contained within them (the 'alveolar gas')

Dead space 150 ml
Respiratory zone 2500 ml (17x)

can exchange through the alveolar walls with the blood. The distance from the terminal bronchiole to the most distal alveolus is only about 5 mm. The respiratory zone has, however, a volume of about 2500 ml and contains most of the gas held in the lung. The combined cross-sectional area of the airways increases extremely rapidly beyond the terminal bronchioles, so that, although inspiration causes bulk movement of gas down the conducting airways, the forward velocity of the gas becomes very small as it enters the respiratory zone. Indeed, in the respiratory zone, ventilation occurs mainly by diffusion, there being very little mass movement of gas. The rate of diffusion of gas molecules is so rapid and the distances are so small that differences in concentration produced by inspiration within the airways and alveoli beyond the terminal bronchioles are abolished in less than 1 second.

The pulmonary arteries run into the lung tissue alongside the branching airways subdividing by way of arterioles to feed the capillary beds which surround the alveoli. The networks of capillaries around the alveoli are very dense and the capillary segments are so narrow and short that there is almost a continuous sheet of blood over the alveolar wall. The resistance to flow through the pulmonary circuit is relatively low—the mean pulmonary arterial pressure being only 15 mm Hg (2.0 kPa)—so that the pressure in the small arteries feeding the capillary bed (as well as in the pulmonary veins draining them) is relatively sensitive to the differences in the hydrostatic pressures which exist, for example, in the lung of upright man, where the apex of the lung is some 20 cm higher than the main pulmonary artery.

The very large area of the alveolar capillary membrane is vulnerable to inhaled particles. The site at which they are removed depends on their size. Large particles are filtered out in the nose. Smaller particles which are deposited on the walls of the conducting airways are removed by the sheet of mucus which is continuously swept up to the epiglottis and swallowed. This mucus is secreted by the glands in the walls of the bronchi and moved by the cilia of the bronchial mucosa. Particles which are small enough to reach the alveoli are engulfed by macrophages which pass into the circulation directly or by way of the lymphatic system.

Lung volumes

The total volume of gas which is held in the lungs at the end of a maximal inspiration is termed the *total lung capacity* (*Figure 4.6*). The total lung capacity of a young healthy male 1.7 m tall is about 6.5 l (BTPS). During normal breathing, however, the volume of gas in the lung is about half the total lung

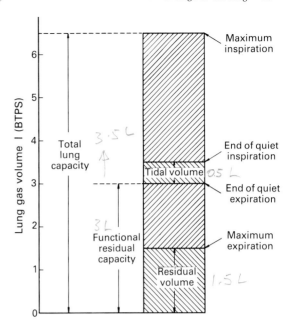

Figure 4.6 The subdivisions of the total lung capacity with normal values for a young male (height 1.7 m).

capacity. The volume of gas in the lung at the end of a normal expiration is termed the *functional residual capacity* and, in our subject, would amount to about 3.0 l (BTPS). At the end of a normal expiration, a further volume of gas can be expelled from the lungs. A considerable amount, termed the *residual volume*, remains in the lungs after a maximal expiration. In our example this would amount to about 1.5 l (BTPS). The total volume of gas which can be expelled from the lungs after a maximum inspiration is termed the *vital capacity*. The vital capacity is equal to the difference between the total lung capacity and the residual volume. In our subject it would be 5.0 l (BTPS).

The *tidal volume*, which is the volume of gas expelled from the lungs during normal expiration, amounts to about 0.5 l (BTPS) in a subject at rest. It should be noted that the tidal volume is only about one-sixth of the volume of gas remaining at the end of expiration, the functional residual capacity. When the tidal volume is increased, either voluntarily or by exercise, a fraction of the increase is accommodated by a reduction of the residual capacity; but there is also an increase in the total volume of gas in the lung at the end of inspiration.

Pulmonary ventilation

Ventilation is the cyclic process of inspiration and expiration in which fresh air is drawn into the respiratory tract and pulmonary gas is expelled from

Lung capa 6.5 L

it. The volume of gas expired is slightly less than that inspired, because with the normal respiratory quotient of less than 1.0, the rate at which carbon dioxide is added to the lung gas is slightly less than the rate at which oxygen is taken up from it. This difference amounts to about 40 ml (STPD) per minute at rest. The total volume of gas expired from the lungs per unit time is termed the *pulmonary ventilation*. It is generally expressed as the volume expired per minute, often called the 'minute volume'.

The ventilation of the lungs is mainly regulated so that it provides the exchange of carbon dioxide between the blood and the air required to match the rate of production of carbon dioxide by the tissues. Over a considerable range of demands for oxygen the pulmonary ventilation increases linearly with the oxygen uptake (*Figure 4.7*). Above a certain level of work, however, a level subject to considerable individual variation, the pulmonary ventilation increases relatively more than the oxygen uptake. The maximum pulmonary ventilation which can be maintained for several minutes by fit young adults varies from 100 to 150 l (BTPS) per minute.

Since pulmonary ventilation is the product of the tidal volume and respiratory frequency, either or both components can contribute to an increase in pulmonary ventilation. At low rates of physical work, pulmonary ventilation is increased mainly by an increase in tidal volume. In moderate or heavy work, the tidal volume amounts to about half the vital capacity; and there is also a progressive rise in respiratory frequency. The respiratory frequency increases from 10 to 20 breaths per minute at rest to 40–45 per minute in maximal exercise.

Alveolar ventilation

Since exchange of gas between the inspired air and the blood occurs only in the alveoli, it is the ventilation of the alveoli rather than the total pulmonary ventilation which determines the gas exchange between the body and the environment. The *alveolar ventilation* is the volume of alveolar gas expelled per unit time. It is acceptable for many purposes to regard the alveolar gas as being of uniform composition. The expired gas consists of alveolar gas diluted with the volume of the previously inspired gas which had remained in the respiratory dead space. In quiet breathing, the average tidal volume of 500 ml (BTPS) will consist of 150 ml (BTPS) of inspired gas mixed with 350 ml (BTPS) of alveolar gas. Although the dead space enlarges slightly with increase of tidal volume, the fraction of the tidal volume which comes from the alveoli rises as the tidal volume is increased.

There is a simple relationship between the alveolar ventilation, the rate of output of carbon dioxide, and the concentration of this gas in the alveolar gas:

$$\text{Alveolar ventilation} = \frac{CO_2 \text{ output per minute}}{\text{Alveolar } CO_2 \text{ concentration}}$$

By the inclusion of a suitable constant this relationship can be transformed to:

$$\text{Alveolar ventilation} = K \times \frac{CO_2 \text{ output per minute}}{\text{Alveolar } CO_2 \text{ tension}}$$

Thus with a constant rate of output of carbon dioxide, the alveolar carbon dioxide tension is inversely proportional to the alveolar ventilation. This relationship is independent of environmental pressure, so that with a constant metabolic production of carbon dioxide, the alveolar ventilation (expressed as volume at body temperature, pressure and saturated with water vapour) required to maintain a given alveolar carbon dioxide tension is the same at all altitudes.

The inspired gas is not evenly distributed to the various regions of the lung. The ventilation per unit volume of lung is greatest in the most dependent part and falls progressively towards the uppermost part. Thus, in erect man, the ventilation of the bottom sixth of the lung is 60% greater than that of

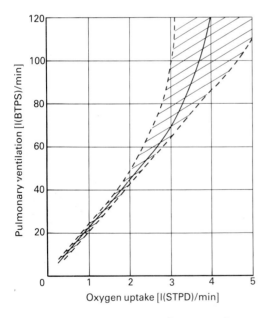

Figure 4.7 The relationship in steady state exercise between pulmonary ventilation and oxygen uptake (metabolic oxygen consumption). The solid curve depicts the mean and the shaded area the variation (± 2 standard deviations) of this relationship for a group of 20 young healthy volunteers.

the top sixth (*see Figure 4.9*). This difference between the bottom and top of the lung disappears in the supine position, when the posterior part of the lung is better ventilated than the anterior regions. The regional differences in the distribution of ventilation are produced by gravity. The weight of the lung causes a progressive increase in the pleural pressure from the upper to the lower part of the lung, so that the alveoli at the top are considerably more distended than those at the bottom. Since the stiffness of the air sacs rises progressively with increase in their volume, the expansion of the alveoli at the bottom of the lung is greater than that of those at the top. Not only do the alveoli in the lower part of the lung expand more during inspiration than those higher up, but the initial volume of the former is less than that of the latter; so that the ratio of volume of gas added to the alveoli during inspiration to their initial volume decreases progressively up the lung. These regional differences in the distribution of inspired gas are abolished in the weightless state and accentuated by exposure to increased accelerative force.

The distribution of inspired gas is also changed markedly at low lung volumes when the intrapleural pressure at the base of the lung exceeds the airway pressure. In these circumstances the lung at the base is compressed, the small airways close and gas is trapped in the distal alveoli. The apical part of the lung is, however, well ventilated. Thus the normal distribution of inspired gas is inverted, the apical regions being better ventilated than the basal regions.

Diffusion

Gases move across the alveolar capillary membrane between the alveolar gas and the pulmonary capillary blood by passive diffusion, obeying Fick's law. The direction and rate of diffusion of a gas across the membrane are determined by the direction and magnitude of the difference between the partial pressures of the gas in the alveolar gas and the blood within the lung capillaries. This difference is greatest at the arterial end of the capillary, since, as gas diffuses across the membrane, the concentration of the gas in the blood comes close to the value at which the partial pressure of the gas in the blood equals that in the alveolar gas. The manner in which the partial pressure of the gas in blood changes along the capillary is a function of the differences between the partial pressures of the gas in the alveolar gas and the pulmonary arterial (mixed venous) blood, its diffusion coefficient, its solubility in blood and the rate of blood flow. At rest it takes about 0.75 s for

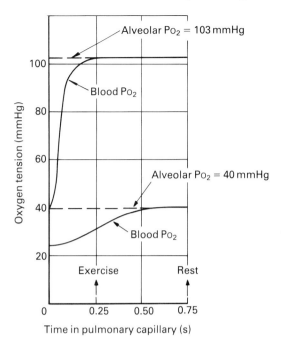

Figure 4.8 The time course of the oxygen tension of the blood as it flows through a typical pulmonary capillary with a normal alveolar oxygen tension (103 mm Hg (13.7 kPa)) and during hypoxia (alveolar oxygen tension, 40 mm Hg (5.3 kPa)). With the higher alveolar oxygen tension the oxygen tension of the blood rises very rapidly reaching that of alveolar gas before it has transversed more than one-third of the length of the capillary. Equilibration of oxygen tension between blood and alveolar gas takes longer at the lower alveolar oxygen tension. Typically, blood transverses the pulmonary capillary in 0.75 s at rest and 0.25 s in moderate exercise.

each red cell to move through the capillary. Heavy exercise reduces this time to about 0.25 s.

The processes involved in the uptake of oxygen by the blood in the pulmonary capillaries are: solution of oxygen in the fluid lining the alveoli; diffusion through the alveolar capillary membrane and through the blood plasma into the red cell; and combination with haemoglobin to form oxyhaemoglobin. Under resting conditions, when a man breathes air at ground level, the difference between the partial pressures of oxygen in the mixed venous blood and the alveolar gas is about 60 mm Hg (8.0 kPa) (*Figure 4.8*), and oxygen passes very rapidly into the blood. The oxygen content, and hence the partial pressure of oxygen in the blood, increases rapidly until, after 0.2–0.25 s, that is, approximately one-third of the way along the length of the capillary, the oxygen tensions of the blood and alveolar gas are very nearly equal (*Figure 4.8*). Thus there is no significant difference between the oxygen tension in the alveolar gas and end-capillary blood. Even in moderate exercise, when the time for which each red cell is exposed to alveolar gas is about one-third of that at rest and oxygen has to cross the membrane at a greater rate, there is still no difference between the oxygen tensions of end-capillary blood and alveolar gas. In heavy exercise, however, when the rate of oxygen consumption rises to 3.01 (STPD)/min the difference between the oxygen tensions of end-capillary blood and alveolar gas is about 15–20 mm Hg (2.0–2.7 kPa). The diffusion properties of the lungs for oxygen are also effective in hypoxia, when the lowered alveolar oxygen tension reduces markedly the oxygen tension difference between the alveolar gas and the blood entering the pulmonary capillaries (*Figure 4.8*). The rate of rise of oxygen tension along the capillary is lowered since the rate of oxygen transfer is slowed. At rest even if the alveolar oxygen tension is lowered to 40 mm Hg (5.3 kPa) the oxygen tension in the blood still rises to this value before it leaves the pulmonary capillary. Moderate exercise with this degree of hypoxia does, however, cause the oxygen tension of the end-capillary blood to be somewhat less than that of the alveolar gas. Thus exercise in moderate hypoxia tends to increase the intensity of the arterial hypoxaemia.

Pulmonary blood flow

The mixed venous blood returning from the tissues is pumped by the right side of the heart through the pulmonary capillary bed. The mean pressure in the main pulmonary artery is only about 15 mm Hg (2.0 kPa) but the pulse pressure is high, the systolic and diastolic pressures being about 25 and 8 mm Hg (3.3 and 1.1 kPa) respectively. The pressure exerted by a column of blood equal to the height of the apex of the erect lung above the main pulmonary artery (20 cm) is 15 mm Hg (2.0 kPa), so that the mean arterial pressure at the apex of the lung is equal to atmospheric pressure. The pulmonary artery pressure increases linearly with distance below the apex to 15 mm Hg (2.0 kPa) at the hilum of the lung and approximately 22 mm Hg (2.9 kPa) at the base. Since the pulmonary veins are very thin, and the pressure in the left atrium is slightly less than atmospheric, the pulmonary veins above the hilum of the lung are collapsed and the pressure within them is effectively equal to atmospheric. Below the hilum of the lung, the pressure in the veins increases above atmospheric pressure, in accordance with the weight of the column of blood from the level of the hilum. Thus the venous pressure at the base of the lung is approximately 7 mm Hg (0.9 kPa).

The pressure around the capillaries of the lung is that of the alveoli, which, during normal breathing, is within 1–2 mm Hg (0.13–0.26 kPa) of atmospheric. The pressure difference controlling blood flow

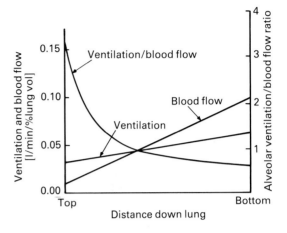

Figure 4.9 The distribution of ventilation and blood flow in the upright lung. Both ventilation and capillary blood flow per unit volume of lung gas increase progressively with descent from the top to the bottom of the lung. The rate of increase of blood flow per unit volume is, however, considerably greater than that of ventilation per unit volume so that the ratio of ventilation to blood flow falls progressively with distance from the top of the lung.

through the capillaries above the hilum of the lung, where the veins are collapsed is, therefore, that between pulmonary artery and the atmosphere. Thus the blood flow increases progressively down the upright lung from the apex to the hilum (*Figure 4.9*). Below the hilum, although the veins are open, so that the difference between arterial and venous pressure is constant, there is a progressive increase in the pressure in the capillaries relative to that in the alveoli. This progressive increase in the transmural pressure of the capillaries gives rise to a graded increase of the diameter of these vessels, so that the resistance to blood flow falls progressively with distance below the hilum. The blood flow, therefore, increases with distance below the hilum (*Figure 4.9*). These regional differences of blood flow are reduced by the increase in the pulmonary artery pressure produced by exercise.

Ventilation–blood flow relationships

The relationship between the ventilation of a group of alveoli (lung unit) and the blood flow through the capillaries in their walls determines the magnitudes of the exchange of oxygen and carbon dioxide between the gas within the alveoli and the blood, and the partial pressures of oxygen and carbon dioxide in the alveolar gas and the end-capillary blood. Only in the weightless state is there uniform distribution of ventilation and pulmonary blood flow to all the alveoli within the lungs. We noted earlier in this chapter that the effects of Earth's gravitational field is to produce a gradient of increasing ventilation and blood flow to each lung unit from the uppermost surface to the lower surface of the lung (*Figure 4.9*). The increase in flow of blood per unit distance down the lung is, however, considerably greater than the corresponding rate of increase of ventilation; so that the ratio of ventilation to blood flow for each lung unit decreases with increasing distance from the top of the lung (*Figure 4.9*). When a man is sitting upright, this ratio falls from 3.3 in the top 7% of the lung to 0.6 in the bottom 10%. The gradient of the ratio of ventilation to blood flow is greatly accentuated by exposure to increased acceleration.

The qualitative effects of the ratio of ventilation to blood flow upon the gas exchange and alveolar gas tension within a lung unit may be seen by considering two extreme values of the ratio. If the lung unit is ventilated but has no blood flow through its capillaries, that is, it has a ventilation–blood flow ratio of infinity, no oxygen will be removed from the inspired air and no carbon dioxide will be added to it. The alveolar gas tensions will therefore be those of inspired air. If, however, blood flows through the lung unit but it is not ventilated, that is, it has a ventilation–blood flow ratio of zero, the tensions of oxygen and carbon dioxide in the alveolar gas will come to equal those in the blood entering the capillary and will therefore be equal to the tensions of these gases in the mixed venous blood. Thus as the ventilation–blood flow ratio of the unit is altered, the composition of the alveolar gas within it approaches that of inspired gas or mixed venous blood. Between these two extremes, a fall in this ratio is associated with a reduction in the tension of oxygen in the alveolar gas, and hence in the end-capillary blood, and a rise in the carbon dioxide tension of the alveolar gas and the end-capillary blood.

The progressive fall of the ratio of ventilation to blood flow from the apex to the base of the erect lung (*Figure 4.9*) gives rise therefore to a progressive reduction of the oxygen tension in the alveolar gas from the top to the bottom of the lung, whilst the alveolar carbon dioxide tension increases progressively down the lung. The magnitude of the changes of alveolar oxygen and carbon dioxide tensions down the lung produced by the changing ratio of ventilation to blood are considerable. Thus in the lung of a man sitting erect and breathing air at ground level, the alveolar oxygen tension falls from about 130 mm Hg (17.3 kPa) at the apex to about 90 mm Hg (12.0 kPa) at the base. The corresponding values of alveolar carbon dioxide tension are 28 mm Hg (3.7 kPa) at the apex and 42 mm Hg (5.6 kPa) at the base. The magnitude of these differences is reduced during exercise when the regional distribution of blood flow is more even, and thus the range of values of the ventilation–blood flow ratio is smaller.

Alveolar–arterial gas tensions

The regional differences of gas exchange within the lung impair the overall efficiency of the lungs. The oxygen tension of the blood leaving the alveolar capillaries varies in exactly the same manner as the alveolar oxygen tension. The lung unit with a high ventilation–blood flow ratio contributes relatively more gas to the expirate than one with a low ratio. However, the lung unit with a low ratio makes a relatively larger contribution to the total blood flow from the lung. Since lung units with a high ventilation–blood flow ratio have high alveolar oxygen tensions, and those with a low ratio have low end-capillary oxygen tensions, the oxygen tension of the mixed expired alveolar gas is higher than that of the mixed blood leaving the lung. The oxygen tension of the mixed pulmonary venous blood is also depressed below that of the mixed expired alveolar gas, because the additional amount of oxygen in the blood from lung units with a high oxygen tension is less than the deficit of the oxygen content of the blood from lung units with a low oxygen tension. This difference is a function of the sigmoid shape of the oxygen dissociation curve of blood (*see* below).

The net result of ventilation–blood flow inequality in the normal upright lungs is that the oxygen tension of the mixed pulmonary venous blood is some 4 mm Hg (0.5 kPa) less than the oxygen tension of the mixed alveolar gas. The effect is less with respect to carbon dioxide, the tension of this gas in the mixed pulmonary venous blood being only 0.5–1.0 mm Hg (0.07–0.13 kPa) higher than the mixed alveolar carbon dioxide tension. The impairment of overall gas exchange in the lungs caused by ventilation–blood flow inequality is, therefore, relatively small in normal man. The oxygen tension of the blood flowing from the pulmonary capillaries is lowered by approximately 4 mm Hg (0.5 kPa) by the admixture of venous blood from the bronchial and thebesian veins (venous shunts) so that the total alveolar–arterial oxygen tension difference amounts to 8–10 mm Hg (1.1–1.3 kPa). Exposure to raised acceleration forces and certain lung diseases which accentuate the ventilation–blood flow inequality causes larger differences between the oxygen tension of the alveolar gas and of the arterial blood.

Control of pulmonary ventilation

The primary function of the lungs is to exchange oxygen and carbon dioxide between the blood and the environment so as to maintain normal tensions of oxygen and carbon dioxide in the tissues of the body in the face of large changes in the rates of oxygen consumption and carbon dioxide production. The ventilation of the lungs is controlled so that the tensions of oxygen and carbon dioxide in the arterial blood are maintained within very close limits.

Neural organization

The activity of the respiratory muscles of the chest wall, diaphragm and abdominal wall is due to the rhythmic discharge from neurones located in the medulla and pons. The primary centre, which is located in the reticular formation of the medulla, exhibits rhythmicity even when completely deprived of afferent impulses. Stimulation of certain neurones within this medullary centre causes inspiration, whilst stimulation of others causes expiration. The activity of this primary respiratory centre is influenced by impulses from the pontine respiratory centres, the reticular activating system and certain peripheral receptors. The important peripheral receptors are the stretch receptors in the lungs, the chemoreceptors and the arterial baroreceptors. The activity of the respiratory coordinating centres is also affected by impulses from the cerebral cortex and hypothalamus. Impulses from the hypothalamus are responsible for the increase in pulmonary ventilation produced by a rise of the temperature of the blood. There is also evidence that afferent impulses arising from contracting muscles and joint receptors during exercise act upon the respiratory centres and the motor neurones of the respiratory muscles.

Chemoreceptors

The most important factors controlling the level of pulmonary ventilation are the carbon dioxide tension, the pH and the oxygen tension of the arterial blood. The rates of discharge of the chemoreceptors, whose impulses impinge upon the respiratory centres, are determined by the composition of the fluid to which they are exposed. The most important receptors which respond to the carbon dioxide tension and pH of the arterial blood, the central chemoreceptors, are situated on the ventral surface of the medulla near the roots of the 9th and 10th cranial nerves. Increases of carbon dioxide tension or hydrogen ion concentration on the surface of this part of the medulla result in an increase in pulmonary ventilation. Changes in the carbon dioxide tension and acidity of the arterial blood are conveyed to these central chemoreceptors by changes in the pH of the cerebrospinal fluid.

Thus when the arterial carbon dioxide tension rises, carbon dioxide diffuses into the cerebrospinal fluid, increasing the hydrogen ion concentration which in turn stimulates the chemoreceptors. When the tension of carbon dioxide in the arterial blood is reduced below normal for several days by, for example, prolonged exposure to hypoxia, the acidity of the cerebrospinal fluid is restored to normal by active transport of hydrogen ions across the brain–blood barrier; and the activity of the central chemoreceptors thereby returns to normal. The central chemoreceptors respond rapidly to changes in tension of carbon dioxide in the arterial blood. Thus it takes only 6–10 minutes to achieve a new steady state of respiration following a step rise in the arterial carbon dioxide tension.

The peripheral chemoreceptors are located in the carotid bodies, which lie in the bifurcations of the common carotid arteries, and in the aortic bodies, which lie around the arch of the aorta. These receptors respond to change in the tensions of carbon dioxide and oxygen in the arterial blood. They are relatively insensitive to changes in carbon dioxide level and contribute little in the steady state to the response of pulmonary ventilation to changes in carbon dioxide tension, which are mediated mainly through the central chemoreceptors. They probably play a larger role in the immediate matching of ventilation to sudden changes in arterial carbon dioxide tension. The activity of the peripheral chemoreceptors is, however, markedly increased by a reduction of arterial oxygen tension. The increase of pulmonary ventilation produced by arterial hypoxaemia is due solely to stimulation of the peripheral chemoreceptors. The central effect of hypoxia is depression of neural activity in the respiratory centres.

Responses to carbon dioxide

There is a very close control of the tension of carbon dioxide in the arterial blood. Changes in the tension of the gas give rise to immediate compensatory changes in pulmonary ventilation. Thus a reduction of the arterial carbon dioxide tension by 5 mm Hg (0.67 kPa) below the normal level removes the drive to breathe until sufficient carbon dioxide has accumulated in the blood to return the arterial tension to normal. Raising the arterial carbon dioxide tension by adding carbon dioxide to the inspired gas causes a rapid increase in ventilation, until a new steady state is attained. There is a linear relationship between the pulmonary ventilation and arterial carbon dioxide tension in these circumstances. The ventilation is increased by about 3 l (BTPS)/min for each 1 mm Hg (0.13 kPa) increase in arterial carbon dioxide tension. The sensitivity of the respiratory centre to carbon dioxide is increased in hypoxia; so that the rise in pulmonary ventilation per mmHg increase in arterial carbon dioxide tension is approximately 91 (BTPS)/min at an arterial oxygen tension of 30–35 mmHg (4.0–4.7 kPa).

The outcome of the sensitivity of the respiratory control mechanism to carbon dioxide is that, under normal conditions both at rest and during exercise, the arterial carbon dioxide tension of a given individual varies by less than 3 mmHg (0.4 kPa) throughout the waking day. There is some variation in the mean arterial carbon dioxide tension between one individual and another. It normally lies between 37 and 42 mmHg (4.9 and 5.6 kPa). The arterial carbon dioxide tension rises slightly above this range during sleep. The relationship between carbon dioxide tension and hydrogen ion concentration and the sensitivity of the peripheral chemoreceptors to the pH of the arterial blood also results in a very close control of the latter. Thus the pH of the arterial blood normally lies within the range 7.36–7.44.

Responses to oxygen

An acute reduction of the arterial oxygen tension does not produce a significant increase in pulmonary ventilation until the tension is reduced below 45–50 mmHg (6.0–6.7 kPa). Below this level of arterial oxygen tension, there is a considerable increase in ventilation, although the latter tends to be reduced by the concomitant decrease of arterial carbon dioxide tension. If the latter is maintained at its normal resting level by adding carbon dioxide to the inspired gas as the alveolar oxygen tension is lowered, the pulmonary ventilation is twice normal at an arterial oxygen tension of about 38 mmHg (5.1 kPa) and 4–6 times the resting value at an arterial oxygen tension of 35 mmHg (4.7 kPa). There are large individual differences in response to arterial hypoxaemia. An increase of the arterial oxygen tension above normal has little or no effect on pulmonary ventilation.

Cortical control

In the short term there is considerable cortical control of pulmonary ventilation. It is relatively easy to reduce the arterial carbon dioxide tension to half its normal value by voluntarily increasing the ventilation of the lungs. Hyperventilation, with a consequent reduction of the arterial carbon dioxide tension, also occurs involuntarily as a result of fear or emotional disturbance. The cortical input to the respiratory centre producing the increase in ventilation in these circumstances may completely override the chemoreceptor control of respiration. The reduction in arterial carbon dioxide tension can be so great that performance and even consciousness are grossly disturbed.

Exercise

It has already been seen that exercise produces a rapid increase in ventilation, the magnitude of which is proportional to the increased oxygen uptake and carbon dioxide output. In all but heavy exercise, the increase in alveolar ventilation is so closely matched to the increased gaseous exchange in the lungs that the arterial tensions of carbon dioxide and oxygen are held very close to the values that exist at rest. The mechanism of this control of ventilation of the lungs during exercise remains largely unknown. The large increases in ventilation occur without an increase in the arterial carbon dioxide tension or a fall in the arterial oxygen tension. The initial increase in ventilation at the start of exercise is probably due to impulses from the exercising muscles and joints.

Gas tension gradients

A valuable expression of the effectiveness of the exchange of the respiratory gases between the inspired gas and the tissues is the magnitudes of the tensions of each gas at various points in the transport system.

Carbon dioxide

The primary factor which determines the tissue carbon dioxide tension is the tension of the gas in the arterial blood. The pulmonary ventilation is normally regulated by the respiratory control mechanism so that the arterial carbon dioxide tension is held constant. The amount by which the tension of carbon dioxide in the venous blood exceeds that in the arterial blood is determined by the carbon dioxide production by the tissues and the blood flow through them. The maximum tension of carbon dioxide in the tissues is only slightly greater than that in the blood flowing from the tissue. Typical values of the carbon dioxide tensions at various points in the carbon dioxide transport system in an individual at rest are presented in *Table 4.5*. The changes in the values produced by light exercise are also given in *Table 4.5*.

Table 4.5 Carbon dioxide tension gradients

	Carbon dioxide tension (mm Hg)	
	Rest	Light exercise*
Maximum value in tissues	48–55	48–50
Mixed venous blood	51	46
Arterial blood	40	40
Alveolar gas	39	39
Expired gas	26	30

*Carbon dioxide production = 0.81 (STPD)/min

The tissues contain relatively large stores of carbon dioxide, mainly as bicarbonate, so that a step change in the tension of carbon dioxide in the blood produces an imbalance between the rate of production of carbon dioxide by metabolism and the rate at which the gas is carried from the tissues by the blood. Thus a sudden sustained decrease of the arterial carbon dioxide tension, such as that produced by voluntary hyperventilation, results in a marked increase in the rate at which carbon dioxide is removed from the tissues and expired from the lungs. Even when the hyperventilation only reduces the arterial carbon dioxide tension by 15 mm Hg, the output of carbon dioxide in the expired gas exceeds that produced by tissue metabolism for 30–60 minutes. During this period, the ratio of the rate of carbon dioxide output to the rate of oxygen uptake measured at the lips, the respiratory exchange ratio, will exceed the respiratory quotient. As the excess carbon dioxide is removed from the tissue and blood stores, the respiratory exchange ratio will fall to equal finally the respiratory quotient.

alveolar vent ∝ O₂ uptake/m

Oxygen

O₂ removed from inspired gas

The difference between the oxygen tensions of the inspired and alveolar gas is proportional to the ratio of oxygen uptake to alveolar ventilation. This relationship is analogous to that for carbon dioxide, the alveolar carbon dioxide tension (in the absence of carbon dioxide from the inspired gas) being proportional to the ratio of carbon dioxide production to alveolar ventilation.

The alveolar tensions of oxygen and carbon dioxide are intimately connected. The relationship between the inspired oxygen tension, the alveolar oxygen tension and the tension of carbon dioxide in the alveolar gas is simplest when the inspired gas is 100% oxygen. Under these circumstances, the alveolar gas consists of oxygen, carbon dioxide and water vapour, and the sum of the tensions of oxygen and carbon dioxide in the alveolar gas (PA_{O_2} and PA_{CO_2} respectively) must equal the tension of oxygen in the inspired tracheal gas (PI_{O_2}), that is inspired

gas saturated with water vapour at deep body temperature (37°C). Thus when the inspired gas is 100% oxygen:

$$PI_{O_2} = PA_{O_2} + PA_{CO_2}$$

and hence

$$PA_{O_2} = PI_{O_2} - PA_{CO_2}$$

This expression is a special case of the alveolar air equation which relates these three gas tensions. When nitrogen is present in the inspired and alveolar gas, it is necessary to introduce a correction factor into the alveolar air equation, since the excess oxygen uptake over carbon dioxide production results in a higher concentration of nitrogen in the alveolar gas than in the inspired gas. The magnitude of this correction factor varies with the respiratory exchange ratio and the concentration of oxygen in the inspired gas. The general form of the alveolar air equation is:

$$PA_{O_2} = PI_{O_2} - PA_{CO_2} (FI_{O_2} + (1 - FI_{O_2})/R)$$

where PA_{O_2} = alveolar oxygen tension; PI_{O_2} = inspired (tracheal) oxygen tension; PA_{CO_2} = alveolar carbon dioxide tension; FI_{O_2} = fractional concentration of oxygen in the inspired gas (dry air); R = respiratory exchange ratio.

When either $FI_{O_2} = 1$ or $R = 1$ the correction factor $FI_{O_2} + [(1 - FI_{O_2})/R]$ reduces to 1.0. The magnitude of this correction factor when a man breathes air and has a normal R(0.85) is 1.14; so that, in these circumstances, the alveolar oxygen tension rises by 0.9 mm Hg (0.12 kPa) for every 1 mm Hg (0.13 kPa) fall in carbon dioxide tension, provided that the respiratory exchange ratio (R) remains unchanged. The respiratory exchange ratio, however, rises towards and even exceeds 1.0 during hyperventilation, so that the alveolar oxygen tension rises by about 1.0 mm Hg (0.13 kPa) for each 1.0 mm Hg (0.13 kPa) reduction in alveolar carbon dioxide tension.

The tension of oxygen in the dry atmosphere, the inspired tracheal gas and the alveolar gas for an individual breathing air at ground level, at rest, during light exercise and whilst hyperventilating to reduce the alveolar carbon dioxide tension to 25 mm Hg (3.3 kPa) are presented in *Figure 4.10*. The alveolar oxygen tension at rest is 103 mm Hg (13.7 kPa) and it remains at this value during light exercise (oxygen uptake of 1.01 (STPD)/min). Hyperventilation, which reduces the alveolar carbon dioxide tension to 25 mm Hg (3.3 kPa) and raises the respiratory exchange ratio to 1.0, increases the alveolar oxygen tension to 114 mm Hg (15.2 kPa).

The oxygen tension of the arterial blood is reduced below that of the mixed alveolar gas by the

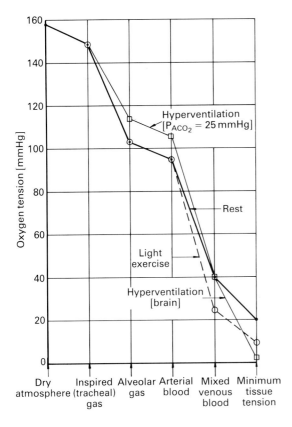

Figure 4.10 Oxygen tension gradients from dry atmosphere to minimum tissue level in an individual breathing air at ground level at rest (curve ⊙—⊙), performing light exercise (curve ◯– – –◯) and carrying out moderate hyperventilation (curve □——□). (See text for further details.)

effects of ventilation–blood flow inequality and the venous to arterial shunts. In all three conditions depicted in *Figure 4.10*, the fall in oxygen tension from alveolar gas to arterial blood is 8 mm Hg (1.07 kPa) so that the arterial oxygen tension is 95 mm Hg (12.7 kPa) both at rest and during light exercise. Hyperventilation, which reduces the alveolar carbon dioxide tension to 25 mm Hg (3.3 kPa), gives an arterial oxygen tension of 106 mm Hg (14.1 kPa).

The fall in oxygen tension between arterial and venous blood is determined by the ratio of oxygen uptake to blood flow in the tissues and the shape of the oxygen dissociation curve of the blood. These relationships are such that, in the resting state, the oxygen tension of the mixed venous blood is 55 mm Hg (7.3 kPa) less than that of the arterial blood, that is, 40 mm Hg (5.3 kPa). In light exercise, the proportional increase in cardiac output is less than the proportional increase in the oxygen uptake by the tissues, so that the fall of oxygen tension from

arterial to mixed venous blood increases to 70 mm Hg (9.3 kPa). The oxygen tension of the mixed venous blood therefore falls to 25 mm Hg (3.3 kPa). The small increase in the concentration of oxygen in the arterial blood associated with the rise of oxygen tension induced by moderate hyperventilation (alveolar carbon dioxide tension of 25 mm Hg (3.3 kPa)) will, because of the shape of the oxygen dissociation curve, have only a very minor effect on the oxygen tension of the mixed venous blood—the latter being raised by about 1 mm Hg (0.13 kPa). So far the tissues of the body have been treated as if they were homogeneous. However, the relationship between oxygen uptake and blood flow varies from one tissue to another, and these differences are accentuated by exercise and hyperventilation. Thus the oxygen tension of the blood flowing from exercising muscle is considerably lower than the oxygen tension of the mixed venous blood during light exercise. The lowering of the arterial carbon dioxide tension produced by hyperventilation reduces the blood flow to the brain, so that oxygen tension of the blood at the venous ends of the capillaries of the cerebral tissues is considerably lower than that of the mixed venous blood. The oxygen tension of jugular venous blood is reduced from 35 mm Hg (4.7 kPa) at rest to 22 mm Hg (2.9 kPa) by hyperventilation to an arterial carbon dioxide tension of 25 mm Hg (3.3 kPa).

Oxygen tension varies from point to point within a tissue, and the concept of mean tissue oxygen tension is of little value. A more meaningful expression of the effectiveness of the oxygen transport system is the minimum oxygen tension in the tissues, although in reality this varies widely from one tissue to another. Estimates of the minimum tissue oxygen tension, assuming uniform oxygen consumption, blood flow and capillary geometry throughout the body, are presented in *Figure 4.10*. In all the three conditions considered in this figure, the minimum tissue oxygen tensions are considerably greater than those required to maintain aerobic metabolism. The reduction in cerebral blood flow induced by hyperventilation to an arterial carbon dioxide tension of 25 mm Hg (3.3 kPa) does, however, reduce the minimum tissue oxygen tension in certain areas of the brain to about 3 mm Hg (0.40 kPa) which may reduce the rate of oxidative phosphorylation and hence impair cerebral function.

Further reading

ASTRAND, P.-O. and RODAHL, K. (1977) *Textbook of Work Physiology*, 2nd edn. New York: McGraw-Hill.

COMROE, J.H., FORSTER, R.E., DUBOIS, A.B., BRISCOE, W.A., and CARLSEN, E. (1962) *The Lung, Clinical Physiology* and *Pulmonary Function Tests*, 2nd edn. Chicago: Year Book Medical Publishers.

COTES, J.E. (1979) *Lung Function: Assessment and Application in Medicine*, 4th edn. Oxford: Blackwell.

DENISON, D. (1981) High altitudes and hypoxia. In *The Principles and Practice of Human Physiology* (Edholm, O.G. and Weiner, J.S., eds.) London: Academic Press.

ERNSTING, J. (1965) Respiration and anoxia. In *A Textbook of Aviation Physiology* (Gillies, J.A., ed.) Oxford: Pergamon Press.

WEST, J.B. (1979) *Respiratory Physiology: The Essentials*, 2nd edn. Baltimore: Williams and Wilkins.

5

Hypoxia and hyperventilation

J. Ernsting and G.R. Sharp, revised by R.M. Harding

Introduction

Living organisms obtain energy for their biological processes by the oxidation of complex chemical foodstuffs to simpler compounds, usually with the eventual formation of carbon dioxide, water and other waste products. Oxygen is therefore one of the most important components required for the maintenance of normal function by living material. The absence of an adequate supply of oxygen to the tissues, whether in quantity or molecular concentration, is termed *hypoxia*. Man is extremely sensitive and vulnerable to the effects of deprivation of oxygen, and severe hypoxia nearly always results in a rapid deterioration of most bodily functions: eventually it will lead to death.

Four different types of tissue hypoxia are recognized, and may be classified according to the primary mechanism involved. These types are:

1. *Hypoxic hypoxia*—Hypoxic hypoxia is the result of a reduction in the oxygen tension in the arterial blood, and hence in the capillary blood. The aetiology includes the low oxygen tension of inspired gas associated with exposure to altitude: so-called *hypobaric hypoxia*. Other causes are hypoventilatory states (e.g. paralysis of respiratory musculature, depression of central control of respiration, airway obstruction and pulmonary atelectasis (including that due to exposure to high sustained accelerations)); impairment of gas exchange across the alveolar-capillary membrane (e.g. pulmonary oedema and pulmonary fibrosis); and ventilation–perfusion mismatches (e.g. chronic bronchitis and emphysema).

2. *Anaemic hypoxia*—Anaemic hypoxia is the consequence of a reduction in the oxygen-carrying capacity of the blood. Thus although arterial oxygen tension is normal, the amount of haemoglobin available to carry oxygen is reduced. The oxygen tension of the blood falls more rapidly than normal as it flows through the capillary beds and so, at their venous ends, it is inadequate to maintain the required minimum level throughout the tissue involved. Causes of anaemic hypoxia include a reduced erythrocyte count (e.g. haemorrhage, increased red cell destruction, decreased red cell production), a reduced haemoglobin concentration (e.g. hypochromic anaemia), synthesis of abnormal haemoglobin (e.g. sickle cell anaemia), a reduced oxygen-binding capability (e.g. carbon monoxide inhalation), and chemical alteration of haemoglobin (e.g. methaemoglobinaemia).

3. *Ischaemic (stagnant or circulatory) hypoxia*—Ischaemic hypoxia is the consequence of a reduction in blood flow through the tissues. Gas exchange in the lungs and the oxygen tension and content of the arterial blood are normal but oxygen delivery to the tissues is inadequate. There is increased oxygen extraction and, once again, the oxygen tension falls to a low level in the venous ends of the capillaries. Local tissue oxygenation is therefore inadequate. Causes of ischaemic hypoxia include local arteriolar constriction (e.g. exposure of digits to cold), obstruction of arterial supply by disease or trauma, and general circulatory failure (e.g. cardiac failure, vaso-vagal syncope, and the fall in cardiac output and blood pressure associated with exposure to high sustained accelerations).

4. *Histotoxic hypoxia*—Histotoxic hypoxia is the result of an interference with the ability of the tissues to utilize a normal oxygen supply for oxidative processes. An example is cyanide poisoning in which the cytochrome oxidase

(among others) of the mitochondria cannot react with molecular oxygen.

Hypoxic hypoxia as a result of a reduction in the oxygen tension in inspired gas is by far the most common form of oxygen-lack which occurs in aviation and is considered in detail in this chapter. The anaemic hypoxia produced by carbon monoxide poisoning, the ischaemic hypoxia produced by exposure to cold, and the anaemic/ischaemic hypoxia produced by sustained accelerations are described in Chapters 9, 17 and 10 respectively.

Hyperventilation is a state in which the level of pulmonary ventilation is in excess of that required by the rate of production of carbon dioxide by the tissues, and hence of its elimination. It is characterized by a reduction in the alveolar and arterial tensions of carbon dioxide; a condition which is termed *hypocapnia*. Moderate hypocapnia produces a significant impairment of the ability to perform psychomotor tasks, whilst an acute reduction in arterial carbon dioxide to about 15 mm Hg frequently causes unconsciousness. Hypocapnia is a normal concomitant of hypoxia, and indeed the two conditions produce almost identical symptoms, although hyperventilation can occur in its own right under certain other conditions of the flight environment: exposure to low frequency vibration, emotional stress, and during positive pressure breathing.

The remainder of this chapter is concerned with a more detailed consideration of the physiological and clinical consequences of hypobaric hypoxia and of hyperventilation.

Acute hypobaric hypoxia: hypoxia in flight

It is generally recognized that the most serious single hazard during flight at altitude is hypobaric hypoxia; that is, the reduction in the molecular concentration (partial pressure) of oxygen in the inspired air produced by ascent to altitude. Even the 25% reduction in the partial pressure of oxygen in the atmosphere associated with ascent to an altitude of 8000 ft produces a detectable impairment in some aspects of mental performance; whilst sudden exposure to 50 000 ft as a consequence of rapid decompression, which reduces the partial pressure of oxygen within the lungs to 10% of its sea level value, will cause unconsciousness within 12–15 seconds and death in 4–6 minutes. In the past, lack of oxygen took a regular toll of both lives and aircraft: many military aircrew were killed by hypoxia in flight, whilst the ability of many more to perform their duties was impaired by the condition. Neither is the world of civilian flying exempt and, although improvements in the performance and reliability of cabin pressurization and oxygen delivery systems have greatly reduced incidents and accidents due to hypoxia, they still occur and constant awareness and vigilance remain essential.

Aetiology

The principal causes of hypoxia in flight are:

1. Ascent to altitude without supplementary oxygen.
2. Failure of personal breathing equipment to supply oxygen at an adequate concentration and/or pressure.
3. Decompression of the pressure cabin at high altitude.

The relative incidence of the various causes of hypoxia in flight over an 8-year period in a military air-force is presented in *Table 5.1*, and it is noteworthy that nearly half the incidents involved student pilots operating unpressurized jet training aircraft.

Table 5.1 Relative incidence of the causes of 400 cases of hypoxia in flight in a military air force

Cause of hypoxia	Relative incidence (%)
Failure to turn on oxygen supply	10
Failure of oxygen supply to demand regulator	6
Failure of demand regulator to deliver correct concentration of oxygen	22
Inadvertent break of connection in hose between regulator and mask	11
Inadequate seal of mask to face	22
Malfunction of mask valves	7
Decompression of pressure cabin	20
Others	2

NB. The demand oxygen regulators used in this air force delivered safety pressure only at altitudes greater than 30000 ft.

The physiological consequences of hypoxia in flight can be considered in three main areas: the respiratory and cardiovascular *responses to* the insult, and the neurological *effects of* those responses and of the insult itself. The clinical consequences will clearly be an admixture of changes in all three areas.

Respiratory responses to acute hypobaric hypoxia

The time course of the physiological changes produced by breathing air at altitude is a function of the manner in which the condition is induced. Thus the changes are usually produced slowly by ascent at the common rate for an aircraft of 2000–3000 ft/min; more rapidly by the reversion to breathing air after failure of oxygen delivery equipment; and fastest following a rapid decompression. Although breathing air during a routine steady ascent is an uncommon cause of hypoxia in professional aircrew nowadays, it does occur regularly in leisure flying (such as in those flying light aircraft, gliders and balloons), and it is convenient to begin by describing the respiratory changes induced by hypoxia in this manner since the relatively slow rate of ascent allows a semi-steady state to be maintained.

Alveolar gases when breathing air

The fall in partial pressure of oxygen in the inspired gas that occurs on ascent to altitude causes a progressive reduction in alveolar oxygen tension. The main determinant of the difference in oxygen tension between inspired gas and alveolar gas is the alveolar carbon dioxide tension. That this is so can be demonstrated by rearranging the Alveolar Air Equation thus:

$$PI_{O_2} - PA_{O_2} = PA_{CO_2} \cdot \left(FI_{O_2} + \frac{1 - FI_{O_2}}{R} \right)$$

where PI_{O_2} is inspired (tracheal) oxygen tension, PA_{O_2} is alveolar oxygen tension, PA_{CO_2} is alveolar carbon dioxide tension, FI_{O_2} is the fractional concentration of oxygen in the (dry) inspired gas, and R is the respiratory exchange ratio.

A fall in alveolar carbon dioxide tension will reduce the difference between the oxygen tensions in the inspired and alveolar gases. But, as is explained in Chapter 4, the tension of carbon dioxide in the alveolar gas is itself determined by the ratio of carbon dioxide production to alveolar ventilation, and this ratio is *independent* of environmental pressure. Accordingly, therefore, alveolar carbon dioxide tension remains constant on ascent to altitude, provided that the ratio of carbon dioxide production to alveolar ventilation is unchanged. In practice, however, on acute exposure to altitude, alveolar carbon dioxide tension remains constant only between sea level and an altitude of 8000–10 000 ft. Above this altitude, arterial oxygen tension falls to a level that stimulates respiration; and so alveolar carbon dioxide tension is reduced by virtue of increased alveolar ventilation. Thus alveolar oxygen tension falls linearly with the decline in environmental pressure associated with an ascent from sea level to about 10 000 ft but, above this altitude, the reduction in alveolar oxygen tension is less than would occur if there was no increase in ventilation and no consequent fall in alveolar carbon dioxide tension. The changes in alveolar gas tensions associated with ascent to altitude when breathing air are shown graphically in *Figure 5.1*.

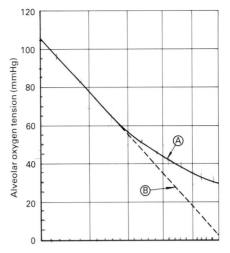

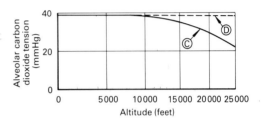

Figure 5.1 The effect of acute exposure to various altitudes, whilst breathing air, on the alveolar tensions of oxygen (curve A) and carbon dioxide (curve C). The curves describe the mean values for a group of 30 subjects seated at rest. The broken lines indicate the values of alveolar tensions of oxygen (curve B) and carbon dioxide (curve D) which would be obtained if the hypoxia induced by ascent to altitude did not increase pulmonary ventilation.

The increase in pulmonary ventilation produced by exposure to a given altitude above 8000–10 000 ft may be regarded as the resultant of two conflicting factors: the lowered arterial oxygen tension stimulates ventilation through its effect on the chemoreceptors of the carotid and aortic bodies, but the increase in ventilation is itself opposed by the respiratory depressant effect of the concomitant reduction in carbon dioxide tension. The compromise struck between these two competing influences is essentially that of the demand for an adequate oxygen supply versus the need to maintain a normal acid–base balance. The magnitude of the increase in ventilation, and hence the fall in alveolar carbon dioxide tension, exhibits considerable individual variation. During acute exposures of subjects at rest, pulmonary ventilation at 18 000 ft is 20–50% greater than that observed at sea level, whilst at 22 000 ft it is 40–60% greater.

The effect of altitude upon the ventilatory response to mild and moderate exercise is a similar but slightly greater proportional increase in pulmonary ventilation, and such an effect can be demonstrated at altitudes as low as 3000 ft. The increase in pulmonary ventilation induced by exercise in moderate hypoxia is, however, such that alveolar carbon dioxide tension is reduced below that produced by breathing air at rest at the same altitude. There is, therefore, a corresponding rise in alveolar oxygen tension, perhaps by 3–5 mm Hg.

The hypoxia induced by breathing air at altitudes of up to about 20 000 ft produces a small, almost insignificant, increase in the total oxygen consumption of the tissues, and in the carbon dioxide production by them. This increase in metabolism is a consequence of the extra work associated with the rise in pulmonary ventilation and in cardiac output. The fall in alveolar carbon dioxide tension produced by the disproportionate rise in pulmonary ventilation, however, liberates carbon dioxide from the very substantial body stores of the gas so that, for a while, the output of carbon dioxide in the expired gas actually exceeds its metabolic production by the tissues. Thus the respiratory exchange ratio (R) is raised at the beginning of an exposure to altitude when breathing air. It slowly returns to the previous resting value as the excess carbon dioxide is removed from body stores and a steady state is regained. For example, R is raised to just over 1.0 on acute exposure to air at 18 000 ft, and its normal resting value of 0.85 is not regained for 30–40 minutes. Clearly, a raised value of R will produce a higher alveolar oxygen tension for a given inspired oxygen tension and alveolar carbon dioxide tension than would otherwise be the case; and so, in the example quoted, with an alveolar carbon dioxide tension of 28 mm Hg, alveolar oxygen tension will fall from about 41 mm Hg at the beginning of the exposure to about 37 mm Hg at the end.

Table 5.2 Mean values for alveolar gas tensions in 30 seated resting subjects after acute (10–20 minutes) exposure to breathing air at altitude

Altitude (feet)	Inspired oxygen tension (mm Hg)	Alveolar tensions (mm Hg) of: Oxygen		Carbon dioxide	
		Mean	SD	Mean	SD
0	148	103.0	5.5	39.0	2.5
8000	108	64.0	5.0	38.5	2.6
15 000	80	44.7	5.0	30.5	2.7
18 000	69	39.5	4.2	28.0	2.5
20 000	63	36.5	4.0	26.5	2.5
22 000	57	33.2	3.0	25.0	2.6
25 000*	49	30.0		22.0	

*After 3–5 minutes' exposure.

The relationship between the alveolar tensions of oxygen and carbon dioxide therefore change progressively throughout an exposure to a given altitude: the alveolar oxygen tension being determined by the level of alveolar carbon dioxide and the value of R, both of which are themselves functions of the intensity of the ventilatory response to hypoxia and of the duration of exposure. The relationship between various altitudes, 10–20 minutes after exposure, and the consequent alveolar oxygen tensions was shown graphically in *Figure 5.1*. The same data are presented numerically in *Table 5.2*, where the considerable individual variability is indicated by the values of standard deviations. In general, the alveolar oxygen tension is reduced, in short-duration exposures, to 45 mm Hg at 15 000 ft, to 40 mm Hg at 18 000 ft, to 35 mm Hg at 21 000 ft, and to 30 mm Hg at 25 000 ft.

Alveolar gases when breathing oxygen

When 100% oxygen has been breathed for several hours, so that virtually all the nitrogen has been washed out of the body tissues and alveolar gas, the relationship between the alveolar tensions of oxygen and carbon dioxide and the environmental pressure simplifies to:

$$PA_{O_2} = (PB - PH_2O) - PA_{CO_2}$$

Where PA_{O_2} is alveolar oxygen tension, PB is environmental pressure, PH_2O is water vapour tension at 37°C (i.e. 47 mm Hg), and PA_{CO_2} is alveolar carbon dioxide tension.

In most situations, however, the time for which 100% oxygen is breathed is only 5–120 minutes, and the alveolar gas still contains a small amount of nitrogen: sufficient to exert a tension of 3–5 mm Hg. Thus in practice the alveolar oxygen tension when breathing 100% oxygen is usually some 3–5 mm Hg less than that predicted by the equation. But, provided that the alveolar carbon dioxide tension remains constant, alveolar oxygen tension will fall linearly with environmental pressure (as it does up to 10 000 ft when breathing air). When breathing 100% oxygen, however, it is not until an altitude of 33 000–33 700 ft that the alveolar oxygen tension falls to 103 mm Hg. that is, to its sea level value (equivalent) when breathing air. And it is not until an altitude of about 39 000 ft is reached that the alveolar oxygen tension falls to 60–65 mm Hg (that is, to a similar value to that reached at 10 000 ft breathing air). Above 39 000 ft, the further fall in alveolar oxygen tension stimulates respiration, even though 100% oxygen is being breathed, just as it does above 10 000 ft when breathing air. The alveolar oxygen tension therefore rises by 1 mm Hg for every 1 mm Hg reduction in alveolar carbon dioxide tension. Thus, for example, the alveolar carbon dioxide tension at 43 000 ft is about 30 mm Hg and the corresponding alveolar oxygen tension is 43–45 mm Hg. *Figure 5.2* is a graphical representation of the changes in alveolar gas

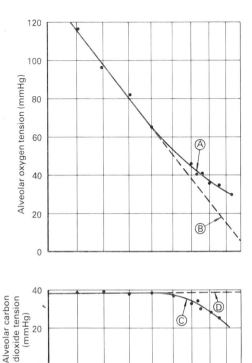

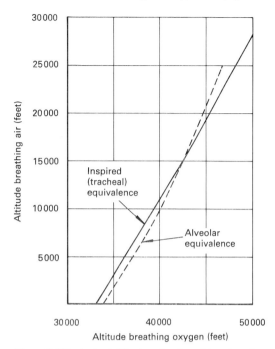

Figure 5.3 Equivalent altitudes when breathing air and when breathing 100% oxygen. The solid curve indicates equivalence based on equal tensions of oxygen in the inspired (tracheal) gas: that is, inspired gas saturated with water vapour at 37°C. The broken curve indicates equivalence based on equal tensions of oxygen in the alveolar gas during acute exposures of seated resting subjects for 10–15 minutes.

Figure 5.2 The effect of acute exposure to altitudes between 30 000 ft and 45 000 ft, whilst breathing 100% oxygen, on the alveolar tensions of oxygen (curve A) and carbon dioxide (curve C). The broken lines indicate the values of alveolar tensions of oxygen (curve B) and carbon dioxide (curve D) which would have occurred in the absence of any increase in pulmonary ventilation.

tensions with altitude when breathing 100% oxygen, and should be compared with *Figure 5.1*.

The concept of *physiologically equivalent altitudes* for a man breathing air or 100% oxygen is of considerable value in the design of protective equipment. But, whilst equivalent altitudes may be stated in terms of equality of alveolar oxygen tension, the latter alone does not completely define oxygenation of the tissues since arterial carbon dioxide tension is also relevant. For most practical purposes, therefore, it is more satisfactory to determine equivalence on the basis of equality of inspired (tracheal) oxygen tension. *Figure 5.3* describes the relationship of equivalent altitudes for both inspired gas and alveolar gas. As a simple example, the effect of the 5000 ft increase in altitude from 40 000 to 45 000 ft when breathing 100% oxygen is equivalent to a 9000 ft increase in altitude from 11 000 to 20 000 ft when breathing air.

Finally, when hypoxia is induced at altitude by a change in the composition of the inspired gas from that containing a high concentration of oxygen to air, the alveolar oxygen tension falls progressively as the concentration of nitrogen in the inspired and alveolar gases rises to 79–80%. During the early part of this process, the oxygen tension of the inspired gas is frequently *less* than that of the blood returning to the alveoli, and so oxygen will pass out of the body *from* the returning mixed venous blood into the alveolar gas (so briefly counteracting the original fall to a small degree) and hence into the expirate. The rate at which alveolar oxygen tension falls in these circumstances is proportional to the alveolar ventilation, but a new steady state is usually attained in the resting subject 2–3 minutes after the reduction in concentration of oxygen in the inspired gas.

Alveolar gases during rapid decompression

The introduction of cabin pressurization systems for aircraft flying at medium and high altitudes brought with it the possibility that the aircraft occupants could be exposed to the risks of rapid decompression should a failure occur in either the structural integrity of the pressure cabin or in the pressurization system (*see also* Chapter 8). The sudden fall in environmental pressure that accompanies a decompression produces almost as rapid a fall in the tensions of the constituents of alveolar gas. Thus such an emergency can produce a very profound fall in alveolar oxygen and carbon dioxide tensions; the magnitude of which will depend upon the gas being breathed at the moment of decompression and the ratio of the environmental pressures at the beginning and end of the event. For example, a rapid decompression from 8000 to 40 000 ft in 1.6 seconds whilst breathing air will cause the alveolar oxygen tension to fall from 65 mm Hg to about 15 mm Hg. Furthermore, since the inspired (tracheal) oxygen tension at that final altitude is only 20 mm Hg, the alveolar oxygen tension will remain below about 18 mm Hg for as long as air is breathed. Under these conditions, the oxygen tension in the blood is considerably higher than that in the lungs and so oxygen passes into the alveoli from the mixed venous blood as it flows through the pulmonary capillaries. The change in alveolar oxygen tension during rapid decompression is illustrated in *Figure 5.4*.

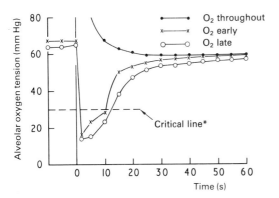

Figure 5.4 Mean alveolar oxygen tensions of four subjects before and after rapid decompression at time 0 from 8000 ft to 40 000 ft in 1.6 seconds. Each subject was decompressed on three occasions: once breathing air before and after the decompression with 100% oxygen delivered to the facemask 8 s after time 0 (O_2 late: o—o), once breathing air before and after the decompression with 100% oxygen delivered to the facemask 2 s after time 0 (O_2 early: x—x), and once breathing 100% oxygen throughout (O_2 throughout: ●—●).
  *Note that if the area described by the alveolar oxygen tension curve below the critical line exceeds 140 mm Hg.s, consciousness will almost certainly be lost.

Alveolar carbon dioxide tension also falls during such a decompression, and may reach a value of just 10 mm Hg. This then partially recovers to a level of 25–30 mm Hg over the ensuing 30 seconds as carbon dioxide passes rapidly from pulmonary capillary blood into the alveolar gas. The inspiration of 100% oxygen during or at some short interval after a rapid decompression will modify the changes described by causing an immediate rise in alveolar oxygen tension (*Figure 5.4*). The rise is rapid at first, but then slows

to reach a value of about 60 mm Hg some 30–40 seconds after oxygen breathing commences. Clearly, the greater the final altitude and the longer the delay in administering 100% oxygen, the greater will be the degree of hypoxia. By implication, therefore, the composition of the gas being breathed immediately *before* the rapid decompression will also influence the severity of hypoxia suffered: a high alveolar oxygen tension in the inspired gas before decompression will minimize the fall in tension seen during and after the decompression. Thus, for example, when 100% oxygen is breathed before, during and after a rapid decompression from 8000 to 40 000 ft, alveolar oxygen tension does not fall below about 60 mm Hg at any time (*Figure 5.4*).

The brief but profound hypoxia associated with rapid decompression has its most marked effects on the central nervous system (*see* below); and specifically on the psychomotor performance of the subject. In order to avoid the potentially catastrophic consequences of hypoxia induced by rapid decompression to a high altitude, alveolar oxygen tension must not fall below about 30 mm Hg. Such a fall is an inevitable consequence of a rapid decompression to a final altitude greater than 30 000 ft when breathing air *even if* 100% oxygen is delivered to the respiratory tract at the moment decompression occurs. The intensity of the hypoxic insult will be correspondingly greater with a greater final altitude, and if delivery of 100% oxygen is delayed. These extremely rapid physiological changes have very important implications for the design of personal oxygen equipment for use at high altitudes since they indicate that, in order to avoid severe neurological disturbances *after* a rapid decompression, an oxygen-enriched breathing gas must be being breathed *before* it. Indeed, the concentrations of oxygen required in the breathing gas in order to maintain an alveolar oxygen tension above 30 mm Hg on rapid decompressions to a final altitude of 35 000 ft, 40 000 ft and 44 000 ft are 30%, 40% and 60% respectively. Even then, in order to prevent significant features of hypoxia developing, 100% oxygen must be delivered within 2 seconds of the start of rapid decompression.

Arterial blood gases

Although the difference between the oxygen tension of the alveolar gas and that of the blood entering the pulmonary capillaries (that is, mixed venous blood) is markedly reduced on exposure to altitude, the diffusion characteristics of the alveolar-capillary membrane are such that the tension of oxygen leaving the pulmonary capillaries still equals that of the alveolar gas when the individual is at rest. Thus in moderate hypoxia the arterial oxygen tension may be some 8 mm Hg less than the alveolar oxygen tension, whilst the carbon dioxide tension of

Table 5.3 Typical values for arterial blood gases of resting subjects acutely exposed to altitude

Altitude (ft)	Arterial blood gases			
	Oxygen tension (mm Hg)	Carbon dioxide tension (mm Hg)	Oxygen concentration (ml (STPD)/ 100 ml blood)	Oxygen saturation of haemoglobin (%)
I. Breathing air				
0	95	40	20.5	97
8000	56	38	18.8	93
12000	43	35	16.9	84
15000	37	30	15.7	78
18000	32	28	14.5	72
20000	29	26	13.2	66
II. Breathing 100% oxygen				
33000	95	40	20.5	97
40000	45	38	16.9	84
43000	36	30	15.4	76

alveolar gas is virtually equal to that of the arterial blood. Typical values for the arterial blood gases of resting subjects, breathing air at various altitudes up to 20 000 ft and 100% oxygen up to 45 000 ft, are presented in *Table 5.3*. It should be noted, however, that there are large variations in the tensions of arterial blood gases in acute hypoxia, both with time in the same individual and between one individual and another. For example, the oxygen saturations of the arterial blood in six resting subjects breathing air at 18 000 ft varied from 65% to 78%. These large variations reflect the sensitivity of alveolar oxygen tension, and so arterial oxygen tension, to the level of alveolar ventilation.

The reduced transit time of blood in the pulmonary capillaries during exercise results in a failure of the oxygen tension in the blood to reach equilibrium with that of the alveolar gas. The alveolar–arterial oxygen tension gradient is therefore increased by exercise in moderate hypoxia from its resting value of about 8 mm Hg to 16–20 mm Hg. And, although exercise whilst hypoxic does produce a small increase in alveolar oxygen tension by virtue of the alveolar hyperventilation, the large rise in the alveolar–arterial oxygen tension difference results in an overall fall in arterial oxygen tension and saturation. This is the explanation for the exacerbation of symptoms and signs of hypoxia when exercise is undertaken.

Cardiovascular responses to acute hypobaric hypoxia

Blood flow

As described in Chapter 4, the rate of blood flow through a tissue bed is a cardinal determinant of the tension at which oxygen is delivered to its cells. The reverse is also the case, however, and the hypoxia produced by a reduction in oxygen tension of the inspired gas will induce both general and regional changes in the circulation. Occasionally, a simple vaso-vagal syncope may also complicate the picture.

General cardiovascular changes

In the resting subject, *heart rate* increases immediately when breathing air above 6000–8000 ft. At 15 000 ft the increase is about 10–15% above the sea level value, it rises to a 20–25% increase at 20 000 ft, and the heart rate is approximately doubled at 25 000 ft. There is a similar proportional increase in *cardiac output*, although stroke volume remains essentially unchanged. Both heart rate and cardiac output are also elevated proportionally during exercise at altitude, although the maximum levels of each (which are the same in moderate hypoxia as when breathing air at sea level) are, however, attained at a lower degree of work under hypoxic conditions. At altitude, the *maximum oxygen uptake* is limited by the cardiac output and the reduced arterial oxygen saturation so that, for example, when breathing air at 15 000 ft, maximum uptake during exercise falls to about 70% of the sea level value.

Despite the increase in cardiac output, *mean arterial blood pressure* during moderate hypoxia is usually unchanged from that of an individual breathing air at sea level. The systolic pressure is usually raised as is the pulse pressure, but there is an overall reduction in *peripheral resistance*, and a redistribution of flow by local and vasomotor mechanisms. Although hypoxia causes vasodilatation in most vascular beds, there are some important features of, and differences in, the responses of certain regional circulations.

Regional cardiovascular changes

Acute hypoxia causes an immediate increase in blood flow through the coronary and cerebral circulations, whereas the peripheral resistance in resting skeletal muscle is unchanged and renal blood flow is markedly reduced. Thus there is a redistribution of cardiac output: flow to essential organs such as the heart and brain is increased at the expense of other less acutely essential organs such as the viscera, skin and kidneys.

Flow through the *coronary circulation* increases in parallel with the rise in cardiac output, in response to the metabolic requirements of the myocardium. Cardiac reserve is reduced, however, and a profound fall in arterial oxygen tension will cause myocardial depression. Occasionally, in such circumstances, there is a severe compensatory vasoconstriction of the coronary vessels which swamps all other reflex responses and causes cardiac arrest. The increase in blood flow through the coronary circulation is such that a subject breathing air at 25 000 ft exhibits no electrocardiographic (ECG) evidence of cardiac hypoxia, even up to the point at which consciousness is lost. In severe hypoxia, myocardial depression is reflected in the electrocardiograph by a depressed S-T segment and a reduction in the height of the T wave. Later, disorders of rhythm and conduction supervene.

The response of the *cerebral circulation* to hypoxic hypoxia is also worthy of further comment since, not surprisingly, the changes in arterial oxygen and carbon dioxide tensions associated with that condition have profound effects. Thus at arterial oxygen tensions above 45–50 mm Hg, cerebral blood flow is exclusively determined by the arterial carbon dioxide tension to which it bears a directly linear relationship over the normal (tolerable) physiological range (20–80 mm Hg). For example, a reduction in arterial carbon dioxide tension from the normal 40 mm Hg to 20 mm Hg will halve cerebral blood flow. A fall in arterial oxygen tension below about 45 mm Hg, however, will induce a hypoxic vasodilatation so that, for example, an arterial oxygen tension of 35–40 mm Hg causes a 50–100% increase in blood flow through the brain. A balance therefore exists between the vasodilating effect of hypoxia upon the cerebral vessels and the vasoconstricting influence of a declining arterial carbon dioxide tension caused by the hypoxic drive to ventilation. Generally, the conflict results in a reduction in cerebral blood flow when breathing air at altitudes up to about 15 000 ft, but an increase (modified by the degree of coexisting hypocapnia) above 16 000–18 000 ft.

Hypoxia of a degree sufficient to desaturate the blood by about 20% causes a rapid reversible vasoconstriction in the *pulmonary circulation*, probably as a consequence of the direct action of oxygen on carotid body-like cells in the walls of the pulmonary blood vessels. (These so-called Feyrter cells are found in increased numbers in the fetus and are believed to be responsible for the diversion of blood away from the lungs *in utero*.) The response is the means by which local blood flow is matched to local ventilation. On ascent to altitude the entire pulmonary vascular bed constricts and, in the presence of a raised cardiac output, this increases pulmonary arterial blood pressure.

Syncope

Heart rate, arterial blood pressure and cerebral blood flow are usually maintained at or above their resting values when unconsciousness occurs as the result of a gross lowering of alveolar oxygen tension (*see* below). In about 20% of individuals, however, the immediate cause of unconsciousness in hypoxia is failure of cerebral blood flow subsequent to a precipitate fall in arterial blood pressure associated with a marked bradycardia. The mechanism underlying the fall in arterial blood pressure in this form of faint is the same as for other types of vasovagal syncope: that is, a loss of peripheral resistance in the systemic circulation brought about by a profound dilatation of arterioles in muscle vascular beds. Syncope is accompanied by pallor, sweating, nausea and, occasionally, vomiting.

Tissue oxygen tension

The minimum acceptable oxygen tension in a tissue depends critically upon the oxygen tension in the blood flowing through its capillaries; and the major factor minimizing the fall of oxygen tension towards the venous ends of capillaries in the presence of hypoxic hypoxia is the relationship, reflected in the sigmoid shape of the oxygen dissociation curve, between oxygen tension and the saturation of haemoglobin with oxygen. A typical oxygen dissociation curve is shown in *Figure 5.5*.

The figure shows that, when air is breathed at sea level, which produces an arterial oxygen tension of about 95 mm Hg, the extraction of 5 ml oxygen from every 100 ml blood flowing through the tissues results in a venous oxygen tension of about 40 mm Hg: that is, a fall of 55 mm Hg. The extraction of the same quantity of oxygen per unit volume of blood when the arterial oxygen tension is reduced to 32 mm Hg by breathing air at 18 000 ft decreases the oxygen tension of the venous blood to 22 mm Hg: thus the fall in oxygen tension as the blood flows through the tissues is reduced to only 10 mm Hg. This most important protective effect of the manner in which oxygen combines with haemoglobin results in a halving of the arterio-venous oxygen tension difference when the arterial oxygen tension is reduced from 95 mm Hg to 65 mm Hg, and to a reduction to a quarter when the arterial oxygen

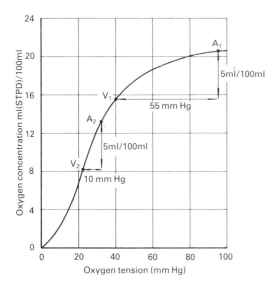

Figure 5.5 Oxygen dissociation curve of whole blood (at a pH of 7.4 and a temperature of 37°C), illustrating the effect of the sigmoid shape of the relationship on the fall in oxygen tension of the blood produced by the extraction of 5 ml oxygen per 100 ml blood by the tissues, as blood flows through them at two different levels of arterial oxygen tension. At an arterial oxygen tension of 95 mm Hg (point A1), the extraction of 5 ml oxygen per 100 ml blood reduces the oxygen tension to 40 mm Hg (point V1); that is, the fall in oxygen tension from arterial to venous blood is 55 mm Hg. In moderate hypoxia, with an arterial oxygen tension of 32 mm Hg (point A2), the extraction of the same amount of oxygen reduces the oxygen tension to 22 mm Hg (point V2); that is, the fall in oxygen tension from arterial to venous blood is only 10 mm Hg.

tension is 40 mm Hg. Although the overall increase in cardiac output produced by acute hypoxia reduces still further the fall in arterio-venous oxygen tension difference, this effect is of much less importance than that associated with the oxygen dissociation curve. For example, the 20% increase in cardiac output induced by breathing air at 18 000 ft, where the arterial oxygen tension is 32 mm Hg, will only raise the oxygen tension in mixed venous blood from 22 mm Hg to 24 mm Hg.

Regional changes in blood flow, and especially the changes in the cerebral circulation described above, are also of importance. The marked reduction in cerebral blood flow, produced by the hypocapnia associated with the mild hypoxia induced by breathing air at 12 000 ft, can result in an appreciable further lowering of the jugular venous oxygen tension. In the more severe hypoxia associated with breathing air at 18 000 ft, the increased arterio-venous oxygen tension difference produced by hypocapnia is more than offset by the concomitant increase in alveolar and arterial oxygen tensions produced by the hyperventilation.

The combined effects of acute hypoxic hypoxia,

induced by a reduction in the oxygen tension of inspired gas, are best summarized by considering the gradient of oxygen tension from the dry atmosphere to the lowest tension in the tissues. *Figure 5.6* illustrates oxygen tension gradients for a man breathing air at sea level and at 18 000 ft.

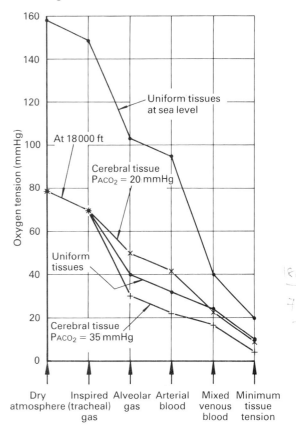

Figure 5.6 Oxygen tension gradients from dry atmosphere to minimum tissue level in an individual breathing air at sea level and at 18 000 ft (curves ·—·), assuming that body tissues are uniform and that the alveolar carbon dioxide tension is 40 mm Hg at sea level and 30 mm Hg at 18 000 ft. The gradients for cerebral tissue in an individual breathing air at 18 000 ft with an alveolar oxygen tension of 20 mm Hg (curve ×—×) and 35 mm Hg (curve +—+) are also shown (*see* text).

The figure shows three oxygen tension gradients at 18 000 ft: the gradient for the body as a whole (assuming that all tissues are uniform), and two gradients for oxygen transport to the brain with mild and severe hypocapnia (alveolar carbon dioxide tensions of 35 and 20 mm Hg respectively). The curves illustrate the effect of hyperventilation upon the fall in oxygen tension between inspired and alveolar gases, and the marked reduction in the fall in oxygen tension along the capillaries in hypoxia due primarily to the relationship demonstrated by the shape of the oxygen dissociation curve. The net effect in this example is that, in the face of a reduction of 79 mm Hg in the oxygen tension of the inspired gas, the oxygen tension of mixed venous blood is only reduced by 16 mm Hg when air is breathed at 18 000 ft. The estimated minimum oxygen tension, on the simplifying assumption that the body is a single uniform tissue, is only reduced from 20 to 10 mm Hg. In the absence of hyperventilation at 18 000 ft, however, the minimum oxygen tension in the brain falls to almost zero, and some decline in oxidative phosphorylation would be expected under these conditions.

Cyanosis

Cyanosis of the skin and mucous membranes, caused by the presence of an excessive concentration of reduced haemoglobin in the capillaries and venules of the hypoxic tissues, is a reflection of the profound desaturation of haemoglobin at low tissue oxygen tensions. There must be at least 5 g reduced haemoglobin per 100 ml capillary blood before cyanosis can be detected reliably and, while this is only an approximation, it does serve to emphasize that the condition cannot manifest in severe anaemia. The central cyanosis of hypoxic hypoxia can be detected reliably only if the oxygen saturation of the arterial blood is less than 75%. Thus normal subjects breathing air are noticeably cyanotic at altitudes above 17 000–19 000 ft.

Neurological effects of acute hypobaric hypoxia

Impairment of mental performance

The impairment of psychological performance produced by lack of oxygen at altitude is of great practical significance in aviation, although there is great variability, both within and between individuals, in the quantitative aspects of the performance of subjects exposed to hypobaric hypoxia. Much of this variation is the result of differences in the respiratory response to hypoxia, with consequently very significant temporal and individual differences in the tensions of oxygen and carbon dioxide in the arterial blood when exposed to a given level of inspired oxygen tension. The hypocapnia induced by the low arterial oxygen tension affects mental performance by reducing still further cerebral tissue oxygen tension, as a consequence of the cerebral vasoconstriction it produces, and by increasing the pH of cerebral tissue (*see* Hyperventilation).

Psychomotor tasks

Simple reaction time is unaffected by hypoxia until the alveolar oxygen tension is below 38–40 mm Hg (that is, above an altitude of 16 000–18 000 ft), but even a reduction of the alveolar oxygen tension to 35 mm Hg increases the simple reaction time by only 50% on average. Performance at pursuit-meter tasks is unaffected until the altitude exceeds 12 000–14 000 ft, although the decrement of performance at this type of task does not become severe until altitudes of 16 000–17 000 ft are exceeded. Choice-reaction time is, however, affected by much less severe degrees of hypoxia: performance at a well-learned choice-reaction time task is usually significantly impaired at 12 000 ft. Tasks requiring complex eye–hand co-ordination, such as instrument flying in a flight simulator, where the task has been well-learned before the exposure, are usually unaffected until the alveolar oxygen tension is reduced below 55 mm Hg (that is, until air is breathed at altitudes above 10 000 ft). If the alveolar oxygen tension falls to less than 50 mm Hg (12 000 ft), there is an approximate 10% decrement in the ability to maintain a given air speed, heading or vertical velocity. This decrement rises to 20–30% at alveolar oxygen tensions of 40–45 mm Hg (15 000 ft).

Psychomotor performance is further compromised by the impairment of muscular co-ordination produced by moderate and severe hypoxia. Above 15 000 ft, for example, a fine tremor of the hand develops so that the ability to hold a stylus or control lever in a fixed position in space is progressively impaired. Muscular incoordination becomes greater with increasing altitude and the subject's writing becomes hard to read.

Cognitive tasks

Performance at previously learned coding and conceptual reasoning tasks is unaffected at altitudes up to about 10 000 ft; that is, for as long as the alveolar oxygen tension remains greater than 55 mm Hg. At alveolar tensions less than this, however, performance declines slowly at first but then with increasing rapidity with increasing altitude. Thus the time taken to complete a simple coding task is increased by 10–15% at 15 000 ft, and by 40–50% at 18 000 ft. The decline in performance at conceptual reasoning tasks is even greater, although the altitude at which impairment of mental ability commences, and the severity of the decrement, varies with the difficulty and complexity of the task. Short-term and long-term memory, as tested by paired word association, and immediate and delayed recall of patterns and positions, is significantly affected when the alveolar oxygen tension is reduced to about 60 mm Hg (that is, when breathing air at 8000–10000 ft). Memory scores may be 25% lower than at sea level at an altitude of 15000 ft. Thus tests of long-term and short-term memory, mental arithmetic, and conceptual reasoning are unaffected below 10000 ft. And indeed, until the early 1960s, it had been assumed that this degree of hypoxia did not produce any effect on human mental performance. It is now recognized, however, that an individual breathing air at 8000 ft may take significantly longer to achieve optimum performance at novel tasks than is the case at sea level. For example, this degree of hypoxia has been found to double the reaction times of initial responses to a complex choice-reaction task as compared with responses at sea level. The intensity of this effect increases with altitude (markedly above 12000 ft) and complexity of the task, and some workers have shown it to be just present at 5000 ft. Others, however, have failed to confirm these findings.

The mechanisms responsible for the cerebral effects of mild hypoxia are not understood, although it is likely that retardation of some oxygenation processes within the brain, leading to disruption of neurotransmitter formation and decay, is involved rather than a failure of oxidative phosphorylation (*see* Chapter 4). This is because the oxygen tension of cerebral venous blood falls by only 2–4 mm Hg on ascent from sea level to 8000 ft, and such a slight fall could not be responsible for the effects seen.

Impairment of the special senses

Even very mild hypoxia, such as that produced by lowering the alveolar oxygen tension to 75 mm Hg (that is, equivalent to breathing air at just 5000 ft), can be shown in the laboratory to impair the light sensitivity of the dark-adapted eye (scotopic or rod vision). The magnitude of the effect, however, is of little practical importance in aviation. The degree of reduction in light sensitivity of scotopic vision only becomes significant when the alveolar oxygen tension falls below about 50 mm Hg (that is, when air is breathed at altitudes above 12000 ft). Retinal sensitivity in relatively bright light (photopic or cone vision) is unaffected by hypoxia until the alveolar oxygen tension is reduced below 40 mm Hg. Finally, moderate and severe hypoxia cause restriction of the visual field, with loss of peripheral vision ('tunnelling') and the development of a central scotoma. And there is frequently a subjective darkening of the visual field, although the subject normally becomes aware of this only after the normal alveolar oxygen tension has been restored when there is a marked apparent increase in the level of illumination.

Auditory acuity is also reduced by moderate and severe hypoxia, but some hearing is usually retained even after the other special senses have been lost.

Loss of consciousness

Provided that vaso-vagal syncope does not occur (*see* above), there is a close relationship in hypoxic hypoxia between the oxygen tension of the cerebral venous blood and the level of consciousness. Consciousness is lost when the jugular venous oxygen tension (*see Figure 5.6*) is reduced to 17–19 mm Hg. The corresponding cerebral arterial oxygen tension varies with cerebral blood flow, which itself depends upon the arterial tensions of oxygen and carbon dioxide. Thus the arterial oxygen tension that produces a jugular venous tension sufficiently low to cause unconsciousness can lie between 20 and 35 mm Hg depending on the degree of hypocapnia. Accordingly, although consciousness is usually lost when the alveolar oxygen tension is reduced to 30 mm Hg or below for a significant period of time, it is possible to lose consciousness with an alveolar oxygen tension as high as 40 mm Hg if there is marked hyperventilation, or to retain consciousness at an alveolar oxygen tension as low as 25 mm Hg if there is no hypocapnia. A subject breathing air on acute exposure to altitude may therefore become unconscious at an altitude as low as 16000 ft or stay conscious as high as 24000 ft.

Effects during rapid decompression

As explained earlier, rapid decompressions to altitudes above 30000 ft when breathing air are inevitably accompanied by a fall in alveolar oxygen tension to 30 mm Hg or less. Such severe falls will have profound neurological consequences if allowed to persist. Thus consciousness will almost certainly be lost if the time course of changes in alveolar oxygen tension on rapid decompression, and the extent of these changes below the level of 30 mm Hg (that is, the area of an alveolar oxygen tension curve below the 30 mm Hg level when plotted against time), result in a relationship of more than 140 mm Hg.s (*see Figure 5.4*).

Even if air continues to be inspired at the final altitude, however, there is no decrement in the performance of a recently learnt sequencing recall task until 12–14 s after the decompression. Thereafter, at a final altitude of 40000 ft for example, the time taken to complete the task increases to about three times its control value 20 seconds after the event. Provided that 100% oxygen is administered within 8 seconds of decompression, performance at the task returns to its control level about one minute later. There is no significant decrement in performance if the severity of the decompression is such that the alveolar oxygen tension remains above 30 mm Hg.

It is the obvious need to maintain alveolar oxygen tension above 30 mm Hg, therefore, and so to ensure that the skilled performance of military aircrew is uncompromised should a loss of cabin pressurization at high altitude occur, that gives protection against rapid decompression such prominence in the design of personal oxygen equipment (*see* also Chapters 6 and 7).

Clinical features of acute hypobaric hypoxia

The clinical picture of acute hypobaric hypoxia is a combination of the cardio-respiratory responses and neurological effects described above, and the symptoms and signs are consequently extremely variable. The speed and order of appearance of signs, and of the severity of symptoms produced by a lowering of inspired oxygen tension, depend on the rate at which, and the level to which, the tension is lowered, and on the duration of exposure to hypoxia. Even when these factors are kept constant, however, there is considerable variation between one individual and another in the effects of hypoxia; although for the same individual the pattern of effects does tend to follow the same trend from one occasion to another.

Several additional factors may influence an individual's susceptibility to hypoxia and so modify the pattern of symptoms and signs produced. These factors include:

1. *Physical activity*—Exercise exacerbates the features of hypoxia.
2. *Ambient temperature*—A cold environment will reduce tolerance to hypoxia by virtue of the additional metabolic workload required to maintain body temperature.
3. *Intercurrent illness*—Similarly, the additional metabolic load imposed by ill health will increase susceptibility to hypoxia.
4. *Ingestion of certain drugs, including alcohol*—Many pharmacologically active substances have effects similar to those of hypoxic hypoxia and so mimic or exacerbate the condition. Those proprietary preparations with anti-histamine constituents are particularly likely to cause problems, as is alcohol.

Clinical picture

Although, in general, the greater the altitude the more marked will be the features of hypoxia, rapid rates of ascent can allow high altitudes to be reached before severe symptoms and signs occur. In such circumstances, however, unconsciousness may supervene before any or many of the classic features appear. For descriptive purposes, therefore, it is convenient to consider the influence of slow ascent to various approximate altitudes on the evolution of the clinical picture of hypoxia.

Up to 10 000 ft breathing air (up to about 39 000 ft breathing oxygen)

The resting subject has no symptoms on ascent to an altitude of 10 000 ft when breathing air (39 000 ft when breathing 100% oxygen), but performance at novel tasks may be impaired, and the sensitivity of the dark-adapted eye may be marginally compromised.

From 10 000 ft to 15 000 ft breathing air (from about 39 000 ft to 42 500 ft breathing oxygen)

The resting subject exhibits few or no signs and has virtually no symptoms. The ability to perform skilled tasks is impaired, however: an effect of which the subject is frequently unaware. A prolonged exposure to the moderate hypoxia at about 15 000 ft frequently causes a severe generalized headache. Physical work capacity is markedly reduced, and exposure to extremes of temperature may induce symptoms and signs of hypoxia.

From 15 000 ft to 20 000 ft breathing air (from about 42 500 ft to 45 000 ft breathing oxygen)

Even in the resting subject, the symptoms and signs of hypoxia appear on acute exposure to altitudes greater than 15 000 ft when breathing air. Higher mental processes and neuromuscular control are affected, and in particular there is a loss of critical judgement and will-power. Because of the loss of self-criticism, the subject is usually unaware of any deterioration in performance or indeed of the presence of hypoxia; and it is this effect that makes the condition such a potentially dangerous hazard in aviation. Thought processes are slowed, mental calculations become unreliable, and psychomotor performance is grossly impaired. Marked changes in emotional state are common. Thus there may be disinhibition of basic personality traits and emotions, and the individual may become elated or euphoric or pugnacious and morose. Occasionally the victim may become physically violent. Tunnelling of vision may occur.

In parallel with this group of cerebral features, disturbances due to hypocapnia commonly occur, and indeed may dominate the clinical picture, as hyperventilation occurs. Lightheadedness, visual disturbances, and paraesthesiae of the extremities and lips may be followed in severe cases by tetany with carpo-pedal and facial spasms. Central and peripheral cyanosis develop, and there is decreased muscular co-ordination with loss of the sense of touch, so that delicate or fine movements are impossible.

Physical exertion greatly increases the severity of all of these symptoms and signs, and may lead to unconsciousness.

Above 20 000 ft breathing air (above about 45 000 ft breathing oxygen)

Resting subjects exhibit a marked accentuation of the symptoms and signs described above. Comprehension and mental performance decline rapidly, and unconsciousness supervenes with little or no warning. Myoclonic jerks of the upper limbs often precede loss of consciousness, and convulsions may occur thereafter. Hypoxic convulsions are characterized by intense, maintained muscular contractions which produce opisthotonos, preceded or followed by one or more myoclonic jerks.

The early (covert) cerebral features of hypobaric hypoxia may be summarized as follows:

1. Visual function:
   (a) Light intensity perceived as reduced.
   (b) Visual acuity diminished in poor illumination.
   (c) Light threshold increased.
   (d) Peripheral vision narrowed.
2. Psychomotor function:
   (a) Choice reaction time impaired.
   (b) Eye–hand co-ordination impaired.
3. Cognitive function:
   (a) Memory impaired.

The overt features of acute hypobaric hypoxia may be summarized as follows:

Personality change	Dizziness
Lack of insight	Lightheadedness
Loss of judgement	Feelings of unreality
Loss of self-criticism	Feelings of apprehension
Euphoria	
Loss of memory	
Mental incoordination	
Muscular incoordination	Neuromuscular irritability
Sensory loss	Paraesthesia of face and extremities
Cyanosis	Carpo-pedal spasm

Hyperventilation

Semi-consciousness
Unconsciousness
Death

Time of useful consciousness

The interval that elapses between a reduction in oxygen tension of the inspired gas and the point at which there is a specified degree of impairment of performance is termed 'the time of useful consciousness'. The length of this interval is influenced by many factors, of which the most important is the accepted degree of impairment. In the laboratory,

this may vary from an inability to perform complex psychomotor tasks to a failure to respond to simple spoken commands. In practice, however, the most useful concept is to regard the time of useful consciousness as the period during which the affected individual can act to correct his predicament. Values for the time of useful consciousness at various altitudes following hypoxia induced by changing the breathing gas from oxygen to air are presented in *Table 5.4*. The large standard deviations at low altitudes serve to emphasize the

Table 5.4 Times of useful consciousness at various altitudes of 50 seated young men following a change from breathing oxygen to breathing air

Altitude (ft)	Time of useful consciousness (s)	
	Mean	Standard deviation
25 000	270	96
26 000	220	87
27 000	201	49
28 000	181	47
30 000	145	45
32 000	106	23
34 000	84	17
36 000	71	16

considerable individual variation in the time of useful consciousness. The variation is a reflection of the influence of many factors including the pulmonary ventilatory response to hypoxia, the general physical fitness of the subject, his age, degree of training, and previous experiences of hypoxia. Finally, it should be noted that the time of useful consciousness at a given altitude is shorter when hypoxia is induced by rapid decompression, rather than by slow ascent (*see also* Chapter 8).

Recovery from hypoxia and the oxygen paradox

The administration of oxygen to a hypoxic subject usually results in a rapid and complete recovery; as is also the case if environmental pressure is increased so that alveolar oxygen tension is restored towards its normal level. A generalized headache is the only symptom that persists, and only then if the exposure to hypoxia was prolonged.

In some subjects, however, sudden restoration of the alveolar oxygen tension to normal may cause a transient increase in the severity of the symptoms and signs of hypoxia for 15–60 seconds. This *oxygen paradox* is usually mild and is manifest only by flushing of the face and hands and perhaps a worsening of performance of complex tasks over the immediate period following restoration of the oxygen supply. Occasionally, oxygen administration may produce a severe paradox with the appearance of clonic spasms and even loss of consciousness. The mechanisms responsible for the phenomenon are uncertain. The paradox usually occurs in subjects who have become hypocapnic during hypoxia, and it is also accompanied by a period of arterial hypotension. Thus the hypotension, in combination with persistent and marked hypocapnic cerebral vasoconstriction which remains for some while after restoration of the arterial oxygen tension, may intensify cerebral hypoxia for a short time. Clearly, it is most important that oxygen continues to be delivered to the victim of a paradox, despite the apparent worsening of the condition on initial administration of the gas.

Hyperventilation

Hyperventilation is a condition in which pulmonary ventilation is greater than that required to eliminate the carbon dioxide produced by body tissues. The consequent excessive removal of carbon dioxide from the alveolar gas, the arterial blood and the tissues results in a reduction in the tension of carbon dioxide all along the chain.

Furthermore, there is a close relationship between carbon dioxide tension and hydrogen ion concentration in the blood and tissues since these substances are in equilibrium according to the equation:

$$CO_2 + H_2O \rightleftharpoons H_2CO_3 \rightleftharpoons H^+ + HCO_3^-$$

A reduction in carbon dioxide tension will drive the equilibrium towards the left and, consequently, there is a fall in hydrogen ion concentration; that is, a rise in pH. Thus hyperventilation also causes an increase in the pH of blood and tissues; that is a respiratory alkalosis.

Aetiology

As described above, hyperventilation is a normal response to hypoxia and is seen when alveolar oxygen tension is reduced to below 55–60 mm Hg. It may also occur as a result of *voluntary over-breathing*; for example, in preparation for a breath-hold dive into water.

Most commonly, however, the condition is produced by *emotional stress*, particularly anxiety, apprehension or fear. Thus a significant proportion of student pilots under instruction exhibit gross hyperventilation in flight; and indeed it has been claimed that 20–40% of student aircrew suffer from hyperventilation at some stage during flying training. The condition is also seen in experienced aircrew when, for example, they are exposed to the mental stress of a sudden in-flight emergency or when they are being trained to operate a new aircraft type. Aircraft passengers who are afraid or anxious frequently hyperventilate.

Pain sometimes induces hyperventilation, as do *motion sickness* and certain *environmental stresses* such as a high ambient temperature and whole-body vibration at 4–8 Hz (as, for example, produced by clear air turbulence when flying at low level).

Finally, hyperventilation is almost invariable in aircrew learning to *pressure breathe* (*see* Chapter 6); and while this tendency may be reduced by training, it cannot be eliminated entirely.

Physiological features of hyperventilation

The hypocapnia of hyperventilation has no significant effect on cardiac output or arterial blood pressure, although there is a redistribution of the former. Thus hypocapnia induces a marked vaso-constriction of the cerebral arterioles and the vessels of the skin, whilst blood flow through skeletal muscle is increased. Although the intense cerebral vasoconstriction tends to minimize the change in hydrogen ion concentration within cerebral tissues, it also markedly reduces the minimum tissue oxygen tension. It is therefore probable that many of the changes produced by gross hyperventilation, and especially the deterioration in performance, the appearance of slow wave activity in the electroencephalogram, and the loss of consciousness are due to a combination of hypoxia and alkalosis in the cerebral tissues.

A reduction in the arterial carbon dioxide tension to below 25 mm Hg causes a significant decrement in the performance of psychomotor tasks, such as tracking and complex co-ordination tests. The reaction time at a two-choice task is increased by about 10% by such a fall, and is increased by 15% at an arterial carbon dioxide tension of 15 mm Hg. The ability to perform complex mental tasks, such as mental arithmetic, is compromised by a reduction in carbon dioxide tension to below 25–30 mm Hg. Steadiness of the hands is also impaired by a reduction in arterial carbon dioxide tension to 25 mm Hg. The ability to perform manual tasks is markedly affected by the muscle spasm which occurs at arterial carbon dioxide tensions below 20 mm Hg. Reduction of carbon dioxide tension below 10–15 mm Hg produces gross clouding of consciousness and then unconsciousness.

The rise in tissue pH induced by hyperventilation increases the sensitivity of peripheral nerve fibres, and reduces the threshold for their response to stimuli. The threshold is lowered by the local fall in hydrogen ion concentration and spontaneous activity occurs, giving rise to sensory disturbances, such as paraesthesiae in the face and extremities, and motor disruption, in the form of reflex firing of proprioceptive fibres via the spinal cord, causing muscle spasm (tetany). Different types of nerve fibres are affected in a consistent sequence: fibres conveying information with regard to touch, position, pressure and vibration being affected first, followed by motor fibres and then cold, heat and (lastly) pain fibres.

Clinical features of hyperventilation

The earliest symptoms produced by hyperventilation become manifest when the arterial carbon dioxide tension has been reduced to 20–25 mm Hg. Usually, there are feelings of lightheadedness, dizziness, anxiety (which, since apprehension is itself a cause of hyperventilation, frequently establishes a vicious circle), and a superficial tingling (paraesthesiae) in the extremities and around the lips. The paraesthesiae are followed by muscle spasms, particularly of the limbs and of the face, when arterial carbon dioxide tension has fallen below 15–20 mm Hg. Contraction of muscle groups in the wrist and hand, and in the ankle and foot, give rise to carpo-pedal spasm. In this state, the thumb is acutely flexed across the palm, the hand flexed at the wrist, the metacarpo-phalangeal joints flexed and the inter-phalangeal joints are extended (the main d'accoucheur). The ankle is profoundly plantar-flexed. Spasm of the facial muscles causes stiffening of the face and the corners of the mouth are drawn downwards (the risus sardonicus). In more severe hypocapnia, when arterial carbon dioxide tension is less than 15 mm Hg, the whole body becomes stiff as a result of general tonic contractions of skeletal muscle (tetany).

The increased irritability of nervous tissue in moderate hypocapnia causes augmentation of tendon reflexes. An example of this lowered threshold can be demonstrated by tapping the branches of the facial nerve as they pass forward over the mandible: such tapping, in the presence of moderate alkalosis, causes twitching of the facial muscles (Chvostek's sign). Finally, as described above, moderate and severe hyperventilation produce a general deterioration in mental and physical performance and this is followed by impairment of consciousness and finally unconsciousness.

It is most important to realize that, in the uncommon event of an individual hyperventilating to the point of unconsciousness as a result of anxiety, the supervention of coma will be followed by a gradual recovery as respiration is inhibited and carbon dioxide tensions regain their normal levels. This is clearly *not* the case, however, if the hyperventilation has been induced by hypoxia. It will be apparent from the previous sections of this chapter that most of the early symptoms of hypoxia are very similar to those produced by hypocapnia (*see also* the overt features of acute hypobaric hypoxia, page 57); indeed, the lightheadedness, paraesthesiae, and apprehension seen during acute hypoxia in a subject breathing air at altitudes between 15 000 ft and about 20 000 ft *are* due to the concomitant hypocapnia. Thus hypoxia should *always* be suspected when symptoms or signs of hypocapnia occur at altitudes above about 12 000 ft, and the corrective procedures *must* be based on the assumption that the condition is caused by hypoxia until proved otherwise.

Further reading

BROWN, E.B. (1953) Physiological effects of hyperventilation. *Physiological Reviews*, **33**, 445–471

CROW, T.J. and KELMAN, G.R. (1969) Psychological effects of mild hypoxia. *Journal of Physiology*, **204**, 248

DENISON, D.M. (1981) High altitudes and hypoxia. In *Principles and Practice of Human Physiology*, edited by O.G. Edholm and J.S. Weiner, pp. 241–307. London: Academic Press

ERNSTING, J. (1963) The effect of brief profound hypoxia upon the arterial and venous oxygen tensions in man. *Journal of Physiology*, **169**, 292–311

ERNSTING, J. (1978) Prevention of hypoxia—acceptable compromises. *Aviation Space and Environmental Medicine*, **49**, 495–502

ERNSTING, J., BYFORD, G.H., DENISON, D.M. and FRYER, D.I. (1973) Hypoxia Induced by Rapid Decompression from 8000 feet to 40000 feet—The Influence of Rate of Decompression. *Flying Personnel Research Committee Report* No 1324. London: Ministry of Defence

HARDING, R.M. (1986) The early symptoms of cerebral hypoxia. In *The Prelude to the Migraine Attack*, edited by W.K. Amery and A. Wauquier, pp. 54–58. London: Baillière Tindall

HARDING, R.M. and MILLS, F.J. (1983) Hypoxia and hyperventilation. *British Medical Journal*, **286**, 1408–1410

LUM, L.C. (1981) Hyperventilation and anxiety state. *Journal of The Royal Society of Medicine*, **74**, 1–4

6

Prevention of hypoxia

G.R. Sharp and J.Ernsting, revised by A.J.F. Macmillan

Introduction

The physiological effects of breathing air at reduced atmospheric pressure must be prevented during flight. One method of achieving this aim is to provide an artificial pressure environment, a pressurized cabin, so that the occupants are not exposed to reduced barometric pressure (*see* Chapter 8). The alternative method is to increase the concentration and hence the partial pressure of oxygen in the lungs by the use of oxygen equipment. In modern military aircraft both methods of preventing hypoxia are generally employed. The altitudes and environmental pressures quoted in the text refer to conditions surrounding the aircraft occupant himself (cabin altitude and pressure) and not those surrounding the aircraft.

The purpose of aircraft oxygen equipment is to maintain an adequate supply of oxygen to the tissues of the body despite a reduction in barometric pressure. At altitudes up to 33 000 feet, the alveolar oxygen tension may be maintained at its ground level value by increasing the proportion of oxygen in the inspired gas. Above this altitude, however, the alveolar oxygen pressure falls, even when 100÷oxygen is breathed. The fall in the alveolar partial pressure of oxygen with increasing altitude above 33 000 feet can be prevented only by maintaining the total alveolar gas pressure. The manoeuvre whereby the pressure in the lungs is raised above the environmental pressure is termed positive pressure breathing. The serious hypoxia that would otherwise occur on exposure to altitudes in excess of 40 000 feet may be prevented by this means.

A secondary purpose of the oxygen system is the exclusion of contaminated cabin air from the gas entering the respiratory tract.

These functions must be achieved with the minimum of physiological and psychological disturbance. In this chapter, the basic physiological requirements of aircraft oxygen systems and the effects of positive pressure breathing required to maintain adequate alveolar oxygen pressure are discussed in detail.

Minimum acceptable concentration of oxygen

To prevent the fall in alveolar oxygen tension that occurs when air is breathed at reduced barometric pressure, the proportion of oxygen in the inspired gas must be increased. The fractional concentration of oxygen required in the inspired gas to maintain a desired alveolar oxygen pressure at any particular altitude may be calculated. *Figure 6.1* shows the relationships between the concentration of oxygen in the inspired gas and altitude required to maintain: (1) the normal ground-level alveolar oxygen tension (103 mm Hg (13.7 kPa)); (2) the alveolar oxygen pressure that exists when breathing air at 5000 feet (75 mm Hg (10.0 kPa)); and (3) the alveolar oxygen pressure that exists when breathing air at 8000 feet (65 mm Hg (8.7 kPa)).

Initially it would seem attractive, on grounds of oxygen economy, to choose an alveolar oxygen partial pressure lower than the normal ground-level value. Thus at 25 000 feet, the inspired gas must contain 63% oxygen to maintain an alveolar oxygen tension of 103 mm Hg (13.7 kPa), but only 41% oxygen to provide an alveolar oxygen tension of 60 mm Hg (8.0 kPa). However, the disadvantages of choosing a relationship between oxygen concentration and altitude that allows the alveolar oxygen tension to fall below the ground-level value are:

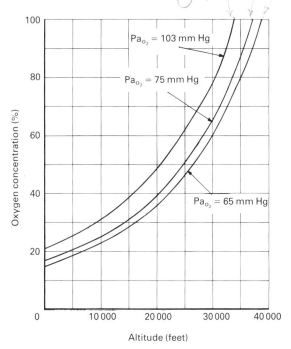

Figure 6.1 handwritten annotations: "To maintain ① ground level = ② 5000' = ③ 8000'"

Figure 6.1 The concentrations of oxygen required in the dry inspired gas at various altitudes in order to maintain alveolar oxygen tensions of 103 mm Hg (13.7 kPa) (equivalent to breathing air at ground level); 75 mm Hg (10.0 kPa) (equivalent to breathing air at 5000 feet) and 65 mm Hg (8.7 kPa) (equivalent to breathing air at 8000 feet).

1. Even the mild degree of hypoxia associated with a lowering of the alveolar oxygen tension to 75 mm Hg (10.0 kPa) impairs the ability to recall recently learned procedures.
2. Lowering the alveolar oxygen tension to the order of 60 mm Hg (8.0 kPa) induces a significant performance impairment which is accentuated by physical exercise.
3. There is a lower margin of safety in the event of either a partial or a complete failure of the breathing equipment to deliver oxygen to the respiratory tract.

Thus, solely on the grounds of preventing hypoxia at altitudes up to 35000 feet, the concentration of oxygen in the inspired gas should not be allowed to fall below that required to maintain an alveolar oxygen tension of 80 mm Hg (10.7 kPa). From a practical point of view, however, the third consideration is probably equally important. When an ill-fitting oxygen mask allows the oxygen delivered to the user to be diluted by the inward leakage of air, the consequent risk of hypoxia is diminished in proportion to the amount by which the concentration of oxygen in the breathing gas supply exceeds that required to prevent hypoxia. For example, at an altitude of 25000 feet an inward leak equal to half the pulmonary ventilation would reduce alveolar oxygen tension from 80 mm Hg (10.7 kPa) to about 65 mm Hg (8.0 kPa) (equivalent to breathing air at 8000 feet); if the oxygen system was designed to maintain an alveolar oxygen tension of 65 mm Hg (8.7 kPa) a similar leakage would reduce the alveolar oxygen tension to 40 mm Hg (5.3 kPa) (equivalent to breathing air at 16000 feet)-a very significant degree of hypoxia.

Thus an oxygen system should be designed to deliver that concentration of oxygen in relation to altitude which will maintain a ground-level alveolar oxygen tension (that is, 103 mm Hg (13.7 kPa)) as indicated by the upper curve of *Figure 6.1* and the minimum oxygen concentration in *Table 6.1*. This ground-level alveolar oxygen tension can only be maintained in this manner at altitudes up to 33000 feet. Above 33000 feet the alveolar oxygen tension falls progressively even when 100% oxygen is breathed.

Table 6.1 Limits for concentration of oxygen delivered to the respiratory tract by an aircraft oxygen system

Cabin altitude (ft)	Concentration of oxygen (%) in dry inspired gas	
	Minimum	Maximum*
0	21	60
5000	25	60
10000	31	60
15000	38	60
20000	49	67
25000	63	80
30000	81	100
33000	95	100
35000	100	100
40000	100	100

*Typical values allowed by current specifications.

Maximum acceptable concentration of oxygen

An oxygen system that provides aircrew with 100% oxygen at all altitudes has the advantage of simplicity, fewer mechanical complications and is cheaper to manufacture than one which supplies a mixture of air and oxygen that varies appropriately with altitude. The objections to breathing 100% oxygen at all altitudes in flight are as follows:

1. It is uneconomical in terms of the consumption of the aircraft oxygen supply since in order to prevent serious hypoxia, 100% oxygen is required only above a cabin altitude of 33000 feet.
2. Breathing 100% oxygen continuously for long periods (12–16 hours) may cause substernal discomfort due to the irritative effect of a high

partial pressure of oxygen on the mucosal lining of the respiratory passages.

3. Breathing 100% oxygen at altitude and during return to ground level frequently gives rise, some hours later, to ear discomfort and deafness (delayed otic barotrauma). This phenomenon is due to rapid absorption of oxygen from the middle-ear cavity into the blood and the intensity of the symptoms is reduced greatly by the presence of nitrogen in the inspired gas and hence in the gas in the middle-ear cavity.

4. Respiratory symptoms, such as coughing, dyspnoea and retrosternal discomfort, occurring immediately after flight in a high-performance aircraft are produced by breathing 100% oxygen prior to and during exposure to $+G_z$ acceleration. The severity of this syndrome is increased by the use of an anti-G suit. The nature of this condition is discussed in Chapter 10, but it should be noted that the symptoms of acceleration atelectasis may be prevented by ensuring that the concentration of nitrogen in the inspired gas is greater than 40%.

For these reasons, an aircraft oxygen system should deliver a mixture of oxygen and nitrogen-derived either from mixing the supply gas with air or by controlling the retention of nitrogen in molecular sieve systems. While the concentration of oxygen should vary with altitude in such a manner that the alveolar oxygen tension is maintained at or just greater than the value (103 mm Hg (13.7 kPa)) which obtains when air is breathed at ground level, the concentration of nitrogen in the gas delivered by the system should be as high as the primary requirement to maintain the ideal oxygen tension will permit. In practice, the concentration of oxygen delivered at a given altitude by an aircrew breathing system varies with the demand, and from one regulating device to another. Thus it is necessary to allow some deviation from the ideal oxygen concentration–altitude curve (*Figure 6.1*, upper curve). Typical maximum oxygen concentrations allowed by current specifications for aircrew oxygen breathing equipment are presented in *Table 6.1*. At altitudes above 40000 feet when 100% oxygen must be delivered at a pressure greater than ambient, the absolute pressure which must be contained within the lungs depends on the degree of hypoxia that is deemed acceptable; and this, in turn, is determined by several factors which will be discussed later in this chapter. Generally, however, most pressure breathing systems maintain an absolute pressure in the respiratory tract of between 120 and 150 mm Hg (16.0 and 20.0 kPa). The relationships between altitude and the positive pressure at which oxygen must be delivered to the respiratory tract (breathing pressure) to maintain various absolute pressures within the lungs are shown in *Figure 6.4*.

Pulmonary ventilation in flight

Oxygen equipment must be capable of meeting the pulmonary ventilation (respiratory minute volume) requirements of the user in a variety of situations both on the ground and during flight. The pulmonary ventilation is determined by the metabolic rate and modified by factors such as hypoxia, excitement and anxiety. Measurements of respiratory minute volume have shown large differences in pulmonary ventilation between one individual and another under similar flight conditions. Typical values of respiratory minute volume obtained under various conditions of flight are shown in *Table 6.2*. The figures are based on data derived from many sources and relate to aircrew who are adequately oxygenated.

Table 6.2 Pulmonary ventilation in various conditions of flight

Conditions	Pulmonary ventilation (litres (BTPS)/minute)
Seated at rest	10–15
Seated active	15–50
Moving about aircraft	25–50
After running to aircraft	Up to 60

The greatest increase in respiratory minute volume occurs when the pilot runs to his aircraft. The mass flow of gas required from an oxygen regulator to meet a given pulmonary ventilation varies inversely with the pressure in the respiratory tract. It follows, therefore, that the sea-level requirement demands most from the delivery system in term of mass flow. Aircrew oxygen breathing equipment should, therefore, be capable of meeting pulmonary ventilations of up to 60 litres (BTPS)/min at ground level.

Respiratory gas flow patterns in flight

During the breathing cycle, the flow of gas in and out of the respiratory tract changes very rapidly. Oxygen equipment must be capable of responding to these changes whilst imposing the minimum of resistance to breathing. Respiratory gas flow patterns related to the various conditions that occur in flight can be measured using a pneumotachograph. Typical records obtained (pneumotachograms) are shown in *Figure 6.2* for:

1. Aircrew seated at rest (curve A).
2. Aircrew performing physical exercise approximating to the effort of moving about an aircraft (curve B).
3. Aircrew speaking aloud whilst seated at rest (curve C).

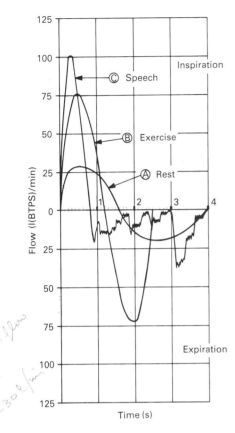

Figure 6.2 Typical respiratory flow patterns
(pneumotachograms) for (1) aircrew seated at rest (trace
A); (2) aircrew moving about an aircraft (trace B) and (3)
aircrew speaking aloud whilst seated at rest (trace C). The
flow throughout a single respiratory cycle is shown for each
of the three conditions.

However, there are very wide individual variations
in the airflow pattern obtained during any particular
activity, and the shape of the pattern depends on the
level of physical activity, the nature of the work
undertaken, the degree of arm movement, posture,
the phase of flight, e.g. level of $+G_z$ acceleration,
etc. In the resting subject (*Figure 6.2*, curve A), the
flow of air increases rapidly at the beginning of
inspiration but then the rate of increase of flow falls
progressively until the peak flow of about 25–30 l
(BTPS)/min is reached. The air velocity falls slowly
and then more rapidly until it reaches zero at the
end of inspiration. The whole inspiratory phase lasts
1–2 seconds and expiration follows without a pause.
This lasts longer than inspiration, and the peak flow
achieved is less than that which occurs during
inspiration. In a resting non-speaking subject, the
peak inspiratory flow is generally about three times
the respiratory minute volume. During moderate
exercise (*Figure 6.2*, curve B), the volume of gas in
each phase of the breathing cycle is increased and

the duration of each phase is shortened. The peak
inspiratory flow also increases, but in these conditions this value amounts to only about 2.6 times the
respiratory minute volume. The duration of the
expiratory phase becomes shorter relative to the
duration of inspiration, and at higher work rates
may be actually less. During speech at rest (*Figure
6.2*, curve C), the volume of gas breathed in each
phase is similar to that during rest without speech,
but the duration of inspiration is very short (0.5–0.6
seconds) and the duration of expiration is lengthened. Speech modulates the flow pattern in the
expiratory phase. In inspiration during speech, the
peak flow and the rate of increase and decrease of
gas flow are very high. Thus speech places one of the
most severe demands on oxygen equipment in terms
of the peak flow delivery and rate of change of flow.

Oxygen equipment must cater for the wide variety
of breathing flow patterns which may occur in
aircrew in flight. In addition, for any given set of
circumstances, there are considerable individual
variations (by as much as 100% between maximum
and minimum peak flow values. The mean values of
gas flow, as typified in *Figure 6.2*, do not provide an
adequate basis for the design of breathing systems.
In practice it is usual to specify the curves given by
the mean values plus twice the standard deviation,
which will include the gas flow requirements of 95%
of normal individuals. Curves of this type show that
oxygen equipment should be designed to meet
inspiratory peak flows of up to 200 l (BTPS)/min.

Imposition of external resistance to respiratory gas flow

Most oxygen breathing equipment imposes additional flow resistance on the respiratory system. This
added breathing resistance must be kept to a
minimum in order to avoid undesirable physiological side-effects.

There have been many experimental studies of
the effects of imposed resistance to breathing, but
the results of many of these studies are difficult to
interpret, in terms of the requirements for oxygen
systems, since the effects vary greatly, depending on
the type and magnitude of the resistance used.
Furthermore, in most studies the external resistance
has been imposed for relatively short periods (10–30
minutes).

However, the general effects of imposing external
resistance to breathing in either or both phases of
respiration may be stated. These effects include the
following:

1. *A change in respiratory rhythm*-Moderate resistances cause slowing and deepening of respiration
   while high resistances cause rapid, shallow
   breathing.

2. *A decrease in pulmonary ventilation*-For a given resistance the reduction is greatest when the resistance is applied both in inspiration and in expiration.
3. *A reduction in alveolar ventilation*-This causes an increase in alveolar carbon dioxide tension.
4. *An increase in functional residual capacity*-This is greatest when a resistance load is applied in expiration alone.
5. *A reduction of the maximum ventilatory capacity.*
6. *An increase in the total respiratory work per minute*-This increases in an approximately linear manner with increasing resistance.
7. *Subjective disturbances*-These range from conscious appreciation of a very slight resistance to breathing to severe resistance to breathing, with sensations of impending asphyxia.

The physiological disturbances induced by the addition of resistance to breathing show great variation of response between different subjects and between the effects on the same subject on different occasions. Thus while reduction in alveolar ventilation and hypercapnia may result from breathing against high levels of resistance, there is no doubt that susceptible subjects (for example, aircrew untrained and inexperienced in the use of oxygen equipment) may hyperventilate and exhibit symptoms of the consequent hypocapnia.

The results of one investigation into the subjective effects of applied respiratory resistance are shown in *Figure 6.3*. In this study, resistance was applied by means of different sized orifices. After a few minutes the subject was asked to comment on the degree of resistance to breathing, with a view to establishing the value of resistance at which mask pressure fluctuations became perceptible to him. During quiet breathing (a peak inspiratory flow of about 30 l/min), an inspiratory suction of 1.6 cm water gauge (160 Pa) was not noticed by the subjects. When inspiratory suction reached 2.8 cm water gauge (280 Pa) resistance was noticed on all occasions. In many aircraft oxygen systems the ability to detect imposition of breathing resistance has been used to provide warning of either supply malfunction or inadvertent disconnection of components of the system. The sensation of resistance to breathing and the physiological disturbances produced by breathing from oxygen equipment depend not only on the total change of pressure in the mask cavity during the respiratory cycle but also on the relationship of these pressure changes to the pressure of the environment. Thus the disturbances induced by the imposition of a given resistance to respiration is less if the mean pressure in the mask is raised slightly (2–6 cm water gauge (200–600 Pa)) above that of the environment than when the mean pressure is equal to or less than the environmental pressure.

Although it is possible to state the magnitude of resistance that will give rise to the described subjective disturbances and undesirable physiological changes, it is difficult to define the acceptable limits of resistance. In general, the aim is to keep the added breathing resistance imposed by the system to a minimum. In practical terms, the maximum acceptable limit for the resistance imposed by aircrew oxygen breathing equipment is that the total changes of pressure in the mask during the respiratory cycle should not exceed 500 Pa (5.0 cm water gauge) during quiet breathing (peak inspiratory and expiratory flows of 30 l (BTPS)/min) or 800 Pa (8.0 cm water gauge) during heavy breathing (peak inspiratory and expiratory flows of 110 l (BTPS)/min).

Prevention of hypoxia above 40 000 feet

To prevent hypoxia above 40 000 feet, oxygen systems must be capable of delivering breathing gas to the respiratory tract at pressures greater than that of the environment.

It would appear from *Figure 6.4* that hypoxia may be prevented at any altitude above 40 000 feet merely by delivering 100% oxygen at appropriate pressure to the respiratory tract. But as the pressure increases, undesirable physiological disturbances may arise. These disturbances are associated with the type of breathing system utilized and thus the manner in which the pressure is applied to the respiratory tract, and the respiratory and circulatory

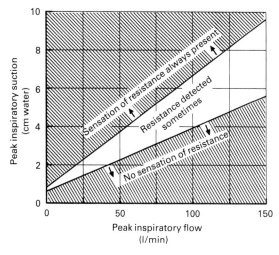

Figure 6.3 Relationships between peak inspiratory flow and peak inspiratory suction at the nose and lips which give rise to a sensation of resistance to breathing. The added resistance was in the form of a sharp-edged orifice and the subject's comments on the presence or absence of the sensation of resistance was recorded after he had been exposed to it for several minutes.

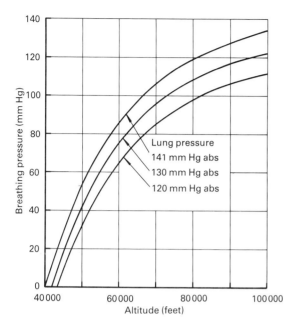

Figure 6.4 The relationship between pressure at which gas must be delivered (relative to that of the environment) and altitude to maintain absolute pressures in the respiratory tract of (1) 141 mm Hg (2) 130 mm Hg and (3) 120 mm Hg.

changes caused by the increased intrapulmonary pressure. Thus it is convenient to consider the physiology of pressure breathing under the following headings: the effects on the head and neck; the respiratory disturbances; the circulatory disturbances; and the acceptable degree of hypoxia.

The effects of pressure breathing on the head and neck

In practice, gas at pressure greater than that of the environment may be delivered to the respiratory tract by means of an oronasal mask. At high breathing pressures, certain drawbacks associated with the oronasal mask may be overcome by the use of a pressure helmet. These two methods of delivering oxygen at pressures greater than ambient are discussed below.

Pressure breathing with an oronasal mask

With an oronasal mask, pressure is applied to the mouth and nose and physical support is given to only a limited area of the face. There are certain mechanical limitations to the pressure that may be delivered in this manner. Thus, some oronasal

masks in current use will not seal adequately when the pressure within them exceeds 25–30 mm Hg (3.3–4.0 kPa). If higher pressures are delivered, the upper part of such a mask lifts off the face and gas streams into the eyes. Other types of oronasal mask have a specially designed reflected edge seal and employ a 'toggle' suspension harness. These types will, when correctly fitted, hold pressures of up to 100 mm Hg (13.3 kPa) without significant leakage. In practice, however, well-defined physiological effects limit the pressure that can be delivered using an oronasal mask since no external support is applied to the floor of the mouth or the neck, the eyes, or the ears. These are as follows.

Distension of the upper respiratory passages

This commences when the breathing pressure exceeds 10 mm Hg (1.3 kPa) and progresses so that with high breathing pressures, there is distension of the mouth, the whole of the pharynx and the cervical portion of the oesophagus. At pressures greater than about 70 mm Hg (9.3 kPa) this distortion causes severe discomfort and it is this discomfort which is the main limitation to the use of an oronasal mask.

Rise of intravascular pressure on the eyes

Increased intravascular pressure caused by the raised intrathoracic pressure dilates the conjunctival vessels. At breathing pressures above 70–80 mm Hg (9.3–10.7 kPa) the conjunctival capillaries may rupture. Contrastingly, the retinal vessels may constrict as a result of hypocapnia induced by the positive pressure breathing.

Spasm of the eyelids

The nasolacrimal ducts open and the gas passes directly into the conjunctival sacs causing blepharospasm. This occurs in a small proportion of people and may seriously interfere with vision.

Ear discomfort

In normal circumstances, the eustachian tubes are occluded during pressure breathing, and unless the subject swallows during the exposure, the tympanic membrane remains in the normal position and auditory acuity is unchanged. Should the subject swallow (a difficult manoeuvre to perform during pressure breathing) the rise in middle ear pressure causes the tympanic membrane to bulge out into the external auditory canal, causing some discomfort and reduced auditory acuity.

Thus, in summary, a suitable oronasal mask may be used to deliver pressures of up to 70–75 mm Hg (9.3–10.0 kPa) to the respiratory tract provided that the length of time for which the pressure is applied is short (that is, about 1–2 minutes). Longer periods at these pressures or the delivery of higher pressures frequently gives rise to severe discomfort. On the other hand, a pressure of 30 mm Hg (4.0 kPa) may be breathed for up to half an hour without undue disturbance or discomfort.

Pressure breathing with a pressure helmet

A pressure helmet may be used as an alternative to the oronasal mask for delivering oxygen to the respiratory tract at pressures greater than that of the environment. Partial pressure helmets give support to the cheeks, floor of the mouth and the eyes, and most of the head and upper part of the neck are also pressurized. Thus the pressure differentials that develop between the air passages and the skin of the head and neck when an oronasal mask is employed are eliminated. In addition, no abnormal pressure differentials are applied to the vessels of the eyes. Some pressure helmets, however, do not increase the pressure in the external auditory meatus: breathing pressures of 110–140 mm Hg may then cause rupture of the vessels in the outer layers of the tympanic membrane, giving rise to haemorrhagic bullae on the surface of the membrane.

The respiratory effects of pressure breathing

Distension of lungs and chest

Pressure breathing tends to distend the chest and lungs; and, in a relaxed subject (when the distensibility of the lungs and thorax is high), the lungs are fully distended by a breathing pressure of 20 mm Hg (2.7 kPa). The maximum pressure that can be exerted and held in the lungs by active contraction of expiratory muscles of the chest and abdominal walls depends on the length of time for which the pressure is operative. Thus during coughing the intrapulmonary pressure may reach peak values of between 200 and 300 mm Hg (26.6–40.0 kPa) for very brief periods. When the pressure is held for about 3 seconds, the maximum expiratory pressure that can be produced is about 120 mm Hg (16.0 kPa). If the lungs are unsupported by the chest wall, they will rupture when the intrapulmonary pressure exceeds 40–50 mm Hg (5.3–6.7 kPa). When, however, the lungs are supported by the walls of the thoracic cavity, intrapulmonary pressures of up to 80 mm Hg (10.7 kPa) can be tolerated without damage. Intrapulmonary pressures above

80–100 mm Hg (10.7–13.3 kPa) cause tearing of the lung parenchyma when the expiratory muscles are relaxed. Gas can pass from the damaged tissue into the tissue planes, causing pneumothorax and surgical emphysema; and into pulmonary blood vessels, causing gas embolism.

Breathing effort

In pressure breathing, the subject must maintain a continuous expiratory effort in order to prevent over-distension of the lungs. Since elastic recoil plays little part in exhaling gas during pressure breathing, the work of breathing is thereby further

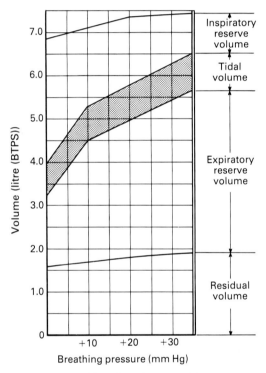

Figure 6.5 The effect of continuous positive pressure breathing on total lung capacity and its subdivisions. The total lung capacity, the residual volume and the functional residual capacity (residual volume + expiratory reserve volume) all become greater with increase of breathing pressure. The greatest increase occurs, however, in the expiratory reserve volume whilst the inspiratory reserve volume is markedly reduced.

increased. A subject experienced in pressure breathing can breathe for short periods at pressures of up to 50 mm Hg (6.7 kPa) although subjects unaccustomed to the procedure are unable to tolerate a breathing pressure of more than about 30 mm Hg (4.0 kPa). Even in experienced subjects, pressure breathing at 30 mm Hg (4.0 kPa) causes quite considerable distension of the lungs and gives rise to increasing respiratory fatigue (*Figure 6.5*). Pressure breathing at 30 mm Hg (4.0 kPa) reduces the inspiratory reserve volume by about 2.51 although total lung volume is increased. This increase in lung volume is associated with expansion of the thoracic cage and descent of the diaphragm.

Increased pulmonary ventilation

In most subjects, pressure breathing causes an increase in the respiratory minute volume, although there is wide individual variation in this response. Pressure breathing at 30 mm Hg (4.0 kPa) causes, on average, an increase in the respiratory minute volume averaging about 50% greater than the resting value. Some individuals double their minute volume at 30 mm Hg (4.0 kPa) positive pressure: others respond hardly at all. Since the increase in pulmonary ventilation during pressure breathing is not accompanied by a corresponding increase in carbon dioxide production, the blood CO_2 level falls. During pressure breathing at 30 mm Hg (4.0 kPa) the alveolar and arterial carbon dioxide tensions are frequently as low as 25–30 mm Hg (3.3–4.0 kPa).

Raised intrapleural pressure

The increase in intrapleural pressure that occurs during pressure breathing is of considerable importance, since it determines the degree of stress that is applied to the circulation. This increase in intrapleural pressure is determined by the applied breathing pressure and the degree of lung distension that it induces. If there is no increase in lung volume, the rise in intrapleural pressure equals the applied breathing pressure. If lung distension occurs, the rise in intrapleural pressure will be less than the applied intrapulmonary pressure by the additional elastic recoil generated in the lung tissue, which is approximately 4 mm Hg (0.5 kPa) per litre distension. Thus if lung volume is increased by 3 litres at the start of pressure breathing, the rise in intrapleural pressure will be approximately 12 mm Hg (1.6 kPa) less than the applied breathing pressure.

Effects of respiratory counterpressure

The major respiratory disturbances that are induced by pressure breathing (that is, lung distension and hyperventilation) may be minimized by applying counterpressure to the surface of the trunk. Counterpressure may be applied by a variety of methods, the most efficient of which is by gas, as in a full pressure suit. Another method, which is almost as efficient, applies counterpressure to the trunk by means of a gas-filled bladder which is connected to the breathing line between the source of breathing pressure and the oro-nasal mask or helmet. In this way, when pressure is applied to the breathing tract, an equal gas pressure is applied in the bladder which covers the trunk. This is the basis of the pressure jerkin, a full description of which is given in Chapter 7.

The circulatory effects of pressure breathing

The circulatory disturbances induced by pressure breathing vary with the magnitude of the pressure applied to the respiratory tract and the time it lasts. The heart and large intrathoracic vessels are normally exposed to the intrapleural pressure: and it is the rise in this, rather than the increase in intrapulmonary pressure, that determines the stress applied to the circulation. Provided that the intrathoracic veins and the heart cavities contain blood, then the diastolic pressures within them are raised by an amount equal to the rise in intrapleural pressure.

Pooling of blood in the peripheral vascular beds

At the start of pressure breathing, the rise in intrapleural pressure is transmitted directly to the large intrathoracic veins and the right atrium. Since the pressure in the extrathoracic veins is normally low the flow of blood from the periphery of the body into the chest is severely impeded and the venous outflow from the limbs ceases completely. Venous return to the heart does not cease at the beginning of pressure breathing since there is a maintained flow of blood from the abdominal viscera and the brain. The flow of blood from the abdomen continues, since the intra-abdominal pressure rises in parallel with that in the pleural space. The jugular venous blood flow is maintained because of the indistensibility of the intracranial vascular bed.

Although the venous outflow from the limbs ceases when pressure breathing commences, the arterial inflow is maintained, and blood collects in and distends the peripheral vascular bed until the peripheral venous pressure exceeds the raised right atrial pressure (*Figure 6.6*). At this point, venous return from the limbs recommences, increasing the systemic venous return to the heart. This initial phase of very marked reduction in venous return to the heart lasts for 10–20 seconds.

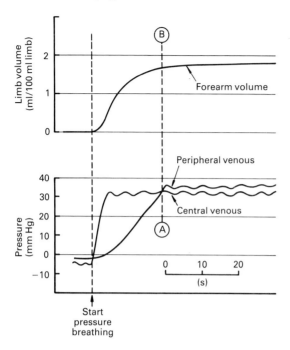

Start
pressure
breathing

Figure 6.6 Effect of pressure breathing at 40 mm Hg with trunk counterpressure on peripheral and central venous pressures and volume of the forearm. The central venous pressure rises rapidly to a plateau value determined by the breathing pressure. The rise of central venous pressure raises it above the peripheral venous pressure and the flow of blood from the limb to the heart ceases. Since arterial inflow continues blood accumulates in the peripheral vascular bed, increasing the volume of the limb (top trace) and progressively raising the peripheral venous pressure. When the capacity vessels in the limb are distended the peripheral venous pressure once again exceeds central venous pressure (at point A-B) so that venous outflow recommences and the volume of the limb stabilizes at a new greater value (continued increase of limb volume is due to accumulation of fluid in the tissues). For clarity, the cardiac fluctuations of venous pressure have been omitted.

The circulation through the limbs is maintained during pressure breathing by displacement of blood from within the trunk into the limbs. The amount of blood thus displaced is determined by the increase in venous pressure and the distensibility of the vessels of the limbs. One of the reflex cardiovascular changes that occurs during pressure breathing is active constriction of the peripheral veins, which tends to reduce the amount of blood displaced from within the trunk. The amount of blood displaced into the limbs of a seated subject by pressure breathing at 30 mm Hg (4.0 kPa) is of the order of 200 ml; at 80 mm Hg (10.7 kPa) 400 ml (*Figure 6.7*).

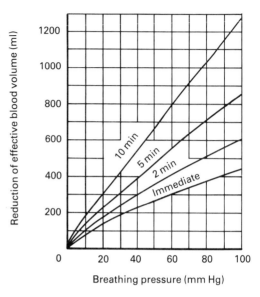

Figure 6.7 Effects of pressure breathing with counterpressure to the trunk on reduction of effective blood volume, in seated subjects. The reduction of blood volume due to displacement of blood into the peripheral capacity vessels is indicated by the curve labelled 'Immediate'. The subsequent further reductions of effective blood volume due to loss of fluid into the tissues are indicated for pressure breathing for 2, 5 and 10 minutes.

Reduction of the effective blood volume

The effective blood volume (the volume of blood that is available for circulatory adjustment) is reduced during pressure breathing by two factors:

1. The initial pooling of blood (described above).
2. The passage of fluid from the circulation into the tissues.

The increase in the pressure within the capillary vessels of the limbs relative to the local tissue pressure, which occurs as a consequence of the raised venous pressure, disturbs the balance that normally exists between hydrostatic and osmotic forces at the blood–tissue fluid interface in the capillary bed. The raised intracapillary pressure drives fluid out of the circulation into the tissues. The rate at which fluid leaves the capillaries depends on the rise of capillary pressure: and this, in turn, is closely related to the increase in venous pressure. Thus, pressure breathing at 30 mm Hg (4.0 kPa) for 10 minutes will result in the loss of about 250 ml of fluid from the circulation whilst pressure breathing for 5 minutes at 100 mm Hg (13.3 kPa) will result in a loss of 500 ml of fluid into the tissues (*Figure 6.7*).

The total reduction in effective blood volume which occurs as a result of these two factors (initial pooling of blood and increase in extravascular fluid) during pressure breathing at 30 mm Hg (4.0 kPa) for 10 minutes is of the order of 450 ml. Pressure breathing at 100 mm Hg (13.3 kPa) for 5 minutes results in a net reduction of the effective blood volume of about 950 ml. This loss of circulating blood into the limbs may be minimized by the counterpressure of inflated bladders (such as those contained in the anti-G suit) on the lower limbs. This principle is used in the design of partial pressure clothing, as described in Chapter 7.

Reduction in cardiac output

The peripheral pooling of blood leads to a lowering of the effective pressure in the right atrium, so that, even when the venous return from the periphery is restored, the cardiac output is less than it was before pressure breathing commenced. During pressure breathing at 30 mm Hg (4.0 kPa) without trunk counterpressure, the cardiac output is reduced by about 30% compared with the resting value. If, however, trunk counterpressure is applied, the same degree of pressure breathing reduces the cardiac output by only 15–20%.

Rise in arterial blood pressure

The arterial blood pressure is raised during pressure breathing, primarily as a result of the transmission of the raised intrapleural pressure to the blood within the left ventricle. If cardiac output and peripheral vascular resistance were unchanged, the pressure within the left ventricle would be increased by an amount equal to the rise in pleural pressure. This rise in intraventricular pressure would be reflected in the systemic arterial blood pressure. In fact, neither cardiac nor peripheral resistance remain unchanged, and the reduction in cardiac output during pressure breathing tends to reduce the rise in arterial blood pressure. This effect is partially counteracted by active constriction of the peripheral resistance vessels-the arterioles.

The net rise in arterial blood pressure that occurs in pressure breathing is an expression of the effectiveness of the compensatory circulatory adjustments that occur in this condition (that is, the increase in heart rate and constriction of arterioles and veins). These reflex circulatory adjustments probably result from the stimulation of volume receptors in the right side of the heart, produced by the displacement of blood from the central part of the circulation into the periphery.

During pressure breathing at 30 mm Hg (4.0 kPa),

the rise in mean arterial blood pressure is of the order of 20 mm Hg (2.7 kPa). During pressure breathing with only trunk counterpressure at 80 mm Hg (10.7 kPa) the mean arterial blood pressure increases by 60–80 mm Hg (8.0–10.7 kPa). If counterpressure is also applied to the lower limbs, the rise in arterial blood pressure is usually greater than the applied breathing pressure. Thus pressure breathing at 80 mm Hg (10.7 kPa) with counterpressure applied to the trunk and lower limbs increases the mean systemic arterial pressure by about 100 mm Hg (13.3 kPa).

Pressure-breathing syncope

As has been described, the cardiac output is maintained during the first 10–15 seconds of pressure breathing by the venous return from the abdomen and head. If the breathing pressure applied to the respiratory tract is very high (for example 80–100 mm Hg), and if no counterpressure is applied to the trunk, the reduction in venous return may be so severe that the arterial blood pressure falls and consciousness may be lost within 10–15 seconds. Normally, however, the venous return to the heart is adequate to maintain a reasonable cardiac output: and this, together with peripheral vasoconstriction, causes the rise in arterial blood pressure already described. Under these circumstances, there is no impairment of consciousness. If, however, pressure breathing is continued for long enough, collapse occurs. The length of time that elapses before syncope occurs during pressure breathing depends primarily on the pressure that is applied to the respiratory tract. Thus most subjects can breathe at 30 mm Hg (4.0 kPa) for 30 minutes without syncope; whilst collapse generally occurs after only 2 minutes breathing at a pressure of 100 mm Hg (13.3 kPa) with trunk counterpressure alone.

Pressure breathing collapse has the following features:

1. Nausea and uneasiness.
2. Dimming of vision.
3. Intense facial pallor.
4. Profuse facial and palmar sweating.
5. Loss of consciousness.
6. Loss of postural tone.
7. Jerky movements of limbs (occasionally major epileptiform convulsions).

The feeling of nausea and facial pallor persist for some time after consciousness returns, frequently for several hours.

Pressure-breathing syncope is accompanied by marked gross changes in the circulatory system. The onset of collapse is heralded by a progressive increase in heart rate and a gradual fall in the arterial blood pressure. A sudden profound brady-cardia occurs, arterial blood pressure falls precipi-tously, and unconsciousness follows within 5–10 seconds. When the pressure breathing is stopped the arterial blood pressure increases slowly over the next 30–60 seconds. Heart rate also increases although both heart rate and arterial blood pressure may remain below resting level for as long as an hour.

Pressure-breathing collapses have many of the features of fainting caused by haemorrhage, pain, etc. The prime cause of the sudden profound hypotension that occurs in fainting is dilatation of the arterioles in muscles. The cardiac output, which usually falls in the period preceding a faint, does not decrease further when the faint occurs and thus does not contribute to the fall in arterial pressure. The disturbances of cerebral function are due to the reduction in cerebral blood flow consequent on the fall in arterial pressure. In pressure-breathing syncope, the extreme peripheral arteriolar vasodi-latation that occurs in muscle is probably produced by vasodilator fibres of the sympathetic outflow. The nausea, abdominal discomfort, facial pallor and skin vasoconstriction are probably humoral in origin (during and following a faint there is an increase in the secretion of posterior pituitary hormone). The receptors and afferent pathways in pressure-breathing syncope are, in all probability, the same as those that are responsible for syncope due to loss of blood (50÷of semi-reclining subjects will faint after about 1100 ml of blood have been withdrawn by venesection). The stimulus in this type of syncope may be the reduction in the intrathoracic blood volume.

The afferent impulses responsible for initiating the cardiovascular changes (bradycardia, muscle arteriolar vasodilatation and secretion of posterior pituitary hormone) almost certainly arise from receptors in the walls of the heart. In trained subjects, the degree by which the effective blood volume must be reduced to produce pressure-breathing syncope (about 800 ml) is similar to that which will cause fainting by venesection. The likelihood of syncope during pressure breathing may be increased by hypoxia, hypocapnia, anxiety, discomfort or pain, intercurrent infection and the post-alcoholic state.

The acceptable degree of hypoxia

The pressure that must be delivered to the respiratory tract at a given altitude above 40 000 feet is determined by the degree of hypoxia that is acceptable. This is because two factors interact: from the point of view of preventing hypoxia, it is

desirable to have a high breathing pressure; from the point of view of the cardiovascular stress imposed by pressure breathing, it is desirable to keep the breathing pressure low. Two aspects of the influence of hypoxia are of interest in the present context. The first relates to the general mental and physical performance of the individual and the second to the modifications of the cardiovascular and respiratory responses to pressure breathing which are induced by the hypoxia.

A complicating feature is the fact that pressure breathing causes a certain degree of hyperventila-tion, even in trained subjects, and if the alveolar oxygen tension is less than 60 mm Hg (8.0 kPa) there is an additional stimulus to increase ventilation. The arterial carbon dioxide tension is therefore usually markedly reduced during pressure breathing at altitude. When 100% oxygen is breathed, a fall in alveolar carbon dioxide tension (caused by hyper-ventilation) gives rise to an equal increase in alveolar oxygen tension. It may initially seem thus to increase the oxygen tension in the arterial blood; but the lowered arterial carbon dioxide tension causes cerebral vasoconstriction, and reduction of blood flow through the brain. The net effect on the oxygen tension in the brain tissue is almost nil. Furth-ermore, as previously discussed, hypocapnia has undesirable effects on the circulation as a whole and renders the subject more liable to pressure brea-thing syncope.

The general mental and physical performance of groups of subjects has been determined whilst pressure breathing for 2–4 minutes with different intrapulmonary pressures at various altitudes. The results of these studies are summarized in *Table 6.3*.

When significant hypoxia is present (alveolar oxygen tension less than 60 mm Hg (8.0 kPa) the cardiovascular responses to pressure breathing are

Table 6.3 The relationship between absolute intrapulmonary pressure and overall performance during pressure breathing

Intra-pulmonary pressure (mm Hg absolute) and equivalent altitude	*Breathing pressure (mm Hg)*	*Applied counter pressure*	*Performance*
141 (40 000 feet)	0–141	Trunk and lower limbs	No significant impairment
130 (41 600 feet)	0–70	Trunk and lower limbs	Mild impairment
120 (43 300 feet)	0–70	Trunk only	Mild to moderate impairment
115 (44 300 feet)	0–30	None	Moderate to severe impairment

modified: the tachycardia and increase in arterial blood pressure are greater. The most striking effect of hypoxia during pressure breathing is, however, the increased incidence of syncope. Thus hypoxia during pressure breathing results in impaired performance and an increased risk of syncope. The effects of varying degrees of hypoxia when different degrees of body counterpressure are applied have been thoroughly investigated. The results of these investigations have led to the development of various partial pressure systems which are discussed in the next chapter.

Further reading

ERNSTING, J. (1963) The ideal relationship between inspired oxygen concentration and cabin altitude. *Aerospace Medicine*, **34**, 991–997

ERNSTING, J. (1966) *Some Effects of Raised Intrapulmonary Pressure*. AGARDograph No. 106. Maidenhead: Techivision Ltd.

ERNSTING, J. (1978) Prevention of hypoxia-acceptable compromises. *Aviation Space and Environmental Medicine*, **49**, 495–502

ERNSTING, J. (1983) *Operational and Physiological Requirements for Aircraft Oxygen Systems*. AGARD Seventh Advanced Operational Aviation Medicine Course. AGARD Report No. 697. Neuilly sur Seine: AGARD/NATO

HARDING, R.M. (1987) *Human Respiratory Responses During High Performance Flight*. AGARDograph No. 312. Neuilly sur Seine: AGARD/NATO

MORGAN, T.R., REID, D.H. and BAUMGARDNER, F.W. (1970) Pulmonary ventilation requirements evident in the operation of representative high performance aircraft. In *Proceedings of 47th Annual Scientific Meeting of the Aerospace Medical Association*, p. 158

SILVERMAN, L., LEE, G., YOUNG, A.R., AMORY, L., BARNEY, L.J. and LEE, R.C. (1945) *Fundamental Factors in The Design of Respiratory Protective Equipment. A Study and Evaluation of Inspiratory and Expiratory Resistance for Protective Respiratory Equipment*. Report No 5339. Washington DC: Office of Scientific Research and Development

7

Oxygen equipment and pressure clothing

R.M. Harding

Introduction

The primary purpose of aircraft oxygen equipment is to maintain an adequate supply of oxygen to the tissues of the body in the presence of the reduction in barometric pressure consequent upon ascent to altitude; that is, to prevent hypoxia. There are, however, a number of other physiological and general requirements, and all of these must clearly be achieved with the minimum of physiological (and psychological) disturbance to the user. The previous chapter dealt at length with the specific physiological requirements of an oxygen system: this chapter is concerned with the means by which these needs, and those of a more general nature, are met in practice. The first section summarizes the various physiological and general requirements of any oxygen system, whilst subsequent sections discuss the principles underlying the design and function of the various components of, and their integration into, a complete oxygen system.

In the United Kingdom, Scale K of the Air Navigation Order requires that equipment that will deliver oxygen-enriched air or 100% oxygen to the crew be installed in all commercial aircraft that fly above an altitude of 10000 feet. Furthermore, if the aircraft is capable of maintaining its cabin altitude below 10000 feet, then oxygen must be available in sufficient quantity to supply all crew members and passengers in the event of a failure of pressurization above 15000 feet, and to supply all crew members and 10% of the passengers if pressurization fails below 15000 feet. In all other aircraft (that is, in those that fly unpressurized), sufficient oxygen must be carried for continuous use by all occupants whenever the aircraft is flying above 13000 feet, and for continuous use by the crew and 10% of the passengers for any period during which the aircraft

flies between 10000 and 13000 feet. In aircraft with high-differential pressure cabins (that is, with a cabin altitude below about 8000 feet at all times during routine flight, such as passenger aircraft and large military transport or bomber aircraft), such (emergency) equipment is not generally used unless the cabin altitude exceeds the safe limits although emergency therapeutic oxygen may be required by ill passengers at low cabin altitudes (*see* Chapter 40). In aircraft with low-differential pressure cabins (that is, with a cabin altitude greater than 8000 feet, such as small military combat aircraft), personal oxygen equipment is worn routinely and used by the aircrew throughout flight.

General classes of oxygen systems

Oxygen delivery systems are classified initially into two major groups: those in which the expired gas is partially or completely rebreathed (closed-circuit systems), and those in which the expired gas is dispersed to the environment (open-circuit systems). Conventional aircraft, both military and civil, employ the latter almost exclusively.

Closed-circuit oxygen systems

Metabolic oxygen uptake, or the degree to which oxygen is taken up by the body from inspired gas, does not have to be complete at sea level to achieve adequate tissue oxygenation. Indeed, expired air at sea level still contains about 16% oxygen. Consequently, although the benefit declines with altitude, considerable savings in the rate of consumption of an oxygen supply can be achieved if expired air is rebreathed from a closed circuit after removal of carbon dioxide.

There are, however, at least three potentially serious disadvantages of such a system. The first is freezing: the expired, and frequently the inspired, gases in a closed circuit are saturated with water vapour, and so ice may occlude hoses and valves if cabin temperature falls below 0°C. The second disadvantage is accumulation of nitrogen: an in-board leakage of air as a result of, for example, an ill-fitting mask, may lead to a progressive increase in the concentration of nitrogen and eventually to hypoxia. The risk of freezing may be overcome by electrical heating of critical components, and a slight overpressure in the system (safety pressure) may be imposed to ensure that any leaks are outboard; but all of this adds to the complexity of the system. The third major disadvantage is the need to remove carbon dioxide: chemical absorbers, such as barium or lithium hydroxide, are heavy and have to be renewed frequently. Recently, however, carbon dioxide permeable membranes have been developed, and these may considerably reduce the bulk and inconvenience of the purification hardware.

Because of these problems, closed-circuit systems are used very infrequently in conventional aviation. They are, however, widely employed in anaesthetic, fire-fighting, and underwater breathing equipment. And, of course, in the manned spaceflight programmes the proven ability of man to survive during free-space or lunar-surface extra-vehicular activity, where the astronaut has to carry all his consumables with him, provides ample evidence of the great *advantages* of closed-circuit systems if sophisticated technology is allowed a free rein (*see* Chapter 32).

Open-circuit oxygen systems

Open-circuit oxygen systems are those in which most or all of the expired gas exhausts to the environment: they are the types that are most commonly encountered in aviation, and they are the types with which the remainder of this chapter is concerned.

Although relatively wasteful of breathing gas, an open-circuit system has the considerable merit, especially in military aviation, of simplicity. There are two main types of such systems: those in which oxygen flows from the supply source throughout the respiratory cycle (*continuous flow systems*), and those in which oxygen flows only during inspiration (*demand flow systems*). In both types, flow to the user from the source passes through a crucial component, the regulator, which essentially governs the delivery behaviour of the entire system. The major disadvantage of continuous flow systems is that the flow of gas from the regulator has to be

pre-set, and so does not vary in response to the respiratory demand of the user. This disadvantage is overcome in demand systems where the flow of gas from the regulator varies directly with inspiratory demand. Whilst a demand regulator is inherently more complex than one providing a continuous flow it can provide the additional automatic facilities required of oxygen equipment fitted to aircraft operating at high altitudes. Accordingly, most high-performance combat aircraft are equipped with open-circuit demand oxygen systems, as are the flight decks of commercial and military transport aircraft.

Physiological and general requirements of oxygen systems

Physiological requirements

The fundamental physiological requirements of an oxygen system were described in detail in the previous chapter, but may be summarized thus:

1. *Adequate oxygen (prevention of hypoxia)*—The alveolar oxygen tension should be maintained at about 103 mm Hg (13.7 kPa). This requirement can only be met at altitudes up to 33 000 feet and is achieved by a progressive increase in inspired oxygen concentration with ascent (airmix). Between 33 000 and 40 000 feet, even 100% oxygen will not prevent a progressive fall in alveolar oxygen tension with further ascent, whilst above 40 000 feet, positive pressure breathing of 100% is required. In certain circumstances, such as when military aircrew are pressure breathing or following loss of cabin pressurization in a military or passenger aircraft, these lower alveolar oxygen tensions are acceptable for short periods. Thus in the case of rapid decompression in a military aircraft, alveolar oxygen tensions of 30 mm Hg (4.0 kPa) may be acceptable (although not desirable) for a very short time provided that 100% oxygen is delivered within 2 seconds of the start of decompression; whilst alveolar oxygen tensions of 75 mm Hg (10.0 kPa) are acceptable for the flight-deck crew and cabin staff of a decompressed commercial aircraft, and tensions of 50 mm Hg (6.7 kPa) are acceptable for seated passengers.
2. *Adequate nitrogen*—Provided that the requirements of protection against hypoxia are not compromised, the inspired gas should contain not less than 40% nitrogen in order to avoid lung collapse on exposure to sustained +Gz acceleration, and delayed otic barotrauma (oxygen ear).
3. *Adequate ventilation and flow with minimal added external resistance*—Personal oxygen systems for use by aircrew should meet the

pressure/flow requirements defined by national and international specifications. Thus such a system should accommodate peak instantaneous flows of at least 2001 (ATPD)/min, with a maximum rate of change of 201 (ATPD)/s^2 at these peak flows; whilst the total change of pressure at the mouth and nose during a respiratory cycle with inspiratory and expiratory peaks of that magnitude should not exceed 30.5 cm water gauge (3.0 kPa). The system should also be capable of delivering a respiratory minute volume required of at least 601 (ATPD).

4. *Disposal of expired carbon dioxide*—The system, whether closed or open, must, respectively, either adequately and safely dispose of the expired carbon dioxide or disperse the entire expirate to ambient. To avoid significant rebreathing the effective additional dead space should be less than about 150 ml.

5. *Appropriate temperature*—The inspired gas should be neither too warm nor too cold for comfort, and its temperature should therefore be within 5°C of cockpit environmental temperature. In practice, no active method is used to achieve this requirement; reliance is placed upon equilibration of temperature during passage of the breathing gas through delivery pipework.

General requirements

Safety pressure

The system should maintain the desired alveolar oxygen tension even in the presence of potential inboard leakage as a result of an inadequate seal between the edge of the mask and the skin of the face. This requirement may be met by providing a slight but continuous overpressure in the mask (safety pressure) above altitudes of 12000–15000 feet, or by enrichment of the gas delivered to the mask.

Protection against toxic fumes and decompression sickness

The user must be able to select 100% oxygen manually at any cabin altitude in the event that toxic fumes or smoke contaminate the cockpit, and when decompression sickness is liable to develop or has done so. The method of delivery must be such as to minimize any inboard leakage of cabin air because of an ill-fitting mask.

Convenience

The operation of the system should as far as possible be automatic and, ideally, the user should only be

required to don a mask (or pressure helmet) and connect it to the remainder of the system. Similarly, facilities such as safety pressure and pressure breathing should be provided automatically. The drills to cope with failures of the system should be simple.

Evaluation of integrity

The equipment should be designed so that failure of the user to perform essential drills is made apparent immediately. For example, it should not be possible for the pilot of a combat aircraft to breathe through his mask until it has been connected, correctly, to the rest of the system; or for him to take off without having turned the oxygen supply on. One satisfactory means of achieving such a requirement is to ensure that inspiratory resistance through the mask is high until it is connected to the system and the oxygen supply is turned on.

The user must also be able to confirm the adequacy of the seal of his mask both before and during flight. This requirement is usually met by providing a manual means of selecting some degree of positive pressure breathing at any altitude (the press-to-test facility).

Indication of supply and flow

The user must have a display of the quantity of oxygen available to him and a positive indication of flow so that he can monitor the correct function of his oxygen system.

Indication of failure

In aircraft where the personal oxygen system provides the primary protection against hypoxia, any failure of the equipment that might lead to that condition must be indicated immediately and clearly to the user. Such warnings may be either objective, as for example in the illumination of a low-pressure warning light, or subjective, as in an increase in inspiratory resistance on inadvertent disconnection of a supply hose.

Duplication

In aircraft with low-differential pressure cabins, in which the personal oxygen system provides the primary protection against hypoxia, a degree of redundancy in the delivery system is essential. Thus many modern oxygen regulators have a secondary or stand-by operating mode which can be selected should the primary regulator fail. In addition, an alternative oxygen supply should be provided in case the main supply system fails or the store becomes depleted. Such an alternative usually takes the form of a small independent source of oxygen (the

Emergency Oxygen (EO)) together with an independent delivery regulator. The volume of oxygen contained in such an emergency supply is generally based on the assumption that failure of the main supply will be followed by selection of emergency oxygen *and* an immediate descent to below 10 000 feet.

There is no requirement for such a secondary oxygen supply in aircraft with high-differential pressure cabins, where the cabin itself provides the primary protection against hypoxia and oxygen equipment is used only if cabin pressurization fails, or if toxic fumes contaminate the cabin.

Protection during high-altitude escape

In military aircraft from which abandonment at high altitude is a possibility, a separate oxygen supply is needed to protect the escapee. Clearly, the equipment must be stowed on the man, in his parachute pack or on the seat itself, in the case of assisted escape systems in which the crew member does not separate from his ejection seat until a low altitude is reached (10 000–15 000 feet). The quantity of oxygen contained in this supply must be sufficient to prevent significant hypoxia during free-fall descent or until man–seat separation. In most military aircraft, the bail-out oxygen supply also serves as the secondary oxygen supply described above.

Independence from the environment

Oxygen equipment must perform satisfactorily under all the environmental extremes that may be met in flight. These include, *ipso facto*, pressure changes, and extremes of temperature, especially cold. With regard to the latter, the equipment must function normally after prolonged exposure to temperatures as low as $-26°C$ in an aircraft on the ground, and to the even lower temperatures likely after a serious failure of cabin pressurization at high altitude (down to $-55°C$). In combat aircraft, the mask or pressure helmet must not be displaced from the face or head by exposure to the maximum sustained accelerations (G forces) produced by the aircraft in normal flight, or by exposure to the accelerations and windblast (Q forces) associated with an escape sequence whilst flying at high speed. Furthermore, the mask valves must continue to function normally under such conditions.

Underwater breathing

Aircraft that ditch in water usually sink rapidly. Oxygen equipment is therefore frequently designed to provide breathing gas down to a certain depth (generally 30 m), and some air forces also require the bail-out oxygen supply to protect a man who has entered water after a parachute descent.

Economy of weight, bulk and cost

The weight and bulk (and cost) of military aircraft installations are critical logistic design features and so must be minimized within the constraints of safety. This is particularly so with regard to conventional oxygen storage systems. Clearly, therefore, physiological requirements should not be met at the expense of wastefully high flows of oxygen. For equally sound ground-logistic reasons, however, replenishment must not be necessary too often.

Oxygen equipment

Figure 7.1 lists the various general components of a typical oxygen system: this section describes each of these in turn.

Oxygen sources

Oxygen may be obtained from a store which is replenished whilst the aircraft is on the ground, or it may be produced as required in flight by some physico-chemical means. In storage it may exist as a gas under high pressure, as a liquid at low temperature under moderate pressure, or as a solid in inert chemical combination. Both gaseous and liquid oxygen stores are in common use in military aviation, whilst gaseous oxygen is the preferred medium for the emergency store on board commercial aircraft. Solid oxygen stores are also used in commercial aircraft, particularly as the emergency supply for passenger use in the event of loss of cabin pressurization. Finally, several methods of concentrating oxygen on board an aircraft, from an air source, have been actively investigated and one of these, the Molecular Sieve Oxygen Concentrator (MSOC), has been successfully installed in several modern combat aircraft.

For rechargeable systems, whatever the source of breathing oxygen, the quality of the gas to be supplied to the man must be of a certain high standard. It must contain at least 99.5% oxygen, be odourless and virtually free of any toxic substances; for example, the carbon monoxide concentration must be less than 0.002%. The maximum allowable levels for various hydrocarbons are specified in relation to the type of storage used since this will influence the potential contamination hazard. In order to avoid the risk of ice formation at low temperature, the stored oxygen must also be very dry: the water content must not exceed 0.005 mg/l at 0°C and 760 mm Hg (101.3 kPa) (that is, under STP conditions).

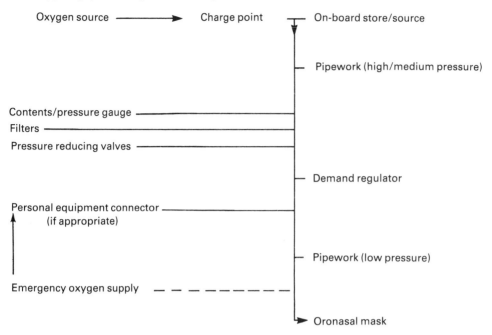

Figure 7.1 Generic components of typical oxygen systems.

Gaseous oxygen storage

Gaseous oxygen is usually carried in steel cylinders at a pressure of 1800 lb/in² (12 411 kPa); although a low-pressure (450 lb/in² (3103 kPa)) storage system is still employed in some aircraft, and a high-pressure (5000 lb/in² (34 475 kPa)) facility has been used in combat aircraft in an attempt to overcome some of the disadvantages of liquid oxygen. The capacities of cylinders commonly used in aircraft vary between 400 and 2250 l (NTP) of oxygen when fully charged to 1800 lb/in² (12 411 kPa).

The aircraft cylinders are charged from large trolley-mounted cylinders, filled with oxygen at a maximum pressure of 3600 lb/in² (24 822 kPa), through a connection, fitted with a sealing cap and an on/off valve, mounted at or just beneath the outer skin of the aircraft. The pressure and flow of gas into the aircraft system is controlled by a regulating device on the charging trolley, whilst the quantity of oxygen on board is indicated by a cockpit pressure gauge connected to the main high-pressure supply pipework. A duplicate pressure gauge is often fitted at the charging point, and both gauges are usually graduated in fractions of Full. The pressure in a gaseous oxygen storage system should not normally be allowed to fall to the ambient level in order to prevent moisture entering the system. The risk of water collecting in storage cylinders is also reduced by regular purging of the entire system, including pipework, with dry gas.

The size and number of cylinders installed, usually outside the pressure cabin, will clearly depend upon the type of aircraft and its flight endurance. In military aircraft, the cylinders are frequently wire-wound to minimize fragmentation should they be punctured. The pipework connecting the cylinders to the delivery system is usually duplicated and, where two or more cylinders are installed, contains non-return valves arranged in such a way that a leak from one cylinder or junction will lead to only a partial loss of oxygen.

Gaseous oxygen storage systems have several clear advantages: they are relatively simple in construction, gaseous oxygen is readily available worldwide, the onboard supply is available for use immediately after charging, and no gas is lost when the system is not in use. The major disadvantage is

Table 7.1 Comparison of typical weights and overall volumes of oxygen storage/supply systems of various types. The figures for gaseous, liquid and solid chemical sources are for systems each yielding 3000 l (NTP) of oxygen: yield figures for molecular sieve systems are not applicable

Storage system	Weight of charged system (kg)	Space occupied by system (l)
High-pressure cylinders containing gas at 1800 lb/in²	19	52
Liquid oxygen converter containing 3.5 l of liquid	8	25
Solid chemical generator containing sodium chlorate	12	10
Molecular sieve oxygen concentrator	19	20

that they are heavy and bulky, and *Table 7.1* illustrates this by comparing typical weights and overall volumes of different types of oxygen storage system.

Despite these logistic penalties, however, gaseous oxygen storage is the system of choice when weight and bulk are not at a great premium, or if the supply is intended only for use in an emergency (and is consequently relatively small). Thus gaseous oxygen storage is commonly used as the emergency supply for the crew and passengers on large transport aircraft, and as the emergency and bail-out supplies in combat aircraft. In addition, portable and therapeutic systems are generally supplied from a small gaseous oxygen storage cylinder.

Liquid oxygen storage

Liquid oxygen (LOX) vaporizes at −183°C, at normal atmospheric pressure, to yield 840 l (NTP) of gaseous oxygen for each litre of liquid oxygen: an expansion ratio almost seven times greater than that for gaseous oxygen stored at 1800 lb/in² (12411 kPa). In addition, the low pressure at which liquid oxygen can be held in its insulated container (typically at 70–115 lb/in² (483–793 kPa)) markedly

reduces the overall weight of liquid oxygen storage devices when compared with gaseous oxygen cylinders (*see Table 7.1*).

An aircraft liquid oxygen converter consists of an insulated container, control valves and connecting pipes (*Figure 7.2*). The converter may be permanently installed in the aircraft or it may be removable, so that there is a choice of either replacement or recharging *in situ*. The liquid oxygen is contained in a double-walled, stainless steel vessel with connections through its walls at top and bottom. The capacity of vessel varies according to the total amount of gaseous oxygen required during flight, but will typically be 3.5, 5.0, 10.0 or 25.0 l. The space between the vessel walls is evacuated to reduce convective and conductive heat transfer to the liquid oxygen to a minimum. Operation of a liquid oxygen converter takes place in three distinct phases, as illustrated in *Figure 7.3*.

1. *Filling phase (Figure 7.3(a))*—The filling inlet of the converter leads, via combined fill-and-vent valves, to the bottom of the container. Connection of the charging hose from the ground liquid-oxygen dispenser opens the fill-and-vent valves, so opening the top of the container to ambient. Gas and liquid can therefore flow freely

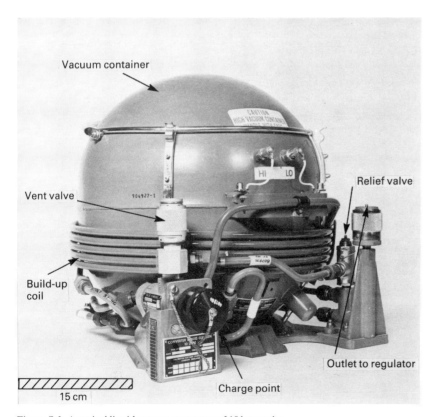

Figure 7.2 A typical liquid oxygen converter of 10 l capacity.

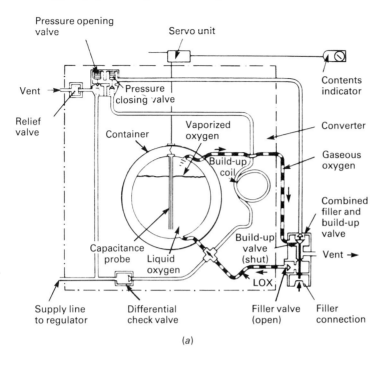

(a)

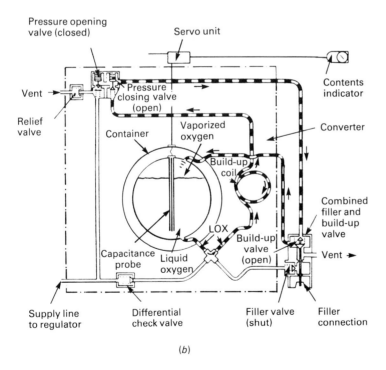

(b)

Figure 7.3 Layout and mode of operation of a typical liquid oxygen system: for details, *see* text. (*a*) Filling phase. (*b*) Pressure build-up phase.

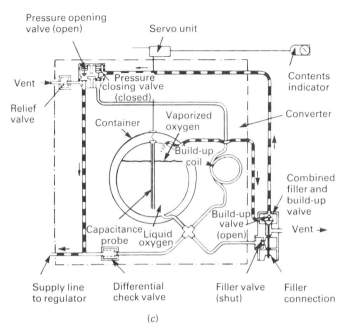

Figure 7.3 (c) Delivery phase.

into the container at the bottom and out again, once full, at the top. As liquid oxygen passes along the charging hose and into the container it evaporates and eventually cools the internal walls of the system to $-183°C$. The liquid then ceases to evaporate and the container rapidly fills with liquid oxygen.

2. *Build-up phase (Figure 7.3(b))*—When the charging hose is disconnected, the fill-and-vent valves close. The top and bottom of the container are then connected via a length of uninsulated pipe, the pressure build-up coil, and a pressure closing valve. Liquid oxygen is now able to flow *from* the bottom of the container into the pressure build-up coil, where it evaporates, and thence into the top of the vessel as a gas. The heat carried in by the gas warms the surface layer of the liquid so that its vapour pressure rises. This process continues until the pressure within the container reaches the operating pressure of the converter (that is, $70–115\,lb/in^2$ (483–793 kPa)). At this point, the pressure closing valve shuts and the flow of liquid oxygen into the pressure build-up coil ceases.

3. *Delivery (Figure 7.3(c))*—When a demand is made upon the system, gas is drawn from the top of the container, via a pressure opening valve, to the delivery supply line and so to the user. Should the demand be so great as to cause the pressure within the container to fall below its level, the pressure closing valve opens once more

to allow liquid into the pressure build-up coil, where it evaporates and carries gas and heat back to the top of the vessel so restoring the operating pressure. In this type of converter, liquid oxygen will only flow from the bottom of the container to the user via the differential check valve when the pressure level in the delivery line falls below a pre-set value. (In other forms of converter, however, gaseous demand by the user is met directly by a flow of liquid from the base of the unit into an evaporating line.)

The insulation of a liquid oxygen converter is never absolute, so that its temperature and hence the pressure of its contents slowly rise. A relief valve is fitted to limit this pressure rise, and this opens at $20–30\,lb/in^2$ (138–207 kPa) above normal operating pressure. Such a pressure is usually attained 10–12 hours after filling, and thereafter up to 10% of the liquid is lost in a 24-hour period.

The amount of liquid oxygen in the vessel is monitored continuously by means of a probe, immersed in the liquid and gaseous oxygen mixture, which measures the electrical capacitance between the two containing shells. The output of this capacitance probe is displayed in the cockpit and at the charging point for use during *in situ* refilling. The pressure at which gaseous oxygen is delivered to the main supply line is usually also displayed to the crew, or there may be a low-pressure warning device.

One major disadvantage of the simple converter described above is that any agitation of the vessel within 6–8 hours of filling will produce a gross fall in delivery pressure as a result of a phenomenon termed *temperature stratification*. The agitation, which may be caused by the vibration of aerobatic manoeuvres or even while taxiing, disturbs the warm layer of liquid at the liquid/gas interface so bringing colder layers of liquid into contact with the gas which then condenses. Pressure consequently falls in the gaseous phase. This drawback may be overcome by adding sufficient heat to the contents of the container immediately after filling to raise the temperature of the liquid to that at which its vapour pressure equals its normal operating pressure: for liquid oxygen with a vapour pressure of 85 lb/in^2 abs (586 kPa), for example, the appropriate temperature would be $-160°C$. The contents of the container are then said to be *stabilized*. The heat required for this stabilization is derived from the evaporation of liquid oxygen delivered to a separate, uninsulated, container during the charging process. As soon as filling is complete, this liquid boils and the gas bubbles up through the liquid in the main container, condenses in so doing and heats all the liquid in the vessel to the required temperature thus eliminating the temperature stratification. Stabilized liquid oxygen converters are installed mainly in combat aircraft.

Liquid oxygen storage systems have two other distinct disadvantages, one of which is real and one of which is potential. Firstly, they are expensive in terms of the quantity of oxygen lost during the various transfer stages from the manufacturing plant to the dispensing containers, and from the dispensing containers to the aircraft; less than one eighth of the liquid produced by a plant reaches an aircraft converter. Further losses inevitably occur from the filled converter as a result of the inherent heat transfer into the vessel, so that frequent recharging is necessary. Secondly, liquid oxygen is potentially at risk from contamination by toxic materials; most commonly the oxides of nitrogen, carbon monoxide, carbon dioxide, hydrogen sulphide, trichloroethylene and hydrocarbons such as methane, ethane, ethylene and acetylene. Such contamination is derived from the atmospheric air from which the liquid oxygen is produced, from plant compression and refrigeration equipment, and from storage, transport and other handling equipment. These contaminants do not evaporate at the same time as liquid oxygen since they usually have higher boiling points, and so can accumulate in the container. Eventually, particles or 'slugs' of contaminant may pass from the vessel into the warming coils where they evaporate and may then be breathed by the user in relatively high concentrations. Great care must therefore be taken to eliminate the entry of contaminants during the manufacture and transfer

of liquid oxygen; and, once in an aircraft converter, control must be exercised to ensure that the concentration of any contaminant remains very low: routine infra-red spectroscopy during ground replenishment is the method employed to achieve this.

All of these considerable disadvantages make liquid oxygen the storage method of choice only when the weight and bulk of the oxygen container must be as small as possible, and when oxygen is used routinely throughout flight, as in combat fighter aircraft. An additional benefit of the use of liquid oxygen converters in this role is that the container, essentially a vacuum flask, is unlikely to explode if punctured by enemy action.

Solid chemical storage

When a mixture of sodium chlorate and finely divided iron is ignited, a proportion of the oxygen contained in the sodium chlorate molecule is released as gaseous oxygen; the reaction proceeding according to the equation:

$$NaClO_3 + Fe \rightarrow FeO + NaCl + O_2$$

The reaction is exothermic so that, once the temperature of the reactants has been raised above 250°C, it is self-generating. The proportion of iron in the mixture controls the temperature, speed of reaction and oxygen yield. The sodium chlorate and iron powder are usually cast or pressed together with an inorganic binder, such as fibre-glass, into a cylindrical mass termed a *candle*. The heat required to initiate the reaction is provided by a small iron-enriched zone at one end of the candle which is activated by a percussion cap, an electric squib, a friction lighter or an electrically heated wire. The reaction proceeds at a temperature of 250–600°C over the cross-sectional area of the candle, and oxygen is produced at a rate that is influenced both by the size of this area and by the degree of insulation of the device. Thus the desired oxygen flow-time relationship can be obtained by shaping the candle. Free chlorine, carbon monoxide and carbon dioxide may all contaminate oxygen produced in this manner, but the inclusion of a small percentage of barium peroxide neutralizes these substances so that the purity of oxygen produced by a candle made of a sodium chlorate/iron/barium peroxide mixture approaches 99.9% with no significant concentration of toxic contaminants.

A sodium chlorate candle, once ignited, provides a continous flow of pure oxygen and is not easily extinguished. This form of oxygen storage is therefore most appropriate for use in situations where a constant flow of oxygen is required for a specified period such as, for example, in emergency oxygen supplies for aircraft passengers. In such cases, the cylindrical candle, with a suitable igniting mechanism fitted to one end, is enclosed in a gas-tight container within a thermally insulated shroud. A unit designed to provide oxygen for ten passengers for 30 minutes (that is, a total oxygen supply of 1300 l (NTP) would be 22 cm in length, 15 cm in diameter, and weigh 5.5 kg (*see also Table 7.1*).

The advantages of this form of oxygen storage include its simplicity (since oxygen can be delivered without the need for reducing valves or regulators), its almost unlimited shelf-life, its relatively small bulk, and the absence of a need for routine servicing. The sodium chlorate candle is also inert at temperatures below 250°C, even under severe impact loads, and so its use is associated with a relatively low fire risk. Once initiated, however, oxygen delivery continues unabated and although it is possible to devise a means whereby a solid system can be used to supply oxygen on demand (by the use of multiple candles and a reservoir), the complexity, weight and bulk of such an arrangement make it unsuitable for use as the primary supply in combat aircraft. Feasibility studies into solid storage systems for use as emergency oxygen stores are being actively pursued.

Onboard oxygen production

The need to replenish the oxygen store of an aircraft imposes considerable operational and logistic penalties on both military and civil aviation. There are also significant fire hazards associated with the production and replenishment of oxygen, especially during military operations. Because of these disadvantages, the onboard production of oxygen is obviously desirable, and several methods of so doing have been explored with varying degrees of success. Virtually all such oxygen systems are driven from a supply of compressed air (usually taken from an engine compressor stage), and require electrical power. Methods of onboard oxygen production include the following.

Electrolysis of water

A prototype system which produced oxygen by the electrolysis of water has been installed in an aircraft and flown, but the purity of the water required, the susceptibility of the electrolysis cell to damage, and the high power consumption needed were such serious disadvantages that the system was not developed any further.

Reversed fuel cell

The normal processes whereby electricity is generated as the energy released when hydrogen and oxygen combine may be reversed by supplying electrical power to a fuel cell. In this so-called 'reversed fuel cell' oxygen is produced at the anode and hydrogen at the cathode. Hydrogen is then oxidized to water by combination with oxygen in the air flowing over the cathode. A reversed fuel cell capable of providing 26 l (NTP)/min of oxygen at 300–400 lb/in² (2068–2758 kPa) would require a supply of clean moist air at 25 lb/in² (172 kPa), would consume about 7 kW of electrical power, and would weigh about 30 kg. A power requirement of this magnitude makes such a system operationally impractical.

The requirement for 26 l (NTP)/min is a perpetuation of the United States specification for a two-man crew, each with a nominal minute ventilation of 13 l (NTP), and based on observations made in the 1940s. Although still used for engineering design purposes, the requirement has little physiological justification in the light of modern knowledge (*see* Chapter 6).

Absorption–desorption processes

Several systems have employed an oxygen absorption–desorption process to extract this gas from compressed air. In such systems, air is passed over a bed of absorbent, which may be heated, at a pressure of about 25 lb/in² (172 kPa). After a time interval, the airflow is stopped and the oxygen which had been absorbed by the bed is recovered by reducing the pressure to a partial vacuum. In practice, two beds of the absorbing material are used alternately to provide a continuous supply of oxygen. Two main chemical absorbents have been investigated for this type of onboard production of oxygen: barium oxide, and fluomine (a synthetic chelate of cobalt). A fluomine system which produces 26 l (NTP)/min of oxygen continuously requires about 1 kW of electrical power and weighs about 50 kg. The oxygen obtained by this type of process is at low pressure and so must be compressed before it can be fed to the breathing regulator. Despite this significant disadvantage, however, a fluomine system was successfully installed in the prototype Rockwell B1 bomber of the United States Air Force. Further evolution of absorption–desorption processes, and indeed of all other onboard oxygen production systems, has now been overtaken by the development of molecular sieve technology.

Molecular sieve oxygen concentration systems (MSOCS)

An alternative method of obtaining a breathing gas containing a high concentration of oxygen is to employ a molecular sieve which adsorbs nitrogen.

Molecular sieves are alkali metal alumino-silicates of the crystalline zeolite family. They consist essentially of very regular tetrahedral structures of

SiO_4 and AlO_4 linked by cations of sodium or calcium to form cages or cavities which are normally filled by water molecules. The size of the cage entrances and cavities varies according to the precise chemical structure of the zeolite. When the sieve material is heated, the water molecules are driven off to leave an open structure with the affinity to adsorb polar molecules. The adsorption of a substance depends not only upon its degree of polarity, but also upon its molecular size: clearly, if the molecule is too large to enter the cage it cannot be adsorbed. The two most common types of sieve material in use at present are the so-called 5A and 13X. The former has some of its sodium atoms replaced by calcium, and this results in a smaller cage entrance ($4.9 \times 10^{-4}\,\mu m$) than that of the 13X material ($1.0 \times 10^{-3}\,\mu m$).

The adsorption process is an exothermic reaction, and is dependent upon both pressure and temperature. An increase in pressure generally enhances adsorption while an increase in temperature causes a decrease. In molecular sieve oxygen concentrating devices, the oxygen and nitrogen are separated by virtue of the fact that nitrogen, despite its slightly larger molecular size, is held more strongly within the sieve cage than oxygen. The cage structure, especially when pressurized, induces a quadrupole moment in the nitrogen molecule so enhancing its adsorption energy and producing an oxygen-rich and argon-rich gas phase around the sieve. Since argon also passes through the sieve, the product gas in such a system contains a maximum of about 94% oxygen: the remainder is argon. By using a pressure-swing technique, whereby the molecular sieve bed is alternately pressurized and depressurized, complete separation can be achieved. Furthermore, the adsorption of nitrogen is reversible and the bed can be purged of the gas during the depressurized phase. The adsorption of more polar

molecules such as water (when in contact with the sieve material for some time) is irreversible, however, and so water contamination will deactivate a molecular sieve.

An oxygen concentrator of this type usually consists of two or more beds of molecular sieve through each of which, in turn, compressed air from an engine bleed source is passed. Thus in the two-bed system illustrated in *Figure 7.4*, one bed is depressurized and purged of its nitrogen (by means of a bleed flow of product gas from the pressurized bed) in readiness for oxygen concentration during its next pressurized phase, while the other bed is producing oxygen-enriched breathing gas. The supply is therefore continuous, although any small fluctuations in delivery pressure are minimized by the presence of a plenum chamber.

A two-bed molecular sieve oxygen concentrator, capable of supplying the breathing requirements of a single pilot, weighs about 19 kg, consumes about 50 W of 28 V d.c. electrical power, and occupies a volume of about 20 l which is less than that of a 3.5 l liquid oxygen converter. Such a device therefore represents an extremely attractive alternative to the liquid oxygen storage devices in common use; and indeed several modern fighter aircraft have had molecular sieves, such as that illustrated in *Figure 7.5*, installed successfully for routine use.

The principal disadvantage of this form of oxygen production is that a failure of engine bleed air supply, as for example during an engine flameout, will clearly result in a failure of the molecular sieve to produce oxygen. This drawback can be overcome by the provision of a small gaseous back-up store of oxygen which can be selected automatically if engine power is lost. Such a back-up supply is also required to provide an immediate source of 100% oxygen to prevent hypoxia following decompression of the cabin to an altitude above 30 000 feet as the speed of

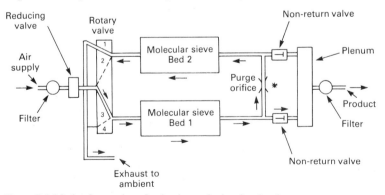

Figure 7.4 Mode of operation of a simple two-bed molecular sieve oxygen concentrator. In this schematic, molecular sieve bed 1 is being pressurized, via line 3, and delivering oxygen-rich product gas to the plenum before passing to the user. A large bleed flow of product gas is diverted to purge nitrogen from molecular sieve bed 2, via orifice * and line 1, in readiness for that bed's pressurization via line 2, when the control valve rotates. Line 4 then becomes the purge route from bed 1 via orifice * .

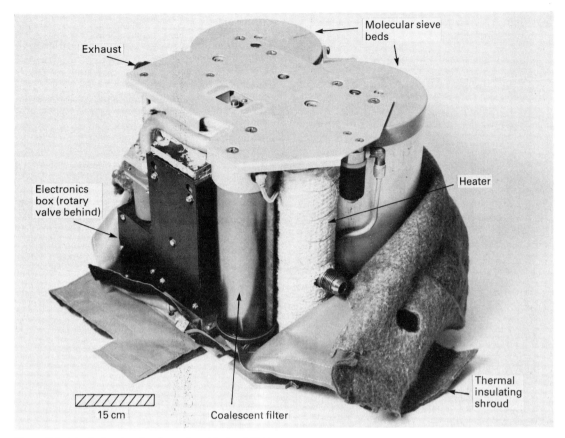

Figure 7.5 A typical molecular sieve oxygen concentrator.

response of the sieve is inadequate in these circumstances. And the same gaseous store, if mounted on the ejection seat, can be used to supply the crew if it becomes necessary to eject from the aircraft at high altitude. In contrast to this potential *lack* of oxygen, a concentration of 94% is too rich for routine flight: thus it is also necessary to provide a means of reducing the concentration of oxygen in the product gas. One way in which this can be achieved is by exploiting another characteristic of molecular sieve behaviour: that is, the concentration of oxygen in the product gas is reduced if the flow demanded through the system is increased. It is preferable, however, to control the concentration of oxygen by varying the operating conditions of the concentrator itself: for example, by adjusting the pressurization cycle time.

The logistic advantages of a molecular sieve oxygen concentrator clearly outweigh any disadvantages, however, and can be summarized thus:

1. Reduction of equipment and manpower costs by eliminating ground manufacture, transport and storage of oxygen.

2. Further reduction of manpower costs and speedier, safer turn around of aircraft by eliminating the need for ground replenishment of the oxygen store.
3. Reduction in frequency of routine maintenance of the oxygen system, as a result of an increase in overall reliability.

Continuous flow delivery systems

From whatever source the breathing gas is derived, the simplest way that it can be delivered to the user is by a continuous flow system, whether by direct flow or via some form of rebreathing or non-breathing reservoir. Although continuous flow systems have advantages in that the accurate prediction of oxygen consumption is possible, and the resistance imposed to breathing is relatively low, direct flow systems are extremely wasteful of breathing gas. Adding a reservoir between the flow regulator and the mask, however, decreases the rate of consumption of the aircraft oxygen store by 50–70%.

Direct flow systems

The most elementary form of continuous flow oxygen system consists of an oxygen store, a regulating device which delivers a continuous flow of oxygen, a flexible delivery hose, and a nasal or oronasal mask. The mask has apertures, which may be valved, through which air can be drawn into the lungs when the demanded inspiratory flow exceeds the flow of oxygen from the system. The same apertures allow expired gas to be expelled to the environment.

This form of oxygen system is very inefficient since oxygen flowing into the mask during expiration, which occupies 50–60% of the total respiratory cycle time, does not enter the respiratory tract at all. Even during inspiration, oxygen flowing into the mask will only enter the lungs when the instantaneous inspiratory flow equals or exceeds the oxygen flow. To ensure that no air is inspired, therefore, the oxygen flow must exceed the maximum inspiratory flow, which is usually about 2–3 times the respiratory minute volume and increases to about 10 times during speech.

Despite their inefficiency, direct flow systems are very simple and are widely used to provide bail-out and emergency oxygen in combat aircraft. A typical oxygen system of this type consists of a small cylinder containing about 50 l (NTP) of gaseous oxygen stored at $1800 \, lb/in^2$ (12 411 kPa), a contents gauge, an on/off valve, a metering orifice, and a delivery pipe to the inlet hose of the mask. The cylinder is turned on manually if the main oxygen supply fails in flight, or automatically during escape at high altitudes. When the cylinder is full, the system generally delivers an oxygen flow of 10–14 l (NTP)/min, expanding to 34–48 l (BTPS)/min at 25 000 feet. To provide inward relief, the connection between the main oxygen supply and the mask hose is usually broken when the emergency flow is initiated. Air is then able to enter the mask whenever the inspiratory demand exceeds the flow of oxygen. Furthermore, if the mask is fitted with a non-return inspiratory valve and a compensated expiratory valve (*see* Oxygen Masks, below), the continuous flow of oxygen into the mask hose will prevent expiration unless it is allowed to vent to the environment during that phase. Consequently, a pressure relief valve is incorporated into the mask hose assembly of this type of mask. It is possible to set the pressure at which the relief valve operates to a high enough value to allow the provision of pressure breathing. In some systems, the excess pressure relief valve is combined with a spring-loaded inlet warning valve so that inadvertent disconnection of the mask hose from the main supply, in the absence of an emergency flow, will be indicated subjectively to the user by an increase in the resistance to inspiration.

Rebreathing reservoir systems

The efficiency of a continuous flow oxygen system is greatly enhanced by incorporating a reservoir between the regulating device and the inlet port of the mask. In *rebreathing* reservoir systems, a flexible reservoir is placed in direct communication with the cavity of the mask, as shown in *Figure 7.6*. The addition of a reservoir ensures that all the oxygen flowing from the regulating device enters the respiratory tract during inspiration provided that, as with direct continuous flow systems, pulmonary ventilation equals or exceeds the flow of oxygen.

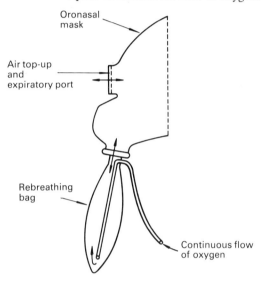

Oronasal mask

Air top-up and expiratory port

Rebreathing bag

Continuous flow of oxygen

Figure 7.6 A simple rebreathing reservoir oxygen mask. Oxygen passes at a constant flow into the distal end of the rebreathing bag. The first portion of the expirate fills the bag whilst the remainder flows out through the expiratory port. The contents of the bag pass into the respiratory tract at the beginning of inspiration to be followed by the continuous flow of oxygen supplemented with air drawn in through the air inlet (top-up) port.

In this type of system, oxygen is delivered continuously from the regulating device into the reservoir bag. The mask usually has a single aperture, which may not be valved, through which air may be drawn into the mask if inspiratory demand exceeds the capacity of the reservoir. Excess oxygen and expired gas are expelled from the mask through the same aperture, which has a resistance to flow deliberately made greater than that acting against flow from the reservoir. Thus the contents of the latter enter the respiratory tract at the beginning of each inspiration before any air is drawn in. Similarly, during expiration, the first part of the expirate passes into the reservoir, and only when this is full is expired gas expelled to the environment. In addition, oxygen flow into the reservoir bag is directed to that part which is furthest from the mask cavity so that oxygen entering the reservoir during expiration displaces any previously expired gas. At the levels of oxygen flow employed, the volume of oxygen that enters the reservoir during expiration is less than the volume of the reservoir, so that a part of the previously expired gas is re-inspired. The gas that is rebreathed clearly includes that which was held in the respiratory dead space during the previous inspiration, and so has a higher oxygen tension and lower carbon dioxide tension than the alveolar gas. Rebreathing using this type of system increases oxygen economy but at the expense of an increase in the effective respiratory dead space.

Rebreathing reservoir continuous flow oxygen equipment was used extensively in American combat aircraft during the early 1940s but its use has several serious disadvantages. These disadvantages are:

1. The system cannot respond to changes in pulmonary ventilation and so, at the flows usually employed, can provide satisfactory alveolar oxygen tensions (and good oxygen economy) only at rest.
2. There is no means of indicating that oxygen is entering the mask.
3. The system cannot integrate conveniently with pressure breathing and pressure suit systems.
4. The need to mount the rebreathing bag on the mask precludes the use of a large reservoir.
5. A poorly fitting mask can destroy the action of the reservoir so that the user receives only the oxygen delivered to the mask during inspiration.
6. Rebreathing introduces moist gas to the reservoir, and so markedly increases the susceptibility of the equipment to freezing: indeed, the minimum environmental temperature at which such systems can be used is about −5°C.

Because of all these drawbacks, rebreathing reservoir oxygen equipment is now used mainly for the administration of oxygen to patients in flight, and to prevent hypoxia following loss of cabin pressurization in transport aircraft. The oxygen flow supplied to this type of equipment is increased from about 2.0 l (NTP)/min at a cabin altitude of 20 000 feet to about 4.5 l (NTP)/min at 40 000 feet; a volume that is adequate to prevent serious hypoxia developing in a seated passenger. Finally, it is assumed that a decompression is very unlikely to be so severe that the cabin temperature cannot be maintained above 0°C: the impaired performance of the system below −5°C is therefore of no consequence.

Non-rebreathing reservoir systems

In non-rebreathing reservoir systems, a non-return valve is placed between the reservoir and the cavity of the mask, so that expired gas cannot enter the reservoir. As in rebreathing systems, the mask has apertures, which may or may not be valved, through which air may be drawn into the respiratory tract, to augment the oxygen supply and expired gas may be expelled to the environment. To ensure that air is not drawn into the lungs until the oxygen reservoir has been emptied, the reduction in mask pressure required to draw air through the air-inlet aperture must again be greater than that required to empty the reservoir. The correct phasing of oxygen and air delivery during inspiration is usually accomplished by a combination of a very low resistance non-return valve placed between the reservoir and the mask, and a spring-loaded, higher resistance air-inlet valve placed in the mask itself.

Although the reservoir may consist of a flexible rubber bag attached directly to the inlet of the mask, the size required makes it more convenient to mount the bag away from the mask. Alternatively, a length of hose attached to the inlet port of the mask can be used as the reservoir. In this arrangement oxygen is delivered into the hose at a point close to the inlet port, so that the hose is filled in the reverse direction to inspiratory flow, and the air-inlet is placed at the opposite end of the reservoir hose to the mask. This configuration ensures that oxygen in the hose is drawn into the mask before air. The most successful non-rebreathing reservoir system employed in military aviation, however, is the RAF economizer system shown diagrammatically in *Figure 7.7*.

The flow of oxygen in this system is controlled by a regulating device which incorporates an on/off valve, a reducing valve, and two or more metering orifices. Flow bobbins indicate that oxygen is passing through the regulator to the economizer (reservoir) itself. An oxygen flow of 3.4–4.6 l (NTP)/min suffices for seated aircrew at cabin altitudes up to 30 000 feet; but this is increased automatically to 5.1–7.4 l (NTP)/min when at higher cabin altitudes, and when moving around the aircraft at all altitudes. The oxygen economizer is a flexible bag with a maximum capacity of 600 ml and fitted with a lightly spring-loaded outlet valve. An external, spring-loaded plate maintains a slight pressure in the reservoir so that when the outlet valve opens because the bag is full, or when inspiration commences, oxygen is delivered to the mask at a low (5–15 mm water gauge (mm wg) (0.07–0.15 kPa)) positive pressure. The outlet of the economizer is connected to the inlet port of the mask via wide-bore flexible hose. The mask itself is fitted with a spring-loaded air-inlet valve which opens when the mask cavity pressure is 15 mm wg (0.15 kPa) below that of the environment. Two small non-return expiratory valves complete the mask ensemble. The design of the economizer and of the mask air-inlet valve, which together ensure that oxygen is delivered at the beginning of

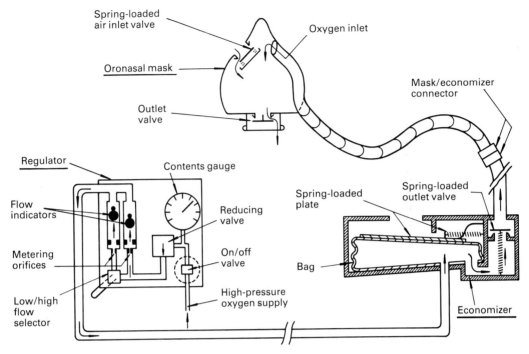

Figure 7.7 The Royal Air Force economizer system. The simple regulator consists of a pressure-reducing valve and a pair of metering orifices which pass oxygen at the selected flow into the flexible bag of the economizer itself. Here the gas is stored until the suction in the oronasal mask, produced at the onset of inspiration, opens the spring outlet valve of the econimizer. Oxygen is then driven into the mask from the economizer bag, under the influence of a spring-loaded plate, at a slight positive pressure. When inspiratory demand exceeds the oxygen flow from the economizer, air from the cabin is drawn through the spring-loaded air inlet valve in the mask.

inspiration with no admixture of air and at a pressure slightly above that of the environment (safety pressure), overcomes one of the serious disadvantages of simpler reservoir systems in which the leak produced by an ill-fitting mask can result in a failure of the reservoir to fill and hence to the development of severe hypoxia at altitude. Several other disadvantages remain, however, and these include:

1. The inability to respond to changes in pulmonary ventilation so that the flow of oxygen has to be set to ensure that alveolar oxygen tension is adequate at the maximum minute ventilation likely to occur in flight.
2. The lack of any indication that oxygen is entering the mask.
3. The inability to accommodate pressure breathing requirements so that the maximum altitude to which the system can be employed is 40000–43000 feet.

Although widely used during the 1940s, non-rebreathing continuous flow systems are now rare. They are of considerable historic importance, however, as an evolutionary step towards current oxygen delivery systems which incorporate demand flow.

Demand flow delivery systems

All of the disadvantages of continuous flow delivery systems are overcome by systems in which the flow of gas from the regulator varies directly with the inspiratory demand of the user. In such systems, it is also possible to provide many of the additional automatic and manual facilities listed earlier, including air dilution, safety pressure, pressure breathing and an indication of flow. The key component in demand oxygen systems is the regulator, although the integration with it of the downstream delivery pipework and the oronasal mask is crucial. A regulator that is capable of delivering gas at increased pressure (that is, of delivering safety pressure and pressure breathing) is termed a *pressure demand oxygen regulator*.

Demand regulators

The principles underlying the design and function of a demand regulator are essentially the same whether the device is panel mounted, seat mounted or man mounted: all are designed to fulfil a number of automatic and manual functions, which include the following.

Breathing gas on demand

In a demand system, the flow of gas from the high-pressure source is controlled by the fluctuations in mask cavity pressure induced by respiration. To achieve this, the regulator is divided into two chambers by a flexible control diaphragm, as shown in *Figure 7.8*. On one side of the diaphragm, the (demand) chamber receives the high-pressure supply from the aircraft oxygen source and also communicates with the user via a delivery hose and the mask, whilst the (reference) chamber on the other side of the diaphragm is open to the environmental pressure of the cockpit.

The pressure changes of respiration are transmitted to the demand chamber where they displace the flexible diaphragm. By means of a connecting lever and pivot, the position of the diaphragm controls the degree of opening of the (demand) valve through which gas from the oxygen source flows into the demand chamber and thence to the user. Thus the reduction of pressure in the mask cavity and in the demand chamber produced by the initiation of inspiration displaces the diaphragm into the chamber and opens the demand valve. The greater the inspiratory demand, the greater will be the reduction in mask cavity pressure transmitted to the demand chamber, and the further will the demand valve open so increasing the flow of gas to the mask. When inspiration ceases, mask cavity pressure increases and so too does pressure in the demand chamber. The diaphragm is restored to its resting position, the demand valve closes and flow of gas to the mask stops. The engineering design of such a regulator is such that flow of gas through the demand valve is equal to the instantaneous inspiratory flow.

The forces needed to open the demand valve are such that a regulator which employs a mechanical link between the control diaphragm and the valve requires the diaphragm to be relatively large if the resistance to inspiration is to be kept within acceptable limits. This type of regulator has therefore to be large enough to accommodate a diaphragm which is typically 8–10 cm in diameter. Alternatively, and especially in modern regulators, the link between the demand valve and the control diaphragm is pneumatic. In this case, the opening of a flexible demand valve is controlled by gas pressure applied to the side of the valve opposite to that exposed to the high-pressure supply line: *see Figure 7.9.*

The controlling pressure is itself determined by a second, pilot, valve the opening of which is governed by a mechanical link to the control diaphragm. As before, movement of the control diaphragm is influenced by the pressure transmitted from the mask cavity to the demand chamber of the regulator. The great advantage of such *servo-controlled* demand regulators is the magnification of the control signal made possible by the pneumatic link. Hence the size of the control diaphragm can be markedly reduced, and the diameter of the control diaphragm in a typical servo-controlled regulator is only 2–3 cm. Furthermore, safety pressure and pressure breathing facilities can be provided by gas loading the control diaphragm; and all of these pneumatic control systems enable the size of the regulator to be reduced significantly.

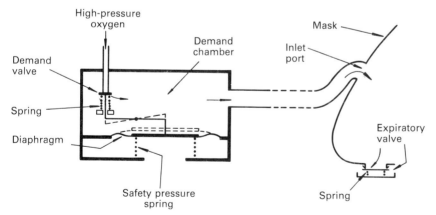

Figure 7.8 Mode of operation of a simple demand oxygen regulator and oronasal mask system. The flow of oxygen to the mask from the high-pressure supply is controlled by the demand valve, which is held in the closed position by the demand valve spring. The reduction in pressure (produced by inspiration) within the mask, the mask hose, and the regulator demand chamber displaces the control diaphragm and opens the demand valve. The rise in mask pressure when inspiration ceases allows the control diaphragm to return to its resting position and the demand valve to close. Biasing the control diaphragm by means of a safety pressure spring raises the mask pressure above that of the environment. The expiratory valve must also be biased (for example, by spring-loading) in order to hold safety pressure in the mask.

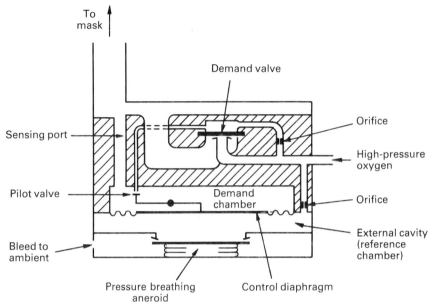

To mask

Demand valve

Orifice

Sensing port

High-pressure oxygen

Pilot valve

Demand chamber

Orifice

Bleed to ambient

External cavity (reference chamber)

Pressure breathing aneroid

Control diaphragm

Figure 7.9 Mode of operation of a typical servo-controlled miniature pressure-demand regulator. The flexible demand valve is held closed by the inlet pressure applied to its rear surface. The suction created by inspiration reduces the pressure within the demand chamber and opens the pilot valve. This allows the reduction in pressure to be transmitted to the back of the demand valve which therefore opens and allows oxygen to flow through it to the mask. Pressure breathing is produced by increasing the pressure within the reference chamber so that the control diaphragm is loaded. This is achieved by an aneroid capsule which progressively increases the resistance to flow to the environment of a small bleed into the chamber (which is itself controlled by an orifice).

Air dilution

The physiological requirements of an oxygen system call for the dilution of oxygen to avoid the consequences (and waste) of breathing 100% oxygen continuously. Such dilution is usually achieved in conventional systems (that is, those based on gaseous or liquid oxygen storage) by mixing cabin air with oxygen in the demand regulator. The degree of air dilution (airmix) decreases automatically and progressively with ascent to altitude in order to maintain adequate oxygenation at all times. Two principal mechanisms are employed to draw cabin air into the regulator: suction dilution and injector dilution.

In regulators employing *suction dilution*, air is drawn into the demand chamber through a spring-loaded air-inlet valve (*see Figure 7.10(a)*), while an aneroid capsule controls the relative resistances to flow through both this valve and the demand valve. Thus as altitude increases and the aneroid expands, flow through the former falls and flow through the latter rises.

Suction dilution cannot provide airmix in the presence of safety pressure, however, and so in systems in which that facility is provided the suction required to induce or entrain a flow of cabin air into the demand chamber is created by passing oxygen

through an injector (venturi) as it flows from the demand valve: *injector dilution*. As with the suction dilution technique, the flow of cabin air is governed by another valve, the opening of which is again controlled by an aneroid capsule (*see Figure 7.10(b)*). The injector dilution technique is widely employed, but does tend to deliver a relatively high (but acceptable) concentration of oxygen during quiet breathing and at low altitudes. For example, a typical injector dilution regulator will deliver 40–50% oxygen even at sea level.

In both forms of air dilution, the air-inlet port can be closed by manual operation of a shutter on the regulator, thus providing 100% oxygen at any altitude in the event of toxic fumes within the cabin, or if decompression sickness is suspected or is likely to develop. (This manual override facility is not required in regulators used in molecular sieve oxygen concentrating systems, where no dilution with cabin air takes place.)

A potential hazard of air dilution is that the user can continue to breathe air through the air-inlet port following a failure of the oxygen supply to the regulator. The development of hypoxia is then a distinct possibility since the increase in resistance to inspiration associated with such a failure may well go undetected even at cabin altitudes of 15 000–18 000 feet. In many modern regulators, the risk of

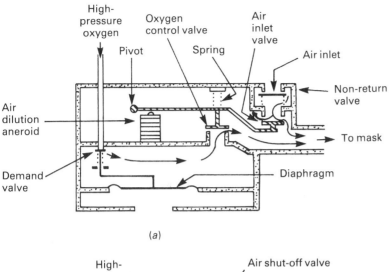

(a)

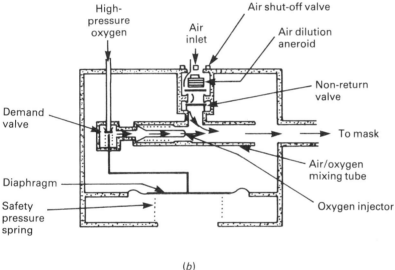

(b)

Figure 7.10 Two techniques for diluting oxygen with cabin air, employed in demand regulator systems. (*a*) Mode of operation for air dilution in a suction demand regulator: *suction dilution*. Air is drawn into the regulator by the inspiratory effort, and the relative flows of oxygen and air are controlled by an aneroid capsule which varies the resistances to flow through the oxygen and air inlet ports to the regulator outlet. (*b*) Mode of operation for air dilution in a pressure demand regulator: *injector dilution*. In this case, air is drawn into the regulator by the suction induced by oxygen flow, from the demand valve, through an injector. The proportion of air to oxygen mixing is controlled by an aneroid capsule which operates a throttle plate in the air inlet port of the regulator.

an undetected failure is eliminated by the incorporation of an additional valve in the air-inlet mechanism which is operated by oxygen pressure. This valve remains shut unless there is adequate oxygen pressure at the inlet to the regulator, and a failure of the oxygen supply pressure therefore results in the immediate occlusion of the air-inlet port with consequent gross impedance to inspiration.

Safety pressure

Since the operation of the regulator demand valve depends upon the transmission of pressure fluctuations produced in the mask cavity by respiration, the mask must seal well against the face and be fitted with an effective non-return expiratory valve (*see* Oxygen Masks, below). An ill-fitting mask will induce an inboard leak of air during inspiration and so will dilute the oxygen contained in the gas delivered by the regulator; and this is a serious potential disadvantage of suction dilution demand regulators. In injector dilution demand regulators, however, this disadvantage may be prevented by creating a slight over-pressure, termed *safety pressure*, in the mask cavity. The pressure in the mask then remains greater than that of the environment throughout inspiration thus ensuring that any leak of gas as a result of an ill-fitting mask is outboard and not inboard.

Safety pressure is delivered by the demand regulator by applying an appropriate force to the control diaphragm by means of a spring which displaces the diaphragm and so opens the demand valve (*see Figure 7.8*). As soon as the pressure in the mask reaches the required level, the rise in pressure within the demand chamber overcomes the force of the spring, the diaphragm returns to its resting position and shuts the demand valve. Clearly, the mask expiratory valve must be modified so that it does not open until mask cavity pressure exceeds the nominal safety pressure. Thus the expiratory valve may either be spring loaded, so that its opening pressure is raised at all times, or it may be *compensated* to the delivery pressure of the regulator, so that the raised opening pressure is only present when safety pressure is being provided (*see also* Oxygen Masks, below). The magnitude of the safety pressure required to prevent inboard leakage around an ill-fitting mask depends on the delivery pressure-flow characteristics of the regulator, and on the resistance to flow from the regulator to the mask cavity. The level of safety pressure, however, generally lies between 15 and 25 mm wg (0.15–0.25 kPa).

The disadvantage of spring loading the control diaphragm to provide safety pressure is that gas will flow from the regulator outlet or from the mask whenever they are open to the environment. Furthermore, consumption of the oxygen supply is increased at all altitudes when safety pressure is being delivered, although hypoxia arising as a consequence of an inboard mask leak is a significant risk only at altitudes above about 15000 feet. In many demand systems, therefore, safety pressure is invoked only when it is required; and is provided automatically by the expansion of a pressure-sensitive aneroid capsule, within the reference chamber, on ascent to cabin altitudes above 10000–15000 feet. A manual switch is also incorporated in some systems so that safety pressure can be selected at a lower cabin altitude if toxic contamination of the cockpit occurs.

Pressure breathing

The increase in regulator delivery pressure required to provide pressure breathing, and the inflation and operation of pressure garments, at cabin altitudes above 40000 feet is achieved by progressively loading the control diaphragm with a suitable spring force, as shown in *Figure 7.11* (*see also Figure 7.9*).

The spring force opens the demand valve and gas flows to the mask until the pressure in the mask and in the demand chamber has built up to the required level. The diaphragm then returns to its resting position and the demand valve shuts. The spring load is applied to the diaphragm either by a spring, which is allowed to expand progressively under the control of an aneroid capsule within the reference chamber of the regulator, or by gas, the pressure of which is also raised by the expansion of an aneroid capsule. The required relationship between regulator delivery pressure and cabin altitude is obtained by appropriate design of the springs and controlling aneroids. As in the case of safety pressure, the pressure breathing mask must be fitted with a compensated expiratory valve. For test purposes on the ground, a means of obtaining one or two set increases in delivery pressure by manual selection is also provided: the test pressures are usually about 20 mm Hg (2.7 kPa) for use with a mask alone, and 40–60 mm Hg (5.3–8.0 kPa) for use with partial pressure garments.

Indication of flow

An indication of the passage of oxygen through the demand regulator serves as means of confirming that oxygen flows with each inspiration, and of detecting outboard leakage in the presence of safety pressure or pressure breathing. Most commonly, the changes in pressure immediately downstream of the demand valve induced by flow through it are used to operate a visual indicator via some form of pressure switch. Thus, for example, pressure variations, as a consequence of flow, may deflect a small diaphragm which completes an electro-magnetic circuit and operates the indicator. In the case of panel-mounted regulators, the magnetic indicator is an integral part of the device; whilst in the case of seat-mounted or man-mounted regulators, the indicator is located elsewhere on the instrument panel. In some systems, the flow sensor may take the form of a spring-loaded slug within the lumen of the oxygen supply line to the regulator. In this case, movements of the slug produced by oxygen flow are transduced electromagnetically or by a light beam, and the indicator is again mounted in a prominent place on the instrument panel. Wherever the indicator is mounted, its regular operation is confirmed throughout flight by the user: it usually displays a white bar in the presence of flow and goes black when there is no flow. The absence of oxygen flow will therefore be readily apparent, as will a continuous flow caused by an outboard leak.

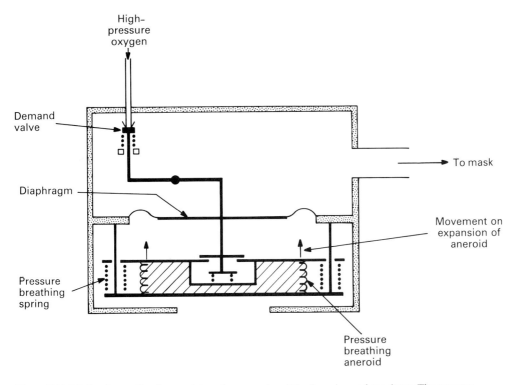

High–
pressure
oxygen

Demand
valve

To mask

Diaphragm

Movement on
expansion of
aneroid

Pressure
breathing
spring

Pressure
breathing
aneroid

Figure 7.11 Mode of operation for provision of pressure breathing by a demand regulator. The pressure breathing aneroid capsule starts to expand at the altitude from which pressure breathing is to commence. This expansion allows the pressure breathing spring to load the control diaphragm and so increase the delivery pressure from the regulator to the mask. The progressive expansion of the aneroid capsule with altitude produces concomitant increases in loading of the control diaphragm and delivery pressure from the regulator.

Indication of contents/pressure

In systems supplied by gaseous or liquid oxygen, a continuous indication of the quantity of gas available is given to the user by means of gauges which display contents in fractions of full or the system operating pressure. In many aircraft, both displays are provided.

Oxygen hoses and personal equipment connectors

The final routing taken by oxygen delivery pipework to the user will depend upon the location within the cockpit of the demand regulator, and upon the presence or otherwise of an ejection seat. Furthermore, in many aircraft in which ejection seats are installed, the usual way in which the user is connected to his personal services is by means of an additional item of equipment: the *personal equipment connector* (PEC). The various ways in which oxygen is delivered from the source to the user are shown schematically in *Figure 7.12*.

As well as the main oxygen supply, the personal equipment connector provides the conduits by which the emergency oxygen supply, the G trousers supply, the air-ventilated suit supply, and the electrical connections for communication can be easily delivered to the user. A personal equipment connector consists of three interlocking parts (the aircraft portion, the seat portion, and the man portion) which enable coupling and uncoupling of services, during routine entry and exit, and during the ejection sequence, to be accomplished in a single simple action. *Figure 7.13* shows a typical personal equipment connector assembly.

Wide-bore oxygen hoses are only used after the delivery pressure has been reduced by the regulator. Such hoses are usually made of natural or vulcanized rubber, reinforced by spirally wound galvanized steel wire and covered with rubberized gauze or stockinette. They are anti-kink and incorporate various end connectors to accommodate the fittings for different aircraft systems. The medium-pressure ($70\,lb/in^2$ ($483\,kPa$)) hoses used in conjunction with servo-operated pressure demand regulators are made of narrow-bore anti-kink reinforced rubber.

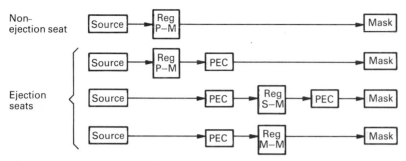

Figure 7.12 Schematic to show the various routes by which an oxygen supply is delivered to the user in demand regulator systems. The routes depend upon the location of the regulator within the cockpit and upon the presence or otherwise of an ejection seat. (Reg P-M: panel-mounted regulator; Reg S-M: seat-mounted regulator; Reg M-M: man-mounted regulator; PEC: personal equipment connector.)

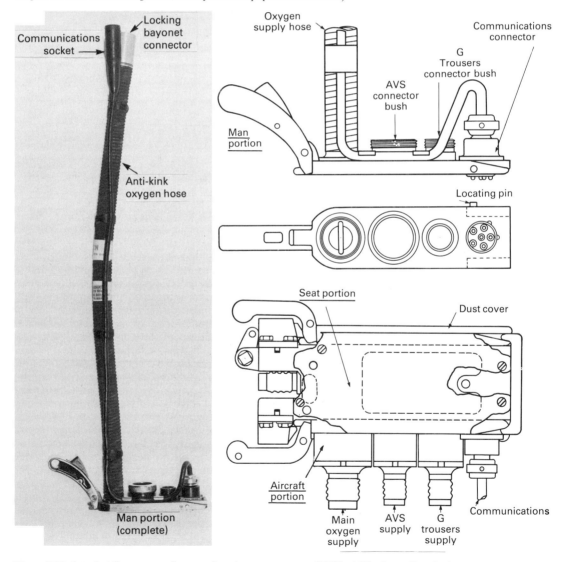

Figure 7.13 A typical (low-pressure) personal equipment connector (PEC). AVS: air ventilated suit.

Oxygen masks

Masks for aircrew

General requirements

A mask for aircrew use must satisfy several interrelated requirements. Thus it must be stable and comfortable to wear for long periods, it must be small, it must fit a variety of facial sizes and shapes, and it must seal against the skin of the face effectively. A typical oronasal oxygen mask, such as is used by British military pilots, is illustrated in *Figure 7.14*.

Comfort demands that the facepiece of the mask should be made of a flexible material which retains that property over the whole range of temperatures in which it may be worn. Natural rubber and silicone rubber are commonly employed for this purpose, but it is important that the sensitizing properties of any rubber mixture used should be as low as possible. It is also clearly desirable that body secretions should not affect the rubber adversely. The flexible facepiece is generally supported by a semi-rigid or rigid exoskeleton which also provides the mounting for the means by which the mask is suspended from a headset or protective helmet. The

mask should be as small as possible in order to reduce any restriction of the visual fields, and to keep limitations on head movement to a minimum. The internal volume or dead space of the mask must be low, typically 120–150 ml, to avoid significant rebreathing. Sizing is much simplified if the lower edge of the mask sits in the sulcus beneath the lower lip rather than beneath the chin itself. Only two sizes of oronasal mask are then required if the line of contact with the skin is over the bridge of the nose, descending just lateral to the mouth and then passing along the sulcus below the lower lip. Four sizes of mask are required if the chin is enclosed.

The most effective and commonly used method of obtaining a seal between the mask and the face is to reflect the edge of the rubber facepiece, so that a thin flap of rubber lies on the surface of the skin within the mask cavity (*Figure 7.15*).

A slight tension in the reflected edge causes it to lie snugly against the skin, and any increase in mask pressure, such as safety pressure or pressure breathing, will tend to improve the seal even further. The flexibility of the mask material and of the seal must be sufficient for comfort and yet rigid enough to prevent deformation caused by accelerative forces which tend to displace the mask. The security of the mask upon the face depends primarily, however, upon the suspension harness by

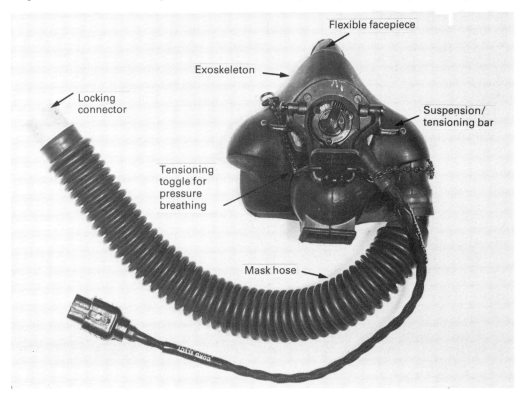

Figure 7.14 A typical pressure demand oronasal mask.

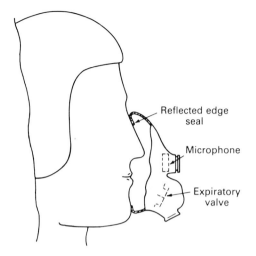

Figure 7.15 An oronasal mask with a reflected edge seal. When gas at a raised pressure is delivered to the mask, the reflected edge of the seal is driven firmly against the skin of the face by the pressure, so preventing leakage.

which it is attached to the headgear, and upon the security of the latter on the head. A relatively rigid suspension system is required if the user is exposed to high levels of acceleration and vibration in flight, and to high levels of acceleration and windblast during an ejection sequence. The suspension system must also incorporate a means of normal adjustment of fit to the headgear, and of rapid tightening for pressure breathing. One method of achieving the former is merely to place the mask comfortably on the face and lock bayonet type connectors on the mask into one of a series of ratchet notches on the helmet. Pushing the mask further onto the face in order to engage the bayonets on a deeper notch provides the means to enhance the seal for pressure breathing. Another method of attaching the mask to the helmet involves engaging chains mounted on the mask exoskeleton over adjustable hooks mounted on the helmet or headset. Tension in this case can be augmented for pressure breathing by drawing the chains over a suspension/tensioning bar on the front of the mask (*see Figure 7.14*). With the advent of routine pressure breathing for enhancement of tolerance of $+G_z$ accelerations, however, it is likely that these simple mechanical methods of mask tensioning will be superceded by automatic mechanisms, such as those already in routine use by several air forces.

Although the valves fitted to an oxygen mask vary with the type of system in which the mask is to be used (*see* below), there are a number of general features that are common to all masks. Thus the delivery hose to the mask usually has an internal bore of 15–20 mm and has a flexible but non-crushable wall. The lower end of the hose carries a

connector by which it is attached (preferably by a locking mechanism) to the supply hose from the regulator. The weight of the hose assembly is often transmitted to the personal clothing by a connecting chain attached to the mask hose connector, in order to eliminate the downwards pull by the hose on the mask. The upper end of the mask hose is attached to the inspiratory port, within which the inspiratory (inlet) valve is located. The inspiratory valve is usually placed high up in the mask to minimize the possibility of its obstruction by particles of debris, and to limit contact with moist expired air. An iceguard is fitted to its internal surface to provide further protection against debris and moisture. The expiratory (outlet) valve is usually fitted in the most dependent part of the mask to allow sweat and saliva to drain effectively. Furthermore, the external surface of the expiratory valve is protected against the effects of low environmental temperatures by an extension of the rubber facepiece, which traps 10–15 ml of relatively warm expired air just beyond the valve. The walls of this extension (or snout) are flexible so that the wearer can break up and remove any ice that has accumulated within it.

The oxygen mask is also used as the carrier for the microphone component of the aircraft communication system (*see Figure 7.14*). The presence of a mask greatly modifies the qualities of speech, and sound pressure levels within the mask cavity during speech may be relatively high: typically 120 dB. Furthermore, speech may be masked by noise generated during the flow of breathing gas through the regulator (particularly when man-mounted), by the flow of gas through delivery hoses and mask valves, and by the direct transmission of cabin noise through the walls of the mask or an open expiratory valve. Finally, the mask forms part of the personal protection of the head, and its stability is therefore especially vital in the event of the cockpit being breached by, for example, a birdstrike; or should the need arise to escape from the aircraft at high speed, with consequent exposure to high windblast (Q) forces.

Particular requirements of demand mask valves

In demand oxygen systems in which the regulator only delivers gas when suction is created at its outlet, the associated mask requires just a single non-return valve in the outlet (expiratory) port. This valve prevents cabin air from being drawn into the lungs and also allows the creation of the suction required to open the demand valve during inspiration. Since there is no way in which gas can be discharged to the environment from the demand chamber of the regulator, expired gas cannot flow back to that chamber and so no valve is required in the inlet (inspiratory) port.

When the delivery pressure of the regulator is capable of being raised above that of the environment (that is, when safety pressure or pressure breathing is being delivered), the non-return expiratory valve must be loaded so that it does not open under the influence of the increased mask cavity pressure. If unacceptable resistance to expiration is to be avoided, however, the setting of the expiratory valve must be such as to allow gas to be expelled from the lungs with only a small additional rise in mask cavity pressure. In those pressure demand systems in which the regulator is capable of delivering safety pressure but not pressure breathing (that is, in systems used only at cabin altitudes of less than 40 000 feet), a simple spring-loaded non-return expiratory valve is fitted to the mask; and the pressure required to open this valve is set at a slightly higher level than that of the safety pressure delivered by the regulator. When safety pressure is present, breathing when using this system is very comfortable but, when safety pressure is absent, the spring-loading of the valve is noticeable as an increased resistance to expiration. Occasionally, therefore, the expiratory valve of the mask is fitted with a control that allows the user to raise the spring-loading manually. Such a variable resistance expiratory valve may be used to hold not only safety pressure in the mask, but also low levels (for

example, 10–15 mm Hg (1.3–2.0 kPa)) of pressure breathing. This technique is not widely used because it requires manual operation and, during pressure breathing, results in excessive resistance to expiration and/or loss of oxygen.

The most satisfactory and extensively employed method of automatically varying the pressure at which the expiratory valve opens is to compensate the device (*Figure 7.16*). A compensated expiratory valve has a gas-loading facility whereby the pressure in the inlet port of the mask is also transmitted, by a flexible diaphragm, piston and spring, to the valve plate on the downstream side of the expiratory valve.

The area of the flexible diaphragm/piston is equal to that of the expiratory valve port so that any increase in the pressure at which gas is delivered to the mask is also transmitted through the compensation chamber to the underside of the valve. The expiratory valve therefore remains shut despite the increase in mask cavity pressure. The additional increase in mask cavity pressure required to open the expiratory valve is unchanged, however, so that the small increase in mask pressure induced by expiration opens the expiratory valve and allows expired gas to flow out. An additional and essential requirement of a mask fitted with a compensated expiratory valve is the need for a non-return

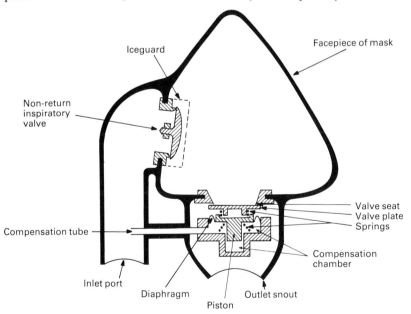

Figure 7.16 The valve system of a pressure demand oronasal mask. The inspiratory valve is a simple non-return device, with a mesh cover which acts as an iceguard. The expiratory valve is compensated, the pressure of gas in the inlet port also being applied along the compensation tube and through a diaphragm and piston to the external surface of the expiratory valve plate. In the resting condition, the expiratory valve is held closed by a spring in the compensation chamber. The valve plate above is separated from the diaphragm and piston below by a second spring which ensures that any reduction in pressure within the inlet port will not allow the expiratory valve to open.

inspiratory valve. If such a valve was not fitted in the inlet port, or if even a small leak was present around a fitted valve, the increase in mask cavity pressure caused by expiration would be free to pass back into the mask hose and thence to the compensation chamber of the expiratory valve. The expiratory valve would then be held firmly shut by the expiratory effort, and the user would be unable to breathe out. In addition, since the inspiratory valve is prone to freezing as a result of expirate flowing over its cold surface, a deflector plate or iceguard must be fitted to the valve to protect it against this hazard. Finally, under certain conditions, such as during excessive head movements, the mask hose may 'pump' and cause the pressure in the inlet port to become less than that of the environment. If this occurs the reduction in pressure is transmitted along the compensation tube to the expiratory valve, which is then free to open and allow the unacceptable likelihood of inspiring air from the cabin. The magnitude of this effect of mask hose pumping can be reduced by installing a restraint cord within the lumen of the hose to prevent excessive lengthening, and can be stopped completely by a further refinement of the compensated expiratory valve: an additional spring interposed between the valve plate and the flexible diaphragm/piston of the compensation chamber. If pressure within the latter falls, and the diaphragm/piston moves downwards, the expiratory valve remains sealed as a result of the valve plate being held against the valve seat by the additional spring (*see Figure 7.16*). A unit that incorporates such a refinement is termed a *split compensated expiratory valve*.

Such a valve will not, however, alleviate the other major disadvantage of mask hose pumping: that is, the rise in mask cavity pressure that it produces. This rise acts to hold the expiratory valve closed so markedly increasing the added external resistance to expiration.

The combination of a non-return inspiratory valve and a split compensated expiratory valve ensures that the mask cavity pressure is controlled automatically to the datum pressure being delivered by the demand regulator, whilst the increase required in mask cavity pressure to open the expiratory valve during expiration remains constant at 15–25 mm Hg (0.15–0.25 kPa).

In those masks used routinely throughout flight by military aircrew, and in association with a personal equipment connector, a third valve is frequently fitted to provide an anti-suffocation facility. The reason for this is that the man portion of the personal equipment connector contains an anti-drowning, self-sealing, 'prop' valve which closes the oxygen port of the connector whenever it is detached from the seat portion (*see Figure 7.13*). Thus should water entry occur after an ejection

escape, or should the connector release inadvertently during flight, the user is able to continue breathing through the anti-suffocation valve. In the case of water entry, the prop valve prevents the inhalation of water through the personal equipment connector. The anti-suffocation valve itself is an inward relief valve which opens when the pressure within the mask cavity falls to 9–13 mm Hg (1.2–1.7 kPa) below ambient pressure; a suction sufficiently high to warn the user that the valve is operative.

Masks for passengers

General features

Although the degree of comfort and standard of seal required of oxygen delivery masks for emergency use by passengers is considerably less than that necessary for aircrew, such masks do have some important design constraints. Thus one size of mask must fit all shapes and sizes of face, and the mask must be easy to don and secure in place by completely untrained passengers. To that end, the mask should be circular in shape to avoid the need to orientate the device on the face, and the harness is usually a simple elastic loop. Passenger masks are not usually designed for use at environmental temperatures below −5 to −10°C.

One very common type of passenger emergency oxygen mask receives a continuous flow of oxygen and incorporates a small reservoir bag in either the rebreathing or non-rebreathing configuration (*see above*). But at least one form of passenger mask has a simple demand valve used in conjunction with a metered oxygen flow. In this case, the intervening hose between the metering orifice and the mask acts as a reservoir for oxygen during expiration.

The masks are usually stowed in overhead compartments or in the back-rest of the seat in front. The doors of the stowage compartment are opened and the masks presented to the passengers automatically should the cabin altitude exceed a pre-determined level: commonly 13 000–14 000 feet. Flow of oxygen to the mask is not initiated, however, until the mask is actively pulled towards the face. A simple, bobbin flow-meter inserted in the supply hose to the mask indicates that flow is occurring. The automatic presentation of the masks, and the magnitude of the subsequent continuous flow of oxygen, is generally controlled from the flight deck by varying the pressure in the ring main which supplies oxygen to all outlets (*see also Figure 7.27*). The pressure in the ring main is itself controlled either automatically or manually by a member of the flight-deck crew.

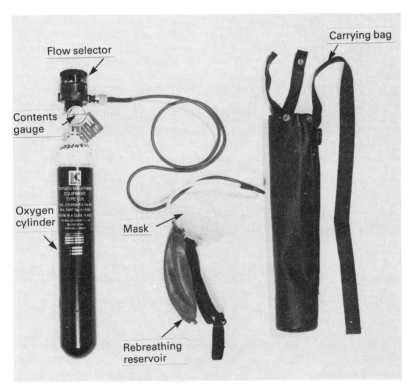

Figure 7.17 A typical portable oxygen set for therapeutic use by passengers or walk-around use by cabin staff. Oxygen is supplied from a 1201 (NTP) capacity cylinder, at one of two pre-set flows, to a simple rebreathing reservoir facemask.

Simple continuous flow systems, usually of the rebreathing reservoir type, are also used to administer therapeutic oxygen to needy passengers; for example, those who have become ill during flight or those for whom flight was predicted to embarrass their cardio-respiratory status (*see* Chapter 40). The oxygen supply is then obtained either from a direct connection to the aircraft's main oxygen store, or from a portable gaseous oxygen cylinder (*Figure 7.17*). National and international regulations determine the number of such therapeutic/emergency oxygen sets that are to be carried.

Smokehoods

Fire and toxic fumes on board an aircraft have obvious, and often tragic, consequences. Even if the aircraft is on the ground when the emergency occurs, or manages a successful emergency landing, the occupants may succumb to smoke and fumes before escape is possible. There is, therefore, a need to provide some form of respiratory protection for crew members and passengers so threatened.

Following several such disasters in civil aircraft during the 1980s, the appropriate regulating authorities have actively pursued the possibility of providing smokehoods for use by the passengers and crew of stricken aircraft. While the small numbers required for crew protection suggest that quite sophisticated devices could be (and, by some airlines, are) provided, the large numbers of passengers carried place severe constraints, in terms of weight, bulk and cost, upon the design of suitable hoods. Furthermore, problems of size roll, the ease of use by untrained subjects, compromised visibility and the ability to communicate must all be addressed; as must the all-important ability of the device to protect the user for the duration of the emergency. Many prototype smokehoods, all of which envelop the head entirely, have been developed *de novo* or adapted from breathing devices used for other purposes. The sophistication of such equipment varies from the simple hood made of transparent plastic and equipped with a charcoal filter through which to breathe, to hoods providing an integral breathing gas supply. The source of supply may be from a chemical candle (such as in the widely used Scott smokehood for cabin staff) or from a gaseous oxygen cylinder combined with active or passive carbon dioxide absorption.

In military transport aircraft, where relatively few people are involved, equipment to allow a crew member to breathe in irrespirable atmospheres (for

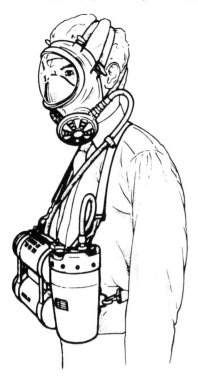

Figure 7.18 A typical military portable oxygen set for use in irrespirable atmospheres. The weight and bulk of such equipment makes it unsuitable for use as a smokehood for passengers.

example, whilst fire fighting) can be provided with little constraint in terms of weight or bulk. A typical smoke set for such a purpose is shown in *Figure 7.18.*

In the system illustrated, breathing gas is supplied as oxygen from two 200 l (NTP) capacity cylinders contained in a unit carried on the chest. Oxygen is supplied on demand via a regulator assembly mounted on the side of a combined mask and visor facepiece, and expiration is through a non-return valve combined with a speech transmitter unit. The system can provide protection in hostile environments, and up to an altitude of 30 000 feet.

Typical oxygen systems

Examples of all the various components described above are integrated to provide a complete oxygen system. The choice of components and their layout will clearly depend upon the type and role of the aircraft in which the system is to be installed, and this section summarizes the general features of some typical oxygen systems both in military and in civil aircraft.

Aircraft with low-differential pressure cabins–combat aircraft

Combat aircraft have low-differential pressure cabins and so the oxygen system provides an essential element of the protection against hypoxia on ascent to cabin altitudes above 10 000 feet. Consequently, those components of the oxygen system that are thought likely to fail in flight are duplicated. Such an installation therefore consists of a primary or *main* oxygen system, and a secondary or *emergency* oxygen system. When the aircraft is fitted with ejection seats, as is nearly always the case in modern combat aircraft, the emergency oxygen system also serves to prevent the development of serious hypoxia following escape from the aircraft at high altitude.

The main oxygen system comprises a store of oxygen, a pressure demand oxygen regulator at each crew position, and a pressure demand oxygen mask. The emergency system comprises a small store of oxygen stowed somewhere in or on the escape equipment, so that it can also provide the bail-out supply, and a separate emergency oxygen regulator.

The main supply in current combat aircraft is virtually always carried as liquid oxygen in converters located outside the pressure cabin, and which can be replaced rapidly when partially used. Single-seat aircraft are typically equipped with a 5 l converter, whilst 10 l converters are usually fitted to two-seat or long-range aircraft. Gaseous oxygen, at an appropriate operating pressure, is led from the converter by a main supply pipe through the wall of the pressure cabin to the inlet of the regulator. The emergency oxygen supply is carried as compressed gas in small cylinders with capacities varying from 50 to 200 l (NTP). The contents of the emergency supply are indicated on a pressure gauge which is checked before every flight, and the cylinder is equipped with a charging point which allows replenishment *in situ*. Emergency oxygen can be selected manually in flight, or automatically during the escape sequence on ejection.

The main pressure demand oxygen regulator for each crew member may be mounted in a variety of positions, and it is convenient to classify the sites used into three groups: the airframe (panel-mounted), the man (man-mounted), and the ejection seat (seat-mounted).

Panel-mounted regulator systems *(Figures 7.19 and 7.20)*

When the regulator is mounted on the airframe, it is usually sited on a front or side console (panel) in such a position that its controls can be reached in flight. Wide-bore, low-pressure hose from the outlet of the regulator passes, via either single in-line

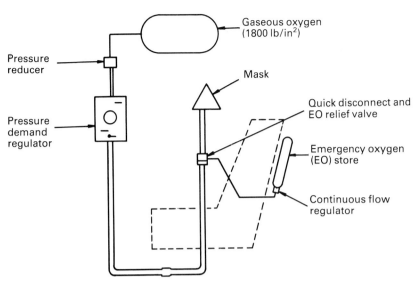

Figure 7.19 A typical pressure demand oxygen system comprising a gaseous oxygen source, a panel-mounted demand regulator, and an oxygen mask. Breathing gas is delivered to the user via a wide-bore, low-pressure hose connected directly to the mask hose by means of a quick disconnect. The continuous flow emergency oxygen supply enters the system at the quick disconnect, which therefore also incorporates an excess-pressure relief valve.

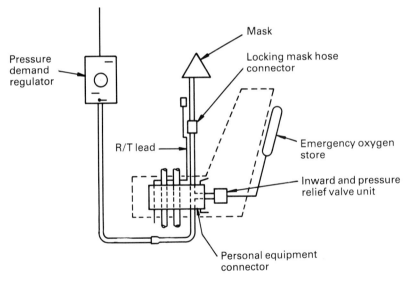

Figure 7.20 A typical pressure demand oxygen system comprising either a gaseous or a liquid oxygen source, a panel-mounted demand regulator, and an oxygen mask. Breathing gas is delivered to the user via a wide-bore, low-pressure hose, passing via the personal equipment connector, to a locking coupling at the mask hose. The emergency oxygen supply, via its own demand regulator, enters the system through the seat portion of the personal equipment connector and thence passes to the user.

connectors (*Figure 7.19*) or a personal equipment connector (*Figure 7.20*), to end in another connector in the region of the user's chest. The inlet hose of the oxygen mask then plugs directly into this connector.

Panel-mounted regulators usually have a large control diaphragm linked mechanically to the demand valve, and are able to provide all the desirable automatic facilities described above. *Figure 7.21* is an illustration of a typical panel-mounted oxygen regulator.

In older aircraft, the associated emergency

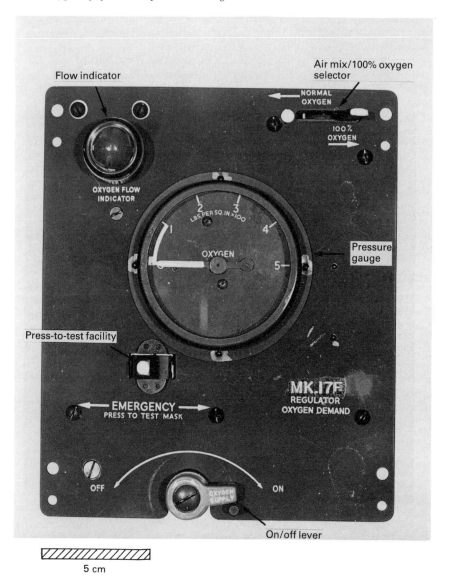

Figure 7.21 A typical panel-mounted pressure demand oxygen regulator.

oxygen system is generally connected to the main system either at, or immediately upstream of, the mask hose coupling (*see Figure 7.19*), and delivery from the emergency supply is regulated by a simple orifice which provides a continuous flow. In more modern systems, however, a small pressure demand emergency regulator may be fitted, which provides 100% oxygen with safety pressure from sea level, and automatic pressure breathing if necessary, delivery being via the personal equipment connector (*see Figure 7.20*).

The major disadvantages of panel-mounted oxygen regulator systems are that the regulator occupies valuable panel space, there is often a long unwieldy length of hose between the regulator and the mask, and the main oxygen supply cannot be routed through the emergency regulator should the main regulator fail to pass gas. The development of pneumatic engineering allowed regulators to be miniaturized, and the consequent reduction in weight and bulk enabled other mounting sites to be utilized.

Body-mounted regulator systems (*Figure 7.22*)

A miniaturized servo-controlled pressure demand regulator can be mounted either on the chest or on the head. The length of delivery hose from the regulator to the mask is therefore short and there is little resistance to inspiration in such systems. Oxygen at medium pressure ($70\,lb/in^2$ ($483\,kPa$)) is carried directly to the inlet of the regulator through narrow-bore (8 mm outside diameter) flexible hose. Routine connection/disconnection between the aircraft supply, the ejection seat and the regulator mounted on the man is accomplished via a (narrow-bore) personal equipment connector. The same device allows automatic separation of supplies during the ejection sequence. Since the main regulator travels out of the aircraft with the seat during such an event, it can be utilized by the emergency supply as well as by the main system. Consequently, the emergency oxygen supply, after passing through a reducing valve which is usually mounted on the emergency cylinder itself, is delivered into the main supply system upstream of the main regulator (*Figure 7.22*).

Mask-mounted or helmet-mounted regulators can be used, in association with an emergency oxygen supply carried in the personal survival pack (*see below*), to provide breathing gas during and immediately after a parachute descent into water, and so reduce the risk of drowning. Considerations of size and weight, however, dictate that a pressure demand regulator mounted in those sites cannot provide air dilution. The additional space on the chest allows a miniaturized air dilution device to be carried. Indeed, some chest-mounted regulators not only provide air dilution, safety pressure and pressure breathing, but also incorporate a second or stand-by regulator which can be used in the event of a failure of the main regulator. *Figure 7.23* is an illustration of a typical chest-mounted miniature pressure demand regulator.

Although body-mounted regulators are readily available for servicing, they are very liable to damage by handling, and are required in greater numbers than for panel-mounted or seat-mounted devices since each crew member must be issued with a regulator. Furthermore, the emergency drills are relatively complicated because separation of the regulator from direct contact with the aircraft or seat services complicates the system, increases the likelihood of problems arising, and lengthens the drills necessary to correct such problems. A final disadvantage is that miniaturization to a marked degree precludes the opportunity to incorporate additional safety features and increase system redundancy (and hence operational effectiveness). All of these disadvantages can be overcome, at the same time as retaining the benefits of pneumatic engineering, by mounting the regulator package on the ejection seat.

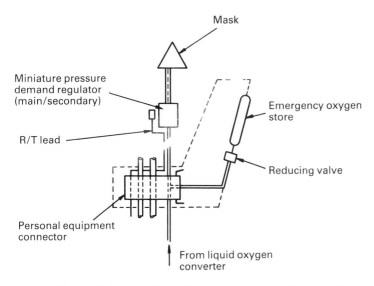

Figure 7.22 A typical pressure demand oxygen system comprising a liquid oxygen source, a chest-mounted demand regulator, and an oxygen mask. Breathing gas is delivered to the user via a narrow-bore, medium-pressure hose, passing via the personal equipment connector, to a locked connection at the regulator. The wide-bore mask hose couples directly to the regulator. The emergency oxygen supply enters the system through the seat portion of the personal equipment connector and then passes to the regulator which is therefore able to provide emergency oxygen on demand.

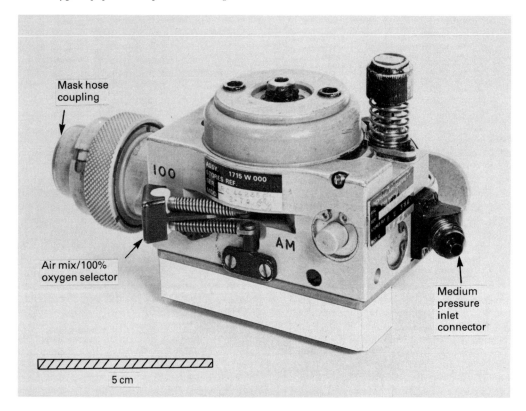

Figure 7.23 A typical chest-mounted pressure demand oxygen regulator.

Seat-mounted regulator systems *(Figure 7.24)*

Seat-mounted regulators may be located either on the seat structure itself or in the personal survival pack. The latter is the site of choice in which to carry the emergency/bail-out supply for the occupants of non-ejection seat aircraft, but the size and weight of emergency regulators to be carried in personal survival packs must clearly be kept as low as possible.

No such constraints apply to ejection-seat-mounted regulators, however, and these provide air dilution with automatic safety pressure from about 15 000 feet and pressure breathing at high altitudes. As with the other systems described, oxygen is usually delivered to the regulator via the aircraft and seat portions of a personal equipment connector. The outlet of the regulator is connected, through the man portion of the personal equipment connector, to wide-bore hose which passes to the coupling by which attachment is made to the inlet hose of the oxygen mask *(Figure 7.24)*. The emergency oxygen supply is usually controlled by a second seat-mounted pressure demand regulator which supplies 100% oxygen, safety pressure from sea level and automatic pressure breathing when required. The emergency regulator can be positioned immediately

adjacent to the main regulator, and indeed may be in the same unit (such an arrangement is termed a *duplex* regulator); it is then possible to arrange for the main oxygen supply to be routed through either the main or emergency regulator, so duplicating the regulator in the main system and improving operational effectiveness. The close association of the main and emergency regulators also allows the corrective drills required in the event of a failure in the system to be simplified. *Figure 7.25* shows a typical seat-mounted pressure demand oxygen regulator.

In the United Kingdom, oxygen systems that employ a molecular sieve oxygen concentrator also incorporate a duplex seat-mounted regulator *(Figure 7.26)*. The technical details of such systems differ markedly from all previous oxygen systems in several fundamental areas.

Since the output pressure from a molecular sieve is usually only about $30\,lb/in^2$ (207 kPa), the regulator must be engineered to function normally (that is, to provide breathing gas on demand, safety pressure and pressure breathing) at this relatively low pressure. On the other hand, the regulator is not required to provide air dilution since that facility is achieved by manipulation of flow through the molecular sieve (*see* Oxygen Sources, above). In the

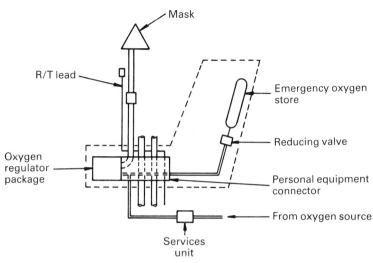

Mask

R/T lead

Emergency oxygen store

Reducing valve

Oxygen regulator package

Personal equipment connector

From oxygen source

Services unit

Figure 7.24 A typical pressure demand oxygen system comprising either a gaseous oxygen or a liquid oxygen source, a seat-mounted duplex demand regulator, and an oxygen mask. Breathing gas is delivered to the user via narrow-bore, medium-pressure hose to the seat portion of the personal equipment connector (to which the regulator package is directly connected) and then via the wide-bore, low-pressure hose of the man portion of the personal equipment connector to a locking coupling with the mask hose. The emergency oxygen supply enters the system through the seat portion of the personal equipment connector and passes directly to the duplex regulator, both elements of which are therefore able to provide emergency oxygen on demand.

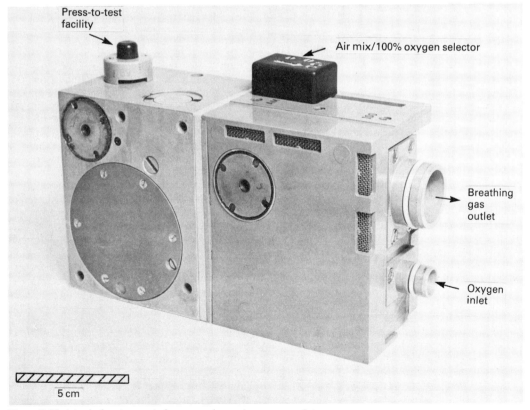

Press-to-test facility

Air mix/100% oxygen selector

Breathing gas outlet

Oxygen inlet

5 cm

Figure 7.25 A typical seat-mounted pressure demand oxygen regulator.

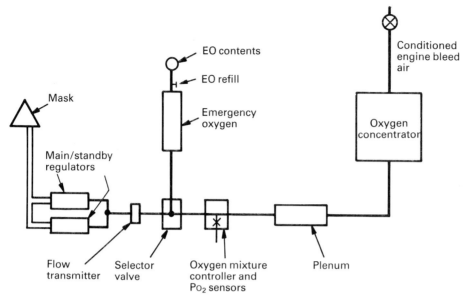

Figure 7.26 An advanced oxygen system employing a molecular sieve oxygen concentrator and a seat-mounted duplex pressure demand regulator. Product gas is delivered from the molecular sieve to the user via the seat portion of a personal equipment connector to which the regulator is directly connected, and thence via the wide-bore, low-pressure hose of the man portion of the personal equipment connector to the locking coupling with the mask hose. In this system, the concentration of oxygen within the product gas is controlled by a sensing device which increases flow through the sieve if oxygen concentration is too high, and decreases flow through the sieve if oxygen concentration is too low. The emergency oxygen supply enters the system through the seat portion of the personal equipment connector and passes to the duplex regulator and thence to the user in the conventional manner. The emergency system also acts to provide a back-up supply of oxygen during temporary reductions in or failures of adequate sieve output. Since these situations may be resolved, the emergency/back-up supply may, uniquely, be turned off.

system illustrated, control of oxygen concentration in the product gas is maintained by continuous monitoring of the partial pressure of oxygen (at the existing cabin altitude) being delivered to an entirely new component of the system: the mixture controller. This device incorporates a sensor which, if the product gas is too rich in oxygen, initiates an increase in flow through the molecular sieve beds and so reduces the concentration of oxygen. Conversely, if the sensor detects that the oxygen content is too low, flow through the beds is slowed to allow oxygen concentration to build up. This controlling sensor thus maintains the partial pressure of oxygen in the gas being delivered to the user at an adequate level at all altitudes. A second partial pressure sensor, set at about 160 mm Hg (21.3 kPa), acts as a warning device should output from the molecular sieve fail altogether (for example, following an engine flameout), or suddenly fall below that required for adequate oxygenation at high altitude (for example, following a rapid decompression), or if there is a failure within the concentrator itself.

Activation of the warning sensor automatically selects the delivery of 100% oxygen from a seat-mounted back-up store of gaseous oxygen. The same store acts as the emergency oxygen supply in

the event of ejection. Since the in-flight emergencies (flameout and rapid decompression) are potentially recoverable, however, a unique feature of the back-up system is that it can be turned off: the initiation of all other conventional emergency oxygen systems in combat aircraft commit the pilot to an immediate descent to below 10000 feet, with obvious operational implications. Thus if the pilot achieves an engine relight after a flameout, the molecular sieve will once again concentrate oxygen and the flight can proceed normally. Similarly, once the molecular sieve and mixture controller have responded to the fall in cabin pressure after rapid decompression, gaseous back-up oxygen is no longer required, so the store can be conserved.

Aircraft with high-differential pressure cabins–passenger aircraft

In aircraft with high-differential pressure cabins, the oxygen system provides the second line of defence against hypoxia and is consequently only used should there be a failure of cabin pressurization, or should toxic fumes contaminate the cabin atmosphere.

Because of its advantages, and especially its world-wide availability, oxygen is usually carried in passenger aircraft in gaseous form at high pressure ($1800\,lb/in^2$ ($12\,411\,kPa$)), although liquid oxygen is used in some aircraft, and sodium chlorate candles in others. The oxygen system for the flight-deck crew is usually separate, with the exception of the oxygen store, from that for the cabin staff and passengers; and the main on/off valve, the contents gauge and all the system controls are situated at the flight engineer's position on the flight deck. In gaseous systems, the high-pressure supply is reduced to the working pressures of the flight-deck oxygen regulators (typically 200–$400\,lb/in^2$ (1379–$2758\,kPa$)) and of the ring main for the passenger circuit (typically 70–$100\,lb/in^2$ (483–$690\,kPa$)).

The flight-deck system must ensure that the crew controlling the aircraft and its subsystems are fully oxygenated at all times, since the well-being of the other occupants depends primarily on their ability to initiate and control a rapid descent to a low and safe altitude. Therefore, the system clearly must provide oxygen for the flight-deck crew for as long as the cabin altitude exceeds 8000–10000 feet, and so demand oxygen equipment is usually fitted to these crew stations. If the maximum cabin altitude on rapid decompression cannot exceed 30000–35000 feet, simple suction demand regulators may be fitted, but the regulators are most commonly of the pressure demand type; and these are always fitted when the cabin altitude can exceed 40000 feet following a decompression. A regulator is mounted at each crew position and carries oxygen, via a

wide-bore hose, to the mask which is placed in a purpose-designed stowage unit from which it can be extracted rapidly when required. The oxygen mask is fitted with a harness system by which it can be attached to a communications headset, and a test of the adequacy of this attachment often forms part of the pre-flight checks (but *see also* Chapter 32). In the event of a rapid decompression, the crew are required to don their oxygen masks, usually within 3–5 seconds, and to continue to use the equipment for as long as the cabin altitude remains above 8000–10000 feet. In certain circumstances, flying regulations require the watch-keeping members of the flight-deck crew to be wearing oxygen masks whenever the aircraft is above a specified altitude such as 43000 feet. The oxygen equipment is also used to protect the respiratory tract if toxic fumes are detected within the cabin.

The performance required of an oxygen system for passenger use is less demanding although, as discussed earlier, oxygen must be available for all passengers when the cabin altitude exceeds 15000 feet, and for a proportion of the passengers (10%) whenever the cabin altitude is between 10000 and 15000 feet. In practice, this means that all passenger aircraft that operate at altitudes above 25000–35000 feet are fitted with a passenger oxygen system. The maximum altitude at which aircraft that are not fitted with an oxygen system for passengers are allowed to operate depends upon the rate of descent that can be achieved following a decompression, and may vary according to national regulations: in the United Kingdom, this maximum altitude is 13000 feet.

The oxygen supply for passengers is usually

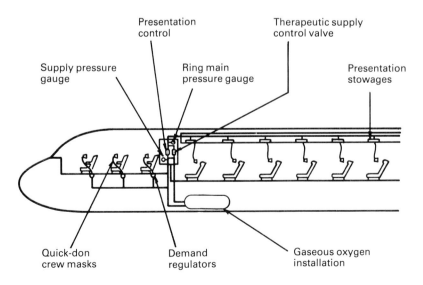

Figure 7.27 Typical arrangement of an oxygen ring-main system on board a large passenger aircraft.

carried around the cabin by means of a ring main (*Figure 7.27*), which feeds the individual mask presentation units.

Pressure in the ring main is controlled automatically so that, should the cabin altitude exceed a predetermined level of between 10000 and 14000 feet, the pressure is increased to about 80 lb/in^2 (552 kPa). This rise in pressure sounds an alarm on the flight deck, opens the doors of the mask presentation units so that the masks drop in front of the passengers, and provides a high flow of oxygen when the passenger pulls the mask onto the face. The flow of oxygen after the aircraft has descended to low altitude can be reduced or turned off by the flight engineer, who can also control the pressure in the ring main manually. Portable (walk-around) oxygen sets, or additional outlets from the ring main, are provided in passenger aircraft for therapeutic purposes; and the cabin staff can use the walk-around sets to provide assistance to passengers when the cabin altitude exceeds 10000 feet (*see Figure 7.17*). Such walk-around/ therapeutic oxygen sets often provide two levels of oxygen flow: a 2.01 (NTP)/min level for use at altitudes below 18000 feet and a 4.01 (NTP)/min level for use at altitudes above 18000 feet. Finally, masks for the cabin crew are, like passenger masks, usually of the continuous flow reservoir type.

Pressure clothing

Aircrew operating modern combat aircraft are normally protected against the hazards of high altitude by a combination of cabin pressurization and a personal oxygen system. In certain circumstances, however, when operating at extreme altitudes, additional personal protection is provided by means of pressure clothing. Such garments are normally worn uninflated and are pressurized only if the cabin altitude exceeds a certain level or if it is necessary to abandon the aircraft at high altitude (above 40000 feet). The extent of this form of emergency equipment ranges from a full pressure suit, which applies pressure to the whole man, to partial pressure garments which pressurize the respiratory tract together with a greater or lesser part of the external surface of the body. Pressure breathing equipment which, via an oronasal mask, pressurizes only the respiratory tract may be considered as the simplest example of partial pressure protection. Full pressure suits are also employed in space flight to provide protection against exposure to the vacuum of space either as a result of a failure of the sealed cabin of the spacecraft or during extra-vehicular activity (*see also* Chapter 32).

In most circumstances, the crew of an aircraft flying at high altitude will initiate an immediate emergency descent in the event of a failure of cabin pressurization. Operational considerations may, however, dictate that a military aircraft must remain at high altitude until the mission is completed. Thus pressure clothing may be used either to provide the wearer with the short-term protection needed to enable a descent to be made to an altitude where such protection is no longer required, or to provide long-term protection so that the aircraft and its crew can remain safely at high altitude.

The major physiological effects of exposure to high altitude are hypoxia, decompression sickness, and hypothermia: effects described in detail in Chapters 5, 3 and 18 respectively. It will be recalled that severe and unacceptable hypoxia occurs within a few seconds of exposure to altitudes above 40000–43000 feet, even when 100% oxygen is breathed. Consequently, protection against hypoxia must be provided whether the duration of exposure to such altitudes is short or long. The relative importance of the other effects, however, depends upon the duration of exposure. Thus a short exposure to high altitude is very unlikely to give rise to serious decompression sickness; and short-term exposure to low environmental temperatures will likewise not cause serious impairment of performance or serious damage to subjects wearing normal aircrew clothing. But if exposure to altitudes above 25000 feet lasts longer than about 5–10 minutes, the risk of developing decompression sickness increases markedly. Similarly, if exposure to temperatures below about −34°C lasts more than a few minutes, uncovered skin will suffer cold thermal injury and general hypothermia may develop. Accordingly, protection against hypoxia, decompression sickness and cold is essential above an altitude of about 25000 feet. Only if there is a reasonable chance that, by virtue of a rapid descent or an ejection, exposure will be limited to a period of less than 2–5 minutes can additional protection against decompression sickness and cold be omitted. These considerations lead to the following conclusions:

1. Prolonged physiological protection against the effects of exposure to very high altitudes can be attained only by means of a garment which maintains a pressure equal to or greater than 282 mm Hg (37.6 kPa) absolute around the body (to prevent hypoxia and decompression sickness), and to which heat can be supplied (to maintain a satisfactory thermal environment). The only form of garment which can fulfil these requirements is a full pressure suit.
2. If the aircraft is able to descend rapidly, however, protection is only needed against hypoxia. In this situation, a full pressure suit is once again the ideal solution since it applies the required pressure evenly to the respiratory tract and to the whole of the external surface of the

body. Pressure differences between different parts of the body do not occur, therefore, and so no serious physiological disturbances arise in either the cardiovascular or the respiratory systems. A full pressure suit is bulky and all-enveloping, however, and impairs routine flying even when uninflated: for this reason, partial pressure garments provide a useful and attractive alternative.

Full pressure suits

Physiological and general requirements

The distinguishing feature of a full pressure suit is that it applies pressure evenly to the entire body surface. The magnitude of the applied pressure is determined by the need to protect against both hypoxia and decompression sickness.

Severe hypoxia can be prevented by delivering 100% oxygen to the respiratory tract and maintaining an absolute pressure within the suit of at least 141 mm Hg (18.8 kPa). But since the suit is also worn in conditions where it is also necessary to prevent decompression sickness, the absolute pressure within the garment should ideally not be less than 282 mm Hg (37.6 kPa): that is, equivalent to an altitude of 25 000 feet or below. However, experience has shown that an absolute pressure within the suit equivalent to an altitude of 30 000 feet (226 mm Hg (30.1 kPa)) is sufficient to prevent serious decompression sickness in seated aircrew, provided that the duration of exposure is no longer than 4–5 hours. If the pressure within the suit is less than 226 mm Hg (30.1 kPa) serious decompression sickness may occur, the severity being directly related to the altitude and duration of exposure. In practice, therefore, the absolute pressure in a full pressure suit may range from as low as 141 mm Hg (18.8 kPa) for short-duration protection, to as high as 282 mm Hg (37.6 kPa) when protection is required for several hours.

Some full pressure suits are inflated with air, oxygen being delivered to the respiratory tract via an oronasal mask mounted within the helmet (*see* below). Consequently, if the suit operating pressure is at the lower end of the range (that is, 141 mm Hg (18.8 kPa)), any inward leakage of air due to a poorly fitting mask will cause severe hypoxia: a risk that is clearly reduced if the pressure in the suit is higher.

Although, if necessary, heat can be *delivered* to a full pressure suit by various means (including ventilation with hot air, electric heating or circulation of heated liquid), its pressure-containing layer is impermeable and the garment therefore imposes a considerable heat load. Consequently, a means of *removing* metabolic heat and perspiration must be

provided throughout the period during which the suit is worn. It is necessary, however, to take special precautions to avoid freezing of valves by the passage through them of moist gas, and to avoid misting of the helmet visor.

When unpressurized, a full pressure suit should not place restrictions on posture or functional movements, and it must provide an efficient oxygen and intercommunication system. It must be compatible with the aircraft escape system, and it should afford protection against any hostile ground environment that is likely to be encountered after leaving the aircraft. Finally, the pressure helmet should also provide some protection against noise and glare.

Technical considerations

Full pressure suits usually consist of an impermeable inner layer of pressure-containing material with an outer retaining layer which prevents over-expansion on pressurization. It is very difficult to match the characteristics of a flexible inflated system to the shape of the human body, and to match the mechanical design of the suit to the natural movement of human joints. Movement is resisted both by friction and by the force required to expel gas from the appropriate part of the suit, and delicate manipulative movements of the fingers may have to be combined with large forces at the shoulder, elbow and wrist.

Consequently, there are many problems associated with the design and construction of full pressure suits, particularly the tendency of the suit to become rigid when it is inflated, with subsequent reduction in mobility, especially at the neck, shoulder and wrist; and the marked tendency of the headpiece to rise from the trunk of the garment. Although the movement of joints may be improved by the use of lightweight metal and gas-tight rotating bearings, the bulk, weight and additional restrictions that these impose limit the value of the full pressure suit as a flying garment in conventional aviation, even when modern fabric manufacturing techniques have been used to reduce the problems of general rigidity.

To maintain the thermal balance of a crewman wearing a full pressure suit, a large ventilating flow of gas is required beneath the impermeable layer, even when the suit is not inflated. Air is taken from the engines to provide gas for ventilation and pressurization, while an oxygen-rich supply for breathing is delivered through an oronasal mask or a helmet. Such suits therefore effectively have two separate gas compartments: one for conditioning and pressurization, and one for the breathing supply. The pressure differential between these compartments must be kept very small to avoid

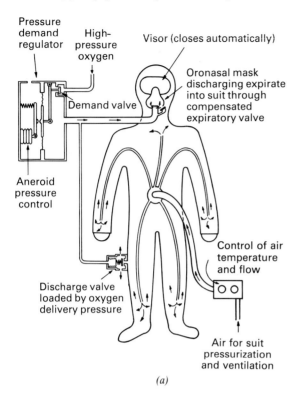

Pressure demand regulator

High-pressure oxygen

Visor (closes automatically)

Demand valve

Oronasal mask discharging expirate into suit through compensated expiratory valve

Aneroid pressure control

Discharge valve loaded by oxygen delivery pressure

Control of air temperature and flow

Air for suit pressurization and ventilation

(a)

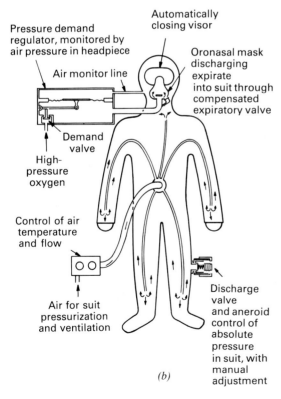

Automatically closing visor

Pressure demand regulator, monitored by air pressure in headpiece

Air monitor line

Oronasal mask discharging expirate into suit through compensated expiratory valve

Demand valve

High-pressure oxygen

Control of air temperature and flow

Air for suit pressurization and ventilation

Discharge valve and aneroid control of absolute pressure in suit, with manual adjustment

(b)

positive or negative pressure breathing. Furthermore, in order to prevent air being drawn into an ill-fitting mask from the remainder of the suit, the pressure within the former must not fall below that of the air inflating the latter. Expired gas from the respiratory tract may be passed either into the air compartment of the suit, or directly to the exterior. There are two common methods of pressure control in full pressure suits, as illustrated in *Figure 7.28*.

In the first method, termed an *oxygen pressure control system (Figure 7.28(a))*, a pressure demand regulator is used to produce the desired absolute pressure in the oxygen compartment of the suit. This oxygen pressure is itself then used to control the air outlet valves so that the desired pressure differential is maintained between the two compartments of the suit. In the second method, termed an *air control system (Figure 7.28(b))*, the pressure of the air in the suit is controlled by a barometrically operated outlet valve. A relatively simple demand valve can then be used to deliver oxygen to the breathing compartment since the absolute pressure delivered by the oxygen regulator is determined solely by the air pressure in the suit.

Finally, in space, where clearly no engine air source is available, and where the astronaut or cosmonaut may leave the spacecraft, a closed-circuit system is required. Breathing gas is circulated around the body, and a backpack unit is employed to remove carbon dioxide, water vapour, heat and odour; and to add the necessary amounts of oxygen to the system. Thermal balance is maintained by a liquid-cooling garment worn under the pressure suit next to the skin (*see also* Chapter 32).

Partial pressure garments and assemblies

Partial pressure garments are less restrictive than full pressure suits and so offer considerable advantages where short-term protection against the effects of hypoxia is all that is required. The basic principle of partial pressure garments is to apply external pressure to parts of the body in order to balance the physiological effects of pressurizing the respiratory tract (*see* Chapter 6). From the physiological

Figure 7.28 Methods of pressure control of breathing oxygen and ventilating air in full pressure suits. (*a*) *Oxygen pressure control system*. The oxygen regulator delivers gas to the oxygen compartment of the suit (oronasal mask) at the required absolute pressure. The pressure of air in the air compartment of the suit (head, trunk and limbs) is controlled by the oxygen pressure fed to the air discharge valve. (*b*) *Air control system*. An aneroid-operated discharge valve controls the pressure of air in the air compartment, and this in turn controls the pressure at which gas is delivered by the oxygen regulator to the oxygen compartment of the suit.

standpoint, the ideal solution is to apply counter-pressure to as much of the body as possible. The advantages of the 'partial' principle, however—(low thermal load, less restriction when unpressurized and greater mobility when pressurized—make it desirable that counterpressure should be applied to the minimum area of the body. Thus the proportion of the body covered by partial pressure garments represents a compromise between physiological ideal and operational expediency. Furthermore, since partial pressure assemblies for high altitude protection are used only for very short exposures, certain compromises with regard to the presence of a moderate degree of hypoxia are also acceptable. Some practical pressure breathing systems, incorporating partial pressure assemblies of increasing complexity and effectiveness, are described below. This discussion does not, however, cover the use of partial pressure garments to provide counterpressure when using pressure breathing as a means of enhancing tolerance to high sustained $+G_z$ accelerations (*see* Chapter 11).

Mask alone

An oronasal mask can deliver oxygen under pressure to the respiratory tract, although there are both physiological and mechanical limitations to using this technique for pressure breathing. Pressures of up to 100 mm Hg (13.3 kPa) can be delivered without significant leakage around the edge of the mask if a reflected edge seal is present: *see Figure 7.15*. In order to achieve this pressure, the tension applied to the mask by means of the harness attaching it to the helmet must be such that it counterbalances the force tending to lift the mask off the face when the delivery pressure is raised. A tension of 6 kgf (58.8 N) is necessary to seal a pressure of 40 mm Hg (5.3 kPa) in the type of Royal Air Force pressure demand oronasal mask illustrated in *Figure 7.14*. Since such a high tension is neither tolerable nor necessary during routine flight, a manual or automatic means of increasing the tension when required is incorporated in the suspension harness. In the mask illustrated (*see Figure 7.14*), this is achieved manually by rotating a toggle over the suspension bar in order to tension the chain harness.

The maximum breathing pressure that can be tolerated using a mask alone (that is, without counterpressure to the body) is about 30 mm Hg (4.0 kPa). If an alveolar oxygen tension of 60 mm Hg (8.0 kPa) is to be maintained (that is, an absolute lung pressure (breathing pressure + environmental pressure) of 141 mm Hg (18.8 kPa)), then this system will provide respiratory protection to an altitude of 45 000 feet. It is practical, however, to accept a greater degree of hypoxia than that associated with an alveolar oxygen tension of

60 mm Hg (8.0 kPa). A breathing pressure of 30 mm Hg (4.0 kPa) at 50 000 feet provides an absolute lung pressure of 117 mm Hg (15.6 kPa) and an alveolar oxygen tension of 45–50 mm Hg (6.0–6.7 kPa). Although this degree of hypoxia gives rise to very marked impairment of performance if it is experienced for any length of time, it is acceptable if a rapid descent is initiated immediately. Typically, the oxygen regulator used in this type of system delivers pressure breathing at altitudes above 40 000 feet, with the breathing pressure increasing from 0.75–7.5 mm Hg (0.1–1.0 kPa) at 40 000 feet to about 30–34.5 mm Hg (4.0–4.6 kPa) at 50 000 feet. Between the altitudes of 40 000 feet and 50 000 feet, breathing pressure increases linearly with the decrease in environmental pressure. The absolute pressure in the respiratory tract therefore falls progressively above 40 000 feet, and produces a gradual increase in the intensity of the hypoxia. Above 50 000 feet, the hypoxia is very severe and unconsciousness supervenes rapidly.

This type of pressure breathing system is widely used throughout the world. The combination of a pressure breathing mask and a suitable oxygen regulator (capable of delivering a pressure of 30–34.5 mm Hg (4.0–4.6 kPa) at 50 000 feet) will provide protection for one minute against the effects of loss of cabin pressurization up to cabin altitudes

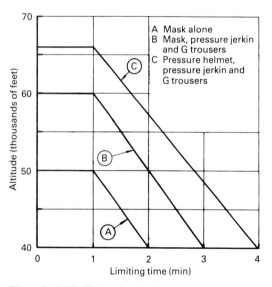

Figure 7.29 The limits of protection against hypoxia provided by pressure breathing systems employing:

(A) A pressure breathing mask alone (maximum breathing pressure of 30–34.5 mm Hg (4.0–4.6 kPa).
(B) A pressure breathing mask with counterpressure to the trunk and lower limbs (maximum breathing pressure of 68–72 mm Hg (9.1–9.6 kPa)).
(C) A partial pressure helmet with counterpressure to the trunk and lower limbs (maximum breathing pressure of 107–110 mm Hg (14.3–14.7 kPa)).

50 000 feet, provided that immediate descent at the maximum rate (10 000 feet/min) is then undertaken to below 40 000 feet. The degree of protection afforded by this system is shown diagrammatically in *Figure 7.29* (curve A).

Mask with trunk and lower limb counterpressure

The most important area of the body to which counterpressure should be applied is the trunk. In the Royal Air Force system, which incorporates both trunk and lower limb counterpressure, full use is made of the pressure sealing properties of current oronasal masks, and a maximum breathing pressure of 70 mm Hg (9.3 kPa) is employed. Trunk counterpressure is applied by a partial pressure jerkin (*Figure 7.30*) which comprises a rubber bladder restrained by an outer inextensible cover.

The bladder extends not only over the whole of the trunk, but also over the upper parts of the thighs to ensure that there is adequate counterpressure over the inguinal canals and avoid the risk of herniation at high breathing pressures. The bladder is inflated to the same pressure as that delivered to the respiratory tract, but pressure breathing at 70 mm Hg (9.3 kPa) with counterpressure to the trunk alone may induce syncope as a consequence of the large displacement of blood to all four limbs.

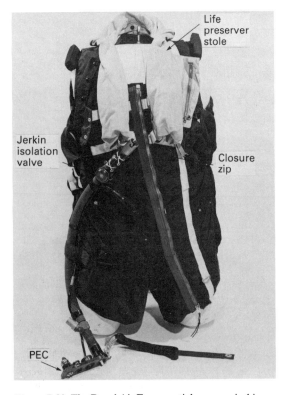

Figure 7.30 The Royal Air Force partial pressure jerkin.

This circulatory disturbance can be reduced by applying counterpressure to the lower limbs via G trousers. Both the jerkin and the G trousers may be inflated at the same pressure, or the latter may be inflated to a greater pressure than that being delivered to the jerkin and mask. There is evidence to suggest that by increasing the pressure within the G trousers to three or four times that in the breathing/trunk counterpressure system, the extent of bladder coverage the counterpressure garment must incorporate for adequate protection at pressure breathing levels up to 70 mm Hg (9.3 kPa) can be drastically reduced (and with it the bulk and weight of the garment) with few additional cardio-respiratory penalties.

If the absolute pressure within the lungs is maintained at 141 mm Hg (18.8 kPa), the mask/partial pressure jerkin/G trousers combination will provide ideal protection to a maximum altitude of 54 000 feet. In practice, however, a certain degree of hypoxia is acceptable, and a breathing pressure of 68–72 mm Hg (9.1–9.6 kPa) can be employed at 60 000 feet, where it will provide an absolute pressure in the lungs of 122–126 mm Hg (16.3–16.8 kPa), and an alveolar oxygen tension of 55–60 mm Hg (7.3–8.0 kPa). The combination of the discomfort of a high breathing pressure in the mask and a certain degree of hypoxia limits the duration of protection afforded by this ensemble. The limit, shown diagrammatically in *Figure 7.29* (curve B), is an interval of 60 seconds at 60 000 feet followed immediately by descent at a rate of at least 10 000 feet/min to 40 000 feet.

Partial pressure helmet with trunk and lower limb counterpressure

In this system, a partial pressure helmet is the means by which pressure is delivered to the respiratory tract, while a jerkin provides trunk counterpressure, and the G trousers provide lower limb counterpressure to reduce the circulatory disturbance induced by high breathing pressures.

The partial pressure helmet is an alternative device for applying positive pressure to the respiratory tract when the pressure at which oxygen is to be breathed exceeds the physiological limits associated with the use of an oronasal mask (*see* Chapter 6). Partial pressure helmets give support to the cheeks, to the floor of the mouth, to the eyes, and to most of the head so eliminating the uncomfortable pressure differentials that develop between the air passages and the skin of the head and neck when an oronasal mask is employed. In most current partial pressure helmets, counterpressure is also applied by oxygen bladders to a limited area of the upper neck but, although the extent of this coverage ensures reasonable head mobility during routine flying, severe neck discomfort may occur during pressure breathing at levels greater than 110 mm Hg (14.7 kPa).

Physiologically, the pressure demand oxygen regulator used with this assembly need only provide an absolute pressure of 141 mm Hg (18.8 kPa) at altitudes above 40 000 feet. In practice, however, the regulator used in the Royal Air Force system can deliver a maximum breathing pressure of 107–110 mm Hg (14.3–14.7 kPa) at 66 000 feet so providing an absolute pressure in the lungs at that altitude of 148–151 mm Hg (19.6–20.1 kPa). The partial pressure helmet/partial pressure jerkin/G trousers ensemble may therefore be used up to a maximum altitude of 66 000 feet, where it will provide protection for up to one minute provided that descent to 40 000 feet follows within a further 3 minutes (*see Figure 7.29* (curve C)).

Pressure helmet with trunk and upper and lower limb counterpressure

It is clearly physiologically advantageous to include the upper limbs in the areas to which counterpressure is applied, and a wide variety of garments have been employed to provide this extensive coverage in combination with a pressure helmet. Many garments, such as those used in Royal Air Force systems, make use of oxygen-filled bladders which cover the body surface to varying degrees. Others, such as the United States Air Force 'capstan' partial pressure garment, utilize a mixture of fabric tensioning by means of capstans and gas-filled bladders (*see* below). The pressure helmets employed vary from the Royal Air Force partial pressure helmet described above (and in which pressure is applied only to the face, part of the head, and the upper neck), to the United States Air Force version in which gas is applied to the whole of the head and neck. Typical combinations include the following:

1. An ensemble comprising the Royal Air Force partial pressure helmet, a sleeved partial pressure jerkin, and G trousers. This system does not apply counterpressure to the lower neck, the axillae, the elbows, the hands, the knees, the ankles or the feet.
2. An ensemble which comprises the Royal Air Force partial pressure helmet and a combined partial pressure suit/air-ventilated suit/G trousers. This single garment consists of one bladder within a fabric restraint layer which covers the trunk, the upper limbs to the wrists, and the lower limbs to the ankles. Separate bladders for the G trousers and a separate air distribution harness are incorporated in the suit.
3. An ensemble that comprises the United States Air Force pressure helmet and capstan partial pressure suit. Counterpressure to the body is applied primarily by the inflation of capstan tubes which are attached externally to the fabric of a close-fitting garment. The capstans are inflated to a pressure five times that of the breathing pressure to produce the appropriate increase in fabric tension. The suit also incorporates a torso bladder which is inflated with oxygen to the level of breathing pressure, but counterpressure is not applied to the axillae or to the hands and feet; although pressurized gloves may be worn as separate items.
4. An ensemble that comprises the United States Air Force pressure helmet and a partial pressure garment. The latter has an oxygen-inflated, one-piece bladder which covers the same areas of the body as the Royal Air Force combined suit (*see* 2 above).

Virtually all of these systems employ oxygen regulators which maintain an absolute pressure in the respiratory tract, and over the pressurized areas of the body, of 145–150 mm Hg (19.3–20.0 kPa). Such combinations will provide prolonged protection against the effects of hypoxia on exposure to altitudes well above 40 000 feet: for example, protection is possible for 30 minutes at 65 000–70 000 feet, and for several minutes at 100 000 feet. Protection against decompression sickness and the effects of low temperature is not provided.

Further reading

ERNSTING, J. (1979) An advanced oxygen system for future combat aircraft. In *Recent Advances in Aeronautical and Space Medicine*. Conference Proceedings CP-265, pp. 2–152–17. Neuilly sur Seine: AGARD/NATO.

ERNSTING, J. (1984) Operational and physiological requirements for aircraft oxygen systems. In *Seventh Advanced Operational Aviation Medicine Course*. Report No. 697, pp. 1–1 to 1–10. Neuilly sur Seine: AGARD/NATO.

ERNSTING, J. (1984) Molecular sieve on board oxygen generating systems for high performance aircraft. In *Seventh Advanced Operational Aviation Medicine Course*. Report No. 697, pp. 3–1 to 3–14. Neuilly sur Seine: AGARD/NATO.

MACMILLAN, A.J.F. (1984) The performance and deficiencies of oxygen systems fitted to current NATO interceptor aircraft. In *Seventh Advanced Operational Aviation Medicine Course*. Report No. 697, pp. 2–1 to 2–7. Neuilly sur Seine: AGARD/NATO.

AIR STANDARDIZATION COORDINATING COMMITTEE (1982) *The Minimum Physiological design Requirements for Aircrew Breathing Systems*. Air Standardization Co-ordinating Committee Air Standard 61/22, Washington, DC.

8

The pressure cabin

A.J.F. Macmillan

Introduction

The physiological disturbances induced by exposure to the low environmental pressures encountered during flight at high altitude must be reduced to a minimum. The most effective way of providing protection against these effects is to raise artificially the pressure in the crew and passenger compartments above that of the immediate environment of the aircraft. Thus the crew and passenger compartments of virtually all modern high-performance combat and transport aircraft are pressurized with air. At first sight there would appear to be great advantages in maintaining the absolute pressure in the cabin at one atmosphere (760 mm Hg) throughout flight. Such a requirement would, however, impose considerable penalties with regard to the weight of the pressure cabin and the pressurization equipment, the power required to pressurize the air and hence the performance of the aircraft. Furthermore, the larger the pressure differential across the wall of a cabin the greater the risk of damage to the aircraft and its occupants in the event of a failure of the structure. In practice, compromises are made between the physiological ideal of a cabin pressure of one atmosphere absolute, the weight and performance penalties of a high cabin-pressure differential and the probability of explosive failure of the cabin. The compromises that have been adopted in the design of pressure cabins can be classified into two groups. Where comfort is of prime concern and the probability of structural damage to the aircraft is very remote, the pressure in the cabin is maintained at a level at which the occupants can breathe air throughout flight. In combat aircraft, where weight is at a premium and there is a risk of failure of the integrity of the cabin due to enemy action, a much lower level of pressurization of the cabin is adopted; the occupants breathe oxygen or an oxygen/air mixture.

There are two methods of maintaining the pressure in the cabin of aircraft above that of the immediate environment. The conventional method, used in virtually all currrent aircraft, is to draw air from outside the aircraft, compress it and deliver it into the cabin. The desired pressure is maintained within the cabin by controlling the flow of compressed gas out of the cabin to the atmosphere. The continuous flow of air ventilates the compartment and, in most aircraft, this flow of air also controls the thermal environment within the cabin, so that the control of pressure and of temperature are closely related. At very high altitudes, the energy required to compress the low-density air to the pressure required in the cabin and the heat generated in the process of compression become excessive. It is impracticable to pressurize the cabin with external air during sustained flights at altitudes above about 80 000 feet. In these circumstances, and in the vacuum of space, the pressurizing gases must be carried within the vehicle. It then becomes uneconomic to condition the cabin with a through-flow of gas which escapes to the environment. Used gases are recycled and loss of gas is reduced to a minimum. The 'sealed' cabin is discussed in Chapter 32. Here we deal with the conventional pressure cabin.

The difference between the absolute pressure within and that of the atmosphere immediately outside an aircraft is termed the cabin differential pressure. The differential pressure is frequently controlled so that it varies with aircraft altitude. Although the pressure in the cabin is generally greater than that of the atmosphere at the aircraft altitude (that is, positive differential) it can, in certain circumstances (for example, during a rapid dive) be less (negative). The absolute pressure in an aircraft cabin is almost always stated in terms of pressure altitude (feet above mean sea level) in accordance with the International Standard Atmosphere (ICAO) scale. The absolute pressure in the cabin equals the sum of the atmospheric pressure and the cabin differential pressure. Thus the cabin pressure of an aircraft flying at an altitude of 25 000 feet (atmospheric pressure, 5.5 lb/in^2 (38 kPa)) with a cabin differential pressure of 4.5 lb/in^2 (31 kPa) gauge is 10.0 lb/in^2 (69 kPa) absolute, which is equivalent to an altitude of 10 200 feet.

Physiological requirements

Three main groups of physiological factors must be considered when defining the requirements for a pressure cabin. The first group are the factors that determine the maximum acceptable cabin altitude: hypoxia, decompression sickness and expansion of gastro-intestinal gas. The second group determines the maximum acceptable rate of change of cabin altitude during ascent and descent of the aircraft: the ventilation of the middle ear cavities and the paranasal sinuses. The third group of factors relate to the magnitude of the effects of a sudden cabin failure.

Hypoxia

The cabin altitude acceptable in an aircraft in which the occupants breathe air is set by considerations of the effects of mild hypoxia on the performance of the aircrew and on the well-being of the passengers.

At altitudes greater than 10 000 to 12 000 feet there is a significant impairment of ability to perform flight tasks; indeed, individuals are detectably slower to react to a novel situation when they are breathing air at an altitude of 8000 feet; at 5000 feet there is just detectable impairment of this type of performance. There is growing acceptance of the fact that the maximum cabin altitude consistent with flight safety is 5000–7000 feet rather than the previously standard 8000 feet. Certain individuals, particularly those suffering from cardiorespiratory disease, may be unable to maintain full oxygenation of tissues above 6000 feet (a matter of considerable importance in civil transport aircraft where passengers cannot be selected for the integrity of their respiratory and cardiovascular systems). Exposure of the standard passenger population to cabin altitudes of the order of 8000 feet for several hours results in noticeable fatigue and sporadic incidents of heart failure which are probably induced by the combination of mild hypoxia, expansion of abdominal gas, lack of movement and the seated posture.

Limitation of the cabin altitude to a maximum of 6000 feet has been shown to eliminate most of these incidents.

If the inspired air is progressively enriched with oxygen, the alveolar oxygen tension (Po_2) may be maintained at the value associated with normal air breathing at sea level up to 33 000 feet. The hypoxia induced in a man breathing 100% oxygen at 40 000 feet is equivalent to that produced when he breathes air at 8000 feet. Since the latter was generally recognized as the maximum degree of hypoxia acceptable, it could be argued that, given 100% oxygen, the cabin altitude could be allowed to rise to 40 000 feet. But this argument ignores the effects of possible malfunction or failure of the oxygen delivery system. The rate at which impairment of judgement and performance develop in a man who has to revert to breathing air increases rapidly above 20 000 feet. Thus the time available to an individual to recognize that his oxygen supply has ceased and to carry out the appropriate corrective action falls from 10–12 minutes at 20 000 feet to 3–5 minutes at 25 000 feet and 1–1.5 minutes at 33 000 feet. Furthermore, the reduction of inspired Po_2 produced by a given fractional inboard leak of air due to an ill-fitting breathing mask increases with rise of altitude. In practice, the incidence and severity of hypoxia become significant at a cabin altitude of about 22 000 feet and rises markedly above that; so that 20 000–22 000 feet is now regarded at the standard limit for regular operations by crews breathing supplemental oxygen. However, some aircraft with a 25 000 feet cabin remain in service in air forces all over the world.

Decompression sickness

Although decompression sickness can occur, when individuals are exposed to an altitude of 18 000 feet, it is very rare below 22 000 feet. A significant, although small number of cases have occurred during exposure to altitudes between 22 000 and 25 000 feet. Since decompression sickness during routine flights is unacceptable, the maximum cabin altitude to which aircrew may be exposed should not exceed 22 000 feet. In some circumstances it may be necessary for aircrew to operate at cabin altitudes as high as 25 000 feet, but unless susceptible individuals are protected by pre-oxygenation occasional cases of decompression sickness will occur.

Expansion of gastrointestinal gas

Gas within the gastrointestinal tract, which expands because of reduction of environmental pressure, only rarely gives rise to anything more than transient discomfort in fit aircrew, provided that the maximum altitude does not exceed 25 000–28 000 feet. Passengers suffering from cardiorespiratory disorders, on the other hand, may be distressed even by the relatively small increase in the volume of gas in the abdomen produced by ascent from ground level to 8000 feet. The maximum cabin altitude of passenger and aeromedical evacuation aircraft should, therefore, be kept as low as possible, certainly below 8000 feet.

Rates of change of cabin altitude

High rates of ascent to altitude, for example 5000–20 000 feet per minute, are very well tolerated, but descent is another matter. The difficulty of equilibration to ambient of the pressures in the middle ear cavities and paranasal sinuses limits the maximum acceptable rate of increase of cabin altitude during descent. A pressure change of $2\,lb/in^2$ $(14\,kPa)$/minute is the maximum that should be permitted for military aircraft if otic or sinus barotrauma is to be avoided. Sudden alterations of descent rates are also undesirable. Inexperienced passengers, who are not trained in the techniques of inflation of the middle ears during descent, will complain of ear discomfort if the rate of increase of cabin pressure (from the 6000–8000 feet maximum altitude) to ground level exceeds about $0.25\,lb/in^2$ $(1.7\,kPa)$/minute that is, 5000 feet/minute. The maximum rate of increase of cabin pressure adopted for most civil passenger aircraft is $0.15\,lb/in^2$ $(1\,kPa)$/minute that is, 300 feet/minute.

Decompression of the pressure cabin

The risk of damage to the occupants of a pressure cabin in the event of a sudden failure of its integrity increases in proportion to the ratio of the area of the defect in the wall to the volume of the cabin and to the ratio of cabin pressures before and immediately after the decompression. The cabins of transport aircraft are designed so that the ratio of the area of the maximum size of defect that could occur in the wall (for example, the loss of a window) to the volume of the cabin is as small as possible. Accesses of larger area—such as doors and hatches—are designed to open inwards. The maximum probable defect will not therefore produce a dangerous rate of decompression, even when the cabin pressure differential is as high as $10–12\,lb/in^2$ $(69–83\,kPa)$ unless there is a major structural failure which would probably destroy the aircraft. In military aircraft, however, battle damage or jettison of a canopy from a small volume cabin could lead to very rapid decompression. To limit the effects of this, the

differential does not normally exceed $4–5\,lb/in^2$ $(28–35\,kPa)$. However, in some combat aircraft a dual differential pressure facility has been adopted in the past. Thus in cruise or patrol conditions a high differential pressure $(8–9\,lb/in^2$ $(55–62\,kPa))$ can be selected thereby permitting aircrew to dispense with wearing oxygen equipment. Reduction of the differential pressure to $4–5\,lb/in^2$ $(28–35\,kPa)$ in danger zones minimizes the effects of sudden loss of cabin pressure but enforces the use of oxygen in combat.

Pressurization schedules

The relationship between cabin altitude and aircraft altitude is termed the cabin pressurization schedule. By convention this is displayed graphically, with the aircraft and cabin altitudes plotted on linear pressure scales (*Figure 8.1*). A straight line through the origin with a slope of 1.0 represents the relationship between cabin and aircraft altitudes when there is no pressurization. A set of straight lines parallel to the zero pressurization curve depicts various constant cabin differential pressures. It is convenient to recognize three types of relationship between cabin and aircraft altitudes. The cabin altitude may be controlled at a constant value over a

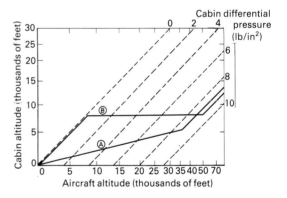

Figure 8.1 Typical pressurization schedules of the high-differential cabins of (1) a passenger aircraft (curve A) and (2) a combat aircraft (curve B). The cabin and aircraft altitudes are plotted on linear pressure scales. The zero pressurization curve (marked $0\,lb/in^2$) passes through the origin and has a slope of 1.0. Constant differential pressures of 2, 4, 6, 8 and $10\,lb/in^2$ (14, 28, 55 and 70 kPa) are indicated by broken lines. The cabin pressurization of the passenger aircraft (curve A) commences at ground level and the maximum differential pressure $(8.8\,lb/in^2$ $(60\,kPa)$ in this example) is reached at 36 000 feet. Contrastingly, in the combat aircraft (curve B) pressurization does not commence until an aircraft altitude of 8000 ft, and the cabin altitude is held at this value until the maximum differential pressure $(9.2\,lb/in^2$ $(63\,kPa)$ in this example) is reached at 50 000 feet.

range of aircraft altitudes; this is termed isobaric control. The cabin differential pressure may be controlled to a constant value as the aircraft altitude varies; this is termed differential control. There is also a form of control intermediate between isobaric and differential, in which the differential pressure although changing with aircraft altitude does not do so to such an extent that the cabin altitude remains constant. In practice, these three types of control are often employed over consecutive ranges of altitudes in the same aircraft. The extent to which the pressurization schedule can be varied in flight by the crew also varies. In high-altitude combat aircraft the cabin pressurization schedule is usually entirely under automatic control and the pilot can only switch on or off the preset schedule: in passenger transport aircraft the flight-deck crew can, within certain limits, vary the pressurization schedule during flight.

High-differential passenger cabins

The cabin of passenger-carrying aircraft operating at altitudes above 5000–8000 feet are pressurized so that the occupants can breathe air throughout flight; they can move freely around the cabin and discomfort and fatigue are minimized. The structure of such aircraft is so robust and the reliability of the cabin pressurization systems so high that the risk of a serious decompression of the cabin is no greater than the risk of other forms of major structural failure. The physiological considerations require that the cabin altitude shall not exceed 6000 feet (or 8000 feet in aircraft designed some years ago) and that the rate of change of cabin pressure with change of altitude of the aircraft shall be as small as possible; the rate of increase of pressure on descent should not exceed 0.15 lb/in² (1 kPa)/minute (approximately 300 feet/minute).

The maximum cabin differential pressure that is used during normal operation of a passenger aircraft is determined by the physiological requirement and the operational ceiling of the aircraft. When the

aircraft is cruising at an altitude below its operational ceiling, the captain decides whether to select the maximum cabin differential pressure, thus maintaining a very low cabin altitude and increasing comfort, or to allow the cabin altitude to rise to the 6000–8000 feet band, thus minimizing the differential pressure and hence prolonging the fatigue life of the cabin structure (*Table 8.1*).

The rate of change of cabin pressure is kept low and within the maximum for comfort of 0.15–0.25 lb/in² (1–1.7 kPa) (300–500 feet)/minute, by pressurizing the cabin from ground level and prolonging the change of cabin altitude for as long as is practicable, taking account of the rate of change of altitude of the aircraft, the pressure altitude at the airports of departure and arrival, and the cruising altitude for the flight. A typical cabin pressurization profile for the flight of subsonic jet-engined passenger aircraft is depicted by curve A of *Figure 8.1*, whilst the behaviour of aircraft and cabin altitudes throughout a typical flight to an aircraft altitude of 40 000 feet is shown in *Figure 8.2*. In such aircraft the flight-deck crew are able to select the desired aircraft altitude at which pressurization of the cabin commences or ceases, the desired rate of change of cabin altitude and the desired maximum cabin altitude. With these variables selected the pressurization system automatically controls the cabin differential pressure to give the required profile of cabin altitude.

High-differential combat cabins

In military aircraft also, it is an advantage to be able to breathe air and so move freely within the aircraft unencumbered by oxygen equipment. Many bomber aircraft are provided with such a cabin pressurization schedule. To minimize the dangers of rapid decompression when the aircraft is liable to damage due to enemy action, a second cabin pressurization schedule similar to that for low-differential combat cabins is usually available. Since trained combat aircrew can tolerate relatively high rates of change

Table 8.1 Typical cabin pressure differentials of passenger aircraft

Type of aircraft	Maximum operating cabin differential pressure		Maximum aircraft altitude (ft) at which cabin altitude (ft) is:	
	lb/in² gauge	kPa	6000	8000
Turbo-propeller-engined	5.5–7.5	38–52	22 000	25 000
			30 500	35 000
Subsonic jet-engined	8.6–9.0	59.5–62	37 000	44 500
			39 500	47 000
Supersonic jet-engined	10.5–11.2	72.5–77	56 000	78 000
			83 000	—

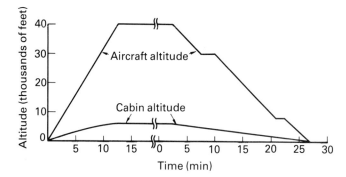

Figure 8.2 The time course of the cabin altitude (lower curve) of a high-differential passenger aircraft during a flight (aircraft altitude, upper curve) up to 40 000 feet and back to ground level.

of cabin pressure (up to $2\,lb/in^2$ ($14\,kPa$)/minute) without discomfort, the control of the cabin pressurization system can be simplified in high-differential combat aircraft by the use of an isobaric control (curve B of *Figure 8.1*). Below a predetermined aircraft altitude, for example 8000 feet, the cabin is unpressurized. Above the aircraft altitude at which cabin pressurization commences, the cabin altitude is held constant until the aircraft altitude at which the maximum operating differential pressure required is reached. Above this altitude the constant maximum differential pressure is maintained so that the cabin altitude rises.

Low-differential combat cabins

In high-performance combat aircraft where weight and performance are primary considerations and there is often a threat to the integrity of the cabin, the crew use oxygen equipment throughout flight and the cabin differential pressure is relatively low. The physiological requirements are that the cabin altitude should not exceed 22 000 feet, in order to minimize the effects of hypoxia due to malfunction or misuse of oxygen equipment and to reduce the incidence of decompression sickness; the maximum cabin differential pressure should not exceed $5.0\,lb/in^2$ gauge ($34.5\,kPa$) in order to reduce the hazard of injury on rapid decompression of the cabin. The maximum cabin differential pressures employed in practice vary between 3.5 and $5.0\,lb/in^2$ (24–$34.5\,kPa$). These differential pressures will prevent the cabin altitude exceeding 22 000 feet at aircraft altitudes of up to 40 000 feet and 57 000 feet respectively. The cabin altitude will not exceed 25 000 feet with differential pressures of 3.5 and $5.0\,lb/in^2$ (24–$34.5\,kPa$) below aircraft altitudes of 46 500 feet and 75 000 feet respectively.

The operation of the cabin pressurization control systems fitted to low-differential cabin combat

aircraft is almost always automatic. Thus cabin pressurization commences at a fixed altitude, the value of which is kept as low as possible in order to minimize rates of change of cabin pressure with ascent and descent of the aircraft but high enough to ensure that the cabin will not be pressurized if the aircraft lands at an airfield with a high elevation. Cabin pressurization generally starts at 5000–8000 feet ambient. An isobaric control schedule may be used until the maximum cabin differential pressure has been achieved. At higher aircraft altitudes this maximum differential is maintained (curve A of *Figure 8.3*). An alternative pressurization schedule (employed in the United Kingdom) allows the cabin differential pressure to increase linearly with reduction of the absolute pressure of

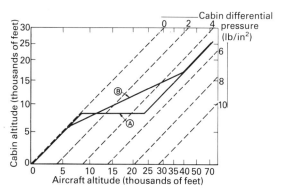

Figure 8.3 Typical pressurization schedules for the low-differential pressure cabins of combat aircraft. The cabin is unpressurized at very low aircraft altitudes. Curve A depicts a schedule in which the differential pressure increases so that the cabin altitude remains constant with further ascent to altitude up to the maximum differential pressure ($5\,lb/in^2$ ($34.5\,kPa$) in this example). Curve B depicts a schedule in which the differential pressure is increased more gradually with ascent to altitude so that the maximum is only operative at aircraft altitudes above 40 000 feet.

the aircraft environment to the maximum differential pressure at about 40 000 feet. Above this height the constant maximum cabin differential pressure is maintained (curve B of *Figure 8.3*). Although the use of isobaric control eliminates changes of cabin altitude over a restricted range of aircraft altitude, the UK schedule results in a significantly lower rate of increase of cabin pressure on descent from high altitude: a distinct advantage when rapid changes of aircraft altitude are required.

Principles of cabin pressurization systems

Source of air

In piston-engined aircraft and some jet-engined aircraft (particularly multi-engined jet aircraft), air for pressurizing and conditioning the cabin is drawn from outside the aircraft and compressed by engine-driven auxiliary compressors. In other jet-engined aircraft, particularly combat aircraft, the air for pressurizing and conditioning the cabin is tapped off the compressor stage of the main engine, upstream of the combustion chambers. In multi-engined aircraft there is generally one auxiliary compressor per main engine; and if directly tapped air is used, it, too, is drawn from each engine. A non-return valve in the duct from each compressed-air source prevents back-flow in the event of a failure of that particular compressor. The flow of air from the engine or compressor is controlled automatically to give the required mass flow of air through the cabin. The total flow of air required is determined primarily by the volume of conditioned air necessary to maintain the desired thermal conditions in the cabin (for the crew, passengers and electronic equipment) and to ventilate the crew and passenger compartments (to remove the carbon dioxide and odours, and replace oxygen). The inflow of air required to maintain the desired differential pressure in the cabin is generally much less than that necessary to condition the cabin. The mass flow of air into the cabin of a two-seat combat aircraft is about 30–40 lb/minute (14–18 kg/minute) (approximately 11 000–15 000 l (NTP)/minute) whilst, in large passenger aircraft, a mass flow of 1.2 lb/passenger/minute (0.55 kg/passenger/minute; 440 l (NTP)/passenger/minute) is commonly employed.

The air passes from the flow controller to the conditioning equipment (heat exchangers and refrigeration system) and through a combined stop valve and non-return valve into the air distribution pipework within the cabin. The non-return valve prevents air escaping from the cabin back through the air supply system in the event of a failure of the source; for example, flameout of the engine of a single-engined aircraft, or rupture of the pipework or conditioning equipment. This valve ensures that the air in the cabin is held there if there should be a complete failure of the supply, so preventing a catastrophic loss of cabin pressure and thus minimizing the increase of cabin altitude in this type of emergency. The stop-valve in the cabin air inlet can be operated from the cockpit to cut off the inflow of air should it be contaminated with smoke or oil. In many aircraft, when the airflow from the engines or compressor is shut off, a ram air inlet to the cabin automatically opens so that it is ventilated with uncontaminated external air. In some aircraft this flow of air into the cabin may be greatly increased in an emergency. This facility, which limits the rise of cabin altitude when there is a large leak, is termed 'flood flow'.

Discharge valve and pressure controller

The air flows out of the cabin through one or more discharge valves, which impose a restriction so as to create the desired cabin differential pressure. The degree of opening of the discharge valve is controlled by either pneumatic or electric signals from the pressure controller. The pressure of the aircraft environment and the pressure of the cabin are fed to the controller which produces an output signal to the discharge valve(s) in accordance with the pressurization schedule for the cabin. In passenger-carrying aircraft, it is possible to set the desired maximum cabin altitude and rate of change of cabin altitude on the pressure controller.

If a discharge valve sticks open, the cabin loses its pressure, so in transport aircraft discharge valves and the pressure controller are duplicated. An independent method of closing a discharge valve that has failed in the open position is also desirable. The discharge valve and pressure controller are not normally duplicated in high-performance combat aircraft where all the cabin occupants have oxygen equipment.

Safety and inward vent valves

The basic cabin pressure control system includes two further valves—safety and inward relief valves. The cabin safety valve prevents the cabin differential pressure rising above a preset maximum if the discharge valve(s) should fail to open. The setting of the safety valve is usually slightly greater (0.2–0.5 lb/in^2 gauge (1.4–3.5 kPa)) than the maximum operating differential pressure. The inward relief valve is fitted to allow atmospheric air to enter the cabin if the pressure in the cabin falls below that of the atmosphere. This condition may arise during a rapid descent if the flow of air into the cabin is reduced or absent. The inward relief valve is usually set to open at a 'negative' differential pressure of $0.2–0.3 \, lb/in^2$ (1.4–2.0 kPa).

In certain circumstances there may be a need to decompress the cabin of an aircraft rapidly. If the cabin is filled with smoke or noxious fumes it may be necessary to decompress and to purge the cabin with external air through the ram air inlet. Although so drastic an action is obviously not desirable in a passenger aircraft flying at high altitude, it can be vital in aircraft carrying passengers at low altitude and at high altitudes in combat aircraft. Another situation in which rapid decompression of the cabin is required is when the crew intend to abandon the aircraft. In low-differential pressure cabins it is acceptable to decompress the cabin by jettisoning the cockpit canopy or door but, except in dire emergencies, a high-differential pressure cabin should be decompressed by fully opening all the discharge valves first.

Indicators and warning systems

The performance of the cabin pressurization system is indicated to the crew of an aircraft by means of a cabin altimeter. In passenger aircraft, the rate of change of cabin altitude and the differential pressure between the cabin and the atmosphere are also presented to the flight engineer. Failure of the pressurization control system to maintain the correct cabin altitude is normally presented to the crew by a warning system. The warning, which may be audible or visual, or both, may be operated by the cabin altitude rising above a preset value, for example 10 000 feet in a high-differential pressure passenger aircraft or the cabin differential pressure falling below that which should exist at the prevailing aircraft altitude.

Causes of failure of cabin pressurization

Whilst pressurization has overcome most of the physiological disturbances induced by exposure to low environmental pressure, decompression of the cabin at high altitude is associated with hazards of its own. Failure of the pressurization of aircraft cabins can be classified by cause, according to whether the fall of the cabin differential pressure is due to a reduction of the inflow of air, excessive discharge, or failure of the cabin structure.

Reduced cabin air inflow

Marked reduction of the air supply from the engine or compressor is much more probable in single-engined aircraft, since in multi-engined aircraft air for pressurization of the cabin is tapped from all the engines or supplied by two or more engine-driven compressors. Loss of the supply of air to the cabin due to flameout of the engine of a single-engined aircraft normally results in rapid aircraft descent, but if the engine fails during the climbing phase of a high-altitude 'ballistic' manoeuvre, the cabin differential pressure may fall to a negligible value before the aircraft starts the descent. Other causes of inflow failure include unserviceable components in the air conditioning system: for example, the cabin inlet valve may stick closed.

The flow of air into the cabin may be turned off by the crew because toxic material or smoke is being carried into the cabin, or as part of the escape drill. However, as long as the outflow of air through the discharge valves is prevented, failure of inflow does not cause a rapid fall of the cabin differential pressure. Pressure cabins are designed to leak very little and serviceability checks are made regularly to ensure that the leak rate remains below a specified maximum.

Failure of the pressure control system

If the pressure controller malfunctions or the cabin discharge valves stick open, the cabin differential pressure falls. If all the discharge valves suddenly go to the fully open position, the differential pressure will fall very rapidly to zero. Such decompressions occur more frequently in single-seat or two-seat aircraft because there is no duplication of the pressure control system. In a passenger aircraft, the duplication of the components and the provision of an independent facility for closing the discharge valves ensure that the cabin differential pressure does not fall significantly.

Structural failure

Failure of the structure can range from impaired sealing of a door, canopy or escape hatch, which may produce a small leak, to disintegration of a transparency, loss of a complete door or cockpit canopy or even a gross structural failure of the wall of the cabin. Failure of a seal or loss of a hatch, door or canopy may be caused by mechanical failure of a component such as an inflatable seal which may not have been identified because of inadequate or faulty servicing or inadequate preflight/take-off checks.

Structural failure of a transparency or part of the wall of a cabin may be due to mechanical fatigue, excessive stress, sabotage or enemy action. Recent government regulations require that the effects of puncture of the cabin wall or a window by a bullet from a personal weapon be taken into account in the design. Gross structural failure of the wall of a cabin in the absence of enemy action or sabotage is extremely unlikely now that the significance of metal fatigue is generally appreciated. The walls may, however, be weakened by corrosion, and frequent inspections are necessary to check that the strength has not deteriorated. In military aircraft, hatches, doors or cockpit canopies may be designed to be jettisoned in flight prior to escape: such mechanism may, of course, also be activated inadvertently.

Incidence

The incidence of accidental decompressions of pressure cabins is relatively low. The incidence over the 6-year period from 1977 to 1983 of all known decompressions in commercial aircraft throughout the world was of the order of 30–40 per year; 40 of the incidents occurred in UK registered aircraft. About one third of these decompressions were performed voluntarily in order to cut off the flow of smoke or other toxic material into the cabin, as a precaution following cracking of a transparency or as a planned drill following receipt of a bomb threat. Most of the accidental decompressions were due to failure of the compressor system, failure of the pressure control system, or opening of a hatch or door. The number of decompressions occurring in military flying even in peacetime is considerably higher than that in commercial operations. An incidence of about 2–3 unplanned decompressions per 100 000 flying hours has been recorded for many years. The major causes of inadvertent decompressions of military aircraft are flameout in those with single engines, malfunctions of the pressure control system, failures of transparencies and loss of canopies. In combat there is naturally a rise in the incidence of decompression due to enemy guns or missiles.

With a few exceptions, crew and passengers survive cabin pressure failure both in commercial and in military operations. Most deaths attributable to decompression have occurred when there was massive disruption of the cabin structure due to metal fatigue. From time to time, individuals are sucked out of a lost hatch, window or door.

Physics of rapid decompression

When air can escape, the pressure falls rapidly at first and then more slowly as the pressure inside and out approach and equalize (*Figure 8.4*). The rate at which air flows through a hole cannot exceed the local speed of sound regardless of the size of the defect or the difference between the pressure in the cabin and that of the atmosphere. The major factors that determine the rate and time of decompression of a pressure cabin are:

1. The volume of the cabin.
2. The size of the opening in the cabin.
3. The pressure in the cabin at the beginning of the decompression.
4. The pressure outside the cabin.

The larger the volume of the cabin the slower the decompression: the larger the defect in the wall the faster the decompression. The ratio of the volume of the cabin to the cross-sectional area of the opening or orifice is one of the main factors controlling the rate and time of decompression. Other factors being constant, the time of decompression is proportional to the ratio of cabin volume to area of the defect in the structure.

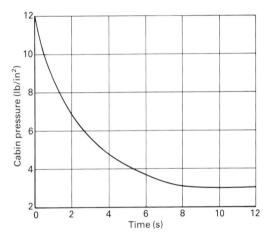

Figure 8.4 The time course of the absolute pressure of the air in the cabin of an aircraft during a decompression from $12\,lb/in^2$ (83 kPa) (5500 ft) to $3\,lb/in^2$ (21 kPa) (38 000 ft). The rate of fall of pressure, which is high at the beginning of the decompression, falls progressively as air escapes from the cabin.

The pressure ratio (cabin/ambient) is the other factor that determines the time of decompression: the larger the ratio, the longer the time of decompression. On the other hand, the actual differential pressure does not directly influence the time but does determine the severity of a decompression: the larger the pressure difference the more severe the decompression. The absolute value of the atmospheric pressure is, of course, the primary factor that determines the physiological consequences after a rapid decompression. These are often of far greater significance than the effect of the fall of pressure itself. For any given cabin pressure differential, the higher the aircraft altitude at the instant of decompression the greater is the ratio of cabin pressure to atmospheric pressure: the higher the aircraft altitude, the longer the decompression time (for a constant ratio of cabin volume to area of defect).

Time of decompression

Several equations have been developed to estimate the time of decompression of a pressure cabin of given volume according to the area of the defect and the cabin and atmospheric pressures. One of the most useful and accurate is that developed by Haber and Clamann. It states that the time of decompression of a cabin is determined by the product of two factors: (1) the time constant of the cabin; and (2) a pressure dependent factor.

Time constant of the cabin

This is calculated as:

$$t_c = V/(A \times c)$$

where t_c = time constant; V = volume of cabin; A = effective area of orifice; c = local speed of sound.

The values inserted into the equation are naturally expressed in consistent units. The effective area of an orifice may be less than its geometric area, in that it may not behave as a sharp-edged orifice. Thus the effective area of a defect created by sudden loss of a complete window or hatch is about 90% of the geometric area. The speed of sound is that at the temperature of the air flowing through the orifice (in practice a value of 1100 feet/second is used). Two examples of calculations of the time constant are given in *Table 8.2*.

The pressure-dependent factor

The pressure factor (P_1) is a complex function of the ratio of the cabin pressure before the decompression to the pressure in the cabin at the end of the decompression. The relationship between these two variables is depicted in *Figure 8.5*. The total time of decompression is given by the product:

$$t_t = t_c \times P_1$$

where t_t = total time of decompression; t_c = time constant of the cabin; P_1 = pressure dependent factor.

Examples of calculated times of decompression for the sudden disintegration of the canopy of a single-seat fighter aircraft and the loss of a window or door of a passenger aircraft are presented in *Table 8.2*.

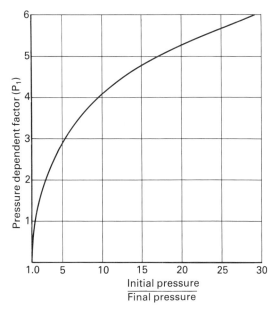

Figure 8.5 The calculation of the time of decompression of the pressure cabin at a constant aircraft altitude. The curve shows the relationship between the pressure-dependent factor of the Haber–Clamann formula and the ratio of the absolute pressure in the cabin before (initial pressure) and after (final pressure) the decompression.

Effect of inflow of air

Where the decompression of a cabin is due to excessive opening of discharge valves or a defect in the wall of the cabin, the flow of air from the engine compressors into the cabin continues. The modifying effect that this inflow will have upon the fall of cabin pressure is determined by the relationship between the flow and the size of the 'orifice' in the cabin wall. If the ratio of flow to the area of the

Table 8.2 Calculated decompression times

	Combat aircraft	Passenger aircraft	
		Loss of window	Loss of door
Cabin volume (ft³)	50	10000	
Nature and area of orifice (ft²)	Disintegration of canopy		
	9	0.5	12
Time constant of cabin (s)	0.005	18.2	0.76
Time of decompression (s):			
(i) from 16000 ft to 40000 ft	0.007	—	—
(ii) from 3000 ft to 25000 ft	—	30.9	1.3
(iii) from 5000 ft to 40000 ft	—	50.0	2.1

orifice is high then this additional flow will create a significant pressure drop across the orifice, thus reducing the rate of fall of cabin pressure and raising the value to which the pressure in the cabin falls at the end of the decompression. In practice, maintained inflow of air from the engine compressors is only of significance when a relatively small defect (for example, loss of a window) occurs in a large aircraft where the inflow is high; it can maintain the cabin altitude 5000–10000 feet lower than aircraft altitude in spite of loss of a window at an aircraft altitude of, say, 35000 feet. In some aircraft the airflow into the cabin may be increased in an emergency so limiting still further the rate of fall of cabin pressure and the final altitude reached in the cabin.

Aerodynamic suction

The pressure immediately outside a defect is seldom the static pressure exerted by the atmosphere at which the aircraft is flying. The movement of the aircraft through the air creates a fall of pressure over much of the external surface of the aircraft. The magnitude of this effect varies with the shape of the aircraft, the position of the defect, the speed and the altitude. The pressure at the external surface of the canopy of combat aircraft and at the windows and doors of transport aircraft is almost always less than the pressure altitude of the aircraft. Consequently, the fall of cabin pressure is accelerated and the final value of cabin pressure reduced below that of the

atmosphere by this Venturi effect of aerodynamic suction. The aerodynamic suction at the windows of transport aircraft cruising at altitude is usually about 0.2–0.6 lb/in² gauge (1.4–4.0 kPa). The aerodynamic suction over the canopy of certain high-performance combat aircraft flying at speed at altitudes between 35000 feet and 45000 feet amounts to between 1.0 and 2.0 lb/in² gauge (7–14 kPa). If the major part or the whole of the canopy of such an aircraft flying at 40000 feet is lost, the pressure altitude in the cabin may exceed the pressure altitude of the aircraft by 8000–10000 feet.

Cabin altitude profiles

The time course of the changes of cabin altitude following a failure of pressurization is complicated by alterations of the flight path of the aircraft during and following the incident. Usually the pilot initiates a rapid descent and so reduces rate of fall of cabin pressure and raises the minimum pressure reached in the cabin. Thus the cabin altitude first increases and then decreases as the aircraft descends. If the rate of decompression is very rapid, the cabin altitude rises to equal, or, if aerodynamic suction is present, to exceed, the aircraft altitude (*Figure 8.6*, curve a). This will then fall as the aircraft descends. In large passenger aircraft, however, the decompression of the cabin is relatively slow, and descent is begun well before the decompression is complete. The maximum cabin altitude attained may be very considerably less than the initial altitude of the aircraft (*Figure 8.6*, curve b).

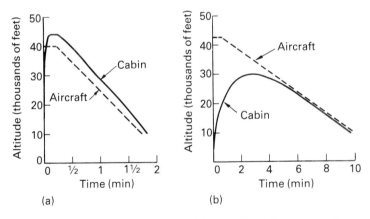

Figure 8.6 The effects of rapid descent of the aircraft and the presence of aerodynamic suction on cabin altitude after a failure of cabin pressurization. (*a*) The behaviour of cabin altitude when the decompression is due to a large defect that allows equilibration of pressure before descent of the aircraft has started. Aerodynamic suction at the site of the defect causes cabin altitude to exceed aircraft altitude. (*b*) The time course of cabin altitude when decompression occurs through a relatively small defect and descent of the aircraft is started 30 seconds after the beginning of the decompression.

Air blast

The sudden flow of air created in a pressure cabin when a decompression occurs raises dust and debris which may markedly reduce visibility. The mist formed by the condensation of water vapour in the expanding air adds to the problems of the crew.

The velocity of the flow of air through the cabin towards a defect in its wall increases rapidly as the air approaches the hole. The air blast can blow loose articles, furnishings and even people out through the defect. Since the force of the blast is only very high close to the hole, the individuals at risk are those in the immediate vicinity; but if there is a major structural failure many or even most occupants may be severely or fatally injured by the associated air blast. The point is usually academic, since such structural failure usually leads to disintegration of the aircraft in the air.

Effects on cabin occupants

Provided the aircraft remains intact, the effect of a failure of the pressurization of a cabin on the occupants depends on three major factors: the rate of the decompression; the pressure change during the decompression; and the pressure in the cabin after the decompression. The rate and pressure range of the decompression determine the magnitude of the effects arising from the expansion of the gas within the various gas-containing cavities of the body. The intensity of the other major effects of decompression—hypoxia and decompression sickness—is determined primarily by the consequent cabin altitude, particularly the maximum cabin altitude and the subsequent pattern of change. A major deficiency in the wall of a cabin also results in a marked fall in cabin temperature, so that the occupants may suffer from cold.

Expansion of gas in body cavities

The physiological consequences of the physical expansion of gas during a decompression occur in the semi-closed cavities such as the lungs, middle ear and paranasal sinuses, and in the closed cavities such as the gastrointestinal tract and teeth. The disturbances that can arise in these organs have been discussed in detail in Chapter 2.

The lungs

Although the lung is potentially one of the most vulnerable organs, in practice tearing of lung tissue and gas embolism due to over-expansion of the lungs are extremely rare outcomes of even a very rapid decompression. If the expanding gas is free to escape from the lungs through an open airway, the risk of lung damage is related to the speed and range of the decompression. The latter are, as has been seen, detemined by the ratio of the cabin volume to the effective area of the defect and the ratio of the pressure in the cabin at the beginning and end of the decompression. The relationship between these variables and the curve dividing safe and potentially dangerous decompressions (*see Figure 2.3*) have been combined in *Figure 8.7*. The risk of damage to the lungs is markedly increased if free venting of gas is obstructed by a closed glottis or by breathing equipment (*see* Chapter 2).

Ears and sinuses

Decompression of a pressure cabin is most unlikely to give rise to symptoms in the middle ears and paranasal sinuses. However, passengers will almost certainly develop pain in the middle ear during the subsequent emergency descent when they are exposed to a large and relatively rapid increase of cabin pressure.

Gastrointestinal tract

Abdominal disturbances are unlikely if the maximum cabin altitude does not exceed 25 000 feet. As the cabin altitude rises above 25 000 feet, an increasing proportion of individuals develop abdominal discomfort and pain due to expansion of gas in the stomach and intestines. The incidence of disturbances is far higher amongst passengers than aircrew.

Hypoxia

By far the most important hazard of the decompression of the cabin of an aircraft flying at high altitude is hypoxia. A rapid fall of the pressure of the immediate environment produces simultaneous decreases of the oxygen tensions of the inspired and the alveolar air in accordance with Dalton's law of partial pressures. There is also a concomitant decrease of the alveolar tension of carbon dioxide. The value to which the alveolar oxygen tension is reduced is determined by the composition of the gas breathed before and during the decompression, by the initial and final cabin altitudes and by the speed of the decompression. The lower the concentration of oxygen in the inspired gas, the greater the range of decompression, the lower the final cabin pressure and the faster the speed of the decompression, the lower is the oxygen tension in the alveolar gas at the end of the decompression. Thus a rapid decompression from 8000 feet to 40 000 feet when a man is

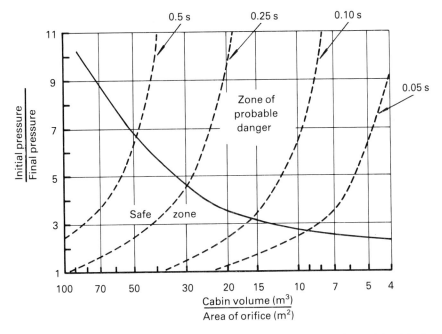

Figure 8.7 The relationship between the speed and range of a decompression and the risk of damage to the lungs as a result of the decompression. The interrupted lines depict the relationships between the ratio of the cabin volume to the area of the defect through which the decompression occurs (the ratio as expressed has the dimension of metres), the ratio of the absolute pressure in the cabin before (initial) and after (final) the decompression and the total time of decompression, according to the Haber–Clamann equation. The solid curve separates decompressions that will not cause lung damage (provided that there is no obstruction to the flow of gas from the lungs) from those that will probably cause pulmonary damage.

breathing air reduces the alveolar oxygen tension to 15–18 mm Hg (2.0–2.4 kPa). Whenever the final cabin altitude exceeds 30000 feet, the alveolar oxygen tension is reduced to below the tension of oxygen in the venous blood flowing into the lungs. In these circumstances oxygen passes out of the blood as the latter flows through the pulmonary capillaries, and, consequently, the blood loses oxygen to the atmosphere. The tension and concentration of oxygen in the blood leaving the lungs fall as abruptly as the alveolar oxygen tension; so that, within 5–6 seconds of the start of the rapid decompression, the blood entering the capillaries of the brain (and other tissues) has a very low oxygen tension. Since the amount of oxygen stored in many tissues, especially the brain, is very small, the tension of oxygen in the tissues also falls rapidly. Thus rapid decompression (1–2 seconds) to a final altitude of 40000 feet produces an impairment of performance in 12–15 seconds and unconsciousness in 20 seconds.

If the aircrew are breathing pure oxygen, the oxygen tension of the alveolar gas is not reduced to below that of the mixed venous blood until the final altitude exceeds 48000 feet. Rapid decompression to altitudes above 52000 feet results in loss of useful

consciousness in 10–15 seconds whether air or oxygen is breathed. The times to impairment or loss of consciousness do not change significantly with final altitudes greater than 52000 feet because the speed of development of cerebral hypoxia is determined primarily by the lung to brain circulation time, the store of oxygen in the cerebral tissue being relatively constant. When the final altitude is less than 52000 feet, the time to impairment of performance and loss of useful consciousness depend on the composition of the breathing mixture and the final altitude as shown in *Figure 8.8*. Although there is always an interval of at least 12–15 seconds between the beginning of a rapid decompression to high altitude and the first impairment of performance, impairment does nevertheless occur even if the duration of the exposure to low pressure is as short as 6 seconds. Thus measures to restore the alveolar oxygen to a near-normal value must be well on the way to completion in less than 5–6 seconds of the beginning of a rapid, severe decompression if an adequate level of performance is to be maintained.

The interval between the beginning of a rapid decompression and loss of useful consciousness when air is breathed increases markedly as the final altitude of the decompression is reduced below

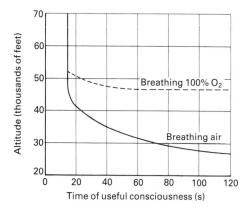

Figure 8.8 Loss of consciousness induced by rapid decompression in 2–3 seconds to high altitude. The curves indicate the effect of the final altitude to which the decompression occurred on the time elapsing from the beginning of the decompression to the loss of useful consciousness. The solid curve shows the relationship for decompressions from 8000 ft while breathing air. The interrupted curve shows the relationship for decompression from 25 000 ft while breathing 100% oxygen.

30 000 feet. Thus useful consciousness is maintained for about 60 seconds after a rapid (3 seconds) decompression to 30 000 feet, and for 120–140 seconds after decompression to 25 000 feet (*Figure 8.8*). Impairment of performance, however, occurs much earlier than loss of useful consciousness. Thus performance at psychomotor tasks is very significantly affected 45 seconds after a rapid (3 seconds) decompression to 25 000 feet.

The emergency action by the pilot of a passenger aircraft when a decompression occurs at high altitude is to initiate a rapid descent. Consequently a plot of the cabin altitude against time assumes a triangular profile (*see Figure 8.6*, curve b). The hypoxia induced by exposure to such a triangular profile with a peak altitude of 25 000 feet is very unlikely to cause seated passengers breathing air to lose consciousness, provided that the time at the peak altitude does not exceed 1 minute and that the total duration of the exposure to altitudes greater than 8000 feet does not exceed 6 minutes. Experiments on monkeys suggest that, while people are likely to lose consciousness when the peak altitude exceeds 25 000 feet, exposure to triangular profiles with peak altitudes of up to 40 000 feet should not be fatal or cause permanent brain damage, provided that the total time above 8000 feet does not exceed 8 minutes. Exposure to higher peak altitudes (with approximately the same total time above 8000 feet) will probably be either immediately fatal or produce severe permanent brain damage.

Decompression sickness

The incidence of decompression sickness only becomes significant when the cabin altitude rises above 30 000 feet and the altitude remains above this value for longer than 5–10 minutes (*see Figure 3.2*). In practice, therefore, decompression sickness will occur only if the aircraft remains at high altitude after the decompression, so that the cabin altitude exceeds 28 000–30 000 feet for some time. Prolonged exposure to altitudes above 28 000 feet does give rise to incidents of decompression sickness unless the crew has breathed 100% oxygen for some time before the decompression.

Cold

The temperature in the cabin following a failure of pressurization is determined by the outside temperature, the nature of the cause of the decompression and the flight path and speed of the aircraft. A large defect in the wall of the cabin of an aircraft at high altitude causes a very large fall of cabin temperature and a high flow of very cold air around the occupants. Such exposure leads to rapid cold injury of exposed skin and to a less rapid fall of body temperature (*see* Chapter 17). Vision may well be impaired by the flow of cold air into the eyes, while the outlet valves and ports of breathing equipment may be obstructed by the formation of ice. Unless an individual wears special protective clothing, such as a full pressure suit, he must descend quickly to increase the temperature of the air entering the cabin through the defect and thus reduce the severity of the cold.

Exposure to altitudes above 63 000 feet

When decompression results in exposure to an absolute pressure less than the vapour pressure of water at body temperature, that is, 47 mm Hg (6.3 kPa) (a pressure altitude of 63 000 feet) the nature of the consequent disturbances differs from that which occurs at lower altitudes. Tissue water vaporizes as the local pressure falls below 47 mm Hg (or a lower pressure if the local temperature is below 37°C). Thus at altitudes between 65 000 and 70 000 feet, vaporization starts in the lungs and in the low-pressure regions of the circulation such as the large intra-thoracic veins. At higher altitudes, water vapour and other gases, such as oxygen and carbon dioxide, escape from the body fluids, a phenomenon termed ebullism. Dogs and monkeys decompressed to near-vacuum conditions (pressure of 1–2 mm Hg) (0.13–0.26 kPa) developed gross swelling of the soft tissues within 5 seconds, became unconscious in about 12 seconds, and quickly progressed to general muscle spasticity, gasping, transitory convulsions and apnoea. The products of ebullism in the veins and atria of the heart rapidly blocked the circulation. Although the electrical activity of the heart continued, the circulation ceased about 10 seconds after the beginning of the exposure. As soon as the pressure increased in descent, the gases were redissolved very rapidly. Provided the duration of the exposure to near-vacuum conditions was less than 2 minutes, circulation and respiration in these animals recovered spontaneously. Studies on monkeys and chimpanzees suggested that exposure to a virtual vacuum for less than 1.5–2.0 minutes is very unlikely to be fatal or to give rise to any neurological damage.

Prevention of hypoxia

Hypoxia is by far the most dangerous disturbance produced by failure of the pressurization of the cabin of an aircraft flying at high altitude. Oxygen delivery equipment which will prevent the otherwise inevitable impairment of performance must be available to the aircrew. A certain degree of hypoxia is acceptable in seated passengers. The primary method of alleviating this hypoxia is the rapid controlled descent of the aircraft to a safe altitude. Where the cabin altitude may rise above 25 000 feet, or where recompression to below a cabin altitude of 15 000 feet in 4 minutes is not possible, passenger aircraft are usually fitted with an emergency system which will provide oxygen for all the passengers for the period that the cabin altitude is above 15 000 feet.

Low-differential cabins

Aircrew operating low-differential pressure cabin aircraft use their oxygen equipment throughout flight. So long as the equipment is capable of delivering 100% oxygen at and above 33 000 feet and pressure breathing above 40 000 feet serious hypoxia is unlikely if cabin pressure should suddenly be lost. The design of the oxygen equipment must be such, however, that the concentration of oxygen in the mask cavity rises rapidly to the required level immediately the decompression occurs. Thus the volume of the breathing system between the air inlet of the regulating device and the mask cavity should be kept to a minimum (less than 500 ml). The required level of pressure breathing must be fully operative within 3 seconds of the time that the pressure in the respiratory tract falls below 141 mm Hg (18.8 kPa) absolute.

High-differential cabins—crew

The flight-deck crew of aircraft with high-differential pressure cabins do not need to use oxygen equipment as long as the pressure cabin is intact. A rapid decompression (decompression time less than 20 seconds) to a cabin altitude above 30 000 feet will, however, produce a significant impairment of performance in those breathing air even if 100% oxygen is delivered to the respiratory tract immediately the decompression commences. This transient hypoxia can be avoided only by breathing 30–40% oxygen (depending on the initial and final cabin altitudes) for some time before the decompression and 100% oxygen immediately the cabin pressure begins to fall. Thus if there is a significant chance that cabin pressurization may fail, the watch-keeping pilot should have his mask secured on his face and be breathing 30–40% oxygen whenever the aircraft altitude exceeds 30 000 feet. When the probability of a fast decompression (decompression time less than about 30 seconds) is very remote, as is the case in virtually all licensed passenger-carrying aircraft, then it is generally accepted that the pilot can breathe air throughout flight provided that he can don a mask and be breathing 100% oxygen within 3–5 seconds of the cabin altitude exceeding 10 000 feet. In certain circumstances, for example, only one pilot at the controls of a subsonic passenger aircraft, government regulations require that he breathes an oxygen–air mixture whenever the aircraft altitude exceeds 41 000 feet. Privately owned, non-fare-paying passenger carrying aircraft need not at present comply with all the regulations concerning oxygen usage. A recent increase in post-decompression fatalities in small cabin volume 'executive' aircraft has led to a reappraisal of the mandatory procedures in all passenger carrying aircraft. The design of the oxygen equipment for the flight-deck crew of high-differential pressure cabin aircraft must be such that 100% oxygen is delivered to the mask directly it is donned.

High-differential cabins—passengers

Minimizing the effects of hypoxia is best achieved by limiting the magnitude and duration of the exposure to low pressure. When decompression can result in a cabin altitude exceeding 25 000 feet, or the duration of the exposure to altitudes above 13 000 feet may be longer than 4–6 minutes, it is current practice to fit an emergency oxygen system to supply all the passengers. Sufficient oxygen is carried to maintain the alveolar oxygen tension of all passengers above 50 mm Hg (6.7 kPa) for as long as the cabin altitude exceeds 13 000 feet. Government regulations also require that enough oxygen should be carried for use by a small fraction (10–15%) of passengers when the cabin altitude exceeds 10000 feet. Although many emergency oxygen systems for passengers present oxygen masks automatically, the proportion of passengers who can be expected to use the equipment correctly is probably less than 50%.

Further reading

CIVIL AVIATION AUTHORITY (1980) *Air Navigation Order—Provision and Use of Oxygen in Public Transport Aircraft, Schedule 5.* London: Civil Aviation Authority

DENISON, D.M., LEDWITH, F. and POULTON, E.C. (1966) Complex reaction time at simulated altitudes of 5000 feet and 8000 feet. *Aerospace Medicine*, **37**, 1010–1013

ERNSTING, J. (1978) Prevention of hypoxia—acceptable compromises. *Aviation, Space and Environmental Medicine*, **49**, 495–502

ERNSTING, J., BYFORD, G.H., DENISON, D.M. and FRYER, D.I. (1973) *Hypoxia Induced by Rapid Decompression from 8000 feet to 40000 feet—The Influence of Rate of Decompression.* Flying Personnel Research Committee Report No. 1324. London: Ministry of Defence (Air)

GREEN, R.E. and MORGAN, D.R. (1985) The effects of mild hypoxia on a logical reasoning task. *Aviation, Space and Environmental Medicine*, **56**, 1004–1008

HABER, F. and CLAMANN, H.G. (1953) *A General Theory of Rapid Decompression.* Randolph Air Force Base School of Aviation Medicine, USAF Project No 21-1201-0008, Report No. 3

MCFARLAND, R.A. (1953) *Human Factors in Air Transportation. Occupational Health and Safety.* New York: McGraw-Hill

MCFARLAND, R.A. (1971) Human factors in relation to the development of pressurized cabins. *Aerospace Medicine*, **42**, 1303–1318

9

Toxic gases and vapours in flight

G.R. Sharp, revised by D.J. Anton

Introduction

Many of the substances used in aviation are toxic to man. The number of potentially toxic substances continues to increase as new materials are used in the construction, operation and maintenance of aircraft. Thermal decomposition caused by over-heating or a fire frequently converts a relatively inert, non-toxic material into toxic gases or vapours. The possibility that such materials may be present and play a part in the causation of any in-flight incident or accident must not be overlooked. Concentration in the cabin air that would not be of significance at sea level may become a hazard, if only by reducing pilot performance, in the air.

Such toxic substances are absorbed into the body mainly via the respiratory tract. Absorption through the skin or gastrointestinal mucous membrane rarely occurs in flight though the conjunctivae may be irritated. The toxic material may be present in the cabin air or in the oxygen supply to the breathing equipment. Oxygen contamination is considered in Chapter 5.

Exposure limits

The Threshold Limit Value (TLV), which is the maximum concentration of a gas or vapour to which individuals may be exposed in the ground environment without any toxic effects, either immediate or delayed, has been agreed for many substances and the limits are continually modified, as new intense. Finally, the continual changing gaseous time-weighted mean which defines the average allowable concentration of the agent for exposure over a 30-year working life consisting of an 8-hour working day, a 40-hour working week and a 50-week

working year. Temporary excursions of the concentration of a toxic agent above the threshold limit value are permissible. A 'ceiling' concentration, which must never be exceeded, is also often useful.

Certain difficulties arise in the application to flight of threshold limit values derived for use in industry. Thus a transient slight impairment of performance that may be quite acceptable in a factory is unacceptable in a pilot. The exposure may occur in combination with stressors common in flight: low pressure, high temperature, sustained acceleration. These can modify considerably the intensity and nature of the effects produced by the noxious substance. More than one agent may be present, so that the combined toxicity must be considered. Furthermore, exposures in flight tend to be short but intense. Finally, the continual changing gaseous environment in the crew compartments of aircraft in flight tends to produce wide and rapid fluctuations in chemical composition of the air. Thus TLVs must be applied with caution in aviation and are no more than a general guide, especially for the relative toxicity of different materials.

Sources of toxic hazards in flight

The main sources of toxic gases and vapours in flight can be classified as follows:

1. Products of combustion: engine exhaust gases; products of overheating or fire.
2. Aviation fuels, lubricants and hydraulic fluids.
3. Anti-icing, anti-detonant and coolant fluids.
4. Fire extinguishing agents.
5. Refrigerants.
6. Ozone.
7. Insecticides, herbicides and agricultural chemicals.

Products of combustion

The products of combustion or heating are the commonest toxic hazard in aviation, whether they arise from the controlled burning of aviation fuel in the aircraft engine, or from overheating or uncontrolled burning of a part of the aircraft structure or contents.

Engine exhaust gases

The composition of the exhaust gases from reciprocating and gas turbine engines is very different (*Table 9.1*): the former contains between 3 and 9% carbon monoxide, the latter less than 0.005%.

There are several ways in which exhaust gases may enter the cabin of an aircraft. In many piston-engined aircraft, exhaust gases are used to provide heat to the cabin by way of heat exchangers. The mechanical integrity of a heat exchanger may fail and exhaust gases pass directly into the occupied compartment. Under some conditions of flight, certain arrangements of the exhaust pipes may allow gases to pass directly into the cabin. A defect in the cabin wall may also allow exhaust gas to contaminate the cabin. The air tapped from the compressor stage of a gas turbine engine for ventilation of the cabin is unlikely to be contaminated by exhaust products since these are formed downstream of the tapping.

Table 9.1 Composition of engine exhausts

Component	Concentration (% wt/wt)	
	Reciprocating	*Gas turbine*
Carbon dioxide	10–15	5.0
Carbon monoxide	3–9	0.003
Total aldehydes	—	0.01
Acetylene	0.37	—
Oxygen, nitrogen, water (approx.)	80	95

Products of overheating or fire

When a material is subjected to excessive heat so that its temperature rises but does not reach the temperature at which rapid oxidation occurs, it may decompose and give off toxic vapours. Electronic equipment is prone to such thermal decomposition.

The materials employed in aircraft structures, equipment and furnishings are extremely varied and the potential toxic hazards of fire are therefore complex. Sometimes oxidation is incomplete and the principal products are intermediate breakdown substances, aldehydes, and carbon monoxide, as well as carbon dioxide and water vapour. Some of the commonest products of combustion, together with the source materials, are listed in *Table 9.2*. All these materials are used in aircraft. Many of them cause irritation to the eyes and the mucous

Table 9.2 Combustion and pyrolysis products with source materials

Toxic gas or vapour	Source material
Carbon dioxide Carbon monoxide	All combustible materials containing carbon
Nitrogen oxides	Celluloid, polyurethanes
Hydrogen cyanide	Wool, silk, plastics containing nitrogen
Formic acid Acetic acid	Cellulose materials, cellulosic plastics, rayon
Acrolein	Wood, paper, oils
Sulphur dioxide	Rubber, thiokols
Halogen acids	Polyvinyl chloride, fire retardant plastics, fluoridated plastics
Ammonia	Melamine, nylon, urea–formaldehyde resins
Aldehydes	Phenol–formaldehydes, wood, nylon, polyester resins
Benzene	Polystyrene
Phenol	Phenol–formaldehyde
Azo-bis-succinonitrile	Plastic foam material

membranes at concentrations below those that produce impairment of mental performance. On the other hand, carbon monoxide, which is a major product of combustion, has very insidious and highly toxic qualities.

Carbon monoxide

Carbon monoxide is a major product of combustion and is invariably produced by fire in an aircraft. It is also present in high concentration in the exhaust gases of reciprocating engines. It is the commonest toxic gas in aviation.

Carbon monoxide is a colourless, odourless gas which produces tissue hypoxia by combining with haemoglobin and thus reducing the oxygen-carrying capacity of the blood. It is absorbed exclusively through the lungs. It diffuses from the alveolar gas into the pulmonary capillary blood where it combines rapidly with the haemoglobin within the red cells to form carboxyhaemoglobin. The affinity of carbon monoxide for haemoglobin is some 210 times greater than that of oxygen for haemoglobin. The ratio of the concentrations of carboxyhaemoglobin and oxyhaemoglobin in blood with specified partial pressures of oxygen and carbon monoxide (Po_2 and Pco respectively) is given by the equation:

$$\frac{\text{Carboxyhaemoglobin concentration}}{\text{Oxyhaemoglobin concentration}} = 210 \times \frac{Pco}{Po_2}$$

Thus at equilibrium, if the Pco is only 0.4 mm Hg in the presence of a Po_2 of 100 mm Hg, the blood contains 50% carboxyhaemoglobin and 50% oxyhaemoglobin, with a consequent severe reduction

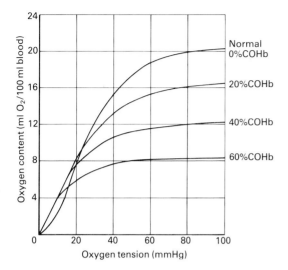

Figure 9.1 The relationship between oxygen tension and oxygen content of blood with a haemoglobin concentration of 15 g/100 ml containing respectively 20%, 40% and 60% carboxyhaemoglobin.

of oxygen-carrying capacity (*Figure 9.1*). When the alveolar Pco is such that the blood contains 40% or more carboxyhaemoglobin, the normal oxygen extraction (fall of oxygen content as the blood flows through the tissues) reduces the Po$_2$ of the blood at the venous ends of the tissue capillaries to a very low value. The consequent hypoxia causes collapse.

The carboxyhaemoglobin concentration in the blood rises rapidly at the beginning of the exposure and then progressively more slowly to an equilibrium (*Figure 9.2*). The equilibrium concentration of

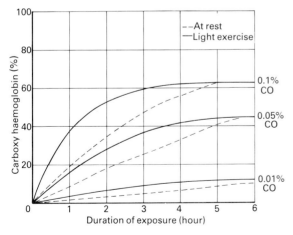

Figure 9.2 The time courses of the concentrations of carboxyhaemoglobin in the mixed venous blood on exposure to breathing carbon monoxide at inspired concentrations of 0.01%, 0.05% and 0.1% in air, at rest (broken lines) and during light exercise (solid lines).

carboxyhaemoglobin is determined by the Pco in the alveolar gas, which depends on the concentration of carbon monoxide in the inspired gas and the environmental pressure. The time taken to reach equilibrium depends on the concentration of carbon monoxide in the inspired gas and the level of pulmonary ventilation. Typical time courses in normal individuals at rest (pulmonary ventilation 6 l/min) and whilst performing light exercise (pulmonary ventilation of 18 l/min) are illustrated in *Figure 9.2*. The rate of rise of carboxyhaemoglobin and the final equilibrium concentration depend on the partial pressure of carbon monoxide in the inspired gas, so that ascent to altitude will reduce the effect of a given concentration of the gas. Although raising the concentration of oxygen in the inspired gas to a high value will reduce the rate of rise of carboxyhaemoglobin, a fall of the inspired oxygen tension induced by breathing air at altitude has no significant effect on this process. On the other hand, the effects of a given level of carboxyhaemoglobin will be markedly increased by the hypoxia induced by breathing air at altitude.

Table 9.3 Symptoms induced by various blood concentrations of carbon monoxide (at sea level with a normal haemoglobin level)

Saturation of haemoglobin with carbon monoxide (%)	Symptoms
Less than 10	None
10	No appreciable effects other than mild headache and slight dyspnoea on vigorous exertion
20	Slight headache, fatigue and dyspnoea even on mild exertion
30	Headache, increasing fatigue, impaired judgement and gross dyspnoea and impairment of vision on exercise
40–50	Severe throbbing headache, confusion, fainting and collapse even at rest
60–70	Unconsciousness

Blood concentrations of carbon monoxide up to 10% saturation rarely cause symptoms at sea level during moderate physical activity if the haemoglobin concentration is normal. The tissues most sensitive to hypoxia, such as those of the nervous system, are the first to be affected. The symptoms of carbon monoxide intoxication are headache, weakness, dizziness, nausea, dyspnoea on exercise, confusion, fainting, coma and respiratory failure. The relationship of symptoms to the carbon monoxide saturation of the blood is given in *Table 9.3*.

Although no symptoms occur at carbon monoxide saturation levels below 10% and although, even at 15–20% saturation, the individual at rest may have little or no indication that anything is amiss, impairment of cognitive and psychomotor performance has been reported at a carboxyhaemoglobin level as low as 5%. Blood carbon monoxide saturation above 10% produces insidious marginal impairment of performance that could affect aircrew performance in flight.

Aldehydes

Aldehydes occur in the exhaust gases from reciprocating engines (*Table 9.1*) and are frequently amongst the toxic products produced by a fire in an aircraft. Acrolein, which is one of the main aldehydes produced in these circumstances, is extremely irritating to the conjunctivae and upper respiratory tract. The threshold limit value is 0.1 ppm. An exposure to an acrolein concentration of 1.0 ppm for 5 minutes causes marked irritation of the eyes, nose and throat. Acetaldehyde, another common combustion product, causes irritation of the eyes and to a lesser extent of the nose and throat. The threshold limit value is 200 ppm (0.02%).

Nitrogen oxides

Oxides of nitrogen are produced when certain substances are burnt (*Table 9.2*). They are also present in high concentration in the exhaust gases from missiles and rockets in which fuming nitric acid is used as an oxidizing agent. Nitrogen dioxide, the most important, produces mild irritation of the eyes and upper respiratory tract at concentrations of 10–20 ppm. Even a short exposure to a concentration of 50 ppm results in pulmonary oedema and exposure to 100 ppm is rapidly fatal. There is virtually no difference in the intensity of irritation or odour at concentrations between 20 amd 100 ppm. It is possible, therefore, to be exposed to lethal concentrations of nitrogen dioxide without serious discomfort.

Aviation fuels, lubricants and hydraulic fluids

Aviation fuels

Servicing crews may frequently be exposed to aviation fuel in liquid or vapour form, but the likelihood of aircrew or passengers coming into contact with these materials in flight is remote. Fuel lines in aircraft are separated by mechanical barriers from the cabin and the cabin ventilation system, so that a leak is very unlikely to contaminate the cabin. On the ground, however, a major spill during refuelling can, in still-air conditions, produce significant contamination of the cockpit and passenger cabin. If aircrew do their own refuelling, they may become exposed to these agents.

Aviation fuels, of which there is a wide variety, are broadly divided into those for piston engines, and those for turbines (*Table 9.4*). All can irritate the skin, but the principal hazard is inhalation of the vapour. The narcosis produced by inhalation (and the contact dermatitis) is due to the aliphatic and aromatic hydrocarbons which are the major constituents of these fuels. Aviation gasoline generally contains tetraethyl lead and tricresyl phosphate, both toxic materials but less important than the hydrocarbons. Frequent exposure to the aromatics (aniline, xylene and xylidine) which are present in aviation gasoline may give rise to methaemoglobinaemia.

Table 9.4 Composition of common aviation fuels

Fuel	Composition
(i) Reciprocating engine fuels	
Aviation gasoline (AVGAS)	A number of varying complex mixtures of aliphatic and aromatic hydrocarbons together with certain additives such as tetraethyl lead, aniline, toluene, xylene and xylidene.
(ii) Gas turbine engine fuels	
AVTAG	A fraction of petroleum distillate close to gasoline.
AVTUR (JP 1)	Mixture of straight run gasoline and kerosene.
JP 3	Mixture of 1/3 fuel oil, 1/3 kerosene and 1/3 gasoline.
JP 4	Mixture of 1/3 kerosene, 1/2 gasoline and 1/6 aromatics (benzene, etc.).

The intensity of the systemic effects produced by inhalation of aviation fuel in the vapour form is determined by the concentration of the vapour and the duration of the exposure. The minimum concentration required to produce a detectable effect is 0.05% and this value is the threshold limit for aviation fuel vapour. A low dose of vapour, such as that resulting from exposure to a concentration of 0.2% for ½ hour, generally causes dizziness, nausea and a frontal headache. Higher doses—for example, that produced by a concentration of 0.25% for 1 hour—give rise to irritation of the conjunctivae with lacrimation, and cerebral irritation with restlessness, excitement and disorientation together with disorders of speech, vision and hearing. Absorption of larger doses of fuel vapour result in unconsciousness, convulsions and death.

It is convenient to include in this section on aircraft fuels the chemical fuel isopropyl nitrate (AVPIN). AVPIN is a yellow, highly inflammable liquid which is used for starting turbine engines. The products of combustion of AVPIN contain high concentration of oxides of nitrogen which are intense pulmonary irritants.

Hydraulic fluids

Hydraulic fluid is carried in pipelines at pressures as high as 3000–5000 lb/in^2 (20.7–34.5 mPa). A leaky union, a defective gauge or a ruptured pipe can produce a mist or stream of hydraulic fluid into the crew compartment. Aircrew may inhale the vapour or get liquid on the skin.

Hydraulic fluids can conveniently be grouped according to the nature of the base from which they are derived. The four major groups are as follows:

1. Petroleum-based hydraulic fluids, which contain esters of long-chain aliphatic acids, tricresyl phosphate and a viscosity polymer. These fluids have a low vapour pressure and are relatively non-toxic unless they are ingested or burnt.
2. Castor-oil-based hydraulic fluids, which contain, in addition to the esters of long-chain aliphatic acids, volatile and highly inflammable compounds including glycols, alcohols, diacetone and butyl cellosolve.
3. Silicon-based hydraulic fluids, which are chemically inert.
4. Phosphate ester-base hydraulic fluids, which consist of the phosphates of triaryl (three benzene ring) compounds. These fluids have a low vapour pressure and are relatively non-toxic unless ingested or heated.

The only constituent of these hydraulic fluids that exhibits any degree of toxicity is the butyl cellosolve contained in the castor-oil-based fluids. Inhalation of vapour containing this compound, which is highly volatile, results in headache, dizziness, impaired vision and confusion. Thermal decomposition of both the petroleum and castor-oil-based hydraulic fluids and those containing triaryl phosphate compounds produce a mixture of aldehydes, carbonyls and carbon monoxide, each of which can produce toxic effects.

Lubricating oils

Although lubricating oil gains entry to the cabin of an aircraft only rarely, it can do so as the result of a mechanical failure in a gas turbine engine. Thus a loose bearing, a cracked oil seal or a leak from an oil supply line may allow oil to mix with the air in the compressor stage of the engine upstream of the point at which air is tapped off to supply the flow of ventilating air to the cabin. The oil may enter the cabin either as a mist or a vapour. In reciprocating engines, oil is frequently in contact with hot engine parts, and the smoke so formed may gain entry to the cabin through a defect in the cabin ventilation system.

Lubricating oils consist of 80–95% base oil which may be derived from petroleum or may be a synthetic ester such as dioctyl or dimonyl sebecate. Both types of oils have a low vapour pressure and are relatively non-toxic. Exposure to oil vapour may cause irritation of the eyes and the upper respiratory tract. Inhalation of the vapour also gives rise to systemic disturbances such as headache, nausea and vomiting. Exposure to oil mist can produce a chemical pneumonitis from direct contact of the aerosol or liquid oil with lung tissue.

Anti-icing, anti-detonant and coolant fluids

It is convenient to consider these fluids together since they contain common chemical substances.

Anti-icing fluids are used to keep windscreens, wings, carburettors and propellers free of ice during flight. They consist of various combinations of isopropanol, ethanol, methanol, ethylene glycol, propylene and water. Anti-detonant (ADI) fluids are used in reciprocating engines to improve performance for short periods, by injecting the fluid into the cylinders as required. ADI fluids are mixtures of various alcohols, such as methanol or equal parts of methanol and ethanol in water. Coolant fluid, which consists of ethylene glycol diluted with water, is used in liquid-cooled reciprocating engines which are now rarely fitted to aircraft. An ethylene glycol–water mixture is used as the heat transport medium in liquid conditioned coverall systems which provide personal thermal conditioning.

Exposure in flight to anti-icing, ADI or coolant fluid usually arises from a break in a pipeline carrying the fluid, so that a spray of the latter enters the crew compartment. Such an exposure produces an inhalation hazard and skin contamination.

Inhalation of vapour or mists containing any of the three commonly used alcohols—methanol, ethanol or isopropanol—produces the same general effects. There is irritation of the mucous membranes and upper respiratory tract with headache, dizziness, tremors, nausea, vomiting, roaring in the ears and eventual narcosis and unconsciousness. Methanol has a greater toxicity than ethanol, the threshold limit values for those alcohol vapours being 0.02% for methanol and 0.1% for ethanol.

Ethylene glycol has a very low vapour pressure, but aircrew may be exposed to high concentrations if it enters the cabin as a spray or mist. High concentrations of ethylene glycol cause mild irritation of the upper respiratory tract and have a narcotic effect. This substance can cause irreversible damage to the convoluted tubules of the kidney. It also causes liver necrosis.

Fire extinguishing agents

A fire extinguishing agent should rapidly extinguish a fire, regardless of the burning material, and both the agent and its thermal decompression products should have a low toxicity. The amount of agent required to extinguish a fire in an aircraft should also be as small as possible. It is difficult to meet all these criteria in practice, and some of the agents used are rather toxic. By their very nature they cause hypoxia since their efficiency depends on the reduction in the concentration of oxygen at the site of burning. Chemicals commonly used in an aircraft include a mixture of water and glycol, carbon dioxide and a variety of halogenated hydrocarbons. A water–glycol mixture has the advantage that it is non-toxic and it is widely employed in hand-operated extinguishers designed to be operated by crew or passengers. It has the disadvantage, however, that it cannot put out fires of liquids. Carbon dioxide, though widely used, is not very effective in dealing with combustile material such as paper and cloth. A variety of halogenated hydrocarbons are contained in aircraft fire extinguisher systems. They vary in their effectiveness and the toxicity of the agent and of its breakdown products. Some, for example, methyl bromide, which is highly toxic, are used in areas such as in engine bays which are remote from the crew and passenger compartments; others, such as bromochlorodifluoromethane (BCF) which has a low toxicity, are used in hand-held extinguishers in the crew and passenger compartments.

Carbon dioxide

Carbon dioxide is carried extensively in aircraft not only as a fire extinguishing agent but also in its solid form (dry ice) as a refrigerant. It is a colourless, heavy gas which acts as a narcotic at concentrations (at sea level) greater than 5%. The threshold limit value for carbon dioxide is 0.5%. Depending on the duration of exposure, increased respiration and air hunger occur at concentrations between 1% and 2.5% carbon dioxide. Concentrations of 3–7% carbon dioxide cause a marked and distracting increase in respiration by raising the partial pressure of carbon dioxide in the respiratory centre, and also impair vision and hearing. Exposure to concentrations greater than 7% results in convulsions, loss of consciousness and death. Unconsciousness may occur within 1 minute at a concentration above 10%.

The effects of carbon dioxide are a function of the partial pressure of the gas in the inspired air. At altitude, the effect of a given concentration of the gas varies inversely with the environmental pressure.

Methyl bromide

Methyl bromide ($CHBr_3$) is a colourless, odourless gas. It is a most effective fire extinguishing agent; but it is also highly toxic and is only employed now in areas where contact with crew or passengers is improbable. The threshold limit value is 10 ppm. Above this concentration it causes sleepiness, headache, nausea and vomiting followed by paralysis and convulsions. Exposure to high concentrations produces rapid narcosis and pulmonary congestion and oedema.

Carbon tetrachloride

Carbon tetrachloride (CCl_4) was widely used in the past as a fire extinguishing agent and may still be found in use in older aircraft. It is a toxic, colourless liquid. The threshold limit value of the vapour is 10 ppm. Exposure to a concentration of 0.02% (200 ppm) produces dizziness, headache, mental confusion and lassitude. The symptoms become more severe as the concentration is raised and unconsciousness, convulsions and death follow exposure to high concentrations. Thermal decomposition of carbon tetrachloride results in the formation of phosgene, inhalation of which produces delayed but very severe pulmonary oedema. Exposure to a concentration greater than 10 ppm rapidly leads to pulmonary damage. Because of its toxicity it has been replaced by other halogenated hydrocarbons, such as bromochlorodifluoromethane.

Chlorobromomethane (CB)

Monochloromonobromomethane (CH_2ClBr) is a colourless liquid with a distinctive odour which has been widely used as a fire extinguishing agent. The threshold limit value is 200 ppm. At higher doses it causes depression of the central nervous system with headache, drowsiness and disturbances of vision and co-ordination. Exposure to very high concentrations may cause pulmonary oedema. The products of thermal decomposition, which include phosgene and carbonyl bromide, are highly toxic to the lungs.

Bromochlorodifluoromethane (BCF)

Monobromomonochlorodifluoromethane (CF_2-BrCl) is a relatively new, highly effective fire extinguishing liquid which has a low toxicity. At very high concentrations—of the order of 4–5%—it acts as a narcotic, causing dizziness, paraesthesia and sleepiness. Thermal decomposition of BCF which, in practice, only occurs to a very limited extent, results in the formation of hydrofluoric and hydrochloric acids, with smaller amounts of phosgene and carbonyl fluoride.

Refrigerants

A variety of very stable, complex, halogenated hydrocarbons containing combinations of chlorine, fluorine, hydrogen and carbon are used in aircraft as refrigerants. They are commonly referred to by trade names, for example, Freon. These agents are not toxic until asphyxiant concentrations are reached. If heated, however, they may decompose to give phosgene, hydrochloric and hydrofluoric acids, all of which are very toxic to the mucous membranes and respiratory tract.

Ozone

Ozone is a triatomic form of oxygen which occurs naturally in the atmosphere where it is formed by the action of the ultraviolet light from the sun on molecular oxygen. The concentration of ozone in the atmosphere increases rapidly with altitude above 40000 feet, reaching a maximum of approximately 10 ppm (by volume) at an altitude of 100000 feet. If the ozone content of the air remained unchanged during passage through the compressor of the aircraft engine and the cabin air conditioning system, the concentration of the gas in the cabin of an aircraft flying at 60000 feet would be of the order of 4 ppm. Ozone is, however, dissociated at high temperature, and the concentration of ozone in the cabins of aircraft flying at 60000 feet has seldom been found to exceed 0.1–0.2 ppm.

Ozone is irritant to the respiratory tract and to mucous membranes. Exposure to high concentrations leads to pulmonary oedema. The threshold for the perception of the odour of the gas is 0.01 ppm whilst exposure to a concentration of 1.0 ppm for an hour causes irritation of the eyes and upper respiratory tract with coughing. Higher concentrations (approximately 10 ppm) have been reported to cause pulmonary oedema in man. The threshold limit value of ozone is 0.1 ppm. Repeated exposure to a concentration of ozone of 0.2 ppm for periods of 3 hours per day does not cause any symptoms or detectable changes in lung function, but a concentration of 0.5 ppm for the same time reduces the timed forced expiratory volume. In flight, therefore, an ozone concentration of the order of 0.2 ppm at sea level is probably acceptable.

Insecticides, herbicides and agricultural chemicals

The aerial application of chemicals is a large industry. The concept can be traced back to a patent filed in Berlin in 1911 by Alfred Zimmerman, a forest officer, who suggested applying lime solution by air to pinewood forests to protect them against the depredations of the 'black-arch' moth. The industry did not come to maturity, however, until after the second world war when a large number of robust, comparatively light propeller driven aircraft were released onto the surplus market. Some of these aircraft were converted to deliver sprays or dusts; subsequent development led to the use of purpose-built aircraft and helicopters. The general requirement of all these aircrafts are that they should be light on the controls, robust and have good low-speed handling performance, as they are flown, frequently overloaded, at the extreme low-speed manoeuvring corner of the flight envelope.

The chemicals employed include pesticides (insecticides, herbicides, fungicides) growth modifiers, and fertilizers. Many of these chemicals are toxic to man and the World Health Organisation (WHO, 1975) has issued classification guidelines, and classifications by hazard for pesticides.

Of all the chemicals employed it is the cholinesterase inhibiting insecticides that give the greatest cause for concern, both because of their acute toxicity and their capacity for inducing chronic cholinesterase depression. The number of accidents attributed to this group of compounds is, however, low, and in the UK only one pilot appears to have died in the last 25 years directly from the effects of insecticide poisoning (Quantick, 1985). This figure should be interpreted with care as subtle behavioural effects may occur with chronic exposure that modify the pilot's ability to conduct the flying task.

In general the risk of pesticide intoxication depends on the following factors:

1. The acute and cumulative toxicity of the chemical used.
2. The concentration after dilution for spraying.
3. Rate of absorption through skin or other routes.
4. The extent of contamination of skin or clothing during handling.
5. Length of time before skin or clothing is washed.

6. Duration of operations with the same or closely related chemical.

Liquid preparations cause greater toxicity problems than granules. Dusts are relatively dilute, although very pervasive, and constitute a risk halfway between that of liquids and granules. The greatest risk of poisoning is run by those handling undiluted material; pilots should not load their own aircraft and are principally at risk only after a crash.

The four major classes of compounds responsible for almost all cases of intoxication of aircrew working in spraying operations are as follows.

Nitrophenols

These are strongly phytotoxic chemicals used as insecticides, defoliants or herbicides. Typical of these compounds is dinitro-o-cresol (DNOC). It is absorbed through the respiratory tract and the skin. They are highly toxic in small concentrations and the effects are cumulative. Early signs of poisoning include sweating, thirst, euphoria and fatigue. A single large dose (2 mg) causes gastric pain and nausea and rapidly produces respiratory distress, cyanosis and death. Chronic poisoning may result from repeated exposure to small doses and gives rise to unexplained constant fatigue, loss of weight and general malaise.

Carbamates

This group includes compounds such as Dimetan and Isolan which have the basic chemical structure $ROC=ONHCH_3$. These are commonly used insecticides and are closely related both chemically and pharmacologically to the therapeutic agents physostigmine and neostigmine. They derive their insecticidal and toxic action from the inhibition of the enzyme cholinesterase. Their toxic action is similar to that of the organophosphates (described below) although the symptoms are less persistent.

Chlorinated, cyclic hydrocarbons

This heterogenous group of compounds is widely used for insecticide purposes: for example, the well-known dichlorodiphenyltrichloroethane (DDT). Some, like DDT, are toxic only when ingested; others, for example Dieldrin, are readily absorbed through skin and are highly toxic. The estimated lethal dose of DDT is 25–30 g whilst that of Dieldrin is only 2–7 g. These compounds owe their insecticidal activity and their acute toxicity to their action on the nervous system. Symptoms and signs of poisoning include nausea, dizziness, headache, tremor, dyspnoea, convulsions and circulatory collapse.

Organophosphates

These compounds are esters or thio-esters of an organic base with phosphoric or thiophosphoric acid. They may be absorbed through the skin or by ingestion. They owe their insecticidal effectiveness and human toxicity primarily to inhibition of the enzyme cholinesterase so that it cannot destroy the acetylcholine released at the nerve endings. As a result, the symptoms of toxicity are many and varied: they include nausea, vomiting, visual disturbance, salivation, bradycardia, hypotension, anal and urinary incontinence, convulsion, coma, respiratory failure and death. Unlike the carbamates and other cholinesterase inhibitors, which have a short period of action, the organophosphates produce irreversible blocking of cholinesterase. The compounds within this group used as insecticides vary markedly with regard to their toxicity in man and also to the speed at which symptoms develop. Thus a dose of between 20 and 100 mg of parathon or TEPP by mouth is fatal, whilst the toxicity of malathion is less than that of DDT.

Action in the event of contamination of cabin air

The first line of defence against toxic hazards in the air is a high standard of servicing; the second is sensible operation of the aircraft.

Action in the air

If contamination of the aircraft cabin should occur, the action that must be taken to avoid the substances reaching exposed parts of the body—and in the case of toxic gases and vapours, to avoid inhalation of the contaminant—depends on whether the aircrew are using oxygen equipment and on the type of oxygen system. The aim is to breathe 100% oxygen as soon as possible and take all action to prevent inboard leakage of contaminated air. The latter actions may include manual closure of the air inlet valve fitted to the oxygen regulator and selection of safety pressure as appropriate. If oxygen is not in use, aircrew should, wherever possible, don any breathing equipment provided and put on goggles or a visor.

Similarly, the skin should be covered as much as possible. If the cabin is contaminated by air delivered from the engine compressors, the inflow into the cabin should be turned off and ram air ventilation selected—provided of course, that hypo-xia can be avoided in the reduced cabin differential pressure that will follow. If no oxygen is available, the pilot will have to reduce altitude.

Action by the medical officer

Individuals who have been exposed to any toxic hazard should be examined as soon as possible after the aircraft has landed so that medical treatment may be given early. The first aim of the investigating medical officer is to try to identify the nature of the toxic substance. This may be revealed by a careful history together with examination of the aircraft cabin and the nature of any materials burned. If CO poisoning is suspected, one must take an immediate blood sample by venepuncture for later analysis. A rapid approximation of blood CO can be obtained by a breath analysis employing a balloon, a commercial gas analysis kit and CO detector tubes (0.001%). The concentration of CO in exposed air can be read from the level of discoloration in the tube, and conversion to blood CO concentration may be obtained from an appropriate chart. This latter test is only an approximation and does not take the place of a full laboratory blood analysis. In the absence of fire, the cabin air of an aircraft which is ventilated by air from the compressor stage of a jet engine is unlikely to contain a significant concentration of CO. By far the commonest cause of toxic contamination of the cabin air of a fast jet aircraft is overheating of a bearing or a failure of a seal of a bearing of a moving part in the environmental control system, which allows lubricating oil and/or the products of heated lubricating oil to enter the cabin air-supply system.

References

QUANTICK, H.R. (1985) *Aviation in Crop Protection, Pollution and Insect Control*, p.57. London: Collins Professional and Technical Books
WORLD HEALTH ORGANISATION (1975). *WHO Chronicle*, **29**, 397, 401

Further reading

DOULL, T., KLAASSEN C.D. and ANDREWS, M.O. (1980) *Casarett and Doull's Toxicology. The Basic Science of Poisons*, 2nd edn. New York: Macmillan Publishing
QUANTICK, H.R. (1985) *Aviation in Crop Protection, Pollution and Insect Control*. London: Collins Professional and Technical Books

Part II

Biodynamics

10

The effects of long duration acceleration

D.H. Glaister

Introduction

The human body is continuously acted on by the force of earth's gravity and is well adapted to an existence in an environment with a force of this magnitude. Modern aircraft are highly manoeuvrable and capable of flying at very high speeds, and during certain periods the occupant may be exposed to accelerative forces of large magnitude.

In aviation medicine, accelerations are usually classified according to their duration and to the direction in which they act on the body. Thus we can consider accelerative forces met with in aviation and spaceflight to be of the following order.

1. *Short duration*—Forces that act on the body for periods considerably less than 1 second. Their effects depend principally on the structural strength of the part of the body on which they act, and are related to the overall velocity change induced. They are usually encountered during ground impact.
2. *Intermediate duration*—Forces that act for about 0.5–2 s. These are encountered in ejection escape from aircraft, but may also occur during catapult launches and deck landings. Tolerance depends not only upon the overall velocity change induced, but also upon the time taken to reach peak acceleration and the peak acceleration level attained.
3. *Long duration*—Forces that act for periods of more than 2 seconds and which may last for several minutes. Forces of this type are met with during various aircraft manoeuvres and during launch and re-entry of space vehicles. The physiological effects of long duration acceleration are produced by the sustained distortion of tissues and organs of the body and by alterations in the flow and distribution of blood and body

fluids. Tolerance depends primarily upon the level of plateau acceleration imposed.

This chapter is concerned primarily with the physiological changes that are induced in man by the inertial forces resulting from long duration accelerations. The effects of shorter duration accelerations and oscillating accelerations (vibration) are dealt with elsewhere.

Physical considerations

A knowledge of elementary mechanics and a clear understanding of the meaning of certain physical terms are essential in the study of acceleration physiology.

Speed, velocity and acceleration

Speed

Speed describes the rate of movement of a body without specifying the direction of travel. Speed is defined as the rate of change of distance, that is, it is the first time derivative of distance. Thus:

$$\text{Speed} = \frac{\text{distance}}{\text{time}} = \frac{\mathrm{d}s}{\mathrm{d}t}$$

where s is the distance, t is the time

Typical units for speed are metres per second (the basic SI unit), miles per hour, knots and feet per second.

Velocity

Velocity describes the rate and direction of travel of an object. Thus it is a vector quantity, having both magnitude and direction. The velocity of a body changes if its speed or its direction of travel change. Velocity is expressed as the rate of change of distance in a specified direction. Units are the same as for speed, with direction specified according to a three-dimensional co-ordinate system which may be based arbitrarily upon the Earth's surface, the aircraft structure, or the aircrew member's spinal alignment.

Acceleration

Acceleration describes a change of velocity of an object. It is defined as the rate of change of velocity and like velocity is a vector quantity having magnitude and direction. Acceleration can result from or produce a change in the rate of movement along a straight line (linear acceleration) or from a change in the direction of travel (radial acceleration) or a combination of both. Acceleration is the second time derivative of distance. Thus:

$$\text{Acceleration (a)} = \frac{\text{velocity}}{\text{time}} = \frac{d^2s}{dt^2}$$

where s is the distance } for the change
$\quad\quad t$ is the time } of velocity

Acceleration can have a positive value (velocity increasing) or a negative value (velocity decreasing). The term deceleration is sometimes employed for a negative acceleration. Typical units for acceleration are m/s^2 (the basic SI unit) and ft/s^2. In aviation, applied accelerations are frequently expressed as multiples of the acceleration due to gravity. The acceleration due to gravity which is termed the gravitational constant and which is indicated by the symbol 'g' (small letter) has the value 9.81 m/s^2 (32.2 ft/s^2). The unit of the ratio of an applied acceleration to the gravitational constant is the 'G' (capital letter). Thus, the G value of an applied acceleration is given by:

$$G = \frac{\text{applied acceleration}}{g}$$

The value of an acceleration of 2 G is therefore $2 \times 9.81 = 19.62$ m/s^2.

Jolt

The rate of change of acceleration is termed jolt. Jolt is the third time derivative of distance, the typical unit being G/s. Jolt is of particular significance when considering the effects of short-duration accelerations on the body, but the rate of onset of acceleration is also of importance in human response to forces encountered in normal flight.

Motion and force

The relationships between motion and force are defined by Newton's three Laws of Motion.

Newton's first law

The first law states that, unless acted upon by a force, a body at rest will remain at rest and a body in motion will move at constant speed in a straight line. Thus a force can produce a change in speed or in direction of motion, that is, a change of velocity. Newton's first law may therefore be regarded as stating that accelerations result from the action of forces.

Newton's second law

The second law states that when a force is applied to a body the body is accelerated and the acceleration is directly proportional to the force applied and inversely proportional to the mass of the body. Expressed mathematically the second law states:

$$a = \frac{F}{m} \quad\quad \text{or} \quad\quad F = ma$$

where F is the force, m is the mass of the body, a is the acceleration.

The mass of a body is the amount of matter in it. It remains constant whatever the acceleration of the body.

Newton's third law

The third law states that to every action there is an equal and opposite reaction. Thus when a force is applied to a body it is resisted by an equal and opposite force, which is termed the force of inertia. For example, when an aircraft accelerates forwards, it is the inertial force that forces the pilot back into his seat. In every case in which man is accelerated (except the gravitational attractions of the Earth), the sensation of increased weight and the redistribution of the blood and displacement of organs occur in the direction of the inertial force.

Weight

Weight is the force exerted by the mass of an accelerating body. A special case is when a body is exposed to Earth's gravitational field, when by definition weight is equal to mass. Thus a body of mass 1 kg exerts a weight of 1 kg when it is accelerated at 9.81 m/s^2 (the gravitational constant). In more general terms the weight (W) exerted by a mass (m) when accelerated at a value of 'a' is given by the relationship:

$$W = m \times \frac{a}{g}$$

Thus, for example, when a mass of 1 kg is acted upon by a force which produces an acceleration of 29.43 m/s^2, that is, an acceleration of 3 G, it weighs 3 kg.

The force exerted by a mass of 1 kg under standard conditions of gravity (an acceleration of 9.8065 m/s^2) is termed the newton, the symbol for which is N. Thus, the definition of 1 newton of force is 1 kg/s^2. The unit of force in the ft/lb/sec system is the pound force (symbol, lbf) which is the force exerted by a mass of 1 lb under standard conditions of gravity (an acceleration of 32.18 ft/s^2).

There is, it should be noted, a difference between the sensation of force (weight) produced by gravity and that induced by other accelerations. Other forms of acceleration produce a sensation of force acting in a direction opposite to the change in velocity. In the case of gravity, however, both the acceleration and the sensation of weight are in the same direction, towards the centre of the Earth. Furthermore, it is only when the acceleration due to gravity is fully resisted by direct or indirect contact with the ground that normal weight is experienced, and a body has no weight if it is allowed to fall with an acceleration of 9.81 m/s^2. Thus gravity is unique in that it can be responsible for acceleration or weight but not for both at the same time.

Prolonged accelerations in flight

Prolonged changes in velocity, that is, accelerations lasting longer than 2 seconds or so, may result from changes in either the speed or the direction of flight.

Linear accelerations

A linear acceleration is one produced by a change of speed without a change in direction. In conventional aviation, prolonged linear accelerations seldom reach a magnitude that will produce significant changes in human performance, as most aircraft do not exert sufficient thrust to produce extended changes in linear velocity. Significant linear accelerations lasting 2–4 seconds are, however, produced during catapult-assisted take-off, arrested landings and when reheat is engaged in certain high-performance aircraft. Large prolonged linear accelerations occur during the launch of spacecraft and when they are slowed upon re-entering the Earth's atmosphere. The magnitude of a linear acceleration may be calculated from various combinations of the total velocity change, the distance over which the velocity change occurred and the time occupied by the velocity change. These equations assume a constant acceleration—a rectangular acceleration pulse gives the lowest value of peak acceleration for a given duration and velocity change. Thus:

$$a = \frac{v}{t} \qquad (10.1)$$

$$a = \frac{v^2}{2s} \qquad (10.2)$$

$$a = \frac{2s}{t^2} \qquad (10.3)$$

where a = the acceleration, v = the velocity change, s = the distance over which v occurred, t = the time during which v occurred

Using SI units and taking g as equal to 10 m/s^2, rough mental estimates of the three variables concerned when accelerations occur can be made using the following relationships:

$$v = 10\,Gt \qquad (10.4)$$

$$s = \frac{v^2}{20G} \qquad (10.5)$$

$$t = \sqrt{\frac{s}{5\,G}} \qquad (10.6)$$

These are particularly useful in considering impact forces, for example in predicting imposed acceleration from estimates of impact velocity and stopping distance (equation 10.5), or in calculating how much padding would be required to prevent injury from a given impact velocity and G tolerance.

Radial accelerations

A radial acceleration is one produced by a change of direction of motion without a change of speed. Such accelerations occur when the line of flight is changed, and, indeed, aircraft manoeuvres are by far the commonest source of prolonged accelerations in flight. Accelerations of the order of 6–9 G or more can be maintained for many seconds by circular flight in agile military aircraft. Centrifuges which are used to study the effects of prolonged accelerations on man also produce radial accelerations.

By Newton's first law of motion, an object constrained to move along a circular path will have the tendency to continue on a straight line which forms a tangent to the circular path. The object is prevented from moving tangentially by a force which pulls it away from the straight line towards the centre of the circle, and is responsible for the change

172

of velocity which accompanies the change in the direction of travel. The magnitude of the radial acceleration of the object towards the centre of its circular path (centripetal acceleration) depends on the circumferential velocity of the object along its circular path and the radius of the path it follows:

$$a = \frac{v^2}{r}$$

where a = centripetal, radial acceleration; v = circumferential velocity; r = radius of circular path

Using this equation it may be calculated, for example, that the radial acceleration of an aircraft travelling at 500 mph (225 m/s) around a circular path with a diameter of 1 mile will be 204 ft/s² (62 m/s²) or 6.3 G. It should be noted that small changes in the speed of the object will have a proportionally greater effect on the radial acceleration than small changes in radius.

Centrifugal forces in flight

The previous section stated that, when an object describes a circular path, it is accelerated radially towards the centre of the circular path. By Newton's third law, the force producing the acceleration of the mass towards the centre of the circular path must be balanced by an equal force acting in the opposite direction—an inertial force which, since it acts outwards away from the centre of the curved path, is termed centrifugal force. The physiological effects of the radial accelerations produced by circular flight are due to centrifugal forces.

The magnitude of the centrifugal force generated by flight in a circular path is given by the equation:

$$F = \frac{mv^2}{r}$$

where F = centrifugal inertial force, m = mass of the body, v = circumferential velocity, r = radius of curved path

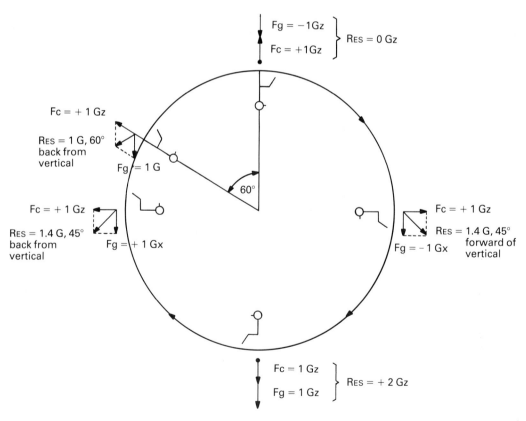

Figure 10.1 The interaction between centrifugal inertial force (Fc) and gravitational force (Fg) on the pilot of an aircraft flown in a loop. The vector diagrams show that the resultant (Res) of the centrifugal and inertial forces varies from +2 G at the bottom of the loop at 0 G at the top. While descending the resultant acts forwards of the long axis of the body and during ascent it acts behind the long axis.

An object in an aircraft executing a circular flight path is not only exposed to the centrifugal inertia forces induced by the radial accelerations but also to the force generated by the linear acceleration due to gravity. The relationship between the centrifugal and gravitational forces frequently changes continuously during the manoeuvre, so that the magnitude and direction of the resultant force acting on the object varies along the flight path. The interactions of these forces may be illustrated by considering the resultant force acting on the pilot flying an aircraft in a loop giving a constant radial acceleration of 1 G. The magnitude and direction of the resultant of the centrifugal inertial force (Fc) of 1 G and that due to gravity (Fg) at several stages in the loop are depicted in *Figure 10.1*. When the aircraft is at the bottom of the loop, the centrifugal and gravitational forces are acting in the same direction along a line at right angles to the longitudinal axis of the aircraft; so that the resultant acceleration will be 2 G and the weight of a mass will be twice its resting value. When the aircraft is inverted at the top of the loop, the centrifugal and gravitational forces are acting along the same line but in opposition to each other, so that the resultant acceleration and the apparent weight will both be zero. At all other points in the loop, the weight lies between 0 and 2, and the angle which the resultant makes with the longitudinal axis of the aircraft changes through 180 degrees during the loop. Thus halfway up and halfway down the loop, the vector

diagrams show (*Figure 10.1*) that the weight of an object will be 1.4 times its resting value. On the ascending loop, however, the resultant force is acting 45 degrees behind the normal vertical whilst it acts 45 degrees forward of the normal vertical midway down the descending loop. When the aircraft is 60 degrees from the top of the loop the magnitude of the resultant is 1.0 Fg so that an object will have its normal resting weight. At this position the resultant is 60 degrees behind the normal vertical on the ascent and 60 degrees forwards of it on the descent. Although perfect loops of the type depicted in *Figure 10.1* are produced in aerobatic flying it is far more usual for an aircraft to fly a track made up of only part of a circular path or several different circular paths. The magnitudes and directions of the accelerative forces acting on the aircraft and its contents can, however, be determined by treating the complex flight path as a series of sections, each with its own radius of curvature.

Terminology of acceleration

When the main interest is the effect of acceleration on man, the direction in which an acceleration or inertial force acts is described by the use of a three-axis co-ordinate system (X, Y and Z), in which the vertical (Z) axis is parallel to the long axis of the body. Considerable confusion can arise if a clear distinction is not made between the applied

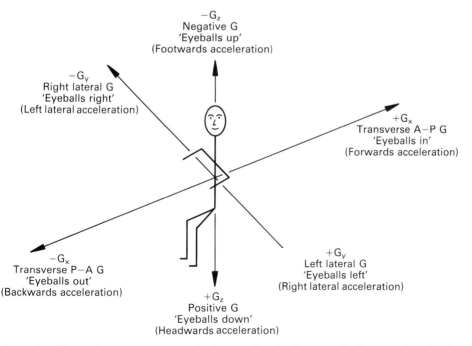

$-G_z$
Negative G
'Eyeballs up'
(Footwards acceleration)

$-G_y$
Right lateral G
'Eyeballs right'
(Left lateral acceleration)

$+G_x$
Transverse A–P G
'Eyeballs in'
(Forwards acceleration)

$-G_x$
Transverse P–A G
'Eyeballs out'
(Backwards acceleration)

$+G_y$
Left lateral G
'Eyeballs left'
(Right lateral acceleration)

$+G_z$
Positive G
'Eyeballs down'
(Headwards acceleration)

Figure 10.2 The standard AGARD aeromedical terminology for describing the direction of acceleration and inertial forces. The vector arrows indicate the direction of the resultant inertial forces.

Table 10.1 Three-axis co-ordinate system for describing direction of acceleration and inertial forces acting on man

Direction of acceleration	Direction of resultant inertial force	Physiological and vernacular descriptors	Standard terminology
Headward	Head to foot	Positive G Eyeballs down	$+G_z$
Footward	Foot to head	Negative G Eyeballs up	$-G_z$
Forward	Chest to back	Transverse A-P G Supine G Eyeballs in	$+G_x$
Backward	Back to chest	Transverse P-A G Prone G Eyeballs out	$-G_x$
To the right	Right to left side	Left lateral G Eyeballs left	$+G_y$
To the left	Left to right side	Right lateral G Eyeballs right	$-G_y$

acceleration and the resultant inertial force as these, by definition, always act in diametrically opposite directions. Thus a headward acceleration tends to displace tissues such as viscera and the eyes footward and the resultant force is termed positive G, $+G_z$. The standard AGARD aeromedical terminology for indicating the direction of accelerations and inertial forces acting on man is listed in *Table 10.1* and illustrated in *Figure 10.2*.

Long duration positive acceleration ($+G_z$)

The crews of agile aircraft are frequently exposed to sustained positive accelerations by changes in the direction of flight either in turns or recovery from dives. The performance of many current combat aircraft is such that the occupants can be exposed to positive accelerations of 5–7 G for 10–40 seconds. The latest generation of air combat fighters can maintain positive accelerations of the order of 8–10 G for periods of up to 60 seconds and 12–14 G is technically feasible with duration limited solely by fuel reserves. These levels may also be attained very rapidly, with onset rates of the order of 10 G/s. For the first time since the development of the anti-G suit, human tolerance becomes the factor limiting aircraft performance.

General effects

Mobility

The increase in the weight of the soft tissues and of the limbs and the body as a whole gives rise to distinctive symptoms and signs even at relatively low levels of positive acceleration. At $+2\,G_z$, there is

sagging of the soft tissues of the face and the increase in the weight of the trunk and limbs is clearly apparent. It is difficult to raise oneself from the sitting posture at $+2.5\,G$ and impossible to do so at about $+3\,G_z$. Unassisted escape from an uncontrolled aircraft is impossible at positive accelerations greater than 2–3 G. Movement of the unsupported limbs becomes progressively more difficult above 3 G until, at 8 G, upward movement of the upper limbs is impossible. Large upward movement such as reaching and grasping the face blind handle of an ejection seat is progressively impaired, the time taken to carry out this operation at 6 G being on average twice that at 1 G, and very few subjects are able to perform it at all at 7 G. If, however, the forearm and hand are well supported, fine control movements and those involving considerable force can be performed with little or no loss of accuracy at positive accelerations of up to at least 8 G (provided that consciousness is not impaired). Even without headgear, a subject cannot raise his head once he has allowed his neck to flex at accelerations above about 8 G. When a typical protective helmet (2 kg wt) is worn, this limitation occurs at $+4$ to $+6\,G_z$. Of particular relevance is the position of the centre of gravity of the head relative to the atlanto-occipital junction and upper thoracic vertebrae. Head-mounted equipment such as helmets, sights, displays, night vision goggles and so forth may bring the centre of gravity forward and encourage forwards flexion of the head under $+G_z$ acceleration.

Vision

Exposure to positive acceleration usually causes deterioration of vision prior to any disturbance of consciousness. Thus exposure to $+4.5\,G_z$ typically produces complete loss of vision, 'blackout', whilst hearing and mental activity are unaffected. At lower levels of acceleration, visual acuity is reduced and there is loss of peripheral vision with retention of central vision—this condition is termed 'grey-out'. There is a large variation in the level of acceleration at which a given loss of peripheral vision occurs. It varies, from one individual to another, with body stature, physical condition, level of illumination of the visual field and target and, in particular, with the degree of relaxation. In one series of experiments, the mean level of acceleration at which the field of vision was reduced to a cone with an angle of 45 degrees was 4.1 G, with a standard deviation of ±0.7 G, whilst the mean value at which blackout occurred was 4.7 G with a standard deviation of ±0.8 G. Whatever the level of acceleration, vision is not disturbed for some 5 seconds after the beginning of the exposure. At moderate levels of acceleration, the intensity of the visual symptoms often decreases 8–12 seconds after the onset of the acceleration. This improvement is due to compensatory cardiovascular responses restoring the flow of blood to the retina. Thus, during exposure to 5.0 G, blackout may occur at 6 seconds but vision be restored some 6 seconds later. Normal vision normally returns in 3–5 seconds after the manoeuvre ends.

Unconsciousness

Exposure to a positive acceleration stress somewhat greater than that required to produce blackout results in unconsciousness. At moderate levels of acceleration, for example, 5–6 G, blackout precedes loss of consciousness; but at higher accelerations, unconsciousness occurs before any visual symptoms have arisen. With very rapid onset rates, the time from the beginning of the exposure to loss of consciousness is 4–6 seconds. As consciousness is lost there is total loss of muscle tone so that the head and trunk slump. Convulsions commonly occur whilst the subject is unconscious. Recovery of consciousness after an exposure has finished is generally slow, with complete incapacitation lasting for 15 seconds or so followed by a similar period of confusion prior to effective recovery. Owing to physiological amnesia and possible psychological suppression, episodes of G-induced loss of consciousness may pass unnoticed. Prolonged exposure to lower levels of acceleration may cause unconsciousness by vasovagal syncope, when there is also pallor, sweating and bradycardia.

Confidential surveys carried out in the US Air Force have revealed that 12% of responding pilots had experienced at least one episode of G-induced loss of consciousness (GLOC), the aircraft concerned being predominantly, but not exclusively, high-performance fighters. In the 2½ year period from January, 1983, seven losses of aircraft and crew were attributed to GLOC. US Navy experience was comparable with 12% of returned questionnaires reporting occurrences of GLOC. Since studies show that 50% of subjects experiencing GLOC on the centrifuge do not recall the event, the real incidence may be closer to 24%, or 1 in 4 of the sampled pilot population.

Cardiovascular effects

The effects of positive acceleration on vision and mental performance are due to decreases of the flow of blood through the vascular beds of the eye and the brain, produced by disturbances of the pressures in the cardiovascular system. Exposure to positive acceleration produces immediate major changes in the distribution of pressure in the arterial and venous systems which, in turn, induce shifts of blood towards the more dependent parts. These initial disturbances evoke reflex compensatory changes which tend to reduce the magnitude of the initial effects.

Initial hydrostatic effects

The pressure exerted by a column of fluid is determined by the height of the column, the density of the liquid and the acceleration to which it is exposed. Provided that the other factors remain constant, the pressure exerted by a column of fluid is directly proportional to the acceleration. The immediate effect of positive acceleration is, therefore, an accentuation of the pressure gradients which normally exist due to gravity in the system in erect man. As during the change from the supine to the erect posture, the pressures in the right and left sides of the heart—since they are created with reference to the pressure in the pleural space and hence the pressure of the atmosphere—remain essentially unchanged at the beginning of an exposure to positive acceleration. The positive acceleration increases the weight of the columns of blood above and below the heart so that the vascular pressures above the level of the heart are decreased and those below the heart are increased by positive acceleration. These changes in intravascular pressures have immediate effects on the size of the blood vessels, since the latter is determined by the transmural pressure (the differences between intravascular and extravascular tissue pressure), the distensibility of the vessel and the amount of blood available to fill it. In turn, the changes in the size of the vessels have major effects on the regional blood flow and blood content. Thus increases in the transmural pressures of small arteries and arterioles below the level of the heart will reduce the peripheral resistance and increase local blood flow, whilst decreases of the transmural pressures of veins above the level of the heart can produce complete collapse of the vessels and cessation of blood flow through them.

The magnitude of the changes of pressure produced in the circulation by positive acceleration is proportional to the vertical distance between the point at which the pressure is measured and the heart, and the level of acceleration. The pressures in the arterial tree of an individual seated erect at $+1\,G_z$ and $+4.5\,G_z$ are illustrated in *Figure 10.3*. The mean arterial pressure at heart level both at $+1$ and $+4.5\,G_z$ is $100\,mm\,Hg$. The mean pressure in the cerebral arteries at eye level, which is $30\,cm$ vertically above the heart, is $100\,mm\,Hg$ less the hydrostatic pressure exerted by the $30\,cm$ column of blood, that is, $22\,mm\,Hg$ at $+1\,G_z$ and $99\,mm\,Hg$ at $+4.5\,G_z$. Thus the mean cerebral arterial pressure

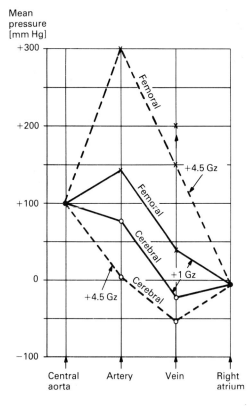

Figure 10.3 The immediate effect of exposure to $+1\,G_z$ and $+4.5\,G_z$ on the mean pressures at the following points in the circulation of a seated individual. (1) Immediately downstream of the aortic valve. (2) In the cerebral arteries and veins at the horizontal level of the eye. (3) In the femoral artery and vein. (4) In the right atrium. Secondary changes in the circulation which occur over the first 30–60 seconds of the exposure to $+G_z$ modify the magnitude of these pressures. The pressure in the femoral vein rises progressively during the first 30–60 seconds of the exposure to $+G_z$ as blood accumulates in the capacity vessels of the lower limbs.

falls from $78\,mm\,Hg$ at $1\,G_z$ to only $1\,mm\,Hg$ at $4.5\,G_z$. The pressure in the femoral artery, which is approximately $60\,cm$ below the heart, is $100 + 44 = 144\,mm\,Hg$ at $+1\,G_z$. The pressure exerted by the $60\,cm$ column of blood is increased to $198\,mm\,Hg$ at $+4.5\,G_z$, so that the femoral artery pressure at this level of positive acceleration is approximately $300\,mm\,Hg$. The corresponding pressures in the venous part of the systematic circulation are also shown in *Figure 10.3*. The pressure in the right atrium of the heart is virtually atmospheric both at $+1$ and at $+4.5\,G_z$. At $+1\,G_z$ the pressure in the cerebral veins at eye level is of the order of $-20\,mm\,Hg$. On exposure to $+4.5\,G_z$ the increase in the weight of the column of blood between cerebral veins and the heart would be expected to reduce the pressure in the cerebral veins to about $100\,mm\,Hg$. The higher transmural pressure across the walls of the jugular veins in the neck produced by positive acceleration reduces the lumen of the veins greatly, increasing the resistance to flow through them; so that, in practice, the pressure in the jugular bulb only falls to about $-50\,mm\,Hg$ on exposure to $+4.5\,G_z$. The pressure in the veins below the heart is increased by the rise in the weight of the column of blood between the point of interest and the right atrium.

Secondary circulatory changes

Although at the moment of the exposure to the positive acceleration the arterial pressure at the level of the heart is unchanged, this pressure falls progressively over the first 6–12 seconds of an exposure. This fall of mean arterial pressure is due to a fall in the peripheral resistance and a reduction in the output of the left side of the heart. The fall of peripheral resistance is caused by the large increase in the transmural pressures of the arterioles in the dependent parts of the arterial tree, whilst the increase in venous pressure in the regions below the heart causes dilation of the capacity vessels and thereby reduces temporarily the flow of blood back to the right side of the heart. If the positive acceleration is maintained, then this progressive fall of pressure, which occurs throughout the arterial tree, persists until 6–12 seconds after the onset of the acceleration. It is then reversed by reflex compensatory changes and an increase in the venous return to the heart as the capacity vessels in the dependent parts of the circulation fill. The reflex compensatory changes occur in response to the fall in pressure in the carotid sinus (the baroreceptive region at the origin of the internal carotid artery at the bifurcation of the common carotid artery). The fall in the transmural pressure in the carotid sinus reduces the activity of the carotid baroreceptors and causes, reflexly, a generalized arteriolar vasoconstriction and a tachycardia. Exposure to $+4\,G_z$

produces a maximum heart rate of 120–140 beats per minute. The venous return to the right side of the heart starts to increase by 10–15 seconds after the onset of the exposure to the positive acceleration, and the output of the left side of the heart increases within a few beats. The venous return and the cardiac output continue to rise over the next 20–40 seconds, although they never regain the pre-exposure level because a significant quantity of the central blood volume remains in the capacity vessels of the lower parts of the body for as long as the exposure lasts. The cardiac output after 30–60 seconds' exposure to $+4\,G_z$ is reduced by about 20% below the resting value. All these compensatory changes tend to restore the arterial blood pressure; so that, after 40–60 seconds, exposure to moderate levels of positive acceleration (up to 3–5 G), the mean arterial blood pressure at heart level is very similar to the pre-exposure level.

The pooling of blood produced by positive acceleration occurs mainly in the lower limbs. Little pooling can occur in the capacity vessels within the abdomen, as, during positive acceleration, the intra-abdominal pressure rises in parallel with the intravenous pressure. Some 60–100 ml of blood are pooled in the lower limbs of a seated subject exposed to $+4\,G_z$ though the circulation is already compromised at $+1\,G_z$ as some 300–800 ml blood is pooled in the lower limbs upon adoption of the upright posture. The rise of pressure within the capillaries in the lower limbs also causes transudation of fluid from the blood to the tissues, so that there is a progressive loss of fluid from the circulation. The rate of fluid loss into the tissues of the lower limbs during a sustained exposure to $+4\,G_z$ is about 200 ml/min. This progressive reduction of the central blood volume due to pooling and transudation eventually causes vasovagal syncope with a sudden fall of arterial blood pressure, due to an intense peripheral vasodilatation, and accompanied by a profound bradycardia.

Retinal circulation

The visual disturbances produced by positive acceleration are caused by ischaemia of the retina. The various degrees of greyout are due to progressive reduction in the flow of blood to the retina: complete cessation of the flow causes blackout. The eye has an internal pressure of 20 mm Hg, so that the pressure in the central retinal artery must exceed 20 mm Hg or blood will not flow through the retina. Blackout occurs during positive acceleration when the systolic arterial pressure at eye level falls below 20 mm Hg. The retinal arteries and arterioles can be seen, with an ophthalmoscope, to be empty when the arterial pressure is less than 20 mm Hg. There is an interval of 4–6 seconds between an abrupt fall of arterial pressure below 20 mm Hg and loss of vision.

The delay is due to a small store of oxygen dissolved in the extravascular fluid of the retina. Similarly, on recovery, the return of vision is delayed several seconds after the arterial pressure at eye level has risen above 20 mm Hg. This delay is due to the time taken to restore the oxygen store and thereby raise the oxygen tension in the retina above the minimum required for normal function. Despite the blackout, consciousness is preserved until the cerebral arterial pressure is reduced to 0–10 mm Hg (*see* below).

The peripheral distribution of the loss of vision in greyout is due to the anatomical arrangement of the blood supply to the retina. The main retinal artery enters the globe of the eye at the optic disc and then subdivides repeatedly as it passes out towards the periphery of the retina. Each of the subdivisions is an end-artery; and, as the branches become increasingly fine towards the periphery of the retina, so the pressure within them falls correspondingly lower. Thus when the pressure in the central retinal artery is reduced by positive acceleration, it is the blood supply to the periphery of the retina that fails first.

Cerebral circulation

The hydrostatic effects of positive accelerations greater than 3.5–4 G on arterial pressure reduce the arterial pressure at the level of the brain to a value that at $+1\,G_z$ would be below that required to maintain an adequate cerebral blood flow, whilst exposure to $+4.5\,G$ reduces the arterial pressure at head level to virtually zero. Furthermore, consciousness is maintained during exposure to positive accelerations sufficient to induce blackout, when the arterial pressure at eye level must be less than 20 mm Hg. Although reflex compensatory changes partially restore arterial pressure at brain level 6–12 seconds after the onset of acceleration, the incidence of unconsciousness is much lower than would be expected. Several mechanisms are responsible for the maintenance of an adequate flow of blood through the brain during exposure to +3 to $+5\,G_z$ even though the arterial pressure is only 0–20 mm Hg at head level. First, the cerebral vessels and brain are enclosed in a rigid bony box and surrounded by cerebrospinal fluid. The pressure of the cerebrospinal fluid falls, owing to hydrostatic effects, during positive acceleration in parallel with the reduction of vascular pressures at head level; so that the pressure differences across the walls of the intracranial vessels remain close to the normal values and the vessels remain open in spite of the fall of intravascular pressure. Secondly, there is active vasodilatation of the arterioles of the cerebral circulation, so that the resistance to flow through them is reduced. Thirdly, the column of blood in the upper part of the veins in the neck creates a siphon effect which maintains the cerebral circulation for as long as the column remains unbroken. Thus a pressure difference between the arterial and venous sides of the cerebral circulation of the order of 50–60 mm Hg is maintained at a positive acceleration of 4–5 G by a pressure in the jugular bulb of −50 mm Hg. With higher levels of acceleration, however, the further lowering of the pressure within the upper part of the jugular veins causes these vessels to collapse completely, thereby breaking the siphon. Blood then ceases to flow through the brain and unconsciousness supervenes in 3–4 seconds. As the siphon breaks, the cerebral vessels are emptied of blood; so that only the oxygen stored as dissolved gas in the cerebral tissue is left to maintain aerobic metabolism. This store is exhausted in about 3 seconds.

Skin capillaries

The high pressure differences across the walls of the capillaries in the skin of dependent parts produced by exposure to positive acceleration not only gives rise to transudation of fluid but may also cause rupture of these vessels with the formation of petechiae. Thus it is not unusual to find showers of petechial haemorrhages on the foot and the forearm after repeated or prolonged exposures to positive accelerations greater than about 4 G.

Cardiac arrhythmias

Benign cardiac arrhythmias frequently occur during and immediately following exposures to high sustained levels of $+G_z$ acceleration. Most common are premature ventricular contractions, but premature atrial beats, sinus arrhythmia with or without junctional block and sino-atrial block have also been described. These changes are probably related to the profound changes in heart rate induced during and following G-exposure. Pathological rhythm disturbances have not, however, been described in human subjects during voluntary exposures to $+G_z$ acceleration.

Pulmonary effects

Pulmonary ventilation and lung volumes

Exposure to positive acceleration at least up to 5 G causes little respiratory embarrassment. Pulmonary ventilation may increase substantially in novice centrifuge subjects, but in trained subjects (and aircrew) it tends to fall, an increase in respiratory rate being more than compensated for by a decrease in tidal volume. This effect is exaggerated by inflation of the abdominal bladder of an anti-G suit. The total lung and vital capacities are unaffected by positive accelerations up to 3 G, whilst exposure to

$+5 G_z$ reduces them by about 15%. Positive acceleration causes descent of the abdominal contents and diaphragm, thereby increasing the functional residual capacity. This capacity is increased by about 500 ml at $+3 G_z$. The descent of the diaphragm produced by positive acceleration is greatly reduced, or even reversed, by inflation of a standard anti-G suit.

Regional lung ventilation

Exposure to positive acceleration accentuates the regional differences in the distribution of ventilation which are present in the lungs of an erect individual

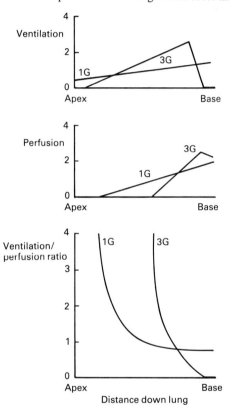

Figure 10.4 The vertical distributions of alveolar ventilation, perfusion and ventilation/perfusion ratio in the upright lung of an individual exposed to $+1 G_z$ and $+3 G_z$ expressed relative to values that would exist if gas and blood were uniformly distributed. Exposure to $+3 G_z$ triples the gradient of ventilation per unit of alveolar volume down the lung that exists at $+1 G_z$. Blood flow to virtually the upper half of the lung ceases at $+3 G_z$ and the gradient of flow per unit alveolar volume is tripled in the lower half. The volume of lung tissue which is ventilated, but not perfused (that which has a ventilation/perfusion ratio of infinity), is markedly increased by exposure to $+3 G_z$ which also increases the spread of ventilation/perfusion ratios in the lower portion of the lung, and produces a region of perfused, but non-ventilated, alveoli at the extreme base.

at $+1\,G_z$ (*see* Chapter 4). The increased weight of the lung magnifies the pressure gradient down the pleural cavity which amounts to about 0.2 cm water per cm of lung per G. Thus, at $+5\,G_z$ the pleural pressure at the base of the lung is 30 cm water greater than that at the apex. The larger gradient of pleural pressure induces, in turn, greater differences in the distension of alveoli down the lung. Alveoli at the apices are more distended, whilst those at the bases are closer to their minimum volumes as compared with their sizes at $+1\,G_z$. These changes accentuate, in turn, the differences in alveolar ventilation down the lung (ventilation per unit alveolar volume) (*Figure 10.4*). Thus at $+3\,G_z$ the gradient of ventilation down the lung is treble that at $+1\,G_z$. Of much greater significance, however, is the effect of positive acceleration in causing cessation of ventilation of alveoli at the base of the lung. Independent of overall lung volume, relative alveolar volumes decrease down the lung to such an extent that alveoli towards the base attain their minimal volume and their associated airways close. The lung volume (on breathing out from total lung capacity) at which this closure can first be detected is termed the closing volume of the lung and increases linearly with acceleration (*Figure 10.5*). Closure of terminal airways in dependent lung tissue will, therefore, occur whenever the lung volume at which a subject breathes is less than his closing volume,

and alveoli distal to the closed airways will contain trapped gas. Since inflation of the abdominal bladder of an anti-G suit raises the diaphragm and reduces the functional residual capacity, its use markedly increases the number of non-ventilated alveoli in the lower part of the lung (*Figure 10.6*).

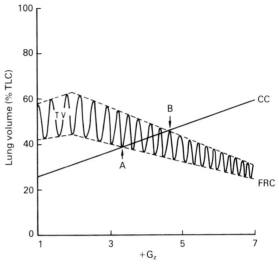

Figure 10.6 Effect of $+G_z$ acceleration on functional residual capacity (FRC) and closing capacity (CC) expressed as a percentage of total lung capacity (TLC) for a subject wearing an anti-G suit which starts to inflate at $+2\,G_z$. The combination of acceleration and anti-G suit inflation causes a reduction in FRC and tidal volume (TV). Terminal airways in the lung bases will start to close at end-expiration at the point marked A, but re-open in the ensuing inspiration until point B, remaining closed thereafter. By increasing the FRC and TV, the performance of an anti-G straining manoeuvre, or breathing under positive pressure, will move points A and B to the right and so increase the level of $+G_z$ at which acceleration atelectasis (absorption of alveolar gas trapped by airway closure) may develop.

Regional pulmonary blood flow

The distribution of blood flow through the lung is greatly affected by positive acceleration, because the external pressure to which the vessels are exposed (that is, alveolar gas pressure) is the same throughout the lung and is unaffected by acceleration, and because the pressures in the pulmonary circuit are relatively low. The mean pulmonary artery and the pulmonary venous pressures at the junction of the middle and lower thirds of the lung are unaffected by positive acceleration. Typical values for these pressures are 15 mm Hg (20 cm H_2O) and 0 mm Hg. The vascular pressures above and below this level are determined by hydrostatic forces; so that, even at $+1\,G_z$, the mean arterial pressure falls to zero 20 cm above the

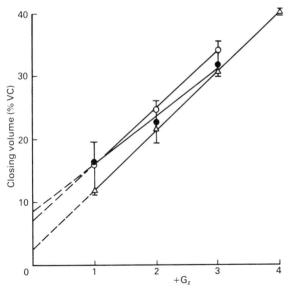

Figure 10.5 The effect of $+G_z$ acceleration on the closing volume of the lung expressed as a percentage of the vital capacity (VC). Values are individual means and the overall range for three subjects. Closure was detected by analysing the expirate to detect a sudden increase in the concentration of a tracer gas, a bolus of which had been inhaled at residual volume during the preceding maximal inspiration.

junction of the middle and lower thirds, that is, just at the apex of the lung. At $+4\,G_z$ the mean pulmonary artery pressure is zero only 5 cm above the junction of the middle and lower thirds, that is, the mean pulmonary artery pressure is zero in the upper half of the lung. Consequently the proportion of the lung which is not perfused increases with increasing acceleration from the uppermost 1 or 2 cm at $+1\,G_z$ to the whole of the upper half of the lung at $+4$ to $+5\,G_z$. Above the level at which the pulmonary venous pressure is zero the blood flow through the alveoli is determined by the difference between arterial and alveolar gas pressures. The progressive rise in the pulmonary artery pressure and, below the junction of the middle and lower thirds, in pulmonary venous pressure as well, with distance down the lung below the non-perfused region, results in a corresponding increase in regional blood flow (*see Figure 10.4*). The rise in blood flow per centimetre down the lung is greater the higher the acceleration. The blood flow decreases, however, in the most dependent part of the lung probably because the rise of interstitial pressure is transmitted to the alveolar gas when terminal airways close, so increasing the resistance to blood flow.

Pulmonary gas exchange and arterial oxygen saturation

Positive acceleration accentuates the increases of both ventilation and blood flow with distance down the lung seen at $+1\,G_z$. The magnitude of the changes in ventilation and blood flow down the lung differ, so that positive acceleration accentuates the ventilation–perfusion inequalities which are present in the normal erect lung (*see Figure 10.4*). In particular, with increasing positive acceleration, there is a progressively larger volume of the upper lung (which amounts to about one-half the lung at $+5\,G_z$) which is ventilated but not perfused, that is, has a ventilation/blood flow ratio of infinity; and a progressively larger volume of basal lung which is perfused but not ventilated, that is, has a ventilation/blood flow ratio of zero. The ventilated but non-perfused region at the top of the lung simply adds to the respiratory dead space and does not, in practice, interfere with the oxygenation of the arterial blood. The considerable spread of ventilation blood flow ratios which is present in that portion of the lung which is ventilated and perfused causes only a small reduction of the oxygen tension of the arterial blood, since, with increasing acceleration, the blood flow is distributed differentially to the better ventilated lower part of the lung. The perfused but non-ventilated alveoli in the lowermost part of the lung do, however, impair the oxygenation of the arterial blood. The oxygen tension of the gas trapped in the non-ventilated alveoli rapidly falls

within a few seconds, by absorption of oxygen into the blood, to equal that of the mixed venous blood. The blood flowing through these alveoli then constitutes a right-to-left shunt. The proportion of the cardiac output shunted in this manner increases with acceleration and, at $+5\,G_z$, amounts to about 50%. This right-to-left shunt of blood reduces markedly the oxygen saturation and tension of the systemic arterial blood. Desaturation of the arterial blood becomes apparent at $+3\,G_z$ and exposure to $+5\,G_z$ reduces the arterial oxyhaemoglobin saturation to about 85% (mean arterial oxygen tension = 6.9 kPa). Breathing 100% oxygen prior to exposure to positive acceleration delays the onset of arterial desaturation, as the alveolar gas trapped in the non-ventilated alveoli has a very high tension, and the oxygen content of the blood flowing through them will only fall to that of mixed venous blood after virtually all this alveolar gas has been absorbed. Inflation of an anti-G suit increases the fall of the oxygen saturation of the arterial blood produced by positive acceleration, as the raising of the diaphragm increases the number of alveoli that are perfused but not ventilated.

Lung collapse

The terminal airways serving alveoli at the base of the lung are occluded on exposure to positive acceleration, so that ventilation of the alveoli connected to them ceases although they continue to be well perfused with blood. The terminal airways open again as soon as the exposure to positive acceleration ends, and so ventilation of these alveoli recommences provided that they contain gas. The number of perfused non-ventilated alveoli at the base of the lung rises with the level of acceleration and is greatly increased by the inflation of the abdominal bladder of an anti-G suit during the exposure (*Figure 10.6*). Since these non-ventilated alveoli are perfused, gaseous exchange continues during positive acceleration between the gas trapped in them and the mixed venous blood flowing through their walls. The blood absorbs the trapped gas from the alveoli at a rate limited by the rate at which the least soluble gas, usually nitrogen, is removed. If little or no nitrogen is present when the positive acceleration is applied, as will be the case if 100% oxygen has been breathed prior to the exposure, the trapped gas will be absorbed very rapidly, and many alveoli will be rendered free of gas whilst the exposure to positive acceleration is in progress. The surface forces holding the walls of the gas-free alveoli together are high and the lung will remain collapsed (atelectatic) after the exposure has ended. Only the high tensions created in the collapsed lung by a deep inspiration will reopen the alveoli.

Exposure to sustained positive accelerations

above about 3 G produces acceleration atelectasis when 100% oxygen has been breathed before the exposure and an anti-G suit used during the exposure. The condition can arise in the absence of the use of an anti-G suit, but the severity of lung collapse is then considerably less. There is a wide individual variation in susceptibility both in the level and duration of acceleration required to produce it and the magnitude of the effect. The symptoms, which are usually not apparent until after the exposure or even the flight in which the exposure occurred, consist of a dry cough, with or without substernal discomfort or pain and exacerbated by a deep inspiration. Chest radiographs reveal basal lung collapse with obliteration of the costophrenic and cardiophrenic angles and shadowing at both lung bases. Radiographic signs of collapse can occur in the absence of symptoms. The symptoms and radiographic signs usually clear completely after several deep inspirations, which often provoke bouts of coughing. In the absence of deep breathing, however, there may be residual basal collapse present 24 or 36 hours after the exposure to positive acceleration. The vital capacity may be reduced by up to 60% of the resting value. The volume of lung collapsed is, however, considerably less than this— the limitation of deep inspiration being reflex in origin. The lung collapse induced by several exposures to moderate levels of positive accelera-tion whilst the subject breathes 100% oxygen produces a right-to-left shunt of the order of 20–25% of the cardiac output. A right-to-left shunt of 25% of the cardiac output will reduce the arterial oxygen tension to 8.0 kPa even when 100% oxygen is breathed at ground level. The minimum concen-tration of nitrogen required in the gas breathed before exposure to acceleration in order to prevent significant acceleration atelectasis is approximately 40%.

Any factor that alters the functional residual capacity of the lung during acceleration exposure will affect the magnitude of the induced right-to-left shunt (and hence arterial oxygen desaturation) and the development of acceleration atelectasis. Such factors include positive pressure breathing during acceleration and the anti-G straining manoeuvre (*see* Chapter 11). Pressure breathing causes a mechanical increase in functional residual capacity (and so should improve arterial oxygen saturation and decrease atelectasis), though the degree of this increase will be reduced, or negated, by the use of chest counterpressure. The anti-G straining man-oeuvre includes an inspiratory gasp prior to the strain so that lung volumes are likely to be greater than when relaxed. It may also be noted that obesity decreases the functional residual capacity while smoking increases the closing capacity of the lung, so these factors may also influence shunting and atelectasis during exposure to $+G_z$ acceleration.

Hormone response

The psychological stress of a centrifuge run, particularly in a novice subject, induces an anticipa-tory tachycardia due to the release of adrenaline and prevented, therefore, by the prior administration of a beta-blocking agent. Acceleration stress, *per se*, induces a specific endocrine response with increases in serum cortisol and catecholamine levels. The cortisol response is too slow to have an effect on tolerance to an acute exposure to acceleration but may be significant in prolonged or repeated exposures. It may, therefore, explain why pilots like to pull G prior to air-to-air combat in order to 'tone up' their physiology. The acute release of catechola-mines and the vasopressor antiduretic hormone (ADH or arginine vasopressin) may also enhance G tolerance by increasing peripheral resistance, heart rate and cardiac contractility. Indeed, release of ADH in response to the sudden hypotension and hypovolaemia invoked by $+G_z$ acceleration may be the trigger for the subsequent production of corticotrophin (ACTH) and the ensuing hormone changes.

Tolerance to positive acceleration

Several problems arise in defining limits of tolerance of positive acceleration. First, the nature of the end-point for tolerance varies with the magnitude of the accelerative stress, from unconsciousness not preceded by blackout at high levels, to blackout at intermediate levels and vasovagal syncope or simply fatigue at low levels of stress. Secondly, the time from the onset of the acceleration to the end-point is a function of the rate at which the acceleration is applied, particularly when this is less than 1 G per second. Thus, the level of acceleration at which blackout occurs is, on average, 1 G higher with a rate of onset of 0.1 G per second as compared with one of 1 G per second. In conventional flight the rate of onset of acceleration for peak accelerations above 4 G is generally greater than 1 G per second, and the duration of exposure is usually defined as the total time for which the acceleration is greater than 1 G (and this convention is followed in *Figure 10.7*). Thirdly, there is a large individual variation in tolerance. Thus in one series of experiments, the positive acceleration required to produce blackout varied between subjects from 2.7 to 7.8 G (mean value = 4.7 G with a standard deviation of ±0.8 G).

A compilation of centrifuge data on tolerance of positive acceleration in relaxed, unprotected sub-jects is presented in *Figure 10.7*. The end-points are unconsciousness or blackout, whichever occurred first. The increase in tolerance beyond 10 seconds is due to the operation of compensatory cardiovascu-lar responses.

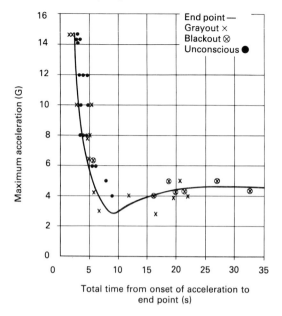

Figure 10.7 A compilation of centrifugal data on the tolerance of $+G_z$ in relaxed, seated subjects (without the use of any protective device). The end points are blackout or unconsciousness, whichever occurred first. The results plotted in this figure were obtained with a variety of rates of onset of acceleration. The increase in tolerance beyond 10 seconds is due to compensatory cardiovascular changes.

Figure 10.7 clearly shows that a subject could be taken to 14 G and brought back to 1 G without any visual loss if the acceleration exposure were completed within a few seconds. However, if he remained at 14 G for more than a few seconds, unconsciousness would occur without premonitory greyout as oxygen stores are exhausted by both eye and brain at about the same rate. A very slow onset of acceleration allows the cardiovascular reflexes to develop and the trough seen in *Figure 10.7* may be avoided. Thus tolerance to $+G_z$ acceleration at an onset rate of 0.1 G/s is about 1 G greater than at an onset rate of 1.0 G/s. The effect on tolerance of G onset rate and run duration is illustrated in *Figure 10.8*.

Heat stress

Exposure to heat reduces the tolerance to positive acceleration. A 1°C rise of deep body temperature reduces the level of acceleration at which blackout occurs by 30–40%. The reduction in tolerance of positive acceleration is due to the cutaneous vasodilatation and shift of blood to the periphery which occurs in response to a rise of body temperature. The lower peripheral resistance and reduced central blood volume enhance the reduction of arterial pressure produced by the positive acceleration.

Hypoglycaemia

Tolerance of positive acceleration is reduced by a falling blood glucose concentration. A 50% reduction of the glucose concentration below the resting value reduces the blackout threshold by about 0.6 G. Once, however, the fall in glucose concentration has produced a hypoglycaemic reaction, with feelings of cold and hunger, sweating and tremor, the acceleration threshold is raised above the normal resting value by about 0.5 G. This increase in the tolerance for positive acceleration is due to the arterial hypertension produced by the adrenalin secreted in the hypoglycaemic reaction.

Alcohol

Ingestion of alcohol reduces the tolerance of positive acceleration. A moderate dose will reduce the threshold by 0.1–0.4 G and will intensify the severity of the symptoms produced by a given level of acceleration.

Hyperventilation

Hyperventilation markedly reduces the tolerance to positive acceleration. Reduction of the arterial carbon dioxide tension to the order of 20–25 mm Hg by 2 minutes' vigorous hyperventilation reduces the

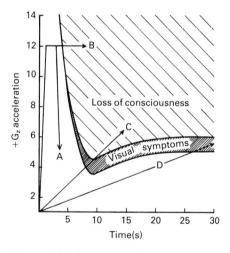

Figure 10.8 Tolerance to $+G_z$ acceleration and effect of onset rate. A brief rapid-onset run (10 G/s) can be tolerated to 12 G without visual loss (A), but if prolonged for more than 4 seconds (B) loss of consciousness may occur without visual warning. Even a moderately fast onset rate (C) beats the cardiovascular reflexes, though loss of consciousness will be preceded by symptoms of greyout and blackout of retinal origin. A slow (0.1 G/s) onset rate allows compensatory reflexes to develop during the application of the stress, symptoms now appearing at a higher G level.

threshold of tolerance by about 0.6 G. Moderate hyperventilation will precipitate unconsciousness in individuals exposed to $+3 G_z$. The increase in cerebral vascular resistance produced by hypocapnia accentuates the reduction in blood flow through the brain caused by the fall in arterial pressure at head level in positive acceleration.

Hypoxia

Whilst mild hypoxia has no significant effect on tolerance of positive acceleration, a reduction of the inspired oxygen tension to 70 mm Hg reduces the threshold for blackout by 0.6 G. More severe degrees of hypoxia (inspired oxygen tension 55 mm Hg) reduce the threshold by 0.8–1.2 G and frequently result in unconsciousness.

Gastric distension

Distension of the stomach increases the tolerance of positive acceleration. The ingestion of 1.5 l water increases the threshold for blackout by 0.6–1.3 G. This effect is probably due to the distended stomach reducing the descent of the diaphragm and heart during the exposure.

Intercurrent infection

Intercurrent infection, such as an upper respiratory tract infection, particularly if it raises body temperature, markedly reduces tolerance to positive acceleration.

Long duration negative acceleration $(-G_z)$

Flight conditions that give rise to negative accelerations are outside loops and spins, and simple inverted flight and recovery from such manoeuvres. Tolerance of negative acceleration is much lower than that for positive acceleration and the symptoms produced by even $-2 G_z$ are unpleasant and alarming. Furthermore, low levels of negative acceleration produce serious decrements of performance. For these reasons, and since many aircraft are not stressed to withstand high negative accelerations, manoeuvres involving negative accelerations greater than 1–1.5 G are seldom experienced in flight.

The physiological disturbances arise primarily in the cardiovascular system. The inertial forces increase the vascular pressures in the upper thorax, head and neck and reduce the pressure in the abdomen and lower limbs, so displacing blood towards the head.

General effects

The feeling of heaviness and the interference with movement in the limbs produced by exposure to negative acceleration are similar to those experienced with positive acceleration. The specific effects of negative acceleration occur primarily in the head and neck. Exposure to $-1 G_z$ produces a sense of fullness and pressure in the head which becomes very disagreeable at $-2 G_z$ and develops to a severe throbbing headache which may persist for some hours after the exposure. There is marked congestion, and exposure for some seconds to 2.5 or greater $-G_z$ produces oedema of the eyelids and petechial haemorrhages in the skin of the face and neck. Congestion of the mucosal lining of the air passages may cause difficulty in breathing and epistaxis may occur. The eyes rapidly become uncomfortable, and at -2.5 to $-3 G_z$, feel as if they are popping out of the head. The conjunctivae are suffused and descent of the lower eyelid and excessive lacrimation can cause reddening and blurring of the vision with subconjunctival haemorrhages. Exposure to negative accelerations greater than 4–5 G for longer than 6 seconds causes mental confusion and unconsciousness.

Cardiovascular effects

Initial hydrostatic effects

The immediate hydrostatic effect of negative acceleration is to increase the vascular pressures in the regions above (anatomically) the heart, and to decrease them below this level. The arterial pressure at head level is immediately increased by the additional pressure exerted by the column of blood between the aortic valves and the head. Thus the mean arterial pressure at eye level increases immediately by 20–25 mm Hg per G, so that it becomes 170 mm Hg on exposure to $-3.0 G_z$. The venous pressure at head level takes several seconds of exposure to rise to a plateau level, as blood has to flow through the capillary bed to fill the capacity vessels before the venous pressure attains the equilibrium value. The venous pressure at eye level at $-3 G_z$ rises to above 100 mm Hg, the effective length of the venous column being from the level of the diaphragm to the head.

Carotid sinus and cardiac output

The rapid and large increase of arterial pressure in the neck stimulates the baroreceptors of the carotid sinus. The response to this stimulation is bradycardia and generalized arteriolar vasodilatation. The intense stimulation of the carotid baroreceptors causes a large discharge of vagal efferent impulses which, in turn, produce bradycardia and a variety of cardiac arrhythmias ranging from simple prolongation of the P-R interval to complete atrioventricular dissociation, with ectopic beats and asystole. Cardiac arrhythmias almost invariably occur on exposures to negative accelerations greater than 1 G. Periods of asystole of 5–7 seconds are not uncommon at $-2.5\,G_z$. The arrhythmias, especially asystole, greatly reduce the cardiac output, so that the mean arterial pressure in the head declines after the initial increase caused by the acceleration *per se*. The generalized arteriolar dilatation also contributes to the reduction of the arterial pressure.

Cerebral circulation

The increases in the pressures in the vessels of the brain produced by negative acceleration are balanced externally by a similar increase in the pressure of the cerebrospinal fluid, so that there is no risk of rupture of vessels within the skull. Although for the first 2–3 seconds there is a large increase of arterial pressure at brain level, the full development of venous engorgement and the consequent rise of venous pressure at this level and the reduction of cardiac output produced by stimulation of the carotid sinus combine together to reduce progressively the arteriovenous pressure difference across the cerebral vascular bed. The cerebral blood flow, therefore, becomes increasingly slower; mental confusion and unconsciousness result. The immediate cause of loss of consciousness on exposure to negative acceleration is generally a prolonged cardiac asystole or a slow ectopic rhythm.

Pulmonary effects

Exposure to negative acceleration produces a headward displacement of the diaphragm and reduces the vital capacity and the functional residual capacity. It also reduces pulmonary ventilation.

The regional distribution of ventilation and blood flow within the lung are changed by negative acceleration in ways analogous to those produced by positive acceleration. In negative acceleration, the apical region of the lung is better ventilated and perfused than the basal region. Since the level at which the pulmonary vascular pressures are unchanged by acceleration is at the junction of the middle and basal thirds, most of the lung remains perfused under negative acceleration. Negative acceleration produces closure of terminal airways, trapping gas in the apical regions; and the continual flow of blood through unventilated alveoli constitutes a right-to-left shunt. Desaturation of the arterial oxyhaemoglobin occurs in negative as in positive acceleration. Acceleration atelectasis produced by exposure to negative accelerations (on 100% oxygen) occurs at the apices of the lungs. As the functional residual capacity of the lung is reduced by negative acceleration, atelectasis occurs more readily than with $+G_z$ and without the intervention of an inflated anti-G suit.

Tolerance

Negative acceleration is not well tolerated. The limit is set by discomfort in the head, oedema of the soft tissues of the face, petechial and sub-conjunctival haemorrhages and loss of consciousness. The maximum negative acceleration that can be tolerated for several seconds is $-5\,G_z$ for a maximum of 5 seconds; $-3\,G_z$ can probably be tolerated by most individuals in the seated posture for 10–15 seconds, whilst $-2\,G_z$ is acceptable for up to at least 5 minutes. A degree of adaptation may develop with repeated exposures, and experienced aerobatic display competitors may tolerate $-6\,G_z$ or more without immediate sequelae.

Long duration transverse acceleration $(\pm\,G_x)$

Accelerations of long duration acting at right-angles to the long axis of the body occur only rarely in present-day conventional flight. They are usually confined to catapult launch, rocket and jet-assisted take-off and carrier landings, though forces in excess of $-2\,G_x$ may build up during flat spins. The forces in these manoeuvres are, however, small relative to man's tolerance and do not give rise to problems. The seats of pilots in future combat aircraft may, however, be inclined back, so as to increase tolerance of accelerations acting at right-angles to the long axis of the aircraft by converting them, as far as the pilots are concerned, from positive accelerations to transverse (forward) accelerations. In early space flights, the accelerations in achieving the velocities required for orbit or escape from earth's gravitational field were such that they could only be tolerated by the occupants of space vehicles if the inertial forces were applied transversely across the long axis of the body. For current manned space vehicles these accelerations act for several minutes and involve peaks of only 3–4 G. Since, both in conventional and space flight, vision of the external world and of instruments and the operation of controls are much easier when the individual lies supine rather than prone on a couch, prolonged transverse accelerations are almost always experienced with the body accelerated towards its anterior (ventral) surface—forward acceleration $(+G_x)$— and seldom with the body accelerated towards its posterior (dorsal) surface—backwards $(-G_x)$ acceleration. Accordingly, the effects of forward acceleration are considered here in greater detail than the effects of backward acceleration.

Since with transverse accelerations the inertial forces act at right-angles to the long axis of the body, gross effects in the systemic circulation do not occur. The major physiological disturbances produced by transverse acceleration occur in the respiratory system, and these limit tolerance of this form of acceleration stress.

Forward acceleration ($+G_x$)

It is unusual for the long axis of the body to be completely horizontal in situations in which exposure to forward accelerations ($+G_x$) occurs. The respiratory discomfort produced by forward acceleration is minimized when the trunk is inclined slightly (15–25 degrees) towards the acceleration vector, and the head is frequently flexed on the trunk to improve all-round vision. In these circumstances, a small but important component of positive acceleration is created which may result in loss of vision and unconsciousness due to the vertical distance (if parallel to the acceleration vector) between the heart and the head. This positive acceleration component may well determine the limit of tolerance for a nominal forward transverse acceleration.

General effects

Increase in the weight of the limbs and in abdominal pressure become apparent at $+2\,G_x$. Difficulty in breathing is usually noted at $+3\,G_x$. At and above $+5\,G_x$ there is a consistent intense dull ache in the chest which is generally most severe at the lower third of the sternum and in the epigastrium and which frequently radiates along the costal margins. The pain is aggravated by inspiration, which becomes progressively more difficult and shallow with increasing acceleration until, at $9–12 +G_x$, there is severe difficulty in breathing. At about $+15\,G_x$, inspiration is extremely difficult and there is a severe vice-like pain in the chest. The limbs cannot be lifted at $+8\,G_x$, although fine controlled movements of the wrist and fingers are possible up to and above $+15\,G_x$, whilst lifting the head is impossible at $9\,G_x$. Petechial haemorrhages may occur in the unsupported regions of the posterior surface of the body. Visual disturbances do not occur when the entire body is truly supine. With the back raised 25 degrees from the horizontal, blackout occurs at about $+10\,G_x$ and consciousness is lost at $14–16\,G_x$. When the angle of the back to the horizontal is only 10 degrees, blackout does not occur until $+16\,G_x$ and consciousness is not lost until the forward

acceleration exceeds $20\,G$. Subjects who are relatively inexperienced may develop dizziness, vertigo and nausea after prolonged exposure to moderate or high transverse accelerations.

Pulmonary effects

Lung volumes and ventilation

The increase in the effective weight of the abdominal contents, which displace the diaphragm into the chest, progressively restricts the inspiratory capacity and reduces the expiratory reserve volume. At $+5\,G_x$ the vital capacity is reduced by 75% and the functional residual capacity becomes equal to the residual volume. The residual volume itself is unaffected by transverse acceleration. The vital capacity becomes progressively smaller with increasing acceleration until, at about $+12\,G_x$, it is equal to the tidal volume. The tidal volume also falls with increasing acceleration, but the respiratory frequency rises to such an extent that the pulmonary ventilation is increased by forward acceleration. The magnitude of the disturbances of respiration and the chest discomfort and pain produced by forward acceleration are reduced by raising the back to about 25 degrees to the horizontal. The position markedly reduces the displacement of the abdominal contents—and hence the diaphragm—into the thoracic cavity which is produced by forward acceleration in the truly supine posture. Respiratory discomfort and difficulty under forward acceleration are also reduced by flexion of the hips and knees to 90 degrees with the long axis of the thighs parallel to the acceleration vector.

Regional lung ventilation

The distribution of inspired gas within the lung in the supine posture is controlled by the same factors as in the upright lung. Exposure to $+G_x$ progressively reduces the ventilation of the alveoli at the back of the lung, whilst ventilation of the front of the lung remains fairly uniform. At $+5\,G_x$ the alveoli in the posterior third of the lungs are unventilated.

Regional pulmonary blood flow

The horizontal level in the supine lung at which the pulmonary arterial and venous pressures are unaffected by transverse accelerations lies approximately one-quarter of the distance from the anterior to the posterior surface of the lung; that is, about 5 cm deep to the anterior surface of the lung. The pulmonary artery pressure at the anterior surface of the lung will, therefore, be of the order of 11 mm Hg (15 cm H_2O) at $+1\,G_x$ and it will be reduced to zero at this point by $+4\,G_x$. With increased forward acceleration, the regional blood flow increases progressively from the front towards the back of the lung. The blood flow falls off somewhat in the most posterior part of the lung due to the rise in interstitial pressure which increases vascular resistance.

Pulmonary gas exchange and arterial oxygen saturation

The absence of perfusion in the very anterior part of the lung and the increased spread of ventilation/blood flow ratios produced by forward accelerations above 3–4 G produce only minor disturbances of the overall gas exchange between inspired gas and blood. The occurrence of a large number of unventilated but perfused alveoli in the posterior part of the lung forms a right-to-left shunt which has a profound effect on overall gas exchanges and produces desaturation of the oxyhaemoglobin of the systemic arterial blood. Exposure to $+6G_x$, breathing air reduces the arterial oxyhaemoglobin saturation to 80–87% whilst exposure to $+8G_x$ reduces it to 72–82%. Desaturation also occurs when 100% oxygen is breathed before and during an exposure to forward acceleration, although the fall of saturation is delayed and its extent reduced. The oxygen trapped in the non-ventilated alveoli must be absorbed before the oxygen tension of blood flowing through them falls to that of mixed venous blood, and the raised oxygen content of the blood flowing through ventilated alveoli reduces the effect of the right-to-left shunt on the oxygen content of the arterial blood.

Lung collapse

Collapse (acceleration atelectasis) of the posterior part of the lung occurs during exposure to forward acceleration when 100% oxygen is breathed before and during the exposure. The mechanism of this collapse is the same as that responsible for the lung collapse that occurs on exposure to positive acceleration of subjects breathing 100% oxygen and using an anti-G suit. In $+G_x$ the closure of terminal airways occurs at the posterior part (most dependent part) of the lung, the elevation of the diaphragm being due to the increased weight of the abdominal contents (cf. the inflation of the anti-G suit in $+G_z$). If there is no nitrogen in the alveolar gas trapped in the posterior lung, there is a rapid absorption which renders the lung atelectatic. The symptoms of lung collapse due to $+G_x$ are similar to those produced by positive acceleration. Breathing 100% oxygen before and during exposure to +6 G for 2–3 minutes produces a 40% reduction of the vital capacity, and the associated right-to-left shunt of blood through the collapsed lung reduces the saturation of the oxyhaemoglobin of the arterial blood to about 75%.

Systemic cardiovascular effects

Since the hydrostatic pressure gradients produced by transverse acceleration are so much smaller than those produced by positive acceleration, there are less pronounced effects on the cardiovascular system than are seen in positive acceleration, with the exception that cardiac arrhythmias occur frequently on exposure to forward acceleration.

Venous and arterial pressures

The pressure in the right atrium is raised by forward acceleration to about 20 mm Hg at $+5G_x$. This increase is due to blood displaced from the periphery—the abdomen and the lower limbs when these are elevated—to the thorax. There is a similar rise in venous pressures throughout the body at the horizontal level of the heart. When the trunk and head are elevated, the rise of venous pressure in the brain will be less than in the right atrium, due to the hydrostatic pressure created by the $+G_z$ component of the acceleration. The increase in right atrial pressure produces a small rise in cardiac output of about 20% at $+5G_x$. The increase in cardiac output produces, in turn, a rise of mean aortic pressure. The mean aortic pressure at $+5G_x$ is increased by 20–30 mm Hg over that at $+1G_x$. When the body is fully supine, arterial pressure in the brain is increased by exposure to $+G_x$. When, however, the trunk and head are elevated in order to reduce respiratory distress, the $+G_z$ component of the acceleration thus introduced reduces arterial pressure at eye and head level. The magnitude of this fall of pressure depends on the posture and the acceleration. It accounts for the visual symptoms and unconsciousness produced by high levels of forward acceleration when the trunk and head are flexed in the direction of the acceleration vector.

Heart

The heart rate is reduced by forward acceleration when the body is fully supine. Forward flexion of the trunk, which introduces a $+G_z$ component, results in an increase in heart rate on exposure to forward acceleration. Cardiac arrhythmias, consisting mainly of premature contractions arising either in the atria or ventricles, are commonly seen on exposure to forward accelerations above 6–8 G. These disturbances of rhythm, which disappear on cessation of the exposure, are probably due to the distension of the right atrium.

Tolerance

Tolerance of forward acceleration is set primarily by the increased difficulty of breathing produced by the increased weight of the anterior chest wall and abdominal contents, the latter acting on the diaphragm. The maximum voluntary tolerance for periods of exposure between 5 and 150 seconds is of the order of 14–15 G, although above $+12\,G_x$ the tolerance depends on motivation and training. The chest pain and difficulty in breathing are reduced by elevating the trunk, but tolerance is then lowered by the occurrence of visual symptoms. Breathing under a positive pressure of 0.7 kPa/G (a pressure of 4.9–5.6 kPa at $+7$–$8\,G_x$) balances the extra weight of the anterior chest wall and restores functional residual capacity, vital capacity and tidal volume to near normal 1 G levels. Additionally, the rise in intra-thoracic pressure increases arterial blood pressure to a comparable degree and enhances G tolerance. Under these conditions an acceleration of $+10\,G_x$ has been tolerated for 30 seconds with little decrement of vision or psychomotor performance. Even without positive pressure breathing, a forward acceleration of $8\,G_x$ with the trunk elevated by 10 degrees can be tolerated for at least 6 minutes.

Backward acceleration ($-G_x$)

The effects of tolerance of backward acceleration ($-G_x$) are considerably influenced by the support afforded to the front of the body. In the seated position this support comes from the restraint harness of the seat, whereas, in exposure in the prone position, the body is usually well supported by a contoured couch. Tolerance to backward transverse acceleration depends critically on the form of support given to the front of the body.

Effects on seated man

Exposure to backward acceleration in the seated position by a conventional restraint harness results in the head being flung on to the chest and the upper and lower limbs being extended forward at right-angles to the trunk. With $-G_x$ acceleration induced in a flat spin this effect makes operation of the ejection seat handle difficult and reduces the effectiveness of the restraint harness's automatic shoulder retraction, so compromising ejection safety. The inertial force displaces blood from the trunk into the head and the limbs. The vascular pressures increase progressively towards the free ends of the limbs. The rise in pressure and distension of the vessels in the head and distal portion of the limbs causes pain (especially in the lower limbs) and petechial haemorrhages. Tolerance of sustained backwards acceleration with a conventional restraint harness is of the order of 10 seconds at $-5\,G_x$ and 300 seconds at $-3\,G_x$. When the head and limbs are

restrained so that the seated posture is maintained, the tolerance is increased to the order of 30 seconds at $-8\,G_x$.

Effects on prone man

When the whole body is supported in the prone position by a contoured couch, exposure to backward transverse acceleration causes difficulty in breathing, nasal drip, salivation, sagging of the lower eyelid and petechial haemorrhages in the dependent parts of the body.

As with forward transverse acceleration, the major physiological disturbances occur in the respiratory system. The reduction of vital capacity and the functional residual capacity produced by backward acceleration is, however, markedly less than that produced by forward acceleration since, with the former, the inertial forces do not force the abdominal contents and diaphragm into the thoracic cavity. Much depends upon the extent to which the weight of the thorax is supported on the anterior chest wall. If support is restricted to the shoulders and hips, respiration is facilitated and the functional residual capacity greater than at a corresponding level of $+G_x$ acceleration. The proportion of dependent lung alveoli (that is, those at the anterior (ventral) surface of the lung) which are not ventilated during exposure to backward acceleration is correspondingly less. This difference in the number of alveoli that are unventilated but perfused results in an arterial oxyhaemoglobin saturation of 94% on exposure to a backwards acceleration of 6 G as compared with a saturation of 80% with a forwards acceleration of 6 G.

The head may be extended on the trunk or the head and the chest raised from the horizontal position in order to improve forward vision. Exposure to backward acceleration then reduces the vascular pressures in the eye and brain. Even with the chest and head elevated to an angle of 25 degrees with the horizontal, vision is unimpaired on exposure to a backward acceleration of 12 G.

Tolerance of sustained backward acceleration by a man supported by a couch in the prone or semi-prone position is in excess of 5 minutes at 5 G and 2 minutes at 10 G.

Lateral acceleration ($\pm G_y$)

With the exception of some experimental aircraft concepts, significant lateral accelerations ($\pm G_y$) do not occur under normal flight conditions. Lateral force control has, however, been demonstrated as a useful flight manoeuvre, particularly during ground attack, and forces in excess of $\pm1\,G_y$ may be generated in some future aircraft. Such levels of acceleration will have little effect other than on head mobility. Greater levels of lateral acceleration (± 3–$4\,G_y$) have profound effects on pulmonary function as the weight of the mediastinal contents acts on the dependent lung to induce airway closure with consequent right-to-left shunting and risk of atelectasis.

Further reading

BURTON, R.R. and WHINNERY, J.E. (1985) Operational G-induced loss of consciousness: something old; some-thing new. *Aviation Space and Environmental Medicine,* **56**, 812–817

BURTON, R.R., LEVERETT, S.D. and MICHAELSON, E.D. (1974) Man at high sustained $+G_z$ acceleration: A review. *Aerospace Medicine,* **45**, 1115–1136

GLAISTER, D.H. (1970) *The Effects of Gravity and Accelera-tion on the Lung.* AGARDograph 133. England: Technivision Services

LEVERETT, S.D. and WHINNERY, J.E. (1985) Biodynamics: sustained acceleration. In *Fundamentals of Aerospace Medicine,* edited by R.L. DeHart, pp. 202–238. Philadelphia: Lea and Febiger

MILLS, F.J. and MARKS, V. (1982) Human endocrine responses to acceleration stress. *Aviation Space and Environmental Medicine,* **53**, 537–540

11

Protection against long duration acceleration

D.H. Glaister

Introduction

There are several methods of raising the threshold to the effects of long duration positive acceleration. Some of these are based on physiological principles while others are based on the experience of aircrew who find that certain measures delay or prevent the onset of symptoms. At present, only the anti-G suit remains in common use, although its protective effect is usually enhanced by certain voluntary efforts on the part of the wearer. It is, however, of interest to examine the other methods of increasing tolerance which have been shown to give varying degrees of protection, and which may be incorporated into future aircraft designs.

Voluntary actions

Avoidance of additive stresses

A number of factors that may affect the tolerance of an individual to positive acceleration were discussed in Chapter 10. For purposes of revision these are listed as follows:

1. Heat and dehydration.
2. Alcohol intake.
3. Hypoglycaemia.
4. Hyperventilation.
5. Hypoxia.
6. Empty stomach.
7. Miscellaneous factors (drugs, fatigue, intercurrent infection etc.).

Avoidance of additive stresses such as those listed above will help to maintain the normal tolerance for positive acceleration manoeuvres. There are, however, various positive measures which may be

taken to increase the tolerance to long duration acceleration, and these will be examined in turn.

Muscle tensing

It has long been recognized that straining and tensing of muscles is an effective method of raising the threshold. Early experiments carried out, in aircraft, showed that voluntary sustained contraction of a large number of skeletal muscles could increase tolerance by 2 G or more. The beneficial action of this manoeuvre is due to a combination of several factors:

1. Pressure on arteries and arterioles increases peripheral resistance by a direct mechanical action.
2. Pressure on veins likewise reduces pooling and increases venous return to the heart.
3. An increase in intra-abdominal pressure assists the upwards passage of venous blood and, by raising the diaphragm, slightly decreases the heart-to-brain distance.
4. There is a slowly developing, reflexly induced, rise in systemic blood pressure.

The merits of this manoeuvre are that it is effective in raising the threshold of tolerance to acceleration without the need for complicated equipment. It suffers from the major disadvantage, however, that the pilot has to make an active effort (which may distract him from his control of the aircraft) and, if it is prolonged, the manoeuvre is fatiguing.

The Valsalva manoeuvre

The Valsalva manoeuvre will provide substantial

protection against blackout during positive acceleration. Forcible expiration against a closed glottis
increases pressure within the thorax and abdomen
and the raised intrathoracic pressure is transmitted
through the heart and great vessels to the arterial
system. The protective effect of this manoeuvre is,
however, short. For the first few heart beats after
the start of the effort, blood pressure is higher than
normal but as the manoeuvre continues, reduction
of venous return leads to a decrease in pulse
pressure and to a systolic pressure that is lower than
the resting value. Since the protection afforded by
this manoeuvre is maintained only while there is a
rise of blood pressure at head level, prolongation of
the manoeuvre, with the resulting fall in blood
pressure and reduction in cardiac output, reduces
the tolerance to acceleration after a few seconds.

The M-1 and L-1 procedures

A more effective method of raising tolerance to
positive acceleration is by a modified form of
Valsalva manoeuvre known as the M-1 procedure.
This is performed by exhaling forcibly against a
partially closed glottis which both increases the
thoracic pressure and allows the diaphragm to
ascend slowly. The forced expiration is interrupted
briefly once every 3 or 4 seconds by a rapid
inspiration. As a protective measure, the M-1
manoeuvre is much more effective than the Valsalva
manoeuvre: although the initial rise of blood
pressure is not so great, a subsequent decline of
blood pressure is prevented since the pauses in the
effort allow venous return to recover. Performance
of this voluntary action in addition to generalized
muscle tensing is effective in increasing the tolerance to positive acceleration by as much as 4 G. The
merits of this procedure are that it requires no
special equipment and it can be used in conjunction
with other forms of protection (for example, an
anti-G suit). The disadvantages of the technique are
that it requires active effort, it is very fatiguing, and
there may be serious interference with
radiotelephonic communication.

The manoeuvre may also be carried out with a
fully closed glottis in which case the periods of raised
intrathoracic pressure are followed by a short
expiratory and inspiratory gasp. This manoeuvre is
referred to as the L1 (for Leverett). Use of either
manoeuvre is a matter of personal preference and
the all-embracing term 'anti-G straining manoeuvre'
(AGSM) is to be preferred. Although these
manoeuvres may be learned at 1 G, a truly effective
manoeuvre must be perfected during exposure to
acceleration when its efficacy can be immediately
related to tolerance. Centrifuges are better than
aircraft in this respect as they offer better control of
pre-set G levels and immediate feedback from a

medical monitor. The use of central and peripheral
lights to monitor the subject's visual field and the
recording of anti-G suit pressure to monitor
abdominal wall contractions (visible as changes in
the pressure trace) further assist the training
process. In conjunction with an anti-G suit, an
effective anti-G straining manoeuvre should allow
most aircrew to maintain effective vision throughout
a 30 second exposure to $+8\,G_z$.

Positive pressure breathing

Another way to achieve a raised intrathoracic
pressure while reducing fatigue is the use of a system
for breathing under positive pressure. Studies have
shown that such a positive pressure is transmitted to
the arterial system on a virtually one-to-one basis so
that, assuming 22 mm Hg/G for the hydrostatic
pressure drop from heart to brain, a mean breathing
pressure of 44 mm Hg should give a 2 G increase in
tolerance. Pressures much greater than this become
relatively less effective and mask leakage poses an
additional problem. The use of a bladder placed
between the occiput and back of the helmet and
inflated to the same breathing pressure has been
found to be effective in providing automatic mask
tensioning and avoids the need for aircrew to
maintain an uncomfortably tight mask or to tension
it manually prior to G exposure.

Positive pressure breathing during G must always
be combined with the use of an anti-G suit as the
raised venous pressures would otherwise induce
excessive pooling of blood in the abdomen and
lower limbs and so reduce venous return. Counterpressure may also be applied over the chest, though
at low levels of breathing pressure (maximum of
35 mm Hg) this has not been found necessary and
flight trials have shown a favourable response with
subjectively improved G tolerance and reduced
fatigue. At higher levels of pressure (50–70 mm Hg),
counterpressure is needed to prevent difficulty with
expiration and over-inflation of the lungs. As with
an effective anti-G straining manoeuvre, the high
vascular pressures lead to petechial haemorrhage
over unprotected areas of skin, the so-called G
measles.

To reduce the occurrence of acceleration atelectasis, the gas breathed should contain a minimum of
40% nitrogen or other insoluble gas. This is difficult
to achieve with conventional diluter demand regulators, but relatively easy with a molecular sieve
oxygen concentrator system, or high pressure
dilution. The chief advantage of positive pressure
breathing as a G-protective measure is that it
reduces fatigue even at levels of acceleration at
which additional pressure must be achieved by
muscular effort (a coincident anti-G straining
manoeuvre). Also the onset of pressure is automatic
and not susceptible to inattention.

Centrifuge training

Many NATO air forces, together with those of Japan and Sweden, which fly high-performance fighter aircraft have introduced centrifuge training programmes for their aircrew. Basic training consists of detailed briefings on the physiological basis for acceleration-induced blackout and loss of consciousness; a demonstration of a good anti-G straining manoeuvre; and individual centrifuge experience at increasing levels to attain a preset goal (for example, $+8\,G_z$ for 15 seconds without loss of vision). The occasional loss of consciousness inevitable in such a programme may be beneficial in drawing attention to the risks and to the slow recovery and confusion that follows. Prior experience of loss of consciousness may shorten subsequent recovery times and it has been argued that such experience should be given to all aircrew much as a hypoxia demonstration is used to acquaint subjects of their individual symptoms. To date there has been no validation as to the effectiveness of a comprehensive centrifuge training programme, nor is it known whether any improvement is permanent, or whether the training should be repeated at regular intervals. However, in individual cases of low tolerance, training has been effective and has allowed aircrew to continue flying high-performance aircraft.

Physical training

Disadvantages of the anti-G straining manoeuvre are the attention required for its initiation and timing together with fatigue induced by sustained muscle contractions. The fatigue can be reduced by appropriate physical conditioning and studies have shown that whole-body strength and aerobic training can significantly increase time tolerance to sustained high-G. For example, a centrifuge exposure which consisted of alternating 15 second periods at $+4.5$ and $+7\,G_z$ could be tolerated for longer (411 s instead of 232 s), an increase of 77%, following weight training. Excessive aerobic fitness may, however, be deleterious to G-tolerance as conventionally measured—visual light loss during brief high-G exposures—since it induces an imbalance between sympathetic and parasympathetic activity, and excessive vagal tone can lead to bradycardia or even to asystole and loss of consciousness. Fitness training should not be pursued so far as to cause the resting heart rate to fall below 55 bpm.

Posture

The methods of protection so far described have depended on raising blood pressure during positive acceleration. A rational alternative is to reduce the height through which the blood has to be pumped in order to preserve cerebral blood flow. Any measure that reduces the vertical distance between the heart and brain will provide a degree of protection against blackout and unconsciousness. Similarly, a change of posture that reduces the tendency for blood to pool in the lower part of the body will help to maintain the circulating blood volume and hence raise the tolerance to acceleration.

Leaning forwards

Leaning forwards from the hips gives limited protection against the effects of positive acceleration. Bending forwards to an angle of 30 degrees will decrease the height of the column of blood (heart-to-brain distance) by about 90 mm and will gain approximately 0.4 G in the relaxed greyout threshold. Crouching in the seat harness may reduce the heart-to-brain column of blood by as much as 200 mm—equivalent to a gain in tolerance of about 1 G. These manoeuvres are not, however, practicable because of reduced vision from the cockpit, risk of head impact on the aircraft structures and difficulties in maintaining adequate restraint by harness.

Raising of the feet

Raising of the feet by the provision of an accessory rudder bar can increase the relaxed greyout threshold by about 0.4 G. This is because of the decrease in dilatation of the arterial tree and of distension of the veins of the lower limbs.

Increasing the back angle

Most relaxed greyout thresholds are estimated with the subject seated in an aircraft seat where the back is at an angle of 20 degrees beyond the vertical and the feet are on the floor. Increasing the back angle increases the relaxed greyout threshold since the vector of acceleration $(+G_z)$ applied to the aircraft structure progressively becomes $+G_x$ relative to the aircrew occupant as the back angle is increased. Increasing the back angle to 75 degrees raises the relaxed greyout threshold by 3 G, but forward visibility for take-off and landing is seriously restricted. The problem of visibility could be overcome by providing an aircraft seat in which the pilot could adjust his sitting position during flight, or by providing a helmet-mounted display of instrument information or forwards view during critical phases of flight.

Drugs

In theory it should be possible to raise the blood pressure or to increase vasomotor tone by means of drugs and thereby raise the tolerance to positive acceleration.

Nikethamide—a central stimulant, has almost negligible effects on blackout threshold, although it appears to diminish fatigue from repeated exposures to acceleration.

Amphetamine sulphate also has negligible effects on tolerance to acceleration, although it may increase the level of awareness and diminish fatigue associated with exposure to positive acceleration. The euphoric side-effects of this type of drug preclude its use in aviation.

Hypertensive drugs—for example, adrenaline. This is so rapidly oxidized in the body that a single dose is unlikely to have any beneficial effects.

Adrenocorticoids—for example, desoxycorticos-terone. This should theoretically increase threshold but is of no practical use owing to its water retaining properties.

Breathing carbon dioxide in certain concentrations will increase the tolerance to acceleration. Carbon dioxide increases blood pressure, causes cerebral vasodilatation and shifts the oxygen dissociation curve to the right (aiding oxygen uptake by brain tissue). Breathing 7.5% CO_2 in air has been shown to increase G tolerance by 1.3 G, independent of the G onset rate. However, the breathing of such a high concentration of CO_2 is extremely unpleasant and interferes with performance so this method is quite impracticable in aviation.

Water immersion

The principle of a rigid suit filled with water had been suggested as a method of protection against positive acceleration by the Germans in 1934. It was shown that blackout threshold could be raised by 2.0 G when the water level was as high as the lower ribs. The pressure exerted on the surface of the body by the water is proportional to the height of the column multiplied by the applied acceleration. Since the entire cardiovascular system is subjected to similar forces distributed in the same way, the two opposing pressures cancel out and the vascular transmural pressures remain unchanged. The tendency for blood to pool in the lower parts of the body and for blood pressure at head level to fall during applied acceleration should be prevented by total immersion, and excellent protection has been demonstrated. Breathing is facilitated by setting the breathing regulator pressure reference in the water at mid-chest level. The method is considered impractical for aircraft application and additionally water immersion cannot protect the lungs so that

ventilation perfusion inequalities still develop and, at very high G levels, there is a risk of lung damage. In centrifuge experiments, however, accelerations of up to $+35\,G_z$ have been sustained for 5 seconds without visual symptoms.

Arterial occlusion

Occlusion of the arterial flow into all four limbs would be expected to increase tolerance of positive acceleration by maintaining peripheral vascular resistance and preventing pooling of blood in the limbs. The protection afforded by an experimental suit with a pneumatic cuff applied to each limb close to the trunk and an abdominal bladder has been investigated. Although this suit gave excellent protection against experimental acceleration, the major limiting factor was ischaemic pain which developed when acceleration was maintained over long periods. An additional disadvantage was that, although arterial occlusion is effective in preventing pooling of blood in the limbs during acceleration, it has no effect on the volume of blood already present in the peripheral vessels at the instant of inflation. This method of protection was abandoned therefore in favour of the anti-G suit.

Abdominal counter-pressure

Early attempts were made to provide protection against positive acceleration by means of abdominal counter-pressure only. This was based on the erroneous belief that pooling of blood in the abdomen was of greater significance than pooling in the legs during acceleration. Several experimental garments were produced of designs varying from a simple elastic abdominal belt to both pneumatic and water-filled belts. None of these garments provided effective protection against the effects of acceleration, and it was quickly realized that better protection could be given if the legs were also compressed. Since there were no technical difficulties in extending coverage to include the lower limbs, attention was concentrated, therefore, on the more efficient garment in the form of an air-inflated anti-G suit.

Anti-G suits

The pneumatically inflated anti-G suit in its present form represents the most suitable and acceptable method of preventing or ameliorating the effects of positive acceleration. The maximum protection that has been claimed for any suit of this type is around 2 G, although experimental studies on a centrifuge indicate a more practical protection of 1.0–1.5 G.

For the sake of historical completeness it should be mentioned that the starting point in the development of pneumatically inflated anti-G suits was the water-filled suit designed by Franks in Canada and used in the early years of World War II. This early form of anti-G suit consisted of a pair of trousers made of inelastic fabric which was filled with water before flight and which provided balanced external pressure during exposure to positive acceleration. The performance of this early form of anti-G suit in protecting against the effects of positive acceleration was excellent although it had many disadvantages. Not only was it bulky and cumbersome but limitation of movement was caused by the weight of water. Complaints were made of loss of 'feel' because of the tendency of the body to 'float' in the water and orientation of the wearer was disturbed. The final demise of the water-filled anti-G suit came when it was demonstrated that the protection given by the suit when inflated with air to a pressure of 1 lb/in^2 (6.9 kPa) per G was equal to or greater than that of the same suit filled with water. The lightness and convenience of an anti-G suit inflated with air represented a considerable advantage over the cumbersome water-filled suit and efforts were concentrated towards the development of the pneumatically inflated suit in its present form.

The modern anti-G suit

A typical modern anti-G suit (*Figure 11.1*) is a trouser-like garment cut away at the crotch and knees to permit greater mobility and to reduce heat load. The outer restraining layer is made of a non-stretch material and within it are contained five interconnecting bladders. The bladders and their outer restraining coverings fit over the abdomen and wrap around the thighs and calves of the wearer. The abdominal portion of the garment is held in position by three waistband webbing straps which may be adjusted to fit the wearer by means of sliding buckles. The girth of the outer restrainer covering the thigh and calves may be adjusted by means of lacing cords, and the lower limb portions of the suit are closed by means of sliding fasteners to facilitate donning. The bladder system is inflated through a flexible hose by means of an anti-G valve which is mounted in the aircraft. The anti-G valve controls the flow of gas, usually air from the engine compressor, into the suit. The valve consists of an orifice, the opening of which is controlled by a mass supported by a diaphragm which is exposed to the pressure in the suit and by a spring. The increase in the weight of the control mass which occurs on exposure to acceleration opens the orifice and allows air to flow into the suit, until the pressure in the latter, acting on the diaphragm of the valve,

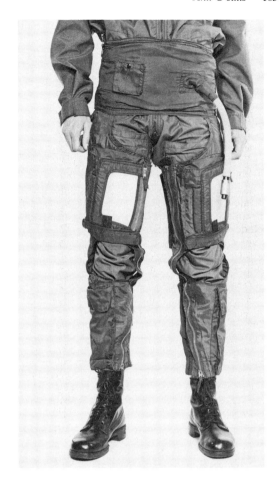

Figure 11.1 A standard Royal Air Force externally worn anti-G suit Mark 4. The bladders over the abdomen, thighs and calves are inflated and deflated through the flexible hose which is attached to the abdominal bladder.

balances the increase in the force exerted by the control mass. As the applied acceleration is decreased the suit pressure opens the orifice and the suit deflates.

The anti-G valve

The anti-G valve controls the pressure in the anti-G suit so that the suit pressure is proportional to the total applied acceleration (in the G_z axis). Most anti-G valves supply a pressure of approximately 1.25 lb/in^2 (8.6 kPa) per additional G. A system in which the pressure is significantly below this optimum will provide less G protection in the relaxed subject. If, however, the pressure in the anti-G suit is much in excess of 1.25 lb/in^2 (8.6 kPa) per G then severe discomfort and even pain will occur. The anti-G valve is designed so that the suit is not inflated until the total applied acceleration exceeds 1.75–2.0 G in order to avoid unnecessary and annoying inflation of the garment during gentle aircraft manoeuvres.

Mode of action of the anti-G suit

The mechanisms whereby the anti-G suit increases the tolerance for positive accelerations include the following:

1. The rise in tissue pressure in the lower limbs and abdomen produced by the inflated suit tends to prevent a large increase in transmural pressure, thereby maintaining peripheral vascular resistance and reducing the pooling of blood into the capacity vessels of the abdomen and lower limbs.
2. The abdominal bladder of the suit supports the abdominal wall and thereby reduces the amount by which the diaphragm is displaced downwards. The anti-G suit tends, therefore, to prevent the increase in the vertical distance between the heart and brain that is normally caused by positive acceleration.

The anti-G suit acts, therefore, to prevent or reduce the magnitude of both the initial and the delayed effects of positive acceleration on the cardiovascular system. Thus the inflation of the suit at the beginning of an exposure produces an immediate increase in peripheral vascular resistance in the lower limbs and prevents the descent of the diaphragm. The anti-G suit also reduces the magnitude of the peripheral pooling of blood that occurs later in the exposure. To ensure that the initial mechanisms are fully effective, the inflation of the anti-G suit must be rapid—within 2–3 seconds of the commencement of the increased acceleration.

Several methods are currently under investigation for improving the protection given by anti-G suits. Valves providing higher gas flows have been developed to speed suit inflation so as to reduce the lag between peak G and maximum pressure. Pre-inflation of the suit to 0.1–0.2 lb/in^2 has the same effect as it reduces the volume of gas subsequently needed to achieve maximum pressure. Electronic anti-G valves are being developed which anticipate gas flow requirements by sensing both instantaneous G and rate of application, so allowing a maximum rate of inflation to the predicted pressure. Suits are being developed that give increased coverage of the lower body, inclusion of the buttocks in the pressurized area giving an additional 0.5 G protection, while complete coverage of the body below the lower ribs appears particularly promising. Finally, systems are being looked at in which a large number of bladders are inflated sequentially with the object of 'milking' blood from the lower extremities towards the heart.

Maximum acceleration tolerance

Studies have shown that the increases in G tolerance afforded by the separate protective mechanisms discussed in this chapter are simply additive when used in combination. Thus, if an anti-G suit gives 1.2 G protection and reclination to a back angle of 65 degrees gives 1.4 G, then suit and reclination together will yield a 2.6 G benefit. The exception to this rule is that positive pressure breathing and the respiratory portion of the anti-G straining manoeuvre each act through the production of a maximal increase in intrathoracic pressure, and so are mutually exclusive. A realistic maximum pressure of 100 mm Hg could be achieved by either means (though effective mask sealing poses a problem with PPB) to give a 4.5 G increase in tolerance (100 ÷ 22 mm Hg/G). However, the same pressure could also be achieved by a 50 mm Hg contribution from expiratory muscle action supported by a further 50 mm Hg PPB. Thus the benefit of PPB is not an absolute increase in achievable G tolerance, but a potential reduction in muscle effort and, hence, fatigue during exposure to sustained high accelerations.

The increases in $+G_z$ tolerance discussed in this chapter relate mainly to changes in relaxed thresholds as judged from peripheral light loss. Studies have confirmed, however, that similar increases are observed using quite different threshold measurements, for example the ability to perform a complex choice reaction time task when straining maximally at high G. The quoted figures may, therefore, be transferred from centrifuge studies to the normal flight environment with some degree of confidence.

The special problems imposed by the high G-onset rates available in agile aircraft were discussed in the previous chapter, and these demand particular protection strategies. The anti-G suit and pressure supply valve should be capable of tracking the imposed G level such that there will not be a significant, and possibly catastrophic, lag in applying counterpressure; but more importantly, the aircrew member must anticipate the G by starting his anti-G straining manoeuvre at G onset rather than waiting to use it to reverse visual symptoms as they develop. As discussed in Chapter 10, the first 'symptom' is likely to be a G-induced loss of consciousness. It follows that a non-pilot aircrew member who may be unaware of an impending G exposure will be at special risk from GLOC.

Given a reasonable level of physical fitness, a correctly fitted anti-G suit and no adverse factors, then an average aircrew member current on high-performance fighter aircraft should be able to sustain $+8\,G_z$ for 15 seconds without losing central vision, or suffering from loss of consciousness. If such a level is not sustainable it is probable that the anti-G straining manoeuvre is not being used correctly and in this case centrifuge training with proper attention to the AGSM should be of benefit. Even $+8\,G_z$ is likely to be exceeded for significant periods in the more agile aircraft types and if aircrew are not to become an increasingly limiting factor to aircraft performance, then additional G protection must be acquired. Possible ways to achieve this are expensive in either time, manpower or cockpit development, and therefore contentious; but include well-planned physical fitness programmes,

centrifuge training, aircrew selection (for G tolerance) and the development of an adequately reclined ejection seat.

Further reading

BURTON, R.R. (1986) Simulated aerial combat manoeuvering tolerance and physical conditioning: current status. *Aviation Space and Environmental Medicine*, **57**, 712–714

GLAISTER, D.H. (1978) *The Influence of Seat Back Angle on Acceleration Tolerance*. Flying Personnel Research Committee Report 1365. Ministry of Defence (Air Force Department)

LEVERETT, S.D. and WHINNERY, J.E. (1985) Biodynamics: sustained acceleration. In *Fundamentals of Aerospace Medicine*, edited by R.L. DeHart, pp. 238–249. Philadelphia: Lea and Febiger

12

Crash dynamics and restraint systems

D.J. Anton

Introduction

The previous chapter dealt with the physiological responses of the individual to accelerations of long duration. This chapter is concerned with the short duration accelerations encountered on aircraft impact with the ground or water. The body response to these accelerations is governed by its mechanical properties.

Decelerations encountered in an aircraft during a crash

By far the commonest cause of injury in aircraft accidents is the very abrupt deceleration that occurs

when an aircraft strikes the ground or water. The kinetic energy of the aircraft is so great that anything but a well-executed crash landing results in the application of damaging forces to the machine and its occupants. These forces are highly variable. They depend on the type of aircraft, the all-up weight and the speed and angle at which the aircraft hits the terrain. Much information has been obtained by experiments in which different types of aircraft were deliberately crashed at various speeds and angles of impact: measurements of acceleration were taken in different sites within the aircraft fuselage. The most recent and sophisticated example of this approach has been the FAA/NASA Full Scale Transport Controlled Impact Demonstration conducted at Edwards Air Force Base at the end of 1984. This

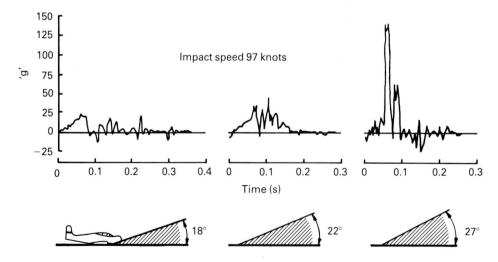

Figure 12.1 Typical recordings of the acceleration profiles measured in the longitudinal direction at the cockpit floor during deliberate experimental aircraft crashes. In each case the impact speed was constant (97 knots). Note how the pattern and magnitude of the recorded deceleration vary with the angle of impact of the aircraft with the ground.

test, which was conducted in part to demonstrate the effects of Anti-Misting Kerosene (AMK) on the propagation of post-crash fire, also carried a comprehensive range of accelerometers and on-board cameras to record the crash environment and its effect on standard and upgraded seating and restraint systems (Hayduk, 1986). *Figure 12.1* shows typical recordings of the acceleration profile measured in the longitudinal direction at the cockpit floor of a jet fighter aircraft deliberately crashed at various angles of impact with the ground and at an impact speed of 97 knots. The pattern of longitudinal deceleration measured at the cockpit floor is very irregular: the profile produced and the magnitude of the acceleration vary with the impact angle.

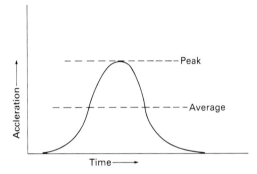

Figure 12.2 Diagram of a half sine-wave 'impulse'.

The deceleration measured at any point in the fuselage is usually defined in terms of magnitude, duration and direction of application—magnitude in units of 'G', duration in fractions of a second, direction as longitudinal, vertical or lateral. Experimentally, abrupt decelerations may be considered as an 'impulse' similar in shape to that shown diagrammatically in *Figure 12.2*. Measurements of the accelerations produced at various sites in the fuselage during experimental crashes of aircraft are usually presented in the form shown in *Table 12.1*, which summarizes data obtained during an experimental helicopter crash. Measurements of the decelerations were made on the floor of the cockpit close to the seats.

The actual profile of deceleration forces obtained during an aircraft crash is governed by the

Table 12.1 Typical deceleration data obtained during an experimental crash in a helicopter

Direction of acceleration	Acceleration (G)		Pulse (sec)
	Peak	*Mean*	
Longitudinal	30	15	0.104
Vertical	48	24	0.054
Lateral	16	8	0.097

diminishing momentum of the aircraft as the terrain resists its forward motion by friction or collision with objects on the ground. If the structures of a crashing aircraft are crushed or deformed progressively, then much of the kinetic energy of the crash is absorbed and the overall deceleration profile is relatively smooth. But if parts of the structure of the crashing aircraft (for example, engines, rigid members, keel structure etc.) plough into the ground during forward motion, then the momentum of the aircraft is reduced more rapidly in peaks of abrupt deceleration of high magnitude which appear on the recorded deceleration profile. Very high peak values of deceleration occur when the crashing aircraft strikes solid objects such as rocks, posts or buildings during its travel across the ground.

When an aircraft ditches, the forces are dependent upon the longitudinal and horizontal velocities relative to the water, the sea state and the site of the aircraft impact relative to the wave front. Little attenuation can be expected from fuselage deformation as impact with the water tends to produce a uniform load distribution across the lower surface of the fuselage.

Forces acting on the occupants of a crashing aircraft

While much information can be obtained by measuring the forces on an aircraft fuselage during experimental crashes it is, of course, the nature and magnitude of the forces acting on the occupants of the aircraft that are important.

In some cases the forces reaching the occupant seated in a crashing aircraft are considerably less than those occurring in aircraft structures immediately surrounding him. This is because of the surrounding structures collapsing and crushing during the impact, so absorbing part of the kinetic energy of the aircraft and attenuating the severity of the force before it can reach the occupant. By careful design, the structures can be made to collapse progressively in a controlled manner and so increase the chances of human survival in an accident. The magnitude of the forces reaching the seated occupant of a crashing aircraft may also be considerably in excess of those that occur in the surrounding structures. This will occur when the occupant, by virtue of poor restraint or inadequate seat design, experiences little deceleration during the early part of the impact. At some point he will, however, strike the aircraft structure or come to full harness extension and be suddenly decelerated to the vehicle velocity in a very short period of time. This 'dynamic overshoot' shows the importance of proper 'coupling' of the occupant to the structure.

Structural damage causing injury

Data obtained from experimental crashes have revealed that certain types of airframe damage are likely to result in injuries to the occupants of the aircraft; these are as follows.

Longitudinal loads on cockpit structures—During a crash in soft earth, nose structures scoop up earth as the aircraft slides in contact with the terrain surface. The scooped earth is accelerated quickly to the same velocity as the aircraft and this produces momentarily high forces which must be supported by the aircraft forward bulkhead. The cockpit structure may collapse, with consequent injury to the legs of the occupant who may then be unable to move. The high levels of acceleration generated in the aircraft structures are also transmitted to the seated occupants. Occasionally, a combination of crushing of the nose section and friction between aircraft structures and the terrain causes the forward structures to be pulled beneath the rest of the aircraft, with rupture of the floor and generation of very high longitudinal acceleration forces.

Vertical (crushing) loads on the fuselage— Collapse of the fuselage shell due to high vertical loads often occurs in accidents where the aircraft hits the ground with a high sink rate. It also occurs in roll-over accidents. Collapse of the shell of the aircraft is often aggravated by large masses, for example, engines, rotors, high wings, etc., positioned above the cockpit. Crash injuries are common.

Transverse (bending) loads on the fuselage— Rupture or collapse of the aircraft protective shell often occurs due to severe bending loads where rapid changes in pitch or yaw develop. This occurs in crashes where the aircraft impacts the ground at a moderate to high impact angle. Rupture of the protective shell exposes the occupants to injury through direct contact with the impact surface, ragged metal edges, etc. Miscellaneous equipment may strike the occupant after the aircraft breaks up.

Deformation (buckling) of the floor structure— Break-up of the floor structure is a common sequel in a variety of aircraft crashes. Since much of the aircraft equipment is mounted on the floor—including, directly or indirectly, the seats—accidents of this type may result in serious multiple injury to the occupants.

Landing gear penetration of the fuselage—Where the landing gear is forced upwards through the floor the occupants may be injured either by direct trauma or through fire caused by rupture of ignitable fluid lines and containers.

From this summary of crash mechanisms, it is clear that much can be done to improve the chances of survival if certain measures are adopted in the design and construction of the aircraft. The following are important in reducing the acceleration loads on the occupants during a crash.

1. The airframe should be such that the structures surrounding the occupant remain reasonably intact and provide a protective shell.
2. The structures, especially those in the immediate vicinity of the occupant, should crush and deform in a controlled and predictable manner so that the forces of acceleration acting on the occupant are absorbed and minimized. These structures should deform without fracture, and materials should crush, twist or buckle without rupture.
3. Aircraft seats should be designed in such a way that they assist in the absorption and distribution of high energy loads before these reach the occupant. Associated restraint systems should provide good coupling of the occupant to the seat so that good 'ride down' characteristics are achieved.

To translate these requirements into practical design requires knowledge of the forces experienced in numbers of accidents, the human tolerance to abrupt deceleration and the engineering cost in terms of increased weight and complexity required to improve crashworthiness to various specified levels.

An example of the statistical approach to crashworthiness is the study conducted by the United States Army into helicopter accidents (Aircraft Crash Survival Design Guide, 1980). Careful analysis of impact data from a series of helicopter accidents led to the definition of percentile survivable velocity changes in the lateral, vertical and longitudinal axes. These figures were then incorporated into specification documents and can therefore be used to quantify design aims. It should be noted, however, that designing to a stated percentile value (say, the 90th) for each axis does not equate to designing to the 90th percentile crashworthiness case. The three-dimensional boundary that encloses the 90th percentile case for each axis would only enclose approximately 73% of the accidents in the original data-base. It should also be noted that changes in helicopter type and in operating procedure would invalidate predictions made from the original US Army data.

Human tolerance to abrupt deceleration

There are still areas of uncertainty concerning human tolerance to abrupt deceleration. For convenience, abrupt deceleration forces are often divided into tolerable, injurious and fatal. 'Tolerable' forces produce trauma such as abrasions and bruising which do not incapacitate; injurious forces produce moderate to severe trauma which may or may not be incapacitating. Given ideal restraint, the accepted limits of tolerance are as follows.

Abrupt +G_z acceleration

It is estimated that an acceleration pulse of approximately 25 G maintained for about 0.1 second is within the limits of tolerability. Minor injuries (including compression fractures of spinal vertebrae) may occur within this level but are not necessarily incapacitating and should not impair the ability of an occupant to extricate himself from a crashed aircraft.

Abrupt −G_z acceleration

Experiments carried out with a subject sitting fully restrained in an aircraft seat indicate that an abrupt −G_z acceleration of about 15 G lasting for approximately 0.1 second is tolerable without producing serious injury.

Abrupt −G_x acceleration

It is believed that the tolerable level of abrupt −G_x acceleration is an acceleration of 45 G sustained for a period 0.1 second, or 25 G for a duration of 0.2 second. These figures were obtained from experimental exposures in which the subject sat in an aircraft seat with optimum restraint. At this level of force some injury may be caused but this is not usually incapacitating.

Abrupt +G_x acceleration

The tolerable limits for acceleration of this type are not accurately defined although it may be assumed that, with the occupant well restrained in a good aircraft seat with an integral headrest, the tolerance will be greater than for abrupt −G_x acceleration. One subject withstood a deceleration of 83 G for 0.04 seconds but was severely shocked by it. For practical purposes similar values may be assumed for human tolerance to −G_x and +G_x impacts.

Abrupt G_y acceleration

Tolerance limits to lateral (G_y) acceleration are not well defined. Experimental studies suggest that an acceleration pulse of 11–12 G with a duration of 0.1 second is tolerated by a man when fully restrained by a harness, but that the survival limit is probably 20 G for 0.1 second.

Factors affecting human tolerance to abrupt deceleration

The following factors are known to affect the human tolerance to short duration acceleration forces.

Magnitude and duration of applied force

A chest-to-back acceleration of 45 G can be voluntarily tolerated by some subjects provided the duration of the pulse is less than 0.044 second. If, under similar conditions, the duration of the pulse is increased to 0.2 second the tolerable magnitude of the force is reduced to about 25 G.

Rate of onset of applied force

Under the same conditions of impact, lower rates of acceleration are naturally better tolerated. For example, in −G_x impact, rates of acceleration about 1000 G/s usually give rise to signs of shock. Impacts of similar magnitude but applied at rates of up to 60 G/s do not. It is believed that, within certain ranges, the effects of the rate of onset of acceleration are related to the natural resonant frequency of the whole body and various organs of the body, and to the compliance of the visco-elastic systems such as bones, joints and ligaments.

Direction of applied force

The body can withstand much greater forces perpendicular to the long axis of the body (forward or backward, G_x) than parallel to it (G_z). In the long axis of the body, greater displacement of viscera in the body cavities is possible and greater strain is placed on the suspensory systems. The skeletal configuration and mass distribution of the body is such that vertical loads cannot be distributed over as large an area as can loads applied in the forward or backward plane.

Site of application of acceleration

In general, parts of the body such as the back and buttocks are more able to withstand a given force than more vulnerable parts like the limbs and head.

Methods of restraint

The more efficient the restraint of an occupant in his aircraft seat the higher is his tolerance to an impact type acceleration. Since this is one of the factors most amenable to control, harness restraint will be considered in some detail.

Principles of restraint and harness design

The purpose of the restraint system is to maintain the man in his workspace during violent manoeuvres of the aircraft and to protect him from the effects of sudden deceleration during impact or escape.

The qualities that a harness restraint system should possess are as follows:

1. *Comfort*—The harness should be comfortable and capable of being adjusted over the required size range.
2. *Efficiency*—It must protect the wearer from injury in the presence of multidirectional forces during impact. The harness should be arranged to provide maximum distribution of these forces and should not cause specific harness injuries. Ideally, it should be capable of being readily adjusted so that little, or no, relative movement can take place between the wearer and the sitting platform.
3. *Ease of use*—The system must be easy to put on and release and should be as simple as possible. A single-point release mechanism is desirable. The operating loads of the harness release

mechanism should be between 66 and 177 Newtons (15–40 lb force) (that is, high enough to avoid inadvertent release, yet low enough to allow single-handed operation). Two separate sequenced actions for release are also desirable in order to prevent inadvertent release.
4. *Minimum restriction*—The system must give the man sufficient freedom to operate all aircraft controls and to carry out his allotted task.

Types of harness restraint systems

Lap belt

This is one of the simplest types of restraint system and is very easy to don. A typical lap belt harness is illustrated in *Figure 12.3(a)*. It requires only two anchorage points, either on the aircraft seat or on the floor, and it provides minimum restriction to the occupant. It has, however, major disadvantages. Firstly, the upper torso is not restrained and will jack-knife on impacts with $-G_x$ or $+G_z$ components. Unless the arc described by the head is free of obstruction, or unless a braced position has been adopted, serious or incapacitating injury may result. Secondly, if the lap belt rises up from the pelvis to lie across the front of the abdomen serious abdominal and lumbar spinal injuries may occur. The retention of lap belts in public transport aircraft owes much to their simplicity of use and their utility in providing restraint under conditions of turbulence. Provided that a proper braced position is

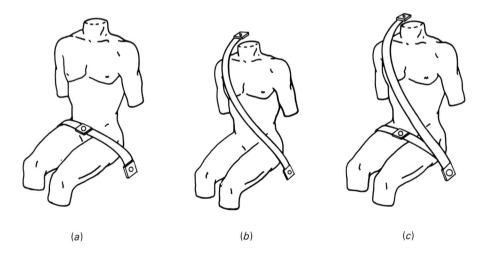

(a)   (b)   (c)

Figure 12.3 Diagram of lap belt restraint harness (*a*) diagonal or 'two-point harness' (*b*) and diagonal and lap combined 'three-point harness' (*c*).

adopted they are probably also appropriate as a restraint device with current aircraft seating systems which are stressed to withstand only low levels of impact.

Diagonal belt

This has the advantage of simplicity but in a crash is probably less efficient than a lap belt restraint alone. A typical diagonal harness is shown in *Figure 12.3(b)*. Since the pelvis is not restrained the seat occupant tends to rotate out of the harness. It can cause a lethal neck 'whip' action of the head and neck during lateral forces. It can also produce internal chest injuries during severe impact.

Diagonal and lap combined harness ('Three-point harness')

This is the most widely used type of harness as a result of its widespread adoption on automobiles. With careful design it gives good restraint for all except lateral accelerations. It is important that the harness should be properly adjusted and that the seat cushions should be reasonably stiff, as otherwise the lap belt component may rise off the pelvis during an impact giving rise to similar abdominal injuries to those encountered with the lap belt alone. Correctly fitted, the harness will give acceptable restraint at accelerations of about $-30\,G_x$. A typical three-point harness is shown in *Figure 12.3c*.

Double lap and shoulder harness ('Four-point harness')

This is a satisfactory assembly and provides better restraint than does the combined diagonal and lap harness. One typical form of double lap and shoulder harness is illustrated in *Figure 12.4(a)*.

Double lap and shoulder harness with a negative G strap ('Five-point harness')

The simple four-point harness is much improved by the addition of a negative G strap (*Figure 12.4(b)*). This strap, also known as 'lap-belt, tie-down strap' or 'harness stabilizing strap', rises from the seat in the mid-line between the legs to join the harness at a central quick-release point. It prevents distortion of the harness by forces imposed on the torso and is extremely effective during aerobatics and aircraft manoeuvres that involve negative G, during vertical vibration in high-speed low-level flight and under crash impact.

Advantages

The advantages of a five-point harness may be summarized as follows.

During aerobatic manoeuvre—Where there is negative G, the pilot must be restrained in all three axes so that all the aircraft controls remain within reach, his protective helmet does not strike the cockpit canopy and his view of cockpit instrumentation and weapons systems (for example, gunsight) is

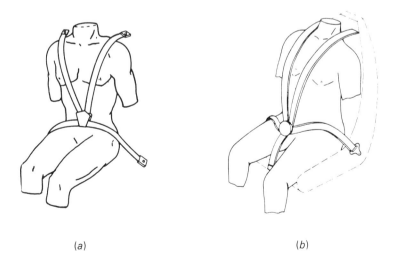

(a)   (b)

Figure 12.4 (*a*) A typical double lap and shoulder harness – 'four-point harness'.
(*b*) A 'five-point harness' which includes a negative G strap.

maintained. It is also important that he should feel secure. The negative G strap ensures good pelvic restraint under these conditions; and, by preventing the quick-release point of the harness moving away from the seat, also restrains the shoulders and prevents excessive extension of the trunk.

During vertical vibration—Vertical vibration that may occur during high-speed low-level fixed-wing and helicopter flight in turbulence can cause such a degree of movement of the pilot in his seat that control of the aircraft is jeopardized. A four-point harness with a negative G strap provides acceptable restraint.

During crash impact—In a forward crash impact $(-G_x)$ the negative G strap is of particular importance. As the torso of the aircraft occupant decelerates, tension is placed on both the lap and shoulder straps. The tension applied to the shoulder straps causes elevation of the central point of a simple four-point harness and this increases the angle at which the lap straps intersect the seat platform. This, in turn, allows the pelvis to rotate underneath the lap strap (so-called 'submarining') so that the lap straps slide upwards off the anterior superior spines of the pelvis and on to the soft tissues of the abdomen. In this way, the spine is allowed to flex and the tolerance of the crashing occupant to the vertical acceleration that often follows initial horizontal impact is greatly reduced. The addition of a negative G strap to a four-point harness prevents rise of the centre-point of the harness on crash impact and maintains the correct angle for the lap straps so that the broadest part of the pelvis bears the major part of the decelerative load.

A final advantage of the five-point harness is that it prevents any movement or displacement of the personal survival pack, which in many fixed-wing military aircraft forms the sitting platform in the ejection seat. Under negative G, the sitting platform is effectively kept in place by the well-restrained occupant without resort to locks and releases on the survival kit itself. Ejection injury to the back is also much less probable if the pilot is firmly anchored to the seat so that minimum relative movement occurs.

Other forms of restraint

The airbag

The airbag or safety cushion system is an alternative means of protecting the occupants of a crashing aircraft from the effects of rapid deceleration. The airbag consists of a strong, inflatable, Neoprene-coated, woven nylon bag stowed in some convenient position in front of the seat. It is fed by a cylinder of compressed air with a device sensitive to rapid deceleration. When the device is triggered, compressed air inflates the bag in less than one-tenth of a second and prevents the aircraft occupant from striking projections on the instrument panel or forward bulkhead. The bag contains porous panels which allow air to leak out slowly, so that after inflation the person protected does not remain immobilized. To prevent 'submarining', the bags are designed so that the legs, knees and torso are fully restrained.

The airbag system has been investigated in the United States for application to passenger-carrying aircraft. Current experimental designs have not so far performed well enough to displace the conventional harness.

Rearward facing seats

Rearward facing seats offer an attractive means of improving passenger restraint in $-G_x$ impacts. It is obviously essential that such seats should incorporate an integral head rest, and should be adequately stressed, but with these provisos, rearward facing seats undoubtedly offer the best impact protection. There has, however, been considerable resistance to their adoption on the grounds of presumed passenger dislike, cost, weight and lack of comfort on take-off and landing. Much of the momentum for the adoption of rearward facing seats was lost around the time of the introduction of aircraft such as the Trident, where the aerodynamic characteristics of the aircraft made it likely that impacts would have a high G_x component against which the rearward facing seat conferred no advantage. A superficial review of survivable airline accidents over recent years suggests that the widespread adoption of rearward facing seats might have resulted in the saving of a few lives.

It is unlikely that rearward facing seats will be adopted in the foreseeable future. At the time of writing the Federal Aviation Authority Notice of Proposed Rule Making (14 CFR Part 25) has proposed a considerable improvement in the requirements for conventional forward facing seats. The widespread adoption of seats to the new standard will reduce further the strength of arguments for retrofitting, rearward-facing seats.

Energy attenuating seating

Mention has already been made that aircraft structures and seats can be designed to collapse progressively when exposed to high impact forces. By this means the loads applied to the seat occupant can be limited. Simple calculation will show that the greatest contribution to load limiting is achieved by the careful design of seating systems. Most practical designs rely on the plastic deformation of metal to achieve energy attenuation and such seats can be retrofitted to existing helicopters using either floor or ceiling mountings. It is difficult to accommodate more than one third of a metre stroke although calculation shows that this is a barely acceptable distance. Assuming a velocity change of 13.1 m/s and an ideal attenuating material giving a rectangular pulse shape, the peak G can be calculated using the formula:

$$G = \frac{V^2}{2gS} \quad (see \text{ Chapter 10, page 141})$$

where G is the peak acceleration in G units,
V is the initial velocity in metres per second,
S is the stopping distance in metres and
g is the acceleration due to gravity (9.81 m/s^2)

Therefore, $G = \dfrac{13.1}{2 \times 9.81 \times 0.33} = 26.5$

It should be noted, however, that simple attenuating devices work at a constant force rather than a constant acceleration. Since force = mass × acceleration, variation in the weight of the occupant or his equipment will cause the lightweight occupant to experience a higher acceleration and therefore use less of the available stroke. Conversely, the heavier occupant will experience a lower acceleration and will require a larger stroke that may result in the system 'bottoming'. To reduce this problem provision has to be made for modifying the force required to operate the energy attenuator according to the boarding weight of the occupant. The reader is referred to the Aircraft Crash Survival Design Guide (1980) for a comprehensive treatment of this subject.

References

Aircraft Crash Survival Design Guide (1980) Fort Eustis, Va.: Applied Technology Laboratory, United States Army Research and Technical Laboratories, USARTL-TR-79-22

HAYDUK, R.J. (1986) *Full Scale Transport Controlled Impact Demonstration*. Washington, D.C.: National Aeronautics and Space Administration Conference. Publication 2395

Further reading

HALEY, J.L. (ed.) (1982) *Impact Injury Caused by Linear Acceleration: Mechanisms, Prevention and Cost*. Neuilly sur Seine: AGARD/NATO. Conference Report CP-322. 1–5

VON GIERKE, H.E. and BRINKLEY, J.W. (1978) Impact accelerations. In *Foundations of Space Biology and Medicine*. Vol. II, Book I, Chapter 6. Edited by J. Calvin and O.G. Gazenko. Joint USA/USSR Publication, Washington, D.C.: National Aeronautics and Space Administration

13

Head injury and protection

D.H. Glaister

Introduction

Head injury is common in all forms of accident trauma. Surveys carried out on aircraft accidents have shown that 40% of injuries sustained are craniofacial, and of all fatalities resulting from aircraft crashes some 14–20% are due to serious head injury.

Interest in the special need for head protection in the military pilot resulted from changes in the design and role of aircraft. Heavy jet-powered aircraft, introduced in the 1950s, tended to sink rapidly when power was lost and many aircrew perished through inability to escape from the crashing aircraft as a result of relatively minor head injury with disturbance of consciousness. Also, as the speed of aircraft increased and operational requirements demanded flight at low level in turbulent conditions, it was feared that both aircraft and occupant might be lost if the pilot lost consciousness as a result of his head striking cockpit structures. Consequently, protective helmets were developed for use by aircrew and since their introduction into military aviation there has been a marked reduction in the incidence of head injury. In many cases the wearing of a protective helmet has proved life saving.

This chapter is concerned with the mechanism of head injury, the principles of head protection and the design of aircrew protective helmets, particularly in rotary-wing aircraft in which the ejection option is not available.

Mechanics of head injury

A number of injuries can occur as the result of the unprotected head striking a hard object or an object striking the head. The common injuries are as follows.

Skull injury

When the human head is subjected to a heavy blow, much of the energy of impact is absorbed by the skull bones which disintegrate in a characteristic way. The outer table of the skull gives way over an area corresponding closely with the shape of the object striking it. It is thrust into the diploë which is compressed and shattered. The force of the blow now spreads into surrounding bone and is borne by the inner table which first bulges, then gives way over an area somewhat larger than that of the outer table. Secondary fissures radiate outwards into surrounding bone along lines dictated by the architecture of the skull.

Broad impacts to the vault of the skull send multiple fissures radiating away from the site of the blow. As these reach the sides of the vault they turn downwards towards the base of the skull and are directed into channels between the thicker buttresses and the floor of the skull. A very heavy blow directed underneath the occupant may lift the upper cervical spine with such violence that it breaks away from its ring base attachments. With skull fractures, the brain and its covering membranes are commonly injured. The skull is also flexible enough under certain conditions of impact to be dented transiently by 10 mm or so, underlying brain damage then being produced in the absence of skull fracture.

Membrane injury

Whether or not fracture of the skull takes place, injury may tear membranes and cause intracranial haemorrhage. Blood accumulates in the epidural, subdural or subarachnoid spaces according to its source. Epidural bleeding normally follows rupture of the middle or posterior meningeal arteries by violent transmitted force. The dura is lifted locally by the haemorrhage, bulges into the interior of the skull cavity and displaces brain. After a 'latent period' during which blood accumulates the injured person may appear dazed or temporarily concussed but soon lapses into unconsciousness as intracranial tension increases. Subdural bleeding is often associated with subarachnoid bleeding and develops by leakage from torn perforating dural veins. Escaping blood following the head injury may remain localized or spread slowly across the brain by its own pressure and by gravity. Symptoms may be quite slow to develop.

Injuries due to movement of the head as a whole

Much more complex brain injuries follow from the general absorption of force as a result of which the head is either displaced suddenly or brought to a sudden stop during impact. Angular acceleration of the head also occurs in impacts of this type and shear forces develop with local or widespread brain damage. With rotational strain, the skull chafes over the surface of the brain and the brain itself undergoes rotation, each lamina twisting over the one immediately below it, stretching and shearing tissues from brain surface to core. The brain stem is especially liable to injury as the spinal column fixes it and acts as a pivot upon which the head rotates. These shear strains cause tearing of membranes and haemorrhage with surface or deep contusion of brain substance. Particularly at risk are the so-called bridging vessels which connect the potentially mobile brain to the fixed skull. A relative displacement in excess of some 10 mm stretches these vessels beyond their elastic limit with resulting rupture and haemorrhage. This type of rotational shearing injury may occur without fracture of skull bones.

Linear strain may give rise to the typical 'contre-coup' type of brain injury where damage or surface bruising of brain is more pronounced in the area exactly opposite to the site of impact than in that immediately under the blow itself. This is due to linear forces causing brain tissue to 'pile up' under the impact and 'rarefy' (with stretching of pial vessels and arachnoid tetherings) over the surface opposite the site of the blow.

Concussion

Head injury, often relatively minor, can cause the clinical state of concussion. This is a transient phenomenon of instantaneous onset and is manifested by widespread symptoms of a purely paralytic kind. It occurs without macroscopic evidence of structural cerebral injury and causes no sequelae although a period of amnesia of variable duration and often retrograde in nature may occur.

The mechanics of concussion are complex. Early workers noted that hydrostatic pressure *per se* had little effect on living tissue which, provided it contained no air, could be considered incompressible. Linear acceleration forces produce both compressional and rarefaction strains within brain tissue and it is now believed that it is rarefaction that causes the injury to brain tissue responsible for concussion. Thus during linear acceleration there is inertia of the brain and a high-pressure zone develops initially at the site of impact with a complementary low-pressure zone at the opposite pole. The low-pressure area of the shock wave leads to cavitation in brain tissue. The subsequent collapse of these microscopic cavities or bubbles damages the cells in the immediate vicinity. Animal experiments and other data have yielded the acceleration–time tolerance curve for human cerebral concussion on which many protective helmet standards are based. Thus the curve shown in *Figure 13.1* relates the onset of concussion in the human subject with a force of impact and its duration. With movement along this curve from left to right there is

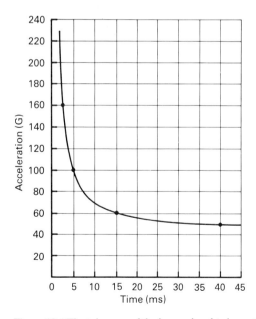

Figure 13.1 The tolerance of the human head to impact acceleration. The curve describes the time for which a given acceleration must be applied to produce cerebral concussion. The four dots, reading from left to right, represent velocity changes of 4 m/s, 5 m/s, 9 m/s and 20 m/s respectively.

a corresponding increase in the product of acceleration × time, or tolerable impact velocity. The potential exists, therefore, for increasing survivability to a given velocity change by increasing the duration of impact with an equivalent decrease in acceleration. However, this curve, developed at the Wayne-State University in the USA, is based on a mixture of data from human cadaver drop tests (skull fracture strength), animal experimentation (concussion mechanisms), and human sled tests (voluntary whole-body tolerance), so cannot be considered definitive. In reality there probably exists a whole series of acceleration–time curves for the many different mechanisms and G vectors, both linear and angular, that can lead to concussion and brain injury.

Tolerance to injury

To consider methods of head protection, a clear understanding of the human tolerance to potential injury mechanisms is essential. One of the problems in quantifying human tolerance to injury is deciding which units one should employ. The deceleration of an impactor or acceleration of the human head is readily measured and can be expressed in the unit m/s² or G. If the head is freely mobile and its mass known, then the force (force = mass × acceleration) can be calculated and expressed in newtons (N).

Similarly, if the contact area is known then the force may be expressed per unit area as a pressure (N/m², or Pa). Finally, the total transfer of energy or work done on the head can be computed and expressed in newton metres (joules). By general convention acceleration (in G) tends to be used when discussing concussion, and energy in joules (J) for head protection requirements.

The relationships between velocity (m/s), acceleration (m/s²) and stopping distance (m) on head impact can be made clear by means of an example. Assume that a human head weighing 5 kg and travelling at a velocity of 10 m/s strikes a solid wall. The frontal bone fractures and is depressed to a depth of 20 mm (0.02 m).

$$V^2 = 2as$$

where V = velocity, a = acceleration, s = stopping distance

Thus $a = \dfrac{V^2}{2s}$

The average deceleration of the head in the example is, therefore:

$$a = \frac{10^2}{2 \times 0.02} = 2500 \, \text{m/s}^2 = 255 \, \text{G}$$

The force acting on the head (or wall) is given by:

$$F = ma$$

where F = force, m = mass

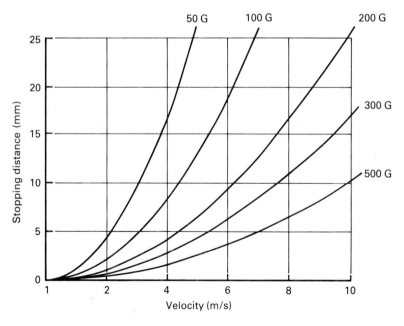

Figure 13.2 Impact of the head. The relationship between velocity at impact, stopping distance and resultant acceleration.

In this example, $F = 5 \times 255 = 1275\,\text{N}$

The kinetic energy of the head before impact is given by:

$$ke = \frac{1}{2}mV^2$$

where ke = kinetic energy

In this example, $ke = \frac{1}{2} \times 5 \times 10^2 = 250\,\text{J}$

If a constant deceleration of the head is assumed the duration of the impact is given by:

$$V = at$$

where t = duration of impact

In this example $t = \dfrac{10}{2500} = 0.004\,\text{s} = 4.0\,\text{ms}$

Since we have defined all the parameters of the head impact used in this example, it should be noted that, if the skull had not fractured, the stopping distance would have been much less (perhaps 3.0 mm). In that case the deceleration would have been 1700 G, the force 8.5 kN and the duration 0.6 ms. The input energy would still have been 250 J. This emphasizes the profound importance of stopping distance on the forces in a given head impact. It also shows how the skull and soft tissues can, as a result of a certain amount of deformation, protect the brain from excessive acceleration. The relationship between stopping distance, impact velocity and acceleration is given in *Figure 13.2*.

Human tolerance to injury mechanisms

The tolerance of the human head to direct impact, linear acceleration and angular acceleration can now be considered.

Direct impact (bone and soft-tissue injury)

The break strength of bone and soft tissue depends very much on the site of impact and ranges from 30 G for the nose, 40 G for the jaw, 50 G for the zygomatic arch, 100 G for front teeth; 50–100 G for an area of $1\,\text{in}^2$ of temporo-parietal bone and 100–200 G for $1\,\text{in}^2$ of frontal bone. The force in the head injury may be calculated (in N) by multiplying the accelerations (G) quoted above, by a factor of 5. Forces required to produce deformation of the cranium without fracture are less well known, but there is evidence that the cranium may be dented up to 12.5 mm without fracture or permanent injury.

Linear acceleration

Numerous animal studies have been carried out in an attempt to measure tolerance to concussion and relate the findings to man. One such prediction is illustrated in *Figure 13.1* which shows the effect of impact duration. This curve has led to some national requirements for protective headgear which specify, for example, that under appropriate test conditions the headform acceleration shall not exceed 400 G, nor 200 G for more than 2 ms, nor 150 G for more than 4 ms. The UK viewpoint is that such detail is unwarranted by the known facts and may even be counterproductive in defining a less than optimum pulse shape. Current British Standards (i.e. BS 6658:1985) specify 300 G (with no time limit) and this simple approach has now been adopted by the Snell Memorial Foundation in the US. Thus it is now generally accepted that the human brain can withstand crash impact forces of the order of 300–400 G without skull bone fracture or concussion, provided that there is no local deformation of the skull.

Angular acceleration

The most extensive estimates of human brain tolerance to angular acceleration have been made by Ommaya and colleagues in the USA and by Löwenhielm in Sweden. *Figure 13.3* illustrates the latter author's tolerance curves for two different injury mechanisms, bridging vein disruption and gliding contusion. Note that both impact criteria—peak angular acceleration and peak angular velocity change—must be exceeded for injury to result.

Methods of preventing head injury

The problem of preventing head injury on impact may be approached in a number of ways.

Provision of adequate restraint system

Restraint harnesses can do much to prevent contact of the head with surrounding structures. However, even with acceptable harness restraint there may be multidirectional flailing of head, arms and legs and to a lesser extent, lateral displacement of the upper torso within the restraint harness during crash impact. A more effective means of preventing contact of the head with surrounding structures during crash deceleration is by provision of a suitable head restraint system.

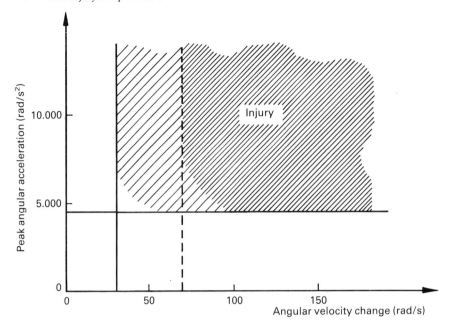

Figure 13.3 Tolerance of the human brain to abrupt rotation. Note that both a peak angular acceleration and peak angular velocity must be exceeded for injury to result. Light hatching, bridging vein disruption; heavy hatching, gliding contusions. (Reproduced from Löwenhielm (1977) by kind permission of author and publishers.)

Adequate space surrounding the occupant

The provision of adequate space in the cockpit within the occupants' immediate environment helps to reduce the injury associated with flailing of the head and contact with surrounding structures during abrupt deceleration. Space is usually at a premium and it is not always possible to site structural parts of the aircraft at a sufficient distance to keep the occupant from striking them. Typical hazards in the cockpit area are window and door frames, instrument consoles, control columns, displays, seat backs, avionic boxes, panels, etc.

Treatment of surfaces

Where it is not possible to design the cockpit in such a way that the occupant's head is prevented from striking surrounding objects on impact, it is often possible to treat surfaces in order to minimize injury. Thus dangerous surfaces or projections within the cabin may be constructed from deformable material which allows a measure of energy absorption when the head strikes it. Although many aircraft cockpits are treated in this manner, the structures and equipment used are far from ideal; though some, for example the parachute-containing

headbox on the Mark 10b ejection seat, have been shown to be effective energy absorbers.

Protective helmets

Although the primary aim should always be to eliminate potentially lethal head impacts, in practice it is usually necessary to resort to personal head protection. Thus provision of a protective helmet for aircrew is now the standard method of reducing the risk of serious head injury in aircraft operations. The mechanics of head protection and the principles of protective helmets are now discussed in detail.

Mechanics of head protection by a helmet

Distribution of impact load and prevention of skull deformities

There are several possible mechanisms whereby a helmet could protect the head during impact. Thus it could distribute the impact load so as to prevent or reduce soft tissue injury. Similarly, a protective helmet could prevent deformation of the skull and so increase tolerance to linear acceleration to the

300 G level. In both cases the requirement is for a strong inflexible shell. However, if the shell is separated from the skull by an appropriate distance, some flexion or distortion of the shell becomes acceptable. In this case the load has to be transmitted to a large area of cranium by a suitable suspension system. A measure of the potential benefit afforded by a rigid helmet shell is given by a simple example.

An aircraft makes a controlled wheels-up landing on a rough field and slows to rest at a modest 5 G, a level of acceleration that would be readily tolerated in terms of whole-body response (*see* Chapter 12). However, at 5 G, the pilot is unable to prevent his head and upper torso being thrown forwards and his head travels some 30 cm prior to striking the top edge of the instrument panel. In the time taken for the head to cover this distance the aircraft velocity will have decreased by 5.4 m/s and it is at this relative velocity that the head strike will occur (assuming no resistance to motion from the neck musculature). Taking head mass as 5 kg, the impact energy will be 73.5 J. Without head protection the 3 mm stopping distance offered by the soft tissues of the scalp will allow an average deceleration to the head of 500 G. Acting over a small area this greatly exceeds the strength of the frontal bone (*see* page 177) so that a fracture will occur with damage to the underlying brain tissues.

The same head, but wearing a well-designed protective helmet, would impact at the same velocity, but the impact energy would be increased by the added helmet mass to some 100 J. However, by distributing the impact over a greater area, skull distortion and fracture are prevented. In addition, the protective padding component of the helmet (*see* below) affords an additional 15 mm of stopping distance. The available 18 mm now allows the head to be brought to rest at an average 83 G, well below the concussion threshold. Thus not only will there be no brain damage, but the avoidance of even transient concussion allows the pilot to extricate himself promptly in the event of a post-crash fire. Note that the same outcome could have been achieved by padding the instrument panel, or by precluding any head contact by the use of effective head restraint.

Provision of finite stopping distance

By providing a finite stopping distance, a protective helmet can reduce the peak acceleration imposed in a given impact. This is an example of a general principle of crashworthiness expounded in the previous chapter. Since the product of acceleration and time (velocity change) is the same, the reduced acceleration will be applied for a longer time. Thus in the example given above, a sixfold increase in stopping distance (from 3 to 18 mm) has afforded a sixfold reduction in average deceleration (from 500 G to 83 G), though the duration of the impact event has also been increased by a factor of six (from 1.1 ms to 6.7 ms). In practice, the maximum stopping distance that can be built in to a protective helmet is about 25 mm—more than this and the device becomes unacceptably bulky. Even this theoretically available 25 mm is reduced by the relatively inefficient energy absorbing materials that can be integrated into a practicable helmet and only some 15 mm is actually available in which to reduce the relative velocity between head and struck object to zero.

There are two basic energy absorbing systems that can be used in protective helmets. Earlier types of RAF helmets employ a fibreglass shell which breaks up on impact. The impact load is transmitted to the head and distributed widely by means of a suspension harness which initially provides an air gap of about 25 mm. Each time a glass fibre ruptures or is pulled out of the resin matrix energy is absorbed by the helmet shell inelastically. In the periphery of the helmet, energy is absorbed by crushable foam materials. This technique implies a compromise with the requirement for a strong, rigid shell.

A second mechanism favoured in the United States and in recent RAF helmets makes use of a layer of crushable foam beneath the shell, which crushes on impact to about 40% of its initial thickness. In this design a stronger shell can be employed.

An important consideration of helmet design is to tune the padding material to human tolerance levels such that the material crushes at a level of transmitted force that is just tolerable. Such padding will appear very hard and will not crush to any significant extent in a minor impact. For comfort, therefore, a double layer of padding may be desirable, the inner layer of which is more yielding. In any event, all materials used should be energy absorbing and this principle can also be applied to other helmet components such as ear cups. This method is widely used for helmets produced in large numbers, for example in protective helmets for motor cyclists, as the major components can be produced cheaply and effectively by injection moulding using thermoplastics. The RAF Mark 4 helmet is a hybrid design which uses a combination of frangible shell, energy absorbing foam and harness suspension, though the reduced air gap means that the harness is used mainly for fitting the helmet to individual heads rather than for energy absorption *per se*. The ALPHA helmet (Advanced Lightweight Protective Helmet for Aircrew) uses a frangible shell and energy absorbing padding, with additional energy absorbing pads for individual sizing. A comparison of the two energy absorbing

Table 13.1 Comparison of two energy absorbing systems for use in protective helmets

A *Helmet employing a frangible shell/suspension harness system*	B *Helmet using a crushable foam liner/hard shell system*
Some stroke lost through elastic extension of suspension tapes	40% of available stroke lost by crushed thickness of foam
Heat load acceptable—can be well ventilated	High heat load unless combined with an air gap and harness
Low coefficient of restitution	High coefficient of restitution
Initial low surface friction may increase following impact	Low surface friction
Easily damaged in routine use (damage visible)	Not easily damaged in routine use (damage invisible)
Poor ballistics protection	Good ballistics protection
Accepts one major impact per site but subsequent load spreading capability is compromised	Accepts one major impact per site *but* load spreading capability remains uncompromised

systems for use in protective helmets is given in *Table 13.1*. Most features of this table are self-explanatory, but mention should be made of the influence of the coefficient of restitution. In a helmet in which energy is absorbed elastically (as to a certain extent by a thermoplastics shell and padding) the helmeted head will rebound on impact and the impact energy will be increased by the addition of a post-impact head velocity. Helmet test methods take this factor into account by measuring the impact forces with an accelerometer mounted within the test headform (*see* below).

Protection against rotational acceleration

A very heavy helmet could reduce head angular acceleration by increasing the inertia of the whole head but only at the expense of excessive weight and an increased risk of neck injury. This mechanism has never been employed deliberately in the design of aircrew protective helmets. However, if it strikes a surface at an acute angle, a head may either slide or roll along the surface, depending on the friction of the contact area. If the helmet shell is made glassy smooth and external protuberances reduced to a minimum, the tendency to slide is increased and rotational acceleration is reduced.

Extent of helmet protection

All the mechanisms for protecting the head that have been discussed above only protect the area actually covered. Overall protection is compromised by the need to provide an adequate field of vision and head mobility. Thus the bones of the face are particularly vulnerable to injury, although the eyes are well protected by the margins of the orbital cavity.

A particular problem arises at the margins of the helmet where the shell is inherently weaker and the discontinuity leads to local concentration of stress. Tape suspensions are ineffective at the helmet margin, and energy absorbing foams have to be used.

Helmet retention

Helmets must be retained following a survivable impact so that protection is available in the event of a second blow. Investigations of RAF aircraft accidents have shown that multiple impacts are not uncommon. Thus, for example, during the ejection sequence the head could strike the canopy, followed by a strike against the separating seat and a final ground strike on landing. Furthermore, aircraft crashes rarely impose a single axis of deceleration and multiple head impacts are likely to occur. However carefully the helmet is fitted and although an adjustable neck strap is provided, helmet losses do occur, especially during high-speed ejection, probably as a result of the high aerodynamic lifting moment that occurs in these conditions.

Windblast protection

In high-speed ejection, the body is suddenly thrust into an airstream which can exert a windblast pressure (q-force) as great as 60 kPa at 600 kt. This pressure on the face may cause petechial and conjunctival haemorrhages, and, if the mouth is open and unprotected, blast damage to the lungs. Face protection in high-speed ejection is essential. The protection can be provided by an oxygen mask and visor of adequate strength mounted to a helmet, which is retained during the ejection sequence. An example of such a helmet which provides blast protection at speeds of up to 750 kt is shown in *Figure 13.4.*

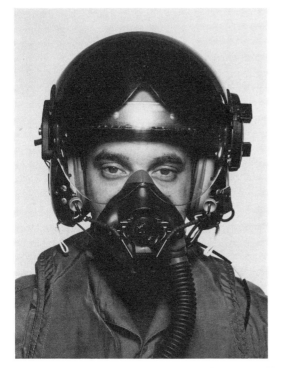

Figure 13.4 A modern aircrew protective helmet worn with a pressure demand mask. The protective helmet is fitted with an outer tinted and an inner transparent polycarbonate visor. The outer visor provides protection against solar glare while either the outer or inner visor will, in the lowered position, protect the face against the high-velocity debris produced by a birdstrike and against the windblast produced by loss of the cockpit canopy or ejection at high aircraft speeds.

Assessment of protection

The various standards used by air forces throughout the Western world for the assessment of protective headgear cover three main aspects of helmet design, as follows, though for convenience and consistency all performance figures quoted refer to the British Standard 6658:1985 specification for type B motorcycle helmets, the minimum legal requirement for riders on public roads within the UK. The

precursors to this standard have been used in developing and evaluating RAF aircrew protective helmets in the past, and the type B helmet specification is the current recommendation for giving the best practicable protection to aircrew at risk from a major head impact.

Penetration resistance

To evaluate a helmet's resistance to penetration the helmet under test is mounted on a rigid headform and struck by a conical striker having a 0.5 mm radius tip. The striker weighs 3.0 kg and is dropped in guided free fall from a height of 2.0 m to give an impact energy of nearly 60 J. Failure is evidenced by penetration such that there is transient electrical contact between the tip of the striker and a soft metal insert at the top of the headform.

Shock absorption

The test helmet, which may have been cooled, heated or soaked to represent environmental extremes, is mounted on an instrumented headform and dropped in guided free fall onto either a flat or hemispherical anvil. The headform, together with its supporting carriage, has a mass of 5 kg and the impact velocities, to be measured just prior to impact, are specified so that the kinetic energies of the impacts are some 105 J and 90 J respectively for the two anvils. Each impact is followed by a second at the same site, but at half the energy, and on no occasion must the acceleration of the headform exceed 300 G. In practice the mass of the helmets adds to that of the headform and carriage so that for a typical helmet weighing 2.0 kg, the impact energies for a first impact against the flat anvil would be of the order of 150 J and a second, 75 J. Impact must still be sustainable without exceeding the 300 G limit. Helmets may be impacted at any point of the crown as well as laterally and posteriorly down to within about 40 mm of the basic plane. On a human head the basic plane is defined as passing through the external auditory meatus and inferior margin of the orbit.

Helmet retention

In this test the helmet is mounted on a rigidly fixed headform and the chin strap preloaded through an artificial chin from which hangs a vertical bar at the lower end of which there is a stop. A magnetically released mass of 10 kg can be slid down the bar so as to impact the stop and produce a sudden jerk load. The preload (of 7 kg) takes the slack out of the system and maximum displacement criteria ensure that a peak load of the order of 3–4 kN must be withstood without failure or excessive stretch of the chin strap.

Rotational acceleration

In addition to the three basic test procedures described above, the current UK motor-cycle specification introduces a test for the helmet's 'sliding resistance'. The helmet is mounted on an anthropomorphic headform which includes a chin and upper neck and is dropped in guided free fall as for the shock absorption test. The anvil, though, is a steeply inclined plane instrumented to monitor the tangential reaction that results from helmet–anvil contact, and pass/fail criteria are based upon the maximum instantaneous force (relatable to peak angular acceleration) as well as its integral with time (relatable to the angular velocity achieved). A flat anvil covered with an abrasive material is used to assess the shell surface material and overall shape, while an anvil which consists of a series of steel bars is used to assess projections. This method is referred to as the oblique impact test.

Other functions of protective helmets

Apart from providing protection against buffet and impact accelerations, protective helmets fulfil other major functions in aviation. Some of these are dealt with in later chapters; they are as follows.

Intercommunication and noise exclusion

The intensity of noise in the cabins of modern high-performance aircraft is so great that unless it is excluded from the intercommunication system both at the microphone and the ears, the overall performance of the system is much impaired. Furthermore, noise levels are frequently such that exposure to them during flight may cause temporary or even permanent hearing loss (*see* Chapter 24). The most important contribution of headgear towards achieving high levels of intelligibility and preventing hearing loss is the reduction of noise that gains access directly to the ear through the headgear structure. The most important factor is the performance of the ear cup and the seal that it provides to the skin around the ear.

Solar glare protection

In high-performance strike or air defence aircraft, frequent interposition of an anti-glare filter is essential in many flight conditions (*see* Chapter 23). The helmet-mounted neutral density filter is placed as close to the eyes as possible. It is adjustable so that it protects from the glare but allows the pilot to see his instruments without the filter. The anti-glare visor must be as light as possible so as to stay in place during high-G manoeuvres.

Protection against birdstrike

The hazard of birdstrike is always present during flight at low level (*see* Chapter 23). To protect the eyes from splinters of broken transparency the headgear can carry a visor made of polycarbonate (3 mm thick) which covers an area of the face and eyes. The lower edge of the polycarbonate visor must abut closely (less than about a 5 mm gap) against the oronasal mask, but must be mounted so that it can be removed at altitudes above which the hazard of birdstrike is negligible (above 1000 feet above ground level). The user must be able to lock the polycarbonate visor in the 'down' position for blast protection, although there is no requirement to select any other position than fully 'up'.

Platform for suspension of oxygen face-mask

The helmet acts as a platform from which to suspend an oxygen mask. The mask must be adjustable so that it may be worn comfortably during routine conditions, yet tightened against the forces of ejection and sealed against escape of oxygen at high pressure during loss of cabin pressure at altitudes above 40 000 feet. The mounting of the headgear on the head and the mode of attachment of the suspension system of the mask must be such that there is no significant movement of the mask on exposure to high levels of maintained acceleration and vibration. The use of positive pressure breathing to increase tolerance to sustained acceleration (*see* page 160) also requires an efficient mask seal, which for comfort, has only to operate during the application of G. The need to tension the mask manually prior to combat can be avoided by means of an automatic tensioning device such as a bladder inflated by mask pressure and lying between the rear of the head and helmet. If the area of the bladder is greater than that of the mask then its inflation will tend to force the helmet, and hence the mask attachment points, rearwards.

Nuclear flash protection and chemical defence

Nuclear explosions in war may result in effects of flash upon the eye (that is, flash blindness or, rarely, retinal burn) from the fireball directly, or indirectly from atmosphere scatter. By night, when the pupil is large, indirect flash blindness is a major hazard and protection of the eye is essential in order to maintain operational efficiency (*see* Chapter 23). Protective headgear may include or be worn with devices that protect against nuclear flash. Similarly, headgear may also be required to integrate with chemical defence respirators or other devices worn by aircrew to protect against chemical agents.

Helmet mounted displays, etc.

An extension of the head-up display principle with an aircraft mounted collimator is to project the display information onto the inside surface of the helmet visor where it may be viewed independent of head position. Similarly, a sight can be placed over a target by moving the head and an appropriate aim angle computed from measured head orientation. Either device requires helmet-mounted electronic and optical components which will add to its mass and need to be mounted so that the centre of gravity of the helmeted head is not unduly displaced. Heavier objects such as night-vision goggles which must be mounted in front of the eyes may be counterbalanced by placing other components to the rear of the helmet, and provision may also be made for the goggles to separate from the helmet prior to ejection or impact.

Other attributes of protective helmets

As with other items of personal equipment, headgear should not be uncomfortable to wear nor impair the efficiency with which the wearer can perform his duties inside or outside the cockpit. It must not impair his ability to board the aircraft and secure himself in his seat.

Weight, size and shape

When the helmet is worn in aircraft frequently exposed to sustained accelerations or vibrations, the total weight of the entire headgear should ideally not exceed 2.0 kg. The weight of the helmet and components should be well distributed over the head, and the centre of gravity (C of G) of the headgear–head combination should be as close as possible to that of the head alone. In particular, the helmet should move the C of G as little as possible above or in front of the natural C of G of the head. The increase in the moment of inertia of the head due to the headgear should also be kept as low as possible; since the weight of the headgear is distributed around the circumference of the head, the moment of inertia tends to increase by a greater proportion than the weight. The helmet should be as compact as possible to keep it away from the cockpit structure, seat, canopy and other items of aircrew personal flying equipment; to improve effective vision; and to allow free movement of the head. The outer surface of the helmet should be kept as smooth as possible as to shape and texture. Any components mounted on the outer shell of the helmet should be of minimal dimensions and smoothly contoured to reduce the effects of glancing blows.

Comfort

Comfort is largely a question of suppressing sources of discomfort. Thus the load of the helmet should be distributed over as large an area of the head as possible. When he puts it on the wearer should be able to alter the distribution and magnitude of the load and have some range of adjustment of the load once he has it on (for example, tension in the chinstrap). The headgear may have to be worn for several hours at a time: pressure points tolerable for 1 hour become highly distracting, annoying and fatiguing after 6 hours.

Security of fit

To be effective the helmet must be firmly clasped to the head. It should not move when the head is moved voluntarily or involuntarily as a result of vibration or sustained accelerations. A stable fit depends on good initial adjustment of the webbing harness so that it fits snugly around the head. The chin strap and an oxygen mask help to keep it in place and the ear cups being clamped on to the sides of the head provide side-to-side stability.

Convenience

The user should be able to put on and take off his helmet easily and without assistance, and he should be able to put on or remove parts of the assembly, or the mask, in the narrow space of a cockpit.

Vision

The helmet should not impose any visual restriction. The wearer should not need to carry out large head movements to see above or behind him in combat or essential cockpit instruments. The lower part of the helmet should not produce any significant restriction of head movement either by preventing full neck mobility or by coming up against items of personal equipment worn on the upper trunk (for example, a life preserver).

References

LÖWENHIELM, C.G.P. (1977) *On Bridging Vein Disruption and Rotational Cerebral Injuries due to Head Impact.* Department of Forensic Medicine and Division of Solid Mechanics. PhD Thesis, University of Lund, Sweden

PEDDER, J.D. and MILLS, N.J. (eds) (1982) *Head Protection— The State of the Art.* University of Birmingham Symposium, 25 September. University of Birmingham

Further reading

BRITISH STANDARDS INSTITUTION (1985) *Protective Helmets for Vehicle Users.* London: BSI. BS 6658:1985

14

Vibration

J.R.R. Stott

Introduction

Any form of motion that repeatedly alternates in direction constitutes vibration. Thus defined, vibration is a widespread physical phenomenon. The motion of tides and ocean waves, the shaking of the Earth's crust during earthquakes, the movement of pistons within the cylinders of engines, the disturbances generated in aircraft flying through turbulent air or in vehicles from the irregularities of the terrain over which they are travelling are all forms of vibration which can be transmitted to man. Vibration is generally transmitted through direct contact between the body and a vibrating structure. In these conditions significant vibrational energy can enter the body with potentially harmful consequences. Vibration may also reach the body by transmission through air. Airborne vibration, if in the appropriate frequency range, is perceived as sound, but at low sonic and subsonic frequencies it may exert other physiological effects.

Much of man's exposure to whole-body vibration occurs through transport in vehicles of various sorts, and although engineering solutions have been found to reduce the physiological hazards of vibration in many types of vehicle undesirably high levels can be encountered in helicopters and in fixed-wing aircraft during low-level flight, as well as in tractors and other off-road vehicles.

Vibration is of operational significance in aviation because it may, among other things, impair visual acuity, interfere with neuromuscular control and lead to fatigue.

Theoretical principles of vibration

The human body is mechanically complex and the pattern of vibration to which it is subjected in, for example low-level turbulence in an aircraft or travelling over a rough track in a road vehicle, is also complex. Some understanding of the effects of vibration can be gained by considering the body as an assemblage of simpler mechanical sub-units and by analysing a complex vibration waveform in terms of its constituent sinusoidal components.

The simplest vibrating system is provided by a mass hanging from a fixed point by a spring. When displaced from its rest position the mass will oscillate about this position for some time before again coming to rest. This vibration involves a repeated interchange of energy between the mass and the spring, the mass having kinetic energy when it is in motion and the spring storing potential energy when it is compressed or extended. In an ideal system, in which no energy is lost from the system, oscillations would continue indefinitely. In practice, the mass encounters some resistance to motion from the surrounding air and further energy is lost within the spring in the form of heat.

If the displacement of the mass from its rest position is plotted against time the resulting graph will be sinusoidal. Sinusoidal motion can be quantified by two pieces of information: the frequency, defined as the number of cycles of motion occurring in one second, the units of which are Hertz (Hz); and the amplitude, generally defined as the maximum displacement in metres from the rest position.

The frequency at which an ideal mass spring system will oscillate when it is disturbed is termed the natural frequency. The natural frequency can be determined from a knowledge of the mass and the spring stiffness according to the formula:

$$f_n = \frac{1}{2\pi} \sqrt{\frac{k}{m}}$$

where f_n is the natural frequency (Hz)

k is the spring stiffness (N/m)
m is the mass (kg).

The formula shows that an increase in spring stiffness will increase the natural frequency while an increase in mass will decrease the natural frequency.

In addition to a mass and a spring, any practical vibrating system possesses a third component, damping. This can be thought of as the means whereby mechanical energy is lost from the system as heat with consequent decay in the amplitude of oscillation. A system having only a small degree of damping continues to oscillate for a long time after an initial disturbance. As the amount of damping is increased so the oscillations that follow an initial disturbance decay more rapidly. With further increase in damping the mass returns to its rest position without any overshoot. The minimum degree of damping required to produce this condition is termed critical damping. Its magnitude can be calculated for a given mass spring system from the formula:

$$C_c = 2\sqrt{k.m}$$

where C_c is the magnitude of critical damping (kg/s), k is the spring stiffness (N/m), m is the mass (kg).

The amount of damping in a system is commonly expressed as a proportion of critical damping, termed the damping factor. A system that has a damping factor of 1 is critically damped, of less than 1 is underdamped, and greater than 1 is over-damped.

As a discrete entity, a damper is exemplified by the shock absorber of a car which typically consists of a piston in a fluid-filled cylinder. Fluid may move from one side of the piston to the other either through orifices in the piston or through an external channel connecting one end of the cylinder with the other. When a force is exerted on the piston it moves at a rate determined by the flow of fluid from one half of the cylinder to the other.

Forced vibration

The previous section has dealt with the behaviour of a mass/spring/damper system when it is left to vibrate following an initial disturbance. It is necessary to consider how such a system behaves when the structure by which it is supported undergoes sustained vibration at various frequencies. *Figure 14.1* shows a mass linked to a base by a spring and a damper. The base is vibrated sinusoidally at increasing frequency. The amplitude of motion of the mass is expressed as a proportion of the motion of the base in the accompanying graph. At low frequencies the mass and the base share the same amplitude of vibration (amplitude ratio = 1).

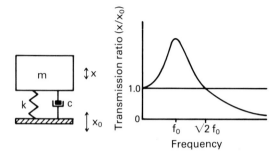

Figure 14.1 A mass/spring/damper system mounted on a vibrating surface. m is the mass (kg), k the spring stiffness (N/m) and c the coefficient of damping (kg/s). The accompanying graph shows the ratio of the sinusoidal motion of the mass to that of the base as the frequency of vibration of the base is increased. f_0 represents the resonant frequency of the system.

As the frequency of vibration is increased the mass begins to vibrate to a greater extent than the base to reach a maximum degree of amplification at what is termed the resonant frequency. With further increase in the frequency of vibration, the relative amplitude of vibration falls until a frequency is reached above which the vibration of the mass becomes progressively less than that of the base.

The extent to which vibration is amplified at the resonant frequency depends upon the amount of damping in the system. *Figure 14.2* shows a set of graphs plotted for different values of damping. With less damping in the system, the amplification of vibration at resonance increases. (It is theoretically

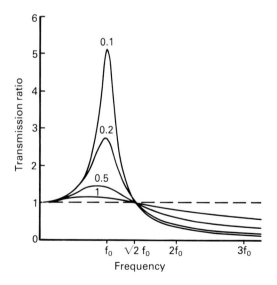

Figure 14.2 Graphs showing the vibration characteristics of a mass spring system with different degrees of damping. The figure adjacent to each graph is the damping factor. f_0 is the undamped resonant frequency.

infinite if there is no damping at all.) It should be noted, however, that even with critical damping there is some amplification of vibration at the resonant frequency, and also that the resonant peak occurs at a somewhat lower frequency in a damped system compared with one having little or no damping.

Irrespective of the degree of damping the response of the mass becomes identical in amplitude with that of the base at a frequency which is $\sqrt{2}$ times the undamped natural frequency. As the frequency of applied vibration is increased above this point the vibration of the mass becomes increasingly small compared with that of the base. In this frequency range the effect of the spring is to isolate the mass from the vibration of the base.

In a system with a low degree of damping the motion of the mass at or near the resonant frequency may be many times that of the external vibration and may result in structural damage. On the other hand, such a system gives a high degree of vibration isolation of the mass at frequencies well above the resonant frequency. In the design of a vibration isolation system, such as the suspension of a motor car, some compromise level of damping (achieved through the vehicle's shock absorbers) has to be found that produces reasonable isolation of the vehicle at vibration frequencies generated by the normal roughness of the road surface but that prevents the vehicle from bouncing out of control if it hits a pothole that excites the resonant vibration frequency of the vehicle. The level of damping factor that best achieves this compromise is generally about 0.7 which limits the amplification at the resonant frequency to about 1.3.

The concept of resonance is particularly important in understanding some of the harmful effects of vibration both in engineering structures and in the human body. The presence of inadequately damped resonances within a complex structure means that comparatively small vibrational accelerations can, at certain frequencies, generate much higher accelerations, and therefore forces, on component parts of the structure, with potentially damaging consequences. A large part of vibration engineering involves the avoidance or the suppression of resonant vibration.

When a structure contains multiple masses resiliently coupled together the behaviour of the system under vibration is correspondingly complex. *Figure 14.3* shows two masses linked in series by springs and dampers to a vibrating base. The accompanying graph shows the motion of the lower mass as a proportion of the vibratory motion of the base when the frequency of vibration applied through the base is changed. Two resonant peaks are now evident at frequencies that differ from the resonant frequencies of each individual mass/spring system. At a frequency between the two resonances the vibration

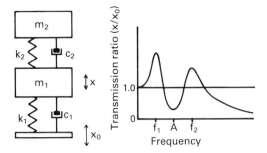

Figure 14.3 The response to forced vibration of two linked mass/spring/damper systems. The graph shows the vibration amplitude ratio of the lower mass with respect to the base. Two resonances are present at f_1 and f_2 with attenuation of vibration at an intermediate frequency. At this frequency the upper mass is resonant relative to the lower mass. The symbols m, k, and c are defined in the caption to *Figure 14.1*.

of the lower mass is much reduced, but at the expense of vibration of the upper mass relative to the lower. This principle is used in the design of the dynamic vibration absorber.

Mechanical properties of biological tissues

While it is of value to identify mass, elasticity and damping in a vibratory system, these constituents are better regarded as properties possessed by a mechanical system rather than as physically discrete entities. For example, no spring exists that does not have a mass associated with the material from which it is made. Similarly, many springy materials (e.g. rubber, connective tissue) possess significant degrees of damping generated by friction at a molecular level within the material.

In the human body it is possible with varying degrees of precision to identify masses that are loosely coupled to the rest of the body by connective tissue which by virtue of its springiness may allow the mass to resonate when vibrated at a particular frequency. Important in this regard are the head, the shoulder girdle, the liver and mediastinum, and the limbs.

The property of elasticity is produced by the spring-like qualities of collagen in muscle and other connective tissues. The mechanical properties of collagen are not so easily modelled as those of an ideal spring. The force required to stretch an ideal spring is proportional to its increase in length. The spring is said to possess uniform stiffness. The collagen of tendon and ligament is non-uniform in stiffness. It becomes stiffer the more it is stretched (*Figure 14.4*). The implication for a vibrating system that has collagen as the spring component is that the

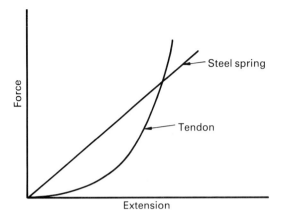

Figure 14.4 The relationship between force and extension for a steel spring compared with that for tendon. Stiffness is given by the slope of the graph. Tendon becomes increasingly stiff as it is stretched.

resonant frequency is dependent on the underlying tension within connective tissue. This connective tissue tension is determined mainly by muscle activity and by the static loading that results from the gravitational environment.

Damping occurs by several mechanisms within the body. In addition to the internal friction within tissue as it is stretched, there is an important damping effect from active skeletal muscle. When active muscle is made to lengthen by the application of an external force the muscle generates an opposing force which, for a given degree of neural activation, is proportional to its rate of lengthening. This is the property of an ideal damper. It is, therefore, not surprising that the state of muscle tension and the consequent body posture are major variable factors governing the mechanical response of the body to vibration. Increased tension in muscles has the effect of stiffening the vibrating system to which they are attached. This tends to raise the resonant frequency and at the same time, by generating increased damping, tends to reduce the degree of resonant amplification.

Vibration sources

In most vehicles there are two principal sources of vibration to be considered. The first originates within the vehicle, in particular the power source; the second is derived from the environment, the terrain over which the land vehicle is travelling, the turbulent air through which the aircraft is flying, or the sea state in which the ship is sailing.

All machinery is liable to generate vibration. In the internal combustion engine the impulse as each cylinder fires and the reciprocating motion of the pistons provide a source of vibrational energy that is propagated to the vehicle through the mountings of the engine and gearbox. Gas turbines and electric motors when in good condition are inherently less likely to generate vibration, but any mass imbalance of a rotating component or looseness in its bearings may result in significant vibration. The detailed analysis of vibration records from accelerometers mounted on the fuselage of a helicopter or on the casing of engines or gearboxes is an important technique for detecting wear in these components during their working life.

The vibration that is generated from an engine is at a frequency that can be predicted from the rotational speed of the machinery. A piston engine rotating at 60 revolutions per second (3600 rpm) is likely to propagate vibration at this frequency (60 Hz). The rotor of a helicopter typically revolves at 4 revolutions/second and, therefore, generates vibration within the helicopter at 4 Hz. The intensity of vibration in helicopters at this frequency is generally low. This is achieved by accurate matching of the mass of each blade on the rotor and by aerodynamically trimming the blades so that they rotate in the same plane. This fundamental rotor frequency is often referred to as the 1R frequency. Generally of greater amplitude is the vibration produced at the blade-pass frequency. This frequency is the 1R frequency multiplied by the number of rotor blades and is usually in the region of 15–25 Hz. In addition, components of vibration are generated at higher harmonics (i.e. integer multiples) of the blade-pass frequency and also at a frequency related to the tail rotor speed. *Figure 14.5* shows the spectrum of G_z vibration recorded in a Chinook helicopter. The repetitive pattern of vibration gives rise to discrete peaks in the spectrum. That at 1R

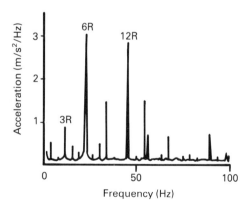

Figure 14.5 The G_z vibration amplitude spectrum of the Chinook helicopter. Peaks labelled 3R, 6R, 12R are harmonics of the fundamental rotor frequency at 4 Hz. In this case the highest peak occurs at the blade-pass frequency (6R), but there is much variation in the relative amplitude of the different harmonics recorded under different flight conditions.

(3.8 Hz) is small: the principal components are at the blade-pass frequency 6R (22.75 Hz) and at the first harmonic of the blade-pass frequency, 12R (45.5 Hz). Other peaks in the spectrum at frequencies unrelated to the main rotor frequency may originate from gearboxes and transmission systems within the aircraft.

Helicopter vibration occurs with broadly similar intensity in all three axes of motion. There may be large differences in the amplitudes of specific harmonics in different modes of flight but the overall amplitude of vibration tends to increase with airspeed and with the loading of the aircraft. Vibration is usually worse during transition to the hover. The measured levels of vibration may differ quite widely between helicopters of identical type operating under similar conditions, though the source of these differences is often elusive.

In fixed-wing aircraft any vibration arising from the power source tends to be at a higher frequency than in helicopters. A single-stage turbine of a fixed-wing jet aircraft typically rotates at about 8000 rpm (130 Hz) and the high-pressure stage of a dual-stage turbine at 14 000 rpm (230 Hz). In a propeller-driven aircraft the blade-pass frequency is in the region of 100 Hz though lower frequencies of vibration may be generated by the beating effect of two propellers running at different speeds.

The main source of vibration encountered in fixed-wing aircraft arises from the atmospheric turbulence through which the aircraft is flying. In consequence the most severe vibration tends to occur during storm cloud penetration or during high-speed, low-level flight. It reflects the random disturbances of turbulent air modified by the aerodynamic characteristics of the aircraft and by the control actions of the pilot (*Figure 14.6*). Most of the vibrational energy of fixed-wing aircraft is found at low frequencies in the vertical axis. In atmospheric turbulence the vertical vibration of the aircraft at 1 Hz may exceed by a factor of 100 that at 10 Hz. The sharp peaks that are characteristics of the spectrum of helicopter vibration are not seen in fixed-wing aircraft though the vibration spectrum may reflect the flexural resonances of the wings and fuselage by showing broad maxima at these frequencies. These features are less evident in the spectrum of high-performance fighter aircraft whose wings and fuselage are more rigidly constructed. However, during buffet, which occurs for example in maximum rate turns that require a maximum degree of aerodynamic lift from the wings, vibration is imposed on the airframe over a narrow frequency range that varies according to aircraft type between about 8 and 20 Hz.

The response of the aircraft as a whole to atmospheric turbulence is determined by the aerodynamic loading on the wings. An aircraft with a large wing area relative to its weight undergoes

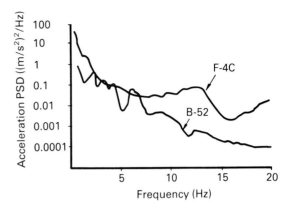

Figure 14.6 Power spectral density (PSD) of G_z vibration from two fixed-wing aircraft, the F-4C fighter and B-52 bomber, during high-speed low-level flight. Note the logarithmic scale on the vertical axis, which emphasizes the lower vibration amplitudes at the expense of the higher amplitudes. The levels of vibration are greater at the low frequencies (<1 Hz) and decline sharply at increasing frequencies (redrawn from Speakman *et al.*, 1971).

greater amplitude low-frequency excursions from level flight as a result of turbulence. Such motion is predominantly in the frequency range of 0.1–1 Hz.

The firing of machine guns from military aircraft transmits to the airframe a series of mechanical shocks. These may be attenuated to some degree by gun mountings that allow the gun to recoil. Such shocks vibrate the airframe not only at the frequency of firing of the gun but also over a broader range of frequencies. The firing of a missile produces a single shock disturbance which evokes a transient vibrational response from undamped resonances within the aircraft.

The measurement and analysis of vibration

Complex oscillatory motion can be described in terms of the changes in position with respect to a fixed point, the changes in velocity relative to a constant or zero velocity, or changes in acceleration in relation to an inertial frame of reference. Displacement, velocity and acceleration are mathematically related and, in principle at least, one may be derived from a knowledge of the other (*Figure 14.7*). Vibration intensity is most frequently quoted in terms of the amplitude of the acceleration in units of m/s^2, but may also be expressed in units of g, the acceleration due to gravity (1 g = 9.8 m/s^2). Vibration at a single frequency can be quantified in terms of its half-peak amplitude, but for a complex vibration containing multiple frequency components

Displacement (m)

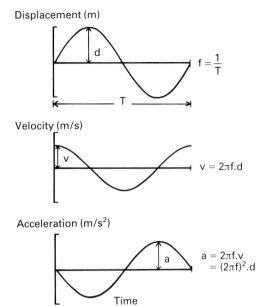

$$f = \frac{1}{T}$$

Velocity (m/s)

$$v = 2\pi f.d$$

Acceleration (m/s²)

$$a = 2\pi f.v$$
$$= (2\pi f)^2.d$$

Time

Figure 14.7 The relationship between displacement, velocity and acceleration for sinusoidal vibration. With respect to displacement, the phase of velocity is advanced by one quarter cycle and acceleration by one half cycle. The duration of 1 cycle of motion, T(s), is known as the period. 1/T gives the frequency, f(Hz). The velocity amplitude, v, is obtained from the displacement amplitude, d, by multiplying by $2\pi f$. Multiplication of the velocity amplitude by $2\pi f$ yields the amplitude of acceleration, a.

the root mean square (RMS) amplitude is used. This can be considered as a type of average amplitude for a complex waveform. The RMS level of a single frequency sine wave is 0.707 of the half-peak amplitude.

A further description of a vibration waveform is provided by the crest factor. If vibration is generated from an impulsive source such as a mechanical hammer or from weapons firing in a military aircraft the recorded vibration will show short-duration high peaks of acceleration, termed mechanical shocks, whose presence makes the perceived severity of vibration much greater than its RMS level would indicate. The crest factor is defined as the ratio of the peak acceleration amplitude of a vibration record to its RMS amplitude. For vibration in which the crest factor exceeds a value of 6 the RMS level of vibration is a poor indicator of its severity and a form of averaging that gives extra weight to the peak levels is used.

The most widely used device in the measurement of vibration is the accelerometer. Accelerometers vary from rugged units designed to measure the high accelerations that occur during an impact to fragile devices that will measure well below the threshold of human perception. Accelerometers are also produced that are insensitive to linear acceleration and respond only to angular acceleration.

When accelerometers are used on the human body the need for high sensitivity and small size are often conflicting requirements. There are very few places on the body surface where good fixation of an accelerometer can be achieved and where the mass of the accelerometer and the springiness of the underlying soft tissue cannot form a resonant system and thereby generate misleading information. The teeth provide a useful fixation point and small accelerometers can be mounted on a dental bite to measure accelerations of the head. Elsewhere on the body, unless fixation is achieved by screwing into bone, accelerometers have to be strapped to the overlying skin. It is often desirable to measure the level of vibration at the point of entry to the body, and this may be achieved in a seated subject by enclosing accelerometers in a seat bar or a thin cushion.

Accelerometers have a directional sensitivity and for a full description of the vibration of a structure three linear accelerometers are needed with their sensitive axes at right angles to each other. Additionally, if angular motion is to be measured a further three accelerometers are required.

The direction of vibration accelerations acting on the body is specified on a three-axis system with reference to the trunk, G_x accelerations acting in the antero-posterior direction, G_y in the lateral direction, and G_z in the cranio-caudal direction. The same system of axes is used in specifying the direction of long-duration accelerations. Rotational accelerations about these axes are referred to in terms of roll, pitch and yaw.

Vibration waveforms can be divided into those that have repetitive or periodic features, the simplest of which is sinusoidal vibration at a single frequency, and those that are irregular or aperiodic such as the vibration of an aircraft in atmospheric turbulence. Any complex vibration waveform can be considered as the summation of a series of increasing frequency sinusoidal components, or harmonics, of appropriate amplitude and phase relationship to each other. The technique of breaking down a vibration signal into its constituent frequencies (Fourier analysis) is important since the effects of vibration on the body are critically dependent on its frequency content.

A plot of the amplitude of each component versus its frequency is known as the vibration spectrum. Periodic vibration generates a spectrum that has narrow discrete peaks with little or no activity in the intervening spectral components. Aperiodic vibration yields a continuous spectrum which may show broad peaks in specific regions of the spectrum.

The biomechanical effects of vibration

Body impedance

When the human body is in direct contact with a source of vibration, mechanical energy is transferred, some of which is degraded into heat within those tissues that have damping properties. A measure of the potential to absorb vibrational energy is provided by the mechanical impedance. Mechanical impedance is defined as the ratio of the peak oscillatory force exerted on an object by a source of vibration to the resulting peak velocity measured at the point of contact with the vibration source. The concept of mechanical impedance is directly analogous to electrical impedance which represents the resistance to the flow of alternating current.

The mechanical impedance of the human body is dependent on the frequency of vibration. If the body were a pure mass without spring or damping components its mechanical impedance would increase linearly with frequency. For a seated human subject this applies only for frequencies of vibration up to about 2 Hz (*Figure 14.8*). Thereafter there is a

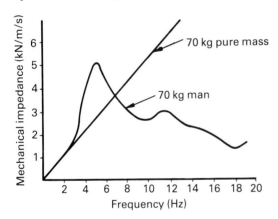

Figure 14.8 The mechanical impedance of a 70 kg seated subject at vibration frequencies up to 20 Hz. The two peaks in the curve occur at the frequencies of the first and second body resonances. Also shown is the impedance of a pure mass of 70 kg.

disproportionate increase in mechanical impedance which reaches a maximum at 4–5 Hz. When vibrated at this frequency a 70 kg man has an apparent mass of 140 kg. This effect is the result of a major resonance within the body. Above a vibration frequency of 7 Hz the impedance of the body falls below that of a simple mass, indicative of the vibration isolation effects of compliant body tissues. Of principal importance is the compression of the soft tissues of the buttocks and flexion of the lumbar

spine which tend to isolate the upper trunk from the source of vibration. Mechanical impedance diminishes with increasing frequency, but this trend is interrupted by a second peak at about 12–15 Hz indicative of a second resonance. The shape of the impedance curve is modified by posture, by the type of seating and restraint system, and by G loading. At 3 *g* the peak in mechanical impedance is shifted upwards to about 8 Hz (Vogt, Coermann and Fust, 1968).

Body resonances

Measurement of mechanical impedance gives little indication of the body structures that are involved in the principal resonances. At least two resonances probably contribute to the impedance peak at 4–5 Hz. Vertical vibration of relaxed, seated, human subjects at these frequencies produces amplification of motion in the shoulder girdle by a factor of 2–3. Less evident, but of greater relevance to human tolerance to vibration, is the resonance of the liver, diaphragm and mediastinum within the body cavity. Animal experiments suggest that this mass moves as one unit against the restraints of compliant connective tissue and of the fluid- and gas-filled abdominal contents. The associated movement of the diaphragm promotes oscillatory airflow in the respiratory tract as well as abdominal wall movement (Coermann *et al.*, 1960), and intra-abdominal pressure changes. All these measures show a peak at 3–4 Hz in man.

The additional energy required to vibrate the body at the frequency of maximum mechanical impedance is absorbed in the supporting connective tissue associated with these resonant structures both by frictional heating and, under more severe vibration, by mechanical disruption of tissues. Animals exposed to lethal levels of vibration (10–15 *g*) at frequencies in the region of their internal body resonance have developed pulmonary congestion with haemorrhage and collapse, diffuse intestinal bleeding and occasional superficial brain haemorrhage. ECG changes indicative of myocardial damage often preceded death (Nickerson and Paradijeff, 1964).

The origin of the second major resonance of the body at 12–15 Hz is less clear. It has been postulated that this resonance is the result of axial compression of the torso controlled by the elastic properties of the spinal column and its supporting musculature, though direct experimental evidence for this is lacking. Both the first and second resonances (4–5 Hz and 12–15 Hz) are evident as peaks in the transmission of vibration from the seat to the head and the shoulders (*Figure 14.9*). However, at 4–5 Hz the amplification of vibration is greater at the

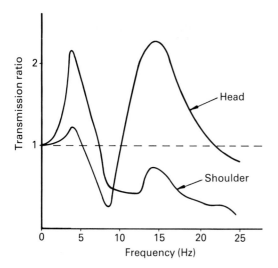

Figure 14.9 The transmission of vibration to the head and shoulders of a seated subject (redrawn from Rowlands, 1977).

shoulders (× 2–3) than at the head (× 1.5) while at 12–15 Hz there is vibration amplification at the head (× 2) but not at the shoulders (× 0.7) (Rowlands, 1977). These findings relate to subjects seated in a chair having a backrest. The presence of a backrest allows vibration to bypass the vibration-attenuating effect of the trunk at higher frequencies. In the absence of a backrest, vibration of the head and shoulders at 12–15 Hz is markedly reduced, but posture has to be maintained by increased muscular activity in the trunk which has the effect of increasing the transmission of vibration to the head at lower frequencies (5–6 Hz).

The mechanical response of the head under vertical vibration involves not only linear but also angular motion, particularly in pitch. This occurs because the centre of gravity of the head lies anterior to the atlanto-occipital joint and the consequent tendency to forward flexion of the head, readily observed in somnolent rail passengers, has in the waking state to be opposed by continuous activity in the neck extensor muscles. The relationship between head pitch acceleration and linear vertical seat acceleration tends to show peaks at 5–6 Hz and at 12 Hz. A further effect is often seen in response to vibration at 3–7 Hz when the oscillation of the head occurs at twice the frequency of the input vibration.

The effect of wearing an aircrew helmet is to increase the mass of the head and, in consequence, the stiffness of the neck muscles that hold the head upright. Measurement of the motion of a well-fitted aircrew helmet shows that it remains well coupled to the head at frequencies of vertical vibration up to about 4 Hz but at 7 Hz the pitch motion of the helmet can be more than twice that of the head.

At different frequencies of vibration other resonances become apparent within the body. Although the maximum oscillatory airflow is produced by frequencies of vertical vibration around 3–4 Hz, speech is not impaired at these frequencies unless vibration levels are severe. From about 6 Hz to 20 Hz the oscillatory airflow produces loudness modulation of speech with possible loss of intelligibility at some frequencies (Nixon and Sommer, 1963).

Subjects vibrated at frequencies between about 2 and 6 Hz experience difficulty in controlling the position of the outstretched hand which may pose problems in the operation of switches and controls in an environment vibrating at these frequencies. Tracking tasks in which the arm is supported and the hand operates a joystick control show most disruption by vibration in the frequency range 4–8 Hz.

As frequencies of vibration are increased progressively smaller structural units in the body may resonate; at lower frequencies (4–8 Hz) the muscle groups in the leg, at higher frequencies (15–20 Hz) the soft tissues of the face, giving rise to a distracting flutter. The possibility of mechanical resonance of the eye has been investigated. Early experiments showed visual acuity to be impaired under whole-body vibration in the frequency range 20–40 Hz and 60–90 Hz (Coermann, 1940). Techniques that involve the tracking of a light spot reflected from the cornea suggest the presence of a small resonance (× 1.2) at around 20 Hz. An indirect method of tracking the retinal image during vibration applied direct to the head has shown resonant peaks at 30–40 Hz (× 1.3) and 70 Hz (× 3) (Stott, 1984). Whole-body vibration applied through the seat at these frequencies is much attenuated within the trunk and relatively little reaches the head. It seems likely that any resonance involves intra-ocular structures rather than movement of the eye globe as a whole. The effect of vibration on vision is considered in more detail in a later section.

The response of the body to vibration transmitted through the feet of a standing subject is little different from that of a seated subject, the straight legs acting as rigid columns. Flexion of the legs brings into play the compliance and damping properties of striated muscle and produces increasingly effective vibration isolation of the trunk to frequencies above 2 Hz, a fact appreciated if not understood by charioteers and down-hill skiers.

When vibration is applied to supine subjects the attenuating effect of the trunk on vibration reaching the head is absent. Measurement of vibration at the head of supine subjects vibrated in the fore–aft direction (G_x) indicates amplification of vibration at frequencies above 4 Hz and a resonant peak with a magnification factor of 2 at 60 Hz. There is also amplification of vibration at around 8 Hz on the abdomen, sternum, and knee.

The effects of vibration on vision

There are two principal requirements to enable the eye to view objects with a maximum degree of visual acuity. The first is that the image formed on the retina is correctly focused, the second is that the eyes should be so directed that the image remains essentially stationary on the fovea. This second requirement of a stable retinal image may have to be achieved when either the object of regard is in motion or when the head itself is moving. Two important reflexes, the vestibulo-ocular reflex and the pursuit reflex, promote stability of the retinal image. The vestibulo-ocular reflex uses sensory information derived primarily from the semicircular canals to generate angular eye movements that compensate for head movements. The pursuit reflex is visually mediated and uses the error of visual fixation to generate eye movements that maintain the retinal image on the foveal region. The shortest neural pathway between the vestibular system and the eye muscles comprises only three neurones and it consequently enables the eye to respond rapidly to changing head movement. By contrast, the pursuit reflex comprises more complex visual processing and is relatively slow in response.

Thus if a stationary subject views an oscillating complex display his visual acuity for details of the display will be reduced if this motion exceeds an angular velocity of 40°/second or if its frequency of oscillation exceeds about 1 Hz. The subject's performance at this task is limited by the pursuit reflex (*Figure 14.10*). By contrast, if a subject who has normal vestibular function undergoes angular oscillation while viewing a stationary display, good visual acuity is maintained up to frequencies of 8 Hz or more. That this ability is dependent on an intact vestibulo-ocular reflex is indicated by the fact that a subject who lacks vestibular function loses visual acuity, both with oscillation of himself or of the display, at frequencies above 1 Hz (Benson and Barnes, 1978). The vestibulo-ocular reflex probably generates compensatory eye movements to angular head movement at frequencies up to 20–25 Hz.

Whole-body vertical vibration generates angular movement of the head principally in pitch. Peak angular accelerations are found at 5–6 Hz and at 12 Hz. Such angular head movement is within the frequency range in which the vestibulo-ocular reflex will promote compensatory eye movements, though with high intensities of vibration at these frequencies subjects may be aware of some visual instability of earth-fixed objects.

The pilot of an aircraft undergoing vibration needs to maintain visual acuity under two principal conditions. The first occurs when he observes the world outside the aircraft; the second when he wishes to read instruments or displays that are, like himself, undergoing vibration. The outside world is at optical infinity and is space stable, though the pilot may need to track objects moving within it such as other aircraft. Under these conditions purely linear movements of the head will produce no retinal image motion and the eye is stabilized to angular head movement by the vestibulo-ocular reflex. Objects that he wishes to track within this field of view are not likely to move so fast that they exceed the angular velocity limitations of the pursuit reflex. It is when viewing objects within the aircraft that the pilot is likely to experience problems. Although the instrument panel and the pilot's seat share approximately the same vibratory motion, the instrument panel is often spring mounted to isolate it from high-frequency vibration. This isolation is achieved at the cost of a resonance at a lower frequency and the consequent possibility of instrument panel oscillation if the aircraft undergoes vibration that has components near this frequency. In addition, the vibration of the pilot's head will be increased at certain frequencies, and at frequencies above 1–2 Hz will be out of phase with the motion of the instrument panel owing to transmission delays through the body. This relative linear motion between the eye and the instrument panel will result in retinal image motion and degraded visual acuity

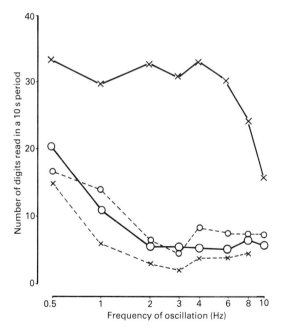

Figure 14.10 Comparison of reading performance (mean of 8 subjects) when subjects undergoing sinusoidal oscillation in yaw read a stationary numerical display (X—X) and when stationary subjects read an oscillating display (O—O). The dotted lines indicate the performance of a subject who lacks labyrinthine function (redrawn from Benson and Barnes, 1978).

since, unlike the outside scene, the instrument panel is not at optical infinity. In these circumstances the eye movements generated by the vestibulo-ocular reflex may not improve retinal image stability. A further circumstance in which the vestibulo-ocular reflex produces inappropriate eye movements occurs in the use of helmet-mounted display systems which generate images that are coupled to and therefore move with the head.

The mechanism by which unwanted vestibular-induced eye movements are suppressed has the same frequency and velocity limitations as the pursuit reflex. (Vestibulo-ocular suppression and ocular pursuit probably involve the same neural pathways.) Thus vestibular-induced eye movements resulting from head vibration at frequencies above 2 Hz cannot be suppressed and may, therefore, contribute to a decrement in visual acuity when both subject and visual target are undergoing vibration. The legibility of a helmet-mounted display is particularly impaired by vibration at frequencies between 4 and 6 Hz (*Figure 14.11*), but it can be improved if the projected visual image of the display is stabilized by moving it in anti-phase to the sensed pitch and yaw rotations of the helmet (Wells and Griffin, 1984).

The legibility of flight instruments in helicopters is a subject that has received insufficient attention. Pilots are often aware that at certain phases of flight, e.g. transition to hover, the levels of vibration render instruments difficult to read. In addition to the relative motion between observer and visual target, many other factors are involved in the legibility of symbolic information—in particular, size, line width, colour, brightness and contrast.

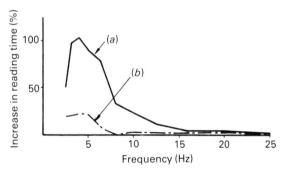

Figure 14.11 The effect of vibration on reading performance from a helmet mounted display (*a*) when the display image is fixed in position relative to the helmet and (*b*) when the image is stabilized in space (redrawn from Wells and Griffin, 1984).

Cardiovascular effects of vibration

Exposure to moderate levels of whole-body vibration produces no highly consistent changes in the cardiovascular system. There may be an increase in pulse rate at the start of vibration exposure but it is not sustained. A rise in blood pressure after periods of vibration lasting 1–2 hours has been reported. In response to whole-body vibration there is an increase in muscle activity both to maintain posture and possibly to reduce the resonant amplification of body structures. This is reflected in an increase in metabolic rate under vibration and a redistribution of blood flow with peripheral vasoconstriction (Hood *et al.*, 1966). More severe levels of vibration have provoked transient cardiac rhythm changes in man and fatal dysrhythmias in cats.

Respiratory effects of vibration

The increase in metabolic rate during vibration is comparable with that seen in gentle exercise and respiration is increased to achieve the necessary increase in elimination of CO_2. However, true hyperventilation may occur leading to reduced carbon dioxide tensions within the body (Ernsting, 1961). The mechanism for this hyperventilation is not fully understood. High levels of vibration may give rise to alarm with consequent hyperventilation. Stretch receptors in the lung may be stimulated by vibration to promote increased pulmonary ventilation.

Vibration over a wide range of frequencies promotes an oscillating airflow superimposed on the normal respiratory air movements. The maximum oscillating volume is found with G_z vibration at 3–4 Hz, corresponding to the frequency of internal body resonance. Although this oscillating volume is less than the anatomical dead-space it has a disproportionate effect on gas exchange on account of the convective mixing of gases promoted by vibration of the air within the bronchial tree. This effect may be maximal at higher frequencies of oscillatory airflow (George and Geddes, 1985).

Individual differences in the degree of hypocapnia induced by vibration may be related to the individual's responsiveness to CO_2. In subjects with a low CO_2 responsiveness minute ventilation is less tightly regulated by arterial CO_2 levels. It has been suggested that the increased ventilation provoked by vibration is not compensated in these individuals by a reduction in CO_2 mediated ventilatory drive (Lamb and Tenney, 1966).

Vibration levels in helicopter operations are generally insufficient to produce overt symptoms of hyperventilation, but end-tidal P_{CO_2} levels of 30 mm Hg have been measured in the laboratory during repeated 2-hour exposures to the simulated noise and vibration environment of the Chinook helicopter (*Figure 14.12*).

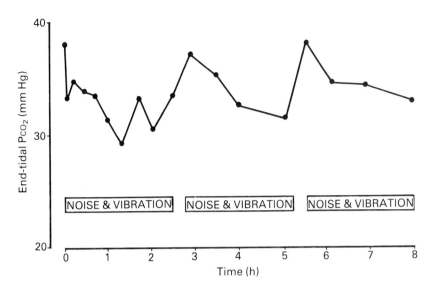

Figure 14.12 Vibration-induced hyperventilation. End-tidal CO_2 levels measured in one subject during exposure to laboratory-reproduced noise and vibration from the Chinook helicopter over an 8 hour period. End-tidal CO_2 levels return to near normal following each 20-minute rest period.

Neuromuscular effects of vibration

Vibration in the frequency range from 20 to 100 Hz when applied direct to a skeletal muscle or its associated tendon provokes a reflex contraction, the tonic vibration reflex, accompanied by an erroneous perception of increased muscle stretch. Local vibration can be regarded as a rapid sequence of mechanical stimuli provoking a succession of stretch reflexes. The effect is mediated through the stimulation of muscle spindles and Golgi tendon organs, whose receptors are responsible for the sense of proprioception. Thus vibration applied to the Achilles tendon or the soleus muscle in a standing subject is perceived as a lengthening of this muscle which is interpreted as ankle dorsiflexion and a forward tilt of the whole body. The subject in an attempt to remain upright generates an inappropriate backward movement of the body to the point where he may fall. Similarly, local vibration applied to the neck extensor muscles provokes an illusion of forward flexion of the head, and vibration to rectus abdominis an illusion of extension of the upper trunk. When vibration is stopped there is a transient illusion of motion in the opposite direction. Furthermore, if during vibration of muscle groups the subject views a stationary light in the dark there is a visual illusion of movement of the light in the direction of the illusory body motion, and it is often possible to record an associated nystagmus (Lackner and Levine, 1979).

In contrast to vibration applied to individual muscles, whole-body vibration provokes a reflex inhibition of tendon reflexes. The effect seems to be peripherally mediated since inhibition of leg reflexes can be as readily produced when vibration is applied through the feet of seated subjects (Roll *et al.*, 1980).

Vibration and motion sickness

Whole-body vibration at frequencies around 0.2 Hz can induce the symptoms of motion sickness in susceptible subjects. This effect occurs to a diminishing extent at frequencies up to about 0.7 Hz. Susceptibility is probably greater for a stimulus in the G_x (fore–aft) direction than for the same stimulus applied in the G_z (cranio-caudal) direction. The frequency range over which motion sickness is provoked lies well below any internal body resonance so that there is no direct mechanical cause for the stomach awareness that characterizes the onset of motion sickness. This stimulus to motion sickness is more fully discussed in Chapter 22.

Infrasonic vibration

Aircraft engines and rocket motors generate airborne vibration over a very broad range of acoustic frequencies. Airborne vibration is, of course, perceived mainly as sound when it lies within the frequency range of the ear. Acoustic frequencies below 25 Hz, nominally the low frequency threshold of hearing, can still be heard if they are of sufficient intensity, but the sensivity of the ear falls off rapidly in this frequency range. Below a frequency of about 18 Hz sounds are no longer heard as a continuous tone but as a series of pulses. At even lower frequencies (5–10 Hz) pressure pulsations are still sensed by the ear though possibly through nerve endings in the tympanic membrane which convey a sense of fullness in the ear and of pain if acoustic vibration is of sufficient intensity (>155 dB at 5 Hz). There is evidence that the feeling of fullness or pressure in the ear is the result of indrawing of the tympanic membrane. It can be relieved, but only temporarily, by venting the middle ear using the Valsalva manoeuvre. The Eustachian tube appears to be acting as a one-way valve so that large excursions of the tympanic membrane force air out of the middle ear more readily than it can be drawn back in. After exposure to intense infrasound, vascular injection of the eardrum may be observed and audiometry may show a small degree of temporary threshold shift (TTS) (von Gierke and Nixon, 1977).

Other symptoms reported by subjects exposed to high-intensity infrasound include nausea and impairment of balance, symptoms that suggest an involvement of vestibular receptors. Vertical nystagmus has been recorded, its onset related to the frequency, intensity, and duration of infrasonic vibration. No objective evidence of equilibratory disturbance has been obtained.

Infrasonic vibration over the frequency range 2–15 Hz can be felt as pressure pulsations on the chest and abdomen often associated with a sense of tightness in the chest. Because of the disparity in density (more strictly, acoustic impedance) between air and body tissues much of the pressure wave is reflected and very little movement is imparted to the chest wall. On the other hand, the fluctuating air pressure generates an alternating mass flow of air in and out of the chest. If the gas flow is measured at different frequencies and constant sound pressure level, a peak in flow is seen at around 50 Hz which is indicative of an acoustic resonance of the chest cavity at this frequency. Dogs exposed to acoustic vibration of 0.5 Hz at 172 dB can cease spontaneous respiration without ill effect. Such observations have led to the use of oscillatory gas flows at frequencies between 0.5 and 6 Hz as a technique for assisting alveolar ventilation in patients with respiratory disease.

It remains to be shown whether, in normal individuals exposed to high-intensity infrasound, the increased elimination of carbon dioxide produced by oscillatory airflow within the respiratory tract tends to lead to hyperventilation in an equivalent manner to whole-body vibration.

Tiredness and an inability to concentrate are also symptoms that may be reported during exposure to infrasound. These effects are indicative of the psychological stressor effects of infrasound.

Human tolerance to vibration and the assessment of vibration severity

Having measured the vibration in a particular environment it is often necessary to assess what effect such levels of vibration will have on a subject who has to operate in that environment; in particular, whether vibration will produce discomfort, reduce working efficiency, or even lead to physical harm.

While animal studies have yielded information on the anatomical sites that are vulnerable to vibration, extrapolation to man leads to uncertainties. The nearest approach to carrying out such an experiment in man required 15 well-motivated volunteers to submit to steadily increasing amplitudes of vibration until they thought they would sustain bodily harm by any further increase (Magid, Coermann and Ziegenruecker, 1960). The results of this experiment (*Figure 14.13*) indicate that the body is least tolerant of vibration between the frequencies of 4 and 8 Hz. The main symptoms for which vibration was discontinued were precordial and mid-abdominal pain. The acceleration levels of vibration that were tolerated at 1 Hz were roughly twice those at 4–8 Hz, and at frequencies between 1 and 3 Hz the

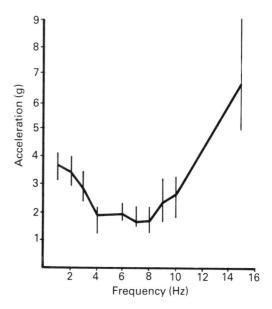

Figure 14.13 Limits of voluntary human tolerance to G_z sinusoidal vibration at frequencies between 1 and 15 Hz. The graph shows the mean of 10 subjects. Vertical bars indicate the range of results at each test frequency (redrawn from Magid *et al.*, 1960).

main symptom was difficulty in breathing. After 1 min exposure to vibration at 8 Hz one subject fainted and was found to have developed a nodal tachycardia.

The general shape of the vibration tolerance curve derived from this experiment has also emerged from psychophysical studies to find the levels of vibration at different frequencies and in different directions that produce equivalent levels of discomfort (Miwa, 1967). From this type of data the International Standards Organisation (ISO) has produced a *Guide for the Evaluation of Human Response to Vibration* (ISO 2631: 1985). The guide sets out levels of vibration acceleration in relation to three criteria:

1. *Safety*—The exposure limit.
2. *Working efficiency*—The fatigue decreased proficiency (FDP) limit.
3. *Comfort*—The reduced comfort limit.

These limits are related numerically: the exposure limit is greater than the FDP limit by a factor of 2 (6 dB) and the reduced comfort limit is less that the FDP limit by a factor of 3.15 (10 dB). The limits are defined over the frequency range 1–80 Hz. They differ in shape for vibration applied in the head–foot direction (G_z) as compared with fore–aft (G_x) and lateral (G_y) directions to take account of the maximum sensitivity of the body between 4 and 8 Hz to G_z vibration and between 1 and 2 Hz to G_x or G_y.

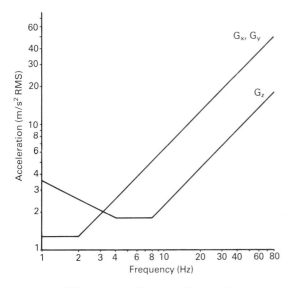

Figure 14.14 International Standards Organisation curves for the assessment of vibration exposure. The curves shown are the Fatigue Decreased Proficiency (FDP) boundaries for vibration of 25 minutes duration in the G_x or G_y and the G_z axes. The reduced comfort and exposure limits are of the same shape, but shifted on the vertical axis. The curves reflect the maximum sensitivity of the body to G_z vibration in the range 4–8 Hz and to G_x or G_y vibration between 1 and 2 Hz.

vibration (*Figure 14.14*). The guide also takes account of the duration of vibration exposure, the limits becoming more stringent as exposure time is increased. The ISO document remains a guide and is not legally enforcible.

Decreased proficiency in a vibrational environment depends on the nature of the task to be performed and on the experience and motivation of the individual. In any given situation in which a subject is exposed to vibration many variable factors have to be considered, only some of which have hitherto been covered by the ISO guide. Recent work has sought to extend the scope of the guide to cover vibration that is occurring over a broad range of frequencies, and vibration that contains repeated shocks—short-duration pulses of force such as might be generated by a mechanical hammer.

In the assessment of vibration measured in a particular environment it is proposed that weighting functions based on the curves of *Figure 14.14* are applied to the vibration spectrum so as to emphasize those frequencies to which the body is most susceptible. Other weighting functions have been derived to assess the disturbance to vision and hand control and to estimate the incidence of motion sickness. From the weighted spectrum can be calculated a Vibration Dose Value, a single figure that takes account of the duration of vibration exposure and is equally applicable to vibration containing repeated mechanical shocks (BS 6841: 1987). Guidelines are also available to evaluate vibration entering the body through vibrating hand-held tools in relation to the occupational risk of vibration-induced Raynaud's disease (vibration white finger) (BS 6842: 1987).

Protection against vibration

The effects of vibration on the body can be reduced by attention to the source of vibration, by modification of the transmission pathway, or by alteration of the dynamic properties of the body. Where the source of vibration is turbulent air this can be avoided by the appropriate routeing of commerical aircraft away from storm cloud activity or by the choice of a different cruising altitude. Reduction of vibration emanating from aircraft engines is a task for the design and maintenance engineers of the aircraft.

Several methods have been used in helicopters to reduce the vibration reaching the aircrew and passengers. Dynamic vibration absorbers are fitted to the cockpit floor in the Chinook helicopter. This device consists of a minimally damped mass/spring system which is fixed to the airframe and has a natural frequency that corresponds to the predominant vibration frequency of the helicopter. Vibration of the aircraft induces relatively large-amplitude resonant oscillation in the mass of the dynamic vibration absorber which in consequence exerts an alternating force tending to oppose and thus reduce the input vibration. Such a device works only over a narrow frequency range, and will amplify vibration at frequencies immediately above and below (*see Figure 14.3*). Another engineering approach to reducing the effects of vibration is by means of vibration isolation of the aircrew seat. This has been achieved in the Lynx helicopter, for example by mounting the seat-pan and backrest on steel springs. Provided the resonant frequency of the system formed by the body mass and the spring seat is at a low frequency relative to the vibration spectrum of the aircraft then increasing attenuation of vibration can be expected at frequencies above 1.4 times the resonant frequency. The resonant frequency of the seat is lower the heavier the occupant of the seat so that the vibration isolation at higher frequencies is more effective for heavier subjects. In practice, the seat and its occupant has a resonance at 3–4 Hz, close to the principal body resonance. Although in flight there is little vibration input at these frequencies, in a crash a spring seat will amplify the impact forces and may consequently worsen the chances of survival. The same principle of vibration isolation is used in the civilian passenger-carrying version of the Chinook helicopter in which the whole floor of the passenger compartment is mounted on a spring suspension.

Mention has already been made of the effects of posture and muscle tension on body resonances. Under severe vibration muscle tensing is an involuntary response tending to increase damping within the body and to stiffen the spring component of vibrating structures and so alter their resonant frequency. Subjects tend to adopt a posture that minimizes vibration reaching the head.

The evacuation of casualties by helicopter has the advantage of speed of access to appropriate medical facilities which is unlikely to be outweighed by the stress of helicopter vibration. None the less, pre-flight assessment should ideally take account of the effects of vibration and, for example, ensure adequate analgesia in patients with fractures. A casualty lying on the floor of the aircraft is exposed to more vibration particularly to the head than is a sitting subject. An air mattress is effective in attenuating vibration at frequencies above about 5 Hz. A degree of vibration isolation is also provided by the compliance of the hanging stretcher mountings installed in some helicopters.

Occupational hazards of vibration

Apart from the hazards of acute exposure to high levels of vibration, long-term exposure to vibration has been suspected as a causative factor in a number of conditions.

The causal link between local vibration to the hand and arm from hand-held vibrating tools and the development of Raynaud's disease (vibration white finger) was first reported in 1911 but has only recently been declared an industrial disease for which in certain groups of workers financial compensation can be paid (Taylor, 1985). The condition is not likely to be seen in aviation medicine but may possibly occur in manufacturing industries related to aviation. Workers who use hand-held grinding and chipping tools for metal finishing and also chain-saw operators are most at risk of developing vibration white finger. Vibration to the hand in the frequency range 20–400 Hz is most liable to lead to the condition. Symptoms appear after months or years of vibration exposure and consist initially of episodes of tingling or numbness in the fingers. Later, attacks of finger blanching, usually provoked by cold, occur with increasing frequency. Touch and temperature sensations are impaired, and the loss of finger dexterity interferes with work and leisure activities. With further vibration exposure blanching attacks are replaced by a more continuous dusky cyanosis. Atrophic changes in the finger pulps may be followed by necrosis of the skin over the finger-tips. Removal of affected individuals from work involving exposure to vibration may halt the progression of the condition but will only reverse it when in its early stages.

Whole-body vibration has been implicated as a factor in the development of disorders of the lumbar spine, particularly in drivers of tractors, earth-moving vehicles, and trucks. Lumbar backache is also a frequent complaint among helicopter pilots. Direct measurement of the movements of the lumbar spine during vibration using markers fixed into the spinous processes indicates that at about 4 Hz not only is there a peak in amplification of vertical motion but also of fore–aft and rotational motion of lumbar vertebrae. The major body resonance occurs at this frequency so that mechanical stress on the lumbar spine is likely to be at a maximum in this frequency range. The epidemiological surveys conducted on drivers of tractors and earth-moving vehicles (reviewed in Dupuis and Zerlett, 1986) indicate that degenerative disorders of the lumbar spine occur at an earlier age in these groups of workers and that vibration is implicated as an aetiological factor. It is not certain whether the same is true for helicopter pilots. The predominant vibration frequency of helicopters tends to be above the major body resonance and the unvarying slightly bent sitting posture that the disposition of cyclic and collective imposes on the pilot may be of greater importance in provoking back pain during flight. Evidence for a greater incidence of radiological abnormalities of the lumbar spine in helicopter pilots is inconclusive. The subject is reviewed by Bowden (1987).

Epidemiological studies have also shown a higher than normal incidence of stomach-related disorders in tractor drivers and drivers of earth-moving vehicles. The relationship to vibration exposure is far from certain though it is of interest that the incidence of stomach ailments in tracked vehicle operators is only half that of wheeled earth-moving vehicle drivers. While the life-style of the two groups of workers could be expected to be similar, the vibration exposure in wheeled vehicles is likely to be much greater.

References

BENSON, A.J. and BARNES, G.R. (1978) Vision during angular oscillation: the dynamic interaction of visual and vestibular mechanisms. *Aviation, Space and Environmental Medicine*, **49**, 340–345

BOWDEN, T. (1987) Back pain in helicopter aircrew: a literature review. *Aviation, Space and Environmental Medicine*, **58**, 461–467

British Standards Institution (1987) *Guide to the Evaluation of Human Exposure to Whole-body Mechanical Vibration and Repeated Shock*. BS 6841: 1987. London

British Standards Institution (1987) *Guide to the Measurement and Evaluation of Human Exposure to Vibration Transmitted to the Hand*. BS 6842: 1987. London

COERMANN, R. (1940) *Investigation into the Effect of Vibration on the Human Body*. Library Translation No 217. Royal Aircraft Establishment, London: Ministry of Defence

COERMANN, R.R., ZIEGENRUECKER, G.H., WITTWER, A.L. and VON GIERKE, H.E., (1960). The passive dynamic properties of the human thorax–abdomen system and of the whole-body system. *Aerospace Medicine*, **31**, 443–455

DUPUIS, H. and ZERLETT, G. (1986) *The Effects of Whole-body Vibration*. Berlin: Springer-Verlag

ERNSTING, J. (1961) *Respiratory Effects of Whole-body Vibration*. RAF Institute of Aviation Medicine Report No.179. London: Ministry of Defence

GEORGE, R.J.D. and GEDDES, D.M. (1985) High frequency ventilation. *British Journal of Hospital Medicine*, **33**, 344–349

HOOD, W.B., MURRAY, R.H., URSCHEL, C.W., BOWERS, J.A. and CLARK, J.G. (1966) Cardiopulmonary effects of whole-body vibration in man. *Journal of Applied Physiology*, **21**, 1725–1731

International Organisation for Standardization (1985) *Guide for the Evaluation of Human Exposure to Whole-body Vibration*. ISO 2631. New York

LACKNER, J.R. and LEVINE, M.S., (1979) Changes in apparent body orientation and sensory localization induced by vibration of postural muscles: vibratory myesthetic illusions. *Aviation, Space and Environmental Medicine*, **50**, 346–354

LAMB, T.W. and TENNEY, S.M. (1966) Nature of vibration hyperventilation. *Journal of Applied Physiology*, **21**, 404–410

MAGID, E.B., COERMANN, R.R. and ZIEGENRUECKER, G.H. (1960) Human tolerance to whole-body sinusoidal vibration. *Aerospace Medicine*, **31**, 915–924

MIWA, T. (1967) Evaluation methods for vibration effect: part 1. Measurements of threshold and equal sensation contours of whole-body for vertical and horizontal vibrations. *Industrial Health*, **5**, 183–205

NICKERSON, J.L. and PARADIJEFF, A. (1964) *Body Tissue Changes in Dogs Resulting from Sinusoidal Oscillation Stress*. Technical Documentary Report AMRL-TDR-64-58. Wright-Patterson Air Force Base, Ohio: USAF Aerospace Medical Research Laboratories

NIXON, C.W. and SOMMER, H.C. (1963) Influence of selected vibrations upon speech III. Range of 6 cps to 20 cps for semi-supine talkers. *Aerospace Medicine*, **34**, 1012–1017

ROLL, J.P., MARTIN, B., GAUTHIER, G.M. and MUSSA IVALDI, F. (1980) Effects of whole-body vibration on spinal reflexes in man. *Aviation, Space and Environmental Medicine*, **51**, 1227–1233

ROWLANDS, G.F. (1977) *The Transmission of Vertical Vibration to the Heads and Shoulders of Seated Men*. Royal Aircraft Establishment Technical Report No.77088. London: Ministry of Defence

SPEAKMAN, J.D. and ROSE, J.F. (1971) *Crew Compartment Vibration Environment in the B52 Aircraft During Low Altitude High Speed Flight*. AMRL-TR-71-12. Wright Patterson Air Force Base, Ohio: Aerospace Medical Research Laboratory

SPEAKMAN, J.D., BONFILI, H.F., HILLE, H.R. and COLE, T.N. (1971) *Crew Exposure to Vibration in the F4C Aircraft During Low Altitude High Speed Flight*. AMRL-TR-70-99. Wright Patterson Air Force Base, Ohio: Aerospace Medical Research Laboratory

STOTT, J.R.R. (1984) The vertical vestibulo-ocular reflex and ocular resonance. *Vision Research*, **24**, 949–960

TAYLOR, W. (1985) Vibration white finger: a newly prescribed disease. Editorial. *British Medical Journal*, **291**, 921–922

VOGT, H.L., COERMANN, R.R. and FUST, H.D. (1968) Mechanical impedance of the sitting human under sustained acceleration. *Aerospace Medicine*, **39**, 675–679

VON GIERKE, H.E. and NIXON, C.W. (1977) Effects of intense infrasound on man. In *Infrasound and Low Frequency Vibration*, edited by W. Tempest, Chapter 6, pp. 115–150. London: Academic Press

WELLS, M.J. and GRIFFIN, M.J. (1984) Benefits of helmet-mounted display image stabilisation under whole-body vibration. *Aviation, Space and Environmental Medicine*, **55**, 13–18

Further reading

BOFF, K.R. and LINCOLN, J.E. (eds) (1986) *Engineering Data Compendium: Human Perception and Performance*. Wright-Patterson Air Force Base, Ohio: Armstrong Aerospace Medical Research Laboratory

GUIGNARD, J.C. and KING, P.F. (1972) *Aeromedical Aspects of Vibration and Noise*. AGARDograph AG-151. Nevilly-sur-Seine, France: AGARD/NATO

HARRIS, C.M. and CREDE, C.E. (eds) (1976) *Shock and Vibration Handbook*, 2nd edn. New York: McGraw-Hill

15

Escape from aircraft

D.J. Anton

Introduction

Unassisted escape implies that egress from an aircraft is effected without the use of any aids other than the muscular power of the escaping individual and the force of gravity. The requirement for escape may arise at any time during flight, but without mechanical assistance it becomes very difficult at aircraft speeds greater than about 200 knots, particularly if the situation is aggravated by an uncontrolled aircraft manoeuvre such as spin or spiral dive. In large aircraft, the occupants may be further handicapped by the difficulty of reaching the escape point if their movement is hampered by the accelerations imposed by such manoeuvres. At high indicated air speeds, aerodynamic forces across the upper surface of the escape hatchway or cockpit may make it impossible for aircrew to abandon the aircraft, and increase the hazard of fouling some part of the aircraft structure.

To overcome these problems, current high-performance, and most military training aircraft, have provision for assisted escape by means of an ejection seat, or capsule. The first part of this chapter is concerned primarily with the principles of unassisted egress from low-flying aircraft in flight, but it is also convenient to discuss parachutes and parachuting.

Techniques of unassisted escape

The precise procedure to be used in an emergency varies with the type of aircraft, its operational role and the configuration of escape hatches, but certain general principles must be observed if the escape is to be successful. The first requirement is, of course, that the aircrew must be properly fitted with appropriate equipment and must understand its operation and use. They must also be familiar with the escape sequence and know the location and method of egress from emergency exits, escape hatches, tunnels or chutes. Unless these drills are known and practised, a man may prejudice not only his own chances of escape but also impede the progress of others who follow him.

Escape falls broadly into three phases: exit from the aircraft, parachute descent, and landing and recovery.

Exit from the aircraft

It is important to enter the airstream cleanly and to avoid striking (or being struck by) the aircraft. This usually implies that the man must propel himself through the door or hatch with as much force as he can muster, and must then assume a compact shape, free from trailing arms and legs. Various techniques have been devised to suit the geometry of different types of exit. For example, to leave by a belly hatch, the escaper usually squats at the rear edge, tucks his knees under his chin, wraps his arms around them and rolls forward into the airstream in a 'cannon-ball' attitude. From narrow side-doors, he will usually crouch slightly, hold both sides of the door, and propel his body outwards and downwards, folding his arms across his chest. To enable escape from large transport aircraft during the initial flight tests, or subsequent to their conversion to some military use, explosive bolts or cord are sometimes used to open hatches. Additional protection from the airstream may then be afforded by deploying a windbreak or even a scoop, to guide the exit from the aircraft. To leave a low-speed light aircraft with a normal canopy, the pilot must first jettison the canopy and lever himself into the airstream, and then dive forwards and downwards as into a swimming pool.

Descent

After successful separation from the aircraft, the man may either fall freely for a while, or open his parachute immediately. At low altitudes, delay is unacceptable, and at heights below 500 feet the interval should be long enough only to allow clearance from the aircraft structure (about 1 second). If the altitude of escape is 200 feet or less, success will be marginal under the best of circumstances, for only about 3 seconds is available for retardation by the parachute. Escape at a height of 100 feet or less is invariably fatal, for the height is lost in less time than that required for full deployment of the parachute.

At medium altitudes (2000–15000 feet) the escaper should wait for some seconds before initiating the opening sequence, both to ensure clearance of the aircraft structure and to allow forward velocity to be lost. The timing of delay can be estimated by counting phrases which take about 1 second to be articulated, and 'one thousand and one, one thousand and two' etc., are hallowed by long usage among parachutists. It is clearly important that the altitude of egress should be known, and death may easily result from blind obedience to the injunction to count slowly to ten and then to pull. It is a useful empirical rule that the first 1000 feet of an unretarded descent takes 10 seconds and that each subsequent 1000 feet occupies 5 seconds.

At altitudes greater than 15000 feet other factors—such as high parachute-opening shock forces, hypoxia and the effects of low temperature—make it important for the deployment of the canopy to be delayed. 'Free fall' is generally advised as the escape technique from these higher altitudes. However, to prevent violent tumbling and spinning of the body it is usual to provide some stabilization by means of a small drogue until the main canopy can safely be brought into operation.

The need for thought and action by aircrew is, in practice, almost invariably avoided by the use of automatic systems. Before leaving the aircraft, the escaper attaches his parachute to a fixed point in the cabin by a static line. When this is pulled during egress, the parachute deployment mechanism is armed. At low altitude, the parachute opens almost immediately (as it should); but if the height at which the escape is initiated requires a time delay, deployment is overridden by a barostatic mechanism. This allows the man to fall freely, or under the control of the stabilizing drogue, until the desired altitude for full deployment of the main parachute is

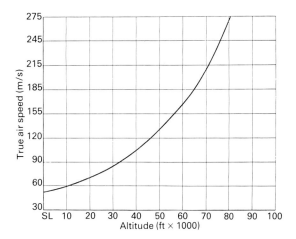

Figure 15.1 The relationship between altitude and true air speed at terminal velocity for a free-falling man.

reached. Sport parachutists will usually descend to 2000 feet before opening their canopy, but military operations may occur over elevated terrain and the barostatic mechanism is accordingly set to operate at 10000–15000 feet. (The same principle is applied to the automatic operation of ejection seats.)

Two opposing forces act upon the body during a free-fall descent. They are (1) that exerted by gravity; and (2) the 'drag' due to air resistance, which tends to oppose the gravitational acceleration.

If the period between egress and deployment of the canopy is sufficiently long, equilibrium between these two forces will be reached. The speed of descent at this time is called the *terminal velocity*. It depends on a number of factors, of which altitude is the major one (*Figure 15.1*). At medium altitude the terminal velocity of a man weighing 90 kg (200 lb) is about 100 knots IAS (approximately 52 m/s). At greater heights, where the air density is lower, the component of drag is smaller and the terminal velocity is correspondingly greater. The posture of the body plays a relatively small but important part in determining the final speed, and expert free-fall parachutists modify the position of their limbs to take advantage of this fact. They are also able to translate vertical speed into horizontal track, and to reach 'opening points' that are considerably displaced laterally from the point at which the aircraft was left. These techniques have no place in escape.

A freely falling man who has reached terminal velocity is, in effect, assailed by a 100 knot wind. He will experience violent flapping of loose clothing and appendages, his limbs may flail, and it may be difficult for him to open or close his unprotected eyes in the face of the gale. Unless by training or by good fortune he has achieved a stable posture, he will be buffeted hither and thither, and runs the risk of being in an unfavourable position when the canopy deploys. If this is the case, the 'opening shock' will be high, and transient violent rotational movements may be applied to the body as it becomes forcibly aligned with the parachute lines.

The extraction of the canopy and its subsequent inflation decelerate the man further, and he eventually reaches a descent speed known as the *reduced terminal velocity*. This also depends on a number of factors, which include the diameter and shape of the parachute, and the characteristics of its fabric. The speed can be calculated from the following simplified formula:

Reduced terminal velocity =

$$\frac{2 \times \text{total weight of man and equipment}}{\begin{array}{c}\text{air density} \times \text{effective area of parachute} \times \\ \text{drag coefficient of parachute}\end{array}}$$

For a man weighing 90 kg descending on a parachute with a diameter of 8.6 m (28 ft), reduced terminal velocity is about 6 m/s. This is approximately equivalent to a jump from a platform 2.5 m high, a fact that is utilized in the training of parachutists.

With a typical parachute deployment time of about 3 seconds, the mean deceleration applied to the body amounts to about 1 G, but the force is not, in fact, applied evenly. It may reach 15–20 G for about 0.3 seconds, although a peak value of 10 G is a more usual figure. Forces of this magnitude lie well within the limits of human tolerance, especially if the body is already aligned with the resultant. Even if it is not, serious injury is improbable, and is likely to be confined to some bruising under the straps of the harness.

Opening shock will be greatly increased if the parachute is operated at a speed greater than the terminal velocity at the altitude of escape. In such circumstances, the body is rapidly decelerated at a rate that varies with the square of the velocity and the density of the surrounding air. Time must, accordingly, be allowed for this deceleration to be completed, lest the very high forces of opening should cause the parachute to fail, or damage the protective equipment and the man. High opening shock will also be experienced if the canopy is deployed at great altitude, even if deceleration to terminal velocity has occurred. It may seem contradictory that such high forces should be experienced in conditions of low air density. The explanation is that the terminal velocity of any freely falling body is at very nearly a constant *indicated* air speed (except at extremely high altitudes). However, the *true* air speed varies inversely as the square root of air density and therefore increases with altitude. For example, at 40 000 feet the atmospheric density is approximately one-quarter that at sea level, and the true air speed at terminal velocity is approximately twice that at 2000 feet; that is, about

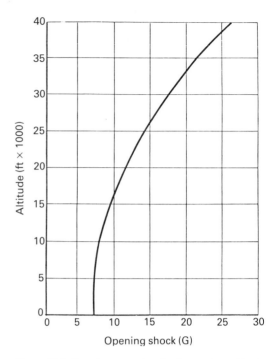

Figure 15.2 Parachute opening shock at various altitudes of deployment. The values shown are typical of those obtained at the terminal velocity of a man using a 8.6 m (28 ft) canopy parachute.

200 knots. The speed of descent on a deployed parachute is also increased at high altitude, but this does not compensate for the higher terminal velocity. At 40 000 feet the descent rate on a fully open parachute is about 30 knots. The change of velocity produced by deployment is thus about 170 knots at 40 000 feet, compared with 85 knots at sea level.

Parachute opening forces at various altitudes are shown in *Figure 15.2*. As with high-speed escape, parachute opening at high altitudes may cause damage to the escape system or injury to the body. The opening characteristics of the canopy depend on the true air speed, and when deployment is carried out at high altitude the canopy will inflate more quickly than at lower heights. The indicated air speed for full development is consequently greater at higher altitudes and the decelerative loads applied to the man and his parachute are correspondingly increased. The size of the canopy also has an effect. Larger canopies are, paradoxically, usually associated with smaller opening shocks, because the time needed for their deployment is greater, and the deceleration is therefore spread over a longer period.

The few aircraft from which unassisted escape is the rule at high speeds and at high altitudes have provision for automatic operation of the parachute at a safe speed and a safe altitude. The probability of damage to the equipment and to the man is, therefore, small although it will be considerably increased if the escaping crew member, through ignorance or fear, operates the manual override that is invariably fitted as a defence against failure of the automatics.

Landing and recovery

About 90% of all non-fatal injuries associated with unassisted escape occur during or immediately following landing. They are largely attributable to unfamiliarity with correct landing techniques, although the inability of the escaper to choose still conditions and flat terrain naturally increases the incidence.

The principles of landing by parachute are simple to state, but sometimes difficult to follow. The final stages of the descent should be as vertical as possible; that is, drift and oscillation should be cancelled. Some control of these unwanted motions can be achieved by pulling down on the appropriate parachute risers, thus distorting the canopy and imparting 'drive' in the required direction to counteract surface wind. Such manoeuvres necessarily increase the rate of descent slightly, but this introduces a much smaller hazard than that of an uncoordinated landing with a high lateral velocity. The hands and arms should be positioned over the head, which should be well tucked into the chest. The feet and legs should be together and the knees slightly bent to cushion the impact of landing. The line of vision should be in the direction of motion to detect obstacles on the ground. The landing shock should be spread over as long a time and as large an area as possible, by allowing the body to collapse in the direction of motion as soon as the feet touch the ground, and rolling from thigh to buttock to shoulder. During the roll, the legs must be kept in apposition. In the light of the limited opportunities for training, and the wide range of conditions (including darkness) under which military aircrew must descend and land, the rate of injury is surprisingly low. Sprained or fractured ankles account for a high proportion of the casualties, and the current overall rate is about 50 per thousand descents.

After landing, the parachute must be collapsed or released as soon as possible to avoid dragging, with the risk of injury from rough terrain. If the descent is made into water, there is a distinct possibility that the man will be dragged by surface winds with his head below water level. To avoid this, parachutists are taught to undo the quick-release fastening of their parachute harness in the last seconds of the descent. They are then supported by the buttock

loop of the harness and by their grasp of the parachute risers. By throwing up their arms and straightening their thighs they can, as their feet touch the water, fall freely from the encumbrance of the parachute and, by inflating their life-preservers, float safely away.

Parachutes and associated equipment

The harness

The design of parachute harness assemblies differs according to the role and performance characteristics of the aircraft and the space available for stowage of the parachute, which may be mounted in the seat or in a separate storage location. In some aircraft the aircrew wear harnesses as part of their personal flying clothing and they attach the parachute pack to the assembly as part of the strapping-in procedure. In others, movement about the cabin forms part of normal flight duties, and the parachute pack is not attached to the harness until

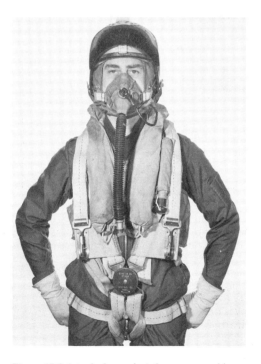

Figure 15.3 A typical parachute harness assembly. Immediately before abandonment, a parachute pack is attached to the hooks mounted on either side of the chest.

the need for egress arises. In yet other systems, the harness forms an integral part of the parachute assembly, which is worn throughout the flight.

Although harnesses vary widely, all consist basically of webbing straps (usually of nylon) arranged to support the man safely and comfortably beneath a deployed canopy. In a typical design, a sling passes under the buttocks and is stabilized by loops around the thighs. Vertical loops pass up the back and over the shoulders to a quick-release fitting mounted on a chest strap. The features of a typical harness are shown in *Figure 15.3*.

The parachute pack

The pack protects the canopy and its accessories and keeps them in the correct position for sequential release when the escape is initiated. The shape of the pack varies with the role, and is different depending on the site of stowage. The requirements for a chest-mounted parachute to be donned at the last moment are obviously not the same as those for a pack that forms the back cushion of a seat, and which is attached to the harness throughout flight. Parachute packing is a skilled procedure, in which a variety of different techniques are employed to suit the conditions of use. In one common method, a 'quarter bag' contains the lower part of the parachute canopy and the suspension lines. The pack contains loops which retain the lines to ensure that they deploy in an orderly manner. The remainder of the canopy is arranged in S-shape folds and contained in the upper part of the pack. The pack is closed by flaps held in place by one or more extractor pins: tie threads are used to reduce the risk of inadvertent opening of the pack. In some assemblies, a small pilot chute is contained in a separate compartment on the main pack.

A 'rip cord' or parachute release line leads from the withdrawal pins of the pack to a handle that is usually mounted on the chest strap of the harness. When the handle is pulled, the pins are released and the pack opens. The pilot chute (if one is fitted) is then ejected into the airstream by a spring. The folded upper part of the canopy is freed, and by its drag it pulls the quarter bag out of the main pack, so releasing the suspension lines. As these tighten, the quarter bag is unlocked, the lower part of the main canopy is freed, and full inflation of the parachute is permitted. The sequence of controlled deployment and inflation provides a smooth and uniform application of force to the body and helps to avoid excessive accelerations. Nevertheless, in adverse circumstances the opening shock of a parachute may be high enough to cause injury.

The canopy

A typical parachute canopy has, when inflated, roughly the appearance of a hemisphere. It is made up of a series of triangular panels (gores) which radiate from an aperture or vent located at the apex. The panels terminate at the circumference, which is known as the periphera or peripheral hem. Nylon suspension lines (shroud lines) run to the periphera from the webbing straps that connect the parachute to the harness assembly. They are continued through the seams connecting the gores, and pass to the opposite confluence point. The webbing providing attachment between the shroud lines and the harness on each side is called the riser.

The material most commonly used for the manufacture of parachute canopies is 45 denier medium-porosity woven nylon, although more recently 'rip-stop' nylon has been used extensively for escape system parachutes. Cotton or polyester fabrics may also be used, although their properties are little different from the more conventional nylon material. Light-duty parachutes used at high altitude or for special purposes may still be made of silk, because silken fabric can be produced at adequate strength and very light weight. The size of the parachute also varies. For paratrooping, the mouth of the inflated canopy may have a diameter of 8.5–9 m, but for emergency escapes, sizes of 5.8–7 m are more usual. The size is dictated in part by the space available for stowage of the parachute pack, and this is often a more important consideration than the marginal increase in descent speed associated with a small canopy.

The properties required of material used for the manufacture of parachutes are as follows:

1. Adequate strength.
2. Adequate porosity. Although the vent provides a funnel for the passage of air, a considerable flow also occurs through the material itself, if the porosity of the fabric is too high, the parachute will open slowly or, under critical conditions, not at all. The sink rate will also be unduly increased. If the canopy is impermeable, the opening shock load will be high, and the parachute will be unstable during descent.
3. Low weight and good flexibility, to avoid excessive bulk and to ease packing.
4. High tear resistance, so that weak points are not produced by stitching or by minor scuffs or abrasions.
5. Good energy absorption. The elasticity of the fabric (and also of the shroud lines) should allow for some of the energy of initial opening and inflation to be absorbed, thus attenuating the forces applied to the body and reducing the risk of damage.
6. Long life. The canopy must retain all the above

properties during all normal handling, storage and operating conditions.

Most parachutes for emergency use are made in the form of a flat disc, although, increasingly, parachutes for assisted escape systems are shaped. Each gore is a plane triangle bounded by straight shroud lines. This type of construction provides efficient distribution of stress, but gives relatively poor stability during descent. The best feature of the flat parachute is its property of rapid opening. However, other designs have been developed, notably for sports parachuting. In some, the gores are shaped, with convex rather than straight sides. The uninflated canopy cannot then be spread onto a flat surface. Shaped gore parachutes are more stable than flat types, and they inflate rather more slowly and smoothly. An extension of the same principle results in guide surface parachutes, which have been developed in an attempt to improve stability further still. They are usually of smaller diameter than the flat canopy, are difficult to construct, and impart a relatively high opening shock.

When the dynamic pressure at which a parachute has to open is increased, the strength of the fabric must also be greater. To avoid excessive bulk and to improve efficiency, the required porosity can be achieved by ribbon construction. In this technique concentric bands of material, separated by gaps, are held together by the nylon cords passing to the apex. The principle is widely used for aircraft braking and for other systems requiring deceleration from high speeds, but it has found little application in escape parachutes. Recently, parachutes incorporating panels of a stretch material of variable porosity have become available for use on emergency escape systems.

One problem with all simple canopies is that they are difficult to steer. Small changes of direction and correction of drift can be accomplished by pulling on one or more risers, thus distorting the shape of the inflated canopy and allowing air to 'spill' from one side. The amount of control that can be achieved by this means is extremely limited, and the requirements of sport parachutists have led to bizarre modifications of the basic hemispherical form. The simplest of these comprises the removal of a part of the whole of one gore, usually at the back of the canopy. The asymmetry of airflow through such a parachute provides forward drive in still air, and can compensate for surface wind. Control is provided by cords attached to the edges of the altered panel, which is normally netted, and the slot may be opened or closed by pulling on the appropriate cord.

In recent years , a family of new devices have been produced. They are known generically as parawings, and consist essentially of sheets of fabric composed of flat or shaped panels. Their relatively small deployed area dictates the use of low porosity fabrics, and if high opening forces are to be avoided maximum deployment speeds must be lower than those acceptable for conventional parachutes.

Assisted escape

The speed and altitude at which military aircraft operate are such that escape can only be achieved by some means of propelling the crew clear of the aircraft structure. Although various forms of closed escape systems (such as capsule or jettisonable cabin) have been developed, the most common method of assisted escape is by an 'open' ejection seat. Over the years ejection seats have undergone many changes and improvements in design and performance, and the reliability of this form of assisted escape has been thoroughly proved by the considerable number of successful ejections from crippled aircraft. Indeed, by the end of 1986, more than 5000 lives had been saved by Martin–Baker ejection seats alone.

This chapter deals only with the principles of a typical escape system and the physiological factors involved.

Requirements for an escape system

An escape system based on the ejection seat should have the following properties.

1. Initial clearance of the ejection path.
2. Sufficient thrust to eject the crew clear of all aircraft structures at all speeds.
3. Adequate trajectory, to allow full deployment of the main parachute before landing, throughout the performance envelope of the aircraft.
4. Fully automatic operation.
5. Adequate restraint for the body, limbs and head.

All these requirements must be met within the tolerance of the human body for the forces developed.

The anatomy of the ejection seat

An ejection seat *(Figure 15.4)* consists of a rigidly constructed framework which provides a sitting platform and the facilities and services for normal aircraft operations. The seat is mounted on one or more rails, attached to the aircraft structure, which provide guidance for the initial part of its trajectory. The seat is also attached to the upper end of a tubular gun, the lower end of which is fixed to the floor of the cabin. In most modern systems the gun is telescopic and contains a number of explosive charges to sustain the thrust as the seat travels up

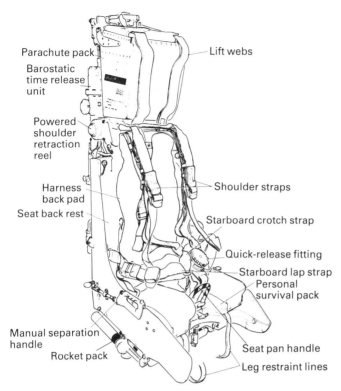

Parachute pack

Barostatic
time release
unit

Powered
shoulder
retraction
reel

Harness
back pad

Seat back rest

Manual separation
handle

Rocket pack

Lift webs

Shoulder straps

Starboard crotch strap

Quick-release fitting

Starboard lap strap
Personal
survival pack

Seat pan handle

Leg restraint lines

Figure 15.4 The main features of a typical ejection seat.

the guide-rail. Other types of ejection seat may also be fitted with a rocket pack, which is ignited at the moment of separation from the gun, and which further increases the final velocity of the seat.

The seat also contains stabilizing and main parachutes, and various secondary explosive and timing devices to ensure the proper sequence of automatic operations. A seat pack (which usually contains survival equipment) and a harness restraint complete the basic anatomy of the seat.

Sequence of operations

The initial sequence varies with aircraft type depending on whether escape path clearance is achieved by canopy jettison, canopy penetration or canopy fragmentation. On most modern ejection seats escape is initiated by pulling a seat firing handle. This fires a cartridge and gas from this is then piped around the seat to initiate:

1. Powered shoulder retraction.
2. Canopy jettison or fragmentation (as appropriate).
3. The ejection gun time delay unit (to allow for canopy jettison), or the ejection gun primary cartridge (for canopy fragmentation or penetration systems).

Canopy jettison is achieved by releasing the canopy locks, freeing the hinge mechanism, and then firing explosive jacks or canopy jettison rocket motors to clear the canopy from the ejection path with sufficient energy to cater for all escape eventualities.

Where canopy fragmentation systems are fitted the initial movement of the ejection seat is used to trigger the detonator that initiates the explosive cord (*see* below).

As the ejection gun extends, the faces of secondary cartridges are exposed. Each cartridge detonates as it is exposed, generating gas which increases the acceleration of the seat. At the moment of ejection gun separation the seat has achieved a velocity of 24–27 m/s for non-rocket assisted seats and approximately 19.5 m/s for rocket-assisted seats. Rocket ignition is timed to start immediately prior to gun separation so that the seat continues to accelerate smoothly away from the aircraft.

At the moment of separation, the seat is travelling forward at the speed of the aircraft, and if the speed is greater than 250 knots it must be slowed down before the parachute can be deployed safely. It must also be stabilized, because it is a free-flying mass with poor aerodynamic properties, exposed to windblast and asymmetric forces. A drogue system is required to give an element of stabilization and deceleration down to a safe parachute deployment

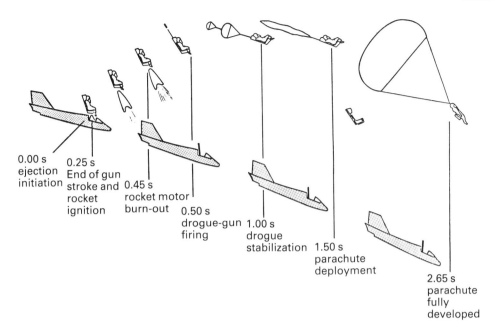

0.00 s
ejection
initiation

0.25 s
End of gun
stroke and
rocket
ignition

0.45 s
rocket motor
burn-out

0.50 s
drogue-gun
firing

1.00 s
drogue
stabilization

1.50 s
parachute
deployment

2.65 s
parachute
fully
developed

Figure 15.5 The sequence of events in a typical high-speed, low-level ejection from an aircraft.

speed. The drogue is extracted from the ejection seat by a drogue gun bullet which is fired by a time delayed drogue gun, the time delay being present to allow clearance of aircraft structure and, for all except the most modern seats, rocket motor burn-out. After a further time delay the locks that secure the occupant's parachute harness to the ejection seat are undone and the pull of the drogue is transferred from the ejection seat to the parachute withdrawal line, producing parachute extraction. The stages of a typical ejection sequence are illustrated in *Figure 15.5*. On the most up-to-date seats sequencing is arranged slightly differently. At low speed and low altitude drogue firing is dispensed with completely and the parachute extracted directly by a rocket extractor (*Figure 15.6*). At higher speeds and higher altitudes a variant of the conventional system is still employed (*Figure 15.7*).

Clearance of the ejection path

Mention has already been made that the ejection path can be cleared by canopy jettison, by canopy fragmentation or by simply ejecting through the

canopy. The method employed depends upon the canopy material, its thickness and its geometry in relation to the man underneath.

Canopy materials

Cast and stretched acrylic are the most common materials used in the construction of cockpit transparencies. On a similar thickness basis, stretched acrylic is the stronger material, and has very different fracture characteristics to cast acrylic. Cast acrylic canopies vary in thickness between 6 and 10 mm. Stretched acrylic canopies can be up to 12 mm thick. The division between the two types is not absolute and depends upon how much the cast material is pulled to get it into shape. Thus considerable caution has to be exercised in comparing the results of ejection through one type of cast acrylic canopy with another, as one canopy may be intermediate between cast and stretched, and hence stronger than expected.

Other materials employed in canopies are polycarbonate, which although immensely strong is relatively soft and deformable and hence must be

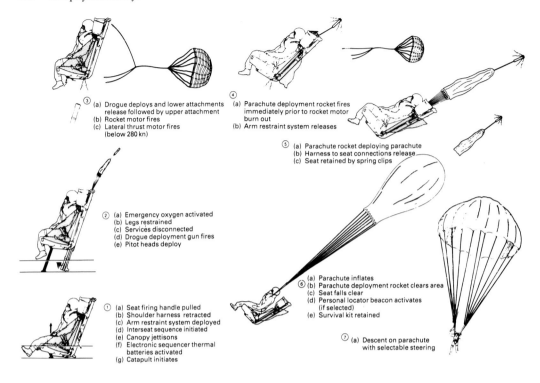

Figure 15.6 Modern ejection seat – low-speed sequence.

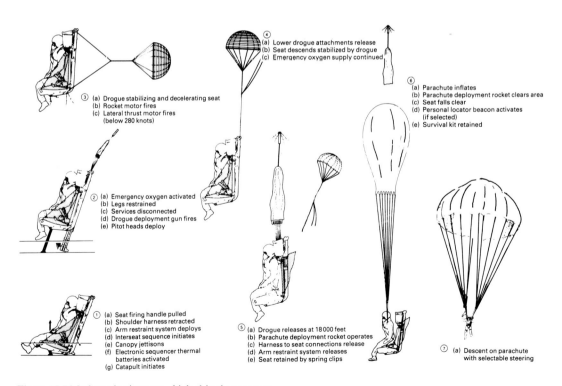

Figure 15.7 Modern ejection seat – high altitude sequence.

jettisoned to permit safe escape; and laminate materials, to which similar considerations as for polycarbonate apply.

Canopy jettison

Canopy jettison is the best way of achieving complete clearance of the ejection path. The jettison mechanism is linked into ejection firing which is inhibited by either an interdictor system or by a fixed time delay to allow time for the canopy to clear the ejection seat path. The jettison process is accomplished by undoing the canopy locks and hinge mechanism and then firing explosive jacks or jettison rocket motors. Typically 0.3 seconds is allowed for clearance of the canopy although with advanced systems this may be accomplished in as little as 0.1 seconds.

Canopy fragmentation

Canopy fragmentation only works satisfactorily on relatively thin (up to 9 mm) cast acrylic canopies. The fragmentation is accomplished by applying a type of explosive cord called Miniature Detonating Cord (MDC) to the inner face of the transparency. The cord consists of an explosive core surrounded by a lead sheath, on the outside of which, on the non-canopy face, are applied a series of backing layers. The rate of propagation of the explosion is extremely high and has the effect of ejecting a shard of material from immediately above the cord and sending shock waves through the transparency that initiate secondary cracking. Complete fragmentation is the design aim as it avoids the possibility of the ejectee colliding with large canopy fragments which may injure him.

Explosive disruption of stretched acrylic is a different matter. This material is much more resistant to the induction of secondary cracking and has the unfortunate characteristic of breaking into relatively large knife-edged pieces. For this reason, the techniques employed have been either:

1. To weaken the canopy by the firing of a single overhead explosive cord.
2. To cut the canopy into two pieces, so-called 'clam-shelling', allowing the ejection seat and occupant to emerge between the halves.

Whether the latter technique is a reliable way of clearing the escape path, particularly from aircraft that have departed from controlled flight, remains to be seen.

On thicker stretched acrylic canopies (9–12 mm) it is necessary to use a chevron-shaped cutting cord to cut and separate the canopy. The effect of shaping is to concentrate the energy of the explosion. These cords have a greater problem of 'back spatter' than MDC. To counter this, silicon elastomeric backings, sometimes incorporating glass microspheres, are applied over the cord to absorb the force of the explosion and contain the 'spatter'.

Through-canopy ejection

Through-canopy ejection is sometimes used as an alternative method in the event of failure of either canopy jettison or canopy fragmentation. Except for the very thinnest of canopies, it is an undesirable way of clearing the escape path as it carries a risk of producing neck injury if the flexed head breaks out the area of canopy above it. There is also an enhanced risk of compression injury of the spine because of the transitory uncoupling of man and seat that is produced as the seat is slowed by breaking through the canopy material.

Initiation of ejection

In early British ejection seats, the pilot had to pull a firing handle mounted in the headbox of the seat. The handle was attached to a shaped blind which was drawn down over the face to give some measure of protection to the head against the effects of windblast. Other advantages of this system were that the head had to be located against the rest and that the act of reaching up for the blind straightened the spine and thus improved the posture for ejection. For tall pilots wearing protective helmets, the firing handle was awkward to reach; and in the presence of positive accelerations difficulty was sometimes experienced in reaching the blind. A secondary firing handle was, therefore, mounted in the seat-pan between the knees of the occupant. Practical experience showed that ejection could be initiated more quickly when the seat-pan firing handle was used, and the advantages of the older method were found to be not as great as had been thought. As a result, use of the so-called secondary handle was recommended as a primary procedure, particularly in situations where time was critical. In later Marks of British seat the face-blind has been omitted and the seat-pan firing handle is the only control. In two-place aircraft, the need for the pilot to tell the navigator to eject introduces a delay that may prove fatal under critical conditions. In some systems, therefore, 'command' ejection has been introduced. When the pilot operates the firing handle, the first action is to tension the harness of the other crew member, drawing him back into his seat. When the canopy has been jettisoned, the navigator's seat is fired automatically, followed by that of the pilot. The rear crew retains the ability to eject independently, without activating the pilot's system. Command ejection has the additional advantage that simultaneous firing of the seats, with a possible risk of subsequent collision, is impossible.

Seat stabilization

The behaviour of the seat after it leaves the guide-rails depends on the indicated air speed at the moment of ejection. At speeds up to about 250 knots IAS, the forward movement of the seat exceeds the backward force exerted by windblast, and the seat tends to tip forward. At ejection speeds greater than about 450 knots IAS, the windblast more than counterbalances the forward thrust, and the seat tips backwards. In the intermediate speed range, the seat will tend to remain more or less upright; but the presence of asymmetric forces may produce rotation and tumbling.

Ideally, the seat should be in a favourable and stable position before the main parachute canopy is deployed. This is not easy to achieve and much

depends on what the ejection seat is doing at the moment of drogue deployment. When the drogue is attached to the seat by a single strop (as is the case in the majority of ejection seats) it is possible for the drogue to deploy anywhere in the upper hemisphere around the ejection seat. If the ejection has taken place below barostat height there is generally insufficient time for full stabilization to occur, and residual seat instability may produce a markedly off-axis parachute deployment. Systems now under development effectively triangulate the seat on a three-strop bridled drogue which is deployed immediately aft of the seat. This has the effect of making the seat fly 'face into wind' in a consistent and reproducible manner.

The forces of ejection

The primary acceleration

The firing of the ejection gun applies accelerations that are primarily in the upward ($+G_z$) direction. Unless a rocket pack is fitted, the duration of the

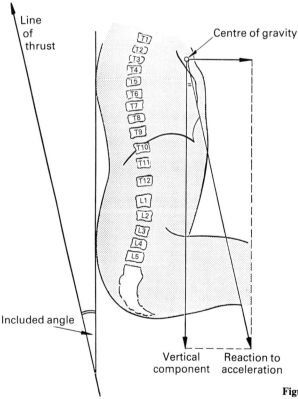

Figure 15.8 The line of thrust of an ejection seat in relation to the long axis of the spine. The centre of gravity is that of the upper torso (above T12).

thrust is limited to the time for which the seat is attached to the gun (usually 0.12–0.15 seconds). The objective must be to attain the greatest possible velocity during this time, and this indicates that large accelerations shall be applied very suddenly. (It will be remembered that velocity is the product of acceleration and time.) The limit of human tolerance for transient forces of this type is set by the structural strength of the body, and particularly of the spine. It has been established by experiment and by practice that the incidence of spinal injury rises markedly if the peak acceleration exceeds 25 G, and if the rate of onset is greater than 300 G/s. These criteria are widely adopted in the design of ejection seats. However, as Chapter 14 shows, the force applied to the body may be considerably amplified by the elasticity and under-damping of the suspension.

The forces of 'overshoot' cannot be entirely avoided but can be greatly reduced by careful attention to the design of seat packs and cushions. Ideally, the man should be rigidly attached to the seat, so that the two move as a single unit. Unfavourable early experience with soft packs led to the development of rigid containers with the upper surface moulded for comfort. A thin cushion of plastic foam may be added, but it is essential that the material is well damped, and that it is almost completely compressed under normal sitting loads. A properly fitted and properly adjusted restraint harness also increases the 'coupling' between the man and the seat: and to ensure that contact is maintained in adverse flight attitudes, harnesses should incorporate a 'negative-G' strap that pulls the man positively downwards.

Although the major component of the ejection acceleration is in the long axis of the spine, significant flexion forces are also involved. As *Figure 15.8* shows, these arise because the line of seat thrust does not coincide with the long axis of the spine. For engineering reasons, the guide-rails are tilted backwards, but to retain full vision and reach the man must be more vertical. The two axes intersect at the seat-pan, but the divergence or included angle between them may then range from about 11 degrees to about 18 degrees, the gap being filled with parachute containers and other equipment. With an included angle of 18 degrees and an applied force of 25 G, the forward component of acceleration is about 8 G. Adequate shoulder restraint is essential, but even so, forward rotation of the head is inevitable.

In rocket-assisted seats, the duration of upward thrust is extended by the time for which the rockets burn; typically, this may be 0.2–0.5 seconds. The final velocity (and hence the altitude gain) of the seat is correspondingly much greater, but it is also possible and advisable to exchange some of this increased speed for a decrease in the initial thrust of

the gun. The rate of application of the force can be reduced to below 250 G/s and the peak value may be reduced to 15 G or less, with an associated reduction in the risk of spinal injury.

Forces of wind-drag and windblast

The seat enters the airstream as a blunt body travelling forward with the speed of the aircraft. It is rapidly decelerated, and the magnitude of the force depends on airspeed, the mass of the system, and the cross-sectional area exposed to drag. If the seat remains stable and facing forwards, the deceleration is wholly in the G_x direction, and the man is well supported by the seat structure. If the seat rotates about its vertical axis, the body is restrained by the harness. For the moderate speeds at which most ejections occur, the decelerative forces of wind-drag and windblast are well within the limits of human tolerance, which are set at about 50 G with a rate of onset of 500 G/s and a maximum duration of 0.2 seconds.

Windblast exerts ram pressure or 'q'-forces on the body. The extent of the pressure varies with the density of the air, and is therefore reduced at higher altitudes. The direct effect of windblast results from the sudden application of force to the chest and abdomen. The situation is akin to that seen in falls into water, and the consequences are also similar. In mild cases, the sufferer may be temporarily 'winded': but if the force is greater, a pulse of high pressure generated in the central blood vessels may be transmitted to the periphery and cause subconjunctival haemorrhages. The threshold of injury for 'q'-forces probably lies at about 31 kPa (4.5 lb/in^2), and serious damage is probable at about 55–62 kPa (8–9 lb/in^2). Theoretically, high 'q'-forces could lead to the rupture of internal organs, and to death.

In the majority of ejections, the more serious effect of windblast is on the limbs and head. At speeds in excess of about 300 knots IAS, unrestrained legs will flail, and may be forced laterally over the side of the seat-pan. Several cases of fracture and of dislocation of the hip were recorded before leg restraint was introduced as a routine. The hands will normally be retained on the firing handle, but at high speeds the force of windblast may tear them free, and allow the arms to fly outwards, upwards and backwards. Positive restraint, particularly at the level of the elbows, is required for ejection speeds in excess of about 500 knots. Unless the head is positively located or actively restrained, it, too, may flail. No satisfactory system of head restraint has yet been devised, and it is fortunate that the majority of ejections take place at speeds that are insufficient to result in serious flail injury to the head.

Forces of drogue and parachute deployment

The drogue parachute is designed to align and stabilize the seat. Despite its small size, at high speed the deceleration forces that it applies can be both severe and applied in an adverse direction. The angular accelerations generated by enforced rotation of the seat to a new attitude may also be very high and despite their brief duration they are acceptable only if the man is firmly supported by the seat.

The factors affecting the 'opening shock' of the main canopy have been discussed earlier in this chapter, which also deals with the forces of landing.

Back injury during ejection

Mechanism and incidence

Individual vertebrae and short segments of the spinal column are able to withstand very large compressive loads applied at right-angles to the plane of the intervertebral discs, but their resistance to forces in other directions is much lower. There is also evidence that damage is more readily produced by dynamic loading than by static compression. In an ejection, the initial thrust is an impulsive load which, even in favourable circumstances, is experienced at an angle of 13 degrees to the long axis of the spine. The natural shape of the column adds another complication. It exaggerates the axial displacement of the applied force in the regions of greater curvature. It is not surprising, therefore, that spinal injury should be a hazard of ejection, despite the attempts to limit the magnitude and rate of onset of the primary acceleration.

The region at greatest risk lies between T10 and L2 and is centred on T12, where the vertebral end-plate has the highest loading per unit area. This part of the spine is subjected to the static load of the trunk and head transmitted through the vertebrae above it and, in the normal sitting posture, it has an unfavourable curvature. Spinal injuries from ejection do occur at other sites. They can often be attributed to forward flexion resulting from a poor posture. Failures are of two types; one consisting of a chip fracture of the upper anterior lip of the vertebra, and the other involving compression collapse of the vertebral body. Two or more vertebrae may be affected; they are usually contiguous, but the fractures are sometimes separated by normal segments. Complete collapse of the

vertebrae with resulting involvement of the spinal cord is, mercifully, almost unknown.

The reported incidence of back injury varies widely, but the use of different criteria makes it impossible to compare data from different sources. However, it is generally accepted that radiographic evidence of fracture can be found in 30–70% of aircrew after ejection, depending upon ejection seat type (*see* Chapter 52).

Although a spinal fracture is usually classed as a major injury, a very high proportion of the cases resulting from ejection make a full recovery and can be returned to full flying duties within weeks. Once healing has taken place the damaged vertebrae need not be regarded as weak points in the spinal column, and there is some evidence that, because of their increased bone density, they are actually stronger. There have been several cases of aircrew who have ejected on more than one occasion, and one has made four successful escapes from crippled aircraft.

Spinal injury is caused primarily by the force of ejection, but the characteristics of the initial acceleration are deliberately restricted to be within the limits of human tolerance. The apparent paradox stems from the definition of tolerance. The design specification of the escape system ensures that the risk of injury to a fully restrained man sitting in an ideal posture will be acceptably small. The amplification of the applied force that can be produced by springy or compressible cushions and by the lack of firm contact between the man and the seat has already been mentioned, but a good posture requires that the spine shall be aligned as closely as possible with the vertical. The flexion permitted by a loose restraint harness tilts the vertebrae, and the ejection force is then applied in an unfavourable direction. For this reason, aircrew are advised to sit well back in the seat, to tighten the harness and to straighten the spine before initiating ejection.

Prediction of the risk of spinal injury

The figures quoted above for the maximum permissible acceleration and the rate of application are derived from experiment and practice, but they embrace two assumptions. These are that the seat and the man form a single rigid unit, so that forces applied to one are experienced by the other without modification, and that the escape system provides an acceleration which rises linearly to a sustained peak value. Neither of these conditions is met by any practical ejection seat, and the translation of data recorded from dummies in test ejections into terms of human hazard is very difficult. One approach that has been used involves the calculation of a Dynamic Response Index, or DRI.

In this technique, a simple computer is used to apply the acceleration waveform, as recorded from the ejection seat, to a model of the man similar to that shown in *Figure 14.1*. Although this procedure makes allowances for spikes and other irregularities in the input waveform it does not, by itself, permit the risk of injury to be predicted. However, the analysis by the same technique of ejection systems known to have caused spinal fracture gives data from which the probability of damage can be estimated. For example, with a DRI of 18 the expected frequency of injury is less than 5%; a DRI of 23 increases this probability to more than 50%.

The DRI has many limitations. It assumes that the man is firmly attached to the seat, and that his body is a simple mass–springer–damper system of known characteristics. In its predictive role it also assumes that the relationship between injury rates and calculated values of the DRI is known and is linear. In practice, the United Kingdom experience has been that the DRI is not an accurate predictor of spinal injury rates. This is a reflection of the many factors in the aetiology of spinal injury on ejection. Nevertheless the DRI is a valuable technique.

Escape under extreme conditions

The requirement that the ejection seat shall operate successfully throughout the flight envelope introduces special problems; these are especially severe at high altitude or high speed. Moreover, the advent of VSTOL aircraft, from which escape may be necessary during rapid descent at very low altitude and with no forward speed, placed new demands on the performance of the escape system. Some of these problems and solutions to them must now be considered.

High-altitude escape

The low air density at high altitude reduces the drag of the seat, which therefore decelerates more slowly on entering the wind-stream. Similarly the 'q'-forces imposed by windblast are lower, for a given aircraft speed, than at lesser heights, and the hazard of limb flailing is correspondingly smaller. These benefits are offset by the greater instability of the seat, and spinning and tumbling may arise in all axes. Rates of rotation up to 250 rpm have been recorded in test ejections and depending on the site of the centre of rotation, the occupant of the seat may be exposed to high degrees of positive $(+G_z)$ and negative $(-G_z)$ acceleration. The stability of the system can be improved by the deployment of drogues, as in the case of lower altitudes, but the reduced 'bite' of the rarefied atmosphere makes them less effective. The forces imposed by the deployment are also greater at high altitude, but they remain well within the

limits of tolerance. The same is not true of the main canopy, and at heights in excess of about 20 000 feet the opening shock of the personal parachute may exceed the structural strength of the fabric, of the body, or of both. It is, therefore, essential to delay the separation of the man from the seat until a 'safe' altitude has been reached. For this purpose, a barometrically operated lock is inserted between the drogues and the timing mechanism by which they are normally released. The seat and the man then fall together to the pre-set height, when the barostat releases its hold and the ejection sequence is resumed. The barostat must, of course, allow separation and canopy deployment to occur well above the ground, and to cater for the range of terrain heights that may be encountered. British seats use a barometric setting of 10 000 feet. In some other countries the preferred value is 5000 m; at that height the opening shock is high without being excessive.

The delay in separation from the seat has purposes other than the reduction of parachute opening shock. After a high-altitude ejection, the man must be protected against the environment, and notably against hypoxia and cold. The emergency oxygen system is frequently mounted on the seat, and premature release of the man would involve immediate interruption of the supply followed by a slow-descent to an altitude acceptable for breathing air. Protection from cold is, or should be, given by the aviation clothing, but the risk of frostbite to exposed areas such as the face cannot be ignored. The combination of the drogues and the barometric device ensures that the period of exposure to these hazards will be as brief as possible, consistent with the need to avoid unstabilized free fall.

High-speed escape

At high altitudes, the hazard of ejection at high speeds is mitigated by the reduced air density and by the availability of time; the former means that the effect of windblast will be less serious, and the latter that deceleration and the operations of the seat automatics can proceed at leisure without undue concern for the loss of height.

High-speed ejection close to the ground, however, involves all the factors that can jeopardize success. The initial thrust must be large to ensure that the seat will clear the rapidly approaching fin; the forces of drag and windblast will be high; time delays within the system must be short to minimize loss of height before canopy deployment and inflation. A compromise must be set between the reduction of delays and premature separation of the man from the seat, for if the latter occurs before sufficient speed has been lost, serious injury is likely to be caused by 'crash' deceleration, and damage to the parachute and personal equipment is highly probable. These dangers are great enough to merit the use of an interdictor that monitors the 'q'-force or the deceleration and halts the automatic ejection sequence until the applied force has fallen below a pre-set value.

The overall situation can also be eased to some extent by the use of rockets to sustain the initial impulse. The additional power gives a higher trajectory and hence more time, both for the slowing of the seat to a safer speed and for the operation of the sub-systems.

Escape from VTOL aircraft

In most phases of flight, aircraft with the capability for vertical take-off and landing can be classified as conventional, though high-performance, machines and the requirements for escape are the same. The one exception is that a number of emergencies leading to ejection occur during the hover and vertical descent. The absence of forward speed presents a minor problem because, in still air, the absence of forward speed for the drogues and main canopy to deploy and inflate less rapidly than usual. However, the need to cater for low-altitude escape dictates that the inherent time delays of the system shall be short, and the sequence may be completed to the stage of release of the man from the seat by the time that the peak of the trajectory has been reached. The deployment of the drogues and the extraction of the personal parachute will thus be assisted by the vertical, rather than the forward, velocity of the seat.

Loss of power at or near the hover leads to a critical situation, because the decisions to eject must then be made when the aircraft is very close to the ground and is sinking rapidly. The rate of descent opposes the thrust imparted by the ejection gun, so that the maximum upward velocity achieved by a standard seat from an aircraft descending at 11 m/s (35 ft/s) will only be about 15 m/s (50 ft/s). In these circumstances the apogee will be insufficient to ensure full deployment of the parachute at a safe height. The only solution is to supplement the ejection gun with a rocket motor – an addition that is of advantage in all escapes, but essential in VTOL aircraft. Even so, it will sometimes be difficult to decide whether to eject or to remain with the aircraft for what may be no more than a heavy landing. It is important, however, to remember that in most combat aircraft head-up displays intrude into the arc through which the head will move in decelerations with a $-G_x$ component. It is, therefore, preferable to eject from such aircraft rather than 'ride it down' through various ground obstructions.

Escape from helicopters

Although considerable research and development effort has been given to ejection seats for 'conventional' military aircraft, there has been no parallel evolution of escape systems for helicopters. This is surprising not only because rotary-winged aircraft have found increasing use both in combat and in civil operations, but because the fatality rate for helicopter aircrew is greater than for their fixed-wing counterparts. Autorotation is the only available method of descent after an in-flight emergency, but its use is limited to the single case of power failure and it cannot be employed during the more common loss of control.

Escape systems based on a standard upward ejection seat are, of course, difficult to integrate into helicopters due to the presence of the main rotor. Proposals have been made for the jettison of the entire rotor or for the explosive disintegration of its blades as the first stage of the escape sequence; it has also been suggested that the rotor could be stopped or folded to allow a clear ejection path. The engineering complexity of these possible solutions is, however, much greater than the interest of air forces in escape from helicopters.

Downward ejection is feasible, but is even less suitable for rotary-winged aircraft than for fixed-wing types. The minimum safe altitude for this method of escape is estimated to be 500 feet under ideal conditions, and about 95% of emergencies in helicopters occur below this height. (More than 50% of them arise at heights of 50 feet or less.)

Sideways ejection offers more promise, but it introduces new requirements for lateral restraint of the crew member and for the stability of the seat when it has left the aircraft. The strength and harness configuration of most helicopter seats are generally poor and considerable improvement is possible and desirable, if only to improve the survival rate in crashes. The angle at which a sideways ejection seat leaves the aircraft is critical, because the clearance between the top of the seat and rotor disc is small; any upward component of force or aerodynamic lift introduces the risk of collision, while a downward trajectory entails a loss of valuable height. For these reasons, a two-stage system has been proposed, in which the lateral thrust that propels the seat clear of the rotors is followed by an upward force to gain altitude. Thus the flight path of the seat is L shaped and safe escape can, in theory, be provided even if the emergency involves a high sink rate.

The mechanical complexity of any system for escape from helicopters is offset to some extent by the relatively modest flight envelope that must be covered. Although the large proportion of emergencies arising near the ground dictates that the system shall gain a considerable amount of height, no provision needs to be made for high-speed operations; indeed, a recent analysis of helicopter emergencies revealed no incidents at speeds greater than 100 knots IAS. The ejection thrust need only be modest; limb and head restraint are unnecessary, and barostats and complex timing devices are not required. A comparatively simple and lightweight escape system could undoubtedly be developed for rotary-winged aircraft, but the effort currently devoted to the problem is small. More attention has been directed to 'crashworthiness' as detailed accident investigation and engineering analyses have shown that the cost benefit of the 'crashworthiness' approach is markedly superior to that of the escape system (*see* chapter 32).

Further reading

GLAISTER, D.H. (1965) The effects of acceleration of short duration. In *A Textbook of Aviation Physiology*, edited by J.A. Gillies. Oxford: Pergamon Press

GLAISTER, D.H. (ED.) (1975) *Biodynamic Response to Windblast.* Conference Proceedings CP 170. Neuilly sur Seine: AGARD/NATO

JONES, M. and JONES, G.M. (1965) Aerodynamic forces and their effects upon man. In *A Textbook of Aviation Physiology*, edited by J.A. Gillies. Oxford: Pergamon Press

Part III

Thermal Stress and Survival

16

The thermal environment and human heat exchange

J.R. Allan

The origins of thermal stress in aviation

Thermal stress arises from an imbalance between a pilot's metabolic heat production and the net result of his heat exchange with the environment. A number of factors influence the latter and these may be divided into three main groups—thermal environmental factors, aircraft factors and aircrew factors.

Thermal environment

All of the four main thermal environmental parameters—air temperature, humidity, radiant heat and air movement—have important effects on man's heat exchange. Aircraft operate over the whole range of naturally occurring climates, from extreme arctic cold to tropical heat, and for much of the time aircrew and groundcrew are exposed directly to the local climatic conditions. The natural environment is particularly important during survival after a crash, ditching or ejection. In flight, the effect of climate is mainly indirect through its influence on the aircraft structure and on cabin conditioning systems with consequent alteration to the cockpit thermal environment.

Cold stress problems in flight are rare these days because of the liberal supplies of hot air available from the engines, but older jet aircraft, flying at high altitude with low engine power settings, can present cockpit temperatures below freezing point. Cold stress problems in flight can arise also when cockpit temperatures are low because passengers are wearing full arctic clothing; for example, troops in helicopters or paratroopers in transport aircraft operated with doors off in winter or at altitude. Cold stress may also be caused by emergency loss of cockpit canopies.

Aircraft factors

Kinetic heating

During flight, the aircraft structure is heated by friction between its surface and the air, and by the rise of temperature caused by air compression in front. The temperature of the skin is a function of ambient air temperature and aircraft speed. During high-speed, low-level flight it may reach 120°C or so.

The structure radiates heat to the pilot and warms the cockpit air during its transit through distributive ductwork and from cabin air outlets to his immediate environment. The effects of kinetic heating may be reduced by insulation of the cockpit walls and the cabin air ductwork.

Radiant heating

Solar radiation through the canopy contributes greatly to thermal stress in aircraft. Owing to differing transmission characteristics for radiation of differing wavelengths the thermal energy can become trapped within the cockpit. This phenomenon is known as the greenhouse effect and is described in detail below.

The requirement for all-round visibility in modern military aircraft offers little hope for major reduction in transmitted solar heat load. However, filter layers—such as a gold film—can assist appreciably.

Electrical heat

With each new generation of high performance aircraft the electrical heat load in the cockpit

Table 16.1 Sources of heat in the cockpit of a Tornado aircraft flying at Mach 0.9 at sea level and 40°C

Source	Heat (kW)
Pilot's heat production	0.06
Aerodynamic heat load	9.0
Electrical heat load (avionics)	1.2
Solar radiation load	2.5
Total	12.76

increases as more and more avionic equipment is fitted. This contributes to the heat stress problem both directly, by heating the cockpit structure and air supply, and indirectly by the cooling load it places on the environmental control system. An example of the total heat input to the cockpit from these sources is given in *Table 16.1*.

Aircrew factors

Physiological responses

Man's own internal heat production from metabolic processes varies from about 60 W at rest to two or three times that figure during vigorous flying activity at low level and high speed. To maintain deep body temperature he must dissipate this heat together with his total heat gain from the environment. Under cold conditions his metabolic heat production must balance his heat loss to the environment.

In response to factors tending to increase temperature, the body reacts first by vasodilatation in the skin and then by active sweating. Similarly, cooling is resisted by vasoconstriction and shivering. These physiological responses are described in greater detail in Chapter 17.

Flying clothing

Flying clothing assemblies contribute to heat stress by interfering with the normal pathways for heat exchange with the environment, partly as a result of the high insulation value of many clothing assemblies, which interferes with convective heat exchange, and partly because of differing water vapour permeability, with several items (for example, anti-G suits and pressure clothing) impermeable to water vapour and thus interfering with sweat evaporation.

Cold stress problems can arise because the extent of clothing insulation required may not be compatible with adequate movement and dexterity, especially of the hands and feet.

The effects of clothing on heat exchange are considered in detail below.

The components of the thermal environment and their measurement

Air temperature

A measurement of air temperature, sometimes referred to as shade temperature or dry bulb temperature, is the obvious starting point for thermal environment assessments. It is important that techniques for measuring air temperature exclude the possible effects of radiant heating or cooling on the sensor. A common example of error from this source is when a mercury thermometer is used for measuring air temperature while exposed to full sunshine. In this situation the readings may be erroneously high due to direct radiant heating of the thermometer.

Traditionally, air temperatures are measured with mercury-in-glass thermometers shielded from radiation by being enclosed in some form of screen. It is also common to measure air temperature in conjunction with wet bulb temperature using an instrument known as a psychrometer (*see* below). Because mercury freezes at about $-50°C$, where extremely low temperatures are anticipated it is advisable to use an alcohol thermometer. A disadvantage of mercury or alcohol thermometers, apart from their fragility, is that they do not lend themselves to automatic measurement or recording. It has therefore become commonplace to use various electrical temperature sensors such as thermocouples or thermistors. The latter are now widely available and are the most generally useful devices for use in aircraft cockpits. They consist of small beads of semiconductor material, the electrical resistance of which varies predictably with temperature. In conjunction with appropriate electronic circuitry they can be used to measure temperature over a very wide range and with accuracies up to 0.05°C or 1% of the range (*Figures 16.1* and *16.2*). Readings can be taken either directly from a suitable meter or stored in a solid state data logger mounted in the cockpit or in a pocket of the flying clothing (*Figure 16.3*).

A modern development of thermocouple technology is the heat flux transducer which enables direct measurement of heat flow from the skin or clothing. The transducer consists of a number of thermocouple junctions arranged close to each face of a disc of waterproof material. Typical dimensions would be radius 14 mm and thickness 3 mm. The discs are calibrated so that the voltage output can be read as heat flow.

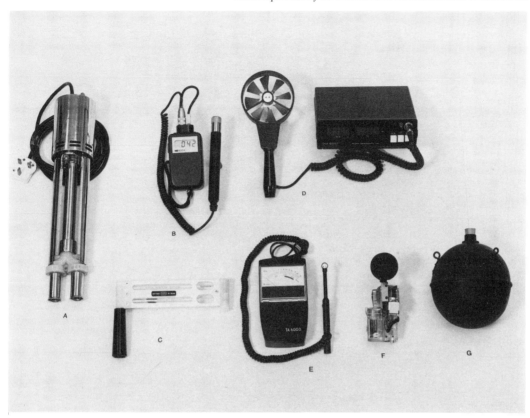

Figure 16.1 Environmental measuring instruments. A = Assmann psychrometer; B = Solid state humidity sensor; C = Whirling psychrometer; D = Vane anemometer; E = Hot wire anemometer; F = Combined 50 mm globe thermometer and psychrometer; G = 150 mm black globe thermometer.

Radiant heat

Radiant heat is given out by all bodies at all temperatures. Radiant exchange between two bodies varies as the difference in the fourth power of the absolute temperatures of their surfaces and is influenced by the geometry of the surfaces and by a characteristic known as emissivity. Matt black surfaces emit and absorb radiant heat in greater quantities than white surfaces.

The wavelength of radiant heat emissions depends upon the temperature of the radiant heat source. When the source temperatures are not particularly high, the radiant heating is in the infra-red range. In contrast, solar radiation comes from a source at very high temperatures and includes a considerable short-wave element in the visible band of the spectrum. In a number of practical situations the distinction can be of some importance. For example, in work areas surrounded by glass or other transparencies, such as aircraft cockpits, greenhouses or vehicles, the short-wave component of sunlight passes freely through the glass or transparency and warms up those structures on which it

falls. The heated structures then re-radiate but the radiation is now in the infra-red region of the spectrum and is not readily transmitted by glass or other transparencies. Thus the heat becomes 'trapped' within the enclosure—a phenomenon that is known as the 'greenhouse effect'.

The mean radiant temperature of the surroundings can be calculated with reasonable accuracy from measured surface temperatures and corresponding angle factors between the source and the individual exposed. This is a complicated procedure and is described in detail by Fanger (1972). It is not suitable for application to aircraft cockpits. A much simpler technique is to measure the globe temperature, T_g, using a black globe thermometer. In its original form this consists of a hollow copper sphere, 150 mm in diameter and painted matt black. The sphere has a thermometer, either mercury-in-glass or a thermistor, placed at its centre. Because of the inconvenience of the traditional globe thermometer, especially in a small cockpit, there has been a tendency in recent times to use smaller globe thermometers with a diameter of 50 mm. Mean radiant temperature may be calculated from globe

222

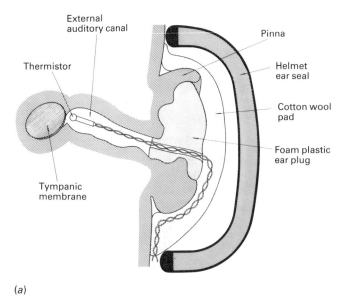

(a)

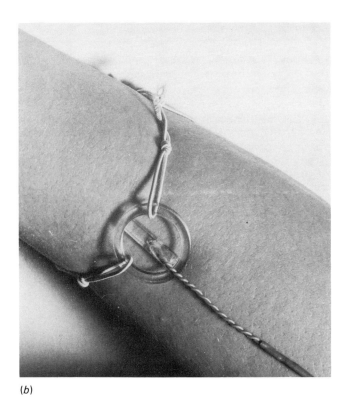

(b)

Figure 16.2 The practical application of thermistors for measuring (a) deep body temperature in the external auditory canal, (b) forearm skin temperature.

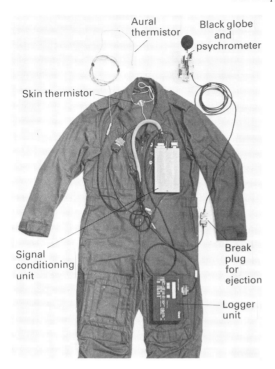

temperature, air temperature and air movement using the following equation:

$$\bar{T}_r = T_g + k.V^{0.5}.(T_g - T_a)$$

where $\bar{T}_r$ is the mean radiant temperature in °C, k = 2.2 for T in °C, V in m/s air movement and T_g is for a 150 mm diameter globe.

If a smaller globe is used then the constant k in the above equation should be substituted by k^d which may be calculated from:

$$k_d = k \left(\frac{0.15}{d}\right)^{0.4}$$

where d is the diameter in metres of the globe used. Most heat stress indices (*see* below) which incorporate T_g use a 150 mm globe and it may be necessary to calculate this from readings of the smaller globe and wind speed (Hey, 1968; Harrison *et al.*, 1978).

It is not always necessary to go to the complication of measuring mean radiant temperatures because the measurements of globe temperature may be used directly in a range of heat stress indices for predicting thermal stress and prescribing control limits. Under very special circumstances where a detailed geography of the radiant surroundings is required, the technique of infra-red thermography may be used for which there are a number of highly effective, if expensive, instruments.

Humidity

Humidity is the concentration of water vapour in the air. It may be expressed in absolute terms either as mass per unit mass of air (kg/kg) or as a partial pressure (mm Hg, torr or kilopascal). There is an upper limit to the amount of water vapour air can hold at any temperature; when this maximum is reached the air is said to be saturated. Saturated air at high temperatures holds more water vapour than at low temperatures. If unsaturated air is cooled, it becomes saturated. The temperature at saturation is called the dew point. If the air is cooled below the dew point, some of the water vapour condenses.

Relative humidity (RH) is the ratio of the actual amount of water vapour in the air to the amount that would be present if the air were saturated at the same temperature—expressed as a percentage. It is often preferable to express humidity in absolute terms; for example, air at 40°C and 50% RH contains much greater quantities of water vapour and will have a greater effect in limiting sweat evaporation than air at 20°C and 50% RH. Saturated air at freezing point contains very small amounts of water vapour. In contrast we know that sweating skin at, say, 30°C has a water vapour pressure at the skin surface of 5.6 kPa. If we know that the environmental water vapour pressure is

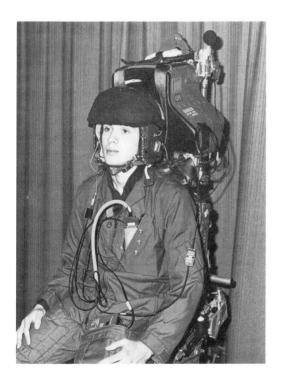

Figure 16.3 Automatic thermal data logging equipment for use in aircraft.

5.6 kPa we immediately know that sweat evaporation is virtually impossible.

Psychrometers

Classically humidity is determined by measuring the wet bulb depression. If the bulb of a thermometer (or a thermistor for that matter) is covered with a wick and kept wet with distilled water and placed in an airstream, the evaporation of the water cools the thermistor which therefore reads below a dry bulb thermometer in the same situation. These measurements are usually obtained by using an instrument know as a psychrometer which includes both the dry bulb and wet bulb sensors. Airflow over the thermometers is induced either by physically swinging them through the air, as in a whirling hygrometer (*see Figure 16.1*), or by mounting the thermometers in tubes through which air is drawn by an electrically driven fan as in the Assman psychrometer (*Figure 16.1*). The readings of dry bulb and wet bulb temperature obtained with a psychrometer are used to enter a psychrometric chart to obtain relative or absolute humidity as shown in *Figure 16.4*.

In recent years the use of psychrometers for the measurement of humidity has become less common due to the advent of a number of solid state humidity sensors. Modern 'solid state' humidity sensors (*see Figure 16.1*) employ a thin film polymer capacitor element specially designed to absorb atmospheric water vapour and whose capacitance varies with ambient RH. They are unsuitable at low water vapour concentrations and extremes of temperature, and must be protected from contamination by pollutant particles especially those containing sulphur. A typical accuracy of ±2% RH can be maintained by regular recalibration. These sensors lend themselves conveniently to automatic data logging techniques.

Air movement

Air movement has an extremely important effect on human heat exchange both at high temperatures, where it affects convection and sweat evaporation, and at low temperatures where it produces the well-known windchill effect (*see* below). In locations out of doors air movement is usually unidirectional

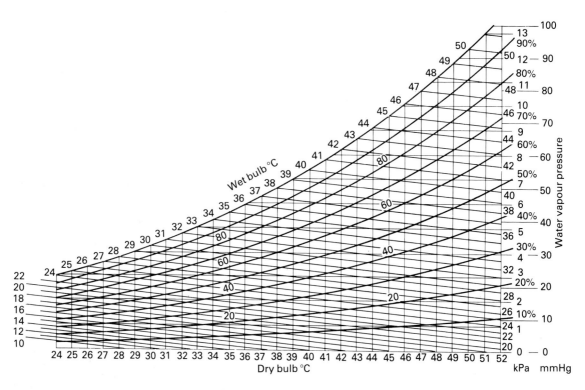

Figure 16.4 A psychrometric chart. The chart is entered with wet and dry bulb temperatures. The point of intersection can be read across to the right-hand scale for absolute humidity. Relative humidity is obtained by interpolation between the lines of equal RH given in 10 per cent steps.

and can be measured using traditional instruments such as vane or cup anemometers. In these instruments the speed of rotation of the cups or vanes is calibrated in terms of wind speed. The speed of rotation is measured either by mechanical means or, in the more modern instruments, by electronic pulse counters. In industrial situations and notably in aircraft cockpits, air movement is frequently omnidirectional and in these circumstances the traditional vane and cup anemometers are liable to errors. Omnidirectional air flow can be measured using devices based on a hot wire anemometer principle which measure the cooling effect of airflow over a heated wire. In modern instruments the heated wire has been replaced by a heated thermistor but otherwise the principle is the same.

A range of environmental measuring instruments is shown in *Figure 16.1*.

Human heat exchange

A naked man exchanges heat with his environment via one or more of four physical pathways: conduction (K), convection (C), radiation (R) and evaporation (E). If body temperature is to remain constant the net result of his exchanges with the environment must be a loss to the environment of an amount of heat equal to his metabolic heat production (H). If this balance is not maintained then the excess heat lost or gained must alter the total body heat content (Q) and lead to a change in body temperature. Man's conversion of food energy into physical work is not an efficient process and for most activities something like 80% of the metabolic energy production appears as heat. Thus for a man in heat balance with his environment we may write an equation as follows:

$$H = M - W = E + R + C + K + S$$

where: H = metabolic heat production; M = metabolic energy production; W = rate of external work; E, R, C and K are the rates of heat loss by evaporation, radiation, convection and conduction respectively; and S is the rate of storage of heat in the body. All quantities may be expressed in Watts per square metre of body surface area (W/m^2). A gain of heat by any channel is a negative loss of heat.

For a given individual any imbalance in his heat exchange with his environment which results in heat being stored or lost in this body will lead to changes in the total body heat content (ΔQ) which are related to his body mass (M), the mean specific heat of human tissues ($c = 3.48 \times 10^3$ J/kg/°C) and changes in mean body temperature, ΔT_b by the equation:

$$\Delta Q = c.M(\Delta \bar{T}_b)$$

Thus for a given imbalance in heat exchange with the environment a heavy man's temperature will change less than that of a light man.

It is a preoccupation of human thermal physiologists and of those interested in developing mathematical models of human thermoregulation to develop mathematical relationships by which heat exchange by conduction, convection, radiation and evaporation may be calculated exactly. The accuracy of these calculations is somewhat controversial and, based as they usually are on naked men, great difficulties arise in predicting the complicated and varied influences of clothing upon these relationships. Most practical aviation circumstances concern clothed men, indeed some of them clothed in highly complicated protective assemblies. However, the value of a short account of the mathematical description of human heat exchange lies in showing the way in which the various environmental components affect each exchange pathway. Beyond that the reader is advised to adopt a healthy scepticism as to the precision and usefulness of these expressions when applied to individuals, although they can be useful when mean responses of large groups are required.

Conduction

Heat is exchanged by conduction between objects at different temperatures in contact with each other. Conduction is relatively unimportant in human heat exchange except in the rather special circumstances of cold water immersion. Conductive heat transfer (K) depends on the temperature difference between the objects in contact and the conductance between them as follows:

$$K = k (T_1 - T_2)$$

The conductance (k) is the property of a material or interface between objects which determines the rate of heat transfer per unit area per unit temperature difference and the normal units are $W/m^2/°C$. It may be convenient to think of conductance as the inverse of resistance.

Convection

When a fluid (liquid or gas) at one temperature flows over a surface at a different temperature heat is gained or lost by convection. In the case of a naked man in air, the rate and direction of convective exchange depends on the temperature difference between the air and the skin surface. The situation is more complicated in a clothed individual and this is dealt with below. Convective heat transfer may be calculated as follows:

$$C = h_c(\bar{T}_{sk} - T_a)$$

where C = the heat exchange by convection (W/m^2), h_c = convective heat transfer coefficient $(W/m^2/°C)$, $\overline{T}_{sk}$ = mean skin temperature $(°C)$, T_a = dry bulb temperature $(°C)$.

The convective heat exchange coefficient, h_c, is not constant under all environmental conditions and depends upon the rate of air movement. It may be calculated from:

$$h_c = 8.3 V^{0.5} \, (W/m/°C)$$

where V is the air movement in m/s.

The important point to note in this relationship is that heat exchange by convection depends both on the temperature difference between the body and the surrounding air or water and on the rate of movement of the air. It matters not whether the latter is naturally or artifically generated.

Evaporation

When water evaporates from a surface, energy is absorbed during transition from the liquid to the gaseous state. This energy is termed the latent heat of vaporization and in the case of the evaporation of sweat it has a value of 2500×10^3 J/kg. This figure emphasizes the extraordinary power of the human sweating mechanism as a heat loss pathway.

In environments where the air temperature is the same or higher than skin temperature then sweating is the sole means available for dissipating the metabolic heat production. In such situations anything that limits evaporation, such as high ambient humidity or impermeable clothing, will rapidly lead to heat storage and a rise in body temperature.

Heat loss by evaporation (E) depends upon the water vapour pressure gradient between the skin surface and the ambient air; it may be calculated from:

$$E = h_e(P_{sk} - P_a)$$

where E = Evaporative heat loss (W/m^2); h_e = the coefficient of evaporative heat exchange $(W/m^2/kPa)$; P_{sk} = water vapour pressure at the skin surface (kPa); P_a = the ambient water vapour pressure (kPa).

The coefficient for evaporative heat exchange (h_e) incorporates the latent heat of vaporization of sweat and the highly important effect of air movement on evaporation. For practical purposes h_e may be calculated from:

$$h_e = 124 \, V^{0.5} \, W/m^2/kPa$$

where V is the air movement in m/s.

It is possible to show (Brebner, Kershake and Waddell, 1958) that for a given air movement there is a constant relationship between the heat exchange

coefficients for evaporation and convection, the ratio h_e/h_c being approximately 15. This relationship holds good for a human subject of given size in air of fixed properties.

As with convection the important point to note from the above is that sweat evaporation is determined by the vapour pressure gradient between the skin and the ambient air and the rate of air flow across the skin.

Radiation

Exchange of heat by radiation between two surfaces depends upon the difference in the fourth powers of the absolute temperatures of the two surfaces. In many practical situations it is acceptable to use a first power relationship as follows:

$$R = h_r(\overline{T}_{sk} - \overline{T}_r)$$

where R = the heat exchange by radiation (W/m^2); h_r = the first power combined radiation coefficient; $\overline{T}_{sk}$ = mean skin temperature $(°C)$; $\overline{T}_r$ = mean radiant temperature of the surroundings $(°C)$.

The coefficient h_r depends upon the temperature of the two surfaces, the geometrical relation between them and such characteristics of the surfaces as emitance and reflectance. Thus it may be seen that heat transfer by radiation depends principally on the temperature of the two surfaces concerned and is unaffected by air movement or the distance between the surfaces. It can take place across a vacuum.

In aircraft cockpits and many industrial situations hot surfaces in the surroundings radiate in the long infra-red. A notable exception to this is the radiation received from the sun in open-air situations or through the canopies of aircraft. Here the radiation is substantially in the visible range $(0.4-0.7 \, \mu m)$. In desert situations the heat energy derived from solar radiation can exceed $1000 \, W/m^2$ body surface area. For practical purposes the value of h_r may be taken as $5.2 \, W/m^2/°C$.

Operative temperature

It will be helpful here to introduce the concept of operative temperature which has some useful practical applications. It will have been noticed above that the processes of convection and radiation have in common that each depends on the difference between skin temperature and an environmental temperature either T_a or T_r. Operative temperature is the result of efforts to combine the air temperature and the mean radiant temperature into a single figure and is defined as the uniform temperature of a radiantly black enclosure in which an occupant would exchange the same amount of heat by radiation plus convection as in the actual non-uniform environment. Operative temperature is numerically the average, weighted by respective heat transfer coefficients (h_c, h_r), of the air and mean radiant temperatures. Thus:

$$T_0 = (h_c T_a + h_r \overline{T}_r)/(h_c + h_r).$$

At air speeds of 0.4 m/s or less and T_r <50°C, operative temperature is approximately the simple average of the air and mean radiant temperatures. It can also be shown that the operative heat exchange coefficient, h_0, is equal to the sum of the heat exchange coefficients for convection and radiation $h_c + h_r$. *Table 16.2* gives the values for these heat exchange coefficients at various wind speeds and will facilitate calculations of likely heat balance in a variety of situations.

Table 16.2 Heat exchange coefficients at various wind speeds

V (m/s)	h_c (W/m²/°C)	h_e (W/m²/°C)	h_0 (W/m²/°C)
0.1	2.6	39	7.8
0.2	3.7	55	8.9
0.3	4.5	68	9.7
0.4	5.2	78	10.4
0.5	5.9	88	11.1
0.6	6.4	96	11.6
0.7	6.9	104	12.1
0.8	7.4	111	12.6
0.9	7.9	118	13.1
1.0	8.3	124	13.5
1.2	9.1	136	14.3
1.4	9.8	147	15.0
1.6	10.5	157	15.7
1.8	11.1	166	16.3
2.0	11.7	175	16.9
2.5	13.1	196	18.3
3.0	14.4	215	19.6
3.5	15.5	232	20.7
4.0	16.6	248	21.8
4.5	17.6	263	22.8
5.0	18.6	277	23.8

h_c and h_e are calculated as $8.3 \cdot V^{0.5}$ and $124 \cdot V^{0.5}$ respectively. h_r is assumed to be 5.2 W/m²/C. $h_0 = h_c + h_r$.

The thermal effects of clothing

The descriptions of human heat exchange given above are related to unclothed subjects. This situation applies to very few everyday practical situations. Aircrew are normally clothed and usually in complicated multi-layer protective clothing. The effects of clothing on human heat exchange are extremely complicated and difficult to describe in

exact mathematical terms but such detailed knowledge is usually unnecessary for the practising occupational physician. He should, however, understand some of the general principles so that he will have a basis on which to formulate practical advice.

In general, clothing impairs the loss of heat to the environment. While this is a considerable advantage under cold conditions it may be a serious disadvantage under warm conditions. The impairment of heat loss effects all four physical pathways—conduction, convection, radiation and evaporation. Impairment through the conductive pathway is of some importance in aviation where it provides the basis for protecting workers from injuries due to contact with very hot or cold surfaces. In terms of overall thermal balance, however, conduction is not of great significance.

The effect of clothing on heat loss by convection and radiation is to decrease conductance between the skin surface and the surrounding air. The general situation is illustrated in *Figure 16.5*. Sensible heat from the skin must first pass through the barrier represented by the clothing, insulation, I_c. At the clothing surface the heat transfer coefficients for convection and radiation, h_c and h_r, may be combined into the operative heat transfer coefficient, h_0, as described above. The reciprocal of h_0 is referred to as the insulation of the environment, $I_a = 1/h_0$. The total resistance or insulation between the skin and the environment in a clothed subject is the sum of the clothing insulation, I_c, and the insulation of the environment, I_a. Thus:

$$I = I_c + I_a$$

This describes the situation in its simplest form represented by a sedentary individual in still air. However, if the individual is working or there is a wind, then the situation may change dramatically. In outdoor conditions where there is a wind, or even in some indoor conditions where there is significant air movement induced by ventilation installations, the effective insulation of a clothing assembly is reduced by reductions both in I_a and I_c. The reduction in I_c will depend largely on the degree of wind penetration into the clothing system. Highly permeable open-weave garments will lose their effective insulation significantly whereas impermeable garments or garments with impermeable outer layers will not do so, although they will be subject to decreases in I_a due to disturbance of the boundary air layers by the wind.

The effect of physical work on clothing insulation arises through two mechanisms. Firstly, physical work such as walking may induce air penetration of the clothing layers in much the same way as wind. Equally important is a phenomenon known as bellows action or pumping. This comes about when the exercise induces exchanges of the air beneath the clothing with ambient air either directly through

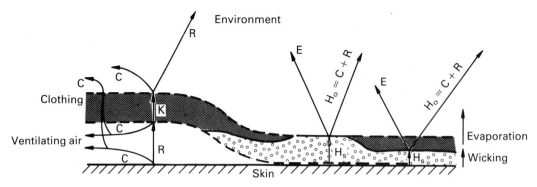

Figure 16.5 Diagram of heat exchange through clothing by convection, radiation and evaporation. C = Heat exchange by convection. R = Heat exchange by radiation. E = Heat exchange by evaporation. H_s = Net heat loss from the skin. H_o = Sensible heat loss = C + R.

the clothing in permeable fabrics or through openings at the wrist, ankles or neck. Bellows action is a useful mechanism for promoting heat loss during exercise in subjects dressed for cold conditions at rest.

With the increasing use of immersion suits or survival suits for the protection of personnel in the aviation world, the offshore oil industry, the fishing industry and the Merchant Marine, the importance of clothing insulation as protection in the event of immersion in cold water has been more widely recognized in recent years. The prime function of the immersion suits or survival suits is to preserve clothing insulation by keeping it dry.

The insulation provided by clothing is determined largely by the thickness of the trapped air layer within the clothing fabrics themselves or between layers of fabric. Very little is contributed by the physical characteristics of the fibres themselves. For this reason it is possible to estimate a mean figure for insulation by measuring the thickness of the clothing including the air layers when the insulation may be calculated as $0.025°C.m^2/W$ per mm of thickness. If the air contained within the clothing is displaced by water leakage during immersion or exposure to rain or spray, then its insulation is dramatically decreased as shown in *Figure 16.6*. Insulation may also be lost as a result of urination following the cold induced diuresis seen in cold immersion.

A wet suit constructed from closed-celled neoprene foam can also provide effective protection in water because the air contained within the cells is not displaced by water during immersion and the suit limits convective heat loss at the skin surface. However, it is interesting to note in passing that a loose-fitting wet suit may exhibit a significant loss of effective insulation due to the water equivalent of the bellows action described for air above. This is known as flushing and the exchange of water

between the layer beneath the suit and the open sea can effectively halve the insulation provided by the wet suit (Wolff *et al.*, 1985).

Clothing insulation may be measured by a number of techniques. Traditionally it is performed by measuring the insulation of samples of the clothing fabric on a device known as a guarded hot-plate (British Standards Institution, 1971). The difficulty with this technique is that it is difficult to compute the overall insulation of a multi-layered clothing assembly from the individual figures for each layer since these do not allow for the variable air layers trapped between the layers of fabric, the compression of the layers or the rather complicated boundary effects. This may, however, be done approximately by multiplying the sum of the individual insulations by 0.8.

Many groups of workers have used heated metal manikins of various kinds for the measurement of clothing insulation and these have the advantage of

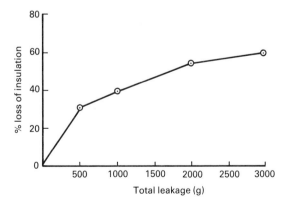

Figure 16.6 Figure showing percentage loss of insulation plotted against water leakage into the insulation worn beneath an immersion suit.

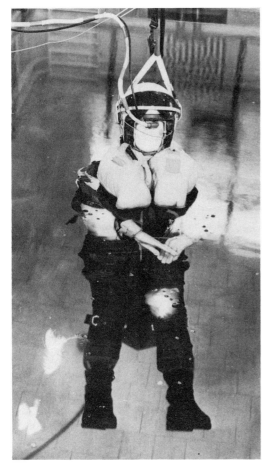

Figure 16.7 An immersible thermal manikin. This manikin is made from aluminium. At equilibrium the measured power input to the internal heaters is equal to the heat lost through the clothing, and the insulation can therefore be calculated.

measuring the overall insulation for whole clothing assemblies rather than for individual items. Modern manikins have the capability of leg and arm movements, thus reproducing realistically the pumping effects of activity (Olesen *et al.*, 1982). Immersible manikins are used for measuring the effective insulation of immersion protective clothing (*Figure 16.7*) when they have the additional advantages of assessing effects of leakage of water into the insulation and of the loss of insulation due to hydrostatic compression on immersion (Allan *et al.*, 1985).

Clothing and radiation

The effect of clothing on radiation heat exchange depends significantly on the wavelength of the radiation. In respect of radiation in the long infra-red, clothing of any colour acts more or less as a black body and absorbs the radiation. Nevertheless, in the case of severe infra-red radiation the clothing may still provide protection against skin burns. In the case of ultraviolet radiation this may be significantly reflected by white clothing which therefore conveys an advantage upon the wearer. This consideration, however, is usually outweighed by the advantages of loose-fitting cotton garments on ventilation and sweat evaporation and this is the explanation why the Bedouin in the desert are not persuaded to exchange their black loose fitting clothing for white.

In military aviation the use of white aircrew helmets can be shown to convey small thermal advantages to the wearer when compared with dark colours. However, white helmets give rise to significant problems in the form of reflections in instrument faces and other equipment and also create an easily visible target. These disadvantages will usually outweigh any thermal advantage.

Clothing and evaporation

Clothing materials impede heat transfer by evaporation more than sensible heat transfer. This restriction to evaporative heat transfer varies over a very wide range, from being virtually total in the case of impermeable fabrics such as neoprene coated nylon, to being insignificant in the case of thin cotton fabrics.

In the case of impermeable fabrics sweat evaporating from the skin will rapidly saturate the micro-environment between the skin and the garment and evaporation will then cease. In practice this is usually not a complete process because openings at the wrist, ankles or the neck permit exchange of the saturated air beneath the clothing with the environment and this allows some evaporation to proceed. Similarly, some exchange takes place around an impermeable anti-G suit or partial pressure clothing. Nevertheless, the wearing of impermeable garments is almost always associated with severe loss of comfort and a significant risk of heat stress due to lack of sweat evaporation.

In recent years a number of new fabrics have appeared on the market which have the property of being permeable to water vapour whilst being waterproof in the sense that droplet water will not pass through them. Somewhat exaggerated claims are sometimes made on behalf of these fabrics but they do appear to reduce the disadvantages of impermeable materials in terms of comfort and sweat evaporation. The fabrics are either constructed as laminations, with a middle layer of microporous PTFE, or are coated with a new modified polyurethane which transports water via a chemical pathway.

When clothing is permeable both to water vapour and to sweat, evaporation may occur at any level from the skin surface to the clothing surface (*see Figure 16.5*). Thus with loose-fitting, thin, cotton clothing and substantial ventilation of the micro-climate, evaporation directly from the skin may predominate. With less permeable fabrics or multi-layered clothing assemblies the sweat may be wicked through the clothing and evaporate either at some intermediate layer within the clothing or from the surface. Clearly when this occurs the cooling effect upon the man will be less effective. In order to develop a method for describing the effect of clothing on evaporation a number of indices have been described, for example the permeability index (Woodcock, 1962) or the permeation efficiency factor (Nishi and Gagge, 1970).

Woodcock's permeability index, I_m, is based on the ratio of the conductance of a clothing system for water vapour, k_e, to that for sensible heat, k_s. The ratio k_e/k_s is compared with a standard for air for which the corresponding ratio is h_e/h_c. The dimensionless permeability index is thus calculated from $(k_e/k_s)/(h_e/h_c)$ and ranges from 0 in the case of impermeable fabrics to unity in the case of air.

Evaporative heat transfer through clothing, where sensible heat and water vapour transfer are at rates well in excess of those possible by molecular diffusion, can be determined from:

$$E = 16.5 \left(\frac{P_a - P_{sk}}{I} \right)$$

where E = Evaporative heat transfer (W/m²); $P_a - p_{sk}$ = vapour pressure difference between the skin and the air (kPa); I = Insulation (m².°C/W); (the constant has the dimensions °C/kPa).

Woodcock (1962) suggested expanding the equation above so as to allow for the water vapour transfer characteristics of different clothing by including his dimensionless permeability index (i_m) to give:

$$E = 16.5 \, i_m \left(\frac{P_a - P_{sk}}{I} \right)$$

From this it may be seen that the ratio i_m/I is highly significant in determining the evaporative heat transfer through a clothing system. It represents the fraction of the maximum evaporation cooling possible in a given environment without wind (insulation (I) being a 'still air' determination).

Indices of thermal stress

It will be appreciated from the above that there are a great many factors that contribute to the overall stress of thermal environments and the resulting thermal strain in individuals exposed to them. These factors include the environmental components (air temperature, humidity, air movement and radiant temperature); physical properties of the body such as shape, size, movement and skin colour; the physical characteristics of the clothing assembly worn; the physiological characteristics of the individual and his work rate. This long list of variables can prove rather alarming to the flight surgeon or occupational physician faced with giving simple, succinct advice for the control of thermal stress.

Many attempts have been made to combine the above factors into simple numerical descriptions or indices, capable of predicting the likely level of thermal stress with some degree of accuracy. The fruits of these endeavours may be divided into three main groups.

Group 1

Indices in this group are based on an analysis of heat exchange and inevitably involve complex mathematical calculations. Examples are the Heat Stress Index of Belding and Hatch (Belding and Hatch, 1955), HSI and the Index of Thermal Stress of Givoni (Givoni, 1964), ITS. On the cold side this group includes the well-known windchill index (Siple and Passel, 1945).

Group 2

Indices in this group are based empirically on physiological observations. Examples are the Predicted 4 hour Sweat Rate (P₄SR) (McArdle *et al.*, 1947), the Wet Bulb Globe Temperature Index, WBGT (Yaglou and Minard, 1957) and the Wet Dry Index (WD) also known as the Oxford Index (Leithead and Lind, 1964).

Group 3

This includes indices based on immediate subjective sensations of warmth on entering an environment. The most common example is the Effective Temperature scale (ET) (Yaglou, 1927) and a derivative allowing for radiant heat which is known as the Corrected Effective Temperature (CET) (Bedford, 1964).

For detailed descriptions of these indices the reader is referred to the references given for each of them. In practice, however, many of them have received minimal practical application, especially in aviation, and they may be regarded as the toys of environmental physiologists. Noteable exceptions, however, are the Effective Temperature scales, the Wet Bulb Temperature index and related derivatives and the Windchill Index. These will therefore be described in greater detail.

Effective Temperature

Effective Temperature scales were developed by Yaglou and his associates in the 1920s (Yaglou, 1927). They are based on the immediate subjective impression of warmth gained when subjects walk from one environment to another. The scales take the form of nomograms, the normal scale being for subjects wearing normal indoor clothing and the basic scale for subjects stripped to the waist. *Figure 16.8* gives the nomogram for the Effective Temperature normal scale. It can be seen that the index allows for air temperature, wet bulb temperature and air movement. The index was originally criticized for not making allowance for radiant

heating and a number of modifications have been proposed to make good this deficiency. The simplest of these is merely to enter the scale using globe temperature in place of air temperature and the resulting index is then referred to as the Corrected Effective Temperature (CET) (Bedford, 1964).

Since the Effective Temperature scale was devised on the basis of subjective sensation, it is hardly surprising that it has proved inaccurate as a predictor of physiological response. It makes no allowance for work rate. Specifically, the Effective Temperature scales tend to overestimate the effect of high humidity in comfortable conditions and underestimate the harmful effects of low wind speed and high humidity in the heat. Its main application therefore has been within the comfort range and since in this range the effect of humidity is relatively small, several authorities have abandoned effective temperature scales in favour of the simpler operative temperature (ASHRAE, 1981). Examples of the use of operative temperature, for individuals doing sedentary tasks in office environments, to define the level of clothing insulation required for comfort and to define acceptable range of operative temperature and humidity for individuals clothed in typical summer and winter clothing are given in *Figures 16.9* and *16.10* respectively.

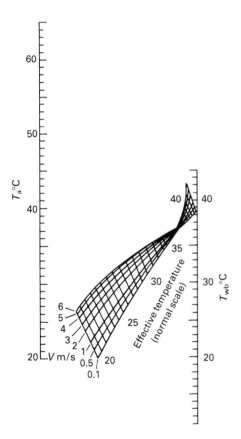

Figure 16.8 Nomogram for effective temperature (normal scale). A line is drawn between the measured dry bulb and wet bulb temperatures. ET is read at the point of intersection of this line with the appropriate curve for the measured wind speed.

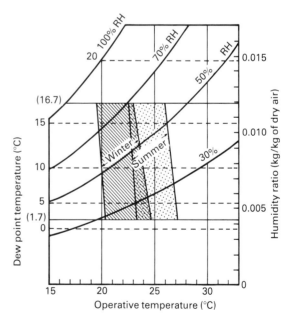

Figure 16.9 Acceptable ranges of operative temperature and humidity for comfort in persons clothed in typical summer and winter clothing undertaking light activities. (After ASHRAE Standard 55-81.)

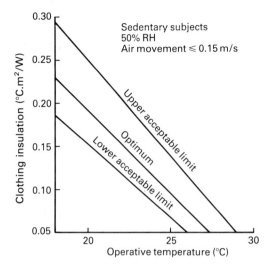

Figure 16.10 Clothing insulation necessary for comfort in sedentary subjects at various operative temperatures. (After ASHRAE Standard 55-81.)

The Wet Bulb Globe Temperature Index (WBGT)

The WBGT was originally developed by Yaglou and Minard (1957) as a simple index for use in controlling heat casualties in the United States Marine Corps during work in the open desert. As originally described it was calculated from measurements of a standard 150 mm black globe thermometer, air temperature and a wet bulb thermometer which was not artificially ventilated as in a psychrometer but merely exposed to the ambient air movement and radiation. The index is calculated as follows:

$$WBGT = 0.7T_{wb} + 0.2T_g + 0.1T_a °C$$

An alternative formula has been proposed for use with a psychometric wet bulb temperature (obtained using an artificially ventilated wet bulb) as follows:

$$WBGT = 0.7T_{wb} + 0.3T_g °C$$

A deriviative of the WBGT known as the wet, dry or Oxford index may be used where radiant heat loads are absent and is calculated from:

$$WD = 0.85_{wb} + 0.15_{db} °C$$

The WBGT has the great advantage of simplicity. It is also capable of being measured directly, with appropriate electronic instrumentation performing the calculation 'on-line'. As a predictor of thermal strain it is most accurate under the conditions for which it was originally devised, that is in the open air with wind movement and a radiant heat load. However, WBGT does not allow *per se* for work rate or clothing and if used to establish limits for environmental control purpose it must be clearly understood that the limits will be related to specific rates of working and specific clothing assemblies. In most industrial situations work rates and clothing are known quantities and recommendations for WBGT limits can be made with this knowledge. The detailed application of the WBGT index in the control of industrial thermal stress is described in International Standard ISO 7243-1982(E).

Fighter Index of Thermal Stress

In military aviation, attempts have been made to use the WBGT Index to control stress in fighter aircraft cockpits and the approach could be developed for other aircraft types and clothing assemblies. The Fighter Index of Thermal Stress (FITS) was developed by Nunneley and Stribley (1979) and is based on predictions of cockpit WBGT from ground conditions in the vicinity. Harrison *et al.* (1978) showed that reasonable accuracy was possible in predicting cockpit WBGT from ground conditions but the relationships are always specific to the type of aircraft and sortie. Body temperature responses can be related to cockpit WBGT but again the relationship will be specific for a given clothing assembly and level of work.

FITS is calculated as follows:

For full Sun:
$$FITS = 0.8281 T_{wb} + 0.3549 T_{db} + 5.08$$
For overcast sky:
$$FITS = 0.8281 T_{wb} + 0.3549 T_{db} + 2.23$$

The wet and dry bulb temperatures are psychromatic measurements of ground ambient conditions.

A caution zone has been suggested as FITS = 32–38°C. When FITS is in the caution zone it is suggested that ground standby in the cockpit should be limited to 90 mins and there should be a minimum of 2 hours between flights. In the danger zone (FITS>38°C) it is suggested that low-level flights should be cancelled, standby limited to 45 minutes and a minimum of 2 hours imposed between flights. Alternative precautions could be devised to deal with each specific situation.

Windchill index and equivalent chill temperature

The index of windchill was originally developed by Siple and Passel (1945) in 1945 from experiments on the time taken to freeze a cylinder of water in a range of temperatures and windspeeds. A windchill chart is shown at *Figure 16.11* from which it may be seen that the chart is entered with inputs of air temperature and wind speed. The centre windchill scale may be read in physical terms as W/m^2 or in subjective terms as indicated.

The windchill index is useful in predicting frostbite for exposed dry skin but is less satisfactory as a basis for deciding suitable clothing for the

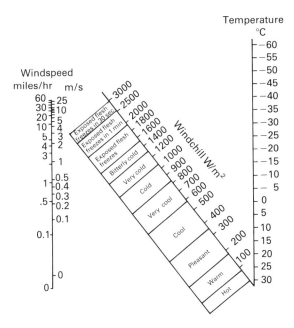

Figure 16.11 A windchill chart. A line is drawn between the measured air temperature on the right-hand scale and the measured windspeed on the left-hand scale. Windchill is read from the centre scale in W/m² or descriptive terms.

Wind speed		Air temperature (°C)																
mph	m/s	−2	−1	−4	−7	−9	−12	−15	−18	−21	−23	−26	−29	−32	−34	−37	−40	−43	−46
1–5	0.5–2.3	−1	−4	−7	−9	−12	−15	−18	−21	−23	−26	−29	−32	−34	−37	−40	−43	−46	−48
6–10	2.6–4.4	−7	−9	−12	−15	−18	−23	−26	−29	−32	−37	−40	−43	−46	−51	−54	−57	−59	−65
11–15	5.0–6.7	−9	−12	−18	−21	−23	−29	−32	−34	−40	−43	−46	−51	−54	−57	−62	−65	−68	−73
16–20	7.2–9.0	−12	−15	−18	−23	−29	−32	−34	−40	−43	−48	−51	−54	−59	−62	−68	−71	−76	−79
21–25	9.5–11.3	−12	−18	−21	−26	−29	−34	−37	−43	−46	−51	−54	−59	−62	−68	−71	−76	−79	−84
26–30	11.7–13.5	−15	−18	−23	−29	−32	−37	−40	−46	−48	−54	−57	−62	−65	−71	−73	−79	−82	−87
30+	>13.5	−15	−21	−23	−29	−34	−37	−40	−46	−51	−54	−59	−62	−68	−73	−76	−82	−84	−90

Little danger or frostbite	Increasing danger of frostbite	Great danger of frostbite

Figure 16.12 Equivalent chill temperature chart. The chart is entered with local air temperature and windspeed. The intersection gives the equivalent chill temperature in ° C *(See text)*.

protection of personnel working outdoors. For this purpose the Equivalent Chill Temperature (or equivalent still air temperature) is more useful. The Equivalent Chill temperature is the still air temperature that would produce the same cooling as the temperature and windspeed actually measured. An Equivalent Chill Temperature Chart is given in *Figure 16.12*.

References

ALLAN, J.R., HIGENBOTTAM, C. and REDMAN, P.J. (1985) The effect of leakage on the insulation provided by immersion-protection clothing. *Aviation, Space and Environmental Medicine*, **56**, 1107–1109

American Society of Heating, Refrigerating and Air conditioning Engineers (1981) *Thermal Environmental Conditions for Human Occupancy*. ASHRAE STANDARD No.55–81

BEDFORD, T. (1964) *Basic Principles of Ventilation and Heating*, 2nd edn. London: Lewis

BELDING, H.S. and HATCH, T.F. (1955) Index for evaluating heat stress in terms of the resulting physiological strain. *Heat Pipes and Air Conditioning*, **27**, 129–136

BREBNER, D.E., KERSLAKE, D.MCK. and WADDELL, J.L. (1958) The relationship between coefficients for heat exchange by convection and by evaporation in man. *Journal of Physiology (London)*, **141**, 164–168

British Standards Institution (1971) BS4745 *Thermal Resistance of Textiles*

FANGER, P.O. (1972) *Thermal Comfort.* New York: McGraw-Hill

GIVONI, B. (1964) A new method for evaluating industrial heat exposure and maximum permissible work load. *International Journal of Bioclimatics and Biometeorology*, **8**, 115–124

HEY, E.N. (1968) Small globe thermometers. *Journal of Scientific Instruments*, **1**, 955–957 and corrigendum p.1260

HARRISON, M.H., HIGENBOTTAM, C. and RIGBY, R.A. (1978) Relationships between ambient, cockpit, and pilot temperatures during routine air operations. *Aviation, Space and Environmental Medicine*, **49**, 5–13

International Organization for Standardization. Standard No. ISO 7243-1982 (E) *Hot Environments—Estimation of the Heat Stress on Working Men, Based on the WBGT-Index* (Wet bulb globe temperature)

LEITHEAD, C.S. and LIND, A.R. (1964) *Heat Stress and Heat Disorders*. London: Churchill

MCARDLE, B., DUNHAM, W., HOLLING, H.E., LADELL, W.S.S., SCOTT, J.W., THOMSON, M.L. and WEINER, J.S. (1947) *The Prediction of the Physiological Effects of Warm and Hot Environments*. RNP 47/391. London: Medical Research Council

NISHI, Y. and GAGGE, A.P. (1970) Moisture permeation of clothing—a factor governing thermal equilibrium and comfort. *Transcriptions of the American Society of Heating, Refrigeration and Air Conditioning Engineers*, **76**, Part 1

NUNNELEY, S.A. and STRIBLEY, R.F. (1979) Fighter index of thermal stress (FITS): Guidance for hot-weather aircraft operations. *Aviation, Space and Environmental Medicine*, **50**, 639–642

OLESEN, B.W., SHIWINSKA, E., MADSEN, T.L. and FANGER, P.O. (1982) Effect of body posture and activity on the thermal insulation of clothing: Measurements by a movable thermal manikin. *Transcriptions of The American Society of Heating, Refrigeration and Air Conditioning Engineers*, **32**, 791–805

SIPLE, P.A. and PASSEL, C.F. (1945) Measurements of dry atmospheric cooling in subfreezing temperatures. *Proceedings of The American Philosophical Society*, **89**, 177–199

WOLFF, A.H., COLESHAW, S.R.K., NEWSTEAD, C.G. and KEATINGE, W.R. (1985) Heat exchanges in wet suits. *Journal of Applied Physiology*, **58**, 770–777

WOODCOCK, A.H. (1962) Moisture transfer in textile systems. *Textile Research Journal*, **32**, 628–633

YAGLOU, C.P. (1927) Temperature humidity and air movement in industries: the effective temperature index. *Journal of Industrial Hygiene*, **9**, 297–309

YAGLOU, C.P. and MINARD, D. (1957) Control of heat casualties at military training centers. *American Medical Association Archives of Industrial Health*, **16**, 302–316

17

Thermal physiology

C.T. Kirkpatrick

Homeostasis and homeothermy

The maintenance of the body's central or 'core' temperature at a more or less constant value (homeothermy) is often cited, in elementary texts, as a prime example of homeostasis—the preservation of a fixed internal environment. There are considerable advantages to the organism if temperature is kept constant, as critical enzyme systems can be developed that work most efficiently at that temperature. The level of the organism's activity is no longer determined by the environmental temperature—a poikilotherm becomes torpid at low temperatures and may not even eat enough food to maintain essential metabolism, but a homeotherm can sustain a constant level of activity whatever the environment. It may even increase its activity in the cold, in an attempt to maintain its body temperature.

Homeostatic mechanisms require a number of components (*Figure 17.1*): one or more detectors to inform the system of the value of the variable which is being controlled; a reference level (set point) to inform the system controller what the correct value should be; a control centre which compares the data from the detectors with the reference level and detects any error, producing an output signal of appropriate magnitude and direction to correct the error; and one or more effector organs which can modify the controlled variable in a manner prescribed by the controlling centre.

The existence of more than one input or effector

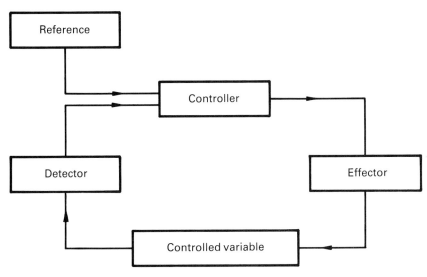

Figure 17.1 Schematic diagram of a simple homeostatic control loop.

pathway is known as redundancy, and the thermo-regulatory system is one in which there is a great deal of redundancy. This is not to suggest that any of the parallel pathways is unnecessary: on the contrary, the efficient working of the whole system requires the integration of information of many types from diverse sources, and the availability of multiple alternatives for effector action.

In mammalian thermoregulation, there is usually a balance between the heat produced internally (in metabolic processes and contracting muscles), and the heat lost to the environment. If the core temperature rises, this is detected centrally and mechanisms such as vasodilatation and sweating are initiated to increase the rate of heat loss. If core temperature falls, mechanisms are brought into play both to conserve heat and to generate extra heat to warm the body. Heat conservation is by vasocon-striction, so that the pathway for heat loss through the skin is given a higher resistance, and the warm blood is retained in the 'core' of the body at the expense of the 'shell' which is allowed to cool. Heat is generated by shivering (the production of heat but no external work by the muscles) or other forms of non-shivering thermogenesis.

Warming the skin often turns on the pathways for heat loss, and cooling of the skin is often sufficient to initiate measures for heat conservation or production, before core temperature has changed.

Detectors

There are at least two main sets of thermoreceptors: the central group and the peripheral group. The central group, located in the hypothalamus and other parts of the central nervous system, are concerned with monitoring the level of the deep body temperature and informing the immediately adjacent thermoregulatory centre. The peripheral group, located mainly in the skin, sample the temperature at the surface and reflect more accurately the influence of the environment on the organism, conveying data about alterations and rates of change of temperature to the central controller. Both types of data are important for the correct operation of the system; gross departures from the preferred core temperature are signalled by the central receptors, but subtle environmental changes can be detected by the peripheral sensors, long before there has been any change in the core temperature.

Although temperature is a single, continuous physical variable, the mammalian nervous system has acquired two distinct types of thermoreceptors, classed as 'warm' or 'cold' receptors, depending upon their dominant mode of action. One approach to the study of thermoreceptors in man is to ask

subjects whether a stimulus applied to the skin feels hot or cold; using this very simple technique it has proved possible to map out the receptive fields of individual warm or cold receptors. There are far more receptors for cold than for warmth, and thermoreceptors are particularly plentiful over the face and the palmar aspect of the fingers, though strangely they are also found in high concentration over the trunk. In animal experiments it is fairly easy to record the impulse traffic in the sensory nerves serving an area of skin while thermal stimuli are applied, and even in man thermosensory nerve activity may be recorded using extremely fine percutaneous needle electrodes.

Both warm and cold receptors operate over a fairly wide temperature range but they differ in the temperature at which their peak activity occurs. For the warm receptors there is a sharp peak at about 40–42°C, with a very rapid decline in activity above this level and a more gradual decline at lower temperatures (*Figure 17.2*). Cold receptors have a much less sharp peak of activity, discharging over quite a wide range of temperatures (some even exhibit a second, 'paradoxical' peak of discharge at high temperature). Individual cold receptors have separate and different temperatures for maximum discharge, and the nervous system can only sense the actual skin temperature by integrating the activity of a large population of receptors, each with a different characteristic profile of discharge with altering temperature. Some cold receptors develop a 'bursting' pattern of discharge over part of their temperature range, and this gives the central nervous system further clues about the skin temperature.

Thermoreceptors have both a static and a dynamic response to temperature. The static response is a steady-state rate of discharge which is more or less constant at a given temperature; the dynamic response is a rapid, transient acceleration or deceleration of discharge at the instant that temperature is changed. For instance, if local skin temperature is suddenly raised, a warm receptor produces a transient overshoot in discharge frequency before settling down to a new, steady discharge rate which is higher than the previous steady rate (*Figure 17.3*). During the same period of temperature increase, a cold receptor exhibits a transient suppression of its discharge and then settles down to a new steady rate of discharge which is lower than before. Since thermoreceptors have a dynamic as well as a static response, they are classed as rapidly adapting receptors.

The function of the central thermoreceptors is almost impossible to study directly in man, but in animal experiments warming or cooling particular regions of the hypothalamus cause thermoregula-tory activity to occur, and a number of groups of cells have been identified in the hypothalamus which

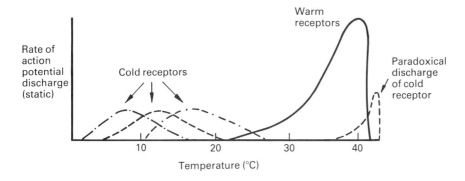

Figure 17.2 Static responses of peripheral warm and cold thermoreceptors.

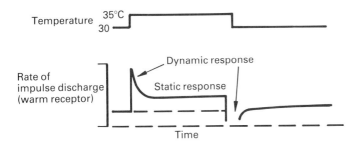

Figure 17.3 Dynamic and static responses of a typical warm receptor to a step change in temperature.

discharge action potentials when they are warmed or cooled. These thermally sensitive cells are situated in the anterior hypothalamus and the pre-optic area; warming this region causes sweating, salivation, polypnoea and vasodilatation while inhibiting shivering; cooling the region increases metabolic rate and shivering, produces vasoconstriction and inhibits sweating. Individual neurones have been identified which have a linear relationship between discharge rate and temperature, with either a positive (warm sensitive) or a negative (cold sensitive) temperature coefficient. The range of temperatures over which these central thermoreceptors operate is much narrower than in the case of peripheral receptors, and the increment in discharge rate for a given change in temperature is much greater: the gain of the receptors is higher.

While the most important central thermoreceptors are in the hypothalamus, groups of thermally sensitive neurones have also been found in the midbrain, medulla and spinal cord; autonomic thermoregulatory responses can be elicited by warming or cooling the spinal cord. Some deep body temperature receptors have also been detected in the visceral area, in the great veins and in the wall of the gut. The receptors have not been isolated, but sensory axons have been found in the nerves supplying these regions, whose discharge patterns have the characteristics of thermoreceptors during warming or cooling.

Effectors

The methods for heat conservation include cutaneous vasoconstriction and increasing metabolic heat production by exercise, shivering or non-shivering thermogenesis; in some animals the erection of hair (piloerection) is also a significant mechanism. The methods available for removal of excess heat include cutaneous vasodilatation, sweating and (in some animals) panting. The mechanisms of piloerection and panting will not be considered further as they are not available for human thermoregulation.

Vascular responses

The skin is endowed with a very rich microcirculation. As well as a dense network of arterioles, capillary loops and venules in the dermis, there are many direct arterio-venous anastomoses which allow large volumes of blood to flow through the skin without traversing the capillary bed. All of these blood vessels (except the capillaries, which have no smooth muscle in their walls) are controlled by autonomic nerves from the sympathetic outflow, which reach the skin in company with the arteries or via the cutaneous nerves.

The blood vessels of the skin are usually under a certain basal level of tonic vasomotor control. Vasoconstriction is achieved by increasing the rate at which impulses pass along the sympathetic nerves thus releasing more noradrenaline from the nerve endings; vasodilatation is generally produced by reducing sympathetic activity, rather than by the liberation of any specific vasodilator substance.

There are, of course, a number of influences that can produce a direct vasodilator effect. When sweat glands are stimulated to secrete by release of acetylcholine from sudomotor sympathetic nerves, the glandular activity results in the production of bradykinin from the tissues surrounding the gland cells. This is a by-product of secretory activity, but has a potent vasodilator effect so that sweating is almost always accompanied by marked vasodilatation. There may be other substances, so-called 'co-transmitters' like vasoactive intestinal peptide (VIP) or adenosine triphosphate (ATP), liberated from sympathetic nerve endings at the same time as the normal neurotransmitters (noradrenaline and acetylcholine), which can cause vasodilatation. There are even substances released from the endothelial cells of blood vessels ('endothelial relaxing factor') which can mediate vasodilatation. However, the most important factor in producing thermoregulatory vasodilatation is a reduction of sympathetic vasoconstrictor tone.

Local factors can mediate vasodilatation or vasoconstriction. Hypoxia or hypercapnia due to tissue activity cause vasodilatation and are important factors in muscles, though of only limited importance in the skin. Local temperature has a very important effect: cooling causes vasoconstriction and heating causes vasodilatation. This effect is clearly demonstrated by immersing the hand or foot in a hot or cold bath. A very clear line of demarcation is seen on the skin between the normal part and the part where constriction or dilatation has taken place. The effect of local heating or cooling can also be shown in isolated blood vessels *in vitro*, which have been removed from all influences of sympathetic nerves.

If the skin is exposed to low temperatures the blood vessels constrict, but below about 5–8°C there is often a secondary or paradoxical vasodilatation which can cause skin temperature to fluctuate cyclically: the so-called 'hunting' reaction of Lewis (*Figure 17.4*). The explanation is probably that although cold provokes vasoconstriction, either reflexly or directly, the low temperature paralyses the contractile mechanisms in vascular smooth muscle and the blood vessels relax. The relaxation allows a little blood to flow, warming the smooth muscle cells enough to allow them to constrict again; then they cool and become paralysed again, and so on. Other explanations postulate the presence of 'axon' reflexes or the release of vasoactive substances from the tissues. The evidence for these is far from clear.

There are some other common patterns of cold-induced vasodilatation, apart from the classical 'hunting' type. In some cases the vessels dilate and remain dilated, with no return of vascular tone until

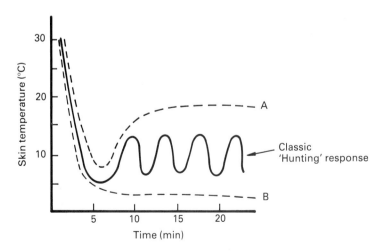

Figure 17.4 Cold-induced vasodilatation (CIVD), Illustrative responses of a finger or toe to immersion in water at around 0°C. Solid line: typical oscillatory or 'hunting' reaction. Dotted lines: A, plateau type of CIVD; B, no CIVD.

the body is warmed. In others no vasodilatation takes place. The ability of an individual to resist cold injury from frostbite or immersion foot can be predicted from his pattern of cold-induced vascular response, as cold vasodilatation protects the extremities from excessive cooling at the expense of some loss of heat from the core.

Cutaneous vasoconstriction or vasodilatation mediated by sympathetic nerves can easily be elicited by cooling or warming the core. They can also be produced by cooling or heating the skin, either near the site of measurement or at a remote site such as the opposite limb. Thus information from both central and peripheral thermoreceptors can initiate the vascular reflexes, and the interaction between these pathways can be quite complex.

The effect of vasoconstriction or vasodilatation is primarily to decrease or increase the thermal conductance of the tissues. The blood flow through skin can vary over a range from 10 to 1000 ml/kg/min; unperfused skin and subcutaneous tissue have about the same conductance as cork, but as blood flow increases the conductance can increase up to four times. Vasoconstricted skin has approximately the same temperature as the environment, while maximally vasodilated skin has a temperature close to that of the core.

The rate of heat loss to the environment depends upon the temperature gradient and conductance between core and skin, and between skin and environment (*Figure 17.5*). If the vessels are constricted in the cold, the gradient between core and skin is large but the conductance is low and little heat reaches the skin; the gradient between skin and environment is usually small and little heat escapes. If the vessels dilate when the body is hot, the gradient between core and skin is small but the conductance is high, so heat is readily transferred to the skin. If there is a large gradient between skin and environment then heat is readily lost, but if the environmental temperature is higher than about 35°C then the gradient virtually disappears and vasodilatation becomes ineffective as a means of heat loss.

The changes in peripheral blood vessels caused by thermoregulatory reflexes can have important effects on the rest of the circulation. Massive cutaneous vasodilatation lowers the total peripheral resistance, and this requires a compensatory rise in cardiac output if arterial blood pressure is to be maintained. The heart rate rises in the heat, and there is also a constriction of visceral blood vessels in an attempt to increase total vascular resistance. If the subject is at rest his muscle blood vessels may also constrict, but if he is exercising then his muscle arterioles will be dilated and the load on the cardiovascular system will be compounded. If cardiac output cannot be maintained, the subject feels dizzy and may faint (heat syncope); falling to

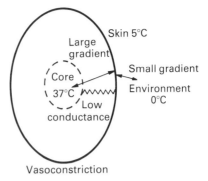

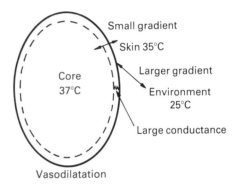

Figure 17.5 Size of core and shell, and temperature gradients in a vasoconstricted body in the cold, and a vasodilated body in a warm environment.

the floor and adopting the recumbent posture is a very effective way of restoring the blood flow to the brain.

During body cooling the peripheral blood vessels constrict, which tends to raise the arterial blood pressure ('cold pressor response'); there is often a compensatory fall in heart rate, but if shivering occurs the circulatory requirements of the muscles increase and the heart rate rises again. The increase in blood flow to the muscles during shivering or exercise reduces the effectiveness of cutaneous vasoconstriction in maintaining heat in the core, and the extra heat loss that results may offset any heat gain due to the muscular activity.

Mechanisms for heat production

The resting metabolism of a human adult produces about 100 W of heat, which is usually in equilibrium with the rate of heat loss. During exercise the heat production can increase to 1–2 kW as a result of increased energy utilization by the muscles and the cardiovascular system. Heat production can also be increased by muscular activity which performs no external work; there may simply be a general increase in tone of all muscle groups, or there may be rhythmic small-amplitude contraction and relaxation of muscle groups (shivering) causing shaking but little overt movement. The maximum heat production during shivering is usually about 500 W.

Shivering can be initiated by a fall in core temperature but also occurs as soon as the body is exposed to cold conditions, before any change in deep body temperature has occurred. In other words, it can be caused by stimulation of skin thermoreceptors. The interaction between core temperature, skin temperature and the respective rates of change are quite complex. Furthermore, shivering occurs in waves which wax and wane during a period of cold exposure; little is known about the drives controlling these variations in activity.

Heat can be produced by increasing the metabolism in organs other than muscle; this is known as non-shivering thermogenesis. The liver is one of the most metabolically active organs, and the rate of breakdown of liver glycogen is increased by circulating adrenaline, so that in cold stress a little extra heat may be derived from this source. The hormones of the thyroid gland raise the metabolic rates of all tissues, and hyperthyroid patients produce excessive heat, but there seems to be little role for the thyroid gland in the extra heat production required for thermoregulation. One of the most important sources of extra metabolic heat in young animals, especially rodents, but also in babies and young children, is brown fat. This specialized adipose tissue is capable of breaking down fat molecules rapidly under the influence of adrenaline or noradrenaline to produce large amounts of heat. Along with the other methods of non-shivering thermogenesis it is of little importance in adult man.

Sweating and its control

The skin contains some 3–4 million sweat glands, with a total mass of 100 g (about the same as one kidney). The apocrine glands of the axilla and groin secrete an oily substance and take no part in thermoregulation. The eccrine glands of the rest of the skin secrete a watery fluid whose evaporation is an extremely effective mechanism for heat loss.

The eccrine glands have a coiled basal secretory portion and a tubular duct which leads to the skin. The secretion is under the control of sympathetic nerves which release acetylcholine as their neurotransmitter. The rate of sweat secretion can be altered by varying the number of sweat glands recruited, by varying the impulse frequency in individual nerves and therefore the rate of secretion of each sweat gland, or by a combination of both.

The fluid secreted by the coiled basal portion of the gland is approximately isotonic with plasma. It is not, however, simply an ultrafiltrate of plasma; there is some active transport of ions and the input of metabolic energy to the secretory process. As the sweat passes up the duct there is active reabsorption of sodium so that the fluid appearing at the surface may be hypotonic; this reabsorption requires time, and as the sweat rate increases the secretion spends less time in the ducts so the opportunity for reabsorption is reduced. At high sweat rates the emerging sweat is nearly isotonic with plasma, so that salt losses are disproportionately higher when sweating is higher.

Sweating is initiated by a rise in core temperature, but can also be caused by heating the skin. It also occurs in response to emotional stimuli such as pain or anxiety. This type of sweating has formed the basis of 'lie-detector' tests since the presence of salty water on the skin reduces its electrical resistance. Sweating occurs at many levels of skin temperature, but when skin temperature is greater than 35°C the evaporation of sweat is the *only* mechanism available for the removal of excess heat from the body.

When the sweat glands are inactive there is still a small loss of fluid from the skin; about 500 ml per day is lost as insensible perspiration. The maximal rate of sweating can be as high as 2 l/hour, though this rate cannot be sustained for long. A more realistic sweat rate is around 1 l/hour, and the evaporation of 1 l of sweat removes about 2.5 MJ of heat. This level of sweating is only useful, of course, if it is allowed to evaporate and does not become trapped under or within the clothing.

Sweating can cause dehydration. The body's thirst mechanism is relatively insensitive, and loss of 1–2% of body weight can occur without symptoms. If the total water content is reduced by 4–5% there is intense thirst, scanty urine and a decrease in blood volume which causes tachycardia. If the water loss reaches 7–10% there is marked impairment of physical and mental capacity with eventual circulatory failure, coma and death.

Treatment for severe depletion of fluid comprises removal of the victim from the hot environment, cessation of activity and enthusiastic rehydration. An intake of 6–8 l water may be necessary in the first 24 hours. The condition is easily prevented by supplying adequate quantities of drinking water together with thorough indoctrination of personnel in the risks of dehydration and the importance of drinking even when they do not feel thirsty.

At high sweat rates the loss of salt is high, and despite the fact that most Western diets contain adequate or excessive amounts of salt one occasionally encounters victims of salt depletion. It most often occurs when sweating has been profuse and the victim has drunk a large volume of water, so diluting his plasma. Since a normal sodium concentration is essential for nerve and muscle function, the salt-depleted individual complains of fatigue, cramps and giddiness. There may be nausea and vomiting, with further loss of water and salt and inability to re-hydrate. This vicious circle can lead to progressive hypovolaemia, circulatory failure and death. The condition can be prevented by provision of adequate salt and encouragement to take it; in the short term any excess will be excreted by the kidneys.

Central control

The seat of thermoregulatory control appears to be in the hypothalamus: not in the anterior or pre-optic areas where the central thermoreceptors lie, but in the posterior hypothalamus. The latter is not sensitive to direct heating or cooling, but electrical stimulation of neurones in this region can produce autonomic thermoregulatory responses, and thermal stimulation of skin or anterior hypothalamus can produce discharge from posterior hypothalamic neurones.

What is the controlled variable? Many would suggest that it is the core temperature which the body attempts to hold constant at all costs, though several of the effector mechanisms are switched on by changes in skin temperature, and others are influenced by rates of change rather than absolute values of temperature. While the simple model shown in *Figure 17.1* gives an overview of the system, it is inadequate to explain all of the features of thermoregulation. No group of neurones has been detected which has the function of a temperature reference, and indeed several observers have denied the existence of a 'set point' for core temperature. Some have postulated that the variable that is being regulated is the total heat content of the body, or the total heat flux across the skin, but it is difficult to understand how such variables can be detected when only central and cutaneous thermoreceptors have been found; there are no known sensors for muscle temperature, and none for thermal gradients across the skin, which would be necessary to detect heat fluxes.

It has been pointed out that the 'set point' of core temperature (if it exists) is not set, in that the normal body temperature fluctuates in a circadian manner and with the menstrual cycle. (However, this behaviour could be explained on the basis of a cyclically varying set point.) It has also been pointed out that during exercise, as heat production increases, the core temperature rises until a new equilibrium is reached where heat loss just balances heat production although the body's total heat content is increased. The existence of thermal

equilibrium at a new steady core temperature has been cited as evidence against a fixed set point. We should note, however, that during the whole period of exercise the body makes full use of its thermoregulatory pathways, and vasodilatation and sweating both proceed at a high rate. This is in contrast to the responses in fever; here the body performs intense heat conservation manoeuvres such as shivering and vasoconstriction during the onset of fever, and then when the new plateau of temperature is reached the activity of the compensatory mechanisms decreases to a level just adequate to maintain a constant temperature. It is not until the recovery phase of the fever, when core temperature is falling, that intense activity of the compensatory mechanisms occurs again, and the patient sweats and vasodilates.

In the hyperthermia of exercise, the body tries but fails to regulate temperature; in fever the body thermoregulates very successfully at its new level of core temperature (*Figure 17.6*). These phenomena are arguments for, rather than against, the concept of a set point.

There are many parallel input pathways, and many alternative effector pathways for thermoregulation. Each effector mechanism may have different and independent thresholds of temperature for its activation, and it is debatable whether one can have a single unifying control centre for the whole system. We could postulate an alternative model

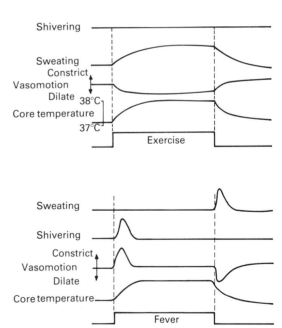

Figure 17.6 Thermoregulatory responses during exercise, and during fever. Note that heat loss mechanisms are maximal throughout exercise, but major regulatory responses in fever occur only at the onset and start of recovery.

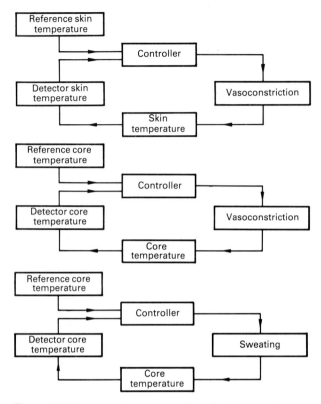

Figure 17.7 Thermoregulatory control described in terms of multiple independent loops. Only a few loops are illustrated; the existence of a large number of additional loops must be postulated.

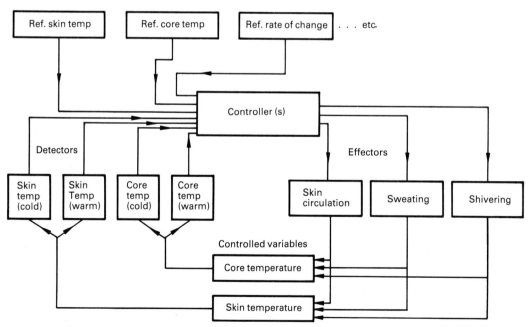

Figure 17.8 Thermoregulatory control expressed as the integration of multiple parallel input and output pathways.

(*Figure 17.7*) in which a number of independent loops occur, one for sweating, one for vascular reactions, another for shivering and so on. There is some evidence for this; cutaneous warm receptors can produce direct effects on the vasodilator control area of the medulla without the intervention of the hypothalamus, whereas cold receptors require the mediation of the hypothalamic centres in order to activate the centre for shivering or the pressor area of the medulla which causes vasoconstriction.

The model with multiple independent loops is probably also inadequate to explain all of the phenomena, as several inputs can interact to influence one effector pathway, while several effector pathways can be affected by a single input channel. A more realistic model may be one with several parallel inputs, several set points and several parallel outputs (*Figure 17.8*). It should be pointed out that all models are merely attempts to understand and explain the system as it exists; the body is not required to conform to any of the cybernetic schemata which we attempt to impose upon it.

Modifications to physiological mechanisms

There are a number of ways in which the physiological responses to thermal stimuli may be modified artificially. Many of these are behavioural. If we are too hot in the sun we can move and sit in the shade or swim in the water; if we are too cold we can swing our arms or take other vigorous exercise, or curl up into a ball to reduce surface area, or move to a place which is warmer. We can use technology to provide a more comfortable artifical environment, building houses, lighting fires or operating air conditioning systems to produce the desired temperature. We can arrange for forced convection to increase heat loss, by manual or automatic fanning of the air.

Another major behavioural mechanism is the wearing of clothes. It provides additional layers of insulation between the skin and the environment; the body's responses are now directed towards exchanging heat between the skin and the microenvironment which exists under the clothing, rather than the external environment. The exchanges between the clothed body and the environment are considered in more detail in Chapter 16.

There is often a conflict between the need to wear clothes as a protection against one type of hazard and the effect that this has on other body systems. Thus the clothes that are donned as a protection against cold or immersion in water may make the wearer very uncomfortable when he exercises in air, and clothing designed to protect against chemicals, infection or the effects of gravitational or hypoxic stress may imposes an additional heat stress upon the body by conferring unwanted insulation.

Some problems with thermoregulation

Heat stress

The thermoregulatory responses to exercise, when the body's rate of intrinsic heat production is increased, have already been discussed. When an extrinsic heat load is imposed upon the body, as when the environmental temperature is high or when the insulation around the body is increased so that heat is lost less easily, there is vasodilatation and sweating. If the normal physiological responses fail to prevent a rise in core temperature, their intensity of action often increases to the point where they can cause serious disturbances in the rest of the body. The effects of massive cutaneous vasodilatation in producing heat syncope and the dehydration and salt depletion produced by excessive sweating have already been mentioned.

As well as disorders arising from excessive action of the normal thermoregulatory mechanisms, there are heat illnesses due to failure of these mechanisms. The most important is failure of sweating. With prolonged exposure to high heat loads (core temperature above about 40.5°C) the sweat glands suddenly stop functioning, for reasons that are poorly understood. The core temperature begins to rise uncontrollably; there may be prodromal symptoms such as headache, dizziness, numbness or drowsiness, or the victim may become restless, uncoordinated, aggressive or confused. There may be a gradual slipping into delirium and coma, or these may occur suddenly without any prodromal signs, and there may be convulsions, incontinence and cardiovascular collapse. This condition is termed heat stroke.

It is essential to reduce the victim's temperature quickly; it should be brought below 39°C within the first hour. There are several effective ways of achieving this, including cold sprays, immersion in cold water and fanning. Too much cooling of the skin may be counter-productive if vasoconstriction and shivering are stimulated; forced convection with warm air is one of the most effective techniques (some victims have been placed in the down-draught of a stationary helicopter!), and spraying with luke-warm water together with vigorous fanning is also useful.

Cardiovascular support and oxygen therapy may be necessary, together with the routine care of very ill or unconscious patients. A careful assessment must be made of the state of hydration, with vigorous re-hydration if necessary.

Cold stress

In a cold environment the body recruits heat conservation and heat production mechanisms; if these fail to maintain the core temperature, in other words if heat production is less than heat loss, then *hypothermia* occurs. Most of the consequences of hypothermia can be explained by the reduced metabolism of critical tissues and organs at lower temperatures.

The ionic pumps at cell membranes are very sensitive to cooling and if their activity is reduced the transmembrane ionic gradients run down. This results in an increase in plasma potassium and an increase in cellular sodium; the cells of the nervous system and muscles become depolarized and as a consequence become more excitable. These changes cause the increased irritability of the myocardium, which develops arrhythmias, and the nervous system which can develop convulsions. Other consequences of brain malfunction include abnormalities in respiration and clouding of consciousness.

While the membranes may be excessively excitable, the contractility of heart and muscles is decreased, and the effectiveness of their function is impaired. Liver and kidney function are also impaired at low temperatures, so that the homeostatic actions of these organs are lost and chemical disarray occurs in the blood.

At low temperatures the peripheral parts of the body can suffer injury and damage even when the core temperature is maintained; the body will sacrifice the peripheries in order to preserve the core. During intense vasoconstriction the peripheral tissues cool very close to the environmental temperature, though they may be spared from damage if there is effective cold-induced vasodilatation. If the temperature falls below the freezing point of skin (about −1.5°C) then frostnip (reversible freezing with no permanent damage) or frostbite (actual damage due to tissue freezing) will occur. Even at temperatures well above freezing the prolonged cooling of peripheries can cause damage, known variously as non-freezing cold injury, immersion foot and trench foot (though the lesions are not necessarily confined to the feet, and one subject suffered injury to the buttock through sitting on the floor of an inflatable dinghy floating in water at 5°C).

The tissue damage caused by freezing is easy to understand. The lesions of non-freezing injury are less easy to explain, and are confined largely to the peripheral nerves. In the simplest cases there is some reversible sensory and motor loss due to degeneration of large myelinated nerves. In more severe cases there is damage to autonomic nerves; on rescue from the exposure to cold the limb appears lifeless and bloodless due to intense vasoconstriction, but on rewarming there is an intense painful vasodilatation and swelling: the limb is effectively sympathectomized. This phase may last for some weeks or months. It is followed by a long phase, possibly lasting for the rest of the victim's life, in which the affected limb is abnormally sensitive to cold, developing painful prolonged vasospasm rather like Raynaud's phenomenon. There may also be hyperhydrosis. The findings are rather difficult to explain, but may represent an incorrect re-innervation of autonomic structures or a state of denervation hypersensitivity.

Acclimatization

It is important to distinguish between acclimatization and acclimation. The untreated person or animal who has not previously been exposed to a particular set of environmental conditions has nevertheless a set of built-in physiological responses which equip the individual to compensate for environmental change such as heating, hypoxia or some other stress. If the subject is repeatedly or chronically exposed, in the laboratory, to an environment which is altered in one particular, such as temperature, then any modification in his physiological responses to the stress is known as *acclimation*; if the individual goes to live in an area where the natural environment is different, and may of course differ in more than one particular, such as temperature and altitude, then the physiological changes are known as *acclimatization*. Acclimation refers to experimental, and acclimatization to natural changes.

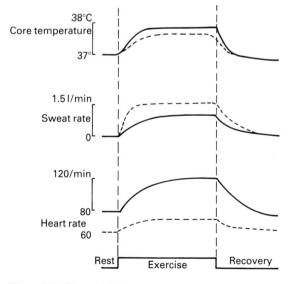

Figure 17.9 Physiological responses to exercise in the heat, in unfit or unacclimatized subjects (solid lines) and in trained or acclimatized subjects (broken lines).

If a person moves from a temperate to a hot region, the first few days are full of discomfort. The individual feels very hot, the heart rate is high even at rest, the exercise tolerance is diminished and there is intense lethargy. After a few days the tolerance of the warm environment is greatly increased, the resting heart rate is lower, and the ability to exercise is improved. The person is not so lethargic, and feels more comfortable.

The response to exercise in the heart is particularly interesting; over a period of about a week the heart rate response to exercise decreases, so that both the resting and the peak heart rate are lower. The amount by which the core temperature rises during exercise becomes less; this is probably explained by an enormous increase in the sweat rate, which is the key to the whole phenomenon of heat acclimatization. The capacity of the sweat glands to produce sweat increases, and sweating is initiated at a lower threshold core temperature than in the unacclimatized subject *Figure 17.9*. The precise mechanisms whereby these changes occur are uncertain, but the change in sweating threshold is probably due to changes in the nervous processing of thermal stimuli; the increase in sweat rate may be partly due to a neural change but also involves an improvement in the secretory performance of the sweat glands themselves.

As well as the increase in sweat rate, there is an increase in the secretion of aldosterone by the adrenal cortex. This hormone aids in the conservation of sodium by the kidney in the face of enormous losses in the sweat, and also slightly decreases the concentration of sodium in the sweat, although with the higher sweat rate the total loss of sodium in the sweat is still considerable.

Acclimatization can be achieved by moving to and working in a hot country; a similar degree of artificial acclimation can be achieved in the laboratory by raising the core temperature to more than 38°C for 1 hour daily for about a week. This can be achieved by exercising at a moderate rate, preferably while wearing a vapour barrier suit (to reduce evaporative heat loss and thus raise the temperature more effectively); it can also be achieved by immersion in a bath of hot water at 41°C for an hour daily for a week.

The changes of heat acclimatization or acclimation have a number of similarities to fitness training; indeed, as exercise during training always raises core temperature there must be an element of heat acclimation during training. However, the reverse does not apply: heat acclimatization by itself does *not* increase fitness!

There is no conclusive evidence for cold acclimatization in humans, though many animals can acclimatize to the cold by increasing their utilization of brown fat or growing extra fur or changing the colour of their fur or feathers. Many human populations living in cold climates, and even explorers going to polar regions are often acclimatized to heat rather than cold, as they wear many layers of warm clothes or live in very warm houses or igloos, and seldom encounter the cold of their environment.

Some groups such as the Ainu women divers of Korea, the bushmen of the Kalahari desert and some Australian aboriginal tribes who are habitually exposed to very low temperatures, seem to demonstrate a certain degree of adaptation. They allow their core temperatures to fall to a level which would switch on vigorous thermoregulatory activity such as shivering in 'normal' people. It is uncertain whether this ability to become cold without shivering is an advantage or a disadvantage, but it is not a response that occurs in a short period of acclimatization.

Repeated exposure to cold usually produces no discernible change in the physiological responses; there is no change in the thresholds for vasoconstriction or shivering, though the subjective ability to tolerate the discomfort of cold peripheries or even a cold core is increased.

Simulation of thermoregulation

Thermal physiologists and their engineering colleagues have made a number of attempts to construct models of the human thermoregulatory system. Some of these have been more or less realistic dummies or manikins, shaped like the human body and constructed of materials with similar thermal properties, and endowed with heat sources and regulatory circuits. Some of the physical models have consisted of simple cylinders of water, and these have often given as valuable information as the more complex models. They are often used to test a very limited range of phenomena, to give a simple answer to a particular question.

In general the thermoregulatory system is too complex to allow the production of a truly realistic manikin; the components can be simulated much more easily in mathematical or computer models. Several early models made use of analogue computers, in which voltages represented temperature, resistances represented insulation, and currents represented heat flux, but with the advent and widespread availability of the digital computer most recent models have relied heavily on the solution of large series of complicated equations using digital numerical techniques.

Some of the computer simulations rely on the empirical approach: a large number of observations are made in actual experiments, and then the data are examined to find the mathematical relationship which best fits the data. The users of such an approach need make no assumptions about the physical laws regulating the system; they simply produce an equation that can be used to predict future behaviour given a particular set of environmental circumstances.

The alternative approach is to start with the physical principles of heat flow and to construct a set of equations based on known physical laws to predict what will happen to the heat content of the body. This is intellectually more satisfying than the empirical approach, but has limitations, because no physical laws are able to predict how the onset of sweating could be regulated by a combination of skin and core temperature, or how shivering would be controlled. Inevitably the constructor of models from first principles has to make use of empirical relationships to describe these variables, so even the most 'pure' of scientific models has to have some empirical components incorporated.

The aim of all the simulations of thermoregulation is to predict the body's thermal behaviour. These predictions have to be validated against experiments on real human beings, but hopefully once the validation is complete, the models can be used with confidence to save the scientist the inconvenience and his subjects the discomfort of performing experiments to test every possible set of environmental circumstances.

Further reading

CLARK, R.P. and EDHOLM, O.G. (1985) *Man and His Thermal Environment*. London: Arnold

EDHOLM, O.G. (1978) *Man—Hot and Cold*. London: Arnold

HENSEL, H. (1981) *Thermoreception and Temperature Regulation*. Monographs of the Physiological Society. London: Academic Press

KERSLAKE, D. MCK. (1972) *The Stress of Hot Environments*. Monographs of the Physiological Society. London: Arnold

STAINER, M.W., MOUNT, L.E. and BLIGH, J. (1984) *Energy Balance and Temperature Regulation*. Cambridge University Press

18

Thermal protection

J.R. Allan

Introduction

Before considering the methods available for protecting aircrew from thermal stresses within their aircraft, it is important to discuss some general measures which can be highly effective in limiting thermally stressful exposures prior to aircraft entry.

The use of buildings

The design and siting of buildings used by aircrew can be important in limiting thermal stress. Even the simplest will provide protection against overhead solar radiation, wind chill and precipitation. They may be equipped with air conditioning systems to provide comfortable conditions at both extremes of environmental temperature. They should be designed and sited so as to limit the amount of physical exertion in walking from room to room, and from the building to the aircraft.

Transport

The judicious use of motor transport can limit both the physical effort and thermal exposure involved in moving from aircrew buildings to aircraft. This is especially important when aircraft are widely dispersed on large airfields, and when aircrew are wearing complicated flying clothing assemblies such as are used for chemical defence.

Aircraft shelters

These are primarily to protect from air or missile attack. They also limit thermal exposures by providing a shield against solar radiation and wind chill and limiting the degree of hot or cold soak of the aircraft prior to aircrew entry and during periods of cockpit standby. The massive thick concrete construction of these shelters has the effect of damping out the usual diurnal variations in temperature so that conditions inside are often cooler than outside during the heat of the day and vice versa at night.

Sun shades and thermal blankets

When aircraft are parked in the open, these simple devices can do much to limit aircraft heating during 'hot soak' conditions. Sun shades specifically designed to cover transparencies are highly effective and their use should be encouraged (*Figure 18.1*). Thermal blankets, large quilted insulating jackets designed to cover that part of the aircraft fuselage occupied by the crew, are also effective but more cumbersome to apply and remove.

Cabin environmental control systems

Environmental control systems, backed up by ground conditioning equipment when required, are the principal means for controlling the internal aircraft environment. Thermal control of the pilot's environment is not, however, their only function: for example, they also provide cabin pressurization, avionic equipment cooling, transparency demisting, rain removal and wing sealing. From the engineer's viewpoint some of these additional functions, particularly avionic equipment cooling, are highly important and have often led to design compromises disadvantageous to the pilot.

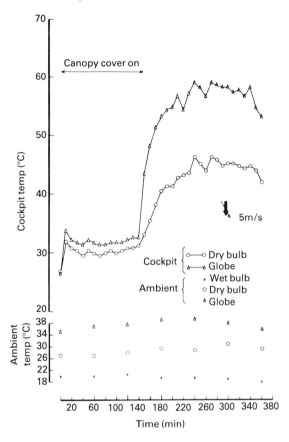

Figure 18.1 Cockpit temperatures during standby in full solar radiation. Note the dramatic rise in globe and dry bulb temperature when the sunshade (canopy cover) is removed. The direction of the wind relative to the aircraft is indicated by the arrows.

Specifications for cabin environmental control

Most current specifications for military aircraft are inadequate with regard to required thermal conditions for the aircrew. They suffer particularly from an almost total disregard for the important influence of radiant heating, particularly solar radiation, and they do not cater for the complex clothing assemblies worn by the aircrew.

Until more is known of the effect of thermal stress on pilot performance, it is unwise to accept any departure from comfortable conditions. One practical approach is to specify that conditions should be such as to maintain a pilot's mean skin temperature close to 33°C. To relate this to the specification of the environmental control system, Hughes (1968) devised a practical means of calculation. The method takes into account the various heat inputs to the cockpit, and also those variables related to the

crew (work rate, clothing insulation, etc.) which affect comfort. The result is a series of design curves which give the required mass flow and cabin inlet air temperature to achieve thermal comfort, defined as a mean skin temperature of 33°C. This approach is thoroughly recommended. In practice the aircraft design team should calculate the cockpit conditions surrounding the pilot for a range of flight conditions—altitude, speed, power setting and ambient environment. The calculations should also be made for taxiing and ground stand-by. Only in this way can a cockpit thermal profile be developed for typical operational sorties. Conditions usually change rapidly over time and it is important not only to assess the overall temperature profile but also to consider the likely impact of transient severe conditions against their magnitude and duration.

Principles of environmental control systems

Figure 18.2 shows a typical environmental control system. High-temperature, high-pressure air is tapped from the engine compressors and cooled initially by being passed through a primary heat exchanger. Here heat is exchanged between the very hot engine air, at perhaps 500°C, and the relatively cold ambient air from outside. The air passes next to the heart of the system which is known as the cold air unit (CAU).

Figure 18.3 is a diagram of a cold air unit. The device consists of a shaft with a compressor mounted on one end and a turbine on the other. When air is driven through the turbine it rotates at high speed and drives the compressor mounted on the same shaft. High-pressure air at high temperature arrives at the compressor from the primary heat exchanger. It is then further compressed, which raises both its pressure and temperature, before being passed through a secondary heat exchanger or intercooler. In the intercooler heat is again exchanged with ambient air, the process being more effective because of the high temperature gradient generated by the work of the compressor. Next the air passes through the turbine. Within the turbine the air expands and this alone would produce a fall in temperature in accordance with the gas laws. However, by causing the air to drive the turbine during expansion, some of the stored energy in the air is converted to work done by the turbine. This greatly enhances the fall in temperature achieved across the turbine. Indeed the greater part of the total fall in temperature is attributable to the conversion of heat energy into work and only a small proportion is due to expansion. A controlled bypass system enables a proportion of hot air to short-circuit the cold air unit and then mix with the colder

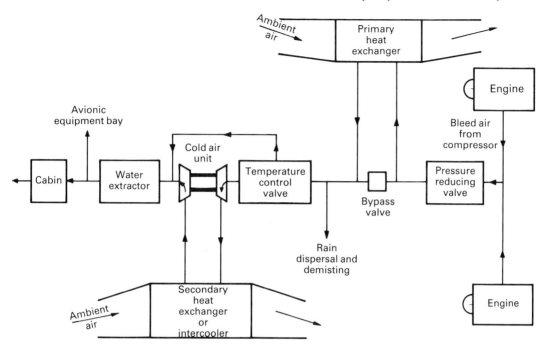

Figure 18.2 A diagram of a typical environmental control system.

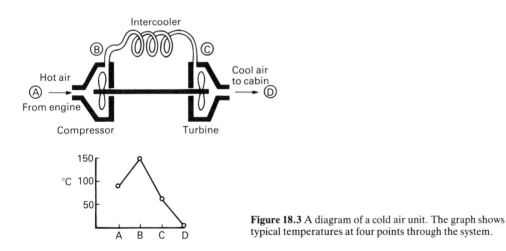

Figure 18.3 A diagram of a cold air unit. The graph shows typical temperatures at four points through the system.

air downstream so as to provide temperature control. During the cooling process much of the water vapour in the air condenses out into droplet form and this is removed by centrifugal action in the water separator.

Figure 18.4 is a simple diagram to show how the various components of the environmental control system are arranged in an actual aircraft.

Distribution ductwork and outlets

In determining the mass flow and temperature requirements for cabin cooling air, the design of the distribution system downstream of the cold air unit is vital. A poor distribution system makes inefficient use of available cold air. In the past it has generally not been possible to produce a mean environmental

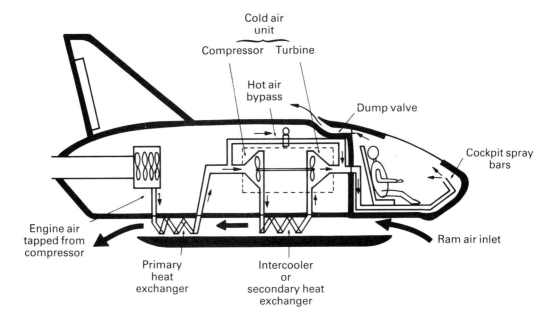

Figure 18.4 Diagram (not to scale) to show arrangement of main components of an environmental control system.

temperature immediately surrounding the pilot that is lower than about the cabin outlet temperature. Thus if inlet temperature is, say, 10°C and outlet temperature 30°C, the mean temperature surrounding the pilot is in the region of 30°C. Careful design of the distribution system can reduce this temperature to a point approximately three-quarters of the gradient from inlet to outlet temperature, that is nearer 25°C in the quoted example.

The distribution system should be designed to produce the maximum cooling in the area immediately surrounding the pilot. This is achieved by careful positioning of the air outlets and by the use of nozzle outlets specially designed to reduce air entrainment. The latter is a feature of poor nozzle design in which warm cabin air is drawn into the outlet cold air jet immediately downstream of the nozzle, and substantially downgrades the quality of cooling air reaching the pilot. The system should also allow personal adjustment by the pilot, particularly with regard to face ventilation.

Insulation

The contribution of high aircraft skin temperature to cockpit thermal stress has already been mentioned. Clearly this can be reduced by careful attention to insulation of the cockpit walls from the cabin air with reduction in both the convective and radiative inputs to the cockpit. It is also important to insulate the distributive ductwork between the cold air unit

and the outlets to reduce the heat input to the cabin cold air supply before it reaches the pilot.

Noise

Cabin conditioning systems can be important contributors to cockpit noise. Careful design can reduce noise generation and transmission in ductwork and outlets.

Water

As a result of the substantial temperature drop across the cold air unit, considerable quantities of water are condensed out of the cabin air supply either as water droplets or ice. Without an adequate system for removal, these droplets or particles of ice can be carried through the distributive ductwork and be blown on to the pilot. This is a common occurrence in several existing aircraft. Even if this does not happen, a lack of effective water separation will lead to reabsorption in the ductwork and a rise in humidity of the cabin air supply.

Design limitations

The high demands for cooling air both for maintaining pilot comfort and for avionic cooling in modern military aircraft present problems to the aircraft designer. The extent of air bleed from engine compressors can have important effects on engine thrust performance and it is not unknown for environmental control systems to be turned off to maintain thrust for high all-up weight take-off. The increasing complexity and insulation of modern aircrew protective clothing systems also provides an increasing barrier to heat exchange with the cockpit air and attempts to solve the problem by further lowering of cockpit temperatures are less and less cost effective. This has led to an increasing interest in personal conditioning for the crew and in alternative means for avionic cooling. The development of liquid cooling systems for both these purposes has proceeded apace.

Ground conditioning equipment

Environmental control systems do not function until the engines are running. Yet the pre-flight period, including any period of cockpit readiness, is probably the most thermally stressful part of a sortie, particularly if the aircraft is parked in direct sunshine. In the absence of an engine-independent personal conditioning system (*see* below), or effective auxiliary power units giving sufficient tapped air to operate the environmental control system, the only practical method for alleviating thermal stress prior to flight is to use ground cooling equipment. This usually takes the form of a large cooling trolley. The cold air from the trolley is piped into the cockpit via specially designed ground connectors. When available, this equipment can be highly effective, although its use increases the work of groundcrew and can present logistic problems. When military aircraft are operated from dispersed airfields, the amount of back-up equipment is usually strictly limited. Heating trolleys can be used in much the same way as cooling trolleys.

Clothing for cold conditions

General principles

The central principle in the design of cold protective clothing assemblies is the provision of clothing insulation (*see* Chapter 16). Additional important attributes are the exclusion of wind and rain in open climate situations and the exclusion of water during water immersion following abandonments over the sea or inland lakes.

Cold weather clothing assemblies are best designed with multiple layers, since this gives additional trapped air between layers and also versatility in

that layers can be added or subtracted to cope with different work rates, or varying environmental conditions. Another practical principle in design is to employ a thick, open-weave undergarment as the innermost layer. When outer layers are sealed at the neck, wrists and ankles, considerable quantities of air are trapped. During physical work these closures can be released to allow free circulation of air through the spaces aided by the bellows action of physical movement. This is known as the Brynje principle.

Wind and waterproofing layers

Clothing insulation is greatly reduced by either wind or water penetration. An external windproof layer is therefore essential for cold protection in windy conditions. Generally this external layer also serves to keep out rain. Nowadays increasing use is made of so-called 'breathable' fabrics which allow the transmission of water vapour but are nevertheless waterproof to droplet water.

A particular cold hazard facing aircrew is water immersion following abandonments over the sea.

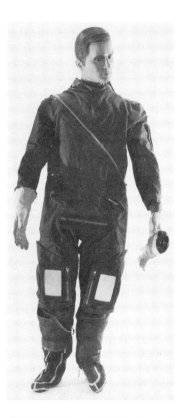

Figure 18.5 A ventile fabric immersion coverall fitted with socks and rubber seals at wrists and neck.

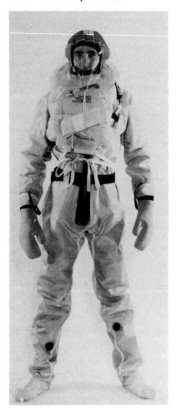

Figure 18.6 A helicopter passenger immersion suit.

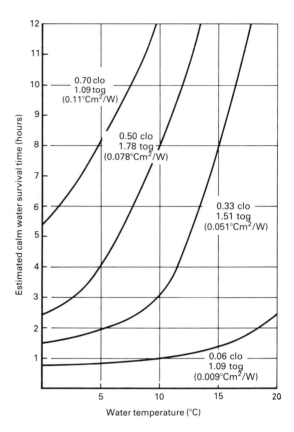

0.70 clo
1.09 tog
(0.11°Cm²/W)

0.50 clo
1.78 tog
(0.078°Cm²/W)

0.33 clo
1.51 tog
(0.051°Cm²/W)

0.06 clo
1.09 tog
(0.009°Cm²/W)

Estimated calm water survival time (hours)

Water temperature (°C)

Figure 18.7 A graph showing predicted survival time against sea temperature for four levels of immersed clothing insulation. The survival time is based on model predictions of the time taken for core temperature to fall to 34°C and the curves are drawn for thin subjects with a 10th percentile mean skinfold thickness.

Water penetration of a clothing system has disastrous effects on clothing insulation (*see* Chapter 16) and death from hypothermia is a real possibility even when rescue responses are relatively quick. The only effective protection is a waterproof immersion suit. The most acceptable type—and none is comfortable—is that made from a ventile fabric. These ventile fabrics allow a degree of air penetration when dry, which facilitates the removal of insensible perspiration and sweat, but the fibres swell when in contact with water and form a waterproof layer. *Figure 18.5* illustrates a ventile immersion suit and shows the rubber seals used at the neck and wrists and also the waterproof socks generally worn in conjunction with these suits. *Figure 18.6* shows a typical immersion suit designed for use by helicopter passengers. Immersion suits do not provide much insulation by themselves but, by excluding water, serve to preserve the insulation of the clothing worn beneath. The total insulation achieved may thus be varied over a wide range by selecting appropriate garments for wear beneath the immersion suit.

Mathematical modelling techniques have enabled the development of predictive curves relating likely survival times to sea temperature and clothing insulation as shown in *Figure 18.7*. A table of clothing insulation for various items of aircrew clothing can be provided, such as the one shown in *Table 18.1* and used in conjunction with *Figure 18.7* to determine an appropriate assembly for given conditions of sea temperature and likely rescue time.

Heads, hands and feet

Heads, hands and feet present special problems in cold protection.

Heat loss from the head can exceed half the metabolic heat production. Aircrew generally wear protective flying helmets, but these may be lost when an aircraft is abandoned. Survival kits should contain additional head protection. For arctic operations, clothing for outside use should include head protection. Anorak or Parka hoods should project well forward of the face, and possess a

Table 18.1 Immersed insulation levels given by various aircrew clothing assemblies. Used with *Figure 18.7*, this allows the correct clothing to be selected for given survival conditions

	Aircrew clothing assembly	Immersed insulation (togs)
No immersion coverall	A Jockey underpants. Aircrew shirt cotton olive drab Mk2. Aircrew coverall Mk15/14A	0.10
	B A + Vest and drawers long cotton ribbed in place of jockey underpants	0.13
Assemblies including Mk10 immersion coverall	D Vest and drawers long cotton ribbed. Aircrew shirt cotton olive drab Mk2	0.50
	E D + Jersey heavy olive drab	0.60
	F D + Coverall aircrew inner knitted Mk1	1.15
	G D + 2 knitted inner aircrew coverall Mk1	1.40
	H D + Inner coverall Mk3	1.20
Assemblies including inner immersion cover	I Vest and drawers long cotton ribbed. Aircrew shirt cotton olive drab Mk1	0.40
	J I + Jersey heavy olive drab	0.50
	K I + Coverall aircrew inner knitted Mk1	1.05
	L K + Jersey heavy olive drab	1.15
	M I + 2 knitted inner aircrew coverall Mk1	1.30

All assemblies include protective helmet, lifepreserver, sweat- or water-resistant gloves, socks terry-loop, aircrew boots and anti-G trousers.

malleable edge to enable them to be shaped around the face. Fur trim improves the protection still further.

The best form of footwear depends on the climatic conditions. In cold/wet environments, footwear must be waterproof and provide adequate insulation. In cold/dry conditions, however, insulation is the more important factor, and, provided aircraft controls can be operated, the Mukluk is ideal (*Figure 18.8*). This consists of a thick, felt inner boot, worn beneath a rubber-soled canvas outer boot. Additional insulation to the sole of the foot can be provided by a felt insole over an incompressible nylon mesh insole.

Good protection of the hands in the cold is generally incompatible with the maintenance of sufficient sensitivity and dexterity. This poses a difficult problem, and it is usually practical to wear only relatively thin flying gloves with fingerless mittens on top. These are adequate in flight so long as the cabin can be maintained well above freezing point. In very cold aircraft, electrically heated gloves (*see* below) should be considered. For non-flight situations the maintenance of sensitivity and dexterity is usually less vital and additional thick gloves or mittens can be worn. For maintenance work, thin contact gloves prevent cold injuries arising from contact with metal objects.

Heated clothing

When it is not practicable to wear enough clothing for adequate protection, additional heat can be supplied through a personal heating garment. Three methods are available: electrical heating; heating by warm air supplied by an 'air-ventilated suit'; or heating by warm liquid circulated through a 'liquid-conditioned suit'.

Heating by warm air was once an attractive proposition in that liberal supplies are usually available from engine tappings and the ductwork systems were sometimes available as part of an air ventilated suit system for cooling. Air has a low specific heat, however, and adequate heat transfer, especially at altitude, is difficult to achieve. It is particularly difficult to heat the feet and hands.

Heating by warm water circulated through a liquid-conditioned suit appears to be a practical proposition although it is unlikely that suitable gloves and socks could be designed. The liquid-conditioned suit or vest (*see* below) is a relatively new concept and to date has not been used in military aircraft except for trial purposes. However, the system shows great promise as a cooling garment and if adopted for this purpose, it is attractive and simple to use it also for heating. The recent development of thermoelectric supply systems enable a cooling system to be converted to a heating system by a simple change-over switch.

Electrical heating is the only personal heating system to have received widespread practical use in aviation. Suits, gloves and socks are available and are manufactured with the electrical elements woven into the fabric (*Figure 18.9*). The total heat input for a full suit is approximately 300 W: 200 W into the trunk and limbs and 25 W to each hand and foot. The extremity heating has proved effective, and the gloves and/or socks are frequently used without the complete suits. However, the gloves are not wholly compatible with the flying task and the system suffers from the disadvantage that it cannot also provide personal cooling.

Future systems for electrical heating include the use of fabrics coated with conducting carbon polymers or woven from conducting epitropic fibres. Both of these methods are under development but, as yet, they have not provided practical alternatives to the knitted wire systems.

254

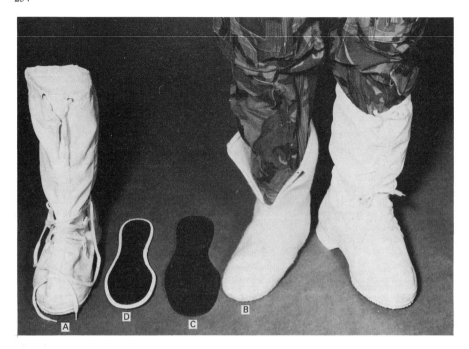

Figure 18.8 The Mukluk. A rubber soled canvas outer boot (A) is worn over a felt inner boot (B). Additional insulation is provided by a felt insole (C) placed over a nylon mesh insole (D).

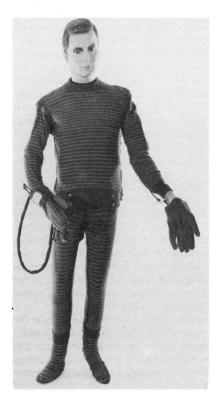

Figure 18.9 A whole-body electric suit with gloves and socks.

Clothing for hot conditions

General principles

General design features for clothing suitable for hot conditions include light weight, loose fit, light colour, good sweat absorption and open weave. For aircrew clothing it is often not possible to provide all these features because of the limitations of cockpit compatibility and because features such as colour are dictated by military necessity. However, attention to these simple requirements can provide some relief from thermal stresses. For example, flying coveralls for wear in summer conditions can be made from open-weave cotton cellular fabric and the waistcoat of a life preserver can be made from an open-mesh, artifical fibre fabric.

Usually the requirement to protect aircrew from the numerous flight hazards involves the use of so much additional special clothing and equipment such as anti-G trousers, life preservers, pressure clothing, chemical protective garments, etc., that relatively little can be achieved through basic clothing design. The effect of this additional clothing, much of which includes impermeable layers, is to render cockpit conditions that might be acceptable for 'shirt sleeve' flying extremely uncomfortable and in some situations unacceptable. To provide alleviation by improving the performance of cabin conditioning systems in these circumstances is difficult and inefficient since cabin temperatures have to be lowered greatly to achieve adequate heat transfer through the complex clothing assemblies.

Furthermore, no alleviation is available from cabin conditioning during cockpit readiness before engine start and it is generally ineffective during taxiing. For these reasons the use of some form of personal cooling system is an increasingly attractive way to maintain thermal comfort.

Personal cooling systems

Personal cooling can be provided using either air or water. In each system the coolant is distributed over the surface of the body by a specially designed personal conditioning garment usually worn next to the skin beneath all other clothing.

Air-ventilated suits

The use of air-ventilated suits was the first practical application of personal conditioning in military aircraft, although they are rarely seen in modern aircraft. Air can be used to cool either by convection or by promoting sweat evaporation. The method selected determines the overall effectiveness of the system, the supply requirements and the detailed suit design.

Overall effectiveness

Cooling by evaporation cannot start until the pilot is sweating; and he will not sweat until his body temperature has increased beyond the level of comfort. For this reason evaporative cooling cannot achieve thermal comfort but simply serves to limit the departure from comfort to the levels required to induce sufficient sweating. Dependence on sweating also entails a risk of dehydration although in most practical cases this is not a significant problem.

By convective cooling, on the other hand, it is possible to maintain a pilot close to thermal comfort with a mean skin temperature near to 33°C and with the usually comfortable thermal gradient of 5–6°C from trunk to the peripheral parts of the limbs. Thus it is clear that cooling by convection is preferable to that by evaporation.

Air supply requirements

The essential feature of an evaporative air supply is that it must be dry, so as to give an adequate vapour pressure gradient from the sweating skin to the air supply. A supply of about 0.5 kg/min evenly distributed over the body surface is usually adequate, and although it is preferable for supply air temperatures to be below skin temperature there is still a net heat loss by evaporative cooling at air temperatures exceeding 45°C. Because evaporative cooling depends on the volume flow of air through the suit, evaporative cooling supplies are easier to maintain at altitude than convective cooling supplies which depend on mass flow.

Air supplies for convective cooling must be sufficiently below comfort skin temperatures to remove the total heat load from metabolism and from the environment. Under severe conditions, suit air inlet temperatures down to 5°C may be required at flow rates of 1 kg/min. Thus for convective cooling, the temperature and mass flow requirements are essential but, subject to the exclusion of overt water droplets, the humidity supply of the air is unimportant.

Either type of air ventilation suit supply requires filtration if operated in a chemically contaminated environment. These filters are large, difficult to incorporate in modern military aircraft, and downgrade the quality of the air supply owing to heat pick-up in the filters. This is a serious disadvantage of air ventilation suit systems and an added advantage of liquid cooled systems.

Suit design

Sweating takes place more or less evenly over the body surface, and a suit designed for evaporative cooling distributes equal volume flow to equal skin areas. A typical evaporative air ventilated suit is shown in *Figure 18.10*.

A suit designed to cool by convection distributes most of the air supply to the arms and legs and only a small amount to the trunk. Thus most of the cooling is over the limbs, and this establishes comfortable skin temperature gradients from trunk to periphery.

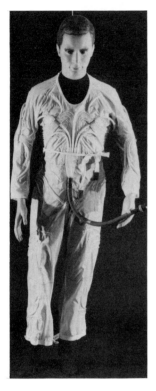

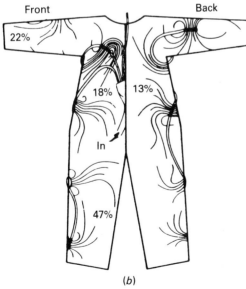

Figure 18.10 An evaporative air-ventilated suit (*a*) and a diagram of the distribution of the ventilating air (*b*).

Liquid-conditioned garments

The liquid-conditioned suit was first developed in the United Kingdom by Burton and Collier (1964) and was successfully used in the Apollo space programme. Until recently it has not been seriously considered for use in conventional military aircraft but its advantages are becoming more widely recognized. Air-ventilated suits have always suffered from poor performance of the aircraft supply systems and now have the serious disadvantage of requiring filtered supplies in a chemically contaminated environment. At the same time the need for personal conditioning has increased as the complication and impermeability of aircrew clothing has increased to meet the protection required in modern aviation environments. Effective supply systems for liquid cooled suits, based on vapour-cycle refrigeration systems or thermoelectric devices, have now been developed to the point where the choice of a liquid-cooled system is a practical option. The increasing use of liquid cooling for avionic equipment offers the possibility of using such systems also for pilot cooling.

The original liquid-cooled garments were whole-body suits as shown in *Figure 18.11*. These consisted of approximately 120 m of small plastic pipes distributed over the body surface and held in place by being incorporated into fabric tunnels stitched to a stretch fabric undergarment. They are worn immediately next to the skin for maximum effect. The supply water was distributed to the wrists and ankles and then flowed centrally to an outlet manifold for return to the supply system. Being a closed-circuit system, protection against chemical contamination is provided without the need for filters.

Recent developments of liquid-cooled garments have included smaller coverage garments such as liquid-cooled vests (*Figure 18.12*) and head-cooling systems (*Figure 18.13*). A vest covering the upper torso and upper arms has been shown capable of extracting heat at 150 W. Although this is significantly less than is possible with a full suit (300–400 W) it has been shown to be sufficient to produce effective control of core temperature. *Figure 18.14* demonstrates the value of a liquid

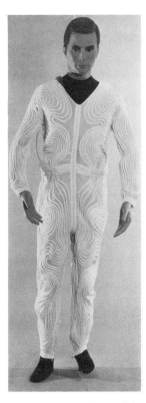

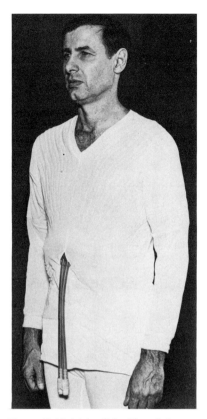

Figure 18.11 A liquid-conditioned suit. The suit has been turned inside out to show the network of small pipes enclosed in fabric tunnels and attached to the inner surface of the suit.

Figure 18.12 A 'piped' liquid-cooled vest.

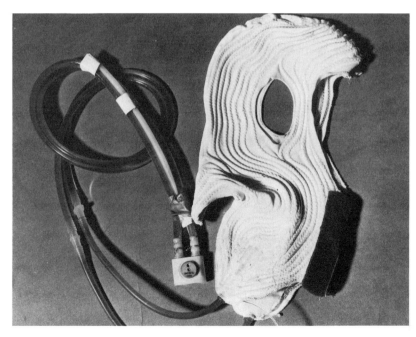

Figure 18.13 A liquid-cooled head and neck cowl.

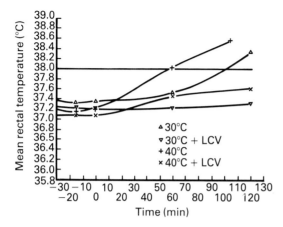

Figure 18.14 Experimental results showing the beneficial effect of a liquid-cooled vest (LCV) when worn with an aircrew equipment assembly including anti-G suit, chest counter-pressure garment and NBC protective clothing and respirator in environments of 30°C and 40°C dry bulb temperature.

cooled vest for a modern clothing system including chemical protection. The vest shown in *Figure 18.12* is a piped version. Other versions have been produced in which the water channels are formed by welding two layers of plastic-coated fabric together so as to form a labyrinth of water channels. The latter system has the difficulties that the chest is covered with impermeable fabric when the vest is not conditioned and the welded channels are more susceptible to occlusion by pressure from overlying harnesses etc.

Head-cooling produces remarkable improvements in subjective comfort and can also provide significant heat extraction to control body temperature. The scalp blood vessels provide a high rate of blood flow and are not subject to the marked vasoconstriction found in other areas when cooled. The chief difficulty with head cooling is to integrate the cooling cowl with the increasingly complicated helmets and other equipment placed on pilots' heads.

Supply requirements for liquid-cooled garments

Because of the close proximity of the pipes to the skin severe vasoconstriction may be induced in cutaneous vessels if inlet temperatures to the garments are lower than about 15°C. Harrison and Belyavin (1978) have shown that a maximum rate of heat extraction is achievable when skin temperature is maintained around 30°C which requires an inlet temperature of 17°–20°C. Thus it is not true to say 'the cooler the better'. Flow rates for whole body

suits using 50% glycol as the transfer liquid should be around 17 g/s (Short, 1976) and little is gained in terms of heat transfer by increases above this figure. Higher flows do, however, help to purge the pipe-work of air bubbles and to produce even flow down the various pipes. Modern piped vests are therefore designed for similar flows as were used in the older whole suits. Pilot control is best achieved by varying inlet temperature whilst keeping the flow constant.

When used for heating it is obviously important to prevent skin burning beneath the pipes and it is therefore essential to have automatic cut-outs limiting inlet temperature to the suit to a maximum of 45°C. With a whole-body suit it is possible to achieve about 400 W of heating but with a vest the heating is limited to about 300 W.

Liquid supply systems

There are a number of possible methods for supplying a liquid conditioned garment:

1. A heat exchanger containing replenishable supplies of latent heat coolants such as ice or CO_2 snow.
2. An air/water heat exchanger in the environmental control system.

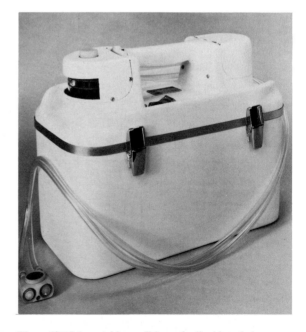

Figure 18.15 A portable conditioner for liquid-cooled garments. The cooling liquid is circulated through cooling pipes in a block of ice which can be re-frozen as required.

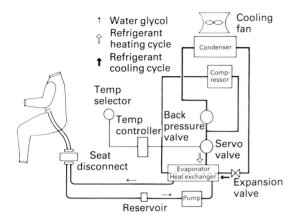

Figure 18.16 A diagram of a supply system for a liquid-conditioned suit. The heating performance of the system could be enhanced by incorporation of electrical heating in the supply.

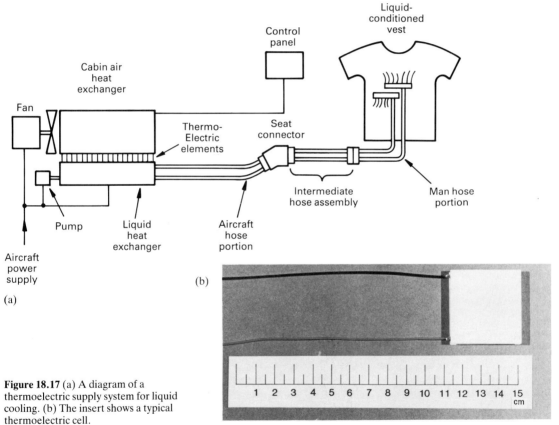

Figure 18.17 (a) A diagram of a thermoelectric supply system for liquid cooling. (b) The insert shows a typical thermoelectric cell.

3. An independent vapour-cycle refrigeration system, separate from the main environmental control system.
4. A thermoelectric system using electrically driven heat pumps.
5. A system using a liquid/liquid heat exchanger in an existing aircraft liquid cooling system provided for avionic cooling; possibly with interface control using thermoelectric devices.

Method 1 presents logistic difficulties, requiring replenishable stores, and is not attractive as an aircraft system. It does, however, provide a useful method for a portable liquid conditioner (*Figure 18.15*). Method 2 is perhaps the simplest but is obviously dependent directly on the environmental control system being in use and cannot therefore work during standby. Method 3 has been developed for several applications both in aircraft and in land vehicles. It is, however, complicated and expensive and may have maintenance difficulties. A diagram is given in *Figure 18.16*. Method 4 is attractive because it involves few moving parts and may be used for cooling or heating simply by reversing the current in the thermoelectric cells. *Figure 18.17* is a diagram of such a system and the insert shows one of the thermoelectric cells employed. Method 5 is also attractive since it shares existing facilities but is obviously dependent on whether a suitable system is available in a particular aircraft.

References

BURTON, D.R. and COLLIER, L. (1964) *The Development of Water-conditioned Suits.* Royal Aircraft Establishment, Farnborough, Hants, UK. Technical Note. No. ME 400.

HARRISON, M.H. and BELYAVIN, A.J. (1978) Operational characteristics of liquid-conditioned suits. *Aviation, Space and Environmental medicine,* **49**, 994–1003.

HUGHES, T.L. (1968) *Cabin Air Requirements for Crew Comfort in Military Aircraft.* Royal Aircraft Establishment, Farnborough, Hants, UK. Technical Report No. 68304.

SHORT, B.D. (1976) *The Effect of Coolant Flow Rates on the Performance of the Liquid-Conditioned Coverall.* Royal Aircraft Establishment, Farnborough, Hants, UK. Technical Report No. 76171.

19

Survival

P.J. Sowood and J.R. Allan

Introduction

Although aviation has made great technical advances over the last 50 years, there is always the possibility that crew and passengers may be forced to abandon their aircraft for various reasons. Since a large proportion of the Earth's surface is essentially inhospitable and uninhabited—covered by ocean, deserts, jungle, or arctic tundra—survival may be necessary in hostile and dangerous conditions. The ability to survive in any given situation and the techniques to be adopted will depend on the local circumstances but certain principles can be described that will apply to a greater or lesser extent in all survival situations. This chapter will describe those principles and, where appropriate, will illustrate them with specific examples of equipment and techniques. In order of priority, survival depends upon protection, location, water and food. Protection from the essential hostility of the environment, followed by rapid location and rescue; if rescue is delayed there will then be the need for the provision of water and food. Survival may also depend upon training and preparedness, fitness, stamina and the psychological resiliance of the survivors.

Protection

Escape from aircraft

Survival commences when the aircrew member or passenger leaves the confines of the aircraft cockpit or cabin. Thus the pilot of a fast jet aircraft forced to eject at high altitude requires protection against the hazards of assisted escape on an ejection seat such as

the G-forces or the lead splatter produced by miniature detonating cord used to break the canopy before ejection. Once out of the aircraft protection is required against the adverse effects of altitude, principally hypoxia and cold. Details of the various equipment provided in association with aircraft

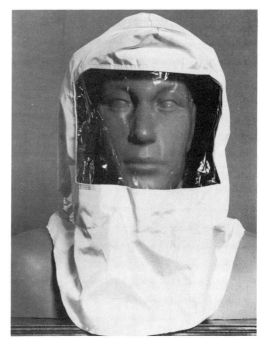

Figure 19.1 A typical smokehood (Scott Aviation) supplying oxygen under low pressure for at least 15 minutes and removing carbon dioxide and moisture in a lithium hydroxide canister.

escape systems, for impact protection and for protection against hypoxia will be found in the appropriate chapters.

Escape from aircraft in an emergency on the ground may involve danger associated with fire and toxic fumes. Passenger-carrying aircraft are designed to comply with regulations concerned with the provision of adequate escape exits. These have to be clearly marked, of suitable size, and access to them maintained at all times. The emergency lighting system must provide sufficient illumination of the escape route in smoke or, in some cases, under water. Cabin attendants are required to receive regular training in the procedures of the evacuation of passenger aircraft, particularly in dealing with panic-stricken passengers who may exhibit irrational and inappropriate behaviour (*see* Chapter 31). Escape under such circumstances may be severely hindered by the effects of toxic fumes produced by the combustion of materials used in the construction of cabin upholstery. Developments in this area should ensure that new aircraft employ materials less likely to produce toxic fumes but meanwhile provision of smokehoods (*see Figure 19.1*) may aid escape in such circumstances.

Survival may also involve escape from an aircraft that is submerged in water, particularly rotary-wing aircraft. Under these conditions there is a conflict between the requirement of the survivor to move underwater to, and exit through, a suitable escape exit and the requirement to provide personal flotation devices and cold protection. Inflated life-preservers will hinder movement underwater and will be too bulky to allow escape through most emergency exits. Similarly, immersion suits may trap excessive air, and attachments to them can cause 'snagging' hazards delaying or preventing escape. Thus the difficulties associated with escape in these conditions have necessitated the establishment of training programmes for military helicopter crews and for the crews and passengers of civil helicopters routinely flying over water. Training is conducted in helicopter 'dunkers', devices reproducing the effects experienced when a helicopter ditches onto water, inverts and subsequently sinks (*Figure 19.2*). An additional problem in such circumstances may be the inability of the occupants to breath-hold for long enough while submerged in very cold water. Equipment exists that allows limited underwater breathing, either using the air contained in a life-jacket or provided from a cylinder and demand valve. This allows the wearer more time to locate the escape route. Escape is aided by adequate illumination of emergency exits and by the provision of goggles to enable survivors to see more clearly under water. The sequence of hazards facing helicopter passengers after ditching is shown in *Figure 19.3*.

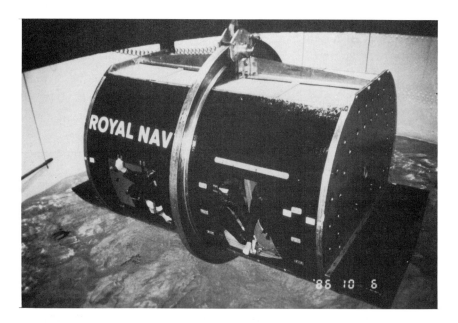

Figure 19.2 Royal Navy Helicopter Dunker. Cabin and occupants strapped into seats are lowered into the water. Once submerged the cabin inverts and the occupants unstrap and swim out through the exits.

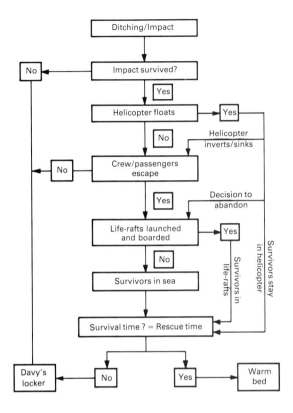

Figure 19.3 Possibilities of survival after ditching.

Protection from drowning

Approximately two-thirds of the Earth's surface is covered in water. There is a significant probability, therefore, that aircrew or passengers leaving a stricken aircraft will land in or on the water. For military aircrew descending into water under a parachute, there is a significant risk of drowning associated with being dragged through the water as the parachute continues to 'fly' over the surface of the sea. Release from the parachute under such circumstances can be difficult and modern parachutes are fitted with water-pockets around the edge of the canopy which fill with water rapidly causing the parachute to collapse.

Protection against drowning is provided by personal flotation devices, life-preservers or life-jackets, which form an integral part of the aircrew equipment assemblies for most military aircrew and are a mandatory provision for passengers in civil aircraft flying over the sea. Liferafts, single or multi-seat, are usually also provided.

Life-preserver design

Personal flotation devices are required to provide adequate buoyancy and maintain the survivor in a safe and stable position in the water, even if unconscious. This means that the mouth and nose must be raised above the surface of the water away from the effects of wave and splash. Detailed specifications of life-preserver design and performance had been described by a number of agencies (for example, International Maritime Organisation, 1974). In principle the buoyancy of the life-preserver should be developed by automatic operation on entry into the water, capable of righting an unconscious survivor from a face-down position, and maintaining him at a flotation angle of about 45 degrees to the vertical with his mouth at least 120 mm above the water. The buoyancy needed can be calculated by consideration of the specific gravity of the largest individual with the highest specific gravity: typically this will be the muscular, athletic male and will be greatest in full expiration. Thus to float the body must displace a volume of water sufficiently large to provide an upward force equal to the body's weight. So for a typical individual additional buoyancy of at least 180 newtons (38 lbf) must be provided to prevent sinking and to maintain the nose and mouth adequately above the water. Current regulations require the 'mouth freeboard' to be at least 120 mm. Additional buoyancy may be needed to ensure self-righting but its distribution is also important for this function. However, adequate buoyancy alone will not prevent waves breaking over the survivor's head under some conditions and therefore the ideal life-jacket should incorporate a method of protecting the face from wave splash.

Self-righting, flotation angle and stability

In order to provide self-righting characteristics and to position the survivor in a stable and comfortable position in the water the buoyancy provided must not only be of sufficient magnitude but must be positioned correctly around the body. Two forces act on a floating body: a downward force due to gravity acting through the centre of mass and an upward force of the buoyancy acting through the centre of buoyancy (*Figure 19.4*). If the centre of mass of the floating body and its centre of buoyancy coincide the body will remain in any position in the water. If, however, these two points do not coincide the body will turn in the water until the centre of buoyancy is immediately above the centre of mass. The further apart these two points are the greater is the turning moment applied to the body. The position of the centre of mass of the unconscious

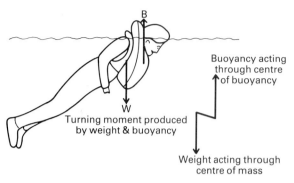

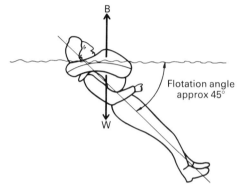

Figure 19.4 Forces acting on a survivor wearing a life-preserver. The turning moment (couple) provided by the weight, acting through the centre of mass, and the buoyancy, acting through a point superior and anterior to the centre of mass, ensures that no matter what position the survivor enters the water the life-preserver will turn him face upwards at approximately 45° to the horizontal.

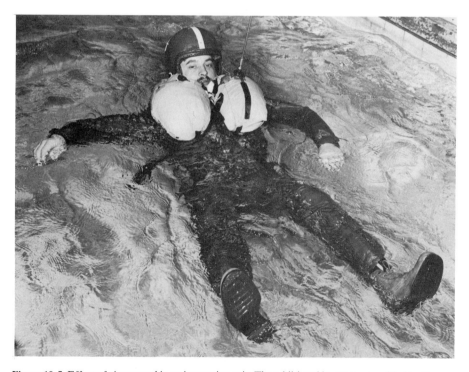

Figure 19.5 Effect of air trapped in an immersion suit. The additional buoyancy provided by the air trapped in the legs of the immersion suit causes the survivor to float horizontally on the surface of the water. In this position he is more susceptible to the effects of waves. In addition, the ability of the life-preserver to turn a survivor from the face-down position is much reduced.

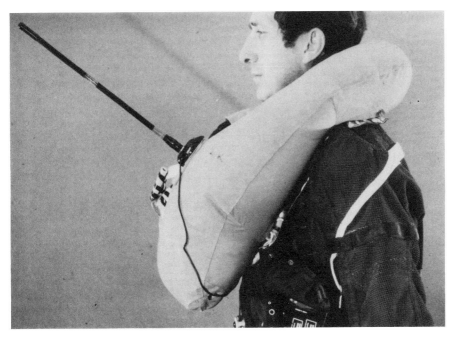

Figure 19.6 Inflated life-preserver showing personal locator beacon in left-hand pocket (bottom edge of the picture), beacon aerial and whistle.

survivor floating in water will be near the logitudinal axis of the body, rather nearer the head than the feet and towards the anterior surface (Macintosh and Pask, 1943).

Thus the ideal life-preserver should provide a centre of buoyancy for the wearer some distance in front of the upper part of the sternum. This will result in a face-up position in the water with the long axis of the body at about 45 degrees to the vertical (Macintosh and Pask, 1957). It is also necessary to provide adequate support to the head to keep the airway clear of the water. This position produces the best wave-riding characteristics with the victim facing the on-coming waves in a stable manner. Unfortunately this ideal position is often compromised by additional, unwanted buoyancy arising as a result of air trapped in the layers of immersion protection, particularly in the lower limbs (*Figure 19.5*). This can lead to a horizontal position on the surface of the water.

Apart from being uncomfortable, this reduces the righting capabilities of the life-preserver and may lead to a stable, face-down position. It also provides less protection from splash and passing waves. The effects can be avoided to a certain extent by incorporating an arrangement of valves in the immersion garment to allow the trapped air to escape but they can allow water to leak into the garment. Trapped air can be reduced to a minimum by ensuring that the garment fits well and by

incorporating elasticated sections in the legs to reduce bulkiness.

A typical aviation life-preserver (*Figure 19.6*) consists of a gas-tight stole fitted to a waistcoat and protected from wear and tear and ejection wind-blast by a durable outer cover. On activation, the stole is inflated by compressed gas, usually carbon dioxide, contained in a pressure cylinder attached to the garment. Once inflated the stole consists of two large lobes securely attached to the front of the chest and connected by a tubular section of smaller dimensions passing from one lobe to the other round the sides and back of the neck. This section serves to support the head so that the mouth and nose of an unconscious survivor are held clear of the water. It is important, however, that this portion should not interfere with self-righting. Double-stole life-jackets are usually used where there is a requirement to be able to wear the life-jacket like a waistcoat. However, this design has the disadvantage that the gap between the two lobes can serve to funnel waves up onto the face, possibly compromising the airway of an unconscious or exhausted survivor. Ideally, the inflatable stole should be a double compartment such that a single point of damage does not render the device useless.

In addition to providing buoyancy, the life-preserver may have stowage for other survival aids such as personal radio-locator beacons, distress flares, a small first-aid kit, a whistle and water operated battery light. Peripheral functions include the provision of attachment for man-mounted oxygen regulations, personal survival packs (PSPs), and personal equipment connectors.

Inflation systems

Inflation of the life-preserver is achieved by release of compressed gas, usually carbon dioxide. When compressed, carbon dioxide liquifies allowing a large quantity of gas to be stored at comparatively low pressure in a small cylinder. Unfortunately, when the pressure is released the phase change so cools the gas that it is prone to freezing, forming carbon dioxide 'snow' or dry-ice, thus prolonging the inflation time. Compressed air does not suffer from this disadvantage but requires compression to much higher pressures to store the same amount of gas in the same size cylinder.

Activation may be either manual or provided by an automatic mechanism activated by immersion in water. Such devices work either by detecting a change in conductivity in an electrical circuit on contact with water or mechanically by dissolving a soluble plug. Both methods activate a cutter which pierces the cylinder releasing the gas. Automatic operating heads require careful design and testing to ensure that they do not operate inadvertently, for example in conditions of rain or high humidity, and that they will function fast enough (typically in under 1 second for electrical devices and under 5 seconds for mechanical heads) to prevent an unconscious survivor inhaling water. In addition, there must be a facility to allow manual operation of an automatic head and oral inflation of the stole should the gas charge be inadequate. The oral inflation valve can usefully provide a means of partially deflating the life-preserver once its buoyancy is no longer immediately required.

Liferafts

More effective protection from drowning is provided by a variety of designs of liferaft ranging from the single-seat liferaft fitted in the seatpan of the ejection seat of a military fast-jet aircraft to the multi-position liferafts provided in passenger-carrying aircraft (*Figure 19.7*).

The liferafts provided for military aircrew are usually contained in the personal survival pack (PSP). This is often fitted in the pan of the crew's seat. Since there is little room in the seat pan and in non-ejection seat aircraft escape may have to be made through small exits, the personal survival pack must be very compact. Although the design of personal survival packs will differ between aircraft

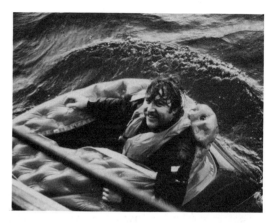

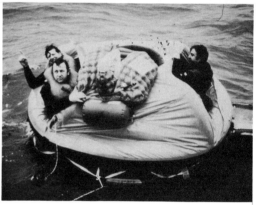

Figure 19.7 Liferafts. (*a*) Single-seat dinghy typical of the type provided in the PSP of ejection seats in fast jet aircraft. (*b*) Four-seat liferaft.

types the liferafts they contain are broadly similar. Annular inflatable chambers provide the principal buoyancy and the occupant sits on a floor which is itself inflatable to improve insulation. A canopy fitted to the top of the raft is erected by an inflatable arch and is closed securely at the front. Single-seat liferafts usually have head cover incorporated into a 2-layer inflatable canopy which is provided with a transparent face cover so that the occupant can see out whilst being totally enclosed and protected from the elements, particularly wind chill and wave splash. The canopy is brightly coloured—usually orange—to aid visual location.

The liferaft may be provided with a sea drogue to prevent the craft capsizing and to orientate the craft downwind to provide some protection from waves and to reduce drift. Because of their small size the incidence of sea sickness in individual liferafts is very high. Most personal survival packs contain a small first aid pack, included in which is some form of anti-motion-sickness medication.

The method of deployment of the liferaft will vary between aircraft types but for fast jet aircrew the personal survival pack containing the liferaft is attached to the parachute harness. During descent the personal survival pack is released from the harness and is suspended below the crewmember on a 5–6 m lanyard to prevent the personal survival pack causing injury, particularly on landing. Once in the water, the survivor pulls the personal survival pack towards him and, if the liferaft has not already inflated automatically, initiates inflation. After boarding and securing the canopy, the liferaft is bailed dry using an integral bailer and the floor and canopy inflated to increase thermal insulation and prevent windchill. The liferaft will usually contain a puncture repair kit, distress flares or rockets, and, in the case of large liferafts, position-indicating radio beacons. In addition, the personal survival pack will contain a limited supply of water, a water desalination kit, a first-aid pack and other survival aids.

Protection from the cold

Immersion garments

The unprotected human subject will lose heat very rapidly and attain a core temperature associated with deterioration both in mental and in physical function when immersed in water as warm as 24°C (Keatinge, 1969). Thus virtually any accidental immersion could result in hypothermia. Protection against heat loss during immersion relies on the provision of an insulating layer around the body either by using a water-impermeable layer worn over insulative garments—the 'dry-suit' concept—

or by using the insulation provided by the air contained in the neoprene foam 'wet-suit'. The latter method is less commonly used for survival protection for aircrew although its use may be associated with some advantages over the 'dry-suit' design.

Immersion suits are made out of either a total water-impermeable material such as a neoprene-coated nylon or materials that have some permeability to water vapour but which are impermeable to droplet water. Thus ventile is a tightly woven cotton fabric the fibres of which, once wet, swell and produce a water-impermeable material. Newer developments include the use of 'breathable' materials which are permeable to water vapour but exclude water. One variety incorporates a microporous PTFE layer laminated between inner and outer fabrics. Other varieties are coated fabrics through which water vapour is transported by a chemical process. Immersion garments (*see Figure 19.5 and 19.8*) are usually a one-piece 'coverall' with seals at the neck, wrists and feet. Often the garment will have water-proof socks or boots fitted and some garments have fitted gloves; the wrists are usually provided with waterproof seals of neoprene rubber whilst a variety of neck seals are manufactured of greater or lesser effectiveness (*Figure 19.8*). In 'split-neck' seals the front opening of the garment is continued up through the neck seal material making donning relatively easy but increasing the probability of leaking.

An improved development of this design incorporates a hood which seals to the face rather than the neck and allows the sliding fastener to be extended higher on the head. Split-neck seals are generally less effective than continuous rubber neck seals.

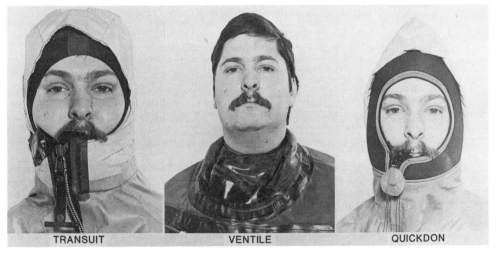

TRANSUIT   VENTILE   QUICKDON

Figure 19.8 Types of immersion suit neck seal. The 'Transuit' and 'Quickdon' suits have 'through the neck' sliding fastener for ease of donning. The ventile suit (centre) employs a continuous butyl rubber neck seal which is more effective although more difficult to put on.

Wet suits do not need to be fitted with waterproof seals or socks and have the advantage that, because they do not trap air, they do not interfere with the buoyancy provided by life-preservers and are less likely to hinder underwater escape through small apertures such as helicopter windows. However, these garments do not provide as much insulation as the 'dry-suit' combined with insulating undergarments and the insulation they provide may be degraded if the wet suit is loose so that water is able to flush in and out of the space underneath the garment (Allan *et al.*, 1986). This flushing can reduce the insulation by up to 50% (*see* Chapter 16).

Testing and maintenance of immersion protection garments

An important aspect of the protection provided by immersion garments is the testing necessary both to prove a new design and as part of the garments' routine maintenance (Allan and Hayes, 1984). The ability of a dry-suit to preserve the insulating properties of the clothing worn underneath depends upon the effectiveness of its water-excluding properties. Although the waterproofness of the fabric, seams and sliding closures can be readily tested by filling the garment with water and the source of any leak pinpointed, the effectiveness of the whole garment including the seals must be tested by an immersion test. In these tests the garment is worn by a subject who either swims at a set rate or floats in a wave tank and the amount of water ingress is measured by weighing. Tests in a wave tank provide a more realistic assessment of the effectiveness of immersion protection than tests in still water but require more sophisticated facilities (Allan, 1984).

The overall insulation provided by a set of immersion protective clothing can be measured on a thermal manikin as described in Chapter 16. The method of predicting likely survival time is described in Chapter 18.

Protocol for the use of immersion protection

Immersion protection assemblies and the insulative garments worn with them may, during routine use, impose a considerable thermal stress in addition to being bulky and uncomfortable. To ensure good compliance it is important that the policies dealing

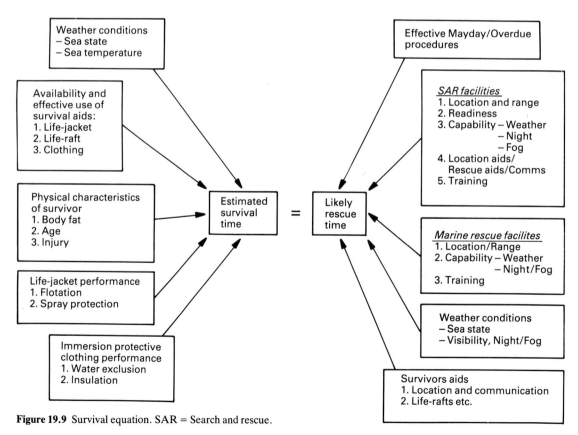

Figure 19.9 Survival equation. SAR = Search and rescue.

with the provision and use of such protection are appropriate (Allan, 1983). The basic approach is to ensure that the survival time is approximately equal to the rescue time by considering all the factors shown in *Figure 19.9*.

Thus for any given area of operation the probable time needed to rescue survivors should be estimated taking into consideration the factors on the right-hand side of *Figure 19.9*. Survival time can be estimated from a knowledge of sea temperature, clothing insulation and body composition using survival curves as described in Chapter 18. Obviously it is prudent to select appropriate insulative clothing so that survival time is comfortably in excess of likely rescue time.

Protection from the cold on land

Protection on land from adverse conditions is aimed at reducing the heat loss caused principally by forced convection. Thus protective garments should be waterproof and windproof. A wind of only 10 knots is equivalent to a fall in air temperature of approximately 3°C (*see* Chapter 16).

Survivors not on the move should seek shelter and this may involve considerable improvisation depending upon the facilities and materials available. Snow holes, snow trenches and igloos require

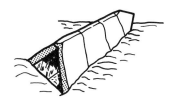

(*a*) Simple snow trench

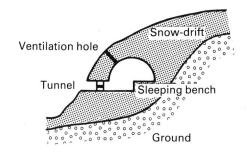

(*b*) Snow hole

Figure 19.10 (*a*) Snow trench. A simple trench about 2 m long covered with slabs of packed snow and designed to accommodate one person. (*b*) Snow hole. Snow holes can be dug wherever snowdrifts of sufficient depth can be found. Adequate ventilation is an important consideration.

suitable snow conditions and despite their simple design, need skill and much effort to construct and use safely (*Figure 19.10*). Small bivouacs may be constructed from the remains of parachutes, brushwood and even spare clothing. The psychological benefit of successfully lighting a fire should not be underestimated apart from its usefulness in drying clothing, melting snow for water and warming food. However, in cold wet conditions the lighting of a fire requires some skill and patience.

Despite extremely low ambient temperatures successful survival may involve work rates high enough to induce sweating. Under these circumstances it is important to adjust the level of insulation being worn to prevent sweating and to stop sweat accumulating in the clothing, thereby degrading the insulation and possibly freezing when the high work rate ceases.

In situations where there are large expanses of snow, the high level of ultraviolet radiation reflected from the snow can be harmful to the conjunctivae. The resulting snow blindness is an incapacitating condition which, should it occur, necessitates complete rest for 24–48 hours with the eyes closed. Prevention is by the use of suitable eye protection, preferably snow goggles.

Prevention of cold injuries

Both frostbite and non-freezing cold injury, should they occur, are a significant threat to successful survival in the cold and ought, therefore, to be carefully avoided. Exposed extremities are particularly prone to such injury especially since the onset is insidious as sensation from the affected part is rapidly lost and the injury only becomes apparent on rewarming. Cold injury can be prevented by maintaining warmth with adequate insulation that is kept dry. Waterproof boots keep out water but also retain sweat; special care of the feet, ensuring good circulation and dry socks, will reduce the incidence of immersion foot. If possible survivors in freezing conditions should adopt a 'buddy–buddy' system and, at regular intervals, systematically check exposed skin for whitening indicating that frostbite might be developing. Each individual may then actively promote warming and insulation in his buddies' extremities.

Protection from heat

In hot conditions there is no less need for protection from the environment. Particularly in the desert it is necessary to shelter from the sun and, if possible, get off the hot sand to reduce the risk of dehydration. Clothing should be light and loose fitting and should cover as much of the skin as possible to protect from sunburn and in deserts from the abrasive action of sandstorms. At night-time the air may be very cold and additional clothing will be needed. Clothing cover also provides some protection against insect bites. Sunglasses or goggles should be worn to protect the eyes from glare and, if available, a suitable ultraviolet filtering sun cream should be used to protect exposed skin.

The jungle environment presents peculiar hazards. For aircrew likely to parachute into jungle, 'tree-scape' devices allow the parachutist to descend from a parachute that may have become tangled in jungle foliage many tens of feet from the ground. Protection will be required from insect bites, and in malarious areas chemical prophylaxis should be taken (*see* Chapter 37). Water is usually more easily obtained in the jungle environment. Wild animals, including snakes, are not usually a threat unless disturbed but some protection may be afforded, particularly at night, by lighting a fire.

Survival packs

In a hostile environment the survivor has only the clothing and material available locally to protect himself. Aircraft and personal survival packs provide additional items including extra clothing, food and water, materials suitable for fire-lighting, and items such as insect repellant, anti-malarial drugs and motion-sickness medication. The comprehensiveness of any particular survival pack is obviously determined by size limitations.

Location

Probably the most effective way of ensuring prompt location and rescue is to file an accurate flight plan with the competent authorities and then to adhere to it. Nevertheless, means of notifying other agencies in the event of an emergency are required and these range from the technically sophisticated (for example, the ability to use radar IFF transponders to transmit an emergency identifying code to the monitoring air traffic control centre) through the 'Mayday' radio call, to the simpler personal locator beacon. Even the personal locator beacon has some technical refinements: one type in use has, in addition to the distress beacon transmission, a facility for voice communication. Personal locator beacons can be activated automatically and, depending on the altitude of the receiver, have a range of up to 60 miles (95 km): the range for voice communication is, however, less and its use limited by battery power. The batteries are replaceable and last for up to 24 hours in the beacon mode.

Short-range means of attracting attention are provided by a variety of pyrotechnic devices. At night rockets and hand-held flares can be used and during the day flares that produce dense coloured, usually red or orange, smoke are available in survival packs. Smoke flares can also be used for 'snow-writing'. Torches can be used for signalling; small electric lights are often provided on life-preservers and liferafts, drawing their power from batteries activated by water immersion. Heliographs are simple mirror devices that use the reflected rays of the sun to attract attention. Life-preservers are often fitted with whistles for very short range signalling and extensive use is made of conspicuous colouring to aid visual detection.

Water and food

The human body continually loses water which must be replaced. In 24 hours, provided no sweating occurs, some 500 ml are lost in insensible perspiration. A further 500 ml is lost through the respiratory tract and nitrogenous waste products require a minimum water excretion from the kidneys of approximately 500 ml. Carbohydrate metabolism will, however, produce approximately 300–500 ml of water every 24 hours, so a daily intake of 1500 ml will maintain positive water balance provided that there is no other significant fluid loss, for example

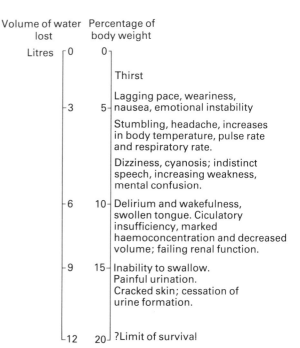

Figure 19.11 Symptoms of dehydration.

sweating, diarrhoea or vomiting. Hot climates or high work loads may produce sweating and, under these circumstances, the water requirement will increase.

Failure to meet this requirement will result in dehydration (*Figure 19.11*). A deficit of about 3 l or 5% of body weight will result in extreme thirst, headache, weariness, a lagging pace, nausea and emotional instability. Further dehydration produces increased heart rate and respiration, and at about a 5 l deficit there is increased weakness, slurred speech, mental confusion, dizzyness and cyanosis. Delirium occurs at a level of dehydration equivalent to 10% body weight and, as renal function becomes impaired, there is a decrease in circulating blood volume and haemoconcentration. At 9–10 l, approximately 15% body weight, swallowing becomes impossible and renal function ceases. Dehydration producing a 20% decrease in body weight is usually fatal.

Water rationing on land

Under survival conditions it may be necessary to ration the supply of water, and the aim here is to limit the water consumed to the safest minimum amount compatible with effective function to make the supply last as long as possible. In temperate climates, and assuming the survivors were adequately hydrated immediately before the incident, it is safe to withhold water completely for the first 24 hours. This will produce mild dehydration without impairing performance significantly. Thereafter rationing will depend upon the size of the supply but should be enough to keep the severe symptoms of dehydration at bay. This will be at least 500 ml per day. Obviously activity must be organized to avoid excessive work rates that might produce sweating and the diet consumed should be water sparing and therefore predominantly carbohydrate.

Water rationing at sea

Water rationing is particularly important for sea survival. Sea water, containing approximately 3.5% sodium chloride, is four times as concentrated as body fluid and if ingested requires additional water to excrete the salts it contains. In addition, drinking sea water will usually result in vomiting and/or diarrhoea and so increase the dehydrating effect. However, the enforced rest associated with sea survival and the usually lower ambient temperatures mean that water requirements are often at a minimum and so the survival time without water may be as long as 15 days, and every 1500 ml of water available will increase this time by one day.

As on land, initially no water should be consumed for the first 24 hours and then at a rate that prevents the symptoms from worsening. Additional fluid replacement will be necessary if sea sickness occurs.

Water rationing in hot climates

In hot climates the danger of dehydration is more immediate. Physical work should be kept to a minimum, preferably undertaken at night, and protection from the heat sought at all times. Water rationing under these conditions is difficult and there is a risk that death by dehydration could occur with some of the water supply still unconsumed. Thirst alone is a poor guide to hydration status. Thus once moderately severe symptoms of dehydration have developed, the available water should be consumed at a rate that prevents the symptoms from worsening. This protocol will ensure that while water remains the survivor will remain reasonably efficient and capable of logical thought and less likely to embark on any foolish course of action.

Sources of drinking water

Survival time will be increased by any available means to provide extra water. Survival packs usually contain a small quantity of drinking water in bottles or foil sachets but the amount is usually limited by the available space. Potable water can be obtained by passing sea water through a desalination kit and similarly water purifying tablets are provided to lessen the danger of infection. In addition, water is available from a variety of vegetation, vines, pitcher plants, coconuts, bamboos etc. Great care should be taken when drinking naturally occurring water and any available means of purification, including boiling if possible, should be used. Other methods of augmenting the water supply include collecting rain water and a variety of methods of condensing water from the atmosphere, but in regions where natural water is scarce the yield is likely to be very small. Sea water may be distilled successfully using solar stills if these are available and there is sufficient strong sunlight.

Energy requirements

Although a person can remain alive without food for many days the debilitating condition that ensues after a modest period of starvation may be incompatible with successful survival activity. Energy is required for the sometimes strenuous work involved in some of the actions promoting survival already described.

In hot environments it is important to ensure that food intake does not increase the requirement for water if this is in short supply. Protein and fat metabolism produce waste products requiring water for their excretion, whereas each molecule of glucose metabolized produces six molecules of water and no other product requiring renal excretion. In addition, a carbohydrate diet minimizes protein catabolism and hence urea production, thereby lessening the excretory load on the kidneys and conserving body water. Therefore, only when water is plentiful may food be taken freely and if water is scarce only carbohydrate should be taken. Satiety is not usually satisfied by carbohydrate alone, and the addition of a small amount of fat will improve the acceptability. Thus toffee sweets are a common inclusion in survival packs.

Although in theory the food content of survival packs can be supplemented with food gathered or hunted in the wild, the ability of civilized man to perform this task successfully is overestimated. Care is required in the selection of wild food since gastrointestinal disturbances can be very debilitating. If there is doubt about the suitability of the food a small quantity should be consumed and then a period of 8 hours allowed to elapse. If no ill effects supervene a further small amount should be eaten and another 8 hour interval allowed. If there are still no problems the safety of the food may be assumed. Sea fish, although an abundant and edible source of food, can be included in the diet only if there is sufficient water. Seaweeds are also edible but present a similar threat of dehydration.

Salt

An important dietary constituent in a hot environment is salt to replace the considerable quantities that may be lost in sweat. As much as 25 g per day may be required although less is required by acclimatized individuals. Care must be taken when administering salt supplements if water is scarce and it is better to err on the side of salt lack rather than risk increasing the requirement for water. If a reasonably normal diet with adequate water is being consumed the addition of salt to food 'to taste' is often adequate to prevent salt deprivation.

Like the provision of fire, the morale boosting properties of food, even if cold, should not be ignored. In addition to this psychological effect, there is a physiological benefit in that metabolic heat production is increased after the consumption of food and so, in a cold survival situation, the main food intake of the day should be taken immediately before sleeping when heat production would otherwise be at a minimum.

Survival training

The strategies for survival described in the preceding paragraphs rely upon a correct appreciation of the hazards and problems confronting the survivor and the adoption of an appropriate course of action. Modern man is not endowed with an innate ability to survive in the wide range of hazardous environments in which he may find himself. Thus training for survival is as essential as the provision of the various survival aids already described. The degree and extent of this training will vary according to the operational scenario. In civil aviation it is essential that cabin crew receive training, for example, in the procedures necessary for rapid aircraft evacuation, sea survival and first aid. The role of cabin crew in emergency situations is crucial since the passengers, apart from the preflight emergencies briefing, will be totally unprepared and likely to react inappropriately. Clear, authoritative and timely direction by confident crew is essential if lives are to be saved.

Passengers travelling under more hazardous circumstances, for example off-shore workers being ferried by helicopter between oil platforms, may need to have specialized training in the use of their survival equipment. Specifically, training is often provided in the techniques of underwater escape from a submerged aircraft, a procedure that requires considerable expertise.

More extensive survival training may be necessary for military aircrew who frequently fly in single or two-seat aircraft often over remote terrain. Air forces provide survival training at squadron level which might include ejection or ditching drills, parachute descent drills, training in sea survival techniques, and first-aid. More specialized courses deal with the techniques necessary for the survival under specific circumstances such as arctic, winter and jungle survival.

Fitness

Survival training increases the psychological fitness of the survivor by helping to dispel the fear of the unknown. Physical fitness is an undoubted aid to survival since considerable stamina may be required to endure the discomforts encountered and to take the steps necessary to implement the principles outlined in this chapter.

Further reading

ALLAN, J.R. (1983) Survival after helicopter ditching: a technical guide for policy-makers. *International Journal of Aviation Safety*, **1**, 191–196

ALLAN, J.R. (1984) *Water Ingress Test for Immersion Suits*. Royal Air Force Institute of Aviation Medicine AEG Report No.504. London: Ministry of Defence.

ALLAN, J.R. and HAYES, P.A. (1984) *The Specification and Testing of the Thermal Performance of Immersion Suits*. Royal Air Force Institute of Aviation Medicine AEG Report No.512. London: Ministry of Defence.

ALLAN, J.R., ELLIOT, D.H. and HAYES, P.A. (1986) The thermal performance of partial coverage wet suits. *Aviation, Space and Environmental Medicine*, **57**, 1056–1160

International Maritime Organisation (1974) *International Convention for the Safety of Life at Sea*, Chapter III (revised 1983). London: International Maritime Organization.

KEATINGE, W.R. (1969) *Survival in Cold Water*, Chapter 1. Oxford: Blackwell Scientific Publications.

MACINTOSH, R.R. and PASK, E.A. (1943) *Floating Posture of the Unconscious Body*. Report No.550 Flying Personal Research Committee. London: Air Ministry.

MACINTOSH, R.R. and PASK, E.A. (1957) The testing of life jackets. *British Journal of Industrial Medicine*, **14**, 168

Part IV

The Special Senses

20

Spatial disorientation—general aspects

A.J. Benson

Introduction

Definition

Spatial disorientation is a term used to describe a variety of incidents occurring in flight where the pilot fails to sense correctly the position, motion or attitude of his aircraft or of himself within the fixed co-ordinate system provided by the surface of the Earth and the gravitational vertical. In addition, errors in perception by the pilot of his position, motion or attitude with respect to his aircraft, or of his own aircraft relative to other aircraft, may also be embraced within a broader definition of spatial disorientation in flight.

Although spatial disorientation, according to the definition given above, includes errors in the perception of aircraft position, such incidents are more accurately described by the term geographic disorientation. The determination of position with respect to fixed co-ordinates on the surface of the Earth is the task of aerial navigation and is one that uses different skills from those used in the perception of aircraft attitude and motion. For this reason the topics of geographic orientation and disorientation are discussed elsewhere in this book.

In some countries, particularly the United States, the term 'vertigo' or 'aviator's vertigo' is synonymous with spatial disorientation, but as vertigo has a more specific meaning of 'a sensation of turning' or 'dizziness' the use of the word should, it is suggested, be confined to this particular kind of sensory experience. A pilot with vertigo may well be suffering from spatial disorientation, but there are many incidents in which the pilot is spatially disorientated but does not have vertigo.

Incidence

Nearly all aircrew experience illusory sensations of aircraft attitude and motion or fail to detect changes in aircraft orientation at some time during their flying career. Such incidents are quite normal for they are due, in general, to physiological limitations of sensory mechanisms. Men's sense organs are functionally adapted to terrestrial life in a stable $1g$ environment. It is, therefore, not surprising that in the aerial environment, where man is exposed to motion stimuli which differ in magnitude, frequency and direction from those experienced on the ground, errors in perception of spatial orientation occur.

The incidence and frequencies of spatial disorientation differ widely between aircrew and are as much influenced by the individual pilot's concept of the term as by the type of flying in which he is engaged. Some will say that they have never suffered from disorientation because they always knew the aircraft's correct orientation by reference to aircraft instruments, even though their 'seat of the pants' sensation did not accord. Others will say that they have some form of disorientation on almost every flight, though they, like their colleagues who ostensibly have never been disorientated, successfully resolve the perceptual conflict and maintain correct control of the aircraft.

Quantitative information on the frequency of disorientation incidents in different types of flight operations is not available but data from a recent questionnaire survey of Royal Navy helicopter pilots is probably representative of the incidence of spatial disorientation in military aviation. Of the 300 helicopter pilots who responded to the questionnaire only 2% denied that they had ever been disorientated in flight, 68% had experienced more than 10 incidents during their flying career, and 61% of pilots had been severely disorientated on one or more occasions. Situations in which both pilots became disorientated simultaneously were reported in 21% of the questionnaire returns.

Table 20.1 Flight experience of spatial disorientation based on a questionnaire completed by 137 fixed-wing pilots in 1956 and 321 pilots in 1970 (from Clark, 1971)

Incident	Pilots reporting incident (%)	
	1970	1956
Sensation that one wing was low although wings were level	60	67
On levelling off after bank, tended to bank in opposite direction	45	67
Felt as if straight and level when in a turn	39	66
Become confused on attempting to mix 'contact' and instrument cues	34	31
On recovery from steep climbing turn felt to be turning in opposite direction	29	55
Feeling of isolation and separation from Earth when at high altitude ('break-off phenomenon')	23	33
On dark night a flare floating straight down appeared to move erratically	21	23
Intent on target, failed to check altimeter and came too close to ground ('fascination')	12	12

Table 20.2 Percentage of pilots who have experienced disorientation of the type described whilst flying helicopters

Rank order		USN	RN1	RN2
1	Sensation of not being straight and level after bank and turn ('The Leans')	91	96	94
2	Misinterpretation of relative position or movement of ship during *night* approach	58	73	74
3	Misinterpretation of true horizon due to sloping cloud bank	47	46	45
4	Misjudgement of altitude following take-off from ship	21	34	38
5	Misperception of true horizon because of ground lights	33	28	15
6	Sensation of being suspended in space	*	19	16
7	Feeling of instability, as if aircraft were balanced on a knife edge	*	-	18

*Incidents described by many pilots at interview but not included in questionnaire.
United States Navy data from 104 pilots (USN) (Tormes and Guedry, 1975), Royal Navy data from 182 pilots (RN1) (Steele-Perkins and Evans, 1978) and 300 pilots (RN2).

Spatial disorientation is also a significant problem in civil transport and general aviation (private) pilots, though the frequency with which illusory perception of attitude and motion occur is not known. Over the period 1982–1986 only 3.1% of the returns made by UK civil pilots in a confidential reporting scheme (CHIRP) described disorientation incidents. This figure is certainly an appreciable underestimate of the frequency with which disorientation is experienced by this pilot population for they are unlikely to report common illusions, such as 'the leans'. Private pilots also suffer from disorientation which in this group is a greater threat to flight safety than in the generally more experienced and better trained military and civil transport pilots. Unfortunately no data, other than anecdotal accounts, is available on the frequency with which spatial disorientation is experienced by general aviation pilots.

Information on the incidence of the many different types of perceptual disturbances, embraced by the definition of spatial disorientation, has been obtained solely from questionnaire studies of military pilots. *Table 20.1* lists the percentage of fixed-wing pilots who reported having experienced particular illusory sensations, and *Table 20.2* shows the responses of helicopter pilots. These data demonstrate unambiguously that, irrespective of the type of aircraft flown, the most common type of disorientation was the false perception of attitude known as 'the leans'; other illusions were less frequently experienced. However, the importance of these statistics is not in the precise percentage of pilots who reported a particular incident but in the demonstration that not all pilots had personal experience of 'common' illusions. The implication of this finding is that aircrew must be told about the varied perceptual disturbances that can occur in flight; not all will learn about such problems and how to cope with them during the course of flying training and subsequent operational duties.

Operational significance of spatial disorientation

The orientation error accident

By far the most important consequence of spatial disorientation is the orientation error accident, for if the pilot bases his control of the aircraft on an erroneous perception of its attitude or its flight trajectory then, by definition, there is an error in the man–machine, closed-loop system which, if not corrected, will almost inevitably lead to impact with the ground. Fortunately, only a small fraction of the disorientation incidents experienced by aircrew has disastrous conclusions. Nevertheless, aircraft crash each year and aircrew and passengers are killed because pilots fail to perceive correctly the orientation of their aircraft. The problem is not a new one; early in the history of powered flight it was recognized that limitations of sensory function could lead to loss of control, particularly when external visual cues for spatial orientation were degraded, as for example when flying in cloud or at night. Yet despite progressive improvements to aircraft instruments and displays which should, and generally do, allow the pilot to maintain correct orientation in all conditions of flight, accidents still occur. The greater proportion of orientation error accidents are associated with flight in poor visibility, technically described as Instrument Meteorological Conditions (IMC), when flight should be by reference to aircraft instruments (Instrument Flight Rules or IFR), but a few accidents occur in good visibility (Visual Meteorological Conditions or VMC) and are due to the misinterpretation of external visual cues.

Orientation error poses a difficult problem of accident investigation; for, if the pilot is dead or is unable to remember what happened immediately before the accident, then the evidence that substantiates the identification of 'orientation error' as a prime cause of the accident, is at best circumstantial, at worst conjectural. In many, perhaps most, accidents where disorientation is considered to be a primary cause an element of uncertainty must remain. Nevertheless, there have been several fatal accidents in which radio communication prior to impact has indicated that the pilot was disorientated. In other accidents, where the pilot survived, his description of his sensations and events preceding the accident could establish, without doubt, that a perceptual error was the primary cause of loss of control.

Over the last decade there has been little reduction in the proportion of accidents attributable to spatial disorientation, in contrast to the reassuring decrease in accidents due to mechanical or structural failure. In the Royal Air Force, of the 130 accidents of fixed-wing aircraft involving human factors that occurred between 1972 and 1986, spatial disorientation was considered to be a major factor in 8.5% and a contributory factor in a further 6.1%. Accident statistics of helicopter accidents in the British Army over the period 1963–1980 reveal that orientation error was a principal cause in 15.1% of all accidents which were responsible for 34% of fatalities (Edgington, 1980). These figures are approximately twice as great as those reported by Hixon *et al.* (1972) for US Army helicopter accidents in which disorientation was the principal cause in 7% of major accidents and 16% of all fatalities.

Orientation error accidents are not confined to military aircraft and in the civil sector it is the private flyer who is most at risk. US general aviation statistics for the period 1968–1975, involving over 35 000 accidents, identified spatial disorientation as a prime cause or contributory factor in 2.5% of all accidents and 90% of the orientation error accidents were fatal (Kirkham *et al.*, 1978). Indeed, it is in the category of fatal accidents that disorientation had greater prominence for it was the third most important factor in this group, accounting for 16% of all fatalities. Orientation error was closely associated with the second leading cause—continued VFR flight into adverse weather—in which it was a cause or factor in 35.6% of fatal accidents.

An analysis of civil air-transport accidents is more reassuring, at least in the UK, where the number in which disorientation was a prime cause has fallen steadily despite the rapid yearly increase in the number of hours flown. Even so, over the last decade disorientation could be implicated in 12% of all accidents to UK civil transports. Of special concern are the approach and landing accidents which, as a group, accounted for some 54% of all hull loss accidents to civil air-transports (ICAO statistics, 1959–1975). Twenty-five per cent of these accidents had as a causal factor the 'visual misjudgement of distance, altitude or speed', hence, by the definition employed in this chapter, the pilots were disorientated. It may be argued that other approach and landing accidents, primarily attributed to 'unprofessional attitude or behaviour' and 'pilot technique', embraced incidents in which defective airmanship also led to disorientation.

Dynamics of the orientation error accident

Just as the illusory perceptions embraced within the term 'spatial disorientation' are protean, so are the ways in which perceptual errors lead to loss of control and orientation error accidents. *Figure 20.1* attempts to illustrate the dynamics of the disorientation accident. The reader's attention is drawn first to the classification of disorientation into two types: Type I, in which the pilot does not appreciate that his perception of aircraft orientation is incorrect; and Type II, the more common form of disorientation, in which the pilot experiences a conflict between what he feels is happening to the aircraft and the correct information on its orientation provided, usually, by aircraft instruments.

Type I disorientation is the greater hazard to flight safety. The pilot who bases his control of the aircraft on false cues may soon lose control and be left with insufficient time or altitude to regain control, even if he has the skill to re-establish his orientation from instruments or other veridical cues. However, loss of control *per se* is not necessarily a

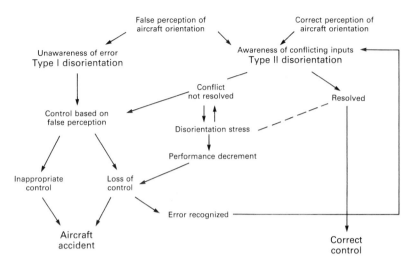

Figure 20.1 Representation of how Types I and II disorientation can affect the pilot's control of the aircraft.

feature of the orientation error accident, though control is inappropriate in all incidents. The pilot who flies his aircraft into the ground because of, say, an erroneous perception of pitch attitude on accelerating during a 'missed approach' manoeuvre, or because of an erroneous perception of ground clearance, has not lost control of his aircraft, for, given the sudden realization of his error, he could take appropriate action. Nevertheless, it is a disturbing fact that many, perhaps the majority, of orientation error accidents are due to Type I disorientation in which the pilot did not realize that he was disorientated.

In contrast, only a small fraction of Type II disorientation incidents lead to an aircraft accident. Commonly, the perceptual conflict is resolved and control of the aircraft is based on the correct interpretation of reliable (usually instrument) cues. Only rarely is the perceptual and motor function of the pilot so impaired by the conflict—'disorientation stress' is perhaps a better term—that control is jeopardized. The manner in which 'disorientation stress' degrades performance is considered in some detail later in this chapter; suffice it to say that it may lead: (1) to the acceptance of erroneous cues and their use in aircraft control; (2) to disturbance of motor function with inappropriate or inadequate control responses; and (3) to impairment of higher mental function so that errors of judgement are made.

Thus infrequently, though not insignificantly, the Type II disorientation may, either of itself or in synergism with other stresses of the flight environment, lead to a Type I incident, with its attendant high probability of an aircraft accident. Disorientation stress can also bring about a complete breakdown in skilled behaviour such that the pilot capitulates and gives up trying to resolve the sensory conflict. Other incidents have been described in which the pilot 'freezes' at the controls and is apparently incapable of making any corrective movement.

Anxiety reactions

Aircraft accidents and impairment of skilled performance are the principal operational consequences of spatial disorientation. Anxiety reactions, although relatively uncommon in relation to the frequency of occurrence of disorientation incidents, are also responsible for some morbidity in flying personnel. In the Royal Air Force about eight aircrew come under medical care each year because of spatial disorientation associated with anxiety.

The interrelationship between perceptual disturbance and neurotic reaction is a close one, so when attempting to unravel aetiological mechanisms in the individual patient it is often difficult to determine whether the disorientation was the manifestation of an anxiety reaction, or whether the perceptual disturbance was the cause of the anxiety. In some aircrew, it is clear from the clinical history that the neurotic reaction is precipitated by an unusually intense vertigo or other illusory perception, such as 'break-off' (*see below*). Typically, the first incident is one that creates apprehension, even frank anxiety, because it is outside the individual's previous experience. On subsequent flights there is heightened introspection and attention to the abnormal sensations. Not surprisingly, disorientation recurs with increasing anxiety and apprehension. The pilot is trapped in a vicious circle, from which escape is likely to come only by admission of his disability and the acceptance of appropriate therapy.

In about 50% of aircrew who come under medical care because of spatial disorientation, the perceptual disorder would appear to be the expression of an anxiety neurosis rather than the precipitant of mental ill health. Not infrequently there is a pronounced phobic element, with symptoms occurring only in specific environmental conditions. If no treatment is given there is, typically, generalization of the anxiety with loss of confidence and development of fear of flying reactions (O'Connor, 1967).

Mechanisms of orientation in flight

The ability of man to sense, or more correctly to perceive, orientation in three-dimensional space depends on his learned ability to interpret the continuous input of signals from many sensory receptors (*Figure 20.2*). Some of these receptors are grouped together to form a specialized sense organ, like the eye or the vestibular apparatus of the inner ear. Others are more generally distributed in the body and are to be found in the skin, the capsules of joints and supporting tissues. The 'seat of the pants' is not endowed with any special sensory receptors! By aircrew usage, this phrase has come to mean not just cutaneous sensations but all non-visual sensory mechanisms that contribute to the perception of spatial orientation in flight.

When we are in our natural environment, that is, when standing, sitting or moving about on the ground, adequate and accurate perception of the spatial orientation of our own body relative to the immediate surroundings is readily achieved by the use of visual cues. These cues along with those from non-visual receptors, also allow us to sense our position, attitude and motion relative to a stable frame of reference, namely, the surface of the Earth and the gravitational vertical (*see* Howard (1982) for a more detailed review of this topic).

In flight, the perceptual task is somewhat more complicated, for the 'immediate surroundings' is the aircraft which has a changing orientation relative to the Earth's surface and to the vertical (*Figure 20.3*). The cues that allow the airman to perceive his orientation with respect to the aircraft are very strong; part of the aircraft is nearly always visible and he is in physical contact with aircraft structures. This close perceptual bond between pilot and aircraft means that the pilot's appreciation of the orientation of his own body in space is rarely separated from his perception of the orientation of the aircraft: the pilot and his aircraft are as one. The motion and attitude of the aircraft, as indicated by cockpit instruments, is perceived by the pilot as motion and attitude of both the aircraft and himself. Similarly, signals from the inner ear which may tell the pilot that he is turning are perceived as angular motion both of himself and of the aircraft (Clark and Graybiel, 1955).

Accurate perception of aircraft orientation, which

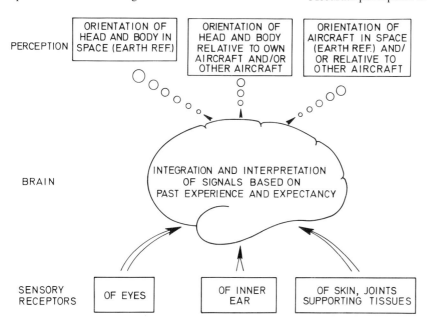

Figure 20.2 Diagram to show the sense organs used by man to determine his spatial orientation and components of his perception of spatial orientation in the flight environment.

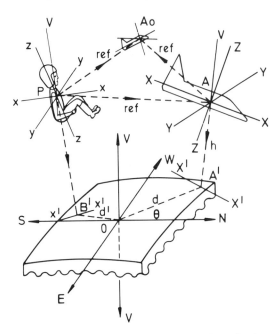

Figure 20.3 Spatial references used during orientation in flight. The pilot has been separated from his aircraft to emphasize the fact that his perception of the attitude of the aircraft relative to the gravitational vertical is determined by his perception of his own attitude relative to the vertical and the orientation of his body with respect to the aircraft. Correct orientation also depends on the correct perception of the height of the aircraft above the surface of the Earth, of the heading of the aircraft and of the projected position of the aircraft on the surface of the Earth with respect to known co-ordinates.

is essential if adequate control of the aircraft is to be achieved, is dependent primarily on the correct interpretation of visual cues, whether these are obtained from outside the aircraft or from cockpit instruments. These visual cues can be supported by information from non-visual sense organs, though in normal flight operations these play a subservient, yet not insignificant, role in the correct perception of aircraft orientation.

The eyes

As noted above, the visual system is of prime importance in spatial orientation. Although the eye is a single sense organ, it is now recognized that functionally there are two visual systems or, more precisely, two modes of processing spatially distributed visual information: one the *focal* mode, the other the *ambient* mode (Leibowitz and Dichgans, 1980).

In everyday life it is *ambient* vision that is used to determine our orientation to our surroundings, usually without conscious awareness of the visual

cues employed. Ambient vision is mediated by relatively large stimulus patterns. Typically, it involves stimulation of the peripheral visual field and is relatively uninfluenced by the brightness or optical quality of the image, indeed, the ambient visual system is part of what may be termed an ambient orientation system for there is convergence at centres within the brain of signals from the peripheral retina with those from vestibular and somatosensory receptors signalling body orientation and movement.

In contrast, the *focal* mode is concerned with object recognition and identification. It requires the resolution of relatively fine detail of the visual image and hence is best represented in the central visual fields (fovea and parafoveal areas of the retina). The information processed by this visual system is usually well represented in consciousness and is critically dependent upon image quality.

The distinction between focal and ambient vision is important when considering the role of vision in determining spatial orientation in flight. When visual cues outside the cockpit are employed, as in VMC, the pilot is primarily employing his ambient visual system. The task requires little conscious processing as it is but an extension of the way spatial orientation is achieved in normal everyday life; a process that is well entrenched from experience since early childhood. However, in conditions of poor visibility, as when flying in IMC, the airman must determine the orientation of his aircraft from flight instruments. These symbolic displays require focal vision, for they have to be scanned, read and interpreted. The task has to be learned and involves considerably greater cortical processing than when external, ambient visual cues are employed. Pilots acquire considerable skill in the use of flight instruments, and, with experience, the task is achieved without undue obtrusion in consciousness, but, by necessity, it involves the focal system which is not the 'natural' orientational mechanism and as such is more susceptible to impairment. Spatial disorientation is thus more likely to occur during flight in IMC than when external visual cues are unambiguous (as in good VMC) and are processed by the ambient visual system.

The inner ear

Even when deprived of vision, man can still sense his orientation to gravity and state of motion during normal activity on the surface of the Earth. The sense organs that allow him to orientate himself, and indeed maintain his balance, are those of the inner ear and other receptors more widely distributed in the body. The sense organs in the inner ear are the most specialized and will be described first.

The inner ear is divided, anatomically and

functionally, into two parts (*Figure 20.4*): (1) organ of hearing, the cochlea; and (2) the organ of equilibrium, the vestibular apparatus. The sense of hearing is of limited importance in the determination of body orientation, though it should not be overlooked that significant information about aircraft position and flight path can be obtained over the R/T during flight operations, and the noise generated by the boundary layer and engine can contribute to the perception of aircraft speed and angle of attack. In contrast, the vestibular apparatus is the sense organ which, by its form and function, is especially adapted to sense linear and angular movements of the head. It provides essential information that allows man to orientate himself and to maintain his equilbrium when standing or moving about on the Earth's surface. In flight, however, the information provided by the vestibular apparatus is frequently erroneous because the magnitude and time course of the motions to which the pilot is exposed are atypical and fall outside the normal dynamic range of this sensory system. In this chapter emphasis is placed on the vestibular contribution to pilot disorientation, but it should not be forgotten that, in certain circumstances, the vestibular system does provide the airman with correct information that can contribute to the maintenance of aircraft control.

Other receptors—kinaesthesis

A variety of sensory endings in the skin, the capsules of joints, muscles, ligaments and deeper supporting structures are stimulated mechanically and hence are influenced by the forces acting on the body. In general, these forces arise from linear accelerations, so the receptors signal the direction of action of the acceleration of gravity as well as the accelerations associated with linear motion. Many of the sensory endings, particularly those in the skin concerned with the sensation of touch and pressure, adapt fairly rapidly, so that they are better at signalling a change in the force environment than steady state conditions. They work in conjunction with the specialized receptors of the inner ear which sense linear accelerations and complement the dynamic rather than the static component of the response of these receptors.

These generally distributed mechano-receptors also provide essential information about the spatial relationships and movement of one part of the body with respect to another. In the absence of vision, man can sense with some accuracy the relative position of his limbs with respect to other parts of his body. This proprioceptive or kinaesthetic sense is achieved mainly by information signalled by receptor in the capsules of joints, though muscle spindles

and other stretch receptors in the tendons may also contribute.

The kinaesthetic receptors thus play an important role in the perception of body orientation relative to external reference. The vestibular apparatus signals the angular movement and attitude of the head with respect to the gravitational vertical; but unless the brain is informed about the position of the head on the trunk, and of the limbs relative to the trunk, man is not able to build up an adequate perception of the spatial orientation of his body and its appendages. Apart from these spatial references, he also needs to know about the structure with which he is in immediate contact. Such information is provided by receptors in and below the skin which respond to touch and pressure. In flight, these cutaneous receptors link the airman to his immediate environment—the aircraft. They are responsible for the close perceptual bond between man and aircraft which ensures that vestibular cues, whether they be true or false, are perceived not only as motion of the head but as motion of the aircraft.

Form and function of the vestibular apparatus

The vestibular apparatus is about the size of a pea; yet within this small volume are sensory receptors which are stimulated by angular accelerations as low as 0.05 degree/s^2 $(0.9\,\text{mrad/s}^2)$ and linear accelerations of less than $0.01\,\text{G}$ $(0.1\,\text{m/s}^2)$. In form and function the vestibular apparatus may be divided into two parts, though not without reason is it called 'the labyrinth'. The semicircular canals contain the receptors responding specifically to angular accelerations; the sac-like utricle and saccule house the otolith organs–the specialized receptors of linear accelerations.

Figure 20.4 is a diagram of the inner ear and shows the arrangement of the membranous structure that forms the vestibular apparatus. Basically there are three ducts, the semicircular canals, which open into the sac of the utricle; below and in connection with the utricle lies the saccule. The membranous labyrinth is filled with a watery fluid, the endolymph, and is attached securely within the labyrinthine cavity of the petrous temporal bone. The space between the membranous labyrinth and bone is occupied by perilymph, a fluid of low viscosity, like endolymph, but having a different ionic constitution. Because the membranous labyrinth is firmly coupled to the skull it experiences the same angular and linear accelerations as the head, and, by virtue of the inertial properties of the sensory apparatus, can signal angular and linear movements of the head.

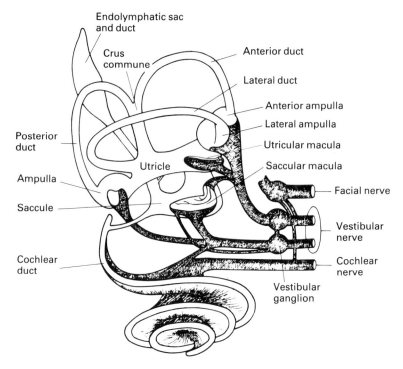

Figure 20.4 Representation of the inner ear on the right side to show the relative positions of the semicircular canals and the utricular and saccular macula. (After Lindeman, 1969.)

The semicircular canals

The three membranous ducts are roughly semicircular and lie in bony canals having an internal diameter approximately four times that of the duct itself; perilymph fills the space between duct and canal. Each semicircular duct has a swelling, the ampulla, where the sensory cells are congregated in a ridge, the crista. These cells have many hair-like projections arising from them, and are covered by a gelatinous structure, the cupula. As shown in *Figure 20.5*, the cupula fills a cross-section of the ampulla, and can be considered as a watertight swing-door which is deflected by movement of the endolymph within the membranous duct. The activity of the sensory cells is determined by the bending of the hair-like processes, which in turn is dependent on the position and movement of the 'swing-door' cupula.

The sensory cells in the ampulla of each semicircular canal are maximally stimulated by angular acceleration in the plane of the canal. As the three semicircular canals on each side of the body are arranged approximately at right-angles to each other (*Figure 20 .6*), then an angular acceleration in any plane will always stimulate the sensory cells of at least two 'canals'. The 'canals' work as functional

pairs in a push–pull type of configuration. The two horizontal canals (h in *Figure 20.6*) work as a pair and sense angular motion in yaw. The vertical canal pairs lie at 45 degrees to the conventional roll and pitch axes so that the forward canal of one side (av) works in conjunction with the rearward canal of the opposite side (pv). Although this arrangement does not correspond with the orthogonal axes in which the airman conventionally appreciates angular motion, the brain is well able to sort out the signals from these three pairs of canals, and can sense accurately the plane, direction and magnitude of an angular movement, provided these parameters of the movement are within the dynamic range of the sense organ.

The way in which the sensory receptors of the semicircular canal provide information about angular motion of the head may best be understood by considering what happens when the head is suddenly turned (*Figure 20.7*). During such a movement the semicircular canals and the whole of the membranous labyrinth will move with the head, but in those semicircular ducts that lie in the plane of the angular movement, the rings of endolymph will tend to remain in their original position because of their inertia. Thus during angular acceleration, a force will develop between the cupula and its associated

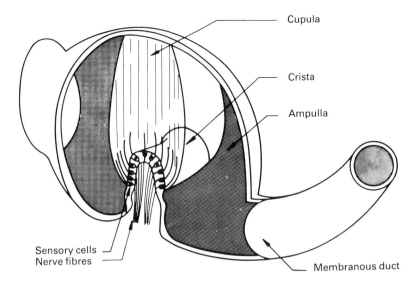

Figure 20.5 A cut-away view of the ampulla of a semicircular canal to show the ridge of
sensory cells (the crista) surmounted by the gelatinous cupula which occludes the
ampulla. (After Lindeman, 1969.)

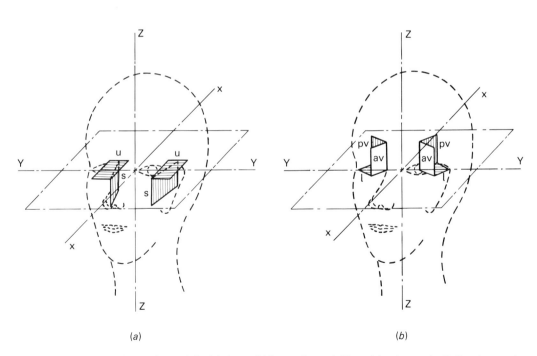

Figure 20.6 The approximate planes of the (*a*) the otolithic maculae and (*b*) semicircular canals. X, Y and Z are the
principal axes of the head; the XY plane is horizontal when Z is vertical. h, av and pv refer respectively to the
horizontal, anterior vertical and posterior vertical canals; u and s indicate the utricular and saccular maculae.

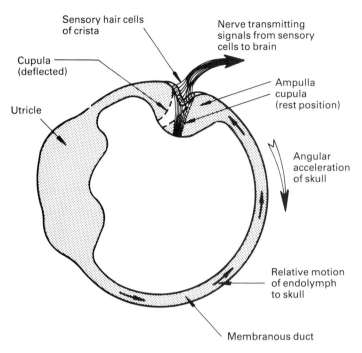

Figure 20.7 How the cupula is deflected by an angular acceleration in the plane of the semicircular duct. The ring of endolymph, because of its inertia, resists angular acceleration and a force is exerted on the flexible cupula which is deflected.

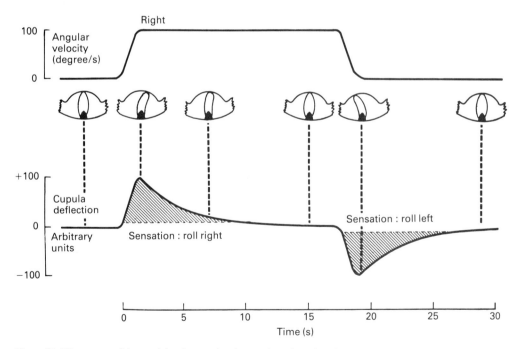

Figure 20.8 Response of the semicircular canal and sensation of turning during prolonged rotation. The upper graph shows the angular velocity during a sustained rolling manoeuvre. The lower graph shows the deflection of the cupula of a vertical semicircular canal stimulated by the angular motion.

ring of endolymph. The cupula 'swing-door' will be deflected, and the activity of the sensory cells altered. During normal head movement, where angular acceleration is followed shortly by deceleration, the dynamics of the hydromechanical system is such that the cupula deflection and the associated signal from the sensory cells closely matches the angular velocity of the head. The semicircular canal acts as a rapidly responding rate of turn transducer, even though the effective stimulus is the angular acceleration of the head movement and not its velocity. Indeed, the transducer works very well for the type of head movement made in normal life on the ground. It has a good frequency response (up to at least 10 Hz) so is able to respond accurately to the rapidly changing angular accelerations of the head that occur during walking, running and jumping etc., as well as to quick voluntary movements of the head.

Although the semicircular canals provide accurate information about angular movements of the head in the natural environment, difficulties arise when the speed of rotation is held steady for several seconds, or when the rate of turn increases or decreases at a steady rate (that is, a constant angular acceleration). In order to illustrate how the semicircular canals provide erroneous information, consider their response to a prolonged rolling or spinning manoeuvre in flight (*Figure 20.8*).

Before the pilot begins a roll, the cupulae of the semicircular canals are in their neutral position, provided that the aircraft has been in a straight and level flight for half a minute or more. As soon as the roll begins, the cupulae of the semicircular canals in the plane of the roll motion will be deflected by the angular acceleration in the roll axis and will generate a signal which reflects accurately the increasing angular velocity in roll. As soon as the rate of roll becomes constant, the cupulae of the stimulated canals begin to return to their neutral position, because there is no longer any angular acceleration and hence no deflecting force. The rate of return of the cupulae and the decay of the evoked sensation of turning is determined primarily by the hydrodynamic properties of the canal-cupula-endolymph system. Typically, in a roll, at say, 100 degree/s (2 rad/s), the sensation of roll dies away in some 10–15 seconds; thereafter, roll at a constant rate can continue indefinitely without any sensation of angular motion in roll being engendered by the semicircular canals, provided the position of the head with respect to the axis of rotation is not altered.

If, after rotating at a constant rate for 20–30 seconds the pilot recovers from the roll, there is an angular acceleration in the opposite direction to that which occurred on entering the roll. The cupulae of the 'roll axis' canals will be deflected and will signal in the opposite direction, with an intensity equal to the change in roll velocity of the aircraft. But once the aircraft is in straight and level flight, the angular acceleration is zero; there is no inertial force to deflect the cupulae so they slowly return to their normal positions. The lack of information about rolling at a constant rate, as well as the erroneous signal of rolling in the opposite direction on recovery from a constant rate of roll, is brought about entirely by the hydromechanical features of the semicircular canals. These are normal physiological responses.

The otolith organs

Two endolymph filled sacs, the utricle and saccule (*see Figure 20.4*), lie below the semicircular ducts and contain plate-like congregations of sensory cells—the maculae (*Figure 20.9*). These cells, like those found in the ampulla, have many hair-like projections which, when deflected, alter the activity of the sensory cells. In both the utricular and saccular maculae, the cells are grouped together in an irregular saucer-shaped area and are covered with a gelatinous layer, the outer surface of which is invested with small calcium carbonate crystals. In life, this has the appearance of a white stony plaque and is called the otolithic membrane; hence the common name for these specialized sense organs-the otoliths. Because the otolithic membrane has a density nearly three times as great as that of the endolymph which fills the utricle and saccule, the sensory hairs are bent as the attitude of the head alters relative to the force of gravity (*Figure 20.10*). Thus the sensory cells signal the position of the head with respect to the gravitational vertical and also changes in the force environment due to linear acceleration of the head.

There are two otolith organs on each side of the head: those of the utricle lie in an approximately horizontal plane when the head is in a normal upright position, and those of the saccule lie in the vertical plane (*Figure 20.6*). This arrangement permits the brain to sense a linear acceleration in any direction, provided the time course and intensity of the stimulus is within the range for which the receptor mechanism is functionally adapted.

Reflex responses to vestibular stimulation—eye movements

So far, the discussion of vestibular mechanisms has been concerned with the sensations produced by signals from the semicircular canals and otolith organs. However, the prime function of the vestibular apparatus is the maintenance of equilibrium, an activity that is normally achieved automatically, without willed or volitional control.

The way the vestibular system controls the muscles of the body to maintain equilibrium is complex and need not concern us here except for the

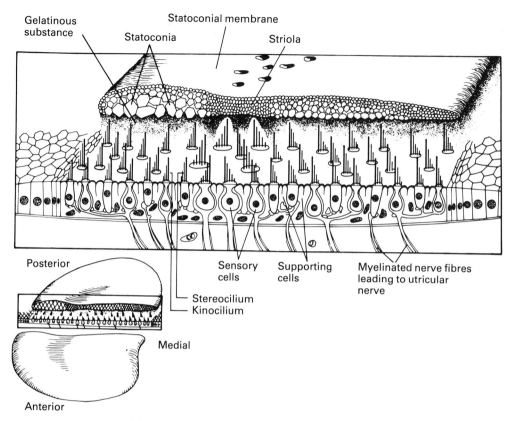

Figure 20.9 The structure of the utricular macula. The lower part of the figure is a general view of the surface of the organ; the upper part of the figure shows details of the sensory cells and the irregular crystalline structure of the otolithic membrane. The saccular macula differs in structure only in shape and in the grouping of the crystals of the otolithic membrane. (Reproduced from Lindeman (1969), by kind permission of author and publishers.)

powerful control exercised over the eye muscles. The function of this vestibular reflex is to stabilize the position of the eye, relative to an object fixed in space, when the head moves. Thus when the head is suddenly turned, the eye is reflexly moved in the opposite direction to that of the head in order to stabilize the image of the outside world on the retina. If the eyes were to move with the head, the retinal image would also move and vision would be seriously degraded by smearing of the image over the retinal mosaic. We know that during natural head movements the semicircular canals correctly transduce the instantaneous angular velocity of the head; therefore the reflex eye movements also have an angular velocity which is approximately equal to but opposite to that of the head. This is true irrespective of whether the motion is in pitch, yaw or roll. Vestibular stabilization is remarkably accurate, particularly for the rapid, small, angular movements of the head that occur during natural movements. Indeed, without a vestibulo-ocular reflex, man is not able to see clearly and resolve fine visual detail when he walks, runs, or is exposed to vibration.

During prolonged angular movement of the head, the compensatory eye movements take on a characteristic form (*Figure 20.11*). When one enters a turn, say to the right, the eyes initially move in the opposite direction (relative to the skull) in order to compensate for the head movement. Once they have deviated about 10 degrees from their initial position they quickly flick in the direction of the turn and then begin another slow compensatory movement. In this way the characteristic vestibular nystagmus is generated. The speed of the slow component of the eye movement—the one that is physiologically significant in the stabilization of the eye with respect to an object fixed in space—is closely related to cupula deflection. Accordingly, during a prolonged spin or rolling manoeuvre, the compensatory eye movement is only correct during the initial change in angular velocity. Once a steady angular velocity is achieved, the signal from the stimulated canals decays and with it the velocity of the nystagmus. On recovery from the manoeuvre, the semicircular canals signal rotation in the opposite direction. The information is inappropriate

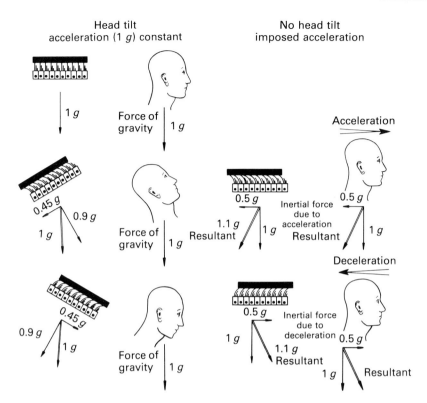

Figure 20.10 A representation of the utricular macula to show how the sensory cells are stimulated by displacement of the otolithic membrane (solid black) when the head is tilted in a fore–aft plane (left side of figure) and under the influence of linear accelerations (G_x) in the fore–aft direction (right side of figure).

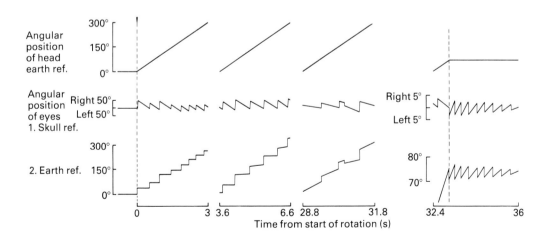

Figure 20.11 Eye movements (nystagmus) during prolonged rotation. At the beginning of rotation the eye movements accurately compensate for the angular motion of the head; after a few seconds the signal from the semicircular canals no longer matches the stimulus and eye stabilization is impaired; after 30 seconds semicircular canal information is all but absent, the eye is not stabilized and there may be impairment of vision for objects outside the aircraft. When rotation stops, nystagmus in the opposite direction develops which, though of low velocity (note change in scale), can degrade the pilot's vision for vision both inside and outside the aircraft.

as is the associated nystagmus which serves only to degrade the vision for objects both inside and outside the aircraft.

Emphasis has been placed on the nystagmus engendered by the semicircular canals, but changing linear accelerations also generate this type of eye movement which, though compensatory in nature, is less accurately matched to the stimulus than the nystagmus produced by angular motion. When the linear acceleration stimulus is constant, as when the head is tilted on one side, a sustained deviation of the eye from its rest position may be observed. These sustained eye movements (called ocular counter-rolling) occur in the expected compensatory direction, but in amplitude are only 5–10% of the angular deviation of the head. The inadequacy of the 'static' vestibulo-ocular reflex stresses the essential dynamic nature of the control of eye movements by the vestibular apparatus. The static aspect of ocular counter-rolling is undoubtedly of significance to perceptual phenomena in flight, though measurement of counter-rolling in the laboratory provide a measure of otolith organ function. (For a more detailed review of the anatomy and function of the vestibular apparatus, *see* Benson (1987)).

Aetiology of spatial disorientation in flight

Aircrew have described many different types of spatial disorientation that occur in different flight conditions and different flight manoeuvres. Not surprisingly, the mechanism underlying the disordered perceptions is commensurately varied. However, in an attempt to bring some order to the diversity of incidents and causal factors, it is convenient to discuss aetiology under two main headings, even though they are not mutually exclusive: (1) when erroneous or inadequate sensory information is transmitted to the brain (an input error); and (2) when there is an erroneous or inadequate perception of correct sensory information by the brain (a central error).

Input error

External visual cues

Disorientation is very uncommon when the pilot has well-defined external visual cues; but when he attempts to fly when sight of the ground or the horizon is degraded by cloud, fog, snow, rain, smoke, dust or darkness he quickly becomes disorientated unless he transfers his attention to the aircraft instruments. The ability to maintain control

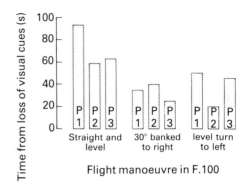

Figure 20.12 Loss of aircraft control following loss of all visual cues, expressed as the time taken to allow the aircraft to assume attitude or flight path requiring 10 000 feet for recovery. (Data from Kraus (1959).)

of an aircraft without adequate visual cues is quite short, typically about 60 seconds, even when the aircraft is in straight and level flight at the time vision is lost, and is shorter still if the aircraft is in a turn (*Figure 20.12*). In such circumstances, loss of control occurs because the non-visual receptors give either inadequate or erroneous information about the position, attitude and motion of the aircraft. These deficiencies are discussed below.

Even in good visibility, the external visual cues provided by ground texture can be poor and may be quite inadequate for the perception of altitude, or, more accurately, height above ground level. Typically, difficulty is experienced when flying over featureless terrain, such as sand or snow, or over water when it lacks wave texture. The difficulty of estimating height when attempting to land on such surfaces, or of maintaining accurate ground clearance in a hovering helicopter, is well recognized by experienced aircrew. At night, the restricted area of ground illuminated by lights on the aircraft exacerbates the problem.

The particular problems of the perception of orientation by external visual cues during that critical phase of flight—the approach and landing—are of special importance and merit more detailed analysis later in this chapter.

Erroneous, as opposed to inadequate, external visual cues less frequently disorientate aircrew, though there is no shortage of anecdotal reports of incidents in which the pilot was confused by atypical visual cues. The pilot who uses the top of a bank of clouds as a horizontal reference or the streamers of an auroral display as the vertical is, by definition, disorientated when these visual references do not accord with the true horizontal or vertical. The perceptual error can be ascribed to an error of expectancy. Cloud tops are commonly horizontal therefore there is a high conditional probability (that is a high expectancy) that a cloud top is horizontal. Accordingly, an error of perception occurs when the pilot uses a familiar cue that may not look atypical but does not accord with the usual rule. At lower altitudes, the trunks of conifers which are commonly vertical may give a false reference when, in response to prevailing wind or local topography, they grow at an angle inclined to the true vertical.

Whereas the preceding examples are associated with errors in the perception of attitude, illusory perception of motion can also be generated by movement of external visual cues. Disorientation of this type is experienced mainly by helicopter pilots who, on attempting to maintain an accurate hover at low altitude, may feel that their aircraft is moving when they look at a precessing wave pattern on water or long grass generated by the ground effect of the rotor. Comparable illusions of vertical motion are produced by the appearance and downward movement of water droplets or snowflakes en-trained in the downwash of the rotor. The moving shadow of helicopter rotor blades cast across the cockpit, or the back-scatter of light from a rotating anti-collision light when flying in cloud, are two further situations in which illusory sensations of motion can be engendered by these so-called vection stimuli.

Disorientation produced by such visual stimuli—whether the essentially static sloping cloud bank or the dynamic, moving shadow of a rotor blade—can be very powerful because the ambient visual system reacts in proportion to the area of retina stimulated. Hence, the larger the angle subtended at the eye by the static or moving stimulus, the more compelling the erroneous sensation (Dichgans and Brandt, 1978).

Visual cues from aircraft instruments

The primary stimulus for the development of flight instruments was the inability of man to sense important variables such as airspeed, heading, altitude, and attitude, in those flight conditions where external cues were degraded by cloud, darkness, etc. Whilst every effort is made by designers and manufacturers to ensure the accuracy and reliability of primary flight instruments, on which the safety of aircraft and occupants depends when flying in IMC, defects do occur. Failure of an instrument is normally indicated by a warning flag, but incidents have occurred in which instruments have failed or the display jammed without indication of malfunction. The pilot fails to realize that his control of the aircraft is based on an erroneous cue. He is disorientated, but may not be aware of the hazardous situation unless the instrument malfunc-tion is detected on cross-checking against other flight instruments.

Neither head-up nor the more conventional, head-down instruments are immune from this type of fault. The problem is, however, usually the more serious when failure of the head-up display occurs. The pilot has to transfer his gaze from the head-up display to the head-down instruments: he loses whatever external orientational cues that were visible and is temporarily unorientated until he has scanned and interpreted the basic flight instruments. In some modern aircraft his task has been made the more difficult because the head-up presentation has been made the primary display of flight information (attitude, heading, air-speed, etc.) and the conven-tional instruments have been relegated to a standby role. Consequently they are small and not optimally positioned with the cockpit, a large movement of head and eyes is required in order to visually fixate on them and even when fixated they are not easily read.

Dynamic limitations of instruments have also been implicated in a few aircraft accidents. Pressure operated instruments, in particular, can be slow to respond and may only indicate correctly some 4–5 seconds after a sudden change in the displayed variable. Such a dynamic error in the vertical speed indicator (VSI) was regarded as a contributory cause of an accident in which an aircraft failed to climb away on a 'missed approach'. It was suggested that, as the aircraft climbed away from the runway, the VSI would have indicated too high a rate of climb and that, as the pilot pushed forward on the stick, several seconds would have elapsed before the instrument would have displayed the loss of altitude.

Impairment of vision

The ability of the pilot to perceive the all-important visual cues, whether these be from the external visual world or from the flight-deck instruments, can be degraded by factors that impair either the quality of the retinal image or the transduction of the image by the sensory cells of the retina (Tredici, 1980).

Unless the retinal image is reasonably stable and fixation of the eye relative to the observed object is preserved for 100 ms or so, then visual acuity is impaired. In flight, vibration is one of the common causes of destabilization of the retinal image and can, in certain circumstances, be of sufficient severity to prevent the pilot from reading the instruments. In helicopters this problem most commonly occurs when maximum power is applied, such as at transition to the hover. In fixed-wing aircraft, the vibration that results from the aircraft entering buffet boundary at high altitude (as in a 'jet upset' type incident) or from high-speed flight at low altitude in turbulence, has prevented pilots from reading their instruments and so potentiated the disorientation engendered by the concurrent changes in the force environment (Martin and Melvill Jones, 1965).

Vestibular nystagmus can also degrade vision when the vestibular response is inappropriate. Like the vibration in 'jet upset', these nystagmic eye movements impair the pilot's only reliable channel of information about aircraft orientation at the very time that false sensations are being evoked by erroneous vestibular signals. Accordingly, on initiating recovery from a spin, the pilot may have a strong sensation of turning in a direction opposite to that of the spin and be unable to see the instruments or even external cues with sufficient clarity to know, unambiguously, that the aircraft has ceased to gyrate. In addition to the nystagmus associated with the onset and recovery from high rates of angular motion, as in a roll or spin, comparable difficulties arise when the vestibular apparatus is stimulated by middle ear pressure change. The sudden, and unexpected onset of pressure vertigo (*see below*) is a potent cause of disorientation where resolution of sensory conflict by reference to aircraft instruments is not aided by the concomitant nystagmus.

Laboratory experiments have shown that the period for which vision is degraded by inappropriate nystagmus is reduced when the brightness and contrast of the observed object is increased (Benson and Guedry, 1971). Consequently, the advice to aircrew, who may find themselves in the unfortunate position of being unable to read the aircraft instruments because of nystagmus, is to increase the level of illumination to the maximum available.

Another factor influencing the period of visual impairment is the plane of the nystagmus. Nystagmus in yaw is suppressed more rapidly than in roll. Hence, during the recovery from a prolonged spin, nystagmus died away more rapidly if the pilot tilted his head backward and tried to look at the horizon during the spin than if he bent his head forward and looked at the ground. On the other hand, if recovery from the spin has to be made by reference to instruments, the movement of the head on transferring gaze from the horizon to the instrument panel can produce a cross-coupled stimulus (*see below*) which potentially disorientates more that the nystagmus engendered by spin recovery.

Amongst the many effects of ethyl alcohol, the way in which it modifies nystagmus has recently come into prominence. Experiments have shown that alcohol increases the duration and intensity of nystagmus by attenuating the suppressive action of the fixation reflex (*Figure 20.13*). A blood alcohol concentration as low as 20 mg/100 ml has been shown to prolong the nystagmic response on stimulating the semicircular canals and to cause a significant impairment of visual performance. With substantially higher levels of blood alcohol, the nystagmus recorded while the subject tries to fixate is hardly of lower velocity or shorter duration than that recorded in the absence of fixation in a subject who has not taken alcohol (Barnes, 1984).

Impairment of vision by glare and dazzle or by the

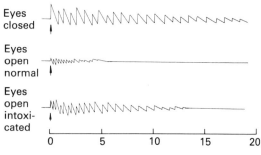

Time after stopping from turning at 100 degrees/s (s)

Figure 20.13 Alterations of post-rotational eye movements by alcohol. The graph shows the nystagmus produced by recovery from sustained rotation at 100 degrees/s. In the dark, or with eyes closed, the eye movements last for 30 seconds or more, but when the pilot fixates on objects inside or outside the aircraft the nystagmus is suppressed, though not abolished until about 5 seconds after the stimulus. Intoxication with ethyl alcohol reduces the effectiveness of the suppressive mechanism and hence prolongs the time for which vision is impaired by inappropriate nystagmus.

reduction in retinal blood flow with $+G_Z$ acceleration has been reported as the primary cause of disorientation and loss of control in a number of aircraft accidents. The specific mechanisms in these derangements of retinal function are described elsewhere in this volume.

Cues from vestibular and other mechanoreceptors

Inadequate cues

The failure of non-visual sensory systems to detect changes in attitude or motion of the aircraft is probably the most important single cause of orientation error accidents, though in accounts of disorientation incidents the absence of sensation is rarely reported; rather, it is the unexpected vertigo or other strong illusory sensation that is described.

Vestibular and kinaesthetic receptors are all mechanoreceptors and transduce motion stimuli only when deformation or deflection occurs under the influence of inertial or reactive forces. The otoliths provide information about the attitude of the head with respect to the specific force (usually gravity), though the perception of attitude is susceptible to modification by adaptive processes. In general, the sensory receptors and their associated central perceptual mechanisms respond only to change. Man has no absolute sense of his position, nor of his velocity, within a spatial co-ordinate system although he can sense change in position and velocity by detecting the angular or linear acceleration associated with the movement. Furthermore, he can perceptually integrate the information provided by the stimulated receptors so that reasonably accurate assessments of the magnitude of the change in position can also be made. However, the foregoing is true only for adequate stimuli; that is, stimuli substantially above the detection threshold and within the dynamic range of the sensory system.

In common with other sensory systems, detection thresholds for motion stimuli transduced by vestibular and kinaesthetic receptors have to be defined in terms of the intensity and the duration of action of the stimulus. For angular movements of short duration (not greater than about 5 seconds) the *angular velocity* must exceed 0.2–8.0 degree/s (3.5–140 mrad/s) (median value 1.5 degree/s or 26 mrad/s) for the motion to be perceived. When a rotational movement is prolonged, then the *angular acceleration* is the more important parameter. The threshold for detection of a sustained (>10 s) angular acceleration has a median value of 0.3 degree/s^2 (5 mrad/s^2), but, in common with other motion detection thresholds, the variation between subjects is large, being 0.05–2.2 degree/s^2 (0.1–38 mrad/s^2) (Guedry, 1974).

The detection of linear movement is determined principally by the magnitude of the change in linear acceleration, though as the response of the otoliths and other mechanoreceptors (in skin etc.) is determined partly by the rate of change of acceleration, i.e. jerk, the threshold of detection varies with the frequency spectrum of the linear motion stimulus. Thus for vertical sinusoidal oscillation in the Z body axis, threshold falls from a mean value of 0.18 m/s^2 at 0.2 Hz to 0.05 m/s^2 at 2 Hz. Thresholds for detection of linear accelerations acting in the X and Y body axes are approximately 50% lower than those for the detection of Z axis stimuli. Although the effective stimulus to the receptors transducing linear motion stimuli is a combination of acceleration and rate of change of acceleration, when subjects are exposed to a sustained linear acceleration of constant magnitude the time (t) taken to detect the stimulus varies with the acceleration (α), such that the product ($\alpha.t$) is a constant. This constant has the dimension of a linear *velocity* and has a mean value of 0.3–0.4 m/s (Young, 1984).

Changes in attitude in pitch and roll (i.e. rotation about the Y and X axes) from the normal upright position (Z body axis aligned with gravity) can involve stimulation of both semicircular canal and otolithic receptors. If the movement is at an angular velocity greater than 1–2 degree/s then the motion is detected by the semicircular canals; if body tilt occurs at a slower rate then detection is dependent on signals from the otoliths. Typically, man can set his attitude with respect to the gravitational vertical with an accuracy of ±2 degrees, but if the rate of movement is very slow (0.1 degrees/s) body tilt of 10 degrees or more can take place before deviation from verticality is detected (Benson, Diaz and Farrugia, 1975).

It is important to recognize that these threshold values have largely been determined in laboratory experiments where the subjects' sole task was to detect the motion stimulus. In flight, the pilot's attention is rarely so restricted and, in addition, he is exposed to a gamut of other sensory stimuli. These factors make it likely that on occasions the magnitude (or time/intensity integral) of the stimulus associated with motion of the aircraft can be substantially greater than the quoted threshold value before a change in attitude or velocity is sensed by the pilot.

Erroneous cues

In this category lie many of the most commonly described disorientation incidents in which the pilot is presented with a perceptual conflict. Signals from vestibular and kinaesthetic receptors give rise to sensations of body, and hence aircraft, motion which do not accord with the correct perception of aircraft orientation obtained from instrument cues. As noted earlier in this chapter, the conflict is usually resolved, but this is not always so. The pilot may, for a number of reasons, accept the false vestibular information and initiate inappropriate control movements with dangerous consequences.

Erroneous vestibular and kinaesthetic cues occur in flight because the pilot is exposed to rotational and transitional motion stimuli which differ in respect of magnitude, direction, or time course from those which man experiences on the ground and for which the receptor systems are functionally adapted. The mechanism mediating the generation of specific illusions of angular motion and of attitude by false vestibular and kinaesthetic cues are described in Chapter 21, but they may be broadly divided, as follows: (1) false information from semicircular canal receptors on recovery from prolonged rotation (somatogyral illusions) and on moving the head during rotation (cross-coupled or Coriolis illusions); and (2) false information from otoliths and kinaesthetic receptors during sustained acceleration (somatogravic illusions) and on moving the head in an atypical force environment (G excess illusions).

In addition, the semicircular canal receptors can be stimulated by changes in middle ear pressure during ascent and descent so that erroneous sensations of turning (pressure vertigo) are produced without there being any angular motion of the aircraft.

Central errors

Disorientation due to the pilot's failure to make optimum use of reliable information about aircraft orientation can arise because of limitations of the brain mechanisms which mediate the perceptual process. In general, the limitations are not caused by disease but are normal behavioural responses to the physical and mental load imposed by the flying task.

Coning of attention or 'fascination'

This most commonly occurs in the student pilot who, under the stress of attempting to perform a demanding and unfamiliar task, allows his attention to be confined to one aspect of his task (Clark, Nicholson and Graybiel, 1953). But with experience and the acquisition of skill, the pilot learns to maintain a regular scan so that all aspects of the aircraft's flight trajectory and systems are adequately monitored. Yet even the experienced pilot, when presented with a high workload, when anxious, or when unduly aroused, can lose efficiency. One aspect of this impairment of performance is a restriction of the field of attention. Thus when flying by instruments the pilot may fix his attention on one instrument, say, airspeed, and fail to notice a potentially dangerous change in attitude or height. The absence of information from non-visual receptors at such a time is of course contributary to the disorientation that occurs with the coning of attention. This type of perceptual limitation most commonly occurs during instrument flight; but it is not unknown for a pilot in good VMC to become 'fascinated' during an attack manoeuvre on a ground target and for him to fail to perceive his height above the ground until dangerously late in the manoeuvre.

Coning of attention should not be mistaken for coning of vision. While it is true that visual events outside the restricted area subtended by a particular instrument are not perceived, this cone of attention is not a solid angle of invariant size. The problem is not overcome by presenting more information within a smaller area, as in a head-up display, for it has been found that coning of attention still occurs, even though the angular subtense of the display is considerably less than that of basic flight instruments.

Error of expectancy

The heuristic nature of the perceptual process has been alluded to in an earlier section where it was pointed out that an individual's perception of a particular sensory event is based on past experience and, hence, on the conditional probability of a particular temporo-spatial pattern of sensory information being associated with that event. The example quoted was one in which the pilot levelled the wings of his aircraft with cloud tops which he thought and expected to be horizontal, but which were inclined to the horizontal. Other incidents have been described in which visual information is misinterpreted and an illusory perception of attitude

results. The pilot flying over the sea on a dark night looks out of the aircraft and sees a number of points of light below him which he perceives as stars, because at night he expects to see stars rather than lights on fishing boats. This misperception leads to another: stars should be above him not below, therefore the aircraft must be inverted. Without checking the attitude display, the pilot rolls the aircraft over in order to bring it to what he mistakenly thinks is the correct attitude. Errors in the perception of distance can occur when ground features are atypical. There have been a number of accidents in which the pilot has overestimated his height above the ground or distance from the side of a mountain because the trees were unusually small. If, for example, the pilot, from past experience, expects birch trees to be 10–20 m tall then his perception of distance from ground covered by stunted trees only 4–5 m high is likely to be in error by a factor of two or more.

Visual information departing from expectancy is the cause of a number of other illusions experienced by aircrew. The 'lean on the sun' illusion is a false perception of attitude that occurs when flying in cloud, particularly when close to the top of the cloud. Though the sun is not visible, the cloud is distinctly brighter in the direction of the sun than in the rest of an amorphous visual scene. In these circumstances the pilot equates the brightest area of cloud with 'up' and the dark cloud below as 'down' and so acquires a false vertical reference. Thus if the sun appears to the left of the flight path, the pilot may bank the aircraft to the left to preserve an apparent straight and level attitude, or, conversely, he may feel that the aircraft is right-wing low when instruments indicate a wings-level attitude. Comparable illusions of pitch attitude have also occurred when flying in cloud on a heading towards the sun.

Expectancy also contributes to the perceptual errors engendered by inappropriate vestibular cues. Years of experience during maturation and normal locomotion and postural activity in a terrestrial environment lead to a high conditional probability that signals from the semicircular canals are an accurate representation of angular movement of the head, and that otolithic signals represent the dynamic component of translational movement and the attitude of the head with respect to the force of gravity. Accordingly, when comparable signals are generated by these sense organs by atypical motion stimuli, there is no reason why the sensation or perception of motion engendered should differ from that which occurs when the receptors correctly transduce a typical stimulus. *A fortiori* when the semicircular canals erroneously signal rotation, say on recovery from a spin, the pilot perceives rotation. Likewise, during sustained acceleration (or deceleration) in the line of flight where the resultant of the imposed acceleration and that of gravity deflects the otoliths, the perceptual process does not distinguish the resultant acceleration from that of gravity alone; errors in the perception of attitude occur because of the high conditional probability that the sustained discharge from the otoliths represents the orientation of the head to the gravitational vertical rather than their response to a sustained acceleration other than that of gravity.

Other disturbances of brain function

The coning of attention that occurs when an individual has to perform a demanding or emotionally stressful task is but one manifestation of the changes in brain function and behaviour that are associated with 'arousal' beyond an optimum level (Easterbrook, 1959). 'Arousal' in this context is used in a somewhat specialized way to identify a behavioural continuum—the arousal continuum—which ranges from drowsiness at one extreme, to acute awareness, even panic, at the other. Although the concept is not perfect, it is useful when one attempts to integrate the varied effects of physical and mental stress on behaviour and brain function.

One important effect of high arousal is that it causes 'regression', a term first used by Head (1920), to describe the reversion to a more firmly established, a more primitive, pattern of behaviour. In flight this may be manifest as a breakdown of the more complex and more recently acquired skills, of which instrument flying is the prime example. When learning to fly by instruments, the pilot is trained to ignore vestibular and kinaesthetic sensations; indeed, the experienced pilot is frequently unaware of such potentially disorientating sensations, even though they may be accessible to introspection. However, when aroused, the pilot is more likely to attend to his endogenous vestibular signals and may even base his control of the aircraft on such inappropriate cues, despite his training to disregard them.

Associated with the loss of recently acquired skills is a 'diminution of cerebral competence'. This term is used to describe the impairment of higher mental function with supra-optimal arousal and embraces the decrement in perceptual integration, decision-making ability, cognitive function and in supervisory activity which can occur in high arousal states. Again, it is when flying on instruments that such disturbances of brain function are most apparent. Pilots who have been highly aroused by, say, sudden and severe disorientation not infrequently report that they were unable to interpret the cockpit instruments, even though they could be seen with clarity. In contrast, aircrew rarely have any difficulty in the interpretation of external visual cues unless vision is seriously degraded.

Although disorientation is more commonly a feature of behavioural states where the level of arousal is high, in a few incidents it is the low level of arousal that is the prime aetiological factor (Clark *et al.*, 1953). Arousal below the optimum also causes a diminution of cerebral competence, and with it a greater probability of perceptual errors. In particular, when the pilot is drowsy or inattentive he is more likely to fail to perceive motion cues and to make an ill-considered response to misinterpreted sensory information.

The 'level of arousal' is far from being the only factor that modifies the process of perception, for this is dependent on the normal function of the central nervous system which, in turn, is dependent on the maintenance of the chemical and physical milieu of the brain within relatively narrow limits. It would be inappropriate to detail here the many factors that, in flight, may interfere with brain function as they range from the classical environmental stresses of flight, like hypoxia, hypocapnia, toxic agents and hyperthermia, to the myriad clinical disorders which, albeit rarely, can impair cerebral competence and disorientate the pilot.

References

BARNES, G.R. (1984) The effect of ethyl alcohol on visual pursuit and suppression of the vestibulo-ocular reflex. *Acta Otolaryngolica Supplement*, **406**, 218–223

BENSON, A.J. (1987) The vestibular sensory system. In *The Senses*, edited by H.B. Barlow and J.D. Mollon, 2nd edn. Chapter 16. Cambridge University Press

BENSON, A.J., DIAZ, E. and FARRUGIA, P. (1975) The perception of body orientation relative to a rotating linear acceleration vector. *Fortschritte der Zoologie*, **23**, 264–274

BENSON, A.J. and GUEDRY, F.E. (1971) Comparison of tracking performance and nystagmus during sinusoidal oscillation in yaw and pitch. *Aerospace Medicine,* **42**, 593–600

CLARK, B. (1971) Disorientation incidents reported by military pilots across fourteen years of flight. In *The Disorientation Incident*. Conference Report CP 95, A1, 1–6. Neuilly sur Seine: AGARD/NATO

CLARK, B. and GRAYBIEL, A. (1955) *Disorientation: A Cause of Pilot Error*. Bureau of Medicine and Surgery Research Report. No. NM 001 110 100. 39. Pensacola, Fla: US Navy School of Aviation Medicine

CLARK, B., NICHOLSON, M.A. and GRAYBIEL, A. (1953) Fascination: a cause of pilot error. *Journal of Aviation Medicine*, **24**, 429–440

DICHGANS, J. and BRANDT, T. (1978) Visual vestibular interactions: effects on self-motion perception and postural control. In *Handbook of Sensory Physiology*, edited by R. Held, H. Leibowitz and H.L. Teuber, Vol. 8, pp. 755–804. Berlin: Springer Verlag

EASTERBROOK, J.A. (1959) The effect of emotion on cue utilisation and the organisation of behaviour. *Psychological Review*, **66**, 183–201

EDGINGTON, K. (1980) Disorientation in army helicopter operations—a general review. In *Spatial Disorientation in Flight: Current Problems*. Conference Report CP 287, B6, 1–6. Neuilly sur Seine: AGARD/NATO

GUEDRY, F.E. (1974) Psychophysics of vestibular sensation. Chapter 1. In *Handbook of Sensory Physiology*, edited by H.H. Kornhuber, Vol. 6, pp. 3–154. Berlin: Springer-Verlag

HEAD, H. (1920) The sense of stability and balance in the air. In *Medical Problems of Flying*. Medical Research Council Special Report. No 53, pp. 215–256. London: HMSO

HIXSON, W.C., NIVEN, J.I. and SPEZIA, E. (1972) *Major Orientation Error Accidents in Regular Army UH-1 Aircraft During Fiscal Year 1969: Accident Factors*. Report NAMRL-1169. Pensacola, Fla.: Naval Aerospace Medical Research Laboratory

HOWARD, I.P. (1982) *Human Visual Orientation*. Chichester: J. Wiley & Sons

KIRKHAM, W.R., COLLINS, W.E., GRAPE, P.M., SIMPSON, J.M. and WALLACE, T.F. (1978) Spatial disorientation in general aviation accidents. *Aviation Space and Environmental Medicine*, **49**, 1080–1086

KRAUS, R.N. (1959) Disorientation in flight—an evaluation of the etiological factors. *Aerospace Medicine*, **30**, 664–673

LEIBOWITZ, H.W. and DICHGANS, J. (1980) The ambient visual system and spatial disorientation. In *Spatial Disorientation in Flight: Current Problems*. Conference

Report CP 287, B4, 1–4. Neuilly sur Seine: AGARD/NATO

LINDEMAN, H.H. (1969) Studies on the morphology of the sensory regions of the vestibular apparatus. *Ergebnisse der Anatomie und Entwicklungsgeschichte*, **42**, 1–113

MARTIN, J.F. and MELVILL JONES, G. (1965) Theoretical man–machine interaction which might lead to loss of aircraft control. *Aerospace Medicine*, **36**, 713–716

O'CONNOR, P.J. (1967) Differential diagnosis of disorientation in flying. *Aerospace Medicine*, **38**, 1155–1160

STEELE-PERKINS, A.P. and EVANS, D.A. (1978) Disorientation in naval helicopter pilots. In *Operational Helicopter Aviation Medicine*. Conference Proceedings CP 255, 48, 1–5. Neuilly sur Seine: AGARD/NATO

TORMES, F.R. and GUEDRY, F.E. (1975) Disorientation phenomena in naval helicopter pilots. *Aviation Space and Environmental Medicine*, **46**, 387–393

TREDICI, T.J. (1980) Visual illusions as a probable cause of aircraft accidents. In *Spatial Disorientation in Flight: Current Problems*. Conference Report CP 287, B5, 1–5. Neuilly sur Seine: AGARD/NATO

YOUNG, L.R. (1984) Perception of the body in space: mechanisms. In *Handbook of Physiology—The Nervous System III*, Part 2, edited by Darian Smith, I. Chapter 22. Bethesda, Ma.: American Physiological Society, William & Wilkins

21

Spatial disorientation—common illusions

A.J. Benson

Introduction

The aetiology of spatial disorientation is discussed in general terms in Chapter 20. The salient features of some of the more frequently reported illusions, together with their causal mechanisms, are the subject of this chapter.

Somatogravic and oculogravic illusions

Errors in the perception of attitude can occur when the airman is exposed to force environments that differ significantly from those experienced during normal activity on the surface of the Earth, where

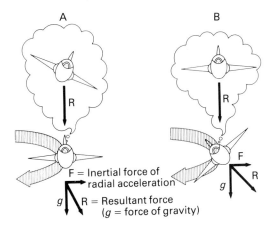

Figure 21.1 False perception of attitude—the somatogravic illusion—in a turn. The pilot equates the sustained resultant (R) with the vertical. Hence in a flat turn (A) he may feel as if rolled out of the turn. In the more usual co-ordinated turn (B) the resultant is aligned with his Z axis and he has no sensation of being banked in attitude.

the force of gravity is a stable reference and is regarded as the vertical. The acceleration of gravity is the same physical phenomenon as a linear (or translational) acceleration, hence the one is not easily distinguished from the other. When the imposed linear acceleration is of short duration or oscillatory, man is able to separate, perceptually, the imposed motion from that of gravity. For example, the motion of a swing or the bounce of a motor car are sensed with reasonable accuracy. But when the acceleration is sustained, as in a centrifuge, or when an aircraft accelerates in response to an increase in thrust or a reduction of drag, the perceptual mechanism is unable to distinguish the imposed acceleration from that of gravity. The two accelerations are combined, and the resultant becomes the 'reference' acceleration which is regarded as the vertical. This occurs because there is a high expectancy that a sustained acceleration is gravity and hence the vertical (Wulfften Palthe, 1922).

The simplest example of an illusory perception of attitude, due to an atypical resultant acceleration (or force) vector, is the inability of the pilot to sense accurately, other than by visual cues, the angle of bank during a prolonged co-ordinated turn (*Figure 21.1*). He does have some information about bank angle from the semicircular canals which are stimulated by the angular motion in roll as the aircraft enters the turn; but once a steady rate of turn and constant bank angle are established, the resultant of the force of gravity and the inertial force due to the radial (or centripetal) acceleration engendered by the curved flight path is normal to the longitudinal and transverse axes of the aircraft and is aligned with the pilot's Z axis. The direction of action of this resultant force does not differ from that of gravity on the body when man is in a normal upright position in a 1g environment. Hence when he is in a co-ordinated turn, vestibular and kinaesthetic cues are not dissimilar to those in level flights, so the pilot is likely to feel that he is in a wings-level attitude. Conversely, in a flat turn, when the resultant vector is not normal to the transverse axis of the aircraft (*Figure 21.1*), he may feel as if the aircraft is banked out of the turn.

These are examples of a group of illusions termed somatogravic illusions in which there is a false perception of attitude on exposure to a force vector that differs in direction and/or magnitude from the normal gravitational force (Benson and Burchard, 1973). More important from the viewpoint of flight safety than the illusory perceptions of roll attitude are those somatogravic illusions where there is an error in the perception of pitch attitude.

Consider the change in the direction of the resultant force vector associated with acceleration in the line of flight (*Figure 21.2*). When the aircraft accelerates, on increasing engine power or reducing drag, the inertial force due to the increase in forward speed combines with the force of gravity to produce a resultant which is inclined backwards. Should this resultant be used as a vertical reference then the airman will feel as if he and the aircraft are in a nose-up attitude. Conversely, when an aircraft undergoes a sustained deceleration, as on applying air-brakes, the resultant vector swings forwards and

the pilot can feel as if the aircraft has pitched nose down.

From laboratory experiments it is known that, on average, the subjective vertical is closely aligned with the resultant vector. However, it has also been shown that it can take a minute or more for the illusion to develop fully and, in common with other illusions, that there are large individual differences in the magnitude of the illusion (Clark and Graybiel, 1963, 1966). Some subjects experience a larger angular deviation of the subjective vertical than is warranted by the change in direction of the resultant, others substantially less. Thus even when the force environment to which the pilot is exposed can be described with mathematical precision, it is not possible to predict with certainty the nature of the erroneous perception quantitatively. *Figure 21.2* is an over-simplification. Qualitatively, however, errors in the perception of pitch attitude do undoubtedly occur when there are changes in aircraft longitudinal acceleration (Graybiel *et al.*, 1979). Even a brief G_x acceleration, such as a catapult launch (5 G or 50 m/s² peak, 2–3 seconds duration), has been shown to give rise to an apparent nose-up change in attitude which, though not large (mean 5 degrees or 0.1 rad), took a minute or more to die away (Cohen, Crosbie and Blackburn, 1973). Conversely, it was shown by Collar (1946) during World War II that a relatively low

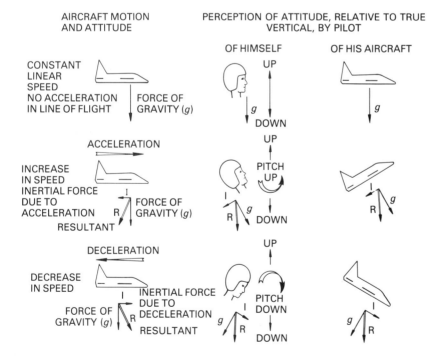

Figure 21.2 Somatogravic illusions during linear acceleration in the line of flight give errors in the perception of pitch attitude.

acceleration of 0.2G, if sustained for several minutes, could delude the pilot into thinking that the aircraft was climbing, or at least was in level flight, when in fact the nose of the aircraft was depressed and height was being lost rapidly.

The somatogravic illusion occurring on take-off and when overshooting is a particular danger, especially at night or in poor visibility. The pilot who at such a time responds to an apparent increase in pitch-up attitude by pushing the control column forwards has little time, and little altitude, in which to rectify his error. The perceptual error is also likely to be intensified by the subsequent flight path of the aircraft which, being curved, introduces a radial acceleration (Martin and Melvill Jones, 1965). The combination of centrifugal force, the inertial force due to the acceleration of the aircraft in the longitudinal axis and gravity produces a resultant force vector with an even larger deviation from the true vertical (*Figure 21.3*). Thus the pilot, on making what he thinks to be an appropriate corrective response, may feel that the nose-up attitude is increasing rather than becoming less, and

he may be tempted to push the stick even further forward. This response increases the tightness of the bunt manoeuvre with further rotation of the force vector, even to the extent of the pilot being exposed to negative G_z. Pilots who have experienced this type of force environment, at a sufficiently high altitude to appreciate and recover from their disorientation, say that the aircraft felt as if it pitched up and flipped over on its back. Recovery was usually made from a near vertical dive, many thousands of feet lower than the height at which the illusion first occurred.

Effect of head movement—'G excess' illusion

It has long been recognized that erroneous sensations of angular motion are evoked when head movements are made in a turning aircraft, and it has been customary to attribute such illusions to cross-coupled stimulation (*see below*) of the semi-

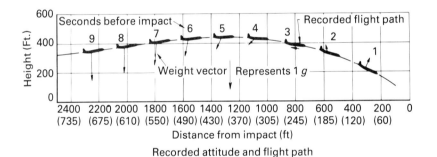

Recorded attitude and flight path

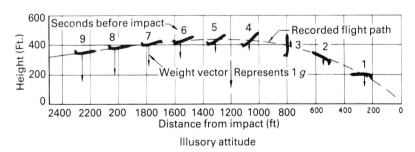

Illusory attitude

Figure 21.3 Recorded flight path and calculated force (weight) vector of an aircraft (Vanguard G-APEE) that crashed after initiating an overshoot. The initial change in the direction of the force vector was caused by acceleration in the line of flight. Later the curved flight path introduced a radial acceleration and was responsible for large changes in the direction and magnitude of the force vector. Over the relatively short time scale in which changes in the force environment occurred it is unlikely that the illusory perception of attitude was as erroneous as indicated in the lower half of the figure, but illusions of the form shown have been reported during comparable bunt manoeuvres. (Distance from impact in m given in parentheses.)

circular canals. However, experiments carried out by Gilson *et al.* (1973) in high-performance aircraft, where a large radius co-ordinate turn was flown with a resultant acceleration of 2G but with a low rate of turn (4 degrees/s), have shown that head movements in pitch, roll or yaw could induce false sensations of aircraft attitude. Commonly, subjects reported an illusory sensation of climb or dive on moving the head in pitch, though neither the direction nor the magnitude of the illusion nor the evocative head movement was entirely consistent between individuals. These false sensations were not caused by cross-coupled stimulation of the semicircular canals, because the plane of the apparent motion did not accord with such a mechanism and the rate of turn was so low. Rather, it is suggested, the sensations are the consequence of a transient and atypical stimulation of otolithic receptors as their orientation to the abnormal force vector changes when the head is moved.

Despite the lack of a clear-cut relationship between head movement and sensation, the illusory sensation experienced by some subjects can be powerful, particularly when the head is moved quickly; others find the sensations confusing and disorientating, yet difficult to describe precisely in terms of aircraft attitude and motion.

Other experiments have shown that a forward head movement in pitch, made during a $+6G_z$ pull-up from a dive, consistently evoked a sensation of tumbling forward in pitch. The illusion is not just an apparent change in attitude but contains an element of rotation in the plane of the head movement, despite the absence of any cross-coupled stimulus to the semicircular canals.

Oculogravic illusions

The illusory perception of attitude engendered by a force vector that is not aligned with the gravitational vertical is in no way dependent on the visual sense: it is an illusion of body orientation—hence the term somatogravic illusion. Unfortunately, the term oculogravic is often, albeit incorrectly, used to describe such illusions, but this adjective should be confined to the apparent movement and false localization of visual targets that may be produced by the same atypical force environments as evoke somatogravic illusions (Graybiel, 1952). Indeed, the oculogravic illusion is best regarded as a visual component of the somatogravic illusion. Thus when an aircraft accelerates and there is a backward rotation of the resultant force vector (*Figure 21.4*), the pilot may experience a somatogravic illusion of a nose-change in attitude which may be accompanied by an apparent upward movement and displacement of objects within his visual field. Conversely, on deceleration, the visual world may appear to move

downwards and be displaced, until the force environment returns to the normal 1 g.

Such changes in the direction and magnitude of the force vector are known to produce compensatory eye movements which, with rapid rotation of the force vector, may be nystagmic and cause transient impairment of vision. These eye movements also accentuate the apparent upward movement of a visual target. Once steady-state conditions are reached (that is, when the force vector maintains constant direction and magnitude) there is a small compensatory deviation of the eye in the pitch-down direction. This causes a displacement of the image of the outside world on the retina and contributes to the apparent displacement of what the pilot sees. However, the angle through which the eye deviates is only about one-tenth of the angle through which the vector is displaced from the true (gravitational) vertical (Lichtenberg, Young and Arrott, 1982). Therefore, it must be concluded that the apparent movement and displacement of the visual scene, brought about by a change in the force environment (that is, the oculogravic illusion), is not due primarily to eye movement but to the perceptual mechanism within the brain which integrates the cues from the otoliths and other receptors stimulated by the linear accelerations (Clark and Graybiel, 1963).

The oculogravic illusion is rarely a problem when external visual cues are well defined, for the illusory movement affects all objects within the visual field so that there is no relative movement between objects in the external visual scene and the frame of reference provided by aircraft structures (for example, cockpit canopy, instrument panel, etc.). In the presence of a resultant force vector that is not aligned with the gravitational vertical, the surface of the Earth may appear to be in a non-horizontal plane, but the position and attitude of the aircraft is not changed with respect to the external visual reference.

At night, however, particularly when only a few stars or isolated lights are visible—conditions in which external visual cues are largely inadequate—the oculogravic illusion can be a significant cause of spatial disorientation (Clark and Graybiel, 1949). The apparent movement and transient displacement of light sources in the external visual scene can be interpreted by the airman as a change in attitude of the aircraft. Alternatively, the apparent movement of an isolated light can lead to the misperception that the light is on another aircraft which he may attempt to follow or, perhaps, to avoid. As an example of an error in the perception of a pilot's attitude produced by the oculogravic illusion, consider the effect of a backward rotation of the resultant force vector (as when accelerating). The illusory movement of an isolated light, say a bright star, will be upwards. This may be perceived by the

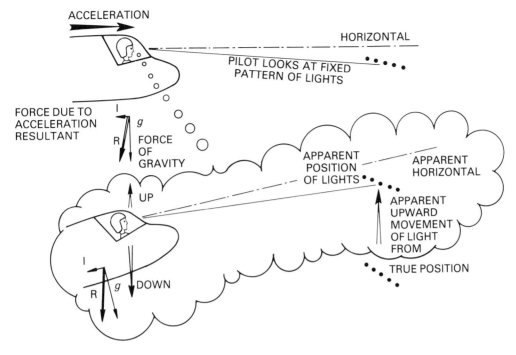

Figure 21.4 The oculogravic illusion. This is the visual component of the somatogravic illusion in which a change in the force environment causes apparent movement and false localization of observed objects.

pilot as a nose-down change in attitude of the aircraft, especially if his attention is confined to the external visual scene and he does not detect the concomitant and equal apparent movement of illuminated displays within the aircraft. The illusory perception is, of course, in the opposite direction to that of the somatogravic illusion produced by the same change in direction of the resultant force vector. Despite this paradox no airman has reported the kind of perceptual conflict that might, in theory, be expected to occur. When there are no external visual cues, the somatogravic illusion is dominant and is supported by the oculogravic illusion affecting the visual scene within the cockpit; when there are isolated cues in the external visual scene and aircraft references are not perceived, the illusory perception of aircraft attitude is dictated by the apparent movement of the external visual target, presumably because the visual percept of spatial orientation carries precedence over one based on non-visual cues.

Visual illusions also occur when there is a change in the magnitude of the force vector without rotation of the vector. These were given the name elevator illusions by Niven, Whiteside and Graybiel (1963) because they were first studied in lifts or elevators, though comparable changes in the force environment occur during flight through an up or down-draught. With an increase in the magnitude of the

gravity vector, such as occurs during vertical acceleration in the upward direction (up-draught), there is a correct sensation of upward movement which is accompanied by an apparent upward motion and displacement of the visual scene. Conversely, when the force vector decreases, as during flight through a down-draught, there is an apparent downward movement and displacement of objects within the pilot's visual scene.

There is apparent motion and displacement of all objects within the visual field so the illusion primarily concerns the perception of external visual references. During vertical translation these should appear to move either in the opposite direction, or not at all, relative to an observer in the aircraft, but the 'elevator illusion' causes objects in the external visual scene to move and be displaced in the same direction as the vertical motion of the aircraft. In contrast, the apparent movement of objects within the visual field that are part of the aircraft (for example, the instrument display) is in the correct sense; the erroneous component of perception is only the apparent displacement of the viewed object which does not move, relative to the observer, during the G_z acceleration.

These visual illusions are relatively easily suppressed and are rarely noticed when flying with good external visual cues. But when external visual cues are sparse the apparent movement of an isolated light may be interpreted as a change in pitch attitude of the aircraft; an upward movement is perceived as pitch nose-down and the converse when there is a reduction in the magnitude of the aircraft's normal acceleration. The hazard from these errors in perception, as in other manifestations of the somatogravic and oculogravic illusions, is that control responses are made by the pilot before he looks at the instruments and checks the orientation of his aircraft.

The leans

A false sensation of roll attitude, colloquially known as 'the leans', is the most commonly reported manifestation of spatial disorientation (*see Tables 20.1 and 20.2*). There are several different ways in which the illusion can be produced but most frequently it is associated with recovery from a co-ordinated turn to level flight when flying by instruments. If the pilot enters the turn gradually and smoothly, the angular velocity in roll as the aircraft is banked into the turn may well be below the threshold of detection (0.2–8.0 degree/s). As discussed earlier in this chapter, the otoliths and other bodily gravireceptors also provide no information about the angle of bank because in a co-ordinated turn the resultant of the radial acceleration (produced by the curved flight path) and gravity remains aligned with the pilot's head–

foot (Z) axis. As depicted in *Figure 21.5* the pilot is, by definition, disorientated because he (or she) feels that the aircraft is in a wings-level attitude when in fact it is in a banked attitude.

If recovery from the co-ordinated turn is made at a sub-threshold rate then by the time the instruments indicate level flight the pilot's sensations will be in accord with the true attitude of the aircraft. If, on the other hand, recovery from the turn is made more abruptly, such that the angular velocity in roll is an adequate stimulus to the semicircular canals, the sensation engendered will be one of a change in roll attitude that is essentially correct with respect to the magnitude and direction of the angular movement in roll. But as the pilot erroneously felt that he was wings level before the recovery manoeuvre, the ensuing perception is one of banking away from the level attitude. Thus one erroneous perception leads to another, and the pilot on recovering from the turn can feel that the aircraft is flying one wing low when the attitude display indicates that the wings are level. There is a conflict of sensory cues—a conflict that has to be resolved. Most pilots in such a circumstance attempt to ignore their own sensations and maintain the correct flight path by instrument reference. Yet once attention has been directed to the false sensation it can be very difficult to ignore, especially when there is no powerful (that is, external) visual cue to tell the pilot that his sensation is in error. The false sensation of bank may persist for many minutes and on occasions much longer;

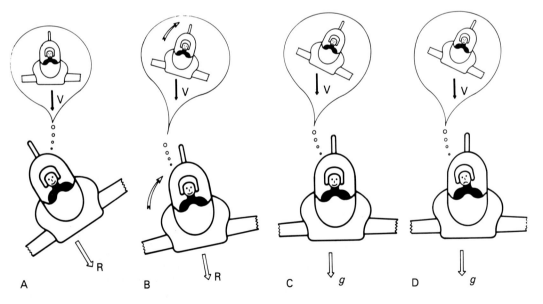

A	B	C	D
Aircraft in co-ordinated turn to right. Pilot feels that wings are level	Pilot rolls out of turn, feels that aircraft is banking to left	Aircraft in straight and level flight. Pilot feels left wing low	Pilot aligns head and trunk to perceived vertical and leans to right

Figure 21.5 Diagrammatic representation of one cause of 'the leans'.

indeed, durations of over an hour have been reported. Control is maintained by instrument reference, but the continued sensory conflict can drain the nervous energy of even the most experienced pilot. The reason why, on some occasions, the illusory sensation should be so persistent is not known, but quite characteristically 'the leans' are dispelled as soon as the pilot has unambiguous external visual cues, such as a well-defined horizon or a clear sight of the ground. Here then is a demonstration of the greater 'strength' of 'ambient' visual cues over 'focal' cues from instruments in determining spatial orientation in flight.

When affected by the 'leans' the pilot may feel compelled to align his body, not with the normal axis of the aircraft, but with the apparent vertical. In doing so he leans in the direction of the original banked attitude (*Figure 21.5*). Alternatively, he may roll the aircraft in order to neutralize the false sensation of bank, so that he may once again feel straight and level. We know that when the pilot leans his head and upper body slightly to one side he also has a tendency to pull the control stick to the side assumed to be the vertical. This, in turn, causes an alteration of aircraft attitude and necessitates further supra-threshold corrections, with possible exacerbation of the 'leans'.

The 'leans' may also be produced by aircraft motion in which a supra-threshold change in the roll attitude is followed by a sub-threshold return to the wings-level position. For example, if a sudden gust induces bank, the change in roll attitude will be correctly sensed by the pilot because the motion stimulus is above detection threshold. But if he recovers only slowly to an indicated level attitude, the sensation of being banked may persist because of the lack of sensory information from vestibular and kinaesthetic receptors during the recovery phase of the manoeuvre.

Another possible cause of the 'leans' is a minor directional asymmetry in the pilot's ability to detect changes in roll attitude. Laboratory experiments and clinical tests have shown that many individuals are more sensitive to angular motion in one direction than the other (Benson, 1973a). Thus in flight, particularly in minor turbulence where the aircraft continuously makes small oscillatory movements in roll, such a threshold asymmetry could give rise to an illusory perception of motion in the direction of greater sensitivity which could be perceptually integrated to give apparent displacement (that is, the 'leans') even though the wings remained more or less level.

Apart from these 'vestibular threshold' mechanisms, the 'leans' can also be caused by the misinterpretation of visual cues. The use of an erroneous horizontal reference—as in 'cloud leans', or the false localization of the vertical during flight in cloud because the brightest part of the cloud is regarded as up (the 'lean on the sun' illusion)—are described in Chapter 20.

False perception of angular motion: vertigo

Vertigo is defined as an illusory sensation of turning, but, as noted in Chapter 20, in aircrew jargon 'vertigo' is applied to any form of spatial disorientation, even when there is no illusory sensation of turning. Accordingly, the adjective somatogyral will be applied to those incidents in which the airman has an illusory perception of angular motion either of himself, or of self and aircraft. The term oculogyral will be restricted to the visual illusions produced by angular motion stimuli, in the same manner as oculogravic and somatogravic are used respectively to identify the visual and non-visual components of the illusions engendered by atypical force environments.

The somatogyral illusion

It was pointed out earlier that the semicircular canal receptors are stimulated only by angular accelerations and hence signal changes in angular velocity. Thus during a prolonged turning manoeuvre at a constant angular speed, whether this be a co-ordinated turn, a sustained roll, or a spin, these receptors only give correct information during the first few seconds of the manoeuvre (*see Figure 20.8*). Once a steady speed of rotation has been achieved the signals from the semicircular canals, stimulated by the initial angular acceleration, die away progressively and fall below the threshold value after about 10–20 seconds. The time taken for the sensation of turning to die away depends on a number of factors: the speed of rotation, the axis of rotation, the nature of cues from other sensory receptors and the extent to which the pilot is familiar with the motion stimuli (level of habituation). But for a typical spin, in which the aircraft may reach a rotational speed of 120–150 degree/s (2–3 rad/s) in 2–3 seconds, it can be reckoned that most pilots will be unable to perceive rotation accurately by purely vestibular mechanisms, after 15–30 seconds. They can, however, detect the continuation of the spin by the erratic pitching rolling and yawing movements that occur in most spinning aircraft and can determine the direction of the spin from the blurred image of the outside world or from cockpit instruments. The task of maintaining an awareness of aircraft orientation is even more difficult during an inverted spin, in part because rolling and yawing movements do not appear to occur in the same sense, as they do in an erect spin, and in part because of the pilot's unfamiliarity with this configuration of flight (Melvill Jones, 1957).

In an erect or inverted spin external visual cues, and, more reliably, the turn indicator display, allow the pilot to determine the direction of the spin and to initiate appropriate recovery action, but as soon as the aircraft begins to come out of the spin there is an angular acceleration in the opposite direction to that which occurred on entering the spin. The semicircular canals are stimulated again and evoke a sensation of turning in the opposite direction (*see Figure 20.8*). This somatogyral illusion occurs at a time when the pilot has to decide when the rotational component of the spin has ceased in order to complete the recovery manoeuvre. The only reliable means of detecting the cessation of the spin is by reference either to instruments or to the appearance of the external visual scene. At this critical time vision may be degraded by nystagmus which is as inappropriate as the concomitant sensation of turning. No matter how hard the pilot may try to 'see', it commonly takes several seconds for the eye movement to be suppressed sufficiently so that instruments can be read.

The presence of false sensations and impaired vision can have serious consequences during spin recovery. On the one hand, the pilot may feel that the spin has been neutralized before this has actually happened and subsequently get into difficulties on attempting to pull out. Alternatively, having recovered correctly, he may feel that the aircraft is spinning in the opposite direction and may make inappropriate control movements to counteract this illusory spin. If he does so, the aircraft can enter a spin in the original direction or even an inverted spin. This can give rise to an even more complex and confusing impression of motion so that, finally, it might be impossible for the pilot to regain control of his aircraft.

Comparable problems arise on recovery from prolonged rolling manoeuvres in level flight, where the illusory sensation in roll may cause the pilot to re-enter the roll. On recovery, the illusory sensations in this axis tend to be of shorter duration than those following rotation in yaw and the impairment of vision less severe. The presence of correct information about roll attitude from the otoliths and kinaesthetic receptors modifies the coupling between the stimulated canals and evoked response, such that the erroneous sensation of angular motion in roll dies away considerably more quickly than the signal from the stimulated ampullae. The nystagmus in roll also has a shorter time constant of decay, though the principal reason why visual impairment is less following roll stimuli than from the predominantly yawing motion of a spin lies in the anisometric distribution of retinal smear. In-

appropriate nystagmus in roll causes little movement of the retinal image close to the visual axis and hence little decrement in foveal acuity; on the other hand, nystagmus in yaw causes movement of the whole retinal image and impairment of acuity over the whole visual field.

Emphasis has been placed on the erroneous sensations (after-sensations) produced on recovery from sustained rotational manoeuvres where sufficient time has elapsed for the cupulae of the stimulated canals to have returned from their deflected to close to their neutral (rest) positions. It should be pointed out, however, that the cessation of rotation after considerably shorter times at constant, or near-constant, speeds also gives rise to illusory after-sensations. As the rate at which the cupula returns to its rest position follows an exponential time course, only a few seconds of steady rotation are required for a significant somatogyral illusion to develop. For example, in *Figure 20.8* the cupular deflection falls to 50% of its peak value after only 4 seconds. Recovery from the roll at this time would, therefore, induce an erroneous sensation of turning in the opposite direction which would have about half the intensity of the after-sensation evoked after a substantially longer time (30 seconds or more) at constant speed.

The rate at which the cupula returns to its neutral position, following deflection by an angular acceleration (a step velocity input), is greater for the vertical canals—that is, those stimulated by roll and pitch motions—than for the lateral (yaw axis) canals (Melvill Jones, Barry and Kowalsky, 1964). Accordingly, the somatogyral illusion is likely to be of greater intensity following just one or two turns in roll than following a rotational manoeuvre in yaw of similar rate and duration; the duration of the after-sensation will, of course, be shorter for the roll motion stimulus than for one in yaw.

The oculogyral illusion

Apart from the impairment of visual acuity caused by nystagmic eye movements, inappropriate signals from the semicircular canals have other effects on visual perception which can disorientate aircrew. These take the form of apparent motion and errors in the localization of visual targets and were called oculogyral illusions by Graybiel and Hupp (1946).

The several components of the oculogyral illusion are best illustrated by considering the nature of visual perception on recovery from prolonged turning, as in a spin. When the turn stops, the nystagmic eye movements are well defined and cause appreciable movement of the visual scene which is cyclical in nature; the more obvious movement, which is in the same direction as the sensation of turning, occurs during the slow phase component of the nystagmus. After several seconds the nystagmus is much reduced in amplitude and velocity so that it becomes possible to fixate on an object within the visual field, but there are still residual eye movements and hence some apparent movement of visual targets, even though these may be seen without appreciable decrement in acuity. If external visual cues are well defined, the sensation of turning (the somatogyral illusion) and the accompanying visual illusions are soon dissipated; but, if external cues are no more than an isolated light or star in an otherwise featureless visual field, illusory perceptions may persist for many seconds, even minutes. Once the initial nystagmus has been suppressed and the target light can be seen clearly, it will appear to rotate with the observer. Furthermore, it will not be correctly localized as it will appear to be displaced in the same direction as the illusory sensation of turn. The displacement becomes less as the vertigo dies away, but these two illusions do not necessarily follow the same time course, so that the target light may be correctly localized when the sensation of turn persists.

Although the oculogyral illusion has been described as part of the visual phenomenon arising from a relatively strong stimulus to the semicircular canals, the apparent movement of an isolated light can be brought about by angular motion stimuli which are close to threshold. Indeed, in laboratory experiments it has been found that the detection threshold of angular accelerations is usually lower when the subject is provided with a discrete visual target and can perceive an oculogyral illusion, than when he is in darkness and can report only on the occurrence of somatogyral sensation (Clark, 1970). In flight, the illusory perception of movement of an isolated light can thus be caused by quite liminal angular motions of the aircraft; the pilot perceives movement of the light, but not of his own aircraft. This error may in turn lead to a further misinterpretation—namely, that the light is not fixed in space but is carried by another aircraft. Disorientation ensues if the pilot accepts this false cue and alters his flight path to join up with the illusory aircraft. Fortunately, the pilot usually becomes aware of his error before an accident occurs; although this type of incident, in common with other manifestations of spatial disorientation, can be a frightening experience.

Illusions due to cross-coupled (Coriolis) stimulation of the semicircular canals

Reference has already been made to the disorientation evoked by head movements in an abnormal force environment, but no less important are the

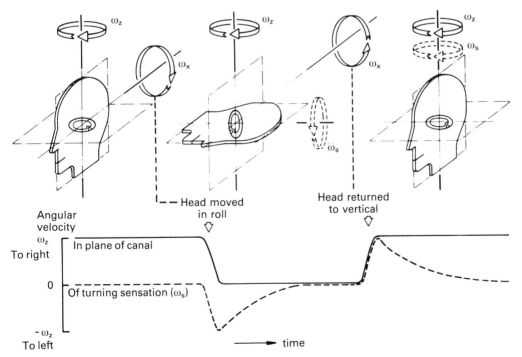

Figure 21.6 Cross-coupled stimulation of an idealized semicircular canal in the transverse (XY) plane of the head. An angular head movement in roll (ω_x) from the vertical to the left-ear down position during sustained rotation in yaw (ω_z) produces an illusory sensation in the orthogonal axis.

illusory and apparently bizarre sensations that can be produced when angular movements of the head are made in an aircraft that is turning. These cross-coupled responses, due to the stimulation of the semicircular canals by the interaction of angular motion in two planes, can be analysed in terms of the Coriolis forces induced by the complex motion. However, it is conceptually much simpler to consider each canal as an angular velocity sensor and to analyse how the angular velocity in the plane of each canal changes with the head movement.

As an initial simplification, let us examine the response of a single yaw axis semicircular canal to angular movement of the head, say in roll, in an individual who is rotating in yaw at a steady speed (ω_z) (*Figure 21.6*). We may further assume that he has been at speed for a minute or more so that the cupula, deflected by the initial angular acceleration in yaw, has returned to its neutral position. If the head is now moved, in a second or so, from the initial vertical position through 90 degrees ($\pi/2$ rad) to, say, the left-ear-down position, the yaw axis canal is taken out of the plane of rotation. The angular velocity in the plane of canal changes from ω_z to zero, and the cupula is deflected in just the same manner as if the yaw axis rotation was stopped without any movement of the head in roll. The sensation is therefore one of rotation in the yaw axis of the head in the opposite direction to that of the sustained rotation. As with the normal post-rotary sensation, this dies away slowly as the cupula returns to its neutral position. Once steady-state conditions are established, if the head is returned to the vertical position, the yaw canal is brought back into the plane of rotation and it 'sees' a change in velocity from zero to ω_z which, of course, stimulates the receptors and gives rise to a correct sensation of rotation in yaw to the right; this subsequently dies away as rotation is at constant speed and there is no force to deflect the cupula. In this example, a head movement through a right-angle in roll to the left was used, but the same effect is produced, for such an idealized yaw axis canal, by a 90 degree ($\pi/2$ rad) head movement to the right, or by movements of comparable magnitude in pitch to the nose-down or nose-up position.

If movements of a smaller magnitude are made, the change in velocity 'seen' by the canal is also smaller. The angular velocity in the plane of the canal is $\omega \sin \theta$, where θ is the angle between the plane of the canal and the axis of rotation of ω. Thus if the head is moved through 45 degrees ($\pi/4$ rad) from the vertical (where θ = 90 degrees ($\pi/2$ rad)) the effective stimulus (ω_e) is:

$$\omega_e = \omega \sin 90 - \omega \sin 45 = \omega(1 - \sin 45) = 0.3\omega.$$

If the head is moved from a left-ear-down position (θ = 0) through 45 degrees towards the vertical:

$$\omega_e = \omega \sin 0 - \omega \sin 45 = -\omega \sin 45 = 0.7\omega.$$

Let us now consider not one canal but three canals. Although in life the vertical canals do not lie in the pitch and roll axes of the skull, the brain is able to resolve the rotation transduced by these receptors into these orthogonal axes, so it is justifiable to represent all six canals as three orthogonal canals in the pitch, roll and yaw axes of the head. *Figure 21.7(a)* represents the angular velocity in the plane of each canal when the head is moved in roll from the vertical to the left-ear-down position while rotating at a steady speed in yaw. During the head movement the roll axis canal 'sees' the rise and fall of angular velocity in roll (ω_x), this movement is executed within a few seconds, so the stimulus is correctly transduced by the receptors. The yaw axis canal is taken out of the plane of rotation and 'sees' a velocity change of ω_z, while the pitch axis canal is brought into the plane of rotation and its receptors are stimulated by the velocity change, also of magnitude ω_z. The sensation evoked by the 'stopping' stimulus to the yaw canal and the 'starting' stimulus to the pitch canal are, with respect to the skull, rotation in yaw to the left and rotation in pitch, forward. The presence of gravity, however, allows the individual to perceive these sensations of angular motion in an Earth reference rather than a head reference system, so the signal from the pitch canal is reported as an increase in the rate of rotation about the vertical (Z) axis, while the yaw canal signal is sensed as a pitching motion about a Y body axis. After the head movement, the sensations of yaw and pitch die away as the deflected cupulae return to their neutral positions, though, characteristically, the distracting and illusory sensation of pitching forward dies away more quickly than that evoked by a simple stopping stimulus to the canals without movement of the head. The principal reason for this accelerated decay is the absence of correlated information from the canals, which signals rotation in pitch, and from the otoliths, which signal no movement of the head with respect to gravity. This conflict between canal and otolith organ cues, whilst it brings about a more rapid attenuation of the illusory sensation, is disturbing and is a cause not only of disorientation but, if repeated, also of motion sickness (*see below*).

Further examples of cross-coupling are illustrated in *Figure 21.7*. A head movement in roll from 45 degrees right to 45 degrees left while rotating at a steady speed (ω_z) about the Z body axis may be shown to be a potent stimulus to the pitch axis canal. When the head is in the tilted position, both the yaw and pitch canals 'see' an angular velocity of 0.7 ω_z: but as the head is moved in roll (ω_x), the yaw canal is brought fully into the plane of rotation and then out of it again to an effective velocity 0.7 ω_z, when the head is tilted 45 degrees to the left. There is no overall change in angular velocity, so there is no sustained cupular deflection. On the other hand, the

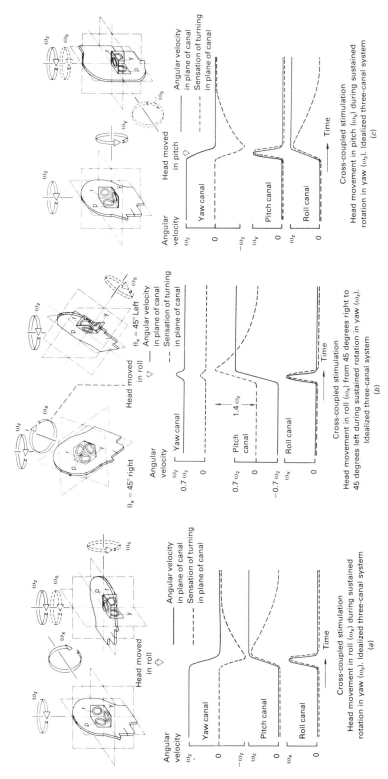

Figure 21.7 Examples of cross-coupled stimulation produced by head movements in roll (*a* and *b*) and in pitch (*c*) during sustained rotation in yaw (ω_z). Note how in each example the illusory sensation is orthogonal to the axis of the two imposed angular movements.

pitch axis receives a stimulus of $2 \times 0.7\ \omega_z$, as it is taken from $0.7\ \omega_z$ in the pitch-back direction to $0.7\ \omega_z$ in the pitch-forward direction. There is thus a strong stimulus in the pitch-forward direction, of greater magnitude than could be achieved by simply stopping rotation from a speed of ω_z in the pitch axis.

Figure 21.7 shows the nature of the stimulus to the semicircular canals when the head is moved in pitch during rotation about the Z axis. This movement takes the yaw axis canal out of the plane of rotation and brings the roll axis canal into the plane of rotation. The illusory sensation is thus one of rotation (roll) relative to gravity, due to the effective deceleration of the yaw axis canal.

Foregoing analysis shows that the principal effect of a head movement in one axis, during rotation about another orthogonal axis, is to produce an illusory sensation of rotation in the third orthogonal axis. It should be emphasized that the effects of dynamic cross-coupling are not due to the presence of endolymph flow in two canals 'inducing' flow in the third, as is suggested in some texts, but to a change in the orientation of the canals with respect to the axis of the sustained rotation. It is important, also, to recognize that the false sensations associated with cross-coupling arise because the imposed rotation is sustained, and that the cupulae of the canals in the plane of the steady turn have had time to return to their neutral positions. When a head movement out of the plane of rotation is made during deceleration from a sustained turn, the erroneous sensations are even more potent and disturbing than when the same head movement is made during the sustained rotation (Guedry and Benson, 1978). In contrast, head movements made during the initial few seconds of the start of rotation in another axis do not give rise to inappropriate sensations because the time course of the rotational stimuli fall within the normal dynamic range of the semicircular canals. Each canal correctly transduces the angular velocity to which it is exposed, so both the imposed rotation and the angular motion of the head are correctly sensed.

So far, attention has been given only to the sensations aroused by cross-coupled stimulation. In an appropriate visual environment oculogyral illusions can also be elicited. These do not differ in any major respect from the illusions evoked by simpler stimuli having only one degree of rotational freedom, in that the illusory movement and displacement of an isolated light is in the same direction as the illusory sensation of bodily rotation. For example, a cross-coupled stimulus that gives a dominant sensation of pitching forward (for example, a head movement in roll to left with steady rotation in Z axis to right) also evokes an oculogyral illusion in which an isolated light in front of the subject appears to move downwards and to be displaced below its initial position. In some circumstances the more obvious component of the illusion is one of displacement rather than rotation. Thus cross-coupling can give rise to erroneous perceptions of attitude as well as to the false sensations of angular motion which are more characteristic of this type of atypical stimulation of the semicircular canals.

In-flight, the disorientation produced by head movement in a turning or spinning aircraft is probably a combination of cross-coupled and 'G excess' illusions (*see below*) for it is rare for the aircraft to execute a manoeuvre involving angular motion without there being an associated change in the force environment. The relative importance of canal and otolithic responses in the disorientation caused by head movement has yet to be resolved, but head movements are undoubtedly a potent cause of perceptual errors in flight. The inappropriate sensations frequently have a sudden and unexpected onset and occur at a time when the pilot's attention is directed to some other aspect of the flying task. The classic situation is one in which the pilot, during a descending instrument turn, has to turn his head to operate controls on the side-consoles in the cockpit, such as the selection of a new R/T frequency. False vestibular sensations produced by head movement occur at the very time that the pilot has no reliable visual cues about the orientation of his aircraft, thereby increasing the probability that aircraft control will be based on these erroneous cues.

Pressure (alternobaric) vertigo

Although somatogyral and oculogyral illusions are usually the consequence of stimulation of the semicircular canals by angular accelerations, it is well established that, in susceptible individuals, pressure change within the middle ear can evoke powerful and quite unexpected vertigo (Wulfften Palthe, 1922). Typically, this is of sudden onset and is related to the equilibration of middle ear pressure as the pilot 'clear his ears' on ascent. It may also appear on descent, though usually in response to a voluntary 'Valsalva' manoeuvre. The vertigo is often initially intense, with blurring of vision and apparent movement of the visual scene, but this is usually short lived and dies away in 10–15 seconds, in much the same way as the vertigo produced by a sudden change in angular velocity. However, the symptoms are not always transient; some aircrew have reported a less intense vertigo which has persisted for many minutes. There is also considerable variability in the plane of the illusory sensation, though it is usually of a consistent and repeatable pattern in any one individual.

Amnestic surveys have shown that some 10–17% of pilots have experienced pressure vertigo at some time or other during their flying career (Melvill Jones, 1957; Lundgren and Malm, 1966). Symptoms are most likely to occur when there is some difficulty in equilibrating middle ear pressure because of a 'stickiness' of the Eustachian tubes, usually due to mild congestion and inflammation brought about by a common cold or other infection of the upper respiratory tract. There are, however, a few individuals who suffer from pressure vertigo even in the absence of infection. Studies by Ingelstedt, (1974) have shown that these individuals require a higher middle ear pressure (> 5.88 kPa above ambient) than the norm (4.31 kPa) to open the Eustachian tube and vent gas to ambient. On the other hand, not all individuals with high opening pressure suffer from pressure vertigo, nor does the lack of Eustachian patency, as indicated by the Valsalva test, correlate well with susceptibility. In some subjects the additional requirement for the induction of symptoms would appear to be an asymmetry in the opening pressures of the Eustachian tubes, such that one ear equilibrates at a low differential pressure the other at a high tubal pressure.

The mechanisms by which the sensory receptors of the vestibular apparatus are stimulated by changes in middle ear pressure is still a matter for conjecture. The dominant symptom—vertigo—strongly suggests that it is the ampullary receptors of the semicircular canals, rather than the maculae, that are stimulated. Furthermore, the transient nature of the disturbance accords with the theory proposed by Melvill Jones (1957), that the cupula is deflected when the overpressure in the middle ear is suddenly relieved on passive venting, or when middle-ear pressure is raised transiently above ambient by a Valsalva manoeuvre. Overpressure in the middle ear may not be transmitted equally to the fluid systems of the inner ear by the round and oval windows, for the stapes footplate might be moved against the pressure gradient by the outward displacement of the tympanic membrane. With the sudden restoration of middle ear pressure there may be a movement of endolymph and perilymph which causes a displacement of the cupula of one or more of the semicircular canals of the affected ear. Unfortunately, little is known about the transient response of the hydrodynamic systems of the inner ear to large-amplitude pressure changes, so it is difficult to explain why some individuals show an altered pattern of end-organ activity with such a stimulus and others do not.

Another mechanism involving a relative ischaemia of the sensory epithelium was proposed by Tjernstrom (1977). He suggested that the overpressure in the middle ear is effectively transmitted to the fluid system of the inner ear because of poor patency of the cochlear aqueduct when there is a rapid pressure change. The estimated pressure in capillaries of the inner ear is <40 mm Hg (5 kPa) above ambient, so if fluids of the inner ear were pressurized to over 40 mm Hg above ambient by an overpressure in the middle ear, then circulatory insufficiency affecting structures within the inner ear is likely to ensue. Although such a mechanism cannot be refuted it must be pointed out that the vestibular reactions induced by the pressure change in the experimental studies of Ingelstedt and Tjernstrom are relatively weak. Vascular insufficiency could well be responsible for the low-grade and sometimes sustained vertigo that is reported by a minority of aircrew with 'pressure vertigo', but it is unlikely to account for the severe yet brief disturbance of vestibular function that can be precipitated by equilibrium of middle ear pressure during ascent or active over-inflation (Valsalva's manoeuvre) during descent.

Despite uncertainties about the mechanism of pressure vertigo and the nature of individual differences in susceptibility, it can be a cause of severe and potentially dangerous spatial disorientation. Apart from the dangers of otic barotrauma, the increased probability of pressure vertigo is another reason why aircrew should not fly when suffering from an upper respiratory tract infection or other conditions that impair ventilation of the middle ear. Aircrew who continue to suffer from pressure vertigo, in the absence of intercurrent infection, should be referred to an otologist for investigation and treatment.

Flicker vertigo

Aircrew have described a number of sensory disturbances that can be attributed to a flickering visual stimulus. Such problems are more common in rotary-wing aircraft where the shadow cast by the main rotor blades passes across the cockpit several times a second. Difficulties have also been experienced when light from a rotation anti-collision beacon illuminates the cockpit either directly or by reflection from cloud or smoke.

The principal complaint is irritation and distraction. Less frequently there is a true disorientation in which the visual stimulus gives rise to a sensation of angular motion of the aircraft in the opposite direction to that of the moving shadow. Fortunately, there is usually little difficulty in determining the true orientation of the aircraft or helicopter, though there is a conflict to be resolved. An associated problem is one of nausea, which must be regarded as a form of visually induced motion sickness in which visual motion cues are not 'matched' by appropriate cues from other sensory receptors. Finally, there remains the possibility of disturbances of consciousness and the induction of epileptiform fits by a photic stimulus which flickers at a frequency close to a dominant rhythm (commonly 8–10 Hz of the α waves) of the electroencephalogram. Fortunately, the incidence of flicker-induced epilepsy is very low in the population as a whole and is negligible in aircrew.

Dissociative sensations ('the break-off phenomenon')

Apart from illusory perceptions of aircraft attitude and motion, aircrew report other incidents in which the disorientation takes the form of an altered perception of the pilot's own orientation with respect to the aircraft and to the ground. Typically, the perceptual disturbance is described by the pilot as a feeling of detachment, isolation or remoteness from his immediate environment and the aircraft he is controlling. Less commonly, the sensory disturbance is more severe and takes the form of an 'outside the body' experience in which the pilot feels that he is outside the aircraft, or at least outside himself, and is watching himself fly the aircraft.

The term 'break-off phenomenon' was coined by Clark and Graybiel (1957) to identify this type of disordered perception because one of the early descriptions came from a pilot who felt as if he had 'broken off from reality'. While accepting the descriptive utility of this term, it must be recognized that comparable sensory disturbances are seen in patients with psychiatric and organic disorders and are called dissociative sensations. However, the occurrence of such dissociative sensations in flight does not *ipso facto* imply that the pilot is psychiatrically ill.

The 'break-off phenomenon' is primarily a sensory disturbance experienced by pilots of single-seat aircraft when flying at high altitudes (*circa* 30 000 feet (10 000 m) and above) during monotonous phases of flight, such as level cruise on a constant heading. In addition, an ill-defined horizon and a lack of external visual cues of relative motion, typified by 'goldfish bowl' conditions in which a dark blue sky above merges imperceptibly into a uniform cloud cover below, are other environmental factors commonly associated with the occurrence of 'break-off'. Although originally described as a problem of high-altitude flight in fixed-wing aircraft, dissociative sensations also occur at very much lower altitudes in helicopters (Benson, 1973b; Steele-Perkins and Evans, 1978). Symptoms have been reported at 500 feet (150 m) when flying over a featureless sea in hazy conditions, though more characteristically break-off is associated with flight at altitudes of 5000–10 000 feet (1500–3000 m), which can be classified as 'high' for a rotary wing aircraft.

The dissociative sensations are usually short lived

and often disappear spontaneously when the pilot directs his attention to some other aspect of the flying task, such as cockpit checks, a change of heading or an R/T message. Less commonly, the pilot has to make a positive effort to redirect attention in order to dispel the illusion. On other occasions break-off may persist until the pilot has a clear view of the ground or is close to clouds which give him unambiguous relative motion cues and a reliable external visual reference.

The results of several surveys (Clark and Graybiel, 1957; Lomonaco, 1958; Sours, 1965) have shown that some 14–35% of aircrew who have flown in a provocative environment (that is, single seat, high altitude) have experienced dissociative sensations. For the majority these have not been a cause for concern; indeed, some pilots find the sensation pleasurable and a contribution to the 'joy of flying'. However, about one-third of the pilots who have experienced break-off find the altered perceptual state to be disturbing and anxiety provoking (Sours, 1965). It is in this group of aircrew that break-off disrupts performance by engendering a high arousal state and by acting as the precipitant of an anxiety reaction. Specifically, such aircrew frequently have an increased awareness of changes in aircraft attitude and motion, with quantitative errors in perception; for example, 5 degrees of bank may feel like 30 degrees of bank. Some also have illusory perceptions of aircraft orientation, such as a false sensation of turn or roll when flying straight and level. These errors in the perception of aircraft orientation are often consistent and are associated with break-off whenever it occurs. Other aircrew do not suffer specific illusions of aircraft attitude and motion, but have a feeling of instability, characteristically likened to the aircraft being 'balanced on a knife edge' or 'as if on top of a pin'. Furthermore, their anxiety is potentiated by the thought that the aircraft will topple from this unstable configuration and will fall out of the sky.

Such unrealistic perceptions are commonly, though not necessarily, the manifestation of a neurotic reaction. However, they do emphasize the role of an unusual sensory experience, like break-off, in the genesis of neurotic reactions. In some cases there is a well-defined phobic element, as the occurrence of anxiety is quite specifically related to the flight conditions in which break-off first occurred, but in others there is generalization of the anxiety with loss of confidence in flying ability and the development of the 'fear of flying' syndrome. It must, however, also be recognized that dissociative sensations may also be the first symptom of a neurosis that develops because of other factors in the individual's work, social life, or constitution. The elucidation of aetiology in an aircrew patient who comes under medical care because of dissociative sensations and anxiety neurosis can be difficult, and may on occasions perplex even the skilled psychiatrist.

Disorientation during approach and landing

The greatest precision in the perception of aircraft orientation is required of the pilot during the approach and landing phase of flight. Apart from correct appreciation and control of arcraft attitude the pilot must determine the spatial position of the aircraft within the 'approach slot', a relatively narrow oblate cone with its apex at runway threshold and its axis aligned with the centre line of the runway and inclined in azimuth at an angle of 2½–3 degrees (45–53 mrad) to the plane of the runway. The task of perceiving spatial position, with three degrees of transitional freedom, depends primarily upon the ability of the pilot to judge distance. More specifically, he is required to judge the distance of the aircraft from the touch-down point in the line of flight, and to judge height which is the distance between the ground and the aircraft. In practice these two judgements are rarely made separately, especially when close to runway threshold, for they are but components of the more general perception of the approach path and glide slope angle.

In addition to determining aircraft position in three-dimensional space, the pilot must also be aware of the aircraft's change in position (that is, velocity) in the approach slot. Judgement of air speed in the line of flight and rate of descent involves the perceptual differentiation (using this word in the mathematical sense) of visual cues of distance, though these are complemented by information from retinal elements that are specificaaly stimulated by movement of objects within the visual field.

In the approach and landing phase of flight the pilot is even more dependent on reliable visual cues to determine spatial orientation of his aircraft than at other times during the flight. During approach, instrument cues may be used to provide necessary information about the spatial relationship of the aircraft to the glide slope, air speed, attitude, height above ground level, and rate of descent; but at some stage, which in poor visibility may be quite late in the approach, the pilot has to transfer from instrument references to external visual references. He has to look at the approaching runway and make optimum use of the visual cues available in order to land the aircraft within a defined area on the runway; he may also have to decide that this manoeuvre cannot be achieved with safety and initiate an overshoot. Alternatively, in good visibility, the whole approach and landing may be carried out using external visual cues almost exclusively, with only a brief instrument check of airspeed during the approach.

Visual cues used during approach and landing

At some stage in all landings the pilot has to make use of external visual cues to judge distance, altitude and derivatives of these variables. These visual cues are essentially monocular cues, for at distances greater than about 10 m (30 feet) binocular cues (stereopsis) do not contribute to the perception of depth (*see* Chapter 23).

A questionnaire survey of 360 commercial airline pilots (Riordan, 1974) revealed that the most important monocular cues are the size and shape of the runway, and the changing perspective, or slant appearance, of the runway as the aircraft approaches on a typical 2½–3 degree glide path. Next in importance is motion parallax. If the aircraft is accurately aligned on the glide slope, the localization of the touch-down point in the pilot's field of view will be constant. Any deviation of aircraft position from the glide slope, or changes in attitude, will be reflected by an appropriate alteration in the apparent position of runway threshold within the frame of reference provided by the edges of the cockpit transparency. Retinal image size is another cue that provides the pilot with information about his distance from the observed object, though this cue is of no value if the pilot has no prior knowledge of the size of the object (for example, buildings, trees, roads, motor vehicles etc.) at which he is looking. Familiar objects or markers along the approach terrain also provide unambiguous and time-honoured cues of distance from touch-down.

In addition to the visual cues that are employed to perceive distance and its derivatives, the movement of object in the parafoveal and peripheral visual fields gives information about speed and altitude, particularly during the final phase of the approach when the aircraft is close to the ground. This 'streaming effect' is a function of the relative angular velocity of objects within the field of view. It increases from zero at the touch-down point to a maximum in the most peripheral part of the visual field, and at any particular point in the visual field the intensity of this 'visual flow' stimulus is a function of aircraft speed and slant distance.

Errors of visual perception during approach and landing

From the foregoing description of the principal visual cues used by pilots during the approach and landing it may be concluded that the perceptual processes are complex and have to be learned by repeated experience in the flight environment. It is, therefore, not surprising that errors of perception of distance, attitude, speed and altitude occur when the visual cues are atypical, when they are degraded or do not accord with expectancy.

Modification of aerial perspective by atmospheric conditions that reduce visibility, such as fog, rain, smoke, haze or snow leads to the over-estimation of distance. In such conditions the runway may appear to be further away than its true distance and the pilot may also think that his height above the ground is greater than in fact it is. Conversely, when atmospheric attenuation is less than that which the pilot has commonly experienced (for example, the clear bright conditions of a high-altitude airfield), distances may be underestimated and as a result he may fly a high approach and have to overshoot.

This tendency perceptually to match what is seen with what experience has led the pilot to expect is also the most likely cause of misjudgement during the approach to runways whose dimensions differ from the runway with which the pilot is familiar. Typically, runways at commercial airports are 45 m (150 feet) wide and 2–3 km (7000–10 000 feet) long. Accordingly, on an approach to a runway that is unusually wide the pilot, understandably, will tend to underestimate distance; conversely, a narrow runway can lead to an overestimation of distance from threshold and increase the probability of landing long or having to overshoot. Even more confusing are those runways that preserve the typical length/width ratio but are wider and hence longer than usual, or narrower and shorter than runways with which the pilot is more familiar.

Other aspects of the local topography may also lead to errors. Featureless terrain, snow-covered ground or a smooth sea are examples of situations where there is a lack of visual texture and insufficient visual cues to allow any reliable perception of height. Sloping terrain also contributes to the false perception of height on the approach in much the same way as sloping runways. It has been found, for example, that ground that slopes up towards the runway or has a similar upward inclination beyond the runway is likely to cause the pilot to over-estimate his height and lead to a lower than normal descent and approach to landing (Kraft, 1978).

Darkness degrades or eliminates many of the visual cues employed during daytime approach and landings. Most accidents during this phase of flight occur at night and characteristically the pilot makes a low approach and lands short (Hartmann and Cantrell, 1968). At night the pilot must rely on the limited visual cues provided by runway and approach lights, and the perceptual task is made even more difficult if the approach is over water or terrain without lights-the so-called 'black-hole'

approach. In simulations of the 'black-hole' landing situation in which only runway and approach lights were visible, it has been repeatedly demonstrated (Mertens, 1981; Mertens and Lewis, 1983) that pilots over-estimated their approach angle, on occasions by a factor of two, and made a low approach. Perrone (1984) has developed a theory of slant perception and presents a convincing argument that the error in judging glide-slope angle during a black-hole approach is due to the lack of perceptive information at distances lateral to the aim-point beyond the runway edge-lights.

Although the factors contributing to errors of visual perception during the approach and landing have been considered in isolation, in practice it is usually a combination of factors that is responsible for the error of judgement and inappropriate control that is the prime cause of an accident. The particular danger of disorientation during this phase of flight lies in the narrow temporal and spatial limits within which the aircraft must be controlled. There is little time and little altitude for errors to be corrected; a decision to execute a missed approach procedure and to overshoot must be made quickly if an accident is to be avoided. The basic problem is neatly summarized by Perrone (1984): 'Humans are not very good at judging the slant of long narrow rectangular surfaces. Pilots must learn to believe their instruments, not their eyes'.

Prophylaxis

Spatial disorientation is disadvantageous to the safety of flight operations, to mission effectiveness and to the mental health of aircrew. Thus every effort should be made to prevent the occurrence of perceptual errors, in particular those that lead to loss of control and aircraft accidents. Prevent is perhaps too strong a word to use when considering disorders of perception caused by natural limitations of sensory function and the fallibility of the central perceptual mechanism but sufficient is known about the aetiology of spatial disorientation to allow rational prophylactic measures to be developed.

Many of the factors that lead to spatial disorientation have already been discussed. These will now be summarized under different headings in order to emphasize the methods, techniques and procedures that may be employed to prevent or at least minimize disorientation.

Aircraft factors

Instrumentation

Spatial disorientation is predominantly a problem of flight in Instrument Meteorological Conditions

(IMC), hence the quality of instrument displays is of vital importance if the pilot is to perceive, both correctly and quickly, the behaviour and orientation of his aircraft so that he may disregard erroneous cues. Ideally, the instruments should provide cues that have the same 'visual strength' as external cues in good visibility conditions, though to date such displays do not exist; indeed, it is unlikely that flight-deck instruments will ever be as compelling as sight of the real world. Every effort should be made to provide the pilot with instruments that can be read quickly and unambiguously, both by day and by night. It is, of course, axiomatic that the instrumentation should be adequate for the manoeuvres and conditions in which the pilot has to fly the aircraft. The impropriety of attempting to fly in marginal weather conditions in an aircraft without an attitude display is obvious, but many accidents to light aircraft and some helicopters are directly attributable to lack of appropriate instrument displays.

Instrument reliability is also of prime importance, for once this becomes suspect the pilot may question the veracity of the display and hence take longer, or even fail, to resolve conflicting sensory cues. By the same token, a clear indication of malfunction is necessary if the perceptual load on the pilot is not to be increased by the display of erroneous information.

The use of the head-up-display undoubtedly assists in the transfer from external visual to instrument cues and should reduce the possibility of disorientation at such times. Likewise, this type of display should reduce perceptual conflict in those flight situations where external visual cues are uncertain, even though the pilot is obliged by operational requirements to look outside the cockpit. However, if the head-up-display is of poor design and lacking in accuracy, clarity or reliability it may contribute to disorientation by increasing arousal or by adding to conflicts.

Cockpit ergonomics

The need to position ancillary instruments and controls so that the pilot does not have to make head movements during critical phases of flight has been discussed in the sections dealing with cross-coupled stimulation and 'G excess' illusions. It should also be recognized that aircrew equipment, such as a flying helmet, can obstruct the field of vision and require head movements to be made in order to see even the primary instrument display.

The configuration of the cockpit canopy is also of significance. The lack of a well-defined aircraft frame of reference undoubtedly contributes to the development of 'the leans' and 'break-off' in those aircraft where the pilot is placed well forward and can see the wings or other parts of the aircraft only

with difficulty. Likewise, the presence of a sloping edge to the canopy, augmented perhaps by an instrument panel in which the dials are not aligned with the transverse axis of the aircraft, does not assist the pilot to maintain a level attitude when flying on external visual reference.

Table 21.1 Principal environmental factors and flight manoeuvres likely to produce or potentiate disorientation

Flight environment	
1 Flight in IMC	Acceptance of erroneous vestibular/kinaesthetic cues especially on transfer from external visual to instrument cues
2 Night	Use of inadequate external visual cues. Apparent movement of isolated lights due to oculogravic and autokinetic illusions. Ground/sky confusion. Inadequate ground illumination, preventing accurate perception of height and attitude for landing and maintenance of hover
3 High altitude	Dissociative sensations (break-off). False horizontal references
4 Flight over featureless terrain	Error in height perception
Flight manoeuvres	
1 Prolonged linear acceleration or deceleration	Somatogravic and oculogravic illusions. 'G excess' illusions with head movement
2 Prolonged angular motion	Turn not sensed. Somatogyral and oculogyral illusions (particularly on recovery). Impairment of vision by nystagmus. Cross-coupled stimulation with head movement
3 Sub-threshold changes in attitude	Change of attitude not sensed. 'Leans'
4 Workload	High arousal enhancing disorientation and reducing ability to resolve conflict
5 Ascent	Pressure (alternobaric) vertigo
6 Cloud penetration	VMC/IMC transfer especially when flying in formation or on breaking formation. 'Lean on the sun' illusion
7 Low altitude in helicopters and VSTOL aircraft	VMC/IMC transfer necessitated by flight into dust, smoke, etc. Illusions of relative motion

Operational factors

Preventive measures in this broad area depend on the recognition of aircraft manoeuvres and flight environments that carry a high disorientation risk. These factors cannot, of course, be considered in isolation, but have to be evaluated in relation to the training and experience of the aircrew. For example, it is but axiomatic that pilots without instrument flying experience will become disorientated if they attempt to fly in cloud or other poor visibility conditions where instrument flying is required. On the other hand, a pilot who is in instrument flying practice is unlikely to suffer from potentially dangerous disorientation in similar flight conditions. Indeed, it is a statement of the obvious that aircrew should only fly those aircraft, those manoeuvres and in those flight conditions that are commensurate with their training, experience and proficiency. Yet each year many orientation error accidents occur, particularly in private aviation, because of a failure to comply with this fundamental rule.

In part, the avoidance of potentially disorientating situations can be achieved by supervisory control, but of no less importance is an awareness by the pilot of his own limitations and of the flight conditions and aircraft manoeuvres likely to induce spatial disorientation. The acquisition of such knowledge is again dependent on the training and the experience of the individual pilot.

The principal environmental factors and flight manoeuvres likely to produce or potentiate disorientation are summarized in *Table 21.1.*

Aircrew factors

It is now necessary to consider what prophylactic measures can be applied to the aircrew to reduce, or better still to prevent spatial disorientation. Training and experience are clearly of paramount importance, but there are other behavioural and clinical factors that should not be overlooked.

Selection

Because of the large differences between individuals in their apparent susceptibility to disorientation in flight, it is logical to assume that selection procedures could be employed to identify the disorientation-prone pilot. More specifically it is necessary to exclude those aircrew, or potential aircrew, whose performance in flight will be disorganized, or who will develop neurotic reactions, because of disorientating perceptions.

Individuals with gross disturbances of vestibular function due to clinical disorders, like Meniere's disease, impairment of equilibratory function due to central lesions, etc., should be recognized at the initial medical examination on the performance of simple tests. A more detailed clinical investigation of vestibular function, such as the use of precise rotational or positional tests, is not, in general, indicated, for they have not been found to have predictive value (Benson, 1973a).

On the other hand, the response of the candidate to strong cross-coupled vestibular stimulation (head movements made when rotating at 180 degrees/s (π rad/s) has been found to correlate quite well with success in flying training (Guedry and Ambler, 1972). Students who reacted badly by the rapid development of autonomic symptoms after only a few head movements showed a significantly higher failure rate than those with a higher tolerance to the vestibular stimulus. However, this test is not specifically one of disorientation susceptibility, as it embraces those students who fail because of airsickness, those with poor air-work as well as those with difficulties in maintaining correct orientation in flight.

Health

It is essential that any trained pilot who suffers a disorder affecting the vestibular and visual sensory systems should not be permitted to fly. There are many disease processes, though few common, that necessitate suspension from flying because they predispose the pilot to disorientation in flight. It is outside the scope of this chapter to discuss them in detail. However, it is important to distinguish chronic disorders, like Meniere's syndrome, where the disability is recurrent and unpredictable, from those that are acute, like labyrinthitis, where complete recovery is to be expected and suspension from flying is only temporary. Pressure vertigo is a specific disability that can be minimized by the restriction of flying of those suffering from upper respiratory tract infections (typically the common cold). Certain individuals may benefit from the limited use of decongestants; but if pressure vertigo is a recurrent problem, specialist advice is required (*see also* Chapter 50).

Apart from the maintenance of physical health, the prevention of disorientation is also dependent on mental health. It is known that perceptual errors are more likely to occur when the pilot is anxious or has a high level of 'behavioural arousal' because of endogenous or environmental factors. Likewise, the pilot who is preoccupied by problems of a social or domestic nature is also more susceptible. It is more difficult to recognize such psychiatric difficulties than the organic disorders mentioned in the preceding paragraphs and, even when they are identified, a high degree of judgement is required to decide whether a particular pilot is fit to fly (O'Connor, 1967). Specialist opinion can always be sought; nevertheless it is the responsibility of the pilot's doctor to pick out, initially, those aircrew whose safety in flight might be at risk because of mental ill health.

Drugs

There is anecdotal evidence that self-medication with 'over-the-counter' drugs increases susceptibility to spatial disorientation (Tormes and Guedry, 1975; Steele-Perkins and Evans, 1978). Indeed, it can be argued that any pharmacologically active substance that is a central depressant or in some way impairs cognitive function is likely to increase the likelihood of the pilot experiencing an illusory perception or of impairing his ability to resolve correctly perceptual conflict. Thus aircrew, and especially pilots, should not be permitted to fly when taking drugs that are known to affect adversely the central nervous system. In particular, aircrew should be made aware of the potential danger of flying after taking certain readily available medications, such as, for example, preparations to allay the symptoms of the common cold, and others containing certain antihistaminic drugs, or hyoscine for reducing susceptibility to motion sickness.

Ethyl alcohol, whether regarded as a drug or a toxic agent, also has a depressant effect on brain mechanisms. In addition, it can cause or potentiate disorientation by its specific action on vestibular mechanisms. The production of positional alcohol nystagmus and vertigo, and the diminution of the pilot's ability to suppress inappropriate vestibular nystagmus, are but two examples. Thus alcohol, even in small quantities, jeopardizes flight safety on several counts and is likely to increase the pilot's susceptibility to disorientation long into the 'hangover' period (Ryback and Dowd, 1970; Oosterveld, 1970). The common custom that flying should be avoided for at least 12 hours after having taken alcohol is probably too lenient. In some circumstances, especially after heavy drinking, more than 12 hours is required for the blood alcohol to fall to a level where there is no impairment of piloting performance or disturbance of vestibular function.

Training

Reference has already been made to the need for flying personnel to have not only an adequate knowledge of the aetiology and varied manifestations of spatial disorientation but also the skill to cope with the problem when it occurs in flight. The specific objectives of training may be summarized as follows:

1. To inform aircrew about those factors that contribute to effective spatial orientation in the flight environment.

2. To familiarize them with the various conditions and flight operations that may lead to spatial disorientation.
3. To inform about the differing manifestations of spatial disorientation and how to detect the onset or existence of spatial disorientation.
4. To explain the mechanisms by which spatial disorientation is produced, and to discuss normal limitations of sensory functions.
5. To inform how disorientation may be overcome and to develop skill so that aircrew can cope with disorientation when it occurs in flight, even when they are subjected to mental and physical stress.

These training objectives are met in part by ground-school lectures and in part by experience in the air. It is most desirable that each student should have personally experienced some form of illusory perception either in a ground-based familiarization device or in an aircraft, for this is the most certain way of convincing him that spatial disorientation is a potential problem to all aircrew and that he is not an exception. The equipment required for classroom demonstration of the physiological limitations of sensory function that are responsible for spatial disorientation in flight need not be complex. A modified bar stool, turned by hand, will suffice to familiarize the student pilot with the fallibility of semicircular canal mechanisms (Collins, 1971). More complex devices, in which the student can be exposed to changes in the force environment, effectively demonstrate somatogravic and oculogravic illusions as well. The possible benefits of a familiarization device having more than one degree of angular freedom are debatable (Benson, 1974), though it can be argued that time spent controlling what is in effect a dynamic flight simulator capable of generating illusory sensations could reduce susceptibility to spatial disorientation in actual flight (Gillingham, 1974).

Ground-based lectures and demonstrations undoubtedly play a part in the 'orientation training' of aircrew, but it is in the flight environment itself that they learn how to cope with the problem of disorientation. Illusory perceptions are much more likely to occur and to distract the pilot when he is, or should be, flying by instruments, hence a high degree of proficiency at this type of flying must be acquired during training (Dobie, 1971). The skill, once acquired, must be maintained by regular practice. One aspect of the maintenance of flying skill, achieved by consistent exposure to the flying task, is that the level of adaptation, or habituation, to the motion experienced in the flight environment is sustained. Aircrew who are in current flying practice, particularly of high-performance aircraft, are in general less aware of vestibular and kinaesthetic sensations than aircrew who have not had recent experience in comparable flight conditions.

The loss of skill associated with prolonged periods of ground duty is well recognized in Service flying, and refresher training with some dual flying is commonly carried out before the pilot returns to operational duties. Yet even after being grounded for only a couple of weeks, some habituation is lost (Aschan, 1954). Surveys have shown that pilots are much more likely to be aware of aircraft motion and to suffer disorientation on the first flight after a period of leave (Melvill Jones, 1957). Such problems can be ameliorated by the gradual re-introduction of stressful flight manoeuvres on return to flying duties. Aircrew must be brought to accept that habituation is lost and that their susceptibility to disorientation is increased after more than a week or so away from flying.

Practical advice to aircrew

Preventive advice may be summarized as follows:

1. Remain convinced that you cannot fly by the 'seat of the pants'.
2. Do not allow control of the aircraft to be based at any time on 'seat of the pants' sensations even when you are temporarily deprived of visual cues.
3. Do not unnecessarily mix flying by instruments with flying by external visual cues.
4. Aim to make an early transition to instruments in poor visibility; once on instruments, stay on instruments until external cues are unambiguous.
5. Maintain a high proficiency and be in practice at flight in IMC.
6. Avoid unnecessary manoeuvres of aircraft or head movements that are known to induce disorientation.
7. Be particularly vigilant in high-risk situations, such as at night and in poor visibility, in order to maintain intellectual command of the orientation and position of the aircraft.
8. Do not fly:
   (a) With an upper respiratory tract infection.
   (b) When under the influence of drugs or alcohol.
   (c) When mentally or physically debilitated.
9. Make your first flight after a period off flying a simple day Visual Meteorological Conditions (VMC) sortie.
10. Remember: experience does not make you immune.

Practical advice to aircrew on how to cope with spatial disorientation when it occurs in flight may be summarized as follows:

1. You can dispel persistent minor disorientations (for example, the leans) by making a positive effort to redirect attention to other aspects of the flying task; a quick shake of the head, provided the aircraft is straight and level, is effective for some pilots.
2. When you are suddenly confronted by strong illusory sensations or difficulties in establishing orientation and control of the aircraft:
   (a) Get on to instruments; check and cross-check; ensure good instrument illumination.
   (b) Maintain instrument reference and correct scan pattern; watch your height at all times.
   (c) Control the aircraft in such a way as to make the instruments display the desired flight configuration.
   (d) Do not attempt to mix flight by external visual reference with instrument flight until external visual cues are unambiguous.
   (e) Seek help if severe disorientation persists. Hand over to co-pilot (if present), call ground controller and other aircraft, check altimeter.
   (f) If control cannot be regained, abandon aircraft with safe ground clearance. Do not leave it too late.
3. Remember: nearly all disorientation is a normal response to the unnatural environment of flight. If you have been alarmed by a flight incident discuss it with colleagues, including your Station Medical Officer. Your experience will probably not be as unusual as you thought.

References

ASCHAN, G. (1954) Response to rotatory stimuli in fighter pilots. *Acta Oto-laryngologica Supplement*, **116**, 24–31

BENSON A.J. (1973a) Use of nystagmography in the study of aircrew with spatial disorientation. In *The Use of Nystagmography in Aviation Medicine*. Conference Proceedings CP 128, A4, 1–12. Neuilly sur Seine: AGARD/NATO

BENSON, A.J. (1973b) Spatial disorientation and the 'Break-off' phenomenon. *Aerospace Medicine*, **44**, 944–952

BENSON, A.J. (ed.) (1974) *Orientation/Disorientation Training of Flying Personnel: A Working Group Report*. Report No R-625. Neuilly sur Seine: AGARD/NATO

BENSON, A.J and BURCHARD, E. (1973) *Spatial Disorientation in Flight: A Handbook for Aircrew*. AGARDograph No 170. Neuilly sur Seine: AGARD/NATO

BULEY, L.E. and SPELINA, J. (1970) Physiological and psychological factors in 'The Dark Night Take-Off Accident'. *Aerospace Medicine*, **41**, 553–556

CLARK, B. (1970) The vestibular system. *Annual Review of Psychology*, **21**, 273–306

CLARKE, B. and GRAYBIEL, A. (1949) Linear acceleration and deceleration as factors influencing non-visual orientation during flight. *Journal of Aviation Medicine*, **20**, 92–101

CLARK, B. and GRAYBIEL, A. (1957) The 'Break-Off' phenomenon: a feeling of separation from the earth experienced by pilots at high altitude. *Journal of Aviation Medicine*, **28**, 121–126

CLARK, B. and GRAYBIEL, A. (1963) Contributing factors in the perception of the oculogravic illusion. *American Journal of Psychology*, **76**, 18–27

CLARK, B. and GRAYBIEL, A. (1966) Some factors contributing to the delay in the perception of the oculogravic illusion. *American Journal of Psychology*, **79**, 377–388

COHEN, M.M., CROSBIE, R.J. and BLACKBURN, L.H. (1973) Disorientating effects of aircraft catapult launchings. *Aerospace Medicine*, **44**, 37–39

COLLAR, A.R. (1946) *On An Aspect of the Accident History of Aircraft Taking Off at Night*. Reports and Memoranda No 2277. London: Aeronautical Research Council

COLLINS, W.E. (1971) Practical techniques for disorientation familiarization and the influence of visual references and alcohol on disorientation related responses. In *The Disorientation Incident*. Conference Proceedings CP 95, A-14, 1-10. Neuilly sur Seine: AGARD/NATO

DOBIE, T.G. (1971) The disorientation accident-philosophy of instrument flying training. In *The Disorientation Incident*. Conference Proceedings CP 95, A15, 1-3. Neuilly sur Seine: AGARD/ NATO

GILLINGHAM, K.K. (1974) *Advanced Spatial Disorientation Training Concepts*. Aeromedical Review No 11-74. Brooks AFB, Texas: USAF School of Aerospace Medicine

GILSON, R.D., GUEDRY, F.E., HIXON, W.C. and NIVEN, J.I. (1973) Observations on perceived changes in aircraft attitude attending head movements made in a 2 g bank and turn. *Aerospace Medicine*, **44**, 90–93

GRAYBIEL, A. (1952) The oculogravic illusion. *Archives of Ophthalmology*, **48**, 605–615

GRAYBIEL, A. and HUPP, D.I. (1946) The oculogyral illusion. *Journal of Aviation Medicine*, **17**, 3–27

GRAYBIEL, A., JOHNSON, W.H., MONEY, K.E., MALCOLM, R.E. and JENNINGS, G.L. (1979) Oculogravic illusion in response to straight-ahead acceleration of a CF-104 aircraft. *Aviation Space and Environmental Medicine*, **50**, 382–386

GUEDRY, F.E. and AMBLER, R.K. (1972) Assessment of reactions to vestibular disorientation stress for purposes of aircrew selection. In *Predictability of Motion Sickness in the Selection of Pilots*. Conference Proceedings CP 109, B5, 1-8. Neuilly sur Seine: AGARD/NATO

GUEDRY, F.E. and BENSON, A.J. (1978) Coriolis cross-coupling effects: disorientating and nauseogenic or not? *Aviation Space and Environmental Medicine*, **49**, 29–35

HARTMANN, B.O. and CANTRELL, G.K. (1968) Psychological factors in 'landing short' accidents. *Flight Safety*, **2**, 26–32

INGELSTEDT, S., IVARSSON, A. and TJERNSTROM, O. (1974) Vertigo due to relative overpressure in the middle ear. *Acta Oto-laryngologica*, **78**, 1–14

KRAFT, C.L. (1978) A psychophysical contribution to air safety: simulation studies of visual illusions in night visual approaches. In *Psychology: From Research to Practice* edited by H.E. Pick, H.W. Leibowitz, J.E. Singer, A. Steinschneiden and H.W. Stevenson, pp. 363–385. New York: Plenum Press

LICHTENBERG, B.K., YOUNG, L.R. and ARROTT, A.P. (1982) Human ocular counterrolling induced by varying linear accelerations. *Experimental Brain Research*, **48**, 127–136

LOMONACO, T. (1958) Il fenomeno del 'Break-Off' in Italia. *Rivista di Medicina Aeronautica e Spaziale*, **21**, 236–242

LUNDGREN, C.E.G. and MALM, L.U. (1966) Alternobaric vertigo among pilots. *Aerospace Medicine*, **37**, 178–180

MARTIN, J.F. and MELVILL JONES, G. (1965) Theoretical man–machine interaction which might lead to loss of aircraft control. *Aerospace Medicine*, **36**, 713–716

MELVILL JONES, G. (1957) *A Study of Current Problems Associated with Disorientation in Man-controlled Flight*. Flying Personnel Research Committee Report No 1006. London: Air Ministry

MELVILL JONES, G., BARRY, W. and KOWALSKY, N. (1964) Dynamics of the semicircular canals compared in yaw and pitch. *Aerospace Medicine*, **35**, 984–989

MERTENS, H.W. (1981) Perception of runway image shape and approach angle magnitude by pilots in simulated night landing approaches. *Aviation Space and Environmental Medicine*, **52**, 373–386

MERTENS, H.W. and LEWIS, M.F. (1983) Effects of approach lighting and variation in visible runway length on perception of approach angle in simulated night landings. *Aviation Space and Environmental Medicine*, **54**, 500–506

NIVEN, J.I., WHITESIDE, T.C.D. and GRAYBIEL, A. (1963) *The Elevator Illusion: Apparent Motion of a Visual Target During Vertical Acceleration*. Flying Personnel Research Committee Report No 1213. London: Air Ministry

O'CONNOR, P.J. (1967) Differential diagnosis of disorientation in flying. *Aerospace Medicine*, **38**, 1155–160

OOSTERVELD, W.J. (1970) Effect of gravity on positional alcohol nystagmus (PAN). *Aerospace Medicine*, **41**, 557–560

PERRONE, J.A. (1984) Visual slant misperception and the 'black-hole' landing situation. *Aviation Space and Environmental Medicine*, **55**, 1020–1025

RIORDAN, R.H. (1974) Monocular visual cues and space perception during the approach and landing. *Aerospace Medicine*, **45**, 766–771

RYBACK, R.S. and DOWD, P.J. (1970) After-effects of various alcoholic beverages on positional nystagmus and Coriolis acceleration. *Aerospace Medicine*, **41**, 429–435

SOURS, J.A. (1965) The 'Break-Off' phenomenon, a precipitant of anxiety in jet aviators. *Archives of General Psychiatry*, **13** 447–456

STEELE-PERKINS, A.P. and EVANS, D.A. (1978) Disorientation in naval helicopter pilots. In *Operational Helicopter Aviation Medicine*. Conference Proceedings CP 255, 48,1-5. Neuilly sur Seine: AGARD/NATO

TJERNSTROM, O. (1977) Effects of middle ear pressure on the inner ear. *Acta Oto-laryngologica*, **83**, 11–15

TORMES, F.R. and GUERDY, F.E. (1975) Disorientation phenomenon in naval helicopter pilots. *Aviation Space and Environmental Medicine*, **46**, 387–393

WULFFTEN PALTHE, van P.M. (1922) Function of the deeper sensibility and of the vestibular organs in flying. *Acta Oto-laryngologica*, **4**, 415–448

22

Motion sickness

A.J. Benson

Introduction

Motion sickness is a condition, characterized primarily by nausea, vomiting, pallor and cold sweating, that occurs when man is exposed to real or apparent motion stimuli with which he is unfamiliar and hence unadapted. Although long recognized as an unfortunate consequence of the use of some artificial mode of transport (nausea from the Greek *nauxia*: sea-sickness; *naus*: ship), the problem of motion sickness was not studied scientifically until World War II when an attempt was made to understand the underlying mechanism of the condition and to develop suitable prophylactic drugs. Yet even to this day, anecdote, hunch, folklore and myth still flourish in the minds of the travelling public and, it must be admitted, in some medical texts.

Motion sickness is a generic term which embraces sea sickness, air sickness, car sickness, swing sickness, simulator sickness, space sickness, etc.—various forms of the malady named after the provocative environment or vehicle. Despite the diversity of the causal environment, the essential characteristics of the provocative stimulus and the response of the afflicted individual are common to all these conditions, hence the use of the general term—motion sickness. Nevertheless, 'motion sickness' is, in certain respects, a misnomer. First, because symptoms characteristic of the condition can be evoked as much by the absence of expected motion as by the presence of unfamiliar motion. 'Simulator sickness' and 'Cinerama sickness' (*see below*) are examples of conditions where the evocative stimulus is the absence of physical motion stimuli. Second, the word 'sickness' carries the connotation of 'affected with disease' and tends to obscure the fact that motion sickness is a quite

normal response of a healthy individual, without organic or functional disorder, when exposed for a sufficient length of time to unfamiliar motion of sufficient severity. Indeed, under severe stimulus conditions, it is the absence, rather than the presence of symptoms, that is indicative of true pathology: for only those individuals who lack a functional vestibular system are truly immune.

It would be better to label the condition as the 'motion maladaptation syndrome', for this term implies the fundamental nature of the disability. But common usage should outweigh nosological pedantry; so, having drawn the reader's attention to its limitations, the term 'motion sickness' will be used in the following discussion of this common disability, which to some may be no more than an inconvenience, but to others it may incapacitate and be a hazard to life.

Symptoms and signs of motion sickness

Principal features

The cardinal symptom of motion sickness is nausea; the cardinal signs are vomiting, pallor and sweating. Other responses are frequently reported, but in general these occur more variably.

Typically, the development of motion sickness follows an orderly sequence, the time scale being determined primarily by the intensity of the stimulus and the susceptibility of the individual (Money, 1970; Reason and Brand, 1975). The earliest symptom is, commonly, the unfamiliar sensation of epigastric discomfort, best described as 'stomach awareness'. Should the provocative motion continue, well-being usually deteriorates quite quickly with the appearance of nausea of increasing severity. Concomitantly, circumoral or facial pallor may be observed, and the individual begins to sweat; this cold sweat is usually confined to those areas of skin where thermal sweating rather than emotive sweating occurs. With the rapid exacerbation of symptoms, the so-called 'avalanche phenomenon', there may be increased salivation, feelings of bodily warmth, a lightness of the head and, not infrequently, quite severe depression and apathy. By this stage, vomiting is not usually long delayed, though there are some individuals who remain severely nauseated for long periods and do not obtain the relief, albeit transitory, that many report following emesis.

If exposure to the motion continues, nausea typically increases in intensity and culminates in vomiting or retching. In the more susceptible individual this cyclical pattern, with waxing and waning symptoms and recurrent vomiting, may last for several days. Those so afflicted are commonly severely anorexic, depressed and apathetic, incapable of carrying out allotted duties, or caring for the safety of themselves or others. Their disability is also compounded by dehydration and disturbances of electrolyte balance brought about by the repeated vomiting.

Associated symptoms and signs

Apart from the characteristic features of motion sickness—pallor, sweating, nausea and vomiting—other signs and symptoms are frequently though more variably reported. In the early stages, increased salivation, belching and flatulence are commonly associated with the development of nausea. Hyperventilation is occasionally observed, while an alteration of respiratory rhythm by sighing and yawning not infrequently precedes the 'avalanche phenomenon'. Headache is another variable prodromal symptom, usually frontal in distribution, though complaints of tightness around the forehead or of a 'buzzing in the head' are not uncommon.

Drowsiness is an important, yet often ignored, symptom commonly associated with exposure to unfamiliar motion, even if not necessarily an integral part of the motion sickness syndrome. Typically, feelings of lethargy and somnolence persist for many hours after withdrawal of the provocative motion stimulus and nausea has abated. However, in certain circumstances a desire to sleep may be the only symptom evoked by exposure to motion, especially when the intensity of the stimulus is such that adaptation occurs without significant malaise (Graybiel and Knepton, 1976). The soporific effect of a repetitive motion stimulus on infants

has long been recognized. It may be that the drowsiness observed in the adult when exposed to appropriate motion is a manifestation of the same mechanism, though it must be acknowledged that the somnolence in an individual who has suffered overt motion sickness is frequently of abnormal intensity and persistence.

Operational significance of motion sickness

Aircrew

From personal experience and observation, most readers will be aware that motion sickness is a debilitating condition which has an adverse effect on performance. In the air, the loss of well-being is, at least, a distraction that interferes with the airman's ability to devote his undivided attention to his task, whether this be piloting the aircraft, navigation, surveillance of engine instruments, monitoring a radar display or any other aircrew duty. At the other extreme, flying personnel can be prostrated by sickness and be completely unable to perform their allotted duty. The man so afflicted is rendered useless and is a liability to other members of the crew. Recurrence of air sickness of such severity necessitates withdrawal of the individual from the specific flight environment, and the possible loss of the services of one upon whom a considerable sum has been expended during training. Severe sickness in a trained individual is unusual, but it is a recurrent if not frequent problem in non-pilot aircrew, such as navigators, who are required to fly in high-performance aircraft after training in more sedate machines.

More commonly, air sickness is a problem during flight training (Dobie, 1974; Hixon *et al.*, 1984). Vomiting interferes directly with the student's ability to control the aircraft and may require the instructor to modify or abort the sortie. Recurrence of sickness delays progress in the training sequence and, if the disability is not controlled, leads to removal of the student from the training programme. When sickness is not overt, the student may suffer in silence. His performance in flight may be impaired and be attributed by his flying instructor to a fundamental lack of skill. In either circumstance, the student may feel humiliated and disgraced by the sickness which he construes as a personal weakness, even a defect, in his constitution. Continued introspection with increasing anxiety and loss of confidence further impair progress and may strengthen the instructor's opinion about the student's lack of aptitude.

Passengers

Air sickness in passengers is also of operational significance when they are required to carry out duties immediately after landing or on leaving the aircraft. Usually, however, the affected passenger has an opportunity to recuperate on arrival at his destination before being required to carry out demanding mental or physical tasks.

Paratroops are likely to suffer more: in the final part of the mission, the aircraft cannot fly at high altitude, above the weather, and hence the occupants may be exposed to the provocative motion of flight through turbulent air. A soldier who is feeling sick and has vomited is less efficient than one who is not so afflicted. Furthermore, morale is not enhanced by the sight and smell of vomiting colleagues. Although anecdotal and circumstantial evidence implies that the air-sick soldier or paratrooper is a less effective fighting man than one who has not suffered from this disability, it must be acknowledged that the magnitude of the decrement in performance has yet to be quantified.

Space motion sickness

Approximately 50% of the men and women who have flown in space vehicles have experienced symptoms similar to those that are characteristic of terrestrial motion sickness. The signs and symptoms of space sickness usually appear within the first few hours in the weightless (or more precisely, microgravity) environment and are frequently precipitated by head and body movements within the vehicle. The severity of symptoms can range from mild malaise and associated anorexia to severe nausea with repeated vomiting. Characteristically, there is a progressive decline in the intensity of symptoms with continued exposure to the atypical force environment and most astronauts have adapted and are symptom free by the third or fourth day in space.

Despite the high motivation and extensive training of space-flight crews, space sickness impairs working efficiency during the first few days in flight; provocative head and body movements are restricted or made more slowly, vomiting interrupts the performance of tasks and the loss of well-being causes a general degradation of performance. Thus space sickness is primarily an operational problem during short space-flights, such as those of the Space Shuttle, in which the operational effectiveness of crew members may be impaired for a substantial proportion of the time in weightlessness. Emesis within the space vehicle may be unpleasant both for the individual who vomits and for other crew members in proximity, but it is not a threat to life.

Vomiting within the pressure suit that must be worn during extra-vehicular activity (EVA) is, however, potentially lethal. It is, therefore, essential that work outside the spacecraft is performed only by those astronauts who either are not susceptible to space sickness or who have recovered from this disability.

Sea sickness

In aviation medicine, sea sickness cannot be ignored, for it is a potentially serious problem to the unfortunate few who have to abandon their aircraft on or above the sea. The motion of a life-raft is a highly provocative stimulus and all but the very resistant succumb in rough seas. Even moderate seas induce symptoms in a relatively short period. In the survival situation, sickness erodes the individual's will to survive; furthermore, it makes him less able and less willing to take positive action to aid survival. In addition to these behavioural consequences, the dehydration and electrolyte disturbances brought about by continued vomiting do not enhance an individual's ability to withstand privation, exposure and other stresses imposed by a hostile marine environment.

Aetiology of motion sickness

An adequate theory of the causation of motion sickness must embrace the fact that this disability can be induced not only by motion in which the individual experiences changing linear and angular accelerations, but also by purely visual stimuli without a changing force environment. Furthermore it should account for the phenomenon of adaptation to the provocative motion as well as the sickness (the *mal de débarquement*) that can occur when man returns to a normal motion environment after having adapted to the atypical one.

Undoubtedly, the vestibular apparatus plays a significant role in the genesis of motion sickness; because, as has been known for more than half a century, patients without vestibular function do not get motion sickness. Nevertheless, the theory that motion sickness is due to vestibular 'overstimulation' alone does not account for the fact that sickness may not be induced by quite strong motion stimuli (for example, vertical oscillation at frequencies above 0.5–1 Hz) yet weaker stimuli (for example, head movement during turns) are highly provocative. Nor does it account for the visually induced forms of motion sickness or the phenomenon of adaptation.

The neural mismatch hypothesis

A more acceptable hypothesis is that motion sickness is the response of the organism to discordant sensory information provided by those receptor systems transducing the motion stimuli. The concept that conflicting sensory cues are of prime importance in the aetiology of motion was suggested more than a century ago, but the *sensory conflict* or *neural mismatch* hypothesis has only gained wide acceptance in recent years, following the publication of studies by Reason (1970, 1978) (*see also* Reason and Brand, 1975), and the elaboration of the hypothesis by Oman (1982). In essence, the *neural mismatch* hypothesis states that in all situations where motion sickness is induced there is a conflict, not just between the signals from the eyes, the vestibular apparatus and the other receptors stimulated by the motion, but that these signals are also at variance with those that the central nervous system *expects* to receive.

Work on sensory-motor processing and adaptation has led to the concept that within the central nervous system there is a 'model' or 'engram' of the afferent and efferent activity associated with body movement and postural control; a model that is built up from continued experience of motor activity in everyday life. In normal locomotor activity, disturbances of body movement, such as when one trips or is pushed unexpectedly, are typically brief and the mismatch between *actual* and *expected* information from the body's motion detectors is employed to initiate corrective motor responses. In contrast, when there is a sustained change in the sensory input, as occurs in atypical motion environments, the continued presence of a mismatch signal indicates to the central nervous system that the internal model is in error and is no longer appropriate. Consequently, the internal model is modified in an adaptive manner, in such a way as to reduce the mismatch to a low level; a process that takes place hand in hand with the development of new configurations of sensory-motor co-ordination.

An essential feature of the *neural mismatch* hypothesis is that the presence of a sustained mismatch signal has two effects: (1) it causes a rearrangement of the internal model; (2) it evokes the sequence of neural and hormonal responses that constitute the motion sickness syndrome. There is clearly benefit in the modification of sensory and motor responses that accompany the updating of the internal model, for this allows the individual to function more effectively in the novel motion environment. Whether motion sickness has survival

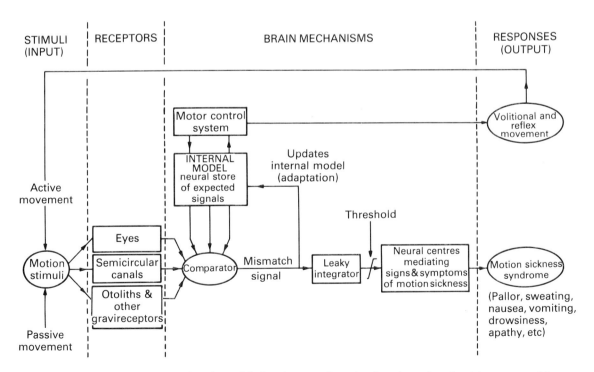

Figure 22.1 Diagrammatic representation of a model of motion control, motion detection and motion sickness compatible with the 'neural mismatch' hypothesis. (Reproduced from Benson (1984) by kind permission of J. Wiley & Sons.)

value, as proposed by Triesman (1977), or is just a design defect, which has only recently (in an evolutionary time scale) become apparent with the use of mechanical aids to transportation, is still a matter for debate.

Figure 22.1 is a diagrammatic representation of the functional components and processes currently embraced by the neural mismatch hypothesis. Active or passive motion of the body is detected principally by the eyes and the vestibular apparatus, though changes in the body's orientation to gravity and imposed linear accelerations also stimulate mechanoreceptors in the skin, muscles, capsules of joints and other tissues. All these sense organs send information to the central nervous system where, it is postulated, there is a neural centre that acts as a comparator of signals from the receptors and of 'expected' signals provided by the internal model.

The output of this comparator is the mismatch signal that, as noted above, updates the internal model and activates the neural centres and pathways mediating the signs and symptoms of motion sickness.

To explain the relatively slow development of symptoms on exposure to provocative motion it is necessary to postulate the presence in the mediating pathway of a mechanism that accumulates the mismatch signal while at the same time allowing it to leak slowly away. In addition to this leaky integrator (the hydraulic analogy is a bucket with a hole in it), there must also be a threshold function in the mediating pathway, for it is known that adaptation to motion can occur, particularly if the stimulus is not intense, without the individual becoming motion sick. A threshold or even several different threshold functions are required to account for the large individual differences in susceptibility and in the order in which the various signs and symptoms develop on exposure to provocative motion.

The manner in which the mismatch signal is likely to change on transfer from one motion environment to another is represented in *Figure 22.2*. In the normal, familiar environment, inputs from the sensory receptors are in accord with those of the internal model, but on initial exposure to unfamiliar motion there is a large mismatch signal. This slowly decays, probably with an exponential trajectory, as the internal model is updated until there is no longer a mismatch between the information from the sensory receptors and that which is 'expected' by the internal model. At this stage the individual may be considered to have adapted to the atypical motion environment, and the signs and symptoms of motion sickness will have disappeared. On return to the familiar, or to some other, motion environment a mismatch occurs initially because the internal model is no longer appropriate and motion sickness (the *mal de débarquement*) may recur. The internal model has to be modified to make it compatible,

once again, with the sensory input. In general, this phase of adaptation proceeds more quickly than the initial adaptation to the atypical environment, because the correlations established by long experience are more easily retrieved than new ones can be acquired. By the same argument, should the individual return to the atypical environment, adaptation is likely to be a more rapid process than on first exposure because the internal model can be rearranged with the aid of retained stimulus patterns acquired during previous exposures to the atypical environment. If transfer from one specific motion environment to another is frequent then a stage is reached when the internal model can be modified quite rapidly, so that the mismatch signal is short lived or of insufficient intensity or duration to engender motion sickness.

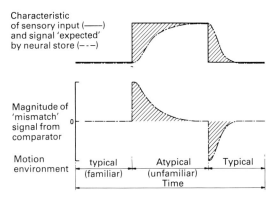

Figure 22.2 Diagram to illustrate the time course of the modification of the 'internal model' on exposure to a new (atypical) motion environment and on return to the normal (typical) environment.

Unfortunately, the neural mismatch hypothesis does not explain why motion sickness should take the particular form that it does, or indeed why motion sickness should occur at all. These are still unresolved problems. However, the hypothesis is a unifying concept, which permits explanation of why sickness should occur in some motion environments and not in others, and explains the basic features of adaptation in the broader context of sensory rearrangement.

The nature of the provocative stimulus

Implicit in the neural mismatch hypothesis of motion sickness is the idea that, in all motion environments where sickness is induced, there is dissonance between the incoming sensory signals and those 'expected' by the neural store. Basically, there are two sensory systems: (1) the visual system; and (2) the vestibular system. The latter is further divided into the angular acceleration receptor system, the ampullary receptors of the semicircular canals, and the linear acceleration or force environment receptor system of the utricular and saccular maculae—the otolith organs as they are more commonly called. Other mechanoreceptors are also stimulated by changes in the force environment, but in general they act synergistically with the otolithic receptors, and need not, in the present context, be considered separately.

Two main types of motion cue mismatch can be specified according to the sensory system involved: (1) visual–vestibular mismatch; and (2) canal–otolith mismatch. In each of these, two types of conflict can occur as follows.

Type 1—When both systems *concurrently* signal contradicting or uncorrelated information.

Type 2—When one system signals information in the absence of the expected signal from the other system.

Examples of these different types of mismatch are summarized in *Table 22.1*, and the characteristic features explained below.

Visual–vestibular conflict

Type 1

In this condition, both the eyes and the vestibular receptors simultaneously signal motion, but of an unrelated or incompatible kind; cues in the two modalities do not accord with expectation based on previous experience. A prime example, in the aerial environment, is the sickness provoked on viewing ground or aerial targets through binoculars from a moving aircraft. Direct observation of the passing landscape from side or rear windows of a vehicle which is changing direction or speed also causes sickness, without the exaggerated apparent motion of the visual field introduced by the use of an unstabilized optical device. Likewise, attempting to read a hand-held map or text in a moving vehicle can be highly provocative, because visual and vestibular motion cues are uncorrelated. In addition, the requirement to scan and maintain fixation on the visual material considerably potentiates the induction of sickness (Guedry, Lentz and Jell, 1979).

Table 22.1 Classification of motion cue mismatch

Type	Identification of motion cue mismatch engendering motion sickness	
	Visual (A)–vestibular (B) mismatch	*Canal (A)–otolith (B) mismatch*
Type 1		
(A) and (B) simultaneously signal contradictory information	(i) Reading hand-held map or text in turbulent flight	(i) Cross-coupled (Coriolis) stimulation. Head movement during rotation about another axis
	(ii) Inspection through binoculars of ground or aerial targets from moving aircraft	(ii) Head movement in abnormal force environment which may be stable (for example, hyper- or hypo-gravity) or fluctuating (during linear oscillation)
Type 2 (i)		
(A) signals without expected (B) signal	(i) 'Simulator sickness'. Piloting of fixed base simulator with moving external visual display (VFA)	(i) 'Space sickness'. Head movement in weightless environment
		(ii) Pressure (alternobaric) vertigo
Type 2 (ii)		
(B) signals without expected (A) signal	(i) Looking inside aircraft when exposed to motion	(i) Low-frequency (<0.5 Hz) linear oscillation
		(ii) Rotation about non-vertical axis

Certain flight simulators, in which there was both a motion base and a visual display of the external scene (visual flight attachment), have also been found to cause sickness during simulated flight manoeuvres that would not have been provocative in actual flight. Disparities, often of a rather subtle kind, between the visual cues of motion and those engendered by the moving cockpit of the simulator are thought to be responsible for the problem. Simulator sickness is, however, more likely to occur in those simulators that have a realistic visual display of large angular subtense, but no cockpit motion and the conflict is of Type 2 rather than Type 1 (*see below* and review by McCauley (1984)).

Type 2

In this category there are two kinds of conflict: (1) when there are visual cues without the expected and normally correlated vestibular signals; and (2) when the vestibular cues are not accompanied by the expected visual cues.

Type 2(i)

The induction of sickness in a Type 2(i) situation is important perhaps as much in relation to theories of motion sickness as in an operational context, because sickness is caused purely by the perceived motion of visual images without physical motion of the observer, and hence without stimulation of vestibular receptors. Such visually induced motion sickness is a problem in some fixed-base simulators fitted with a display of the external visual world which moves in accord with the computed attitude and flight path of the aircraft. In 'simulator sickness', the principal mismatch is between the visual input and the absence of those signals from semicircular canals, otoliths, and other mechanoreceptors, which the pilot expects to accompany the flight manoeuvre executed in the simulator. The argument that simulator sickness is due to the unfulfilled expectations of vestibular and somatosensory inputs is supported by the finding that pilots with considerable experience of the real aircraft are more susceptible to this disorder than those with little or no previous experience of actual flight in the aircraft being simulated. This difference presumably reflects the greater entrenchment of the association between specific visual and vestibular cues in the former group than in the latter, and hence the greater severity of the conflict when they are confronted with the 'rearranged' sensory inputs in the simulator. Sickness is usually less when the simulator cabin is given some motion, even though the linear and angular acceleration experienced by the pilot are but a caricature of the real motion of the aircraft. Sickness may be exacerbated, however, if there is not good concordance between the

physical motion of the simulator and that of the visual display, especially in the temporal relationship between visual and vestibular motion cues.

The sickness (Cinerama or Imax sickness) that can be induced by viewing a motion picture shot from a moving vehicle (for example, from a helicopter manoeuvring at low level) and displayed on a large screen is another example of the same type of visual–vestibular mismatch.

Type 2(ii)

In this condition there is an absence of the expected visual signal when the vestibular receptors are stimulated by the motion of the vehicle. This kind of conflict is present in all modes of passive transport where the passenger lacks a clear view of the visual scene outside the vehicle. In the air, for example, the linear and angular accelerations associated with flight in turbulence are signalled by vestibular receptors, but there is no correlated visual information when the individual looks at aircraft instrument displays, or indeed any part of the interior of the aircraft that moves with him and hence provides a relatively stable visual input. It is well known, both from practical experience and laboratory experiment, that the incidence of sickness is lower when one has a clear view of the outside world than when vision is confined to the cabin or structure with which one moves. Thus, pilots, typically, suffer less sickness than navigators, except when the pilot becomes a passenger and is deprived of familiar external visual cues.

It should be clearly recognized that motion sickness can occur in many situations when the individual experiencing motion has his eyes closed and the basic mismatch is of the intravestibular kind (*see below*). However, the nature of the visual input can materially augment or decrease the intensity of the conflict, and, in the less severe motion environments, can determine whether the man does, or does not, become sick.

Intravestibular (semicircular canal–otolith) conflict

During natural postural and locomotor activity in a stable, $1g$ environment, a correlated pattern of vestibular activity is established. For example, angular movement of the head in pitch and roll is associated with the concomitant stimulation both of the vertical semicircular canals and of the otolith organs, as the position of the head with respect to the gravitational acceleration changes; on the other hand, rotation of the head in yaw about a vertical axis is not accompanied by an alteration in the signals from the otoliths. This normal, established, association between semicircular canal and otolith organ information is disturbed by certain volitional yet natural head movements when made in an abnormal motion or force environment as well as by atypical passive motion itself.

Type 1

This is the situation where both canals and otoliths signal contradictory information when the head is moved, either voluntarily or passively, in the presence of some other angular motion or an abnormal force environment.

Cross-coupled (or Coriolis) stimulation of the semicircular canals occurs when an individual, who is being rotated about a particular axis, moves his head other than in the plane of the imposed rotation. One configuration of canals is taken out of the plane of rotation and they are stimulated by the apparent reduction in rotational speed: while another set of orthogonal canals is brought into the plane of rotation and they receive a stimulus equivalent to an increase in the rate of turn. The

result of this cross-coupled stimulus is to produce an erroneous signal of turn about an axis that accords neither with that of the imposed rotation nor with the axis in which the voluntary head movement is made (*Figure 22.3*). (A more detailed description of cross-coupled stimulation of the semicircular canals is given in Chapter 21.) Furthermore, the signal from the stimulated canals persists after the movement has been completed, for the deflected cupulae commonly take 10 seconds or more to return to their neutral positions. During this time, the otoliths correctly sense the true attitude of the head with respect to gravity; hence there is a mismatch between the otolith signal and that from the canals. This is a potent form of stimulation for inducing sickness to which all individuals with an intact vestibular system may succumb provided the speed of rotation is high enough, the head movements are repetitive and they are of sufficient amplitude.

Head movements made in an abnormal force environment also cause sickness, though in this situation the canals—being essentially insensitive to

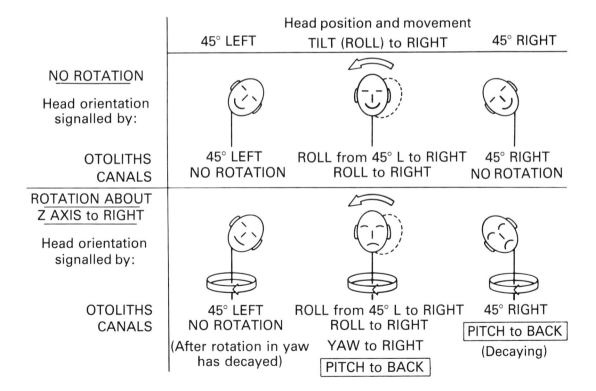

Figure 22.3 Comparison of signals generated by vestibular receptors when the head is moved in roll through 90 degrees in a stable 1 g environment (upper part of figure), and when there is a sustained rotation about a vertical (z body) axis (lower part of figure). Note how, in the latter condition, the cross-coupled (Coriolis) stimulus generates a false signal of rotation in pitch which is not accompanied by concordant signals from the otoliths.

linear accelerations—correctly transduce the angular movement of the head while the otoliths give inappropriate and hence conflicting information. It is known that information about the attitude of the head with respect to the gravitational vertical is derived from the deflection of the sensory hairs of the maculae by the component of the acceleration acting in sheer (that is, parallel to the plane of the maculae). Experiments have shown that, in a hypergravity force environment, the perception of a change in head attitude is exaggerated; conversely, in a force environment of less than $1g$ it is reduced (Ormsby and Young, 1976). Accordingly, in an abnormal force environment, any head movement that alters the orientation of the head with respect to the force vector will be associated with atypical signals from the otoliths. There will be a mismatch between the signal from the semicircular canals, which correctly transduce the head movement, and that from the otolith organ which will not accord with the signal 'expected' by the neural store.

Type 2 (i)

There are a number of situations and conditions occurring in aerospace flight in which motion sickness is induced by stimulation of the semicircular canals in the absence of expected and correlated signals from the otolith organs and other gravireceptors. Spacesickness is one example, for in the weightless environment of spaceflight angular movements of the head are transduced correctly by the semicircular canals but the otoliths do not signal the change in orientation of the head in pitch and roll, as they do on Earth. Whereas most voluntary head and body movements can be provocative on initial exposure to weightlessness, the finding that head movements in pitch and roll are the most nauseogenic strengthen the argument that spacesickness is caused by a canal–otolith mismatch (Oman *et al.*, 1986). With head movements having high angular accelerations and velocity there is likely to be atypical stimulation of otolithic receptors, and the mismatch is of Type 1; a Type 2 conflict is present when the head is moved slowly at rates that stimulate the semicircular canals but not the otoliths.

Another problem, common both to divers and to aircrew, is pressure or alternobaric vertigo (described in Chapter 21). In this condition, asymmetric stimulation of semicircular canals is brought about, without apparent involvement of the otoliths, by changes in ambient pressure. The vertigo is usually transient and motion sickness is not a common feature, although, in some individuals, the stimulus can be quite intense and may engender nausea but rarely vomiting.

Atypical stimulation of the semicircular canals, without disturbance of otolithic function, is seen in a number of other pathological or toxic states in which vertigo and nystagmus are accompanied by the signs and symptoms of motion sickness. Specific mention should be made of the positional vertigo associated with the consumption of ethyl alcohol (positional alcohol nystagmus) and benign paroxysmal vertigo. Both of these conditions cause symptoms on the ground, but in flight they can be intensified by linear accelerations greater than $1g$ produced by high rate turns and other flight manoeuvres.

Type 2 (ii)

The converse to the Type 2 (i) canal–otolith mismatch occurs when the otolith signal is not accompanied by the expected signal from the semicircular canals. Provided the individual does not move his head, sustained rotation at a steady speed about a vertical axis does not cause sickness, because once the effect of the initial velocity change has died away, neither the semicircular canals nor the otoliths signal rotation. However, when the axis of rotation is not vertical, or, in the worst case, it is horizontal (as in a barbecue-spit) then there is a mismatch between canal and otolithic signals. The otoliths are stimulated by the continued reorientation of the body to the force vector and signal rotation, but the canals fail to signal rotation as rotation is at a constant speed and there is no angular acceleration stimulus. Sustained rolling manoeuvres in level flight are associated with this kind of intravestibular mismatch, though in general the period of exposure is brief and is usually executed by pilots who have acquired some adaptive immunity.

Much more significant is the motion sickness induced by linear oscillation, typically the heaving motion of a ship, or the repetitive linear accelerations experienced in an aircraft flying through turbulence and vertical gusts. In such a motion environment, the force vector (that is, the resultant of the gravitational force and that due to the imposed linear acceleration) is continually changing in magnitude and direction without the expected correlated signal from the semicircular canals. Furthermore, when the oscillation is of low frequency ($<0.5\,\text{Hz}$), there is a phase error in the signalling of the linear motion by the otoliths which can be in conflict with the transduction of the changing force by pressure receptors in the skin or with visual information.

In a number of experiments carried out on four-pole swings, vertical oscillators or modified lifts it has been shown that the incidence of sickness increases as the frequency of oscillation falls (*Figure 22.4*). This clearly defined laboratory relationship between the frequency of the stimulus and sickness rate accords with observations made in flight. Aircraft whose modal frequency of oscillation is

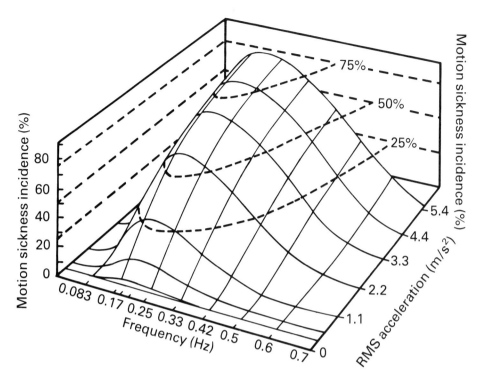

Figure 22.4 Incidence of motion sickness as a function of frequency and acceleration, evoked by 2 h exposure to vertical (z body axis) sinusoidal oscillation. (After McCauley *et al.* (1976).)

high (0.8–0.9 Hz) when flying through turbulence tend to produce less sickness and less impairment of performance than an aircraft that oscillates at a lower frequency (0.4 Hz). Similarly, a large motor car with a soft suspension and low natural frequency causes more sickness in passengers than one with a stiffer suspension and a more rapid dynamic response.

Neural centres and pathways in motion sickness

The neural mismatch hypothesis provides an adequate explanation of why certain motion stimuli cause sickness and of adaptation to a changed sensory environment. It argues for the presence, within the central nervous system, of integrative and co-ordinating centres, but it provides little insight into the neurophysiological processes or the location of the centres and pathways mediating the protean signs and symptoms of the motion sickness syndrome. Work on experimental animals has yielded some information on the relevant neural mechanisms, but the picture is far from complete and has, if anything, become more uncertain as the result of

more precise ablation studies carried out over the past few years.

Figure 22.5 summarizes the principal elements and pathways that can be implicated in the genesis of motion sickness and relates these to the physiological and behavioural responses that characterize the syndrome. There is good evidence that the vestibular apparatus, and hence the vestibular nuclei and their central projections to the cerebellum, have to be intact for motion sickness to be induced (Money, 1970). Removal of the entire cerebellum confers immunity to swing sickness in the dog, though which part of the cerebellum is essential is less certain. Previously the nodulus and uvula were considered to be critical structures but work by Miller and Wilson (1984) has shown that ablation of these structures did not prevent vestibularly induced vomiting in cats. Convergence of vestibular, visual, kinaesthetic and cerebellar afferents occurs at the level of the vestibular nuclei, so the comparison of actual and expected motion cues could take place within these brain stem nuclei. It is, however, more likely that the cerebellum is the locus of both the comparator and the internal model. It receives the necessary afferent signals about body motion from retinal, vestibular, kinaesthetic and somatosensory receptors; in addition, the

328 *Motion sickness*

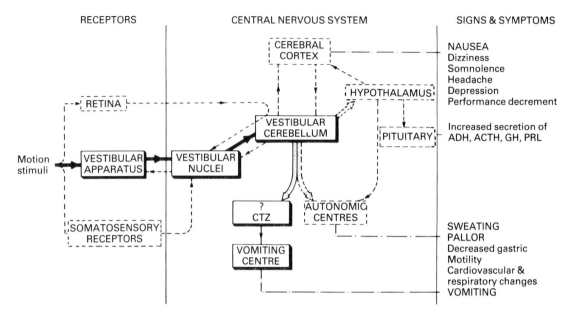

RECEPTORS CENTRAL NERVOUS SYSTEM SIGNS & SYMPTOMS

Figure 22.5 Neural structures in motion sickness. CTZ = Chemoreceptor trigger zone. (Modified from Benson (1977).)

cerebellum is known to be an important integrative centre in the control of motor activity and movement.

The way in which the cerebellum, or some other neural centre, initiates the sequence of sensory and autonomic responses that characterize the motion sickness syndrome remains a matter for speculation. The slow development of the syndrome and the persistence of signs and symptoms after the withdrawal of provocative stimuli suggests that there is some neuro-humoral mechanism. The identity of neurotransmitters or the possible accumulation of a substance within the cerebro-spinal fluid that stimulates the vomiting centre in the medulla oblongata have yet to be determined. It was thought that the chemo-receptive trigger zone (CTZ), close to the area postrema on the floor of the fourth ventricle, was an essential link in the descending pathway mediating motion sickness; but precise ablation studies have shown that this is not so (Borison, 1985). It would appear, however, that a neuronal centre, close to the area postrema and CTZ at the level of the calamus scriptorius, is a vital element coupling higher centres to the neuro-anatomically ill-defined vomiting centre in the region of the fasciculus solitarius.

Modification of the activity of hypothalamic nuclei is manifest by the increased secretion of antidiuretic and other pituitary hormones that accompany motion sickness (Eversmann *et al.*, 1977). However, neither hypophysectomy nor partial destruction of the hypothalamus prevent the

development of motion sickness in dogs. Indeed, decerebrate dogs and, anecdotally, decerebrate man are not immune.

Incidence of motion sickness

Motion sickness is a normal response to an abnormal environment, but there are very considerable differences between individuals in their susceptibility to the condition. Nevertheless, provided the motion stimulus is of sufficient intensity and duration, only those without a functioning vestibular system are truly immune. The incidence of sickness in a particular motion environment is governed by a number of factors, notably:

1. The physical characteristics of the stimulus (i.e. its frequency, intensity, duration and direction).
2. The intrinsic susceptibility of the individual.
3. The nature of the task performed.
4. Other environmental factors (e.g. odour).

The incidence of air sickness ranges from a fraction of 1% in large civil transport aircraft to 100% during 'hurricane penetration flights, in those who had no previous experience of such severe turbulence; and a 90% incidence in those who had flown in such conditions before (Kennedy *et al.*, 1972). In military aviation, air sickness is most manifest during flying training, where the disability at least impairs training, and at worst leads to

Aetiology of motion sickness   329

attrition with all its economic and social consequences. A survey (Dobie, 1974) of the incidence of air sickness in Royal Air Force trainee pilots, based on instructor reports, revealed that 39% of the students suffered from air sickness at some time during training, usually in the early stages, and that in 15% of students it was sufficiently severe to lead to disruption or abandonment of the flight. An extensive review of the problem (Hixon, Guedry and Lentz, 1984) in US Navy flight officers being trained to perform various non-pilot duties (navigators, radar operators, etc.) produced a mean incidence of air sickness in 13.5% of all flights. This was associated with vomiting on 5.9% of flights and led to a performance decrement (as assessed by both instructor and student) on 7.3% of flights. Some 59–63% of the students experienced symptoms on their first flight, 55–83% were sick on more than one flight and 15–30% were never air sick. (The ranges quoted reflect the differing incidences in the several categories and stages of training studied by Hixon *et al.*)

Typically, air sickness is most troublesome during the initial training flights. Thereafter the incidence of sickness falls as the student becomes adapted to the motion of the aircraft, but often rises again when aerobatic and high-G manoeuvres are introduced in the training programme. Much can be done to ease the student's problem by the instructor grading the flight manoeuvres during the first few hours of instruction. The initial demonstration of general handling should not be a test of the student's resistance (or susceptibility) to air sickness. The induction of symptoms early in training does not accelerate adaptation; indeed, it may impede this process by engendering anxiety and erode the student's confidence in his (her) ability to be a successful pilot.

Once trained to an operational standard it is rare for pilots to suffer from air sickness, though they sometimes experience symptoms when they are passengers and not in control of the aircraft. Non-pilot aircrew, in particular navigators, in high-performance aircraft and those working within the body of maritime reconnaissance aircraft may, however, continue to be troubled by air sickness. The proportion so afflicted is low but, anecdotally, there are a few aircrew who continue to vomit on nearly every flight, yet stoically and effectively carry out their operational duties.

Troops being transported by air are very much at risk; paratroops, in particular, are likely to be exposed to provocative motion during low-level approaches to dropping zones. In-flight studies have revealed sickness rates as high as 75%, though an incidence of 10% is perhaps more typical. Unfortunately, paratroops rarely fly with sufficient frequency to allow substantial adaptation to occur; furthermore, in flight they are usually closeted in the fuselage without sight of the ground or other external visual reference.

The incidence of sea sickness is no less variable

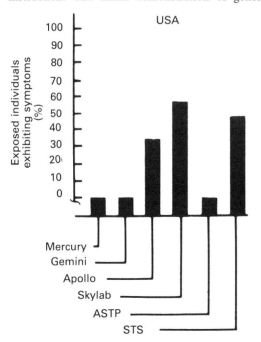 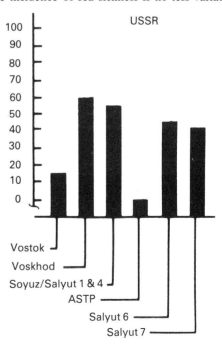

Figure 22.6 Incidence of space sickness. ASTP = Apollo–Soyuz joint mission; STS = space shuttle. (Reproduced from Reschke and Vanderploeg (1984), with kind permission of authors and publishers.)

than that of air sickness, though in terms of the number of people affected it is much more common, for the motion is generally more severe and more prolonged than in other forms of transportation. The motion of inflatable life-rafts is probably the most provocative, for in rough seas all but the very resistant succumb; an incidence of 99% has been reported (Money, 1970). Even moderate seas induce symptoms relatively quickly. For example, in a life-raft trial 55% of subjects had vomited and only 24% were symptom free after exposure for 1 hour to artificial wave motion (Brand, Colquhoun and Perry, 1968).

Space sickness like other types of motion sickness varies in severity and frequency. Symptoms were not reported by early US astronauts who flew in the small Mercury and Gemini spacecraft, but with the advent of the larger Apollo vehicle and the greater freedom of movement within the capsule, 11 of the 33 Apollo astronauts experienced symptoms comparable with those first reported by Titov. As may be seen from *Figure 22.6* the incidence of sickness in subsequent programmes, with the exception of the Apollo–Soyuz (ASTP) flight, has varied between 40% and 60%, despite attempts to reduce susceptibility by training, the administration of anti-motion sickness drugs and other procedures. Some 50% of all the astronauts and payload specialists who have flown on the Space Shuttle over the period 1981–1985 suffered from space sickness of 1–4 days' duration with symptoms ranging from mild malaise to repeated vomiting.

Prediction of the incidence of motion sickness

Despite the large number of factors that play a part in the aetiology of motion sickness, the few quantitative studies that have been carried out, both in the laboratory and in the field, have yielded reasonably concordant data from which a procedure for predicting the incidence of motion sickness has recently been developed (Lawther and Griffin, 1987). In essence, calculation of the effective stimulus dose, to which the incidence of vomiting is linearly related (*Figure 22.7*) takes into account three factors: (1) the intensity of the periodic motion; (2) the frequency spectrum of the motion; and (3) the duration of exposure.

Expressed mathematically, the percentage incidence of vomiting (*V*) and the stimulus dose (*D*) are given by:

$$V = K \cdot D = K \cdot \left[\int_0^T a^2_{(t)} \cdot dt \right]^{1/2}$$

where K is the dose constant (estimated at 1/3 for the general population), T is the duration of exposure in seconds (*Tmax = 6h*), $a_{(t)}$ is the

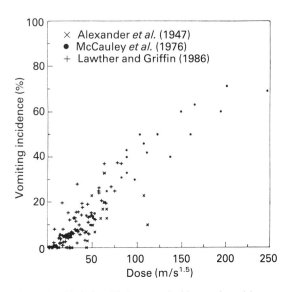

Figure 22.7 Relationship between incidence of vomiting and stimulus dose, calculated by the procedure described in the text. (Reproduced from Lawther and Griffin (1987) by kind permission of the authors and publishers.)

weighted acceleration in m/s². (The weighting is achieved by a filter having characteristics similar to the frequency dependence shown in *Figure 22.4. See* Lawther and Griffin (1987) for details.)

Prediction of an 'illness rating' (*I*) on a scale of 0 (I feel all right) to 3 (I feel dreadful) may also be made by using the formula:

$$I = (0.045 \times V) + 0.1$$

Where *V* is the predicted percentage of subjects who will vomit.

The procedure is probably valid for a fairly wide cross-section of the population as it is based on data obtained both from fit young men in enclosed small cabins and from a more heterogeneous group of passengers on sea-going ferries. Such factors as age, sex and degree of adaptation all influence susceptibility and modified values of K would be required to estimate the incidence of motion sickness in specific populations.

Factors influencing susceptibility

The considerable variability between subjects in their response to provocative motion is an important feature of motion sickness. The broad dispersion of susceptibility is illustrated in *Figure 22.8* which shows the number of subjects who developed well-defined signs and symptoms as a function of the intensity of the cross-coupled (Coriolis) stimulus to which they were exposed. The distribution is even more asymmetric than shown in the figure, for the

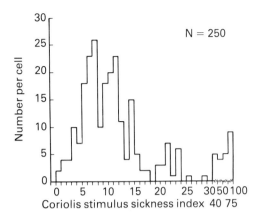

Figure 22.8 Distribution of susceptibility to cross-coupled (Coriolis) stimulation in 250 normal subjects. (Reproduced from Miller and Graybiel (1970) by kind permission of authors and publishers.)

measure of stimulus intensity is non-linear: the speed of rotation was increased incrementally throughout the test until definite signs and symptoms were elicited. Individual differences in the rate at which the subjects adapted to the stimulus also influence the shape of the histogram. Those having a low tolerance to the stimulus had little time to adapt, whereas those who were less sensitive were able to make a larger number of head movements and hence had a greater opportunity to adapt to the stimulus. The 'high tolerance' tail of the distribution embraces the fortunate few who probably have low intrinsic susceptibility and are fast adapters.

An adult's susceptibility to motion sickness appears to be a relatively stable and enduring characteristic for there is evidence that those who are sensitive to one type of provocative motion are likely to succumb when exposed to another (Kennedy and Graybiel, 1962; Money, 1972). Susceptibility to space sickness is, however, an exception to this general rule, for no significant correlation has been established, despite considerable effort to do so, between astronauts' responses to provocative stimuli, both on the ground and in aircraft, and their malaise in orbital flight (Reschke *et al.*, 1984).

Susceptibility changes with age (Reason and Brand, 1975). Motion sickness is rare below the age of 2 years, but with maturation susceptibility increases rapidly to reach a peak between the ages of 3 and 12 years. Over the next decade there is a progressive increase in tolerance which continues, albeit more slowly, with increasing age. This reduction in susceptibility with age has been recorded both for sea sickness and air sickness, but the elderly are not immune; 22% of those suffering from sea sickness on a Channel Island ferry were over the age of 59 years (Lawther and Griffin, 1986).

Females are more susceptible to motion sickness than males of the same age. This is evidenced by the highly significant difference between men and women in the distribution of a measure of susceptibility based on questionnaire responses, and by the higher incidence of vomiting and malaise, reported by female passengers than by male passengers on Channel Isle ferries. The incidence data suggest that the difference in susceptibility between men and women is in the ratio of approximately $1:1.7$, thus the value of K in the prediction equation (*see* page 300) is 0.25 for men and 0.42 for women. The reason for this sex difference, which applies both to children and to adults, is not known. It may be that females are more ready to admit to having had symptoms. In the adult, hormonal factors may also play a part, as susceptibility is highest during menstruation and is increased in pregnancy.

In a group of men or women of the same age, large differences in susceptibility exist; differences that reflect a basic characteristic, a dimension of personality, of the individual. However, Reason has shown that at least three factors can be recognized that contribute to inter-subject variability in susceptibility (Reason and Graybiel, 1972).

One of these factors is 'receptivity', a term that refers to the way in which the individual processes the stimulus within his nervous system. It is suggested that the man who has high 'receptivity' transduces the sensory stimulus more effectively, and that it evokes a more powerful subjective experience, than in a person of low 'receptivity'. Hence, according to the hypothesis, the 'receptive' has a more intense 'mismatch' signal and is therefore more likely to suffer from motion sickness than the non-receptive when exposed to provocative motion. Another factor is adaptability, which describes the rate at which the individual adapts to an atypical motion environment or, in more general terms, adjusts to the conditions of sensory rearrangement. A number of studies have shown wide and consistent differences in the rate at which individuals adapt when exposed to an unfamiliar motion stimulus. Those who adapt slowly suffer more severe symptoms and require a longer period for adjustment to the motion than the fast 'adaptor'. Slow 'adaptors' are more susceptible to motion sickness than the fast 'adaptors', but this does not mean that slow 'adaptors' are also 'receptives'. Indeed, it has been shown that these two factors are essentially unrelated.

Concepts of receptivity and adaptability permit explanation of how an individual will react on first exposure to an unfamiliar motion environment; but there remains one more factor: the manner in which adaptation is retained between exposures to the provocative motion. Anecdotal reports and laboratory experiments have shown that there are wide interindividual differences in the retention of adaptation. Also, it has become clear that this attribute does not correlate closely with measures of receptivity or the rate of initial adaptation (that is, adaptability). Poor retention of adaptation is illustrated by the airman, typically a navigator, who is troubled by motion sickness when flights are separated by several days of ground duty, but is symptom-free when he is able to fly regularly with not more than one or two days on the ground between flights. The man with better retention is not so afflicted; so that, once having adapted to the provocative motion of a particular flight environment, he remains symptom free even when flights are quite spasmodic.

These factors—receptivity, adaptability and retentivity—all influence susceptibility (*Figure 22.9*) but are not of equal importance when one attempts to assess if air sickness is likely to be a problem to a particular airman or potential airman. Evidence of high receptivity implies that sickness will occur on initial exposure to unfamiliar motion; but, if the individual is a fast adaptor and has good retention of adaptation, air sickness is unlikely to be a persistent problem. On the other hand, a person with low adaptability and poor retention is likely to continue to be afflicted by sickness when exposed to provocative motion. Knowledge of these constitutional factors can thus be an aid in the prediction both of motion sickness susceptibility and the likely benefit to a particular individual of desensitization therapy (*see below*).

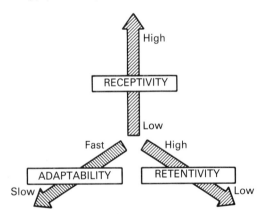

Figure 22.9 Diagram to illustrate three factors that determine motion sickness susceptibility, once allowance is made for the age and sex of the individual. The susceptibility to motion sickness increases with the length of the arrow.

Mental activity

In addition to the perceptual factors described in the previous section, there is another psychological (or behavioural) factor that influences susceptibility— the nature of mental activity during exposure to provocative motion. Laboratory studies and observation aboard ship and aircraft have shown that, when the individual concentrates his attention and mental effort on some task, he is less likely to become sick than when he is not so occupied. When he relaxes and has more time for introspection, or is asked to describe how he is feeling, then the appearance of symptoms and, more significantly, signs of motion sickness are not so long delayed.

The mechanism underlying the role of cognitive processes in the aetiology of motion sickness is not understood. Nevertheless, if aircrew and passengers can be kept occupied by tasks that take their minds off 'the state of their stomachs', then the incidence of sickness is likely to be decreased.

Anxiety and neurotic reactions

The similarity of the cardinal signs and symptoms of motion sickness with those engendered by fear and anxiety has fostered the opinion, held by a number of writers, that such psychogenic factors are of prime importance in the aetiology of motion sickness. The weight of evidence (*see* review in Reason and Brand, 1975) favours the conclusion that the physical characteristics of the motion stimulus and dimensions of personality other than anxiety traits are the principal factors determining the incidence of motion sickness; fear and anxiety are only of secondary importance. Nevertheless, significant correlations have been found in a number of studies between susceptibility and several personality characteristics (referenced by Collins and Lentz, 1977). The most consistent finding was a relationship between neuroticism and susceptibility; but, in addition, susceptible subjects tended to score higher than non-susceptibles on measures of introversion and anxiety, and they had more medical and emotional problems. The 16 Personality Factors (16PF) test, in conjunction with the other psychometric tests administered by Collins and Lentz (1977), led to the general conclusion that non-susceptible individuals tended to be tough and aggressive and are better able to cope in a non-emotional manner with stressful situations. Susceptible individuals are more likely to manifest autonomic emotional responses under stress, whether this be a physical (e.g. motion) or a mental stress.

The aetiological significance of these relationships between dimensions of personality and perceptual style is difficult to determine. There is some evidence that introversion and neuroticism are associated with slow adaptation (Reason and Graybiel, 1972), so this is one mechanism by which tolerance to provocative motion may be impaired. It must also be recognized that the neurotic individual is more likely to be aroused and made anxious both by the unpleasant symptoms of motion sickness and by the motion environment itself (e.g. aerobatic flight). Hence he, or she, will adapt less rapidly, or perhaps not adapt at all, to the provocative motion.

Anxiety can be considered both as a potentiator of susceptibility and as a consequence of motion sickness. Anxiety can also produce symptoms that are essentially indistinguishable from those evoked by provocative motion. The differentiation of *fear* sickness from *motion* sickness is relatively straightforward when nausea and vomiting occur in the absence of provocative motion. Examples are, the student pilot who develops symptoms after a certain time in the air irrespective of the intensity of the motion stimuli experienced, or the passenger who becomes sick as soon as she (rarely he) steps aboard the aircraft. On the other hand, when symptoms are consistently produced by certain flight manoeuvres, such as aerobatics, it is much more difficult to determine whether the symptoms are the expression of a neurotic reaction or are a 'normal' response to discordant motion cues. Typically, the airman with air sickness reports a diminution in the severity of symptoms with repeated exposure to the provocative motion. The individual with anxiety characteristically does not show such adaptation; indeed, symptoms may become worse on successive flights, particularly when there is a strong phobic element to the neurotic reaction or when a conditioned behavioural response is established. However, when the severity of symptoms remains relatively constant on repeated exposure to the provocative motion, anamnestic evidence is rarely sufficient to differentiate whether the air sickness is caused by low adaptability and poor retentivity, or is the manifestation of a neurotic reaction.

Prevention and treatment

Behavioural measures

Passengers in an aircraft can minimize motion cue conflict by restriction of unnecessary head movement, for example by pressing the head firmly against the seat or other available support, preferably in a reclined position. If space permits, they should lie down on their backs, as this posture has been shown in laboratory trials to reduce the incidence of motion sickness by approximately 20%. Visual–vestibular conflict is decreased by closing the eyes, unless of course the passenger has a clear view of the horizon or other stable visual reference outside the aircraft. Attempting to read a book, while a desirable means of occupying the mind and diverting attention from a lack of well-being, more commonly accentuates discordant visual cues and is rarely helpful.

Aircrew are not usually able to lie down and close their eyes when engaged on operational duties, yet they can still organize their activity so that unnecessary movements are not made. In particular, head movements should be reduced to a minimum, though not to the extent that either scan or look-out are impaired. Where possible, discordant visual cues should be minimized, as noted above. When aids to vision are employed for target recognition (for example, the use of binoculars for identification of ground targets), sickness is reduced and visual acuity enhanced if the optical image is stabilized.

Adaptation

The most potent therapeutic measure, at least in the long term, is adaptation to the provocative motion. This is 'nature's own cure' and is the preferred method of preventing sickness, particularly for aircrew who should not fly under the influence of anti-motion-sickness drugs.

The basic philosophy governing the acquisition and maintenance of protective adaptation is that aircrew should be gradually introduced to the provocative motions of the flight environment, and that adaptation, once achieved, should be maintained by regular and repeated exposure to the motion stimuli. Student pilots and those returning to flying after ground duties should have a graded introduction to the more stressful flight manoeuvres so that adaptation may be acquired, preferably without severe malaise. The wide differences between aircrew, both in initial susceptibility and rate of adaptation, make it difficult to lay down firm guidelines. Nevertheless, instructors should be advised to grade the duration of exposure and intensity of provocative motion stimuli in a manner commensurate with the tolerance of the aircrew under training.

The maintenance of protective adaptation is best assured by regular flying duties, though such factors as interindividual differences in the retention of adaptation, variations in weather conditions and operational roles, preclude temporal definition of the word 'regular'. Some aircrew are troubled by motion sickness if 2–3 days elapse between flights; others, with better 'retentivity', may not be more susceptible even after several weeks on the ground.

'Desensitization' therapy

Despite the high incidence of air sickness during the initial phases of flight training most aircrew adapt with repeated exposure to the provocative motion of flight, sometimes aided by a short course of an anti-motion sickness drug. There is, however, a small percentage of aircrew (estimated at about 5%) who fail to develop sufficient protective adaptation and in whom the continued sickness may necessitate suspension from flight training or, more rarely, operational duties. Most of the aircrew with what may be called intractable air sickness can be helped by a programme of treatment of a type initiated in the Royal Air Force more than 20 years ago by Dobie (1974). In its current form (Bagshaw and Stott, 1985) this 'desensitization' therapy involves first a 2–3 week period of twice daily exposure to cross-coupled (Coriolis) stimulation of progressively increasing intensity that may be alternated with low-frequency vertical oscillation or a provocative visual–vestibular interaction stimulus. The ground-based phase of therapy is followed by 10–15 hours of dual flying in which there is incremental exposure to progressively more provocative flight manoeuvres. This procedure has effectively prevented the recurrence of air sickness on return to flying duties in all but about 15% of those who have undergone therapy.

The desensitization programme, outlined above, places considerable emphasis on exposure and adaptation to physical motion stimuli. There is, nevertheless, a psychotherapeutic element in so far as the 'patient' is reassured that air sickness is a normal response and that it is not the manifestation of a personal weakness or 'lack of moral fibre'. Furthermore, as treatment progresses, he is made aware of his increasing tolerance which serves to allay any anxiety that he may have had about his ability to cope with provocative motion in the flight environment.

In the United States Air Force the desensitization therapy employs biofeedback and relaxation techniques in addition to passive Coriolis stimulation (Giles and Lochridge, 1985; Jones et al., 1985). The underlying concept is that by learning to control autonomic responses and allay anxiety evoked by motion stimuli, susceptibility to motion sickness will be decreased and the rate at which protective adaptation is acquired will be enhanced. Laboratory studies (Cowings and Toscano, 1982) have demonstrated that a significant increase in subjects' tolerance to motion stress can be achieved solely by autogenic and biofeedback training. It would appear, however, that in the absence of repeated exposure to provocative motion stimuli, biofeedback and relaxation techniques coupled with supportive psychotherapy was effective in returning only 40% of referred aircrew to flying duties. In contrast, when these behavioural techniques were combined with 20 sessions of incremental Coriolis stimulation and were followed by five 'reorientation' flights 85% of the aircrew were returned to flying duties (Jones et al., 1985).

Selection

A variety of techniques are available for assessing an individual's susceptibility to motion sickness (*see*

Lentz, 1984). Most widely used is some form of cross-coupled (Coriolis) stimulation, but tests in which there is visual–vestibular mismatch (the Visual–Vestibular Interaction Test) or stimulation of the otoliths (e.g. tilted axis rotation, parabolic flight, linear oscillation) have also been employed. In an extensive longitudinal study, carried out by Hixon et al. (1984), significant correlations were found between the incidence of air sickness during flight training and the student's responses to cross-coupled stimulation and to visual–vestibular conflict. Motion sickness questionnaire data also correlated highly with susceptibility to sickness in flight. It should be noted, however, that the questionnaire of Hixon et al. was administered after the personnel had been accepted into the Navy. Questions about previous history of motion sickness presented during the pre-entry medical are not answered with objective honesty. For example, Dobie (1974) found that only 3.6% of potential aircrew admitted to having suffered from motion sickness before selection; but subsequently, when the same questions were posed in a confidential questionnaire to the same group during aircrew training, 59% gave affirmative responses.

Because of the essential role of the vestibular system in the aetiology of motion sickness attempts have been made to relate indices of vestibular function to susceptibility. Most of these studies have failed to show any correlation, though Bles, de Jong and Oosterveld (1984) did find a higher frequency of labyrinthine imbalance (on caloric testing) in a group suffering from chronic sea sickness than in the control group.

As discussed earlier, susceptibility is associated with certain dimensions of personality (neuroticism, anxiety and introversion) but the correlations, though significant, are relatively weak. Even the highly significant correlations found by Hixon et al. are not high enough for the results of provocative test and motion sickness questionnaire scores to be used as selection determinants, for they do not reliably identify those individuals in whom sickness will be a continuing problem during flight training or subsequent operational duties.

Whereas correlations have been established between data from various laboratory tests and susceptibility to motion sickness in a number of terrestrial environments, no consistent relationship has yet been found between such measures and susceptibility to space sickness, despite considerable research effort.

Aircraft factors

Although it is known that the incidence of motion sickness increases as the frequency of oscillation decreases, this fact has not apparently been considered by the aircraft designer or others concerned with aircraft dynamics. An aircraft that responds to a gust perturbation by low-frequency (<0.5 Hz) movement is clearly less desirable, from the air sickness viewpoint, for long duration sorties at low level or for 'hurricane hunter' type operations, than one with a higher characteristic frequency. In some aircraft, low frequency oscillation, usually of a 'dutch roll' type, is induced by the autopilot control system. A reduction in the incidence of air sickness, particularly in passengers and non-flight-deck aircrew of such aircraft, can be achieved by improvement of control dynamics.

Other relevant aspects of aircraft design concern the postural stability of the aircrew or passenger within the aircraft. Thus restraint harnesses, the provision of head support, and seat design in general all play a part. The arrangement of instruments and displays can also contribute to a reduction in the incidence of air sickness, as can the siting of work stations within the aircraft. Such factors are of particular concern to non-flight-deck aircrew who should, whenever possible, be seated close to the centre of gravity of the aircraft. Furthermore, they should be provided with displays and controls that do not require large-amplitude head movements to be made in the course of normal operations.

Environmental factors such as heat, unpleasant odours, etc., are usually over-emphasized in the aetiology of motion sickness, though it must be acknowledged that comfort is enhanced and sickness perhaps less likely if they are adequately controlled. A feeling of warmth is a common feature of motion sickness; hence, it is not surprising that fresh air or a cooling breeze causes symptomatic improvement. However, the belief that a hot oppressive atmosphere increases susceptibility, though understandable, has not been supported by several objective studies.

Drugs

Over the years many medicinal remedies have been proposed for the prevention of motion sickness. The number of drugs that have been tested is large (Brand and Perry, 1966; Wood, 1970), but relatively few are effective (*Table 22.2*) and none can completely prevent the development of signs and symptoms in everyone in all provocative motion environments.

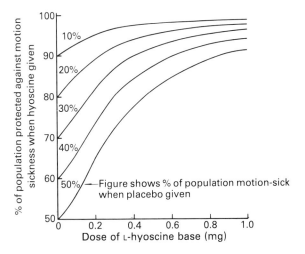

Figure 22.10 Protection against motion sickness afforded by L-hyoscine, at five levels of 'placebo sickness'. Note the logarithmic shape of the curves, and the lack of complete (100%) protection, even with a large dose of the drug. (After Brand and Perry (1966).)

Figure 22.10 shows the protection afforded by differing doses of one of the most effective drugs, L-hyoscine hydrobromide (L-scopolamine hydrobromide in the USA). When the motion is relatively mild and only 10% of the unmedicated population suffer from sickness then use of the drug can increase protection so that all but 2% of the population are not sick. But when the motion is of such severity and duration that 50% are sick when no drug is given, a large dose of hyoscine (1.0 mg) still leaves 8% of the population unprotected. In

Table 22.2 Adult dose regimen for anti-motion sickness drugs

Drug	Dose (mg)	Time of onset (h) (approx)	Duration of action (h) (approx)
1. Hyoscine hydrobromide (Kwells)	0.3–0.6	½–1	4–6
2. Cyclizine hydrochloride (Marzine, Valoid)	50	1–2	4–6
3. Dimenhydrinate (Dramamine, Gravol)	50–100	1–2	6–8
4. Cinnarizine (Stugeron)	30	1½–2	6–8
5. Promethazine hydrochloride (Phenergan) Promethazine theoclate (Avomine)	25	1½–2	24–30

Trade names of British proprietary products given in parentheses.

life-rafts, sickness rates approaching 100% have been reported, so it is not surprising that a significant proportion of the occupants will still suffer from sea sickness even when the dose of drug given is sufficient to cause side-effects.

None of the drugs of proven efficacy in the prophylaxis of motion sickness is entirely specific and all have side-effects. Both the anti-histaminics (such as promethazine and dimenhydrinate) and the anti-cholinergic, hyoscine, are also central depressants and can cause impairment of performance. Hyoscine, at all therapeutic doses, has been shown to cause a performance decrement on tasks requiring continuous attention and memory storage for new information (Parrott, 1986), but only at doses greater than 0.8 mg does it interfere with performance of a pursuit tracking task. Promethazine 25 mg has also been shown to impair psychomotor performance (Wood *et al.*, 1985). Other side-effects of hyoscine—notably blurred vision, sedation, dizziness and dry mouth—may also contribute to performance decrement (Brand *et al.*, 1968).

There is thus good reason for the general rule that anti-motion sickness drugs should not be taken by aircrew, and under no circumstances taken by a pilot when he flies solo. There is a place, however, for the administration of prophylactic drugs to susceptible student aircrew, particularly during the early stages of flying training when accompanied by an instructor. There is no evidence to suggest that hyoscine or the other specified drugs interfere with the acquisition of protective adaptation; rather, it may be argued, they aid adaptation by allowing greater exposure to motion stimuli and also by decreasing anxiety. On the other hand, the continued exhibition of anti-motion sickness drugs to aircrew is to be deprecated because such a pharmacological 'crutch' is not compatible with operational duties.

No such restrictions apply to the use of drugs by passengers for the alleviation of motion sickness. Paratroops and other personnel who must operate at peak efficiency on leaving the aircraft or at the end of a flight are a possible exception, though the putative performance decrement attributable to motion sickness and that due to drug side-effect is a dilemma to be assessed only with detailed knowledge of all facets of the operational situation.

The choice of prophylactic drug is, in part, dependent upon the foreseen duration of exposure to provocative motion and, in part, upon differences between individuals both in the efficacy of a particular drug and the severity of side-effects (Graybiel *et al.*, 1975). So if, in practice, one drug is not effective or not well tolerated, then it is justifiable to give another drug or combination of drugs. Where the therapeutic objective is to provide short-term protection, oral ʟ-hyoscine hydrobromide (0.3–0.6 mg) is the drug of choice. This acts within ½–1 h and provides protection for about 4 h.

Side-effects can be troublesome and tend to be accentuated if repeated administration (at 4–6 h intervals) is required for more prolonged prophylaxis. With the development of trans-dermal, drug-transport techniques it is now possible to provide a loading dose of 200 µg hyoscine and its controlled release at 10 µg/h for up to 60 h by means of a patch placed behind the ear (the Trans-Dermal Therapeutic System or TTS). The protection afforded by TTS is reported to be comparable with that achieved by oral hyoscine, but there does appear to be greater inter-subject variability in both the efficacy and in the incidence of side-effects than found with repeated oral administration of the drug (Homick *et al.*, 1983). When hyoscine is administered transdermally, peak blood levels are not reached until 8–12 h after application of the patch, so it is necessary to anticipate a requirement for prophylaxis by at least 6 h.

The antihistamines promethazine and meclozine, when taken by mouth, are absorbed more slowly than hyoscine and are not effective until about 2 h after administration, but they provide protection for at least 12 h. Other drugs in the same group, such as cyclizine, dimenhydrinate and cinnarizine, are absorbed at about the same rate though their duration of action is shorter—about 6 h.

The demonstration that ᴅ-amphetamine increases subjects' tolerance to cross-coupled stimulation led to an evaluation of the use of this analeptic in combination with the established anti-motion sickness drugs. It was found that there was a synergistic increase in prophylactic potency and a decrease in the sedation which is a common side-effect of hyoscine and the antihistamines. Ephedrine is almost as effective as amphetamine in enhancing the efficacy of the anti-motion sickness drugs and should be used in preference to amphetamine when prescription of this potentially addictive drug is contra-indicated.

Assessment of therapeutic potency both in laboratory and in field trials has indicated that the combination of ʟ-hyoscine hydrobromide (0.3 mg) with ephedrine sulphate (25 mg) or ᴅ-amphetamine sulphate (5 mg) is most effective for short-term (4 h) protection. In situations requiring more sustained prophylaxis the combination of promethazine hydrochloride (25 mg) with either ephedrine sulphate (25 mg) or ᴅ-amphetamine sulphate (5 mg) is recommended.

Management of established vomiting

Vomiting that is severe and repeated can lead to dehydration and loss of electrolytes. If this occurs in a survival situation (for example, on a life-raft) it may cause breakdown in morale, loss of interest in surroundings and a loss of ability to co-operate with rescue attempts. In such cases attention should be given to the following:

1. *Maintenance of intake* of fluids, electrolytes and calories.
2. *Use of drugs*—these must be given parenterally. If given by mouth they may not be absorbed or will be returned with the vomit. The following preparations are recommended.

Drug	Dose (mg)	Route
L-Hyoscine hydrobromide	0.3	Intramuscular injection
Cyclizine hydrochloride	50	Intramuscular injection
Cyclizine hydrochloride	50–100	By suppository
Promethazine hydrochloride	25	Intramuscular injection

3. *Supportive measures*—make the patient lie down, attend to general comfort and give reassurance.

References

BAGSHAW, M. and STOTT, J.R.R. (1985) The desensitisation of chronically motion sick aircrew in the Royal Air Force. *Aviation Space and Environmental Medicine*, **56**, 1144–1151

BENSON, A.J. (1977) Possible mechanisms of motion and space sickness. In *Life-sciences Research in Space*. Report SP-130. Paris: European Space Agency

BENSON, A.J. (1984) Motion Sickness. In *Vertigo*, edited by M.R. Dix and J.D. Hood, pp. 391–426. Chichester: J. Wiley & Sons

BLES, W., de JONG, H.A.A. and OOSTERVELD, W.J. (1984) Prediction of seasickness susceptibility. In *Motion Sickness: Mechanisms, Prediction, Prevention and Treatment*. Conference Proceedings 372, 27, 1–6. Neuilly sur Seine: AGARD/NATO

BORISON, H.L. (1985) A misconception of motion sickness leads to false therapeutic expectations. *Aviation Space and Environmental Medicine*, **56**, 66–68

BRAND, J.J., COLQUHOUN, W.P. and PERRY, W.L.M. (1968) Side-effect of L-hyoscine and cyclizine studied by objective tests. *Aerospace Medicine*, **39**, 999–1002

BRAND, J.J. and PERRY, W.L.M. (1966) Drugs used in motion sickness. *Pharmacological Review*, **18**, 895–924

COLLINS, W.E. and LENTZ, J.M. (1977) Some psychological correlates of motion sickness susceptibility. *Aviation Space and Environmental Medicine*, **48**, 587–594

COWINGS, P. and TOSCANO, W.B. (1982) The relationship of motion sickness susceptibility to learned autonomic control for symptom suppression. *Aviation Space and Environmental Medicine*, **53**, 570–575

DOBIE, T.G. (1974) *Airsickness in Aircrew*. Report - 177. Neuilly sur Seine: AGARD/NATO

EVERSMANN, T., GOTTSMANN, M., UHLICH, E., ULBRECHT, G., von WERDER, K. and SCRIBA, P.C. (1977) Increased secretion of growth hormones, prolactin, antidiuretic hormone and cortisol induced by the stress of motion sickness. *Aviation Space and Environmental Medicine*, **49**, 53–57

GILES, D.A. and LOCHRIDE, G.K. (1985) Behavioural airsickness management programme for student pilots.

Aviation Space and Environmental Medicine, **56**, 991–994

GRAYBIEL, A. and KNEPTON, J. (1976) Sopite syndrome: A sometimes sole manifestation of motion sickness. *Aviation Space and Environmental Medicine*, **47**, 873–882

GRAYBIEL, A., WOOD, C.D., KNEPTON, J., HOCHE, J.P. and PERKINS, G.F. (1975) Human assay of anti-motion sickness drugs. *Aviation Space and Environmental Medicine*, **46**, 1107–1118

GUEDRY, F.E., LENTZ, J. and JELL, R.M. (1979) Visual vestibular interactions: 1. Influence of peripheral vision on suppression of the vestibulo-ocular reflex and visual acuity. *Aviation Space and Environmental Medicine*, **50**, 205–211

HIXSON, W.C., GUEDRY, F.E. and LENTZ, J.M. (1984) Results of a longitudinal study of airsickness incidence during naval flight officer training. In *Motion Sickness: Mechanisms Prediction, Prevention and Treatment*. Conference Proceedings, 372, 30, 1–13. Neuilly sur Seine: AGARD/NATO

HOMICK, J.L., KOHL, R.L., RESCHKE, M.F., DEGIOANNI, J. and CINTRON-TREVINO, N.M. (1983) Transdermal scopolamine in the prevention of motion sickness: evaluation of the time course of efficacy. *Aviation Space and Environmental Medicine*, **54**, 994–1000

HOMICK, J.L., RESCHKE, M.F. and VANDERPLOEG, J.M. (1984) Space adaptation syndrome: incidence and operational implications for the Space Transportation System programme. In *Motion Sickness: Mechanisms, Prediction, Prevention and Treatment*. Conference Proceedings, 372, 36, 1–6. Neuilly sur Seine: AGARD/NATO

JONES, D.R., LEVY, R.A., GARDNER, L., MARSH, R.W. and PATTERSON, J.C. (1985) Self-control of psychophysiologic response to motion stress: using biofeedback to treat airsickness. *Aviation Space and Environmental Medicine*, **56**, 1152–1157

KENNEDY, R.S. and GRAYBIEL, A. (1962) Validity of tests of canal sickness in predicting susceptibility to airsickness and seasickness. *Aerospace Medicine*, **33**, 935–938

KENNEDY, R.S., MORONEY, W.F., BALE, R.M., GREGOIRE, H.G. and SMITH, D.G. (1972) Motion sickness symptomatology and performance decrements occasioned by hurricane penetrations in C-121, C-130 and P-3 Navy aircraft. *Aerospace Medicine*, **43**, 1235–1239

LAWTHER, A. and GRIFFIN, M.J. (1986) The motion of a ship at sea and the consequent motion sickness amongst passengers. *Ergonomics*, **29**, 535–552

LAWTHER, A. and GRIFFIN, M.J. (1987) Prediction of the incidence of motion sickness from the magnitude, frequency and duration of vertical oscillation. *Journal of the Acoustical Society of America* (in press)

LENTZ, J.M. (1984) Laboratory tests of motion sickness susceptibility. In *Motion Sickness: Mechanisms, Prediction, Prevention and Treatment*. Conference Proceedings, 372, 29, 1–9, Neuilly sur Seine: AGARD/NATO

LENTZ, J.M. and COLLINS, W.E. (1977) Motion sickness susceptibility and related behavioural characteristics in men and women. *Aviation Space and Environmental Medicine*, **48**, 316–323

MCCAULEY, M.E. (1984) *Research Issues in Simulator Sickness: Proceedings of a Workshop*. Washington DC: National Academy Press

MCCAULEY, M.E., ROYAL, J.W., WYLIE, C.P., O'HANLON, J.F. and MACKIE, R.R. (1976). *Motion Sickness Incidence:*

Exploratory Studies of Habituation, Pitch and Roll and The Refinement of A Mathematical Model. Technical Report No. 1733-2. Goleta, Cal.: Human Factors Research

MILLER, E.F. and GRAYBIEL, A. (1970) The semicircular canals as a primary etiological factor in motion sickness. In *4th Symposium on the Role of the Vestibular Organs in Space Exploration.* SP-187, 69–82. Washington: NASA

MILLER, A.D. and WILSON, V.J. (1984) Neurophysiological correlates of motion sickness: role of vestibulo-cerebellum and 'vomiting centre' reanalysed. In *Motion Sickness: Mechanisms, Prediction, Prevention and Treatment.* Conference Proceedings, 372, 21, 1–5. Neuilly sur Seine: AGARD/NATO

MONEY, K.E. (1970) Motion Sickness. *Physiological Reviews,* **50,** 1–38

MONEY, K.E. (1972) Measurement of susceptibility to motion sickness. In *Predictability of Motion Sickness in the Selection of Pilots.* Conference Proceedings. 109. B.2, 1–4, Neuilly sur Seine: AGARD/NATO

OMAN, C.M. (1982) A heuristic mathematical model for the dynamics of sensory conflict and motion sickness. *Acta Oto-laryngologica,* Supplement, 392

OMAN, C.M., LICHTENBERG, B.K., MONEY, K.E. and McCOY, R.K. (1986) M.I.T./Canadian vestibular experiments on the Spacelab-1 mission: 4. Space motion sickness: symptoms, stimuli and predictability. *Experimental Brain Research,* **64,** 316–334

ORMSBY, C.C. and YOUNG, L.R. (1976) Perception of static orientation in a constant gravitoinertial environment. *Aviation Space and Environmental Medicine,* **47,** 159–164

PARROTT, A.C. (1986) The effect of transdermal scopolamine and four dose levels of oral scopolamine (0.15, 0.3, 0.6 and 1.2 mg) upon psychological performance. *Psychopharmacology,* **89,** 347–354

REASON, J.T. (1970) Motion sickness: A special case of sensory rearrangement. *Advance Science,* **26,** 386–393

REASON, J.T. (1978) Motion sickness adaptation: A neural mismatch model. *Journal of the Royal Society of Medicine,* **71,** 819–829

REASON, J.T. and BRAND, J.J. (1975) *Motion Sickness.* London: Academic Press

REASON, J.T. and GRAYBIEL, A. (1972) Factors contributing to motion sickness susceptibility adaptability and receptivity. In *Predictability of Motion Sickness in the Selection of Pilots,* Conference Proceedings 109, B4, 1–15, Neuilly sur Seine: AGARD/NATO

RESCHKE, M.F., HOMICK, J.L., RYAN, P. and MOSELEY, E.D. (1984) Prediction of the space adaptation syndrome. In *Motion Sickness: Mechanisms, Prediction, Prevention and Treatment.* Conference Proceedings, 372, 26, 1–19. Neuilly sur Seine: AGARD/NATO

TRIESMAN, M. (1977) Motion sickness an evolutionary hypothesis. *Science,* **197,** 493–495

WOOD, C.D. (1970) Anti-motion sickness therapy. In *5th Symposium on the Role of the Vestibular Organs in Space Exploration.* Report SP-314: Washington DC: NASA

WOOD, C.D., MANNO, J.E., MANNO, B.R., REDETZKI, H.M., WOOD, M.J. and MIMS, M.E. (1985) Evaluation of anti-motion sickness drug side-effects on performance. *Aviation Space and Environmental Medicine,* **56,** 310–316

23

Vision in flight

D.H. Brennan

Anatomy and physiology

General

Each eyeball is roughly spherical, approximately 2.5 cm in diameter and lies within the bony orbit suspended in fat. It is protected against damage from all directions except at the front where protection is limited to that provided by the eyelids.

The eyeball is hollow and depends on its own internal pressure to maintain its shape and integrity. It is composed (*Figure 23.1*) of three coats which are modified at the front to admit light. The outermost coat (or sclera) is tough, supportive and relatively avascular; its anterior transparent region is called the cornea. The middle coat or uvea is vascular, its prime function being nutritive; anteriorly this middle coat becomes the ciliary body and iris; posteriorly it forms the choroid. The innermost coat

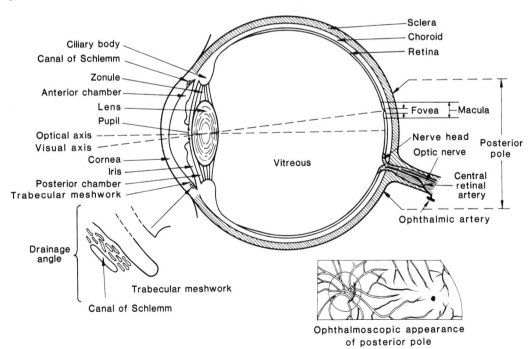

Figure 23.1 The essential features of the eye.

is the retina which is light sensitive and in extent corresponds to the choroid. The globe is divided into two main compartments by the lens-iris diaphragm: a large posterior compartment filled with a clear jelly called the vitreous and a smaller anterior chamber filled with a clear liquid called the aqueous.

Extra-ocular muscles

The globe rotates about its own centre in response to the pull of the three pairs of extra-ocular muscles. The medial and lateral recti act solely in adduction and abduction. The superior and inferior recti act primarily in elevation and depression but have secondary functions as adductors and in torsional movements. The superior and inferior obliques act primarily in depression and elevation but are secondary abductors and also contribute to torsional movements. The two eyes are 'yoked' together and their axes remain parallel in all conjugate movements. Their axes are of necessity not parallel in the disjunctive movements of convergence and divergence.

Cornea

The anterior transparent window, or cornea, is approximately 1 mm thick at its junction (limbus) with the sclera, thinning to about 0.7 mm at its centre. It is composed of four layers; a thin outer epithelium which rapidly regenerates when damaged, a thick layer of fibrous lamellae called the substantia propria, a thin inner elastic structure called Descemet's membrane, and an endothelial coat of single-cell thickness which covers Descemet's membrane and is continuous with the endothelium of the anterior surface of the iris.

The corneal stroma is composed of collagen surrounded by mucopolysaccharide. It acts like a gel and will thus rapidly hydrate. Excess hydration and loss of transparency is prevented by the endothelium which actively 'pumps' sodium ions and associated water into the aqueous. This process requires oxygen. A secondary mechanism preventing excess hydration is the corneal epithelium which acts as a partial barrier to lacrimal fluid.

The cornea is avascular and only minimal quantities of oxygen are obtained by diffusion from the pericorneal plexus of vessels at the limbus. The oxygen supply to the epithelium is derived primarily from the atmosphere, whereas the supply to the endothelium is obtained mainly from the aqueous. At sea level when the oxygen tension at the corneal epithelium is 150 mm Hg, it is 100 mm Hg at the mid-layer of the cornea and only 55 mm Hg at the aqueous surface of the cornea (endothelium). Contact lenses that reduce oxygen tension at the corneal epithelium may well have profound effects on vision at altitude (*see* Chapter 51).

Uveal tract

The iris is a pigmented contractile tissue which has a hole in its centre called the pupil. The colour of the iris is a function of the degree of pigmentation, brown eyes being heavily pigmented whilst blue eyes are relatively lightly pigmented. The pupillary diameter varies with the contraction of the iris musculature; the normal excursion is between 3 and 7 mm. Drugs can increase the range to 1.75–8 mm. The pupil varies according to ambient lighting and regulates the amount of light entering the eye, this being proportional to the square of the pupillary diameter. When the diameter is large, some rays of light enter the eyes obliquely, and these oblique pencils of light do not stimulate cones as efficiently as central pencils (Stiles Crawford effect). Although measured pupillary diameters may be 8 mm, the maximum 'effective' pupil diameter in cone vision is 5.5 mm.

The ciliary body is roughly triangular in section and when viewed from behind is seen as a ring. Around the ring are numerous processes, which secrete the aqueous humour. The aqueous is a fluid which is similar in composition to blood plasma but the protein content of the aqueous is lower. The aqueous is constantly formed by the ciliary body and drains through the trabecular meshwork of the canal of Schlemm, which lies in the angle formed by the cornea and iris root. The normal intra-ocular pressure of between 10 and 20 mm Hg is maintained by the rate of formation and the resistance to outflow of the aqueous.

The ciliary muscle, which is unstriated, is contained within the ciliary body and consists of three groups—the longitudinal, circular and radial muscles. The aggregate contractile force of these muscles slackens the tension in the suspensory ligament of zonule and permits the lens to assume a greater convexity and thus increase its refractive power.

The choroid is the continuation backwards of the uveal tract, separating the retina from the sclera. It is composed of three vascular layers and an inner layer, comprised mainly of collagen and connective tissue, called Bruch's membrane, which is in apposition with the pigment epithelium of the retina. The choroid supplies the nutritional requirements of the outer retina and macula. The apparent anomaly that the light-sensitive receptors are furthest from the light is because they need to be close to the choroid which nourishes them.

Lens

The lens is approximately 9 mm in diameter and 4 mm thick. It is transparent, elliptical and biconvex; the anterior radius of curvature is 10 mm and the posterior radius of curvature 6 mm. It is supported around its equator by fibres, the zonular fibres, which are inserted into the lens capsule. The anterior surface of the lens is bathed in aqueous and is in apposition with the pupillary portion of the iris. The small irregular space between the posterior surface of the iris and the anterior surface of the lens, which varies in size as the lens shape alters during accommodation, is known as the posterior chamber. The large vitreous filled space is called the posterior compartment. The lens is enclosed in a capsule and consists of a central nucleus and a thick cortex, composed of elongated cells which are laid down in onion-like layers by the anterior epithelium throughout life.

With age, the lens loses some of its plasticity and cannot assume the same convexity as it did in youth. This causes a progressive inability to focus near objects. In addition, the nucleus increases in size, may become yellow and loses some of its transparency.

The lens is the second refracting structure. The majority of the refractive power of the eye is at the air–corneal surface and the total corneal refractive power averages +43 dioptres. A dioptre (D) is a convenient measure of positive or negative lens power. It is defined as the reciprocal of the focal length expressed in metres. Thus a 1 D lens has a focal length of 1 m, a 2 D lens has a focal length of 0.5 m and a 0.5 D lens has a focal length of 2.0 m. A further advantage of this notation is that the total power of a combination of lenses in apposition is the sum of their positive or negative dioptric powers. The eye lens continues the refraction started by the cornea and brings rays of light to a focus on the retina. The average power of the unaccommodated lens is −20 D. The accommodative power, as mentioned, falls with age, being approximately +14 D at 10 years, +4 D at 40 years and +1 D at 60 years.

The stimulus for accommodation might be considered to be solely a blurred retinal image. If this were the case, accommodation would be a slow process, as the lens focused backwards and forwards around the point of true focus until a sharp image was 'tuned'. Chromatic aberration may play a large part in rapid focusing. The eye, unlike a good optical system, is not corrected for chromatic aberration. When the eye focuses in white light, the red component of the object is subject to less refraction than the blue. This results in the production of colour fringes on the retina, which in practice are largely ignored. The magnitude of the fringes is greater at night owing to pupillary dilatation. When one accommodates in white light, if the object is too close, red fringes predominate; if too far away there is a predominance of blue fringes. The eye/brain is thus provided with a clue as to whether accommodation should be increased or relaxed. The importance of colour fringes in rapid accommodation is an argument against monochromatic lighting systems such as red cockpit lighting. In monochromatic light, greater reliance must be placed on spherical aberration for accommodative clues. A further argument is that red light requires greater accommodative effort than white light; the extra accommodation may cause difficulty for presbyopes and hypermetropes. It is not uncommon for aircrew who are over the age of 40 years and are becoming presbyopic to complain of difficulty in focusing on instruments illuminated by red light.

Retina

The retina is a thin transparent membrane which covers most of the posterior compartment. The outermost layer of the retina is the pigment epithelium, and this lies on the choroid. Next to the pigment epithelium are the light-sensitive receptors called rods and cones. Next to the rods and cones are the bipolar cells and their synaptic layers; innermost of all are the ganglion cells and their axons which converge on the optic disc (the exit of the optic nerve). As can be seen from the retinal structure, light must pass through the nerve layers of the retina before reaching the light-sensitive receptors. The neural retina functions by sending impulses, generated by the action of light on receptors back towards its inner or vitreal surface. The ganglion cells on this side of the retina pass the visual information onwards to the optic nerve and thus to the brain. There is, however, considerable horizontal processing, the retina itself modifying the data to enhance the visual information before it reaches the ganglion cells. There is a specialized area of retina known as the macula about 600 μm in diameter with the fovea at its centre. This area lies approximately 3 mm temporal to the optic disc and is used for tasks demanding high visual acuity, both form and colour, and is an area composed entirely of cones. The trick of looking off-centre to see faint lights is to allow the rods to be stimulated. The rods are used for night vision and are highly light sensitive when dark adapted. They cannot differentiate colours or provide a good form acuity. If one considers foveal acuity as unity, at 5 degrees eccentric from the fovea the acuity has dropped to 0.25, at 20 degrees eccentric to the fovea this figure has fallen to 0.05 (*Figure 23.2*). This fall in acuity reflects the increasing ratio of rods to cones. At the fovea, each cone is connected to a single optic nerve

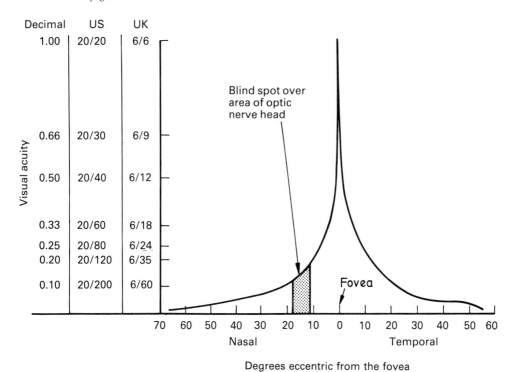

Figure 23.2 The variation of visual acuity (expressed in decimal, British and USA notation) at retinal sites eccentric to the fovea. The acuity at 5 degrees eccentric to the fovea is only one-quarter that at the fovea.

fibre, and the one-to-one relationship between receptors and nerve fibres contributes to the foveal ability to discriminate fine detail. Peripheral to the fovea the number of cones connecting to a single ganglion cell progressively increase, with a consequent fall in visual acuity. The rods are functionally connected into large groups, and the convergence of many rods on to one nerve fibre helps to give the rods their sensitivity to light. It is also one reason for their inability to discriminate detail.

Visual function

It is conventional to compare the human eye with a camera, but this analogy is too facile. The eye is self-focusing; it can adjust over an enormous range of luminances, it is capable of fine hue discrimination, and it can distinguish detail that subtends visual angles of less than 30 seconds of arc.

The optical system of the eye is, however, relatively crude and its sophisticated performance is principally due to the co-ordination between eye and brain. The brain and the neural retina process visual information, adding and subtracting as necessary, to improve the image incident upon the retina.

It is convenient to separate visual function into its three component senses, namely, light, form and colour.

Light sense

The eye is capable of functioning over a wide range of luminances. The luminance of an object is a measure of its brightness; it is the product of the illumination falling on the object and its reflectance. In the SI system it is expressed in candelas per square metre (*Figure 23.3*). The threshold stimulus may be as low as 10^{-6} cd/m² , corresponding to faint starlight; and the maximum limit, where discomfort is evident, as high as 10^6 cd/m² , corresponding to bright sunlight on snow. Two mechanisms function over this range. Scotopic or rod vision operates from threshold to approximately 10^{-3} cd/m². Over this range, form acuity is poor and vision is monochromatic. Above 1.0 cd/m², photopic or cone vision takes over, giving, with increasing luminance, the advantages of good form acuity and the ability to discriminate colours. The transitional stage when both rods and cones are functioning is known as mesopic vision and corresponds very roughly to full moonlight.

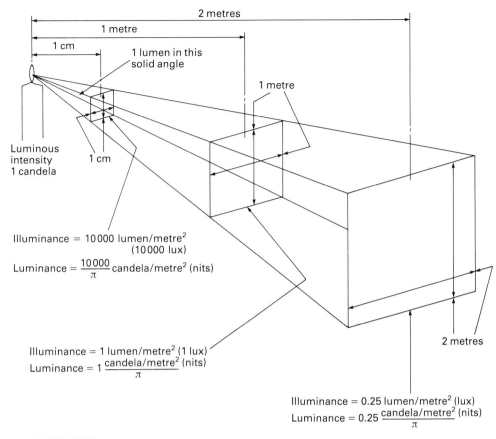

Illuminance = 10000 lumen/metre^2 (10000 lux)

Luminance = $\dfrac{10000}{\pi}$ candela/metre^2 (nits)

Illuminance = 1 lumen/metre^2 (1 lux)

Luminance = 1 $\dfrac{\text{candela/metre}^2 \text{ (nits)}}{\pi}$

Illuminance = 0.25 lumen/metre^2 (lux)

Luminance = 0.25 $\dfrac{\text{candela/metre}^2 \text{ (nits)}}{\pi}$

SI BASE UNIT
  Candela: A unit of luminous intensity. Approximately equivalent to the intensity of a domestic candle.

SI DERIVED UNITS
  Lumen: A unit of luminous flux. A point source of 1 candela emits 1 lumen per unit solid angle (steradian).

  Lux: A unit of illuminance (illumination). It is the distribution of light incident upon a surface in lumen/metre^2.

Candela/metre^2 (nits): A unit of luminance (brightness). It is the product of illuminance and reflectance

Figure 23.3 A photometric diagram illustrating the optical quadratic law and defining the relevant SI units.

The eye requires time to adjust to varying luminances because the mechanism is photochemical. When it adapts from dark to light, this adjustment is rapid; but in adapting from light to dark the adjustment is slow. As can be seen from the dark adaptation curve (*Figure 23.4*), there is not a steady increase in sensitivity; the curve is in two portions, the initial rapid adaptation being that of cones and the slower adaptation that of the rods. A further feature of rod and cone vision is their different spectral sensitivity. Rods are maximally sensitive to blue–green light at about 500 nm and cones to yellow–green light at about 560 nm (*Figure*

23.5). This differing sensitivity is called the Purkinje phenomenon. It is evident at dusk, when red objects appear relatively darker whilst blue objects retain their subjective luminance.

A result of this double mechanism for light appreciation is that, to detect dim lights, one must look off-centre. It used to be customary, also, to wear red goggles in lighted crewrooms and to use red cockpit lighting, since rods, unlike cones, are insensitive to the longer red wavelengths. The advantage of preserving rod adaptation is, however, to a large extent illusory as few flight tasks can be performed with rod vision. In most instances good

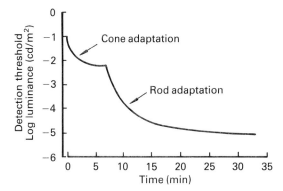

Figure 23.4 The dark adaptation curve of the eye showing the change of sensitivity to light with time in the dark.

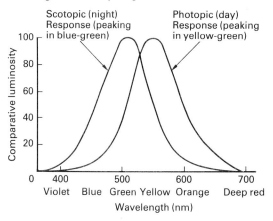

Figure 23.5 The special sensitivity of the eye at high and low levels of luminance. The maximum sensitivity of the cones is to yellow–green light while that of the cones rods is to blue light. The difference is the basis of the Purkinje phenomenon.

cone acuity is imperative and the disadvantages of red cockpit lighting systems in colour discrimination, the reduction in accommodative clues and the distortion in the relative luminance of coloured objects far outweigh any theoretical advantage.

A valuable feature of rod vision is its ability to detect movement as an image traverses the retina. It is useful, therefore, in search procedures at night not to allow the rod image to stabilize within the range of involuntary eye movements but to scan the area in small arcs, inducing on the retina a moving image of a stationary object.

Form sense

The ability to discriminate details is a measure of the resolving power of the eye, in particular of the fovea. Visual acuity may be expressed as the reciprocal, expressed in minutes of arc, of the angle subtended at the eye, by the point of detail registered. The conventional notation is to state normal vision as 6/6. This means that the test eye can see at 6 m that which the normal eye should be able to see at 6 m, which is one minute of arc: 6/5 means that the test subject sees at 6 m that which the normal eye would only see when 5 m from the chart or 30 seconds of arc. Conversely, 6/12 means that the subject can see at 6 m only that which the normal eye could recognize at 12 m. The US notation is similar but is expressed in feet, 20/20 being the equivalent of 6/6 (*see Figure 23.2*).

Under good conditions the eye can resolve detail that subtends a visual angle of 30 seconds of arc. As the diameter of a cone is between 1 and 2 μm two points of detail fall on to separate cones with an unstimulated cone lying between. If the points fell on to adjacent cones they would be registered as one large point and there would be no discrimination. The resolving power of the eye is not, however, entirely limited by the size of a retinal cone: under some special circumstances much finer resolution appears possible. A single line may be differentiated against a plain background when it subtends a visual angle as small as 0.5 seconds of arc. This is more a measure of contrast than of resolution, but is important in aviation, as aircraft or wires may first be appreciated by their contrast against sky.

A number of factors may influence the resolution of the eye: atmospheric conditions; the optical quality and cleanliness of interposed transparencies; refractive errors; and pathological change. The large pupillary diameters that occur in darkness reduce the depth of field of the eye, rendering more evident the visual decrement caused by refractive errors; myopes, in particular, may find they need corrected flying spectacles at night though their vision is adequate by day.

Recognition of targets is profoundly influenced, also, by the inductive state of the retina. One part of the retina modifies the function of another part, and this is known as spatial induction. A stimulus on a portion of retina will also affect function of that portion to a subsequent stimulus, and this is known as temporal induction. In aviation, spatial induction or simultaneous contrast will enhance the recognition of aircraft against the sky. The bright sky diminishes retinal sensitivity and a grey aircraft therefore appears darker, with a consequent increase of the contrast between the target and the sky. Temporal induction or successive contrast, on the other hand, may reduce target recognition. If a bright object such as the sun forms an image on a portion of the retina, the sensitivity of that portion will be depressed for a considerable period of time. This may cause low-contrast targets to remain unseen.

Visual acuity is largely by contrast between target and background and also by the prevailing luminance of the target. Acuity improves with increasing

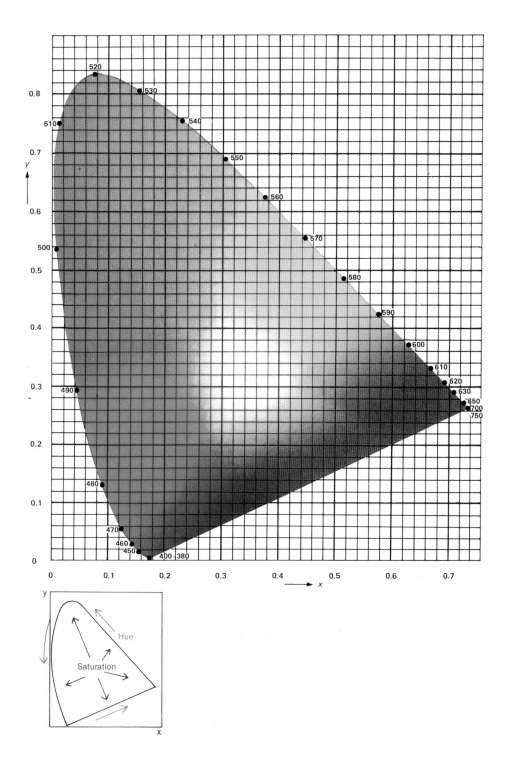

Plate 1 CIE 1931 (x,y)-chromaticity diagram. (Reproduced from *Precise Color Communication* by permission of Minolta (UK) Limited.)

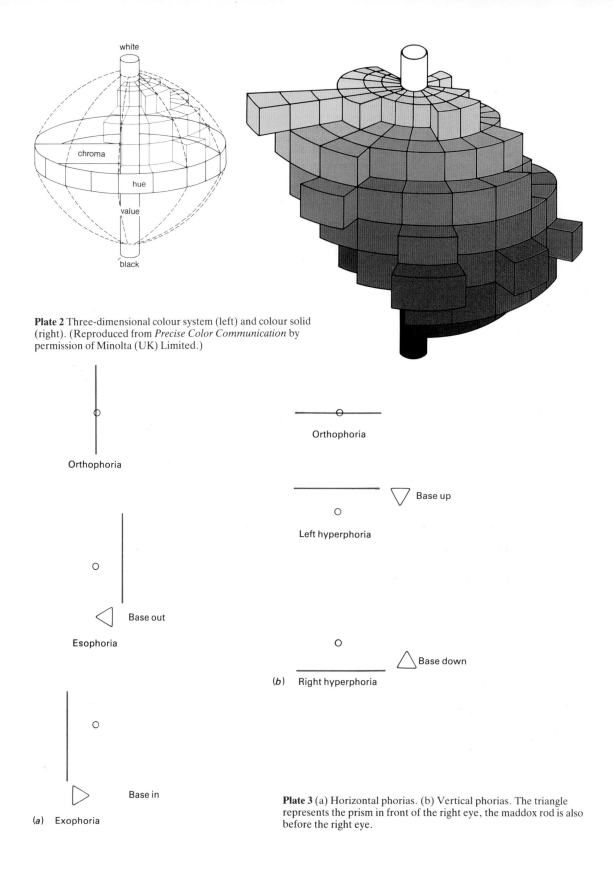

Plate 2 Three-dimensional colour system (left) and colour solid (right). (Reproduced from *Precise Color Communication* by permission of Minolta (UK) Limited.)

Orthophoria

Orthophoria

Esophoria

Base out

Base in

(a) Exophoria

Left hyperphoria

Base up

Right hyperphoria

Base down

(b) Right hyperphoria

Plate 3 (a) Horizontal phorias. (b) Vertical phorias. The triangle represents the prism in front of the right eye, the maddox rod is also before the right eye.

luminance up to a level of about 10^3 cd/m^2, beyond which no further increase occurs.

The best resolution is achieved when the luminance of the target and the ambient lighting are similar. If an airman is placed in a dark cockpit with only a small window on the world, the resolution of bright external targets will suffer. When the cockpit illumination is increased, resolution improves. The converse of a bright cockpit and a dim target also impairs resolution.

Colour sense

Colour sense is a function of the cones and therefore of photopic (day) vision. According to the Young–Helmholtz theory of colour vision, there are three classes of cone present maximally at the macula, in the ratio of 1:10:10. These cones have absorption peaks at about 420 nm (blue), 534 nm (green) and 564 nm (red) (Bowmaker, 1981). A combination of these three primary colours in the correct proportions is seen as white light, and by varying the proportions and saturation any other colour can be matched. According to the work of Walraven (1966), information from the three types of cone is analysed into three channels: a brightness channel, which is the summation of brightness information from each cone; and two chromatic channels, a red–green and a yellow (red + green)–blue channel.

Colour defectives are generally subdivided into three main groups.

1. *Monochromats*—Complete absence of colour sensation:
   (a) Rod monochromats do not possess functional cones, the deficiency occurs with a prevalence of 1 in 30 000 of the population.
   (b) Cone monochromats are exceptionally rare, occurring with a prevalence as low as 1 in 100 000 000. The condition is associated with good visual acuity. The deficiency is probably central rather than within the photoreceptors.
2. *Dichromats*—These require only two primaries to match all colours:
   (a) Protanopes: 1 in 100. These lack red cones. They suffer a loss of brightness as well as absence of red sensation. This gives rise to red/green confusion.
   (b) Deuteranopes: prevalence 1 in 100. Do not possess separate red and green cones but a single cone, presumably containing red and green pigments. There is no loss of brightness, but red/green confusion.
   (c) Tritanopes: prevalence 1 in 65 000. Very rare, lack blue cones. The normal individual is tritanopic if the field of vision is small enough as the fovea centralis does not contain blue cones. This foveal tritanopia precludes the use of blue

as a signal colour where the signal may be seen as a point source.
3. *Anomalous trichromats*:
   (a) Protanomalous: prevalence 1 in 100. Require more red stimulation for a match than normal.
   (b) Deuteranomalous: prevalence 1 in 20. Require more green stimulation for a match than normal.
   (c) Tritanomalous: rare, but prevalence suggested to be 1 in 4000. Require more blue stimulation for a match than normal.

As can be seen from the relative prevalence values, we are usually concerned with red/green defectives.

The signal colours of red and green in both lights and flares could be made more obvious to the protanope and deuteranope if the red were more orange and the green were more blue. To make confusion even less likely, further cues could be added, such as a bar across a green light, but not on a red; or, in flares, by using a two-star red and a one-star green. The lattice lines in Decca, Loran or Consol charts could have an added shape coding.

If, however, the red signal colour were made more orange, it would be necessary to abandon yellow light signals as these could be confused with the new red standard. It would also be necessary to ensure that white light is of a high colour temperature, as discrimination between a dim white light and the new red signal colour could be difficult.

If the green signal colour were made more blue it would be necessary to increase the power of the illuminating source. This would be necessary as the new filter would have a greater absorption factor, and in order to maintain visibility at its present level power consumption would have to be increased two or three times.

Yellow is not a vital signal colour in aviation, and the power of illuminating sources can be increased, but it is unlikely that the gain in recruits would justify the international effort and cost.

Visual perception is dependent on a great variety of different visual cues supplemented cortically by experience and intelligence. Much of the visual information may be duplicated by different cues, and it is this abundance of information that gives an individual confidence in what one sees.

Any colour, using the Munsell system, may be defined by specifying the levels of three variables. The first of these is the hue or dominant wavelength and this determines whether we call a colour blue, green, yellow or red, etc. The second is the chroma which can make hues either vibrant or weak and this depends on the saturation or admixture of white light to the hue. A red hue may be a spectral and saturated vivid colour; add white light and it becomes a desaturated pink. The final variable is the value or how light or dark a hue appears and this is related to a grey scale in equal steps from white to black. The blue of the sky appears lighter than the blue of the sea and the green of a lawn appears lighter than the green of a forest even though their hues and chroma may be similar. If we numerically label each of these three variables we can define precisely a colour as in the CIE L* a* b* system in which L* represents value and a* and b* represent hue and chroma respectively (*Plate 2*), or by a combination of letters and numbers as in the Munsell system. Another system is the CIE chromaticity diagram on which we define hue and chroma in terms of their x and y coordinates and express lightness in terms of Y (*Plate 1*). The variable Y denotes the brightness of a colour in terms of the ratio of the primary colour Y, which is a green colour with a wavelength of 555 nm, in the specimen when compared with a pure specimen of Y.

Current vision testing, in many nations, only requires potential aircrew correctly to interpret the pseudo-isochromatic plates such as those by Ishihara. Should they fail this test, they must correctly identify red, green and white when presented in a lantern test such as the Holmes–Wright or Farnsworth. These tests generally do not monitor blue defects and present red and green colours in a moderately saturated form. Aircrew are now being presented with cathode ray tube (CRT) displays which use unsaturated colours and also present various hues of blue some of which are also desaturated. It follows that the testing of colour vision is in need of review so that red, green and blue discrimination and the chroma required for hue recognition are monitored. Such testing would be valuable not only for the interpretation of CRT displays but also for general colour requirements when many colours, such as traffic lights, may be desaturated by atmospheric conditions. It may be that a CRT generated test will be developed, but

until this or another task-related test is available, the Farnsworth Munsell 100 hue test may prove valuable.

The Farnsworth Munsell 100 hue test is composed of caps of various hues which together form a colour circle spanning the visible spectrum. The subject is presented with four boxes containing the caps with a fixed coloured cap at each end. The subject is required to sort the caps into their natural hue orders. Any errors can be recorded both in terms of their frequency and magnitude and can be related to wavelength.

Visual function in flight

There are several visual problems that are peculiar to aviation.

Empty field myopia

During flight, particularly at night or in cloud, the external scene is often featureless. Without visual cues to attract attention the eye frequently exercises a degree of accommodation of between 0.5 and 2.0 D. This brings the focus of the eye to a point in space perhaps 1–2 m away, making the pilot functionally short sighted. Should another aircraft enter his visual field it may well not be seen, as objects at infinity are blurred. It is important, therefore, that aircrew be instructed to look periodically at objects, such as wing tips, at virtual infinity in order to relax their accommodation.

High-speed flight

Large distances may be travelled during the time taken to perceive and react to objects appearing in the visual field. This problem may become critical in the high-speed, low-level role, especially when vibration may increase pilot stress. *Table 23.1* lists

Table 23.1 Distance travelled by an aircraft whilst the pilot is perceiving and reacting to an object approaching in his visual field

Stage in avoidance of an object		Distance travelled in nautical miles by an aircraft flying at:		
		500 kt	1000 kt	1500 kt
(1)	Time taken from image first falling on peripheral retina to focused central fixation and recognition = 1.0 s	0.14	0.28	0.42
(2)	Time taken for decision and subsequent action = 2.5 s	0.35	0.70	1.04
(3)	Time taken for aircraft to change course = 1.5 s	0.21	0.42	0.62
	Total time elapsed = 5.0 s	0.70	1.40	2.08

The above distances must be doubled when two aircraft travelling at the same speed are on a head-on collision course.

the estimated times required for the various steps from an image falling on the peripheral retina to perception, reaction and the start of aircraft manoeuvre. These periods may not be reduced, and indeed they may be extended under adverse conditions. When a pilot transfers his attention from scanning the external field to reading an instrument and returns to the external field, there is a time interval of up to 2.5 seconds, during which time the aircraft covers considerable distance. It is therefore important to present vital information in a collimated form, either by head-up or helmet-mounted displays, in order that all attention need not be removed from the external scene. Less important instruments should be so designed, sited and lighted that the information they give may be rapidly extracted.

Dynamic visual acuity

In the previous section, where the form sense was discussed, it was assumed that the object of interest was stationary. Where a target moves across the visual field the eye must track it to maintain foveal fixation. The ocular pursuit mechanism is capable of maintaining steady fixation where the angular velocity does not exceed a value much greater than about 30 degrees/s. At an angular velocity of about 40 degrees/s, visual acuity may drop to half its static value, the decrement increasing further as the angular velocity increases.

Depth perception

The binocular cues of accommodation and convergence have a limited value in depth perception at the visual ranges important in aviation. This limitation is due largely to the short inter-pupillary distance of about 6 cm. The binocular cue of stereopsis is, however, considered to be the single most important depth cue available to aircrew. Stereopsis is the third stage of binocular vision, the first and second being simultaneous perception and fusion. The interpupillary separation between the two eyes produces disparate images at both maculae. These differing retinal images can be fused to produce a three-dimensional effect. In depth perception if two points are at different distances from the observer, each point, as seen by both eyes, will subtend different binocular angles (binocular parallax). The angles are dependent on the distance of each point from the observer and his interpupillary separation (*Figure 23.6*). The difference between these values of binocular parallax is the measure of the binocular disparity. The generally accepted minimum values

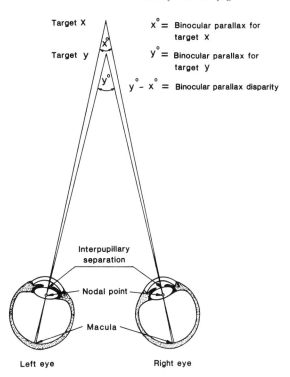

Figure 23.6 Stereoacuity. Derivation of values for binocular parallax disparity.

of binocular parallax disparity which can be detected are 2–24 seconds of arc. For example, let targets X and Y be 500 and 550 m distant from the observer respectively and let the observer's inter-pupillary separation be 65 mm (0.065 m). The binocular parallax disparity in this example is approximately 2.5 seconds of arc, and the targets may thus be discriminated in depth.

Monocular cues

1. *Parallax*—Head movements cause targets which are at different distances from the observer to move in opposite directions relative to each other. The nearer target moves in reverse direction to the head movement.
2. *Perspective*—Converging parallels such as runways and railway lines show the recedance of these terrain features.
3. *Relative size*—Objects the size of which is known are able, by virtue of the visual angle they subtend, to provide information as to their distance from the observer.
4. *Overlapping contours*—Objects that overlap others must be closer.

5. *Aerial perspective*—Objects at greater distances appear bluer, owing to the scattering of light. White aircraft lights may appear more red when seen at distance because the red component is less subject to scatter than the blue component; this is a further reason to exclude blue signals in aviation.

Visual illusions

The most important illusions—Coriolis, oculogravic and oculogyral—are discussed in Chapter 21.

An illusion that is solely ocular is autokinesis. A light, such as a star or aircraft tail-light, seen against a black background will, after a short time elapse, appear to wander in different directions. These apparent movements occur because the background does not provide sufficient information about the involuntary eye movements that are occurring. These eye movements are then interpreted as movements of the light. Autokinesis is one reason for the abandonment of ultraviolet instrument lighting. The glowing phosphors on the numerals and pointers when seen against a black cockpit provided the conditions necessary for the illusion. In modern aircraft, some degree of general lighting is usually provided to give a visual reference.

Flicker, produced by helicopter rotors or strobe-lighting systems, has been found to cause epilepti-form episodes. The problem arises when the frequency is between 5 and 20 Hz being maximal at about 12 Hz. Modern strobe-lighting systems, which are favoured for their conspicuity, have a flash frequency of around 100 flashes per minute and should be harmless.

Protective devices in military aviation

Solar glare

Glare, from direct, reflected or scattered sunlight causes discomfort and reduction in visual acuity. Spectacles suffice in transport aircraft, but in high-performance aircraft where the crews wear protective helmets, an adjustable tinted visor, integral with the helmet, can provide simultaneous protection against external glare and an undiminished view of the flight instruments. In the fully lowered position the visor should be capable of cutting out all unfiltered light.

Sunglasses and visors should have a luminous transmittance of the order 10–15%. In temperate climates this aims to reduce the level of bright ambient light reaching the cornea to approximately 3000 cd/m², the region in which form acuity and contrast discrimination are maximal. A fixed density that is attenuating variable light levels must always

be a compromise but variable density filters have problems of their own particularly related to their photodynamics and fabrication into visors.

Sun filters have a protective role as well as that of improving visual acuity and increasing comfort. They should attenuate harmful radiation in the CIE photobiologic band ultraviolet B [UV(B)] 280–315 nm and UV(A) 315–400 nm. UV(B) radiation can cause photochemical changes resulting in an acute kerato-conjunctivitis or a delayed catarac-togenesis from longer wavelength UV(B) 295–315 nm; over-exposure to UV(A) radiation may also result in the formation of cataracts. Both UV(B) and UV(A) should be attenuated to a maximum transmittance of 1%. The short-wavelength visible light (400–500 nm), owing to the more energetic nature of blue photons and the absorption spectrum of melanin, is also hazardous to retinal cones and the retinal pigment epithelium. Prolonged exposure to the blue component of bright white light can result in accelerated retinal ageing and the development of macular dystrophies; a common cause of blindness in the elderly. It is important, therefore, that the spectral transmittance in the band 400–500 nm does not exceed that for the remainder of the visible band and, preferably, should be slightly lower and free of any spikes in transmittance. Gross attenuation of the band cannot be permitted because of resulting errors in blue–green hue discrimination. The attenuation in the remainder of the visible band 500–760 nm should be as spectrally neutral as possible to enhance colour discrimination. Although desirable, attenuation in the infra-red (A) 760–1400 nm is difficult to achieve with plastic filters and is not as important as short-wavelength attenuation.

The densities of the filter(s) before each eye should be matched to avoid false spatial projection (Pulfrich effect). This effect results from the differing reaction times between eyes when they view the same target through filters of varying density or colour. These different reaction times may cause a target, which is moving at 90 degrees to the direction of gaze, to appear in different positions to each eye. When fused the target may assume a false position in space.

The field of view of sunglasses and visors, as worn, must be as wide as possible. The physical and optical properties should be within ISO standards and it may be advisable to consider the application of a quarter wavelength anti-reflection coatings, anti-abrasion coatings, or both.

Protection of the face against birdstrike

The hazard of birdstrike is always present during flight (both day and night) at low level. Approximately 85% of incidents in the UK occur at

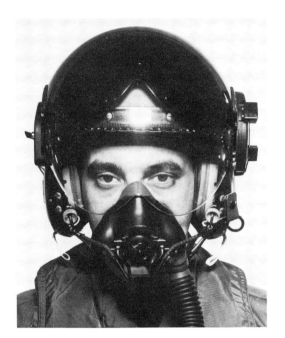

Figure 23.7 A double visor assembly fitted to an aircrew protective helmet. The inner visor is of clear polycarbonate and the outer visor is of tinted polycarbonate.

altitudes below 500 feet agl, whilst only 7% occur at altitudes above 1000 feet agl. The incidence of birdstrikes in low-level high-speed flight is such that a hit in the cockpit area is a not uncommon emergency. Ideally, cockpit transparencies should be strong enough to withstand bird impact, but the cost in weight may be prohibitive. If practical, secondary protection to the aircrew should be provided by a tough screen mounted within the cockpit; but this requirement may be incompatible with adequate external vision or a clear ejection path. In the absence of other forms of protection, a helmet-mounted visor made of a strong transparent material, such as polycarbonate (3 mm thick), is essential. The visor should protect all the uncovered area of the face as well as the eyes. Thus the lower edge of the polycarbonate visor should abut closely (less than 5 mm gap) against the oronasal mask. As there is virtually no hazard of birdstrike over 2000 feet agl. the aircrew should be able to remove the polycarbonate visor since any layer in front of the eyes can produce a small but significant impairment of vision. Whilst it is desirable that the user should be able to lock the polycarbonate visor in the down position for blast protection, there is no requirement to be able to place it in any position other than fully up or fully down. Although it would simplify and lighten the headgear if the strong polycarbonate visor could also act as the anti-glare visor there are many flight conditions in which

birdstrike protection is required without the anti-glare function; for example, low-level flight at dusk and night. A dual visor system is considered essential (*Figure 23.7*).

Blast protection

During a high-speed ejection, the head is exposed to very high aerodynamic forces. These aerodynamic forces impart angular accelerations to the head and thrust it hard against the seat. In addition, the wind blast may damage the tissues of the face, in particular the eyes, by causing gross displacement and rupture of tissues. The headgear may well be lost altogether. It is important to guard against all these hazards by ensuring that the helmet, visor and mask are so integrated that they remain in place throughout the ejection. Current systems provide adequate protection against blast up to 600–650 knots Indicated Air Speed.

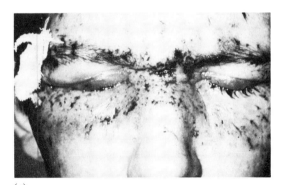

(*a*)

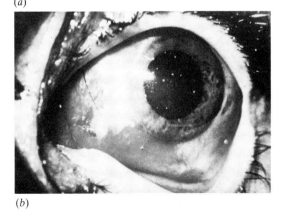

(*b*)

Figure 23.8 Damage to the eyes and face caused by lead spatter from a miniature detonating cord. (*a*) shows superficial damage to the skin of the face and eyelids. (*b*) Retraction of the eyelids. Note the presence of lead particles on and within the cornea and conjunctiva (white spots). A slit-lamp examination also revealed the presence of lead within the crystalline lens.

Canopy fragmenting devices

Where there is no reasonable certainty that the canopy can be clear of the aircraft before the seat moves, explosive devices are fitted to shatter the transparencies and permit the seat and occupant to pass safely through. There have been a number of occasions on which lead-spatter from the explosive charges has caused superficial damage to the face and eyes (*Figure 23.8*). The most severe damage has been ocular penetration through cornea and lens to the vitreous. In one incident the lens became opaque and the cataract required surgical removal.

It is unlikely that any significant ocular damage will result if the visor is lowered or the eyes closed or preferably both. Various guards—some metal, some in foam plastic—have been developed to prevent lead-spatter tracking down the inner surface of the visor. There is the risk that they may increase misting.

Lasers

Lasers are devices that produce beams of monochromatic light, usually of small diameter,

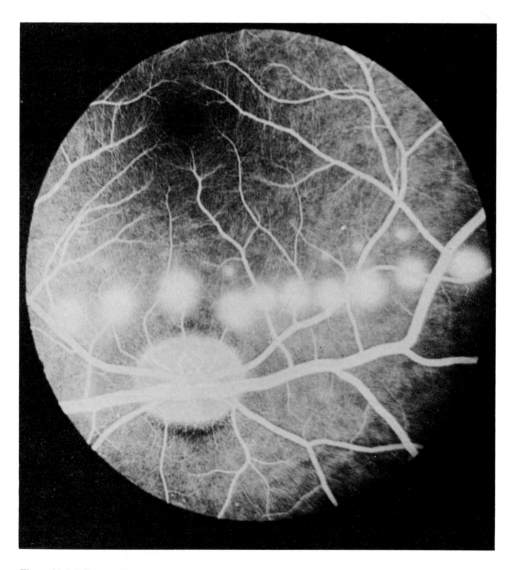

Figure 23.9 A fluorescein angiogram of the retina of a rhesus monkey showing lesions produced by a 'Q' switched neodymium laser operating at various energy levels.

intense and highly collimated. The energy density within the beam only decreases slowly with increasing distance from the laser. The eye has the ability to focus the collimated beams of some lasers and to concentrate the energy into small image sizes on the retina (*Figure 23.9*). Thus lasers can damage eyes at a considerable distance from the source.

Neodymium, gallium arsenide and ruby lasers which emit at 1060 nm, 900 nm and 694.3 nm respectively are the most important lasers encountered in military aviation. The applications of these lasers include ranging and target illumination.

Protection is best provided by distance. Codes of practice, such as the current issues of ANSI Z136 and BSI 4803, give guidance on the method of calculating the Nominal Ocular Hazard Distance (NOHD), the distance within which the laser may be hazardous. The calculation is based on knowledge of the maximum safe corneal energy or power density for the particular laser system together with the beam divergence and maximum output of that system. It must, however, be realized that the calculated NOHD does not make allowance for atmospheric conditions that may give rise to 'hot spots', nor for intra-beam viewing through optical instruments with a magnifying effect. The necessity for protection of a pilot from his own laser is debatable. The likelihood of a specular reflector in the range area orientated normal to the beam must be very small, the probability being less than 10^{-6}. Should such a reflector be present, its reflectivity at the laser wavelength is not likely to be high.

Where it is considered necessary, protection may be provided by goggles or visors with the requisite optical density at the laser wavelength. Care must be taken to ensure that the luminous transmittance, effect of the tint on colour recognition and optical properties of any protective device are adequate for the task.

Nuclear flash

The fireball resulting from a nuclear explosion is capable of producing direct and indirect flash blindness and indeed may cause a retinal burn. By day, the small pupillary diameter and the optical blink reflex should prevent retinal burns at distances at which survival is possible. Similarly, indirect flash blindness from scattered light within the atmosphere and the globe itself does not pose a problem. Direct flash blindness from the image of the fireball is difficult to avoid, but again at survival distances the irradiated area is likely to be small. Even in the worst case, the fireball imaged on the macula, para-macula vision should allow all vital flight procedure to continue. At night, when the pupil is

dilated, the situation is much worse. Retinal burns are possible and, more important, indirect flash blindness may deprive the pilot of all useful vision for periods exceeding 1 minute. In short, protection against nuclear flash is desirable by day but vital at night.

A number of protective measures have been proposed. If an exterior view is not required, or only required infrequently, all transparencies may be covered with opaque blinds. Another suggestion has been an eye patch which may be removed when one eye has been affected, but this is essentially only a two-shot device entailing all the disadvantages associated with uniocular vision, e.g. absence of stereopsis and a reduced field of view. What is required is a visor which could be worn at all times when nuclear flash is a possibility. This visor should have a very high luminous transmittance when 'open' and a very low transmittance when activated by a nuclear flash, clearing rapidly when the flash is removed. The visor should, preferably, be made of polycarbonate or other high-impact resistance material so that it may replace the one intended for birdstrike protection in the dual visor system. Another approach is to use an electro-optic shutter consisting of a ceramic wafer of lead lanthanum zirconate titanate (PLZT) sandwiched between two polarizers with their axes of polarization set at 90 degrees with respect to each other. When electrically activated the PLZT wafer rotates the plane of polarization of light transmitted by the first polarizer. When a photo-diode is triggered by a nuclear flash the voltage to the PLZT wafer ceases and the rotation of the plane of polarization is reversed so that light is not transmitted by the second polarizer. This switching is effected in microseconds and produces high optical densities and thus attenuation of the flash. Although these characteristics appear ideal the PLZT device has disadvantages, it is complex and thus expensive and the open state luminous transmittance is low, about 20–22%.

Reference

BOWMAKER, J.K. (1981) Visual pigments and colour vision in man and monkeys. *Journal of The Royal Society of Medicine*, **74**, 348

Further reading

ABRAMS, J.D. (1978) *Duke-Elder's Practice of Refraction*, 9th edn. Edinburgh: Churchill-Livingstone

BRENNAN, D.H. (1987) Non ionising radiation. In *Hunter's Diseases of Occupations*, edited by W.R. Lee, Chapter 15. London: Hodder and Stoughton

DAVSON, H. (1980) *The Physiology of the Eye*. Edinburgh: Churchill-Livingstone

LERMAN, S. (1980) *Radiant Energy and the Eye, 1, Functional Ophthalmology Series*. New York: Macmillan

SLINEY, D. and WOLBARSHT, M. (1980) *Safety with Lasers and Other Optical Sources*. New York: Plenum Press

WALRAVEN, P.L. (1966) The fluctuation theory of colour discrimination. In *Studies in Perception*. Soesterberg, Netherlands: The Institute for Perception RVO/TNO, National Defence Research Organisation

24

Noise and communication

G.M. Rood

Introduction

Noise may be defined as a sound which is unpleasant, distracting, unwarranted or in some other way undesirable. The definition is entirely subjective, and this subjectivity, this reliance on man as a measuring instrument recurs throughout most of the attempts to assess and quantify auditory effects.

The human hearing mechanism has a wide range and is fairly tolerant; but this tolerance is exceeded in many aircraft, with the following potential effects:

1. Communications, both speech and other auditory signals inside the aircraft, air-to-air and air-to-ground, may be degraded.
2. The sense of hearing may be damaged, temporarily or permanently.
3. Noise, acting as a stress, may interfere with the flying task.
4. Noise may induce varying levels of fatigue.

This chapter deals primarily with the problem of noise within the aircraft; the almost as important but different problems of the effects on the environment are dealt with only briefly.

Physical characteristics of sound

Production of sound

Sound is, physically speaking, any undulatory motion in an elastic medium (gaseous, liquid, or solid) which is capable of producing the sensation of hearing. Normally the medium is air. A simple sound may be produced by a piston vibrating in a tube (*Figure 24.1*). The movement of the piston produces variations of the pressure of the air in the tube, so that the molecules of air at any given point are alternately compressed and rarefied. A simple sound in which the pressure fluctuations follow a sinusoid is known as a pure tone. The velocity with which the waves of compression and rarefaction pass along the tube is the velocity of sound. The frequency of the sound is the number of times with which each complete cycle repeats itself in unit time, whilst the wavelength is the distance between two corresponding points in successive cycles (*Figure 24.1*). These quantities are related by the expression:

$$\text{Wavelength} = \frac{\text{Velocity of sound in the medium}}{\text{Frequency}}$$

Sound pressure

In a pure tone the sound pressure fluctuates so that, for half the time of a complete cycle, it is above, and for the remainder of the time it is below the prevailing atmospheric pressure. This average ure can be specified in terms of the amplitude, which is the peak value of each half cycle. Sound pressure is normally specified, however, as the average pressure throughout the cycle, notwithstanding the fact that the pressure is fluctuating about the prevailing atmospheric pressure. This average pressure is obtained from the squares of the values of the sound pressure at a large number of instants throughout one or more cycles (this eliminates the negative values). From this one calculates the mean square, and finally the root mean square (RMS) or 'effective' value. For pure tones the RMS value is 0.707 of the amplitude of the wave. The standard

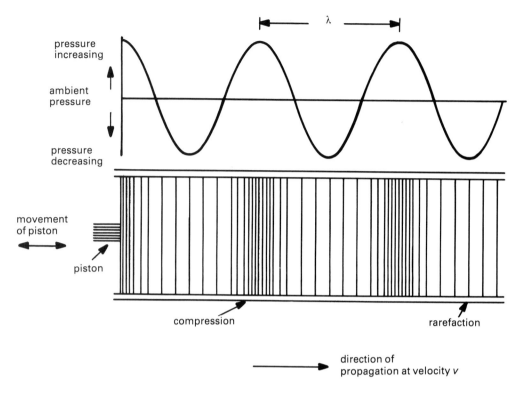

Figure 24.1 Production of a simple sound by oscillation of a piston in a tube. The sinusoidal movement of the piston at the left-hand end of the tube produces regular compression and rarefaction of the gas immediately adjacent to it. These pressure fluctuations are transmitted through the gas in the tube. The distance between two consecutive peaks or troughs of pressure is the wavelength (λ) of the tone.

unit of pressure which is used in measuring sound is the Pascal (Pa).

The threshold of human hearing at a frequency of one kilohertz (1 kHz) is a sound pressure of about $20\,\mu\text{Pa}$ ($2 \times 10^{-5}\,\text{N/m}^2$ or $2 \times 10^{-4}\,\mu\text{bar}$). This is a pressure of only 2×10^{-10} atmosphere. At the other end of the scale, a sound pressure of 200 Pa may be accommodated by the ear before the onset of pain. The ear is thus capable of responding over a very wide dynamic range from 2×10^{-5} to $2 \times 10^2\,\text{Pa}$ (140 dB).

Sound pressure level

Since sound essentially comprises a series of pressure fluctuations, then it follows that measurement of sound pressure level involves measurement of an absolute pressure. The unit of sound pressure level, however, is the decibel, which is a dimensionless unit.

The dB is often uniquely associated with noise measurement, but it was borrowed originally from electrical communications engineering and represents a relative quantity. When used to measure noise, for example 94 dB, it means 94 dB above a reference quantity. This reference level is $20\,\mu\text{Pa}$ and is referred to as 0 dB (zero dB), which is, in fact, about the weakest sound that can be heard by a person with good hearing in a very quiet location. The relationship between SPL and dB is:

$$\text{Sound pressure level in dB} = 20\,\log\left(\frac{p}{p_0}\right)$$

where p = measured pressure
p_0 = reference pressure ($20\,\mu\text{Pa}$)

It is now possible to see that a doubling of pressure from the reference pressure of $20\,\mu\text{Pa}$ (that is to say $40\,\mu\text{Pa}$) may be described in dB:

$$\text{SPL (in dB)} = 20\,\log\frac{40}{20} = 20\,\log 2$$
$$= 20 \times 0.3010 = 6\,\text{dB}$$

Thus each increment of 6 dB represents a doubling of sound pressure. Similarly a tenfold increase in pressure to $200\,\mu\text{Pa}$ can be defined as:

$$dB = 20 \log \frac{200}{20} = 20 \log 10 = 20 \ dB$$

Hence it can be seen that as the decibel levels increase linearly, the actual sound pressure levels increase logarithmically (6 dB = twice; 12 dB = four times; 18 dB = eight times, etc.).

The reason why this seemingly complicated logarithmic method is used is because noise is nearly always exclusively related to human hearing or human response and the human ear is a detector of un-paralleled quality in relation to dynamic range. From the quietest sound which can be heard (the threshold of hearing), to the loudest sound which can be tolerated before the onset of pain (pain threshold), the range is more than one to ten million. The direct applications of linear scales to the measurement of sound pressure would therefore lead to the use of very high and unwieldly numbers.

Conveniently, the response of the ear to sound stimuli is also logarithmic, not linear. That is to say the ear is at its most sensitive at low sound levels and responds progressively less sensitively as the sound level increases. It has therefore been found most practical to express acoustic parameters as a logarithmic ratio of the measured value to the standard value.

Use of the decibel scale thus reduces a dynamic range of sound pressure levels of 1: 10 000 000 to a more manageable range of 0 to 140 dB (dB = $20 \log 10^7 = 140 \ dB$). It is also useful because 1 dB is about the smallest value of significance, in that under normal circumstances a change of 1 dB may just be detectable by the human ear.

It is worth noting that zero dB does not mean an absence of noise, it merely implies that the level in question is equal to the reference level. Thus if the measured sound pressure level is 10 μPa, then the level in dB would be 20 log 10/20 = 20 log 0.5 = 20 × −0.3010 = −6 dB. Hence it can be clearly seen that negative dBs are possible—it may not be possible to hear them but it is possible to measure them with sensitive measuring devices.

A further point worthy of note, but not of prolonged explanation, is that if two sound sources having the same sound pressure level, say 70 dB, are measured together, then the overall sound pressure level will not be 140 dB, but 73 dB. Doubling the number of sources raises the sound pressure level by 3 dB, a further doubling (to four equal sound sources) raises the sound pressure level by 6 dB to 76 dB, and so on. Conversely, of course, any measure which reduces the measured dB value by 3 dB signifies a reduction of no less than half in sound energy.

Similarly, if there are two sources at say, 80 dB and 86 dB, then the overall level is only 1 dB up on the higher source, in this case 87 dB overall. It follows that if one source is 10 dB quieter than

Table 24.1 Sound pressures and sound pressure levels of various sound environments

Sound pressure (Pa)	Sound pressure level (dB)	Environment
200	140	Turbojet at 50 feet
20	120	Jet take-off 500 feet
		Inside low-level fighter
		Large jet landing
		Inside helicopter
2	100	
2×10^{-1}	80	
		Street corner traffic
		Normal speech at 3 feet
2×10^{-2}	60	
		Office
		Living-room
2×10^{-3}	40	
		Library
2×10^{-4}	20	
		Broadcasting studio
2×10^{-5}	0	Threshold of hearing at 1 kHz

another source, it does not significantly contribute to the summed overall sound pressure level.

The absolute sound pressures and equivalent sound pressure levels for a number of noise environments are presented in *Table 24.1*.

Complex sounds and frequency analysis

A finite signal, no matter how complex, may be considered to be made up of a number of simple sine waves (Fourier series). The sine wave components of a signal constitute the frequency spectrum. The frequency spectrum of a sine wave (*Figure 24.2*) clearly consists of only one line; that of more complicated but periodic waves consists of harmonically related discrete lines, and that of statistically distributed signals—such as random noise—shows a continuous spectrum. There is a subjective significance here. It is that if two pure tones are played together, they are heard as a chord rather than as a single sound (that is, the ear appears to be performing some sort of Fourier analysis on the signal). The analogous effect does not prevail in the visual system—a red light mixed with a green light produces a perception of yellow light indistinguishable from that produced by a pure yellow light source.

The noises in real life that are usually measured, however, are rarely simple acoustic waves of single frequency (pure tones), but are usually a jumble of sounds which vary from a low-frequency rumble to a high-frequency screech. Human reaction to such sounds depends not only on the overall level, but also on the composition of the noise in terms of frequency. To measure this composition, frequency analysis is carried out which provides a curve showing how the sound energy is distributed over a range of frequencies (*Figure 24.2(c)*). The noise is electronically separated into its frequency bands such as octave bands, each of which covers a 2 to 1

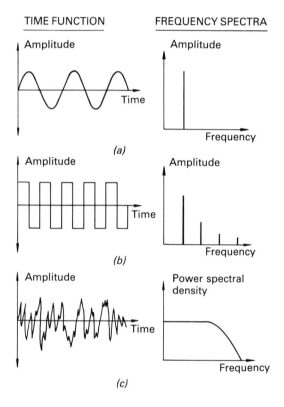

TIME FUNCTION   FREQUENCY SPECTRA

Figure 24.2 The frequency spectra of (*a*) a pure tone, (*b*) a complex periodic and (*c*) a complex non-periodic signal.

range of frequencies. Such analysis yields a level for each band, called appropriately band level. For octave band analysis these are called octave-band levels.

If a more detailed analysis is required, narrower bands are used. By splitting an octave band into three parts, one-third octave bands are produced, and these represent to a much greater degree the way in which man hears; in one-third octave bands the bandwidth is about 23% of the centre frequency.

For some purposes, however, still narrower bands are necessary (for noise control purposes for example) and it is possible to use analysers with

one-tenth octave bands (about 7% in width); analysers with 1% bandwidths are also available.

Finally a point is reached where the bandwidth is no longer a percentage of the band centre frequency, but is actually 1 Hz wide. This is called the spectrum level.

Propagation of noise

Sound generated from a noise source does not remain at constant sound pressure level as the distance from the source increases. The further the distance from the source the lower the level. The energy in the sound wave is proportional to the area that the wavefront occupies, and thus as the distance increases the sound pressure levels decrease.

There are essentially two types of noise source:

1. A point source, where the source is small compared with the measuring distance from that source. An analogy could be a loudspeaker in a field.
2. A line source, which is a source, or series of sources, spread in a line which is longer than the measuring distance from it. For example, a train with a number of carriages emits noise that may be regarded as a line source. However, as the distance from the line source increases, it can be seen that the line source begins to approach a point source.

These two definitions are important as the propagation of noise from a point source occurs with a spherical wavefront and the sound pressure levels decrease by 6 dB each time the distance from the source is doubled, whilst a line source has an attenuation of 3 dB per doubling of distance. As the distance increases, finally to a point where the line source may be regarded as a point source, then the attenuation of sound changes gradually from 3 dB to 6 dB at these points.

A reasonable analogy for visualizing point and line sources is the dropping of a stone or series of stones in a pond. A single stone will result in spherical propagation, whilst a series of stones, dropped in line, will result in line propagation—the result of a series of spherical propagations.

To this natural attenuation must be added the additional attenuations, or amplifications, due to atmospheric influences or contact with solid objects.

Atmospheric influences include air absorption (including fog and rain), the effects of temperature gradients, of wind, and changes in the product of air density and speed of sound. In addition to these small changes in attenuation must be added the effects of ground absorption, which differs for propagation over hard surfaces (e.g. concrete) or soft surfaces (e.g. vegetation)—as on an airfield, due to obstructions such as walls, buildings, clumps of trees etc., and the fact that at a point the total sound pressure level may consist of a direct acoustic path plus a reflected path—which can be high or low depending upon the relative phases of the two sound waves.

Thus it is clear that the noise measurement of, say, a jet aircraft running up on an airfield, depends not only on the distance from the aircraft but also on the environmental conditions between the source and receiver and the prevailing meteorology conditions, and this may change from day to day, and even from hour to hour. Single, simple measurement is rarely enough to provide an adequate description of noise exposure under these conditions.

Mechanism of hearing

The outer ear

The outer ear has long been regarded as unimportant in hearing, but it plays a part in localizing sound sources. For mammals with limited visual acuity, such as man, it is, or was, essential to have a pinna presenting a wide mobile surface to enable both

detection and localization of any danger sounds. The pinna in man is essentially limited to the production of high-frequency reinforcement for directional effects in localization of sound. The process of monaural hearing allows detection whilst binaural hearing enables spatial location. Unlike a horse, which has ten vestigial mobilizing muscles for its pinna or auricle, man is limited to three and must compensate for this deficiency in aural mobility by making movements of the head and neck.

The beginning of the process of auditory transduction, however, can be said to start at the tympanic membrane, which vibrates in response to changes in air pressure in the auditory canal. The tympanic membrane has a certain resistance to movement or 'impedance'. The auditory canal, about 36 mm in length, performs significant 'matching' of this impedance to the air. This matching is somewhat frequency dependent, being poor at frequencies below about 400 Hz.

The middle ear

The air-containing middle ear is vented to atmosphere via the Eustachian tube so that atmospheric pressure variations do not cause maintained pressure differences across the tympanic membrane. The important function of the middle ear is that of

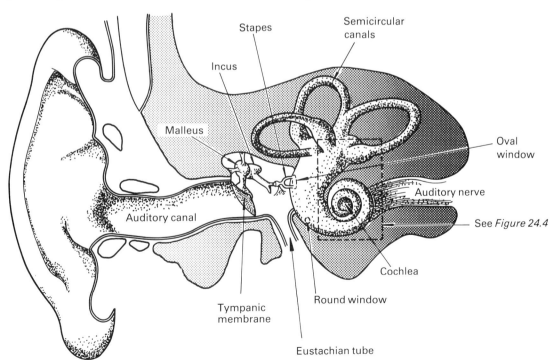

Figure 24.3 A diagram of the ear. An enlargement of the part of the cochlea outlined by the dotted rectangle is shown in *Figure 24.4*.

impedance matching. Because the inner ear is filled with fluid while the eardrum is a membrane driven by changes of gas pressure, there is a large impedance difference caused by the difference of acoustical impedance in the two media (i.e. fluid and air). The specific acoustic resistance of air is approximately 42 acoustic ohms whilst that of a small body of water is 9000 ohms. A loss of some 30 dB is apparent which must be regained. Two processes in the middle ear effect this process. One is a leverage effect, the other hydraulic.

The ossicles provide a leverage ratio of only 1:3:1, giving only 2.3 dB gain and it is left to the area ratio of the tympanic membrane to the stapes base to provide the major gain path (*Figure 24.3*). The malleus, connected to the tympanic membrane, experiences large excursions; but these are transformed to much smaller amplitude at the stapes, which is connected to the relatively much smaller area (compared with the tympanic membrane) of the oval window, generating much higher pressures suitable for driving the fluid-filled inner ear. The diameter of the tympanic membrane is approximately 9.5 mm giving an area of 71 mm^2, only two-thirds of this area being effective (47 mm^2).

The area of the stapes base is in the region of 3.2 mm^2, giving an area ratio of 14.7, which provides 23 dB of gain. This combination of leverage and area ratios compensates to a major extent for the losses due to impedance mismatch. The ossicles are not, therefore, acting as an amplifier, as no energy is gained in the process; they simply modify the nature of the vibration, in order to maximize the efficiency of the transfer of energy between outer and inner ear.

The other main function of the middle ear is that of protecting the inner ear against particularly large amplitude vibrations (loud noises) which could be damaging. This is achieved in two ways, as follows:

1. *The acoustic reflex*—This reflex changes the impedance of the middle ear so as to discriminate against large-amplitude, low-frequency vibrations. It works by contraction of the stapedius and tensor tympani muscles which act on the bones in the middle ear. Though primarily a brainstem reflex, this response is affected by the state of the subject's attention.
2. *Subluxation of the ossicles*—The articular portions of the malleus, incus and stapes move in and out of joint. The subluxation reduces the efficiency of the ossicles as a transmission system and protects the inner ear.

The inner ear

The functions of the outer and middle ear are to 'condition' the auditory signal arriving at the pinna

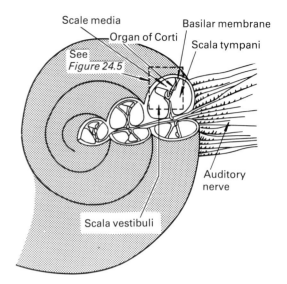

Figure 24.4 A cut-away diagram of the cochlea of the inner ear. The details of the arrangement of the internal structure of the cochlea outlined by the dotted rectangle are shown in *Figure 24.5*.

to make it suitable for the inner ear, the function of which is to transduce this signal (which still consists of rapid pressure changes) into a neural code.

The cochlea is a coiled tube which is divided longitudinally into three main compartments: the scala vestibuli; scala tympani; and scala media or cochlear duct (*Figure 24.4*). The scala vestibuli and scala tympani contain perilymph and are in communication with one another as the cochlear partition does not completely divide the cochlea. The pressures are equalized via the orifice, the helicotrema, at the end of the cochlea furthest from the oval window. A structure called the basilar membrane (*Figure 24.5*) performs a mechanical frequency analysis on the incoming signal. The membrane runs almost the length of the cochlea and is narrow at the basal (oval window) end of the cochlea and gradually widens towards the apex. Running along the basilar membrane are rows of hair cells. The short processes of hairs of these cells extend to touch the lower side of the tectorial membrane—a gelatinous shelf which overlies the basilar membrane. Movement of the basilar membrane relative to the tectorial membrane deforms the hairs. This deformation initiates the nerve impulse.

When the stapes causes pressure changes in the endolymph of the scala vestibuli (these are at the same frequency as the sound arriving at the ear and proportional in amplitude), a travelling wave is produced in the basilar membrane. This travelling wave appears initially as a bulge at the basal end of the membrane, and over the course of the next 4

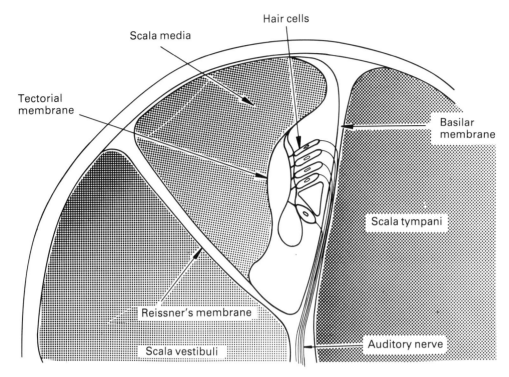

Tectorial membrane

Scala media

Hair cells

Basilar membrane

Scala tympani

Reissner's membrane

Scala vestibuli

Auditory nerve

Figure 24.5 A diagram of a cross-section of the basilar membrane and the organ of Corti, the hair cells of which are stimulated by movement of the tectorial membrane relative to the basilar membrane.

milliseconds it travels along the membrane, waxing and then waning. The point at which the maximum amplitude of vibration occurs on the basilar membrane depends on the frequency of the stimulating sound. Low tones produce maximum excitation at the basal end of the membrane and high tones at the apex. The information relayed to the brain by the auditory nerve is not only a function of the location of maximum vibration on the membrane; the frequency of impulses in any fibre or collection of fibres corresponds to the frequency of the stimulating sound. This relationship holds for frequencies up to 3–4 kHz, the highest frequencies used in speech. Thus there are two ways in which the frequency of a sound is indicated to the brain; the rate of firing in the auditory nerve, and the locus of maximum displacement of the basilar membrane.

Subjective sensation

Loudness and noisiness

Objective or physical methods of measurement are defined in terms of sound pressure level and frequency, while the corresponding subjective

sensations (what we actually hear) are expressed in terms of loudness level (phons) and pitch respectively. Loudness may be defined as the subjective magnitude of a sound, while pitch is the subjective sensation of frequency.

Since a sound at a particular frequency depends on the ear to translate its level into loudness, the response of the ear is of paramount importance in this translation. Unlike most hi-fi equipment the ear does not have a frequency response which is flat, but one which varies with both frequency and level. Thus the loudness of a sound depends not only on its sound pressure level but also on its frequency. *Figure 24.6* shows the pure tone frequency response of the ears, taken from the ISO/R 226-1961 standard. These curves are known as the equal loudness contours, or phon curves. Each curve plotted has equal loudness and it can be seen that, for example, a loudness level of 50 phons requires a sound pressure level of 50 dB at 1 kHz, while at the lower frequencies, where the ear is less sensitive (say 60 Hz) a sound pressure level of 70 dB is required to maintain this loudness. Alternatively, at the higher frequency of 4 kHz (very close to where the ear is maximally sensitive) an SPL of only 44 dB is needed to maintain the loudness level of 50 phons.

The curves have been constructed from a number of psychoacoustic experiments, in which large

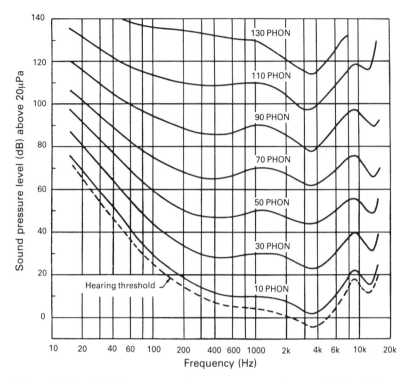

Figure 24.6 Equal-loudness contours for pure tones at sound pressure levels of 10, 30, 50, 70, 90, 110 and 130 dB (phon). The broken curve is the normal hearing threshold for pure tones.

numbers of subjects judged loudness against the physical parameters of sound pressure level and frequency, using a frequency of 1 kHz as a reference. Additionally it can be clearly seen that as the SPLs rise, the response of the ear flattens. For example at low levels the difference on the 50 phon curve between 60 Hz and 1 kHz for equal loudness is 20 dB, while at the higher loudness level of 110 phons the difference reduces to only 7 dB.

Loudness level is measured in phons, phons being the subjective sensation of SPL. The loudness of a pure tone of 1 kHz is said to have a value in phons equal to its SPL; this is simply how phons are defined.

During the psychoacoustic experiments subjects were also asked to judge what represented a doubling of loudness and this was judged as 10 phons. Thus 60 phons is twice as loud as 50 phons. So, in terms of human response, loudness doubles with every 10 phon increment in stimulus. To some extent this can be related to sound pressure levels since at 1 kHz an increase of 10 phons loudness level is the same as an increase of 10 dB. This is reasonably true across the frequency band generally, except at low frequencies, where the phon curves are more closely spaced and a lower decibel increase corresponds to a 10 phon increase.

While it is relatively easy to deduce how much louder a sound of 76 phons is than a 66 phon sound (10 phon—twice as loud) it is more difficult to deduce a difference of say 14 phons. Hence another scale has been devised, known as the sone scale. This is a ratio scale where the number of sones doubles as the loudness doubles—hence a sound of 6.4 sones is twice as loud as one of 3.2 sones.

To match the phon and sone scales, 1 sone is arbitrarily defined as equal to 40 phons. Thus if 1 sone = 40 phons, then 2 sones = 50 phons, 4 sones = 60 phons, etc. Mathematically this may be expressed as

$$P = 40 + 33\log_{10} S$$

where P is in phons and S is in sones.

Loudness expressed in phons is strictly called 'loudness level', whereas expressed in sones it is simply called 'loudness'. However, in many cases these strict definitions are not adhered to, and some care is required.

To calculate loudness or loudness level of a sound more complex than a pure tone, data must be available in the form of a sound spectrum—either in octave band or one-third octave band. The one-third octave band method was formulated by Zwicker (1960), while the octave band method results from

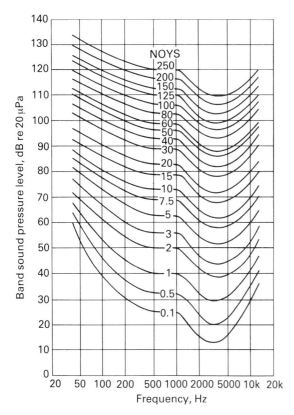

Figure 24.7 Equal noisiness contours (from Kryter, 1970). The curves show equal impression of noisiness related to frequency and noise level—a pure tone at 50 Hz and 70 dB SPL is equally noisy as a corresponding pure tone at 2 kHz but only at 43 dB SPL (i.e. a 27 dB difference in level but equally noisy).

work by Stevens (1956). Often the loudness levels calculated from Zwicker's method will be followed by the suffixes GF or GD—this means either calculated from free-field frontal sound (GF) or from diffuse field data (GD). Stevens' method is only valid for diffuse fields and may be suffixed by OD (octave diffuse).

A further aspect of human sensation is the related concept of noisiness and annoyance. Like the equal-loudness (or phon) curves, similar curves may be constructed for noisiness (*Figure 24.7*), with noisiness being measured in noys. Comparison of the two types of curves shows that the noy contours dip more sharply between 2 kHz and 5 kHz, indicating that sounds in this frequency range do not have to have a very high SPL to be considered noisy.

The unit of noisiness, the noy, is the counterpart in noisiness of the sone in loudness. Perceived noise level (PNL), which is given the unit of perceived noise decibel (PNdB), is the counterpart of the loudness level in phons. Thus where 40 phons = 1 sone, 40 PNdB = 1 noy, and, of course, a doubling of noisiness to 2 noys = 50 PNdB, etc.

Perceived noise level (PNL) may be applied directly to aircraft external noise; in the USA methods have been devised of evaluating the noisiness of aircraft, using as a basis the equal-noisiness contours.

Although it is necessary to understand the concept of subjective loudness, the phon is seldom used in normal measurements of, for example, cockpit noise—which is usually quoted in dB SPL or dB(A).

Measurement of noise

Physical measurement of noise and its relation to subjective impression is most important. Measurement is generally enabled by a sound level meter, which measures the sound pressure levels through a microphone, the microphone changing the sound pressure levels measured to a voltage in a controlled manner, and these voltages being read on a voltmeter, usually calibrated in decibels (dB). When measuring sound pressure level the instrument is set up such that the meter responds to all frequencies equally (i.e. there is no frequency weighting involved). As has been shown previously the ear does not respond to all frequencies equally and if it is necessary to use a sound level meter to provide an indication of human response to a noise field, then between the process of taking the voltage from the microphone and reading a level on the voltmeter, some frequency weighting must be included to take account of the response of the ear. Since the ear has a different frequency response with differing sound pressure levels then, in theory at least, an infinite number of weighting curves would be required for each noise level. In practice, this is successfully reduced to three, which follow three of the equal loudness contours.

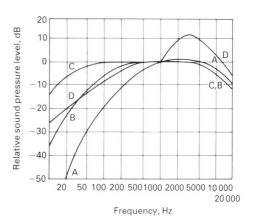

Figure 24.8 'A', 'B', 'C' and 'D' weighting scales for sound level meters. The relative responses for the four characteristics at different frequencies are shown.

For sounds which are judged 'not loud', the 40 phon contour was smoothed and used as the 'A' weighting. For moderately loud sounds the 70 phon contour was used as a basis for the 'B' weighting, whilst the 'C' weighting was for 'loud' sounds and based on the 100 phon contour. These weightings are written as dB(A), dB(B) and dB(C) respectively. *Figure 24.8* shows these weighting curves as well as the 'D' weighting curve. The 'D' weighting originated from the fact that dB(A) gave such a widely usable correlation of subjective response to physical measurement over a wide range of intensities and a wide range of human sensations, that the 40 PNdB (1 Noy) equal noisiness contour was used in the 'D' weighting as a simple correlate of noisiness. However, the 'D' weighting has not shown itself to be sufficiently superior to the 'A' weighting to be used generally and the 'A' weighting is now the most widely used method of correlating subjective impression and measured levels—even over the whole of the loudness range. Thus 'B', 'C' and 'D' weightings are rarely used.

Sound level meters which have these weighting networks built into them may be used to give some indication of the frequency constitution of the noise being measured. Thus if the measurement on the A scale is 70 dB (A) and on the C scale 77 dB (C) it is clear from *Figure 24.8* that the noise has a large low-frequency component.

Noise and aircraft

Noise generates problems both outside and inside aircraft. People who live near airfields understandably do not wish to be disturbed by the intrusion of aircraft noise into their homes. Groundcrew working on aircraft do not wish to be deafened; and aircrew, naturally, would like a quiet working environment in which communication is not only possible but easy.

Noise sources

The sources of noise and consequently the associated noise fields differ with the type of aircraft. In military flying the worst noise problems generally occur in the high-performance jets and the helicopters. These are both troublesome principally because of the high levels of internal noise which cause difficulty not only with aircrew communications but may, over a period, cause a degree of permanent hearing loss.

The major sources of noise in aircraft are:

1. Power sources, transmission systems, propellers and jet efflux.

2. Interaction between the aircraft and the medium through which it flies (flow of air over aircraft surfaces).
3. Subsidiary noise arising from cabin conditioning and pressurizing systems, hydraulic systems, and communication equipment.
4. Sonic booms.
5. Armament discharge.

Jet-powered aircraft

The operational requirement to be able to fly fast and low has increased the problems due to internal cabin noise. Over the years there have been gradual increases in cabin noise levels of fast jets and it is now not uncommon for aircrew to be exposed to noise levels of between 115 and 120 dB when flying at operational speeds and heights—typically 420–480 knots at 250 ft.

The major source of noise in these cases is from the turbulent flow across the aircraft canopy and structure, and from the cabin conditioning flows into the cockpit which are used for cooling, demist and pressurization. The contribution from the boundary layer turbulent flow depends essentially upon the structure and shape of the canopy and its relation to the remaining aircraft structure, as well as the speed and height of the aircraft.

Additional sources are from cockpit-mounted equipment, in some aircraft from the engines and from other mechanical/hydraulic systems within the aircraft structure; although these are generally of secondary nature. A cabin noise spectrum obtained during high-speed low-level flight in a fast jet is shown in *Figure 24.9*. As the aircraft climbs to altitude, however, and the air density decreases, the pressure fluctuations in the turbulent flow decrease in intensity and the contribution to the overall cabin

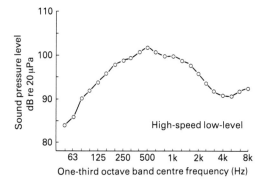

Figure 24.9 Typical cabin noise spectrum for a fast jet aircraft flying at high speed (450 knot) at low altitude (250 feet).

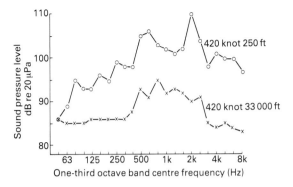

Figure 24.10 Effect of altitude of flight on cabin noise spectrum of a fast jet aircraft flying at 420 knot.

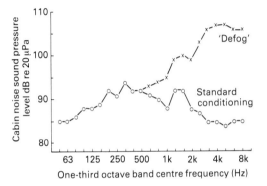

Figure 24.11 Effect of selection of defog or emergency demist on cabin noise spectrum in a fast jet aircraft.

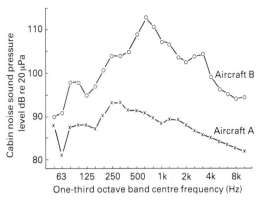

Figure 24.12 Cabin noise spectra of a 'quiet' (aircraft A) and less 'quiet' (aircraft B) fast jet aircraft flying at high speed (500 knot) at low level (500 feet altitude).

noise level from the external aerodynamic sources is diminished. *Figure 24.10* shows the extent of the decrease for the same aircraft in flight at high and low altitudes. As the contribution from the external sources decreases, so the contribution from the cabin conditioning source will increase and, depending upon the quality of design of the conditioning system and the outlet sprays, may dominate the noise spectrum at higher altitudes—albeit at generally lower overall cabin noise level.

Normally as air mass flow to the cabin conditioning system increases the noise levels increase. In most aircraft, even quiet examples, conditioning noise will dominate when it is necessary to use 'defog' or 'emergency demist' and in these types of cases (*Figure 24.11*) substantial increases in high-frequency noise levels occur.

Further differences occur between aircraft of the same type, and, in multi-seat aircraft, between seat positions. Thus noise levels may be different between the pilot and navigator positions, especially

in tandem seat aircraft, and it is commonly accepted that within aircraft types some aircraft are noisier than others.

Depending upon the design, noise levels between different types of aircraft can vary greatly and the difference between a noisy and 'quiet' aircraft operating at the same speed and height is depicted in *Figure 24.12* to illustrate the range.

Whilst it is difficult, for many operational reasons, to design aircraft structures and transparent canopies to ensure low noise levels, it is considerably easier to design cabin conditioning systems which do not contribute strongly to cabin noise.

The external sound field from a jet-powered aircraft is filled with distributed noise from the jet engine with some harmonic contribution from rotating parts of the engine. At high indicated air speeds in flight, aerodynamic noise can also contribute to the external sound field. The intensity of jet noise heard at any given distance from the aircraft varies with the listener's position with respect to the jet axis. *Figure 24.13* shows the noise level distribution around a single jet aircraft for engine run-up on the ground. The highest noise is not directly in line with the jet but on the quarters.

Conventional turbojet engines produce thrust by heating a relatively small mass of air to a high temperature and thus accelerating it to a high velocity. This high-velocity air, mixing turbulently with the surrounding air, generates the noise. The same amount of thrust can be produced, however, by imparting a lower velocity (thereby causing less noise) to a larger mass of air. This occurs in jet engines with a high by-pass ratio, where a cowled fan is fitted to the front of the engine. The fan acts almost like a propeller to accelerate a large mass of air, only a fraction of which passes through the combustion chamber of the engine.

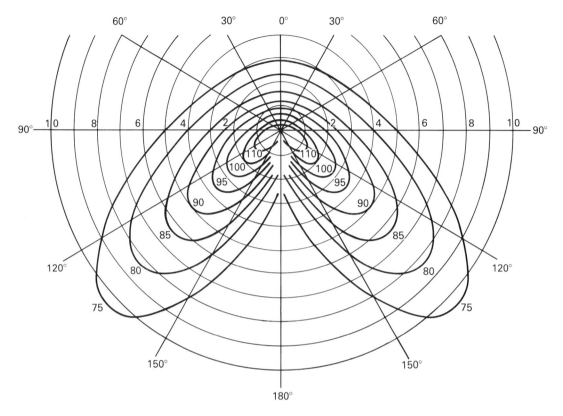

Figure 24.13 The distribution of noise levels around a single-engined jet aircraft on ground run-up. The concentric circles indicate distance from the aircraft, the radii of the circles increasing from 1000 feet to 10 000 feet at intervals of 1000 feet. The long axis of the aircraft is indicated by the vertical 0–180 degree axis of the diagram. The heavy lines join points of equal perceived noise level (PNdB). The value of the perceived noise level is indicated for each contour by the number immediately below the contour. Note that the perceived noise level contours form lobes at an angle to the jet axis.

Rotary wing aircraft

Helicopters have a totally different noise spectrum which comprises essentially of aerodynamically induced noise from the main and tail rotor and mechanically induced noise from the main gearbox and various transmission chains, all of which produce dominant narrow band noise peaks. Consequently the spectrum is built up from a combination of deterministic discrete and random broad-band noise components. A typical spectrum for a single rotor helicopter is shown in *Figure 24.14* indicating the contributions from the rotor, gearbox and ancillaries. The rotor frequency is a product of the rotational speed of the rotor and the number of rotor blades, and on most major single rotor helicopters is around 20 Hz. The gearbox frequencies are directly related to the gear-meshing ratios of the power input/output gears and are generally in

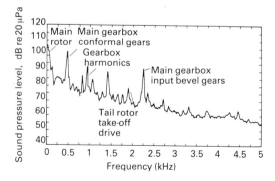

Figure 24.14 Cabin noise spectrum of a helicopter with a single rotor (Lynx) showing the various aircraft components contributing to the cabin noise levels.

the higher frequency range around 400–600 Hz. For twin rotor helicopters of the Chinook type, the rotor frequencies are generally lower, partially due to fewer rotor blades, and generate discrete noise at around 12 Hz at levels of up to 125 dB. In most cases these levels of infrasonic noise will cause no problems, but some noise-induced symptoms may occur in a few people.

Owing to these high-level 'spikes' of noise from the various components, operational problems may occur when tasks involving listening for low-level signal returns are necessary, such as detecting or classifying sonar or electronic surveillance measures and electronic countermeasure returns. The high levels of discrete noise may cause frequencies above and below the dominant noise source to go unheard as well as at the particular source frequency. This phenomenon is known as auditory masking and is, very simply, the occlusion of one sound by another. It is possible to calculate the auditory threshold below which the detection of sounds is improbable, and it is similarly possible to show, using the human psychometric function, that 15 dB above this threshold, 100% detection is possible. Thus it is possible to predict the levels and frequencies of signals which may be detected and the probability of detection. *Figure 24.15* shows noise levels at the ear for a Lynx helicopter with the auditory threshold

calculated and plotted. The curve shows the levels at which 100% detection will occur.

The external sound field of the helicopter is created predominantly by a combination of rotor noise and by the engine exhaust which is maximum close to the exhaust outlets. This type of aircraft may be a noise nuisance to people on the ground because it operates at low speed and low altitude and consequently remains within earshot for long periods.

Turbo-prop and piston-engined aircraft

Generally the major source of noise in these type of aircraft is the propeller. In the same way as the helicopter, the dominant frequency is a function of the propeller rotational speed and the number of blades. As these aircraft fly at higher speeds than helicopters there is a higher contribution from boundary layer noise, although it does not approach the levels generated by the jet transport types. The internal noise is generally at its highest levels in the plane of the propellers. *Figure 24.16* shows cabin noise spectra for two typical aircraft. It clearly shows the dominant effect of the propellers.

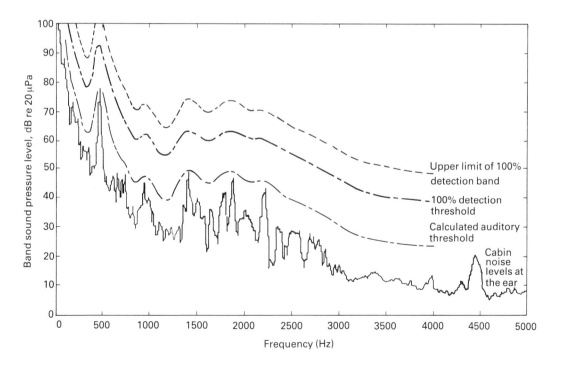

Figure 24.15 Calculated pure-tone threshold and noise at the ear (10 Hz resolution) in the Lynx.

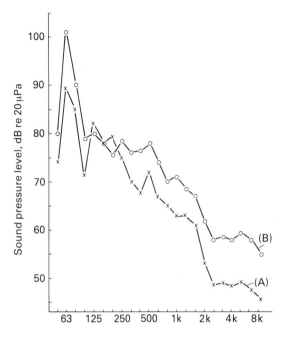

Figure 24.16 Typical cabin noise spectra for turbo-propeller (curve A, 78 dB(A)) and propeller (curve B, 82.5 dB(A)) aircraft.

Jet transport aircraft

Similar to fast military jets, the major contributors to passenger jet internal noise are from the boundary layer turbulent flow and from cabin conditioning. The noise spectrum is normally broad

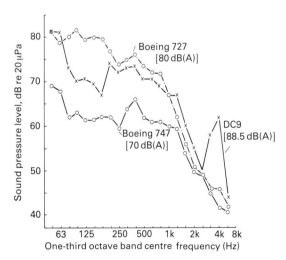

Figure 24.17 Cabin noise spectra for Boeing 727, DC-9 and Boeing 747 aircraft. Total sound pressure levels (dB(A)) are given in parentheses.

band and varies down the length and across the width of the aircraft. Noise levels at the cabin side-wall may be up to 6 dB higher than at the centre of the cabin. Noise also emanates from such sources as hydraulic or mechanical systems (flaps, slats etc.), although generally these only occur during specific phases of flight (landing, take-off etc.). Typical values are depicted in *Figure 24.17* for wide- and narrow-bodied jets.

VTOL, V/STOL and STOL aircraft

Aircraft of these types are either intended to take off or land vertically, have short take-off and/or landing runs or may be a combination of both (e.g. short take-off, vertical landing—STOVL).

The majority of STOL aircraft in current use are propeller driven and utilize special wing designs such as high aspect ratio wings, slotted flaps and leading edge slots/slats to achieve lift coefficients which are high enough at slow speed to provide sufficient lift. A further group, aimed mainly at military use, utilize powered lift devices such as under-wing or over-wing blowing, augmentor wings and deflected slipstreams. A further technique is used in the Harrier type of aircraft which utilizes vectored thrust alone to provide vertical transition during take-off or landing (VTOL).

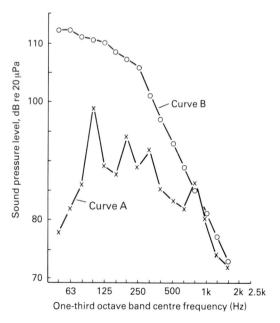

Figure 24.18 Typical cabin noise spectra for conventional short take-off and landing aircraft (curve A) and short take-off and landing aircraft with wing-blowing devices (curve B).

Noise problems generally occur only during the landing or take-off phase of flight when the high lift or vectored thrust devices are in use. During all other phases of flight the aircraft may be viewed as a standard aircraft of the appropriate type.

Typical spectrum shapes for STOL/VTOL vehicles are shown in *Figure 24.18* which shows clearly the increases in low-frequency noise that is apparent when using powered lift devices, and the propeller dominated noise of civil type aircraft.

Supersonic aircraft

When a supersonic aircraft is operating at subsonic speeds, the internal and external sound fields are similar, in nature and intensity, to those produced by a conventional jet aircraft. When flying at supersonic speeds, aircraft of this type generate shock waves in the atmosphere and although these do not intrude into the internal sound field (indeed, the aircraft is remarkably quiet, since boundary layer noise is reduced and jet noise is left behind) the generation of 'sonic boom' creates a problem in the external sound field.

When air, flowing past an aircraft flying at a speed exceeding Mach 1, decelerates slowly, shock waves are formed which spread out from the leading and trailing edges of the aircraft. These waves are propagated through the atmosphere, forming a characteristic 'N' wave of pressure which can be heard and felt at great distance (*Figure 24.19*). The shock wave coming from the aircraft forms a cone, and the intersection of the cone of disturbance with the ground circumscribes an area within which the sonic boom is registered. As the aircraft flies at supersonic speed it trails a cone of disturbance along a track or 'boom carpet', the width of which depends on the size of aircraft and its height above ground (the track may extend up to 50 km or more behind a large aircraft). The noise of a sonic boom is predominantly low frequency (less than 100 Hz), but the leading edge of the shock wave may have a rise time to peak pressure of 1 ms and thus higher frequency content produces the sharp 'crack' characteristic of some sonic booms. Depending upon the time interval between the positive and negative peak pressures (which is directly related to the length of the aircraft), the sonic boom may be heard as either two booms in quick succession (as from Concorde) or as a single boom (as from most military jet fighters). The sonic boom signatures are essentially the same in pressure–time history but if the time interval between peak pressure is less than approximately 70 ms, the integration time of the ear prevents a subjective impression of two separate events. Outside the 'boom carpet' the shock, having become degraded by distance and lost

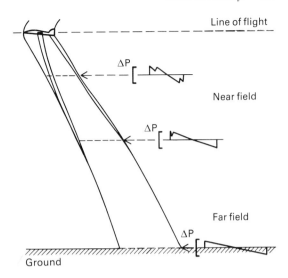

Figure 24.19 The pressure fields created by an aircraft flying at supersonic spped. Shock waves arise from the bow and tail of the aircraft and from individual parts of the structure including the wings and engine nacelles. The complex pressure patterns close to the aircraft (near field) gradually coalesce as they travel through the atmosphere to form the two-shock N-wave of the far field.

its high frequency content, is heard as a low-pitched rumble-like thunder.

Much has been written on the effect of sonic booms on people and their property on the ground. It is sufficient here to say that, while there may be concern over structural damage to old and poorly constructed buildings, sonic booms of intensities likely to be generated by commercial operation of supersonic transport aircraft may disturb but not harm people or animals and do not constitute a hazard to hearing.

Reduction of cabin noise levels

The sound fields inside aircraft can vary from the quiet to intensely noisy. There are certain engineering means of reducing the noise levels at source, but, except for certain dramatic changes (for example, the introduction of high bypass ratio engines) reducing the noise at source by engineering means has met with only limited success. Reduction of noise at the aircraft structure normally requires the addition of mass or bulk, both of which are generally unacceptable to the operator. Some possible ways of reducing cabin noise are as follows:

1. Increasing the canopy thickness. This would undoubtedly help reduce aerodynamic noise in strike aircraft, but it would also increase weight and possibly impede the ejection path.

2. Damping the walls of the cockpit. This may be possible again to reduce aerodynamic noise—but in fact the large amounts of avionic equipment already attached to the cockpit walls provide reasonable damping. It is certainly the case that damping could be used to quieten the interior of helicopters, in which structural vibrations are an important noise factor, but the weight penalty associated with providing such damping is usually felt to be unacceptable, certainly for military operations.

3. Smoothing the boundary layer by removing unnecessary excrescences or by reshaping surfaces. This is not an important problem in slow aircraft; and in fast aircraft it may be taken for granted that, because of aerodynamic considerations, all excrescences are necessary ones. Nevertheless, improvements have been occasionally brought about by this means.

4. Redesigning the conditioning system or reducing the air flow through the system. In the past the conditioning system has seldom been designed with noise in mind, and redesign may well be possible. It is also true that mass flows of air have sometimes been found to be in excess of that required and that a reduced flow has produced a reduction of cabin noise without affecting thermal conditioning.

It is scarcely necessary to add that a properly maintained aircraft is likely to be less noisy than a neglected one.

Communication

In many aircraft the only form of communication is speech; non-verbal methods of communication (gesticulation, facial expression) are not possible where the aircrew are physically separated. This may represent a very significant loss.

The physical nature of speech

Speech sounds are not steady or continuous through time. Although speech is composed, from a perceptual point of view, of 'phonemes', these phonemes do not precisely correspond to any physical pattern of sound. (Phonemes do not precisely correspond to the letters used in a word. 'Meaty' is phonemically written /m/,/i/,t/,/i/.) The pattern of sound associated with a given phoneme depends on the age, sex and personal idiosyncracies of the speaker as well as on the location of the phonemes in the word. The /p/ in 'spoon' is physically very different from the /p/ in 'pan', yet it is perceptually identical. The perceptual system is not, therefore, performing a simple decoding of the incoming signal but is performing a complicated pattern recognition task in which many cues, including the context in which the sound occurs, are being utilized.

Each sound consists of various combinations of different frequencies, and in fact some sounds (for example the s in sea) contain almost all the speech frequencies and approximate to white noise in which all frequencies are equally represented. Vowels consists of high-amplitude sounds. All vowels are 'voiced' (that is, the larynx is used in their production) as are some consonants (for example, /b/). However, many consonants (for example, /t/) are unvoiced and of lower amplitude than vowel sounds, and this has some consequence in the testing of equipment.

The energy content of speech is widely distributed. The information content of speech is, however, not so widely distributed, a matter of primary importance in the design of communication systems. The way in which the information content of speech is distributed is discussed on page 371.

The amplitude of the speech is often not great enough for good intelligibility in a noise environment. This is due to a complicated phenomenon known as 'masking': suffice it to say that it is obviously difficult to comprehend quiet speech in a loud noise environment. Many sorts of physical distortion and clipping of speech peaks can occur, and, in aircraft, various protective devices and communication systems are used to protect and preserve the speech. The effectiveness of these devices can be assessed only in terms of intelligibility.

Intelligibility

The most straightforward form of intelligibility test is one in which a single word is read to a listener. The listener writes down the word which he believes that he has heard and his response is marked for correctness. This is basically the method used in the Harvard phonetically balanced (PB) word lists, against which other tests are compared. The 50 word lists used in the Harvard PB test are supposed to have a phonetic constitution similar to that of spoken English.

The Harvard PB word lists are, however, open to many sorts of error and need practice. Intelligibility assessments can be made more easily by means of one of the forms of Rhyme test. In these tests the listener is provided with a multiple choice answer sheet. Thus the response alternatives given to the stimulus word 'hat' might be 'bat', 'cat', 'fat', 'rat', 'hat' and 'mat', from which the listener deletes the one which he hears. The response list generally contains words varying in only one phoneme from one another (in the example given here a consonant

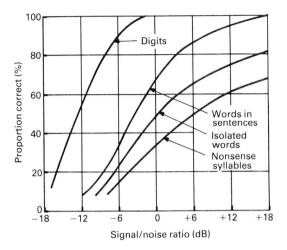

Figure 24.20 The effect of the signal:noise ratio and the nature of the signal on its intelligibility. The intelligibility of the signal increases with signal:noise ratio, with size of the vocabulary employed, with the internal 'redundancy' and the context of the signal.

phoneme). Consonant phonemes are generally used, as vowel phonemes are, on the whole, louder and consequently not so readily affected by poor signal to noise ratio (the difference in decibels between the level of the signal and that of the masking signal). Other types of distortion (such as that produced by over-driving an inadequate transducer) may require a vowel test and suitable tests do exist.

A further type of two choice intelligibility test is the Diagnostic Rhyme Test (DRT) which uses two rhyming words where the initial consonants differ by a single attribute. Detailed analysis of the responses will indicate in which area a communication system will need to be improved.

These types of test are important in the assessment of narrow band digital speech channels (secure speech transmissions) where plain speech is encoded, transmitted in 'scrambled' digital form and decoded back into plain speech at the receiver's end.

The intelligibility of a signal is affected not only by the masking noise in which the signal is heard (*Figure 24.20*), but also by the size of the vocabulary from which the signal is taken (see digits compared with isolated words), the internal 'redundancy' of the signal or words (see how poorly totally non-redundant nonsense syllables fare) and the context of the signal (isolated words compared with words in sentences).

Some speech is intelligible at negative signal/noise ratios, that is, when the 'average' (long-term root mean square) level of the speech is less than that of the noise. An example may be drawn from *Figure 24.20* where, at a signal to noise ratio of −12 dB,

digit intelligibility is around 55%, whilst for isolated words (where intelligent guesses are not as productive) it requires an increase of around 15 dB in the signal to a +3 dB signal to noise ratio to obtain a similar level of intelligibility. This is because the level of speech varies in time, and for very 'probable' words (drawn from a small vocabulary or where contextual information is given) enough information is still present above the ambient noise to provide the perceptual system with data on which to base an identification.

It is fortunate, because of the poor quality of many aircraft commmunications systems, that the speech used in aircraft is fairly redundant. 'Redundant' is used here not in the true sense of 'unnecessary' but in the incorrect but common jargon sense that, in any individual utterance, more speech sounds are present than are necessary for the unambiguous detection of a digit, letter or word. For example, when it is wished to use the letter I (pronounced EYE) which contains only two vowel phonemes (/a/ as in father, /i/ as in meat), the word INDIA is used instead, which contains five phonemes—with a consequently higher probability of recognition. However, the problem remains that any perceptual process relies to a very large extent on the experience of the listener, and if message A is probable, but message B arrives (which is acoustically similar), then B will be heard as A. This sort of mishearing has often had serious consequences but is best illustrated by the apocryphal story about the pilot who, during the take-off run, noticed that his co-pilot was looking unhappy. 'Cheer up' he said, whereupon the co-pilot lifted the undercarriage ('gear' up), to the detriment of the aircraft.

The final test of the quality of any communications system must remain the intelligibility test: but the inconvenience of using large numbers of people to test systems has led to the adoption of physical methods of assessment. It was noted that, although the energy of speech is distributed widely, the information content is not, that is to say, although there are a large number of speech sounds in the part of the speech spectrum below, say, 300 Hz, these do not contribute a great deal to the intelligibility of the speech. It is generally correct to say that only 20% of intelligibility is contained in 80% of the energy of speech—the vowel sounds— whilst 80% of the intelligibility is found in 20% of the total energy—the consonants. Large numbers of experiments have been performed in an attempt to assess the relative contributions of different parts of the spectrum to intelligibility and as a result of these calculations such as those presented in *Table 24.2* have been developed allowing a predictive and calculable method of assessing probable speech intelligibility.

This method of dividing the speech and noise spectrum into a number of bands and assessing the

Table 24.2 **The method of calculating the Articulation Index (AI) which uses the weighted and summed speech signal to noise ratios to enable an AI figure to be determined. The speech signal to noise ratio is taken at the output from the microphone. This AI figure is then related to *Figure 24.21* which gives the level of intelligibility for particular types of text material (i.e. sentences, limited vocabularies, nonsense syllables etc.)**

(a) Measured values

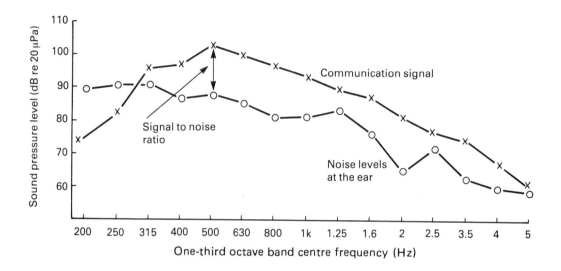

(b) Calculation of Articulation Index

Frequency (Hz)	Signal to noise ratio (A) (dB)	Weighting factor (B)	Product (A × B)
200	0	0.0004	0.0000
250	0	0.0010	0.0000
315	5	0.0010	0.0050
400	10	0.0014	0.0140
500	16	0.0014	0.0224
630	14	0.0020	0.0280
800	15	0.0020	0.0300
1000	12	0.0024	0.0288
1250	6	0.0030	0.0180
1600	11	0.0037	0.0407
2000	16	0.0037	0.0592
2500	6	0.0034	0.0204
3150	11	0.0034	0.0374
4000	7	0.0024	0.0168
5000	2	0.0020	0.0040

AI = 0.3267

(c) Calculated intelligibility (from Figure 24.21)

AI = 0.33 = 85% intelligibility for sentences for first presentation to listeners
= 94% intelligibility for sentences known to listeners

contribution of each band to the overall sum is called the Articulation Index (AI). Depending upon the relative accuracy required, the overall spectrum can be divided into a greater or lesser number of bands. Generally it is preferable to use the larger number and in the example (*Table 24.2*), the spectrum is split into 15 bands, each one-third of an octave wide. For a smaller number of bands, octave bandwidths may be used. The signal to noise in each band is multiplied by its weighting factor, which indicates its relative contribution to the overall speech intelligibility, and the resultant figures summed to give the articulation index figure. This AI figure is then related to an intelligibility figure proper by use of the curves shown in *Figure 24.21*, which is similar to the approach of *Figure 24.20* in respect to changes in intelligibility due to contextural information, redundancy, size of vocabulary, etc.

Thus a measure of subjective intelligibility may be obtained from direct physical measurement. The method must, however, be used with care since it is subject to many caveats and qualifications. This AI method is used with aided communication systems; that is, using an aircraft crew communication system in conjunction with headsets or flying helmets. In many aircraft or other vehicles face-to-face communication is necessary without resort to an aided system. In this case a simpler method called Speech Interference Level (SIL) is used. In this method, the cabin noise levels are measured in octave bands and the three bands centred on 500, 1000 and 2000 Hz are summed arithmetically and the average taken. This average figure is compared with a set of figures which will indicate the level of communication possible. This method may be illustrated with the following example. It is useful to note that this method may be used over a wide range of transportation vehicles (buses, cars etc.) as well as in the industrial environment.

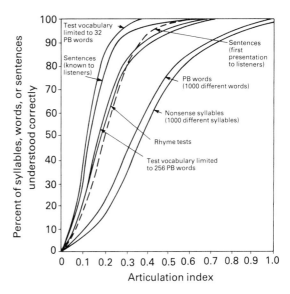

Figure 24.21 Relationships between articulation index and intelligibility. These relationships vary with the type of material and the skill of the talkers and listeners.

The results of an octave analysis of noise levels on the flight-deck of a jet transport aircraft were:

Octave band frequency (Hz)	125	250	500	1000	2000	4000
Sound pressure level (dB)	100	88	84	85	74	63

Speech interference level (dB) = (84 + 85 + 74)/3
                                = 81

The particular problem is to assess whether a pilot can talk to his co-pilot or engineer, who are seated at a distance of 1.2 m, with normal voice levels.

Table 24.3 shows that at a separation distance of 1.2 m the SIL would have to be 56 dB for normal speech effort, and rise to 74 dB for a shouting voice. In this example the pilot would be unable to talk to his crew, even using a shouting voice, and aided communications would be necessary. The cabin noise levels would have to be reduced to a level where an SIL of 56 dB could be obtained to just allow communication.

Communication in aircraft

There are two interface sites between the man and the aircraft communications system, namely, the human output device (mouth, throat, nose) and the human input device (ear). The goal at both these locations is to transduce the signal as faithfully as

Table 24.3 Speech interference levels (SIL) of steady continuous noises at which reliable communication is barely possible. The values apply to male vocal effort and to speaker and listener facing each other (subtract 5 dB for female voices)

Separation distance (m)	*Preferred speech interference level (dB)*			
	Normal effort	*Raised*	*Very loud*	*Shouting*
0.15	74	80	86	92
0.3	68	74	80	86
0.6	62	68	74	80
1.2	56	62	68	74
1.8	52	58	64	70
3.7	46	52	58	64

Source: Beranek (1971)

possible and maximize the exclusion of ambient noise; the acoustic merit of a mask or helmet will depend on how well it performs these two functions.

Output from the man

Speech may be transduced into electrical signals by a microphone built into an oronasal mask, by a throat microphone or by a 'noise-cancelling' boom microphone.

Mask-mounted microphones

The acoustic attenuation properties of oxygen masks are similar to the attenuation properties of flying helmets—poor at low frequencies and improving with rising frequency. Like most acoustic systems the mask system may have resonances which are a function of interactions between different parts of the mask structure and will reduce attenuation, sometimes to the point of producing higher sound pressure levels inside the mask than outside. However, as *Figure 24.22* clearly shows, the speech signal to noise ratio is generally more than adequate to provide good intelligibility at the mask microphone output. Even in the noisiest aircraft the quality of the signal from a microphone mounted in an oronasal mask is good. Nevertheless, because of matching imperfection and other distortions introduced downstream of the mask, aircrew frequently and unjustly put the blame for inadequate communications on this piece of equipment.

Throat microphones

A throat microphone is inherently less sensitive to airborne noise and can generally provide a better signal to noise ratio than the noise cancelling type. However, the overall frequency response is limited and the microphone output has a preponderance of low-frequency components, which whilst giving good signal to noise ratios, do not contribute significantly to a high intelligibility.

The transducer of the throat microphone is pressed against the pharynx and is sensitive to the powerful vibrations which occur here in 'voiced' phonemes. If the reader places his fingers on his larynx and says 'aaaa' these vibrations can be felt clearly. However, if he does the same and says 'sss' or any other 'unvoiced' consonant he will feel nothing. Similarly, the throat microphone does not respond to 'unvoiced' phonemes. Because of this, a throat microphone leaves a lot of speech to be 'filled in' or inferred by the listener. The throat microphone does, however, have excellent rejection of normal airborne sound, so that what is lost in quality

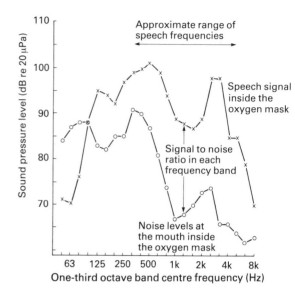

Figure 24.22 Sound pressure levels in the cavity of an oronasal oxygen mask, due to transmission of noise from the cabin through the walls and valves of the mask and to speech.

of speech transduction may be gained in terms of noise rejection. This form of transducer is commonly worn in helicopters where the rejection of noise is invaluable in some situations (for example, the winchman).

'Noise-cancelling' boom microphones

This form of microphone transduces speech very well, and generally performs its function perfectly satisfactorily. The noise-cancelling properties of these microphones are a function of frequency and provide better cancelling properties at low frequencies than at high. Depending upon the quality of design and the type of construction some microphones have better noise rejection than others, which enables some microphones to have noise discrimination (or rejection) of up to 10 dB at 4 kHz, whilst others have none. At lower frequencies noise rejection can be up to 30 dB with a theoretical maximum of 45 dB at 100 Hz.

Owing to the low-frequency content of helicopter noise, noise-cancelling boom microphones are well suited to this type of vehicle and generally provide an acceptable solution for noise reduction. However, there is one highly critical point that enables the microphone to work efficiently—the microphone must be placed close to the lips; in fact, it be should as close to touching the lips as possible. Even minor movement away from the lips, in the order of 2–3 mm, will significantly degrade the speech signal to noise ratios.

Input to the man

In principle, it should be possible to provide a satisfactory signal/noise ratio at the ear by simply turning up the gain of the communications system until the signal is loud enough to hear above the ambient noise. Several factors make this solution impractical. Firstly, speech at or greater than 125 dB causes discomfort and pain. Secondly, listening to speech at sound pressure levels considerably less than 125 dB for any significant period of time poses a distinct threat of damage to the hearing. Thirdly, physiological changes take place in the ear at high sound levels, and it is not clear that a given signal/noise ratio or articulation index at a high noise level would produce the same intelligibility as that produced at more moderate levels. It is undesirable to present speech at levels much in excess of 100 dB. If a 15 dB ratio is required, the ambient noise at the ear must not be greater than 85 dB. Thus in general terms if the ambient sound pressure level inside the aircraft cabin is 115 dB, the helmet or headset should provide an attenuation of at least 30 dB. By applying the same reasoning in more detail across each frequency band the amount of attenuation required throughout the frequency spectrum may be defined.

Helmets and headsets

Acoustically, an aircrew helmet consists of two parts, the shell and the ear muffs. The contribution of the shell to the overall attenuation of the helmet is small and will consequently be disregarded for the purposes of this chapter. Helmets and headsets are thus identical in that they attempt to protect the ear by placing around it a sound-proofed cavity which is sealed by some means to the head and which contains a transducer for transmission of speech and non-verbal signals. Some lightweight headsets produced for quiet environments are little more than transducers. Other headsets, which are really ear defenders with a built-in transducer, provide very good attenuation. The ear muff is composed of four basic parts—the shell, the seal, the internal damping and the transducer. Similarly the attenuation characteristics of the headset can be split into three distinct regions—low, medium and high frequencies.

At low frequencies, below 400 Hz, the attenuation of the earshell is controlled by movement of the earshell against the head. Thus the important parameters of the earshell are shell volume, the spring stiffness of the earshell seals and the air volume, and the fit of the earshell on the head. Increasing the volume of the shell will invariably increase low-frequency attenuation, but at the cost of increases in bulk. A doubling of volume will result in a general increase of low-frequency attenuation of the order of 6 dB maximum. A further doubling is needed (four times the original volume) to gain up to another 6 dB.

In the intermediate frequency range, from 400 Hz to around 2 kHz, it is the transmission loss of noise through the shell walls that is important and thus the type and mass of shell material are the overriding factors. The greater the mass, the greater the attenuation, all other factors being equal.

Above 2 kHz the noise field inside the earshells becomes considerably more complex and it is the damping material within the shell which absorbs the high frequency noise. Typical materials are plastic foam or glass-wool, and a change of material will change the attenuation characteristic.

A further factor which is rarely considered is the inclusion of any subsiduary structures within the earshell such as telephones or a structure or plate to contain the damping materials. Improper support of these devices can be highly detrimental to attenuation between 500 Hz and 2 kHz, and sometimes above.

Transmission of sound to the inner ear occurs not only by airborne means through the auditory system, but also by direct transmission through the body, generally through the skull and bony parts of the head and hence is described as bone conduction. Normally the body-conducted or bone-conducted sound is negligible below 500 Hz. The transmission is greatest around 1–2 kHz, where the useful attenuation of conventional hearing protectors may be limited to around 45 dB.

However, whilst it is possible to state those parameters which may, or may not, improve headset attenuation, headset design is a series of compromises (e.g. weight versus bulk versus subjective acceptability). As such, the optimum headset, whilst possible to design in general terms, may not be acceptable for normal use.

The importance of the noise attenuation provided by the aircrew helmet is not to be underestimated. This is a function that it is required to perform daily, while other functions, for example protecting the wearer against impact, may never be needed. Within the size and weight constraints placed on the helmet, the attenuation using conventional techniques is probably as good as it could be—given current materials (*Figure 24.23*).

Only little attenuation is provided at low frequencies for the aforementioned reasons, but since the amount of information in speech is small at frequencies below 300 Hz, little gains in speech intelligibility can be made by reducing noise levels at these frequencies, apart from in very noisy aircraft. However, the noise levels under the flying helmet in a fast jet (*Figure 24.24*) peak at around 250 Hz and

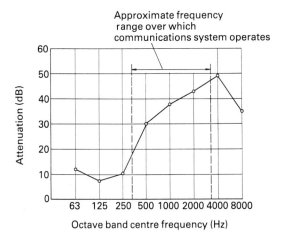

Figure 24.23 Attenuation of external noise provided by a modern protective helmet. Note that the attenuation is low at low frequencies. The approximate frequency range over which aircraft communication systems typically operate is also shown.

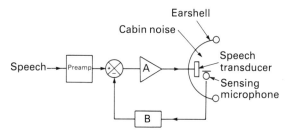

Figure 24.25 Schematic diagram of an active noise reduction system. The diagram shows how the noise inside the earshell is collected by the sensing microphone and fed back in a negative feedback loop via amplifier B, to be inverted in phase and fed through amplifier A back into the earshell via the speech transducer. The inverted phase noise from the feedback loop and the in-phase noise already in the earshell are mutually destructive and the sound pressure levels in the earshell are consequently reduced. Since speech is also reduced in level, it is preamplified from its source and fed into the shell at an increased level, thus compensating for the active reduction of the speech levels.

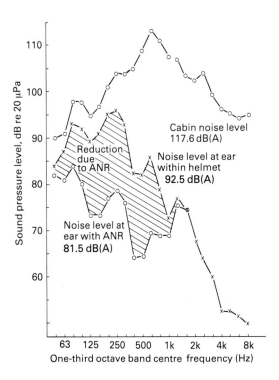

Figure 24.24 Effect of aircrew helmet (RAF aircrew helmet Mk 4) and active noise reduction (ANR) upon the noise spectrum at the ear in a fast jet aircraft flying at high speed at low altitude. The cabin noise (top curve) is attenuated by the aircrew helmet giving the noise spectrum indicated by the middle curve. Active noise reduction reduces the noise level at the ear (bottom curve) by the amount indicated by the shaded area.

these high noise levels increase considerably the risk of hearing damage. Further reduction in noise levels are necessary at these lower frequencies, which, by passive means, are not practical—and, in some cases, not possible.

However, by using newly developed active noise control techniques, generally described as Active Noise Reduction (ANR), considerable increases in low frequency attenuation without the attendant disadvantages of passive solutions can be achieved.

In simple terms, ANR is achieved by continuously sampling the noise in the earshell with a small microphone (*Figure 24.25*); this signal is inverted in phase and then reintroduced into the shell by the telephone transducer, reducing the noise levels inside the earshell by destructive interference of the acoustic field. The reduction in levels currently attainable are shown in *Figure 24.24* and illustrate the reductions achieved at the ear of aircrew. Reductions of 10 dB(A) or more are possible which significantly reduces the risk of noise-induced hearing impairment. Current ANR systems in the UK are fully compatible with current and future helmet design, and *Figure 24.26* shows an active system contained within an existing helmet earshell with no increase in earshell mass.

Measurement of attenuation

The overall acoustic performance of a helmet or headset is best measured by an intelligibility test; but it is frequently measured directly.

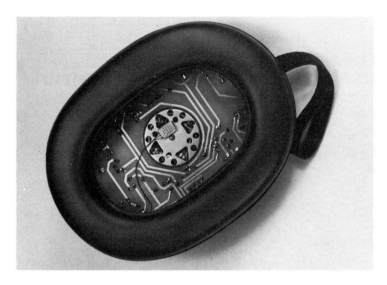

Figure 24.26 An active noise reduction system fitted to the earshell of an RAF aircrew helmet Mk 4. The system only requires a 28 V aircraft supply to be fully operational.

A helmet *per se* achieves no attenuation. It excludes noise only when mounted on a head. The attenuation of the device will therefore have properties which, as has been shown in the discussion on bone conduction, is frequency dependent, and may be as low as 45 dB in the 2 kHz region. It also follows that the attenuation of the helmet will be affected by how well it fits and this may vary from one day to another. This variance in fit, and hence acoustic attenuation, is relatively small within subjects—normally a standard deviation of less than 1 dB—but the variance between subjects is considerably larger and would typically reach standard deviations of 4–5 dB. This variance is predominantly due to anatomical differences causing slight differences in fit. *Figure 24.27* gives an indication of the resulting spread of acoustic attenuation and shows the mean attenuation bordered by upper and lower values which represent the spread across 97% of the population. The distribution across this spread is Gaussian.

There are two basic methods of measuring attenuation. The best standardized method is known as the measurement of real ear attenuation at threshold (REAT). In this technique a group of subjects are tested audiometrically with either pure tones or one-third octave bands of noise to find their sound thresholds at different frequencies with and without the helmet or headset. The difference between the values is taken to represent the amount of sound excluded by the protective device, that is, its attenuation. Objections to this method are that it is laborious and prodigal of subjects; moreover the measurements are taken only at isolated frequencies or frequency bands so that if the device exhibits

bizarre properties between these points, this will go undetected. Furthermore, the evaluation is conducted in extreme quiet and the device may exhibit different properties when exposed to higher levels of noise; and large amounts of variance exist in the data. The alternative method is to use miniature microphones. One microphone is inserted under the ear muff (that is, at the ear), and the other is placed outside. The difference between the outputs of these two calibrated microphones is taken to represent the attenuation. The method is quick, easy and accurate, all frequencies may be measured and analysed in any form, the measurements are made in high levels of ambient noise and can even be made in an aircraft while the aircrew are at work.

The two methods are not wholly incompatible, but significant differences occur at the lower frequencies (*Figure 24.28*). These can be attributed to auditory masking at low frequencies caused by the blood flow in the carotid artery resulting in low-frequency pressure pulses in the ear canal which mask the incoming acoustic detection signal and require higher levels of signal to allow satisfactory detection.

Hearing loss

When exposure to high noise levels ceases a number of after-effects may be manifest. These include ringing in the ears (tinnitus), caused by continued firing in the auditory nerve (apparently a sort of irritative after-effect), and a partial deafness, or

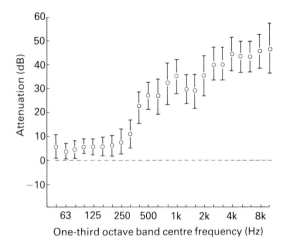

Figure 24.27 Noise attenuation provided by an aircrew helmet (RAF aircrew helmet Mk 4) on a population of subjects (mean ± 2 standard deviations).

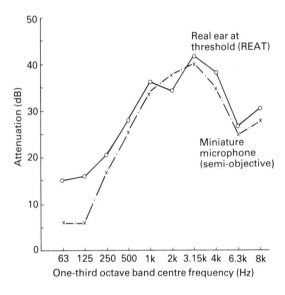

Figure 24.28 Sound attenuation provided by a helmet measured by real ear at threshold (REAT) technique and using a miniature microphone inserted beneath the ear muff.

reduced sensitivity to sound known as 'noise-induced temporary threshold shift' (TTS). If exposure to loud noises is continued, then a permanent form of deafness or permanent threshold shift (PTS) (*see also* Chapter 50) is manifested. Although permanent deafness is of more practical interest than TTS (TTS may, however, be important, for example to combat troops being discharged from a noisy troop-carrying aircraft), there is a relationship between the two quantities.

Temporary threshold shift

The degree of temporary threshold shift is measured by subtracting the threshold data measured for an individual at a given time after a noise exposure from his resting (unexposed) threshold data. Since recovery of hearing after the exposure is fairly rapid, the time between the end of the exposure and the measurement of the hearing level is important. The frequency at which the maximum TTS is manifested is not necessarily that of the sound exposure. The maximum TTS generally occurs at a higher frequency than that of the sound which caused it (*Figure 24.29*). The greater degree of shift is found in the 3–6 kHz band. It is also this band which shows the greatest permanent loss due to continued exposure, in particular at 4 kHz. The magnitude of the TTS following exposure to a sound of a given pressure level is determined by the logarithm of the exposure time. When the length of the exposure is fixed, the magnitude of the TTS is determined by the SPL of the sound producing the TTS. The pressure level of the sound and the exposure time may be combined to describe the overall noise exposure or noise 'dose'. In a changing noise environment, this quantity is difficult to assess by independent measurements of sound pressure level and duration of exposure; and, consequently, noise 'dose meters' are commercially available to give a direct read-out of the integrated dose.

There is some evidence that there is a relationship between the temporary threshold shift produced by a short exposure to a noise and the permanent threshold shift brought about by continued exposure. It is suggested, for example, that if the temporary threshold shift is measured 2 minutes after an 8-hour exposure, this is equivalent in dB to

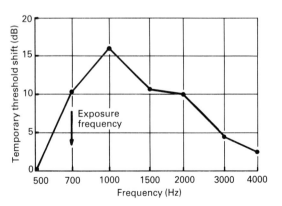

Figure 24.29 Temporary threshold shift measured 5 minutes after the end of an exposure to a pure tone of 700 Hz for 5 minutes. The maximum shift occurred at a frequency of 1000 Hz.

the 10-year permanent threshold shift produced by exposure to the noise for 8 hours per day. This is a statistical relationship which cannot be applied to the individual. Temporary threshold shift measured on a large number of individuals can be used, however, to make some predictions about the long-term hazards presented by the noise to that population.

Acceptable noise levels

Acceptable noise depends largely upon the reason for the need for acceptability. Acceptability for good speech communications is liable to be very different than that for the reduction of hearing damage risk.

In, for instance, aircraft cabin noise specifications, some compromises are made to the varying requirements but, generally, if the aircraft cabin noise, in both fixed- and rotary-wing aircraft, meets the recommended levels then the majority of criteria for acceptable noise levels will be satisfied.

For hearing damage alone, it is difficult to establish an 'acceptable' or 'safe' noise level whether by retrospective or prospective means, because such a survey depends on a population that has been exposed to a reasonably constant source of noise for a long time. In a retrospective survey, some assumptions must be made about the original audiograms (which will almost certainly be unavailable). It is generally agreed that exposures to noises of less than 75–80 dB(A) produce no increase in deafness in a population. (A population becomes deafer as it grows older because of normal ageing processses. When the effects of noise are referred to, what is meant is the increased incidence or level of deafness in a population, over that occurring by normal ageing (presbyacusis).) Above this level, there is a relationship between the degree of permanent threshold shift, the duration of the exposure and the sound pressure level and the frequency constitution of the noise.

The methods of calculating the hearing 'damage risk' in specific conditions is simplified, but not degraded, by the requirements to measure the noise on the A weighting scale only.

Different daily exposures can be converted to a standard exposure by adjusting the effective sound pressure level (that is, producing a 'loudness equivalent'—Leq), and thus the increased risk of deafness can be determined from a table (*see* ISO document R1999).

In industry it is common practice, for safety's sake, to make the simple, easily supervised rule that all personnel should wear ear defenders whenever they work in an environment where the ambient noise is in excess of 85 dB(A). Military aircrew regularly wear the best ear protection available, and yet during normal operational flying they may be exposed to levels well in excess of 85 dB(A) despite their protection. Since the cochlea does not distinguish between noise, speech, music etc.—this function is performed by higher centres in the brain—damage may occur not only by cabin noise but also by high communication levels or non-verbal signals. The noise dose may be measured at the ear directly by means of miniature microphones placed beneath the ear muff. This technique has shown that the contribution to the overall dose made by the communications signal is a significant one; but one cannot yet be certain whether the modern helmet worn properly in modern military aircraft sufficiently protects the hearing. Final conclusions on this point can only emerge from the study of regular audiograms of aircrew and controls over a long period.

It is important to be aware that since individuals vary greatly in their susceptibility to hearing damage, there is no method for predicting individual risk of hearing damage. Current predictions are for groups of humans exposed to a given noise immission (a product of level and time of exposure) and will only allow prediction as to the percentage of the group that will suffer impairment—not the individuals within that group that will suffer.

Personal audiograms, however, will allow an assessment of an individual's hearing loss directly and should be taken on a regular basis for aircrew, groundcrew or others regularly exposed to high noise levels.

Psychological effects of noise

No one likes noise. Aircrew operating noisy aircraft state that the noise causes fatigue, makes them irritated, and effectively increases their workload. They all regard it as some sort of flight safety hazard. It may be that these effects are direct consequences of the noise acting as a stressor, but this is unlikely. The effects that aircrew report probably arise from the increased difficulty in interpreting communications. Listening to speech is work in the sense that it is a form of information processing; it requires mental capacity and it takes time.

Identification or response time to speech is related to the intelligibility of what is said. While intelligibility cannot, for practical reasons, be used as a convenient index of the workload generated by communications, response time can be. *Figure 24.30*

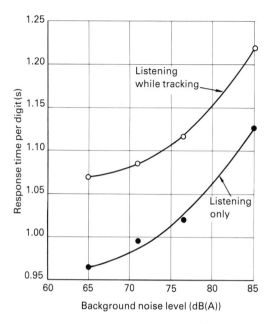

Figure 24.30 Effects of level of environmental noise on time taken to respond to a rapidly presented series of digits. The higher the background noise—that is, the lower the signal:noise ratio—the longer the response time. When the subject had to perform a tracking task as well as the listening task the response time at a given signal:noise ratio was increased.

shows the result of an experiment in which a subject was required to respond to a rapidly presented series of digits at various signal/noise ratios, both when he was concurrently performing a tracking task and when he was not. The time to respond to a list of digits is affected both by the signal/noise ratio and by the addition of the other task. That is, there is competition for the available mental capacity between the man's normal piloting activities and his communications processing requirements. This competition is aggravated by reduced intelligibility (increasing the noise level) and it should not be regarded as surprising that the result is fatigue and irritation produced by this effective increase in workload.

In the laboratory, noise may certainly be shown to act as a stressor, affecting the performance of tasks, producing 'narrowing of attention' as well as making other tasks (for example, the memorizing of some sort of material) more difficult, though it is not easy to design experiments which are free of extraneous influences. There are, however a number of generalized statements that can be made on noise levels, the task involved and the individual characteristics of the operator.

For the noise field the following parameters may affect task performance:

1. Continuous noise with specific meaning to the task involved will not generally impair performance below 90 dB(A).
2. Intermittent noise and impulsive noise are generally more disruptive than continuous noise at the same level.
3. High-frequency components of noise generally have a more adverse affect on performance than the lower frequency content.
4. Noise tends to increase errors and variability rather than directly affect work rate.

It has been shown that greater performance decrements are attributable to noise where the task involves continuous operation, requires prolonged vigilance or where two tasks are performed simultaneously than tasks that require simple repetition. In fact, in simple repetitive tasks, the overall performance may be enhanced by noise. Tasks that involve perception of auditory cues are, *per se*, most susceptible to noise impairment.

Where individual differences are concerned, identical levels of noise and exposure will affect different operators in (sometimes radically) different ways. This will essentially depend upon the operator's previous experience in performing the task under conditions of noise, the levels of arousal and motivation, and generally the personality—introverts may be more affected than extroverts.

Other stressors, such as vibration, heat, hypoxia, loss of sleep etc., are known to interact with noise and result in synergistic effects (i.e. the combined effect is greater than the sum of the individual effects). An example is in the perception of ride quality in aircraft where ride quality is assessed more severely under conditions of noise and vibration together than an assessment using the sum of the two individual stress contributors.

A further parameter is duration of exposure, since the adverse effects of noise appear to be cumulative, involving a large decrease in performance at the end of the task period—particularly important if the period of exposure is prolonged.

In many ways, defining the effects of noise on human performance is like trying to define annoyance. Both are a function of many parameters, human and environmental, and research results, generally available on a statistical basis, again apply only to groups of people; not to individuals.

The psychological effects of noise are weighted differently under different conditions. Much effort, ingenuity and skill may be needed to carry out tasks under adverse noise conditions. There are innumerable ways of completing a task and even under ideal conditions humans vary in the way they approach and deal with each phase of the problem. Welford

(1978) notes that 'performance and workload appear, therefore, to depend upon the interaction of four factors: the demands of the task; the capacities of the performer; the strategies used to relate demands to capacities; and, when a range of strategies is available, skill in choosing the most efficient.' He then goes on to look at each variable and, when discussing strategy, notes 'the precise strategy adopted on any one occasion for a particular task involves a synthesis of various generic strategies, all of which are necessary for the particular performance, but none of which is sufficient alone. This is true for familiar activities repeated on different occasions, and is even more true of the strategies adopted when tackling an entirely novel task.'

All of these problems point strongly to the wide range of difficulties in producing a general model of human performance, but there remains general agreement that high levels of noise in the crew compartment have a deleterious effect on performance, and this is supported by increasing anecdotal and empirical evidence drawn from comparisons of the quieter combat aircraft, such as the Tornado, with the less quiet aircraft.

Aircraft noise in the environment

The noise created by subsonic aircraft only affects the general population during take-off and landing

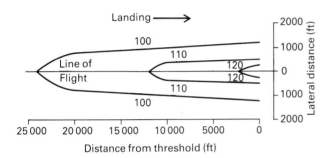

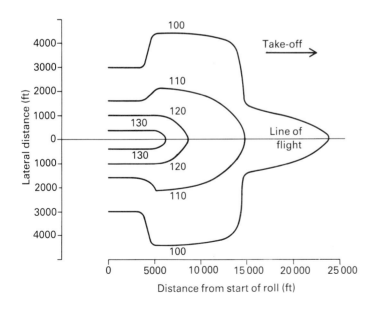

Figure 24.31 Peak values of perceived noise level for a heavy jet aircraft at indicated points during landing and take-off. The figures alongside the contours indicate the values of PNdB.

phases. There are also other phases of flight during which military aircraft obtrude upon the population—low-flying practice and weapons practice, for example, though the ranges and routes are deliberately located as far away as possible.

Noise around airfields is not primarily a health hazard. There is some evidence of increased psychiatric morbidity, or increased recognition of morbidity among the population living in the areas around noisy airports. Any social stress of course may manifest itself in psychiatric symptoms among the susceptible; and there is a social problem of noise around airfields as is made clear by the number of complaints. It is not easy to correlate the social problem with physical measurement of the noise level, because the degree of disturbance to any individual will depend on many factors: how loud it is; the pitch; its quality; whether there are discrete bands in broad-band noise; irregularites of pitch; whether it is continuous or intermittent; how unexpected it is; at what time of the day or night it comes; whether it is particularly inappropriate to one's activity; individual susceptibility; and, finally, emotional 'overtones' which colour one's attitude.

It is clear that it is difficult to take all these factors into account in attempting to assess the subjective effects of airfield noise in physical terms. Research has shown that the most important factors that determine the annoyance of aircraft noise are the 'noisiness' of the exposure and the frequency of its presentation (i.e. the number of aircraft movements). The number of movements is easy to measure, and the most accepted measure of noise to give an indication of 'noisiness' is Kryter's measure of 'perceived noise level' (PNL) which is measured in 'perceived noise dB' (PNdB).

Perceived noise level is a subjectively based scale. The PNL of a noise is defined as the level of a reference noise judged by normal observers as being equally noisy. The reference sound used is a band of random noise between one-third and one octave wide centred on 1000 Hz. The method is standardized and the PNdB may be calculated from an octave band measurement of SPL. The scale has been evolved with the measurement of aircraft noise specifically in mind. The shape of the PNL contours in the vicinity of a typical airport is shown in *Figure 24.31*.

Results from a number of surveys, but in particular in the vicinity of Heathrow Airport, have shown that the degree of annoyance complained of varies in a regular way with both noisiness and number of aircraft movements. It has been found that increases of both PNL and movements cause an increase in annoyance; and, moreover, that the effect of annoyance of a 9 PNdB increase is the same as the effects of a four-fold increase in numbers of aircraft. A simple relationship may thus be described—the noise and number index (NNI)—

which gives an overall indication of annoyance level. This NNI is defined as:

$$NNI = (PNdB)_N + 15\log_{10}N - 80$$

where $(PNdB)_N$ = average peak noise level of an aircraft operating during a day; N = number of aircraft operations over a 24 hour period.

Table 24.4 indicates the conditions produced by different values of NNI. Values of around 40 NNI are only moderately annoying in general but are annoying in terms of intrusiveness. In the same way that PNdB contours may be drawn around airports, NNI contours may be constructed for an airport or any other location, and will indicate the numbers of people liable to suffer some form of annoyance.

The NNI method generally involves assessment of the annoyance involved in civil aircraft operating normally from a civil airport. Military procedures are often different in form for operational reasons and the Royal Air Force has evolved a criterion based on equivalent continuous noise level (Leq) used in conjunction with the 'A' weighting. This index, and the maximum sound level in dB(A), are used to assess environmental noise around airfields.

The criteria are:

1. Dwellings exposed to a maximum sound level in excess of 125 dB(A) should be purchased by use of compulsory powers if necessary.

Table 24.4 Annoyance caused by aircraft noise – population response for various values of the noise and number index (NNI)

NNI value	Examples of conditions
10	Occasional aircraft flying overhead producing noise levels which cause disturbance out of doors but not within houses
35	Regular overflights by aircraft, noise levels intrusive inside houses
55	Continual overflying at noise levels which can interfere with conversation within houses – this is the level above which soundproofing grants are available around London (Heathrow) Airport
65	Incessant overflying by aircraft at noise levels which can interfere with sleep and conversation even within soundproofed houses
75	This very high value can occur beneath intensively used flight paths when departing aircraft are still low and using full power. No residential accommodation in the UK is subjected to such NNI levels

2. Dwellings exposed to maximum sound levels of between 117 and 125 dB(A) on a recurring basis (or a 12 hour Leq of 83 dB(A) or more) should be purchased if owners or occupiers wish, but no compulsory purchase should be exercised.
3. 12-hour Leq in excess of 70 dB(A) qualifies for grant assistance.
4. Additionally, dwellings falling within the maximum single event footprint of 82 B(A), where more than 20 aircraft movements per night occur regularly, also qualify for grant assistance.

Reducing environmental noise levels

Ideally, aircraft noise should be reduced at source, and this approach has paid dividends in that current civil jet aircraft are significantly quieter than their predecessors by virtue of improved engine design. Generally, however, aircraft—particularly military aircraft—are still noisy, and it seems to be the verdict of society that the penalty suffered by the relatively few people who experience the problem is justified by the provision of high-speed travel for large numbers of people and defence of the realm. The lot of these people can be improved in a number of ways. These include: siting (airfields and airports should be kept away from populated areas); noise abatement procedures which limit the use of engine power to the minimum consistent with safety; insulation of roofs, walls and windows; and restrictions on the operating hours of airfields so as to reduce the NNI to a minimal level at night and early morning.

Similarly for military airfields, purchase of properties exposed to unacceptable levels and grants for acoustic insulation schemes for the lower levels of noise exposure assist in preventing annoyance and lead to better coexistence between the military operators and the exposed public.

References

BERANEK, L.L. (ed.) (1971) *Noise and Vibration Control*. New York: McGraw-Hill.
ZWICKER, E. (1960) *A Method for Calculating Loudness*. Acoustica. Akustiche, Beihtfte

Further reading

ANSI S3.5 (1969) *Methods for the Calculation of the Articulation Index*. American National Standards Institute.
ANSI S6.4 (1973) *Definitions and Procedures for Computing the Effective Perceived Noise Level for Flyover Aircraft Noise*. American National Standards Institute.
ANSI S3.14 (1977) *For Rating Noise with Respect to Speech Interference*. American National Standards Institute.
ANSI S12.6 (1984)/ASA STD 1 (1975) *Method for the Measurement of Real Ear Protection of Hearing Protectors*. American National Standards Institute.
ANSI S1.42 (1986) *Design Response of Weighting Networks for Acoustical Measurements*. American National Standards Institute.
ASA S3.2 (1960) *Measurement of Monosyllabic Word Intelligibility*. American Standards Association.
BERANEK, L.L. (ed.) (1960) *Noise Reduction*. New York: McGraw-Hill.
BROCH, J.P. (1971) *Acoustic Noise Measurement*. Naerum, Denmark: Bruel and Kjaer.
BS 5330 (1976) *Estimating the Risk of Hearing Handicap Due to Noise Exposure*. British Standards Institution.
BS 5108 (1983)/ISO 4869 (1981) *Measurement of Sound Attenuation of Hearing Protectors*. British Standards Institution.
BS 5108 (1974) *Method of Measurement of Hearing Protectors at Threshold*. British Standards Institution.
BS 2497 (1972) *The Normal Threshold of Hearing for Fine Tones by Earphone Listening*. British Standards Institution.
BS 3045 (1958) *The Relation Between the Sone Scale of Loudness and the Phon Scale of Loudness Level*. British Standards Instituion.
BURNS, W. (1973) *Noise and Man*. London: John Murray.
IEC 179 (1900) *Specification for Precision Sound Level Meters*. International Organisation for Standardisation.
ISO R 131 (1959) *Expression of the Physical and Subjective Magnitudes of Sound or Noise*. International Organisation for Standardisation.
ISO 2204 (1973) *Guide to the Measurement of Airborne Acoustical Noise and Evaluation of its Effects on Man*. International Organisation of Standardisation.
ISO R 226 (1961) *Normal Equal Loudness Contours for Pure Tones and Normal Threshold of Hearing under Free Field Listening Conditions*. International Organisation for Standardisation.
ISO R 1996 (1971) *Assessment of Noise with Respect to Community Response*. International Organisation for Standardisation.
ISO 1999 (1975) *Assessment of Occupational Noise Exposure for Hearing Conservation Purposes*. International Organisation for Standardisation.
ISO R 266 (1975) *Preferred Frequencies for Acoustical Measurements*. International Organisation for Standardisation.
KRYTER, K.D. (1970) *The Effect of Noise on Man*. New York: Academic Press.
MAY, D.N. (1978) *Handbook of Noise Assessment*. New York: Van Nostrand Reinhold.
MILLER, R.D. (1971) *Effects of Noise on People*. Washington, DC: US Environmental Protection Agency.
MIL-STD-1294 (1981) *Acoustical Noise Limits in Helicopters*. Washington, DC: US Department of Defense.
MIL-S-00806B (1970) *General Specification for Sound Pressure Levels in Aircraft*. Washington, DC: US Department of Defense.
PETERSON, A.P.G. and GROSS, E.E. (1972) *Handbook of Noise Measurement*. Concord, US: General Radio.

STEVENS, S.S. (1956) Calculation of the loudness of a complex noise. *Journal of the Acoustical Society of America,* **28**, 807–832

WELCH, B. and WELCH, A.S. (eds) (1970) *Psychological Effects of Noise.* New York: Plenum Press.

WELFORD, A.T. (1978) Mental workload as a function of demand, capacity, strategy and skill. *Ergonomics,* **21**, 151–167

Part V

Aviation Psychology

Introduction to aviation psychology

R.G. Green

If, as Eysenck asserts, psychology is about people, then aviation psychology is about people who fly—pilots, navigators, engineers, cabin crew, and passengers. Defining the population of interest to the aviation psychologist is, however, easy in comparison with providing the reader with an introduction to the roots and territory of modern psychology.

The function of these psychology chapters is not to attempt to turn the reader into an aviation psychologist, but to provide him with a background knowledge of the subject.

Airlines and air forces employ relatively large numbers of doctors to fulfil essential practical functions. It is therefore inescapable that the man on the spot (whether it is an airline office or fighter base) who will be consulted about all problems related to the 'human factor' in the aviation system will be the doctor.

What follows is written to enable the doctor to give opinions on problems not previously familiar to him, or, at least, to be aware of the area covered by aviation psychology and thus to know whether help should be sought. However, an attempt will first be made to give some idea of the nature of modern psychology.

Psychology as a science

Some readers may feel that psychology is based on speculation rather than evidence, lacks precision, or is simply commonsense rendered incomprehensible with jargon. Such arguments may be sustainable in some areas of psychology, and some would say that the reason for this is that psychology is a relatively recent science still awaiting its Newton and Einstein.

This would not be entirely fair, for the essential problem of psychology is the modelling and explanation of behaviour, and behaviour is variable and subject to many influences. Some headway has, however, been made. During this century there have been two disparate general approaches or schools of thought that have dominated the development of psychology. The first is *Psychoanalysis*, or the psychodynamic approach, which was developed by Freud. He was a clinician who realized (in working with those termed, at the end of the last century, hysterics) that not all his patients' symptoms could be attributed to organic disease. He developed an initial model in which he accounted for the problems of his patients in terms of the ways in which their personalities had developed and the ways in which they responded to events, especially traumatic events, in their past.

Freud saw what he termed psychosexual development (a core concept in his theories) as falling into three main phases—the oral, anal, and genital phases—and believed that the adult personality depended on the ways in which development might have become fixated in one of these phases. Freud suggested, for example, that those orally deprived as infants will grow to be exploitive of others, aggressive, and jealous, whereas those who experienced an opposite kind of oral phase will be over-optimistic and dependent. Later in life Freud developed his well-known tri-partite model of the 'psyche' which comprised the 'id', the seat of all animalistic impulses driven only by the pleasure principle, the 'superego', that mental policeman that incorporates moral teaching and restraint, and the 'ego' which is the real you, mediating the conflicting demands of the id and the superego.

If the popularity of ideas were a good test of their truth, then psychoanalysis would easily pass. The terms coined by Freud have become part of everyday language, his philosophy has affected twentieth century thinking in many ways, and the practice of fairly classic psychoanalysis as a treatment for the depressed and dissatisfied is still widespread.

But it is easy to criticize Freud's entire approach. The models that Freud developed can be seen as responses to his own rather unusual upbringing by a doting mother (giving rise to the developmental ideas) and to the First World War (which caused him to ponder the worst of which man is capable). Nowhere does Freud subject his ideas to experimental test; he simply believed from his experience that they worked. In this important sense, Freud's approach can be described as pre- or non-scientific. Eysenck, a modern personality theorist, has described Freud's work as having set back the treatment of mental illness by 150 years. Some current applications of Freudian notions within aviation are almost certainly totally misguided (Chapter 28 discusses a bizarre selection test based on the idea of ego defence mechanisms that is, nevertheless, in current use), but some are capable of integration in a more rational approach (for example, the 'actions not as planned' described later are closely related to the 'Freudian slip').

Even at the turn of the century, there were those who took an entirely different approach to the study of mental life. Perhaps the most notable of these was Ebbinghaus, principally remembered for his pioneering work on the study of human memory. If Freud was concerned with why people forget things, Ebbinghaus was more concerned with how. His experimental findings on the apparent decay of information in human memory still stand, but more importantly he paved the way for the growth of the second approach to psychological investigation, the experimental approach.

It cannot be escaped that the most influential school of thought within the experimental approach has been *Behaviourism*, and that the most notable behaviourist is Skinner. All pure behaviourists believe that the only legitimate matter for scientific study is that which may be objectively observed. Such an approach leads directly to the sort of experiment in which a definable stimulus is presented and observable behaviour (the response) recorded. Many experiments along these lines have been conducted in the 'Skinner box', a piece of equipment in which an animal may be placed in order to see how its behaviour is modified by a regime of rewards (such as food) and punishments (such as electric shock). Results from experiments such as these were used directly in the construction of programmed learning courses and in the development of 'teaching machines' which may be regarded as open-plan Skinner boxes. Behaviourist ideas have also been applied in attempts to rehabilitate young

offenders, to treat sexual deviants, and to socialize schizophrenics. Of particular interest in the present context are the 'behaviour therapies' that have been adapted to treat those suffering from motion sickness or from flying phobia (*see below*). The importance of behaviourism to psychology in general, however, is that it did not rely on dreams and introspection, but adopted a strictly experimental approach to the evaluation of psychological ideas.

The strength of behaviourism, its rejection of the necessity to consider mental events, is also its weakness. It pays no regard to individual motives or feelings, and leads to the notion that people perform badly not because of intrinsic weaknesses but because they are victims of a less than optimal environment; all their behaviour and personality is seen as a set of responses produced by the stimuli to which they happen to have been exposed.

Behaviourism may have been an important influence in bringing a scientific approach to psychology, but there have been other shaping factors, and these have tended to stem from the technology of the day. When telephone exchanges represented the height of technological achievement, the nervous system was frequently likened to them; but a more important influence on psychological thought came from the telecommunications industry—information theory. It became important to be able to quantify information so that the channel capacity of a given link could be measured objectively. It was possible not only to compute, for example, how many telephone conversations equated to one television picture, but it enabled psychologists to develop models of how humans process information. The information processing approach to human cognition is dealt with in some detail in this book. In dealing with humans in this way, it will become apparent to the reader that the most recent influence on psychology has been the computer.

Although the comparison between the most basic function of the nervous system—the firing or non-firing of a single cell—and the binary states that exist within a computer is tempting, the physical mechanisms of brains and machines are clearly very different. The analogy exists at what might be termed a system level. Computers and brains both appear to have central elements that are crucially necessary, that have to be supported by short- and long-term memory stores, and that may be used to control other, apparently autonomous, devices. To give a banal example, the reader will be able, simultaneously, both to think and walk, the computer both to calculate and drive a printer. The processors and buffer stores required for one may have something to tell us about the mechanisms required for the other. At this system level, we may represent a memory as a labelled box without regard for its physical reality; it is of no relevance whether its physical location is in the cortex, cerebellum, or hippocampus. The important consideration is whether our model of labelled boxes appears to describe the ways in which people are observed to behave, and whether the model yields predictions that may be tested by experiment or simulation.

The testing of theories by experiment will be familiar, but the advent of small yet powerful computers has enabled the models of human information processing to exist not just on paper, but in such machines. The creation of such artificial intelligence has enabled human problem solving not only to be simulated in very sophisticated ways, but has already started to pay for itself in the development of the computer systems used in pattern and voice recognition, and in the 'expert' systems already used, for example, in medical diagnosis.

Aviation psychology

Today, the range of topics tackled by psychologists is wide. At one extreme, social psychology and sociology merge indistinguishably in attempting to study the ways in which people relate to one another, and, at the other extreme, the physiological psychologist and physiologist enjoy an equal identity. Psychologists are not simply concerned with the conduct of research but have found themselves filling vocational careers in society. Educational psychologists are to be found assessing children who are slow learners or behaviourally difficult, clinical psychologists both assessing and treating the psychologically sick, and industrial psychologists providing support in a wide variety of ways to many government and commercial bodies.

Aviation psychology has been distinguishable from other applications since the Second World War, and, in keeping pace with the technology of aviation, can fairly be said to have been in the vanguard of applied psychology since then. World War II created a large demand for aircrew, and this acted as the spur for the consideration of problems of selection and training. The problem of deciding whether a given individual possessed the qualities that would give him a reasonable chance of successfully completing training was crucial then and is still important today.

If the problem has remained, the conditions have changed. The pilot is no longer flying a machine with manual controls and direct displays. Today's military aircraft cannot function without complex electronics connecting the controls to the control surfaces. The pilot's information displays are generated by other computers that acquire and evaluate vast quantities of data before deciding what

the pilot should be made aware of. How can we tell whether we need the same sort of pilot to fly traditional and modern aircraft? Do we need the same sort of pilot to fly a military aircraft in combat for an hour as is needed to fly 400 passengers in a 14-hour cruise?

Pilot training has always been expensive but today, in keeping with the cost of aircraft, it is astronomically so. These costs are wasted if the pilot and aircraft are lost in an accident, and this has provided the spur for aviation psychologists to participate in the investigation of human error. Although this study has become the sole activity of some psychologists, it is not dealt with separately in this book. This is because accidents happen for many reasons; they may be caused by personality problems, poor social relationships on the flight deck, failures of perception or skill, domestic or environmental stress, or by poor design of equipment. The following chapters attempt to address these problems, since an understanding of all of them is necessary if the psychologist is to make a useful contribution to the safety and efficiency of flight.

Beyond the scope of the following chapters is an attempt to provide an understanding of the investigative or research techniques in psychology, though the teaching of these techniques may comprise a large part of an undergraduate psychology course. It is sometimes said that the important thing about a psychologist is not what he knows, but his know-how. There is a good deal of truth in this, but it has already been observed that the object of this book is not to turn the reader into a psychologist but to provide a background knowledge. He should thus be aware that interviews, questionnaires, laboratory experiments, and field trials constitute the routes for the acquisition of psychological knowledge, but need not concern himself with the details of these procedures or the statistics required for their analysis.

A difficulty in producing a text that is both a theoretical introduction and an applied primer is in knowing how to organize the material since some will be concerned with psychological models of personality, human perception and information processing, social interaction, and behaviour under stress; and some with the applied problems of equipment design, selection, training, and accident prevention. An essentially pragmatic approach has been adopted in which some chapters address principally theoretical issues and some the applied problems, but, throughout, attempts have been made to illustrate the interdependence of these approaches.

This introduction has attempted to put aviation psychology into its historical and contemporary context: the thinking and techniques used clearly stem from identifiable roots but it is a modern discipline tackling a wide variety of safety and efficiency problems in a technology-based industry. The authors of the following chapters have a genuine enthusiasm for the subject—we hope that the reader will find himself sharing it.

Further reading

COLEMAN, J.C. (1977) *Introductory Psychology: A Textbook for Health Students*. London: Routledge and Kegan Paul
MILLER, G. (1966) *Psychology: The Science of Mental Life*. Harmondsworth: Pelican Books

Glossary of terms used in aviation psychology

Achievement test   A test of the individual's current ability to perform a particular activity (cf. APTITUDE TEST).

Action not as planned   'Absent-minded' behaviour particularly likely to occur during skilled activity for which MOTOR PROGRAMMES have been developed.

Ambient visual system   The visual system responsible primarily for the acquisition of orientation information (cf. *FOCAL VISUAL SYSTEM*).

Aptitude test   A test that attempts to predict the efficiency with which an inexperienced individual will be able to perform a particular activity after practice (cf. ACHIEVEMENT TEST).

Arousal   The degree of activation or alertness, controlled by impulses from the ascending reticular activating system to the cortex.

Attention   The allocation of MENTAL RESOURCES to particular information sources or activities. Selective and focused attention involve restriction of the information sources to which resources are applied, the former under voluntary control but the latter imposed by environmental conditions; divided attention involves the allocation of resources to two or more information sources.

Behaviourism   The school of psychological thought that rejects the validity of covert mental processes as useful concepts in the explanation of behaviour, relying solely upon observable responses to stimuli.

Bottom-up processing   Information processing that is driven by the nature of environmental stimuli.

Cocktail party phenomenon   An everyday example of a selective ATTENTION task, in which an attempt is made to listen to one speaker in the presence of other competing conversations.

Cognitive dissonance   A mental state produced by conflict between the individual's beliefs and the evidence before him. The individual strives to reduce dissonance by changing his beliefs or by ignoring or re-interpreting the evidence.

Cognitive failure   A lapse of perception, memory, or action during well-practised activity (*see* ACTION NOT AS PLANNED, MOTOR PROGRAMME).

Cognitive processes   The mechanisms underlying the acquisition, transformation, and storage of information, and the execution of responses.

Conditioning   A learning procedure whereby a response (the 'conditioned response') comes to be elicited by a previously neutral stimulus (the 'conditioned stimulus'). In classical conditioning, the response to be conditioned is initially made instinctively to an 'unconditioned stimulus', e.g. salivation at the sight of food. After repeated juxtaposition of the conditioned and unconditioned stimuli ('reinforcement'), the conditioned stimulus becomes effective in eliciting a similar response (the 'conditioned response'). In instrumental conditioning, the conditioned response is made in order to obtain a goal; positive reinforcement involves a reward, e.g. food presented after pressing a lever, whereas negative reinforcement involves punishment, e.g. an electric shock on turning into the wrong alley in a maze. Extinction occurs when reinforcement is withheld. During extinction, episodes of 'spontaneous recovery' of the conditioned response are likely after rest periods. The conditioned response may be elicited by stimuli similar to the conditioned stimuli–stimulus generalization.

Consolidation   The process by which information is laid down in long-term MEMORY.

Correlation coefficient   An index of the closeness of the relationship between two variables.

Culture-free, culture-fair   Ideally, scores on mental tests, such as those measuring intelligence, should be unaffected by the individual's cultural background (culture-free); in practice, this objective is unattainable, and it is more realistic to attempt to minimize the advantage of one culture over another (culture-fair).

Dichotic listening task.   A task in which pairs of stimuli are presented, one to each ear, in rapid succession.

Distal stimulus   The stimulus as it exists in the external world (cf. PROXIMAL STIMULUS).

Ergonomics   The study of work, particularly in relation to man–machine systems (*see* HUMAN FACTORS).

Extraversion   One of Eysenck's three dimensions of PERSONALITY, the major components of which are sociability and impulsiveness.

Factor analysis   A statistical technique used to reduce a complex table of inter-correlations between variables to a small number of factors, each representing a fundamental source of variation in the data. Some PERSONALITY tests were constructed using this method.

Feedback Information about the effects of an action that is used to control later action.

Focal visual system The visual system that is concerned primarily with the identification of objects (cf. AMBIENT VISUAL SYSTEM).

General adaptation syndrome Selye's notion that any stressor produces a fixed pattern of physiological adaptation, in three phases: the alarm reaction, the stage of resistance, and the stage of exhaustion.

Human factors An American term to denote the study of man in his working environment, roughly equivalent to ERGONOMICS.

Hygiene factor In Herzberg's theory, a job context factor that prevents dissatisfaction, but cannot produce satisfaction (*see* MOTIVATOR).

Idiographic An approach to psychological enquiry that emphasizes the uniqueness of the individual and the sources of individual differences (cf. NOMOTHETIC).

Intelligence quotient (IQ) Defined as (MENTAL AGE/chronological age) × 100. This is a true ratio IQ. Some intelligence tests use a deviation IQ based on the number of standard deviations by which the individual's score deviates from the sample mean.

Interference In MEMORY, forgetting produced by new information (retroactive interference) or by old information (proactive inhibition).

Leadership styles The behaviour of leaders varies along several dimensions. A fundamental distinction may be drawn between 'task-oriented' leadership (concern with achieving the group's goals) and 'relationship-oriented' leadership (concern with maintaining group morale).

Memory The storage of information. Three major memory systems can be distinguished: sensory memory acts as a very brief buffer for information arriving at the sensory receptors; short-term memory has a duration of a few seconds, and its functional aspects are emphasized by the alternative term 'working memory'; long-term memory is the system responsible for effectively permanent storage of knowledge about the world, two facets of which are semantic memory (for information such as word meanings) and episodic memory (for incidents in the individual's personal history).

Mental age The chronological age for which the individual's performance on intelligence tests is representative (*see* INTELLIGENCE QUOTIENT).

Mental capacity, mental resources Virtually synonymous terms referring to the processing facilities that the information processing system has available to perform its activities. It is clear that mental capacity is limited; a more controversial issue is whether there are separate resource pools specialized for particular types of processing (*see* SINGLE CHANNEL THEORY, MULTIPLE RESOURCES).

Mental workload The total demand upon the operator associated with the attainment of a particular level of task performance.

Motivation The needs and drives that determine behaviour.

Motivator In Herzberg's theory, a job content factor that helps to satisfy the need for self-actualization, and produces job satisfaction (*see* HYGIENE FACTOR).

Motor programme A behavioural 'subroutine', developed after practice on a skill, that requires minimal central processing resources. Activities controlled by motor programmes are characterized by 'open-loop' processing, in which little use is made of FEEDBACK concerning the effects of actions, rather than the 'closed-loop' processing of activities to which attention is directed.

Multiple resources The notion that there exist separate, specialized pools of MENTAL RESOURCES (cf. SINGLE CHANNEL THEORY).

Neuroticism One of Eysenck's three dimensions of PERSONALITY, reflecting the individual's level of trait anxiety.

Nomothetic An approach that attempts to discover general laws or principles of behaviour (cf. IDIOGRAPHIC).

Perception The interpretation of sensory information.

Perceptual constancy The relatively unchanging PERCEPTION of an object, despite variations in the pattern of stimulation received by the sense organs. For example, the retinal image of an object moving away from an observer becomes progressively smaller, but the object's size is perceived as constant. Constancies of shape, brightness and colour can also be demonstrated.

Performance operating characteristic (POC) A function depicting the level of performance attained on two concurrent tasks, as the priority assigned to each is varied. If performance on a task is found to vary with allocation of processing resources, it is said to be resource limited; if not, it is said to be data limited.

Personality Enduring predispositions to behave in particular ways. The traits that comprise personality can be distinguished from states, which represent transient changes in behaviour or mood.

Projective technique A method in which the subject's interpretation of a vague stimulus is assumed to reflect his PERSONALITY.

Proximal stimulus The stimulus as it is received by a sensory organ (cf. DISTAL STIMULUS).

Psychoanalysis An influential school of psychological thought founded by Sigmund Freud. One of the major contributions of psychoanalytic theory is the notion of unconscious motivation of behaviour.

Psychoticism One of Eysenck's three dimensions of PERSONALITY, reflecting the individual's level of tough-mindedness.

Rehearsal Maintenance rehearsal refers to rote vocal or sub-vocal repetition of information to avoid its loss from short-term MEMORY; elaborative rehearsal involves extraction of the meaning of information to facilitate transfer from short-term to long-term memory.

Reliability In mental testing, the consistency of a test's scores. Split-half and alternate-forms reliability reflect the test's internal consistency, whereas test–retest reliability is a measure of consistency between separate administrations of the test.

Risky shift The riskier decisions made by a group than by the members of the group in isolation.

Selection ratio The ratio of number of selected applicants to total number of applicants.

Shadowing task A selective ATTENTION task in which the individual must repeat a message presented to a particular sensory channel, despite the presence of competing messages.

Single channel theory The notion of a central processor of limited capacity that processes information serially and acts as a 'bottleneck' in the human information processing system.

Social influence The pressure exerted by the group upon the individual to conform to social norms, comply with direct requests, or obey authority.

Stereopsis A binocular cue to depth provided by the slightly different image of a given scene on each retina.

Stress, stressor Stress is a response to unfavourable environmental conditions. These conditions are referred to as stressors.

Success ratio In personnel selection, the ratio of the number of selected applicants who pass the training phase to the total number of applicants selected.

Top-down processing Information processing that is guided by hypotheses concerning the nature of the incoming data (cf. BOTTOM-UP PROCESSING).

Tracking task A dynamic task in which the subject must minimize the discrepancy, introduced by a 'forcing function', between the desired and actual position of a display element. In pursuit tracking, a subject-controlled cursor must follow a moving target; in compensatory tracking, the target is stationary, and only the error (distance between the cursor and the target) is displayed.

Transfer functions In dynamic systems, the relationships between operator input and system output.

Transfer of training The effect of learning a particular task on performance of a later task. Later performance may be either facilitated (positive transfer) or hindered (negative transfer).

Type theory A theory of PERSONALITY that assigns individuals to distinct categories, exemplified by the ancient classification of individuals as phlegmatic, choleric, sanguine, or melancholic.

Validity In mental testing, the degree to which a test measures what it purports to measure.

Yerkes–Dodson Law A law that suggests (a) that there is an optimal AROUSAL level for the performance of any task, performance declining as arousal is increased or decreased from this level (the 'inverted-U' relation); and (b) that the optimal level of arousal is inversely related to task difficulty.

25

Perception

R.G. Green

The five senses of sight, hearing, taste, smell, and touch are familiar to every child. This chapter does not attempt to address these qualities in turn for they do not all present either special difficulties or especially useful attributes to aircrew. For example, the sense of touch is used by the pilot in much the same way that it is used in everyday life. The pilot who is required to wear special, protective, gloves may wish that he had greater tactile sensitivity in his fingers, and it may be by the sense of smell that he first detects noxious fumes in his cockpit; but these are not problems or attributes peculiar to flight.

The visual environment in which the pilot finds himself is, however, very different from that which prevails for the terrestrial observer. He is immediately surrounded by the visual world of his cockpit or flight deck which is both close to him and physically locked to him; when he rolls, it rolls, when he pitches, it pitches. Beyond this is the real world. If he is in cloud, the world is opaque, and if he is in clear conditions there is a gap, sometimes of several miles, between the pilot and the next object, usually the ground. Such a visual gap can never be experienced by the ground-based observer—unless, of course, he looks up.

Hearing is also a sense that is of special importance in the air. Many pilots fly alone, and auditory communication is their only means of contact with any other individual. In the military fighter the only link between the pilot and his navigator is acoustic, and even in the largest airliner the pilot can do nothing but speak to the air traffic controller. In addition to speech, the auditory channel is used as the medium for coded displays and warnings of considerable complexity. Maximizing the effectiveness of this channel is obviously a prime consideration.

Interestingly, the remaining senses of importance to the pilot are not those of which the terrestrial layman is particularly aware. The vestibular and somatosensory systems do not figure at all in the list given at the beginning of this chapter, and the layman is likely to know little of them beyond the fact that his inner ear has something to do with balance. These senses are, however, crucially important in allowing us not just to maintain posture and move but also to control eye movements and preserve a stable visual image of the world. In flying, these senses of orientation remain important but are often sources of difficulty rather than assistance. They can produce profound disorientation in the pilot, they cause problems in the utilization of advanced-technology head-mounted displays, complicate the design of simulator motion systems, and interact with vision to cause motion sickness.

The hearing and vestibular systems are dealt with elsewhere and for this reason, and because of the central importance of vision in flight, this chapter is devoted largely to the problem of visual perception.

Visual perception

On Saturday, 16 July 1983, a British Airways S61 helicopter undertook a normal transit across the sea from Penzance to the Isles of Scilly. The visibility was not good but was greater than that specified as the minimum by the company and the Civil Aviation Authority (CAA). The flight was executed at 2000 feet and the ground was clearly visible to the crew before the aircraft crossed the coast. On approaching the Scillies the aircraft commander let down to 250 feet, intending to stabilize at this height. The co-pilot was busy looking at the radar and navigation equipment, but the captain remembers looking forwards out of the windshield, possibly to identify the islands on which they were closing. While the pilots were engaged in these activities the aircraft lost height and crashed into the water, killing most of those on board.

The reason for noting this accident here is that a serviceable helicopter was flown into the water without the handling pilot having perceived, visually, any height loss, even though he was looking out of the aircraft prior to its impact with the water. Clearly, before any rules or guidelines may be drawn to regulate the visibility requirements for flight, some understanding of the way in which the human visual system works, and the sort of information that it requires, is necessary.

The psychophysiology of vision

The eye is a device that is used to transduce the light radiated and reflected by the external visual world and to generate the neural code that eventually arrives at the visual cortex. An image of the world is formed on the retina by the front elements of the eye. Most of the refraction necessary to form this image is effected by the cornea; the lens is used to make the adjustments required to bring near or far objects into focus on the retina (*see* Chapter 23). The image on the retina is not of good quality as the optical elements of the eye are poorly corrected by comparison with a modern camera lens. There is, thus, a disparity between the nature of the actual image on the retina and the well-corrected picture of the world that we perceive.

That our perception is not isomorphic with the retinal image is easily demonstrated. The retina contains a blank section, the blind spot, where the optic nerve leaves the eye, yet we do not see the world with a section missing. The blind spot may readily be made apparent, however, by locating an image on it. A simple technique for doing so is shown in *Figure 25.1*. If the left eye is closed, and the right eye is used to fixate the cross, the circle will disappear when the page is viewed from the distance (probably about 150 mm) at which the circle falls on the blind spot.

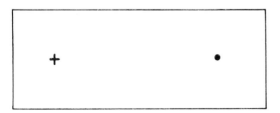

Figure 25.1 Demonstration of the blind spot. With the left eye closed, fixate the cross using the right eye from a distance of about 150 mm. The circle will disappear.

The visual illusions provide further examples of the distinction to be drawn between the 'percept' and the 'data' or the retinal image. The illusion shown in *Figure 25.2* demonstrates the considerable disparity that can exist between the world and the percept, but begs the question of how such a disparity can come about. Clearly, some idea of the way in which the internal model of the world is formed is called for.

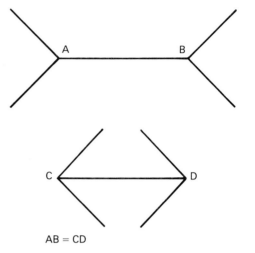

AB = CD

Figure 25.2 The Muller–Lyer illusion. Line CD is the same length as line AB, but appears shorter.

The encoding of visual information begins at retinal level. Recordings from single ganglion cells in the retina show the sort of results shown in *Figure 25.3*. Ganglion cells receive their input from a number of receptors, and the cell illustrated has excitatory synapses between itself and the receptors in the centre of its retinal field, but inhibitory synapses between itself and the receptors in the outside of its retinal field. Such a cell is said to have an 'on' centre with an 'off' surround, and will be maximally stimulated by a light source that exactly covers the centre of its field. Ganglion cells have also been identified that have fields exactly opposite to that described above; i.e. they have 'off' centres with 'on' surrounds.

The firing of ganglion cells habituates if the pattern of stimulation is constant; in common with many types of receptor, it is change in the nature of the stimulus that produces the greatest response. This is not of practical significance as the pattern of retinal stimulation is changing constantly because of eye movements, though if an image is artificially stabilized on the retina, it does disappear. This is why the retinal blood vessels are not perceived even though they are present on the retina and positioned between the lens and the retinal receptors. Their shadows are stabilized and hence are not perceived, but interestingly they may be destabilized, and

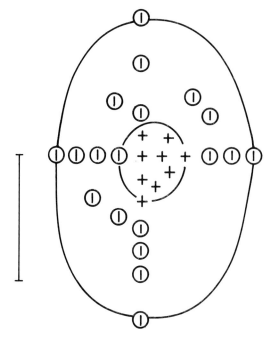

Figure 25.3 A ganglion cell. The cell has excitatory synapses (+) with receptors in the centre of its retinal field, but inhibitory synapses (−) with receptors in the outside of its retinal field. Bar = 1 mm.

hence made observable, by shining a vibrating light into the corner of the eye.

To return to the analysis of the visual image; if the outputs of cells that have concentric receptive fields were combined appropriately (*Figure 25.4*), then clearly a cell could be imagined that would function as a 'line detector'. Furthermore, appropriately more complex combinations could be designed that would function as edge, angle, and end detectors.

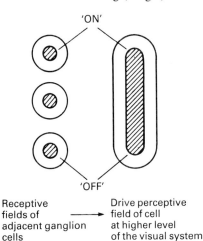

Figure 25.4 A 'line detector' formed by adjacent ganglion cells.

Micro-electrode studies have demonstrated the existence of just such combinations of cells in the visual cortex, and this form of pattern analysis of visual stimuli undoubtedly represents the first step of the perceptual process.

It is tempting to suppose that perception could be entirely driven in this 'bottom up' way and that our percept (the output of the system) is generated deterministically by the hierarchical process described. Clearly, however, neither the 'distal' stimulus (the 'real world' stimulus) nor the 'proximal' (or retinal) stimulus it produces are invariably sufficient to drive an accurate percept. *Figure 25.5*, the well-known Necker cube, and *Figure 25.6* illustrate that one distal stimulus can be the source of more than one percept, though interestingly only one percept may be entertained at a time. It must also be noted that the ambiguity of both of these stimuli occurs only at a late stage of processing. The cues provided by the bottom-up processes to the central synthesis or model building process are constant. It is only when our internal model is being

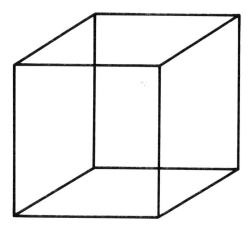

Figure 25.5 The Necker cube: a figure ambiguous in depth.

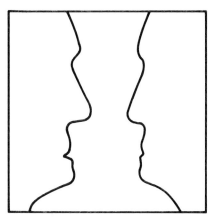

Figure 25.6 One urn or two faces?

built, and when our experience of the world (in these cases, in terms of our categorized information store of the cues that make up various views of cubes, or of urns and faces) is taken into account in attributing visual meaning to these stimuli that two possible hypotheses or interpretations of the data appear. Since in *Figure 25.6* neither urns nor faces are intrinsically more probable, vacillation between models (or percepts) results; but if the viewer had lived in a world without urns, there would surely be little chance of this figure appearing in any way ambiguous.

Figure 25.7 is a well-known trick that relies on the power of top-down processes to produce the percept 'BIRD IN THE HAND' from a stimulus containing two 'THEs'. It is interesting to speculate on the fate of the second 'THE'. It clearly forms an image on the retina and is passed up the sensory chain to the visual cortex, i.e. it is obviously sensed. It is only when this sensory information is being utilized in the formation of a mental model of the world that our expectations have the opportunity to produce a percept that is highly probable in terms of the experience of the native English speaker.

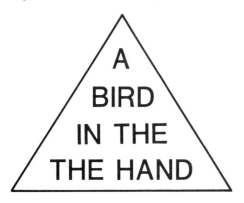

Figure 25.7 Top-down processes may produce a probable but inaccurate percept.

Thus our internal image, or model, of the external world is formed as a result of the analysis of incoming stimuli, but these stimuli are dealt with very much in terms of our existing experiences of the world, and the visual perception of depth illustrates these points.

A good illustration of the variety of bottom-up information that may be used in the construction of our mental model is provided by the study of depth perception. We perceive only a structured, three-dimensional model of the world, yet we form this model from two, two-dimensional proximal images. Although it appears useful to have two images of the world in order to perceive depth, the world does not suddenly appear two- rather than three-dimensional if we close one eye. There is clearly a variety of cues that we may use, and the main ones are as follows:

1. *Convergence*—When any object is viewed, the eyes are rotated such as to place the images of the object on the foveas. Obviously, when a near object is so viewed, the optical axes of the eyes will converge to a greater extent than when a far object is viewed, and the degree of convergence may thus be utilized as a cue to depth or range.

2. *Stereopsis*—Although the interocular distance is not large, it is sufficient that slightly different images of a viewed object are produced on each retina. This is simply because each eye has a slightly different view of the object. The disparity between the images produced on each retina decreases with range, and the degree of this disparity may consequently be used as a cue to depth.

3. *Accommodation*—The lens changes shape in order to bring objects at different ranges into focus on the retina; these accommodational changes are used as cues to depth.

4. *Retinal versus actual size*—As an object's distance from the eye increases, its retinal size (and the visual angle that it subtends) reduces. However, in a static scene the retinal size of an object may be used as a depth cue only if the actual size of the object is known to the observer. If it is not known, then no distinction is possible (in terms of this cue) between a near but small object and a large but distant object.

5. *Overlap*—It goes without saying that if an opaque near object is in front of another object, then part of the observer's view of that far object will be occluded. It is less obvious that in order to use this overlap as a depth cue, the observer must have a stored notion of the integrity and shape of the objects that he is viewing. Thus in *Figure 25.8* the observer will assume that he is viewing a square in front of a circle, though it is possible that he is, in fact, viewing the two objects shown in *Figure 25.9*, in which the 'circle' is actually the nearer object.

6. *Position in visual field*—It is not invariably true, but is sufficiently true to be useful as a cue, that as an object's range increases, it becomes closer to the horizon (which we may define as being at the observer's eye level). Thus in *Figure 25.10* the circles will tend to be perceived as more distant than the squares because of their greater proximity to the horizon.

7. *Aerial perspective*—As objects become more distant, dust and pollutants in the air reduce the 'clarity' with which they are seen because brightness and colour contrasts are eroded.

8. *Relative motion*—If two objects are moving at the same speed, parallel to the horizon (i.e. at right angles to the viewer's line of sight), then the angular velocity of the near one will be greater than the angular velocity of the far one.

The angular velocity of an object at the eye is thus determined both by the object's velocity and by its range, and a knowledge of either one of these will enable a subjective estimate to be made of the other.

Interestingly, none of the above cues has been labelled 'perspective', because this word is used to mean the global impression of depth that can be

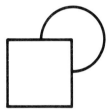

Figure 25.8 Overlap as depth cue: the viewer assumes that a square is in front of a circle.

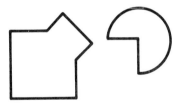

Figure 25.9 The viewer's assumption concerning the objects in *Figure 25.8* may be erroneous.

portrayed in a plane. It is sometimes used more specifically to mean the way in which parallel lines appear to converge to a vanishing point at the horizon, but it may be seen that this effect is actually a special case of the phenomenon described under 'retinal *v.* actual size' above. While addressing the problem of 'perspective', however, it is also interesting to observe that although all the cues described above may appear self-evident, the technique of using a change in size to represent the third dimension in art is a relatively recent innovation. In traditional Chinese and Egyptian art (and in children's drawings), overlap, and to some extent location in the field, are the only indicators of depth used; objects at all ranges are drawn the same size.

Another point that should be noted about the depth cues described above is that some of them derive from the image and some from physiological feedback (for example on eye position). The physiological cues are generally short range; accommodation and convergence operate over distances measured in metres or a few tens of metres, and the cue of stereopsis operates over larger but still limited distances. The image-derived cues work over almost limitless ranges: overlap and retinal *v.* actual size are quite usable if a mental model of two differently distanced mountains is being created. It is generally true that the visual model created by the pilot is based on ranges over which the physiological cues are of little help; the image-derived cues are important for him. Lastly, it is reiterated that all of

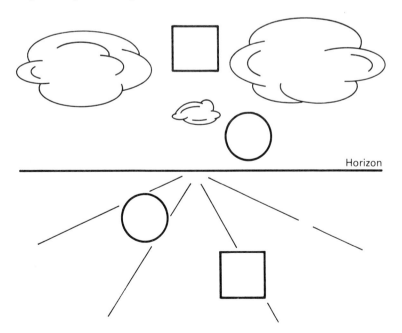

Figure 25.10 Position in visual field as a cue to depth. The circles are closer than the squares to the horizon, and are therefore perceived as more distant.

these image-based cues require some top-down input for their interpretation.

Before leaving this most basic introduction to visual perception, the perceptual constancies of size, shape, and colour must be mentioned. The term 'size constancy' refers to the phenomenon that changes in the retinal size of a known object are not perceived as being as great as they actually are. A demonstration of this effect is shown in *Figures 25.11* and *25.12*. The smaller rectangles in each picture are of identical size, yet may not appear so.

'Colour constancy' refers to the phenomenon that the colours of objects in the world are perceived in a

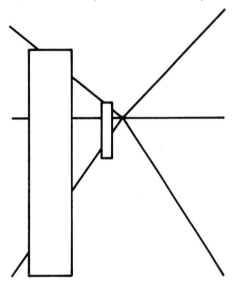

Figure 25.11 Compare the smaller rectangle to that in *Figure 25.12*.

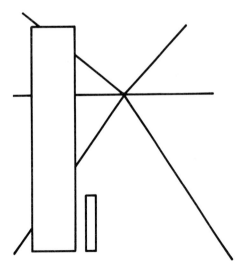

Figure 25.12 The smaller rectangle is the same size as that in *Figure 25.11*.

remarkably constant way under grossly different illuminations. It is readily demonstrated that the perception of colour depends more on the colour context in which an object is seen than on the precise wavelengths that it reflects, but the most commonplace example is the constancy with which colours are seen under artificial light or daylight. Colour photographs taken under these different light sources demonstrate forcefully their different spectral compositions, yet the natural observer will appreciate little subjective difference.

'Shape constancy' refers to the tendency of observers to regard a figure as maintaining its known shape even when viewed from distorting points of regard. Thus if a subject is asked to view a circle obliquely such that the circle's retinal image is an ellipse, and he is then asked to choose a real ellipse which would match that retinal ellipse, he will choose a figure that is more circular than the retinal shape.

In summary, we have established that perceptions are based on both bottom-up and top-down processes, that we can identify and experiment with the cues used to help generate our perceptions, and that there are mechanisms that are clearly basic to the perceptual process yet of which most people remain totally unaware. Some perceptual problems in aviation will now be examined in terms of the type of mechanism already discussed.

The example given at the beginning of this section illustrated how a shortage of visual cues enabled a helicopter to be flown into the sea with a resultant loss of life. There are many other similar incidents which are at least as informative but attract little attention because a dramatic outcome was avoided. The following is such an example written in the pilot's own words:

> In the descent to our destination airfield at night (the weather being reported good), we requested a visual left-hand circuit. Whilst attempting to keep the runway in sight, unreported stratus was encountered over the sea. The aircraft was allowed to descend beneath the cloud, and we looked for the runway to the left. The Ground Proximity Warning triggered but positive action was not taken because the surface of the sea could be seen clearly and the height LOOKED OK. This caused us to misread our altimeters and mistake 200 feet for 1200 feet. We were still some way from the airfield and heading for rising ground. Fortunately, we realized our mistake and rapidly climbed to a safe altitude.

Two main perceptual points are made in this report, which was provided by the pilot in confidence. The first is that sea, or any other surface that is either featureless, or textured with visual grain (e.g. waves or bushes) of unknown actual size, can produce profoundly inaccurate judgements of range, in this case, height. Even more remarkable instances of retinal *v.* actual size cue problems occur. Thus a navigator who had ejected was concerned, during his descent, that he would crash through the roof of one of a number of caravans that were parked in a field. He believed that he still had some way to descend when the ground appeared suddenly to rush up to meet him. Only after landing did he realize that the caravans had, in fact, been beehives, and that he had misjudged his height because of this top-down error (his incorrect assumption of the actual size of the stimulus).

The second point of interest in the above report is that once an inappropriate model had been constructed, the pilot saw, to some extent, what he expected to see. Top-down influences were so strong in his perception of the altimeter that an incorrect percept resulted. It seems that once we make our model of the world we are reluctant to change it, perhaps particularly when we are fatigued or busy and do not have the mental resources available to take a step back and re-evaluate the incoming information. A similar pattern of misperception, but in this instance auditory, occurred in a well-known incident to a Boeing 747 landing at Nairobi. The controller had cleared the aircraft to descend to 'seven–five–zero–zero' feet. The crew failed to detect the 'seven', and thus sensed (bottom-up) only the 'five–zero–zero'. Since 500 feet was not a reasonable clearance for them, they perceived (by virtue of top-down influence) 'five–zero–zero–zero', 5000 feet. The altitude of Nairobi is greater than 5000 feet above sea level, and the aircraft warning system indicated that it was descending below the instrument glide slope (going too low): but all of the warnings were accommodated into the captain's existing mental model by interpreting them as spurious. This incident occurred very early in the morning (at the bottom of the crew's circadian cycle) after a long night flight when they would have been poorly placed to re-evaluate the sensory data.

The visual approach

The most demanding visual task, and perhaps the best researched, concerns the visual approach to land. Though many landings are made as a result of circuit flying in which landmarks may be used as a check against height to provide the pilot with an artificial aid to acquiring the correct glide slope, it is also true that the pilot must be able visually to judge his glide slope from a straight-in approach without any cues other than those that he derives from the surface of the world.

Since pilots occasionally misjudge approaches and land in the runway's undershoot, it is important to understand what cues are available to be used in this operation and how pilots may best be taught the

visual 'skill' required. It is reasonable to call the judgement of the visual approach a skill because it has the skill characteristics of developing with practice, and of the possessor of the skill being unaware of its components. Indeed, if skilled pilots are asked what visual cues they use in the judgement of approach slope, they are likely to refer to the 'aspect' (retinal shape) of the runway. Many flying textbooks and instruction courses throughout the world teach that the runway will look long and thin if viewed from too high and broad and flat if viewed from too low. However, the runway shown in *Figure 25.13* indicates that range from the runway also changes its retinal shape, and consequently the usefulness of the aspect cue is almost certainly very limited.

There is, however, a constant and unchanging cue present in the retinal image of an approaching runway, and this is the visual angle subtended at the eye between the horizon and what might be termed the visual touchdown point. This is illustrated in *Figure 25.14*.

If a flat Earth is assumed (and the effect of the Earth's curvature is small at low altitudes) then the line passing through the horizon and the pilot's eye will be parallel to the surface of the Earth. It may then be seen that the line joining the pilot's eye and the visual touchdown point makes an angle with the surface of the Earth which is the angle of approach (angle A in *Figure 25.14*), and that the angle, at the eye, between the visual touchdown point and the horizon (angle B) is, by simple geometry, the same. *Figure 25.14* also clearly shows that angle B remains equal to the angle of approach throughout the approach to land.

If pilots are to use this cue, they must be aware of the location of the horizon, but they will often be required to carry out visual approaches in poor visibility, or at night, when the horizon cannot be seen. In these circumstances, the location of the horizon must be implied—top-down processes must be brought to bear—and there are at least three distinct cues that may be used to do so. The first derives from the runway itself. So long as the runway is level, then its extended sides will meet at the horizon. If, however, the runway slopes upwards, then its sides will meet above the actual horizon, angle B will appear too large to the pilot, and he may be seduced into making a low approach. The second derives from the texture gradients in the terrain. These also act to indicate the location of the horizon. Should the terrain slope upwards, the pilot who has learned to use this cue may make the same low approach as the pilot discussed above. The runway shown in *Figure 25.13* is in fact preceded by up-sloping terrain which, in some pilots, undoubtedly produces low approaches. The third possible cue to horizon location derives from the pilot's experience of horizon position on his canopy. Aircraft

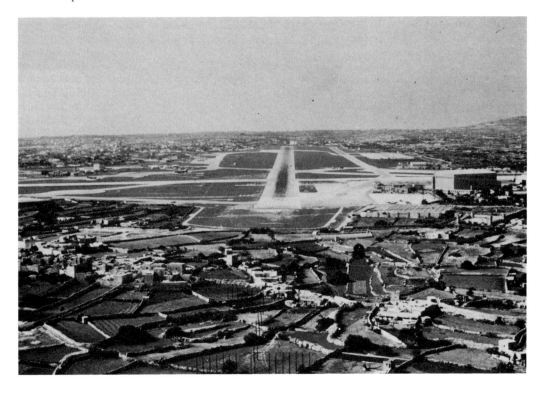

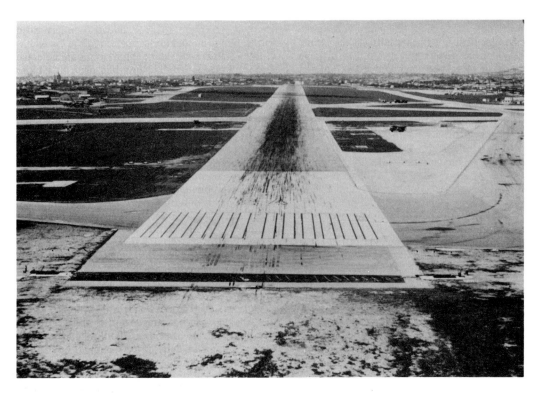

Figure 25.13 The retinal shape of the runway changes with range.

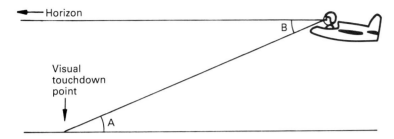

Figure 25.14 The visual angle between the horizon and the 'visual touchdown point' remains constant.

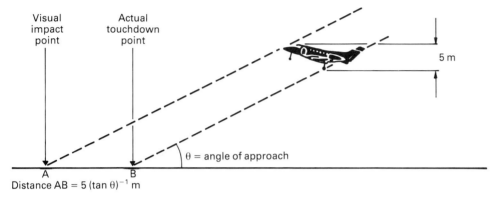

Figure 25.15 The actual touchdown point precedes the 'visual impact point'. Low angles of approach produce short landings if the pilot fails to appreciate his height in the late stages of the approach.

generally have a fairly stable pitch attitude during an approach, which will place the horizon and visual touch-down points at familiar canopy locations. If, however, our pilot is used to flying an aircraft that has a fairly level approach attitude, and then transfers to a different type of aircraft with a more pitched-up attitude on the approach, he may infer a familiar canopy position for the invisible horizon which will make angle B appear much too large and produce the perception of a very steep approach. Correcting for this will again produce a low approach.

It would require difficult experimentation to discover which of the cues to horizon location any particular pilot uses, and it may fairly be suggested that different pilots use different combinations of them. If so, then this would make sense of the observation that at certain runways, such as that illustrated in *Figure 25.13*, most pilots (using a good combination of cues) have no difficulty (most of the spin-up marks in this photograph being in the normal position). However, some pilots (those who, in this instance, have learned to depend too heavily on terrain cues) produce spin-up marks dangerously near the threshold of the runway.

The reason why low angles of approach produce short landings is that the undercarriage does not

impact the runway at the visual impact point, but (if the descent is unchecked) some way before it. *Figure 25.15* shows that the gear will touch down before the visual impact point at a distance approximately equal to the vertical separation between the eye and the gear divided by the tangent of the approach angle. If the gear/eye distance is 5 m and the approach angle 2 degrees then the gear will touch down more than 140 m before the visual impact point. Normally, of course, the pilot will, in the very late stages of the approach, begin to appreciate his height above the ground and check his descent such that the undercarriage lands on the runway. If, however, he misjudges his height above the ground because of a lack of range cues (e.g. at night, or just after snowfall), or if the available range cues are misleading (e.g. where the runway is of abnormal width) then he may permit the aircraft to impact the ground too early. A considerable number of accidents are probably caused by this effect.

The mid-air collision

Most commercial airliners operate on airways or in controlled airspace and the separation between them is maintained by radar or procedural control.

Even in such airspace mistakes can occur and lead to appalling mid-air collisions such as that which occurred at Zagreb between a DC9 and a Trident in 1976. It is therefore important that the crew of such aircraft should maintain a good visual look-out for other aircraft. It is even more important for the pilots of military and private aircraft to do so. Indeed, visual look-out is one of the most important tasks of any pilot.

There are, however, a number of effects that conspire to make the identification of a colliding aircraft difficult for even the conscientious pilot, and the first of these is the problem of constant relative bearing. *Figure 25.16* shows that if two aircraft are to collide, then each aircraft maintains a relative bearing to the other aircraft that is constant until the moment of impact. The subjective effect of this is that the colliding aircraft stays in the same place on the pilot's canopy unless he makes a head movement. This has two unfortunate consequences. The first is that no other aircraft that the pilot has ever seen (unless he has been involved in a previous mid-air collision or air-miss) will have possessed this characteristic, and he may not therefore have

learned to use movement relative to his canopy as a cue to detection. The second is that the peripheral retina drives what is sometimes termed the 'ambient' rather than the 'focal' visual system. The ambient system is concerned with using motion of the proximal stimulus to provide a percept of orientation, and to attract the attention of the focal system (concerned with the detailed and conscious interrogation of the world) to items of interest in the peripheral retina—particularly items that change by moving or flashing. Movement is thus a very important attention-getting stimulus to the ambient system, but the colliding aircraft is the only one that fails to provide it.

As a colliding aircraft grows nearer, its retinal size naturally increases, and it may be supposed that this should act as a cue to detection. The rate at which this increase in size occurs is not, however, linear. *Figure 25.17* shows that the image of the colliding

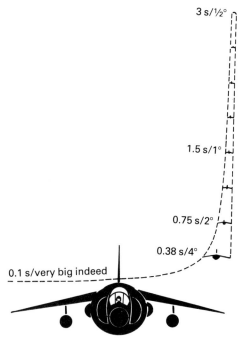

Figure 25.17 The retinal size of the colliding aircraft remains relatively small until very shortly before impact.

aircraft stays relatively small until very shortly before impact since, roughly speaking, the retinal size of the aircraft will double with each halving of the separation distance (separation distance changing linearly with time). It is probably for this reason that conversations with pilots who have experienced close air-misses or who have survived collisions characteristically contain the assertion that a good visual look-out was being maintained, with the offending aircraft suddenly looming large, and apparently from nowhere.

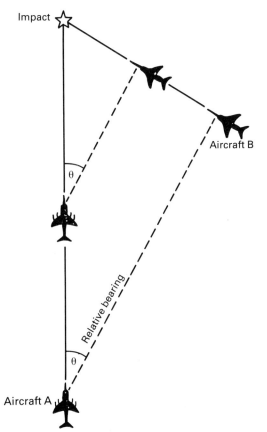

Figure 25.16 If two aircraft are going to collide, each maintains a constant relative bearing to the other.

Nevertheless, it may still seem surprising that colliding aircraft go unseen since they should represent targets that are well above minimal acuity levels for some time before impact. *Figure 23.2* makes clear, however, that acuity is not distributed evenly across the retina. As the eccentricity from the fovea increases, acuity drops dramatically. Experimental work (Harris, 1973) has shown that the probability of detecting an aircraft target is closely related to the local retinal acuity. It is therefore true that colliding aircraft will be perceptible so long as they are acquired at or near the fovea. Many pilots, however, experience the effect of seeing an aircraft, only to look away from it and be unable to spot it again even though they search the part of the sky where they know it to be. It may then re-appear as if from nowhere when, by virtue of a chance eye movement, its proximal image is placed close to the fovea.

The efficiency of a visual search is thus likely to be governed by the way in which the proximal image of each part of the external world can be placed on the fovea and surrounding retinal area. Visual searches may be conducted only by using saccades with intervening rests, and it is largely true to say that the world is interrogated only during the rests. Many pilots believe that they make visual searches by means of smooth and continuous eye movements, but such eye movements may be made only when a smoothly moving target is being tracked. The percept may be of a smooth scan, but this percept is constructed from a succession of stationary images. The pilot must unconsciously decide the density with which to distribute his fixation points on the outside world. If the distribution is dense, the probability of detecting the presence of an aircraft in the search area increases, but the overall size of the area searched decreases. If our pilot chooses to space his fixation points by 20 degrees, and has a visual world that subtends 200 degrees in azimuth and 60 degrees in elevation, then a total of 30 saccade/rest cycles will be required for the search. Since each cycle occupies about one third of a second, the complete search will consume about 10 seconds. This is clearly more than enough time for an aircraft that went undetected during the first fixation to become sufficiently close to be a hazard or even to collide.

The foregoing suggests that if pilots are to continue to fly relying only on vision to separate them from other aircraft, then collisions will continue to occur, however diligent the pilots may be. Fortunately, the probability of a mid-air collision is low, but an understanding of the processes may enable pilots to improve their search and should prevent legislative authorities from censuring those pilots who are unfortunate enough to be confronted dramatically by the limitations of their perceptual systems.

The two main examples of visual problems discussed here—the visual approach and the mid-air collision—represent the two most critical · visual situations in flight. Nevertheless the importance of vision in all flight must not be forgotten. It is the only sense that may be relied upon to provide reliable information on orientation, and is the source of the vast majority of other information that enables the pilot to build his internal model of the external world.

The essential point to understand about all perceptual processes is that our percept is a model or hypothesis about the external world which is built both from incoming information and from our expectations. Indeed, we are able to make sense of the world only because of our experience and expectations. It is, however, just these essential expectations that can sometimes lead us to make our model more in terms of the way that we would like the world to be, think that it ought to be, or in the way it always has been, than in the way it actually is.

Reference

HARRIS, J.L. (1973) Visual aspects of air collision. In *Visual Search*, pp. 26–50. Washington: National Academy of Sciences

Further reading

BOFF, K.R., KAUFMAN, L. and THOMAS, J.P. (eds) (1986) *Handbook of Perception and Human Performance. Volume 1, Sensory Processes and Perception*. New York: John Wiley

26

Cognitive processes

E.W. Farmer

Introduction

A central objective of aviation psychology is to ensure that the demands of the flying task do not exceed human information-processing capabilities. Apparently diverse activities such as selection and training, equipment design and accident investigation all share this underlying objective. It is therefore important to consider the fundamental mechanisms, or cognitive processes, that determine the limitations upon human performance.

Experimental studies of cognitive processes were pioneered in the nineteenth century by researchers such as Donders, who attempted to dissect reaction time (RT) to a stimulus into its constituent components; and Ebbinghaus, who conducted a long series of studies on human memory. With the emergence of behaviourism as a dominant school of psychological thought, particularly in the United States, it became unfashionable to investigate cognitive processes, or even to assume their existence, since observable responses were considered to be the only valid psychological data. During the Second World War the limitations upon operator performance became increasingly apparent, and interest in human information processing was renewed. Neisser (1967) coined the term 'cognitive psychology' for this rapidly developing area of psychological inquiry.

Attempts to distinguish the major components of the human information processing system have tended to result in a collection of 'black boxes' arranged in flow diagrams resembling those depicting a computer system. This 'black box' approach is a useful means of depicting the interrelationships between mental processes, but should not be interpreted literally; the boxes represent distinct functions rather than distinct physiological structures.

In this chapter, two major aspects of human information processing, memory and attention, are considered.

Memory

Human memory refers to the storage and retrieval of information. Three memory systems can be distinguished, each with different functions and properties.

Sensory memory

If subjects are presented with three rows of four letters for 50 ms, their memory of the display decays so rapidly that they can report only about four letters. Sperling (1960) devised an ingenious method of estimating the amount of information available in the period immediately after the display is erased. He modified the 'full report' technique, in which subjects attempted to report all that they had seen, to a 'partial report' technique, in which a cue appearing soon after the offset of the display indicated which subset of items was to be recalled.

When an auditory cue to recall a particular row of items was presented immediately after the display was erased, about three of the four letters in any row could be reported, indicating that about nine letters were available. However, performance declined rapidly as the delay between display and cue increased, and reverted after only 1 second to that obtained using the full report technique. A similar initial advantage of partial report over full report was later observed when subjects were cued to recall items on the basis of colour, shape, or size, but not when the cue referred to more abstract stimulus qualities such as the distinction between letters and digits (Coltheart, 1972).

These results have two major implications. One is that there is a storage system for visual information that decays within about 1 second. A second is that this 'iconic memory' stores only the gross physical characteristics of the stimulus.

The icon is susceptible to disruption by a later visual stimulus (visual backward masking). Turvey (1973) showed that the masking produced by a flash of light differed from that produced by presentation of a second patterned stimulus, apparently reflecting the existence of retinal and more central components of iconic memory.

Iconic memory is only one of a number of modality-specific sensory memories. In audition, for example, it is 'echoic' memory that permits one to begin to count clock chimes after the first one or two have rung. The function of sensory memory, regardless of modality, is to act as a temporary buffer from whose contents 'interesting' information may be selected for more detailed analysis. Selection is facilitated by gross physical differences between display items; practical implications of this finding will be discussed later.

Short-term memory

After one has dialled an unfamiliar telephone number, it is then likely to be forgotten. The system that permits retention of information for a few seconds is called short-term memory, and is distinct from the sensory memory described above.

The duration of short-term memory was demonstrated in a classic study by Peterson and Peterson (1959), who presented three consonants to subjects and required them to recall the letters after a particular time interval. The interval was filled by counting backwards in threes from a specified number. In this experiment, recall declined very rapidly. Indeed, after only 9 seconds, the probability of recalling the letters correctly was reduced to about one in three.

If the subjects had not been required to perform the counting task, their performance would have been far superior. The counting task was introduced to eliminate rehearsal (vocal or sub-vocal repetition), which provides fresh input to short-term memory and thus prevents information loss. Even if the opportunity is given to rehearse, however, there is a limit to the amount of information that can be maintained in short-term memory. In a famous paper, Miller (1956) estimated the capacity of short-term memory to be 7 ± 2 items. Memory performance may be improved by 'chunking' the stimulus (separating it into meaningful segments,

each of which acts as a single unit). For example, the following sequence of letters and digits:

$$VC10F16747B52$$

may easily be remembered by anyone familiar with aircraft types. It has been shown that chunking can enable remarkably large sequences to be memorized.

Acoustic coding appears to play an important role in short-term memory. For example, acoustically similar items are remembered rather poorly (Conrad and Hull, 1964), and confusion errors during recall from short-term memory are similar to listening confusions for items presented in a background of noise (Conrad, 1964). There is some evidence that acoustic recoding of information may occur automatically. Corcoran (1966) showed that when subjects are asked to cross out every letter *e* on a page of text (a task in which acoustic properties are irrelevant), they are more likely to miss the silent *e* (as in 'take') than the pronounced *e* (as in 'send').

The memory search paradigm devised by Sternberg (1966) indicated the way in which the contents of short-term memory are accessed. A fundamental issue is whether all of this information is available simultaneously (parallel access), or whether it is necessary to search through the items one at a time (serial access). Sternberg presented subjects with a list of items called the memory set, followed by a probe item, and required them simply to indicate whether the probe item had appeared in the memory set. Sternberg found that RT increased linearly with the number of items in the memory set, at a rate of approximately 40 ms per item. Thus it appeared that search through short-term memory was conducted in a serial fashion, the probe item being compared with items held in memory at a rate of about 25 comparisons per second. The identical slopes of the functions for 'yes' and 'no' responses suggested that subjects searched the contents of memory exhaustively, despite locating the probe, if it were present, after searching on average only half of the items.

It has been seen that information is rapidly lost from short-term memory if rehearsal is prevented. One possible source of this forgetting is that the information simply decays over time; another is that items in memory are displaced by the arrival of new items (the interference hypothesis). Experimental evidence supports the latter hypothesis. For example, when subjects are presented with a probe item from a memorized sequence, and are required to report which item followed it in the sequence (the serial probe technique), performance declines as a function of the number of interfering digits following the probe, but not as a function of the intervening time interval (Waugh and Norman, 1965).

The experiments described above reflect the interest during the 1950s and 1960s in the *structural* properties of short-term memory such as its duration and capacity. More recently, however, attention has been directed towards the *function* of short-term information storage. Clearly, this faculty has not developed simply to enable the temporary storage of telephone numbers. The work of Baddeley and his colleagues since the mid-1970s (*see* Baddeley, 1983, 1986) has indicated, indeed, that short-term memory plays a major role in many everyday practical tasks—such as reading, mental arithmetic, reasoning, and comprehension—that include temporary storage of information but would not conventionally be considered 'memory' tasks. To emphasize the importance of the functional aspects of short-term memory, Baddeley has coined the term 'working memory'.

In one of the experiments that helped to establish the concept of working memory, subjects were required to remember six digits while performing a verbal reasoning task based upon grammatical transformation. The time taken to perform the verbal reasoning task was substantially increased by the concurrent memory load, an indication that the memory and reasoning tasks placed demands upon the same system.

Experiments such as this, often including the requirement to perform two tasks simultaneously, led Baddeley to propose a model of working memory comprising a 'central executive' and two slave subsystems. The central executive is a limited-capacity attentional system that controls and coordinates the activity of the system. The articulatory loop comprises both a passive phonological input store, with a capacity of 2–3 seconds' worth of speech, and an active subvocal rehearsal buffer. This subsystem therefore plays an important role in the perception of speech, and can be used as an active memory store by the optional process of rehearsal discussed above. The visuo-spatial sketchpad is considered to be analogous to the articulatory loop but serves to store visuo-spatial rather than verbal material.

Support for this model was provided by Farmer, Berman and Fletcher (1986). Prevention of verbal rehearsal by the technique known as articulatory suppression (repetition of irrelevant speech sounds such as '1,2,3,4,1,2...') interfered with verbal, but not spatial, reasoning. However, an analogous spatial suppression technique (continuous tapping of four metal plates) produced the opposite pattern of interference with reasoning.

Long-term memory

Thus far, two distinct types of memory have been distinguished: sensory memory, and short-term (or 'working') memory. Neither of these, however, can account for the permanent storage of information. To extract meaning from the sequences of visual patterns comprising this sentence, it is necessary to call upon a vast amount of stored knowledge. Such knowledge is stored in long-term memory.

Clearly, both knowledge and skills may be retained on a more or less permanent basis. There appear to be two types of knowledge-based long-term memory system. The present discussion will be concerned primarily with the more extensively researched of these, semantic memory, which is responsible for general knowledge such as the meanings of words. The second system, called episodic memory (Tulving, 1972), is concerned with retention of specific incidents in the individual's personal history.

It remains unclear whether these different types of long-term memory should be considered separate memory systems, or whether they essentially comprise a single system. Indeed, even the distinction between short-term memory and long-term memory has been challenged by some researchers, who favour a unitary view. However, sufficient evidence has accumulated to suggest that these are separate systems (*see* Baddeley, 1976). During free recall of word lists, a recency effect is noted in which recall of the last few items, still in short-term memory, is superior to that for the earlier items that are represented only in long-term memory. Variables that affect recall of the material in long-term memory, such as presentation rate, have no effect upon the recency component.

The study of amnesia has provided further evidence against the unitary view. For example, patients exhibiting Korsakov's syndrome have a severely limited ability to learn new information, although their short-term memory is unaffected and they are able to recall events that occurred before their illness. The converse pattern of disruption (impairment of short-term memory with apparently normal long-term memory function) has been reported in some brain-damaged patients.

A further distinction between short- and long-term memory concerns the types of coding characteristic of each. We have already seen that verbal material tends to be coded acoustically in short-term memory and that acoustic similarity therefore leads to poor short-term retention. Baddeley (1966) showed that semantic similarity was much more disruptive of recall from long-term memory than acoustic similarity. Thus, information in long-term memory appears to be coded by meaning.

Although search through short-term memory appears to occur serially, such a procedure is obviously inappropriate for the retrieval of information from the vast amount of material stored in long-term memory. As an analogy, consider the task of finding a specific book from one of seven lying on a desk. A strategy of examining each in turn is probably as efficient as any other. But this would be an extremely time-consuming method of locating a book in a large library. Fortunately, librarians do not arrange the items on their bookshelves simply in the order in which they are received. Rather, they use a hierarchical classification system that greatly facilitates retrieval of a particular item. There is evidence that long-term memory is structured similarly, in an arrangement called a semantic network.

The role of semantic relationships in the organization of long-term memory is demonstrated by category clustering during free recall: subjects tend to recall together items belonging to the same category, even if the items are presented randomly (Bousfield, 1953). Moreover, recall is facilitated by cuing subjects with category names (Tulving and Pearlstone, 1966).

The notion of a semantic network was formally introduced by Collins and Quillian (1972) on the basis of differences in the time required to decide the truth or falsity of statements such as 'a canary is a bird' and 'a canary is an animal'. It appeared that RT reflected the time required to find an appropriate pathway through a semantic hierarchy. Difficulties in the original model led Collins and Loftus (1975) to propose a revised model of the semantic network. New information is assumed to be laid down in an appropriate area of the network, and to form associations with relevant nodes. The revised model retains the notion of hierarchical organization. For example, canary and ostrich are both associated with bird, which in turn is associated with animal. However, the importance of 'semantic distance', represented by the distance between nodes, is also recognized: it takes longer to verify that an ostrich is a bird than to verify that a canary is a bird, because canary is a more typical example than ostrich of the category bird.

The memorability of information in the semantic network is determined by the 'breadth' or richness of encoding (e.g. Baddeley, 1978). To continue the library analogy, material that is richly cross-referenced will be more easily retrievable. Thus, the rote 'maintenance' rehearsal used to remember a novel telephone number for a short period seldom leads to its long-term retention. 'Elaborative' rehearsal, involving extraction of semantic content and integration with existing knowledge, is much more effective.

In contrast to the clear constraints upon the capacity of short-term memory, there are no known limits to the amount of information that may be stored in long-term memory. Forgetting, in the context of long-term memory, is best considered a failure to retrieve, rather than loss of information. Two major sources of forgetting are retroactive interference, in which the acquisition of new material interferes with the recall of previously learned information, and proactive inhibition, in which previous knowledge interferes with later learning. The familiar tip-of-the-tongue phenomenon appears to support the notion that forgetting is often a matter of inability to retrieve information that is present in memory. It has been verified that subjects in the tip-of-the-tongue state are able to provide information about the particular word, such as the number of syllables it contains, despite their failure to recall the word itself (Brown and McNeill, 1966).

Levels of processing

Increasingly permanent storage is accompanied by more abstract and economical encoding. Thus sensory, short-term, and long-term memory represent distinct 'levels of processing' in human information processing. Sensory memory comprises a relatively unprocessed description of the physical characteristics of a stimulus, whereas short-term memory utilizes acoustic coding, and long-term memory semantic coding. This arrangement is an efficient means of processing the large amount of information arriving at the sensory receptors. During reading, for example, there is little need to retain detailed information concerning the physical characteristics of the individual letters, or even of the exact words used by the author; it is the meaning of the information that should be remembered.

Memory of accidents

The events immediately prior to an aircraft accident are of particular interest to the accident investigator. However, survivors' memory of this critical period is likely to be affected by a number of factors.

Emotion, for example, has been shown to influence recall (Baddeley, 1982). The poor immediate recall of unpleasant stimuli, attributed in Freudian theory to the ego defence mechanism of repression, appears in reality to be a consequence of the associated state of high physiological arousal. Interestingly, the recall of such stimuli in the longer term (after, say, 1 month) is superior to that of neutral items. Thus the survivor may find that an initially hazy recollection of the accident becomes considerably clearer over a period of time.

Memory may be permanently lost, however, if concussion is suffered during an accident. Retrograde amnesia induced by trauma may extend over a considerable period before the accident. Typically, memory for the earlier part of this period returns, leaving permanent loss of memory for the events immediately prior to concussion. This enduring amnesia, according to Baddeley (1976), is probably attributable to a failure of the memory trace to be consolidated (transferred to long-term memory).

The witness to an accident may also experience systematic distortion of memory. A classic study by Carmichael, Hogan and Walter (1932) demonstrated that subjects' memory of an ambiguous shape was influenced by the particular verbal label with which it was presented (*Figure 26.1*). Thus an individual's initial interpretation of an event is likely to influence his later recall, a fact that may help to explain the considerable discrepancies sometimes noted between different accounts of the same event.

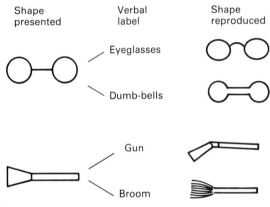

Shape presented	Verbal label	Shape reproduced

Figure 26.1 The effects of language on the reproduction of shapes. (After Carmichael, Hogan and Walter, 1932.)

Memory for stimuli and events is also subject to distortion at the time of recall. Loftus (1979) reported a series of 'naturalistic' studies on eye-witness testimony. In a typical experiment, subjects were presented with a film of an automobile accident and then asked carefully constructed questions concerning the events depicted. Loftus showed that misleading questions, which referred to objects or events not actually witnessed, led subjects to incorporate this false information in their memory of the film. Moreover, the way in which a particular incident was described had a profound effect on memory. Subjects' estimates of the speed at which cars were travelling when they collided were influenced systematically by the verb used in the question. The verb 'smashed' produced the highest estimate of speed, whereas 'contacted' produced the lowest. Loftus' findings indicate the ease with which unintentional distortion may be introduced during the post-accident interview (Knight, 1983).

Attention

It is generally recognized that man has limited capacity to process information. Since the amount of information arriving at the sensory receptors considerably exceeds the processing capacity of the system, available mental resources must be allocated selectively. The study of attention is concerned with the process of resource allocation.

Early experimental work on this topic, during the 1950s, concentrated on man's ability to attend exclusively to one of several concurrent sources of information. This is known as *selective* attention. More recently, the emphasis has shifted towards *divided* attention, which refers to the sharing of attentional resources between two or more information sources.

A familiar example of a selective attention task is the 'cocktail party phenomenon' described by Cherry (1953). This refers to the attempt to listen to one particular speaker despite the presence of several other distracting conversations. The ability to attend selectively to a particular information source in a complex environment is important in activities such as flying. Indeed, a test of selective attention has been developed for the selection of Israeli Air Force pilots (Gopher, 1982). Although efficient selective attention is often demanded by the flying task, it may have adverse consequences if an inappropriate aspect of the task is selected. As an example, Wickens (1984) cites an Eastern Airlines accident that occurred because the crew, preoccupied with a malfunction, failed to notice loss of altitude.

In complex tasks, it is often necessary to share attention between several information sources. For example, a pilot may have to make and respond to R/T transmissions while controlling the attitude of his aircraft. Laboratory studies have indicated the ease with which particular types of task may be combined, and have permitted the construction of models of the attentional system that may be used both to guide the design of aspects of the flying task and to estimate aircrew workload. Moreover, it has become apparent that there are individual differences in the efficiency with which resources may be allocated between tasks. For this reason, tests of time-sharing ability are incorporated in many aircrew selection programmes.

Selective attention

Several fundamental questions may be asked concerning our ability to attend selectively to particular sources of information. For example, what conditions affect the efficiency of selective attention? At what point in the information processing system does selection occur? Is the information on unattended information sources ('channels') completely filtered out, or does it proceed through the system in attenuated form?

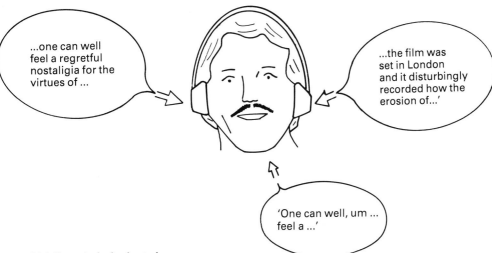

Figure 26.2 Cherry's shadowing task.

The work of Cherry (1953) clarified some of these issues. Cherry presented subjects simultaneously with two spoken messages, and required them to 'shadow' (repeat aloud) one of the messages but to ignore the other (*Figure 26.2*). This task was performed with ease if the two messages were presented to different ears, but with some difficulty if both messages were presented to each ear. Under the latter conditions, the use of disconnected phrases rather than continuous prose made selection almost impossible.

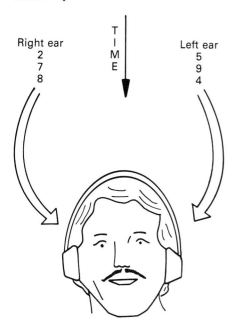

Figure 26.3 Broadbent's dichotic listening task.

Cherry found that little information was extracted from the unattended message. Subjects could detect only gross physical characteristics of this message, such as a transition from male to female speakers; they did not, apparently, extract semantic information, and often did not notice when the unattended message was played backwards.

Broadbent (1958) devised another type of task, called dichotic listening, to investigate selective attention. He presented subjects with a series of three pairs of digits, and then tested recall. Each pair was presented simultaneously, one digit to each ear (*Figure 26.3*). Broadbent found that typically only four or five digits were recalled, and that subjects preferred to organize their recall by ear, rather than by the order in which they had heard the digits.

To account for findings from shadowing and dichotic listening studies, Broadbent (1958) proposed a filter model, in which an input selector (filter) operated early in processing (*Figure 26.4*). Thus all sensory input was held in a brief memory store (corresponding to sensory memory), after which the information on a particular channel was selected for further processing. It was assumed that switching between channels was time consuming, taking about 0.25 seconds. Hence subjects in dichotic listening tasks performed better if they organized recall by ear (requiring only one switch between channels), and their recall of items from the second channel was poor because of the rapid decay of information in the sensory store. Moreover, because the filter was located at the periphery of the system, only the gross physical characteristics of unattended information were retained.

Filter theory was significant because it provided a set of assumptions that could be tested empirically.

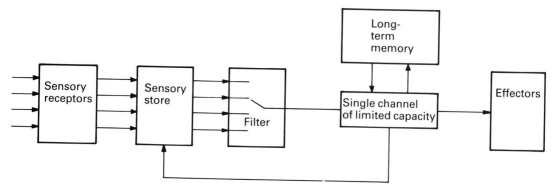

Figure 26.4 The filter model. (After Broadbent, 1958.)

Many of these were quickly refuted (Moray, 1969). For example, it was noted in shadowing tasks that subjects often recognized their own name when it was presented on the unattended channel, and that they tended to follow a message that was switched between the ears, rather than merely shadow the information presented on a particular channel. Moreover, when two phrases were alternated between the ears, subjects could switch attention to follow the semantic content as efficiently as they could attend to the contents of each channel in turn. Such findings were contrary to the notion of selection prior to semantic analysis, with relatively effortful switching between channels.

Treisman (1964) produced a refined version of filter theory that could account for semantic processing on the unattended channel. She proposed that a series of tests was performed on the content of the sensory channels, initially on the basis of physical cues, as in Broadbent's model. However, selection at this level was not absolute: the filter was 'leaky' and permitted unattended material to proceed through the system in an attenuated form, where its more abstract qualities, such as semantic content, were tested. The model further assumed that recognition thresholds were variable. Items of particular meaning to the subject, such as his own name, had a permanently lowered threshold. Moreover, the context of messages produced transient variations in threshold. For example, presenting 'the cat sat on the' would lower the threshold for recognizing 'mat'. This model could account for subjects' ability to hear their own names on the unattended channel, and their tendency to recognize information on the unattended channel that was semantically related to the attended message, since in both instances even an attenuated signal would provoke recognition.

Deutsch and Deutsch (1963) suggested that the notion of a filter was redundant. In their model, selection occurred late in processing (i.e. after semantic analysis), and recognition was determined both by the strength of the sensory signal and by its 'pertinence' (that is, its significance to the individual). According to Deutsch and Deutsch, therefore, the subject's own name is recognized on the unattended channel because of its high pertinence.

In summary, it can be suggested that man's ability to attend selectively to aspects of his environment is fairly efficient, particularly when selection is on the basis of a gross physical distinction. Under such conditions, little awareness of the content of unattended material is noted. Nevertheless, this material is clearly subject to semantic analysis, since an 'interesting' event on an unattended channel is often recognized.

A practical example of selective attention research of relevance to aviation concerns the optimal design of displays. The extraction of information from a visual display often involves search for a particular item or class of items. Findings from selective attention studies suggest that a coding dimension based upon gross physical display characteristics will be a more efficient aid to search than a more abstract coding method. Colour, for example, has been shown to be a potentially useful coding dimension. If the colour of the target item is known, irrelevant items may be rejected rapidly. Nevertheless, it should be noted that the use of colour may introduce costs as well as benefits. Irrelevant variation in colour within a class of target items is likely to impair performance (Christ, 1975). Moreover, although search time decreases as a function of the colour difference between target and non-target items, it increases as a function of the colour difference within the set of non-targets (Farmer and Taylor, 1980). Since, in most real-life displays, the same item may assume the role of target or non-target, the excessive heterogeneity introduced by over-enthusiastic use of colour coding may produce a net decrement in performance.

Man's ability to attend selectively must also be considered in the design of warning signals. Clearly, the efficiency of warning signals depends in part upon their likelihood of entering a sensory channel. Wickens (1984) points out that auditory warnings are often preferable to visual, since the latter may be missed if the gaze is averted. Nevertheless, shadowing and dichotic listening experiments indicate that recognition of a message is by no means an inevitable consequence of its reception by a sensory channel; the message must possess attention-getting properties. Modulated tones are more attention-getting than those of a continuous nature, and loudness is similarly important. In the visual modality, factors such as size, location, brightness and movement influence the likelihood that a signal will successfully gain attention (Morgan *et al.*, 1963; Wickens, 1984).

Wickens (1984) distinguished between selective and focused attention. The former is consciously controlled by the individual; the latter is induced by environmental conditions. In a later chapter, it will be seen that environmental stressors produce changes in attentional focus that may have profound implications for flying performance.

Divided attention

In Cherry's shadowing experiments, one message was defined as relevant and the other as irrelevant. Although the ability to ignore distracting messages is important in the flying task, it is seldom appropriate to devote attention to a single task element. There is therefore considerable interest in the limits of man's ability to perform more than one activity at a time, a topic central to the practical problem of mental workload.

One of the fundamental issues of divided attention concerns the nature of the limited processing capacity. Broadbent's model, discussed earlier, assumes that there is a single central processing channel that acts as a 'bottleneck'. In this model, it will be remembered, there is a filter early in the system that selects inputs for further processing. The single channel can process only one input at a time, and so dual-task performance depends upon time-sharing (alternating attention) between two inputs. A second class of model, suggested by Moray (1967) and Kahneman (1973), assumes the existence of flexible, general-purpose resources that can be allocated to any task. According to this type of account, any number of tasks may be performed simultaneously, provided that their total demand for resources does not exceed the capacity of the system.

In practice, the bottleneck model, and the alternative allocatable resource conception that allows for parallel processing, make similar predictions concerning performance, since they each assume that all tasks draw upon the same limited capacity (McLeod, 1977). For convenience, both can be regarded as single-channel models (although only the former corresponds to the strict interpretation of this term), and can be contrasted with models that postulate separate, specialized resource pools (e.g. verbal and spatial) responsible for particular types of processing. Examples of multi-processor or multiple-resources models include those proposed by Allport, Antonis and Reynolds (1972), McLeod (1977), and Navon and Gopher (1979).

The major distinction between single-channel and multi-processor models lies in their predictions concerning the effects of task similarity on concurrent performance. The former suggests that similarity will have little effect on dual-task performance, whereas the latter predicts that two quite dissimilar activities, which draw upon different processors or resource pools, may proceed with no apparent mutual interference.

It is sometimes found that two quite dissimilar tasks interfere. For example, Phillips and Christie (1977) reported that mental arithmetic disrupted the visualization of complex patterns. This finding might be taken as evidence for the single-channel conception. However, McLeod (1977) demonstrated that a two-choice auditory reaction time task interfered with tracking when manual responses, but not when vocal responses, were required. Thus it appeared that the requirement for manual responses placed demands upon a specific resource pool used by the tracking task. McLeod further showed that performance on the tracking task was unaffected by variation in the difficulty of a concurrent mental arithmetic task, a result that is also difficult to reconcile with single-channel theory.

Clearly neither the single-channel nor the multiple resource approach can account for all of the experimental findings. It seems likely that a compromise position may prove more fruitful. Such a compromise is represented by Baddeley's model of working memory discussed earlier. This model postulates the existence both of a general-purpose 'central executive' and of specialized subsystems. It can account for the interference between dissimilar but demanding tasks by assuming that their combined demands exceed the capacity of the central executive; it can also account for task-specific patterns of interference by assuming that only similar tasks will require access to the same specialized subsystem.

To summarize: it appears that man may indeed be able to perform more than one activity at a time, provided (1) that the combined demands of these activities do not exceed central processing capacity, and (2) that the activities do not overload any of the subsystems of working memory.

Norman and Bobrow (1975) suggested that task performance typically improves as more and more resources are applied; under such circumstances, the task is said to be *resource limited*. However, a limit is reached beyond which the allocation of further resources no longer influences performance. The task is now *data limited*, since its performance is influenced only by the quality of the sensory data available. For example, some benefit may result from devoting attention to a transmission on a noisy radio channel, but a point will be reached at which recognition can improve further only by improving the clarity of the signal.

Norman and Bobrow (1975) devised the Performance Operating Characteristic (POC) as a means of depicting performance on two concurrent tasks as the amount of resources applied to each is varied. Points on the POC are generated by varying the relative priority of each task. Resource limitation is indicated by change in performance as a function of task priority; data limitation is indicated by insensitivity to increased resource allocation (*Figure 26.5*).

Green and Farmer (1985) used POC methodology to compare the demands of an ambient attitude indicator and those of the conventional indicator. The ambient display is intended to indicate the location of the horizon by means of the pattern of illumination of a series of light-emitting diodes (LEDs) mounted on the canopy arch of suitable single-seat or tandem-seat aircraft. In its simplest form, only the LEDs above the pilot's horizon would be illuminated.

Under normal circumstances, the ambient rather than the foveal (central) visual system is responsible for processing orientation information. It was therefore considered likely that the ambient display would be superior to the small conventional attitude indicator, particularly since the former could be interrogated without fixation and might therefore interfere less with concurrent activities. In the laboratory, subjects were required to perform a tracking task, using either the ambient or conventional display, in which the object was to maintain a straight and level position. Concurrently, they performed a visual reaction time task. Variation in the priority assigned to the tracking and reaction time tasks permitted the construction of POCs (*Figure 26.6*), which indicated that performance on both tasks was superior when using the ambient attitude indicator, and that tracking with this display was less adversely affected than with the conventional display by withdrawal of resources. There is therefore reason to believe that the ambient attitude indicator may help to reduce workload.

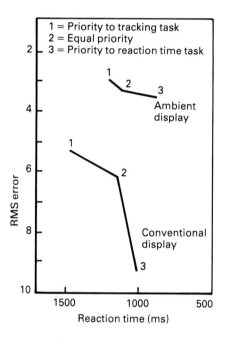

Figure 26.6 Control of an ambient and a conventional attitude indicator while performing a concurrent reaction time task. The data are plotted in the form of a Performance Operating Characteristic. (After Green and Farmer, 1985.)

The ability to perform two tasks simultaneously is a function not only of the nature of the tasks, but also of the individual's level of experience. Learner drivers, for example, often find it difficult to listen to directions given by an instructor, whereas experienced drivers can converse with ease under normal circumstances. Allport, Antonis and Reynolds (1972) provided experimental evidence of the apparently low resource demands of complex but well-practised tasks. They found that experienced pianists could sight-read and play unhindered an unfamiliar musical piece while performing a concurrent auditory shadowing task. Spelke, Hirst, and Neisser (1976) gave two subjects extensive practice of reading short stories whilst writing dictated word lists. Eventually, these subjects were able both to write and to extract the meaning of the words simultaneously with reading and comprehending the

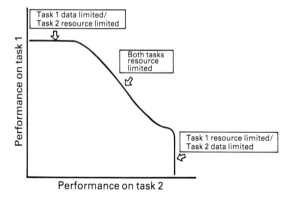

Figure 26.5 A Performance Operating Characteristic, showing areas of resource limitation and data limitation. (After Norman and Bobrow, 1975.)

stories at normal speed. Because of the similarity of these tasks (both required semantic analysis), it is difficult even for a multiple resources model to account for such findings.

Practice on a task apparently produces a decrement in its resource demands. After considerable exposure, task performance may become automatic. The initially demanding task of changing gear while driving is eventually performed with little or no awareness. In motor skills such as driving or flying, behavioural subroutines are developed that require minimal processing resources. These subroutines are known as 'motor programmes' (Keele, 1968). Whereas activities under conscious control rely heavily upon feedback concerning the effects of previous actions (closed-loop processing), motor programme activities apparently do not use feedback (open-loop processing).

Comparable development of automaticity has been noted in perceptual skills. Schneider and Shiffrin (1977) reported findings from visual search

tasks that the use of a consistent, rather than varying, set of targets enabled subjects to develop automatic processes that permitted them to search at the same rate through displays of different sizes for varying numbers of targets.

Failure of attention

Although the development of motor programmes during skill learning frees attentional resources, it paradoxically increases the likelihood of error. Reason (1981) argued that, even when the control of skilled performance is delegated to motor programmes, attentional resources must intervene at critical points to ensure that the correct behavioural sequences are called into action. From a diary study in which volunteers recorded 'actions not as planned' (i.e. absent-minded behaviour) in their everyday life, Reason established that such errors almost always constituted well-practised but in-

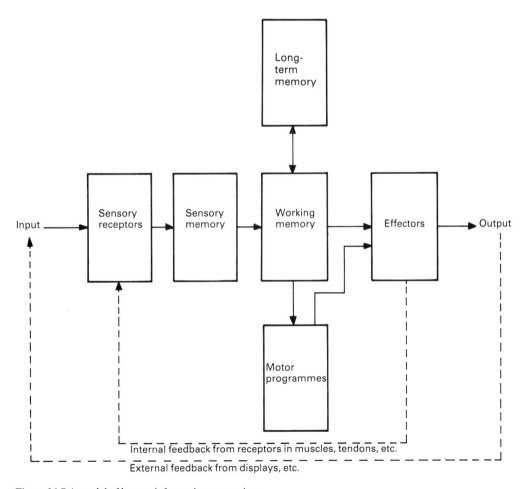

Figure 26.7 A model of human information processing.

appropriate behavioural sequences. One respondent reported that he intended to get his car out of his garage, but that when he stepped out onto the porch he proceeded to don his gardening clothes; another answered his office telephone and shouted 'Come in' into the receiver.

Reason postulated that the more well established the motor programme, the more likely it is to be activated, particularly when attentional resources are directed elsewhere. Since the actions controlled by the motor programme are performed without feedback, and seldom reach conscious awareness, the individual often fails for some considerable time to become aware that his behaviour is not as planned. As Norman and Shallice (1980) noted, errors in skilled performance often lie in the initiation rather than the execution of actions.

Although most of the action slips noted in the diary study had trivial consequences, Reason (1976) found that some accidents to civil aircraft were almost certainly attributable to similar slips during well-practised activity. These included instances in which aircrew had shut down a healthy engine rather than the one in which a fault had developed. Reason refers to actions not as planned as 'the price of automatization'.

Individuals probably differ in their liability to action slips. Broadbent *et al.* (1982) developed a 'Cognitive Failures Questionnaire' (CFQ) which asked subjects to report their liability to failures of perception, memory and action. These types of failure were correlated together, and with other measures of absentmindedness, suggesting a general tendency towards slips.

A model of human information processing

The 'black box' approach can be used to depict the relationships between the major components of the information processing system discussed in this chapter (*Figure 26.7*). As stated earlier, these 'black boxes' represent functional distinctions rather than physiological entities.

References

ALLPORT, D.A., ANTONIS, B. and REYNOLDS, P. (1972) On the division of attention: A disproof of the single channel hypothesis. *Quarterly Journal of Experimental Psychology* **24**, 225–235

BADDELEY, A.D. (1966) The influence of acoustic and semantic similarity on long-term memory for word sequences. *Quarterly Journal of Experimental Psychology*, **18**, 302–309

BADDELEY, A.D. (1976) *The Psychology of Memory*. New York: Harper and Row

BADDELEY, A.D. (1978) The trouble with levels: A re-examination of Craik and Lockheart's framework for memory research. *Psychological Review*, **85**, 139–152

BADDELEY, A.D. (1982) *Your Memory: A User's Guide*. London: Sidgwick and Jackson

BADDELEY, A.D. (1983) Working memory. *Philosophical Transactions of the Royal Society of London*, **B302**, 311–324

BADDELEY, A.D. (1986) *Working Memory*. Oxford University Press

BOUSFIELD, W.A. (1953) The occurrence of clustering in the recall of randomly arranged associates. *Journal of General Psychology*, **49**, 229–240

BROADBENT, D.E. (1958) *Perception and Communication*. London: Pergamon Press

BROADBENT, D.E., COOPER, P.F., FITZGERALD, P. and PARKES, K.R. (1982) The Cognitive Failures Questionnaire (CFQ) and its correlates. *British Journal of Clinical Psychology*, **21**, 1–16

BROWN, R. and MCNEILL, D. (1966) The 'tip of the tongue' phenomenon. *Journal of Verbal Learning and Verbal Behaviour*, **5**, 325–337

CARMICHAEL, L., HOGAN, H.P. and WALTER, A.A. (1932) An experimental study of the effect of language on the reproduction of visually perceived form. *Journal of Experimental Psychology*, **15**, 73–86

CHERRY, E.C. (1953) Some experiments on the recognition of speech with one and two ears. *Journal of the Acoustical Society of America*, **25**, 975–979

CHRIST, R.E. (1975) Review and analysis of colour coding research for visual displays. *Human Factors*, **17**, 542–570

COLLINS, A.M. and LOFTUS, E.F. (1975) A spreading activation theory of semantic processing. *Psychological Review*, **82**, 407–428

COLLINS, A.M. and QUILLIAN, M.R. (1972) Experiments on semantic memory and language comprehension. In *Cognition in Learning and Memory*, edited by L.W. Gregg, pp. 117–137. New York: Wiley

COLTHEART, M. (1972) Visual information processing. In *New Horizons in Psychology: 2*, edited by P. Dodwell, pp. 62–85. Harmondsworth: Penguin

CONRAD, R. (1964) Acoustic confusions in immediate memory. *British Journal of Psychology*, **55**, 75–84

CONRAD, R. and HULL, A.J. (1964) Information, acoustic confusion and memory span. *British Journal of Psychology*, **55**, 429–432

CORCORAN, D.W.J. (1966) An acoustic factor in letter cancellation. *Nature (London)*, **210**, 658

DEUTSCH, J.A. and DEUTSCH, D. (1963) Attention: Some theoretical considerations. *Psychological Review*, **70**, 80–90

FARMER, E.W., BERMAN, J.V.F. and FLETCHER, Y.L. (1986) Evidence for a visuo-spatial scratch-pad in working memory. *Quarterly Journal of Experimental Psychology*, **38A**, 675–688

FARMER, E.W. and TAYLOR, R.M. (1980) Visual search through colour displays: Effects of target–background similarity and background uniformity. *Perception and Psychophysics*, **27**, 267–272

GOPHER, D. (1982) A selective attention test as a predictor of success in flight training. *Human Factors*, **24**, 173–183

GREEN, R.G. and FARMER, E.W. (1985) Attitude indicators and the ambient visual system. In *Report of the Sixteenth Conference of WEAAP, Helsinki*, edited by M. Sorsa, pp. 114–121. Helsinki: Finnair Training Centre

KAHNEMAN, D. (1973) *Attention and Effort*. Englewood Cliffs, NJ: Prentice-Hall

KEELE, S.W. (1968) Movement control in skilled motor performance. *Psychological Bulletin*, **70**, 387–403

KNIGHT, S. (1983) The post accident interview. In *Flight Operations Symposium*, edited by N. Johnson. Dublin: Irish Air Line Pilots' Association/Aer Lingus

LOFTUS, E.F. (1979) *Eyewitness Testimony*. Cambridge, MA: Harvard University Press

MCLEOD, P. (1977) A dual task response modality effect: Support for multiprocessor models of attention. *Quarterly Journal of Experimental Psychology*, **29**, 651–667

MILLER, G.A. (1956) The magical number seven, plus or minus two: Some limits on our capacity for processing information. *Psychological Review*, **63**, 81–97
a model. *Acta Psychologica*, **27**, 84–92

MORAY, N. (1969) *Attention: Selective Processes in Vision and Hearing*. London: Hutchinson Educational

MORGAN, C.T., COOK, J.S., CHAPANIS, A. and LUND, M.W. (1963) *Human Engineering Guide to Equipment Design*. New York: McGraw-Hill

NAVON, D. and GOPHER, D. (1979) On the economy of the human processing system: A model of multiple capacity. *Psychological Review*, **86**, 214–255

NEISSER, U. (1967) *Cognitive Psychology*. New York: Appleton-Century-Crofts

NORMAN, D.A. and BOBROW, D.G. (1975) On data-limited and resource-limited processes. *Cognitive Psychology*, **7**, 44–64

NORMAN, D.A. and SHALLICE, T. (1980) *Attention to Action: Willed and Automatic Control of Behaviour*. San Diego: University of California Centre for Human Information Processing. Report No. 8006

PETERSON, L.R. and PETERSON, M.J. (1959) Short-term retention of individual items. *Journal of Experimental Psychology*, **58**, 193–198

PHILLIPS, W.A. and CHRISTIE, D.F.M. (1977) Components of visual memory. *Quarterly Journal of Experimental Psychology*, **29**, 117–133

REASON, J.T. (1976) Absent minds. *New Society*, **November 4**

REASON, J.T. (1981) Actions not as planned: The price of automatization. In *Aspects of Consciousness*, edited by G. Underwood and R. Stevens, pp. 67–89. London: Academic Press

SCHNEIDER, W. and SHIFFRIN, R.M. (1977) Controlled and automatic human information processing: I. Detection, search and attention. *Psychological Review*, **84**, 1–66

SPELKE, E., HIRST, W. and NEISSER, U. (1976) Skills of divided attention. *Cognition*, **4**, 215–230

SPERLING, G. (1960) The information available in brief visual presentations. *Psychological Monographs: General and Applied*, **74**, 1–29

STERNBERG, S. (1966) High-speed scanning in human memory. *Science*, **153**, 652–654

TREISMAN, A.M. (1964) Selective attention in man. *British Medical Bulletin*, **20**, 12–16

TULVING, E. (1972) Episodic and semantic memory. In *Organisation of Memory*, edited by E. Tulving and W. Donaldson, pp. 282–402. New York: Academic Press

TULVING, E. and PEARLSTONE, Z. (1966) Availability versus accessibility of information in memory for words. *Journal of Verbal Learning and Verbal Behaviour*, **5**, 381–391

TURVEY, M.T. (1973) On peripheral and central processes in vision: Inferences from an information processing analysis of masking with patterned stimuli. *Psychological Review*, **80**, 1–52

WAUGH, N.C. and NORMAN, D.A. (1965) Primary memory. *Psychological Review*, **72**, 89–104

WICKENS, C.D. (1984) *Engineering Psychology and Human Performance*. Columbus: Charles E. Merrill

27

Individual differences

E.W. Farmer

Introduction

Many psychological studies seek to discover general laws or principles of human behaviour. Care is taken to minimize the effects of variation between subjects, and such variation is regarded merely as a source of error. This is known as the nomothetic method. The idiographic approach, in contrast, is based upon the premise that human behaviour is best understood in terms of the characteristics that define the uniqueness of the individual and the differences between individuals. Sir Francis Galton, a pioneer of intelligence testing, was one of the earliest proponents of this viewpoint.

Both of these approaches have a place in aviation psychology. Questions such as 'Does the use of colour facilitate the extraction of information from visual displays?' are typically addressed by means of nomothetic research; however, questions such as 'Is this individual suitable for fast jet training?' require an idiographic solution.

The major sources of individual differences in mental function are considered in this chapter. A later chapter will discuss the relevance of these idiographic variables to the applied problem of aircrew selection.

Personality

In everyday life, intuitive judgements about the personality of others are commonplace. There are at least 17 000 words in the English language that describe behavioural characteristics. The scientific assessment of personality requires that intuition be replaced by an objective means of identifying and measuring its fundamental components.

The term 'personality' refers to enduring predispositions to behave in particular ways. These *traits* can be distinguished from *states*, which are transient responses to environmental circumstances. Thus anxiety attributable to a specific stressful stimulus would be considered a state, whereas a generalized proneness to anxiety would be considered a trait.

One of the earliest systems of personality classification was proposed by Galen, and was based upon the Hippocratic notion of four fundamental body 'humours'. In Galen's system, the balance of these humours determined whether an individual was melancholic, choleric, phlegmatic, or sanguine. Galen's classification is an example of a *type* theory, since it is based upon the assumption that there are discrete categories of personality. A modern theory in which the notion of types appears is that of Eysenck. The cornerstone of Eysenck's approach is the statistical technique known as factor analysis.

Factor analysis reduces a table of inter-correlations between items to a small number of factors. Each factor can be considered to be a vector in a multidimensional factor space, and represents a fundamental source of variation in the item scores. The nature of the factor is inferred from the pattern of factor loadings (the correlation of each item with the factor). Some researchers, such as Eysenck, favour factor-analytic solutions that yield orthogonal (uncorrelated) factors; others, such as Cattell, prefer to derive oblique (correlated) factors, which can themselves be subjected to further factor analysis.

In the construction of personality inventories, the correlation matrix for responses to a large number of questions is subjected to factor analysis. An item is chosen for inclusion in the inventory if it loads strongly onto a particular factor and is not strongly associated with other factors.

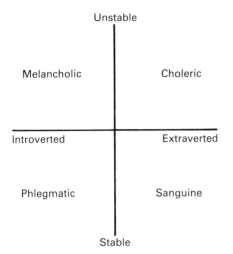

Unstable

Melancholic   Choleric

Introverted ———————————————— Extraverted

Phlegmatic   Sanguine

Stable

Figure 27.1 Eysenck's personality dimensions of extraversion and neuroticism. Each quadrant is equated with one of Galen's personality types.

During research spanning several decades, Eysenck has presented evidence for three fundamental personality dimensions: *extraversion*, *neuroticism*, and *psychoticism* (Eysenck and Eysenck, 1969, 1976). Since these factors are orthogonal, an individual's score on any factor is independent of his scores on the other factors.

The major components of extraversion (E) are sociability and impulsiveness. Thus the extreme extravert is outgoing, sociable, and uninhibited; whereas the extreme introvert is reserved, shy, and cautious. According to Eysenck, E is related to the excitability of the central nervous system. The dimension of neuroticism (N), which extends from emotional stability to extreme anxiety and worry, may be associated with the lability of the autonomic nervous system. The four combinations of introvert/

extravert and stable/unstable appear to correspond quite closely to Galen's types. For example, the unstable extravert can be identified as the 'choleric' temperament (*Figure 27.1*).

Eysenck's final dimension of psychoticism (P), which indicates degree of tough-mindedness and antipathy, is the least well established. As might be expected, P scores are elevated in psychotics and criminals. Normal samples, however, show much less variation than is observed for E or N. Psychoticism appears to be related to maleness, and its physiological basis may be androgen level.

An alternative approach to the study of personality, also drawing heavily upon factor analytic techniques, is that of Cattell, who has proposed the existence of 16 major personality factors (*Table 27.1*). Since these factors are considered to be fundamental to behaviour, they are described as *source* traits, to be distinguished from the *surface* traits that represent the behavioural manifestation of patterns of source traits.

The major difference between the theories of Eysenck and Cattell is the level of personality description (type or trait) that each considers appropriate, as illustrated in *Figure 27.2*. In practice, this distinction is related to the 'depth' of the factor–analytic procedure. Eysenck's dimensions of E and N appear in Cattell's scheme as 'second-order' factors produced by further factor analysis of the 16 primary factors.

Although there are many other types of personality theory, those based upon the factor–analytic method are particularly important within experimental psychology because they permit comparison of individuals on clearly defined and objectively derived dimensions of personality. Kline (1983) provides an excellent introduction to the work of Eysenck and Cattell. Other theoretical approaches are discussed by Fransella (1981).

Table 27.1 Catell's sixteen personality factors

Factor	Low score description	High score description
A — Warmth	Reserved	Outgoing
B — Intelligence	Dull	Bright
C — Ego strength	Unstable	Stable
E — Dominance	Submissive	Assertive
F — Impulsivity	Sober	Impulsive
G — Group conformity	Expedient	Conscientious
H — Boldness	Shy	Bold
I — Emotional sensitivity	Unsentimental	Sensitive
L — Suspiciousness	Trusting	Suspicious
M — Imaginativeness	Practical	Imaginative
N — Shrewdness	Forthright	Shrewd
O — Guilt proneness	Self-assured	Apprehensive
Q1 — Radicalism	Conservative	Radical
Q2 — Self-sufficiency	Group dependent	Self-sufficient
Q3 — Ability to bind anxiety	Uncontrolled	Controlled
Q4 — Free-floating anxiety	Relaxed	Tense

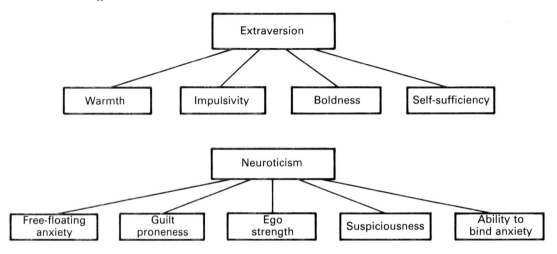

Figure 27.2 The relationships of Eysenck's dimensions of extraversion and neuroticism to Cattell's personality factors (type versus trait approach).

Personality assessment

Any psychological test is useful only if it satisfies the basic psychometric criteria of reliability, validity and discriminability (Anastasi, 1968). It must give consistent results, measure what it purports to measure, and be sufficiently sensitive to discriminate between individuals.

The consistency of results obtained when a test is used on different occasions is known as *test–retest* reliability. The test's internal consistency must also be high, and this can be assessed by *split-half* reliability in which scores on half of the items are correlated with those on the other half.

High reliability is a necessary, but not a sufficient, condition for high validity. Several types of test validity may be distinguished:

1. *Content* validity describes the extent to which the test samples the range of behaviour to which it is addressed. Thus a test of flying aptitude would have high content validity only if it incorporated all of the activities representative of the flying task.
2. *Predictive* validity refers to the ability of the test to predict a criterion score. For example, success in flying training could be used as a criterion for aircrew selection tests.
3. *Construct* validity incorporates the ability of test scores to confirm hypotheses generated on the basis of the nature of the abstract psychological construct (such as intelligence) that the test purports to measure.
4. *Concurrent* validity refers to the correlation between test scores and measures of the same attribute obtained by other means.

5. *Face* validity refers to the extent to which the test appears to measure the intended attribute. Low face validity does not necessarily undermine the soundness of the test, but may influence the subject's attitudes and motivation.

A test with high reliability and validity would be of little practical benefit if it could not discriminate between the individuals studied. When applied to populations of highly intelligent individuals, for example, intelligence tests designed for use with the general population often prove to be rather insensitive. In such an instance, it may be necessary to use a test, such as the AH5 (Heim, 1968), developed specifically for intelligent groups.

Interviews and observational methods

In some personnel selection procedures, an attempt is made by means of interview, or of observation of groups of applicants performing a task, to gain information concerning personality. However, these methods are extremely subjective and are therefore susceptible to distortion. Vernon (1964), although acknowledging that the selection interview has several important functions, dismisses it as a method of inferring fundamental personality characteristics.

More formal techniques for personality assessment may be divided into three major groups: questionnaires, projective tests, and objective tests (Kline, 1983). These are discussed below.

Personality questionnaires

Two of the most well-known personality questionnaires, or inventories, are those based on the work of Eysenck and Cattell. In the Eysenck Personality Questionnaire (EPQ), a series of statements is presented, each requiring the response 'yes' or 'no' depending on whether it describes the subject's usual way of feeling or behaving. The items of the Cattell Sixteen Personality Factor Questionnaire (16PF) each permit three possible responses, such as 'true', 'uncertain', and 'false'. In both of these tests, each item is included on the basis of its strong loading on a particular personality factor. Raw scores on the 16PF are converted into 'stens' (standard tens) which allow direct comparison of the individual with a particular population.

An alternative method to factor analysis in the construction of personality tests is known as criterion keying. This method comprises identification of questions that discriminate between particular groups, such as neurotics and normals. It is entirely empirical and atheoretical, and there is no requirement to understand *why* a particular item is a good discriminator. The Minnesota Multiphasic Personality Inventory, constructed using criterion keying, has important clinical applications.

The best-known personality inventories satisfy the psychometric criteria discussed above to a reasonable degree. However, there are problems associated with the use of such questionnaires. It is often difficult to disguise the purpose of the questions, and this transparency permits the subject to fake his responses. In personnel selection, for example, applicants may dissimulate by providing answers that they believe to be the most socially desirable. Fortunately, the degree of dissimulation may be estimated by the inclusion of 'lie' questions that describe standards of behaviour that could not reasonably be expected to be attainable (for example, 'I have never told a lie'). The number of such statements that the subject endorses provides a measure of dissimulation.

A further factor that the constructor of personality questionnaires must consider is acquiescence—a tendency to agree with any statement. The likelihood of such a 'response set' being created can be minimized by varying the mapping of 'yes' and 'no' responses onto the personality scale.

Questionnaires constructed with due regard to the problems mentioned above represent a useful means of assessing personality. One of their greatest advantages is that they can be scored without subjective interpretation. In contrast, projective techniques, which are considered next, depend almost entirely upon subjectivity.

Projective tests

The Rorschach test, in which a subject is asked to interpret ink-blots, is an example of a 'projective' technique, so called because the subject is assumed to project his own personality onto the stimulus. A further example in common use is the Thematic Apperception Test (TAT), devised by Murray, in which the subject is asked to construct a story around each of a series of pictures.

A common feature of projective tests is the presentation of vague, ambiguous material, since well-defined stimuli would presumably inhibit the process of projection. In contrast to questionnaire methods, the subject is given freedom to respond as he chooses. The advantage of this arrangement lies in the richness of data that it elicits; the major disadvantage is that scoring depends largely upon intuition.

As might be expected, there are serious doubts concerning the reliability and validity of projective techniques. There is little consistency either within or between scorers. Furthermore, the mood and attitudes of both subject and experimenter influence the results of these tests (Vernon, 1964; Kline, 1983). In their defence, Kline (1983) has discussed attempts to develop objective scoring methods that would greatly enhance the usefulness of projective techniques.

Objective tests

The major features of objective personality tests are that they are scored objectively, and that their purpose is not apparent to the subject. The latter characteristic distinguishes them from the questionnaire method.

The leading proponent of objective tests is Cattell, who has described more than 800 possible objective tests (Cattell and Warburton, 1965). Some objective tests are based on performance measures such as reaction time; others measure the subject's behaviour in natural settings. For example, the fidgetometer, a chair fitted with sensors to measure any movements made by the subject, could be used during an interview.

Although objective tests may prove to be extremely effective, much research is needed to establish their validity. Meanwhile, rigorously developed questionnaires appear to offer the most convenient and sound approach to the scientific measurement of personality.

The pilot personality

There is considerable evidence that the personality of the average pilot is distinct from that of the general population (Farmer, 1984). US Navy jet pilots were found by Fry and Reinhardt (1969) to exhibit 'active-masculine' personalities. Comparable, but less extreme, deviation from the profile characteristic of the general population was noted for male pilots in US general aviation (Novello and Youssef, 1974a). The personality profile of their female counterparts was rather similar (Novello and Youssef, 1974b), and indeed resembled more closely that of the average male than of the average female. In the framework of Eysenck's dimensions of personality, pilots tend to present as considerably more stable than the general population, and somewhat more extraverted (e.g. Bartram and Dale, 1982).

It can be concluded, therefore, that there is an identifiable 'pilot personality'. The characteristic differences between the pilot and the general population are probably more extreme in military than in civil groups. Nevertheless, the pilot personality appears to transcend even sex differences.

The 'accident-prone' personality

If the common conception that some individuals are more error prone than others could be substantiated, this aspect of personality would be useful during aircrew selection. However, although certain personality characteristics appear to be associated with increased likelihood of accident involvement, the notion of a single, clearly defined, accident-prone personality is probably untenable.

Levine *et al.* (1976) reported that attitudes to risk taking were predictive of injuries and accidents aboard an aircraft carrier. Sanders and Hofmann (1975) obtained evidence that scores on some scales of the 16PF were correlated with accident involvement among US Navy aircrew, but a later study (Sanders, Hofmann and Neese, 1976) failed to replicate these findings.

Alkov and Borowsky (1980) found that social maladjustment appeared to be associated with accident involvement. Although this conclusion is of uncertain validity, since personality assessments were obtained from flight surgeons who were aware of the individuals' accident histories, it is consistent with findings from studies of automobile accidents implicating aggressive, anti-social, or non-conforming behaviour (Farmer, 1984).

There have been several attempts to relate the dimensions of extraversion and neuroticism to accident involvement. One of the most common conclusions is that the neurotic extravert is most at risk (e.g. Shaw and Sichel, 1971). However, there is considerable variation between studies (Farmer, 1984), and it has sometimes been found, for example, that introverts are more likely than extraverts to be in accidents.

These fundamental discrepancies may reflect the ultimate futility of the search for a unique accident-prone personality. Different personality characteristics will probably predispose individuals towards different types of error. The sensation-seeking behaviour of the extravert and the caution of the introvert may both present risk in particular circumstances. Only a finer analysis of the nature of accidents will reveal their relationships to personality.

Intelligence

In its broadest sense, intelligence comprises the ability to use knowledge to adapt effectively to the environment. The measurement of intelligence has assumed great importance in modern society. Its relevance to aviation is primarily associated with selection and training.

In the early years of the twentieth century, Alfred Binet was presented with the task of identifying mentally subnormal Parisian schoolchildren. Binet devised a series of problems which varied in difficulty, and could therefore discriminate between children of different ages. From a given score, *mental age* could be calculated in terms of the chronological age for which the individual's performance was representative.

Binet's tests were developed by Terman, and became known as the Stanford–Binet tests. Terman introduced the notion of the *intelligence quotient* (IQ), defined as:

$$IQ = (mental\ age/chronological\ age) \times 100$$

Thus a child of 6 years with a mental age of 7 years and 6 months was said to have an IQ of 125. This type of IQ is known as a *ratio* IQ, and can be distinguished from the *deviation* IQ used in many modern tests, such as the Wechsler Intelligence Scales. The deviation IQ is a standard score (a score expressed in terms of the number of standard deviations by which it deviates from the mean); since it is not a true 'intelligence quotient' based on the ratio of mental to chronological age, it can be interpreted as a traditional IQ only if the distribution of scores is matched to that obtained using the Stanford–Binet's ratio method (Anastasi, 1968). To satisfy this requirement, scores on most tests, including the Wechsler scales, are therefore rescaled to produce a distribution with a mean of 100 and a standard deviation of 15.

One source of controversy concerning intelligence tests is their possible unfair discrimination against individuals of certain socio-economic or cultural backgrounds. The ideal solution to this problem would be the development of a *culture-free* test, in which there is no possible influence of past experience. However, since test taking is itself culturally determined a more reasonable approach is to recognize the existence of cultural biases and to develop *culture-fair* tests in which these biases are minimized. For example, items may be selected that can be assumed to be novel or, conversely, to be extremely familiar to every individual likely to take the test. However, no intelligence test can be said to have achieved complete cultural fairness, and this problem must be acknowledged when comparing scores from different cultural groups.

Most well-known intelligence tests have demonstrated reasonable reliability. For example, scores on alternate forms of the Stanford–Binet test are highly correlated, and each form has high internal consistency as measured by the correlation of scores on individual items with total score. Validity is a rather more controversial topic. A major aspect of the construct validity of intelligence tests is that scores should increase during childhood and adolescence, and this principle guided the construction of the Stanford–Binet test. The predictive validity of intelligence tests is less well established. Although they are highly correlated with most measures of scholastic achievement, they perform poorly in the prediction of job success and in other practical applications. These shortcomings, however, may be partly attributable to the fact that intelligence interacts with other factors, such as personality, in most real-life situations.

The nature of intelligence

Two important issues concerning the nature of intelligence are whether it is a unitary attribute or a collection of specialized abilities; and whether it is determined primarily by genetic or environmental factors.

The development of correlational and factor-analytic methods played a major role in the construction of theories concerning the components of intelligence. Spearman (1904, 1927) noted that scores on many different types of test were positively correlated, but that the degree of correlation was often rather low. To account for these findings, he proposed a two-factor theory of intelligence, in which a general ability (g), responsible for the correlations between tests, was supplemented by a variety of specific (s) factors. Thus the ability to perform a particular test would be a function of g and of the s factor appropriate to that test. Modern research relating intelligence to information-processing concepts suggests that g may be identifiable as attentional resources (Hunt, 1980).

The fundamental importance of g, or general intelligence, was challenged by Thurstone (Thurstone, 1938; Thurstone and Thurstone, 1941), who established by factor analysis a small number of distinct 'primary abilities' (for example, verbal, numerical, and spatial). Guilford (1967) extended this notion by postulating the existence of 120 separate abilities, defined in terms of task materials, processing requirements and the type of solution required (*Figure 27.3*). The major source of the

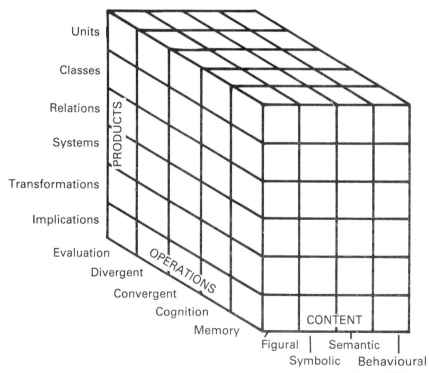

Figure 27.3 Guilford's model of the structure of human intellect. (After Guilford, 1965.)

discrepancies between these theories is the depth of factor analysis considered appropriate. For example, Spearman's g can be recovered by further factor analysis of Thurstone's primary abilities (cf. the personality theories of Eysenck and Cattell discussed earlier).

In general, intelligence tests are concerned primarily with the measurement of g rather than of specific abilities. Tests of the latter are more properly called aptitude tests, and are useful in applications such as personnel selection.

Cattell has proposed the existence of two distinct g factors: fluid ability (*gf*) and crystallized ability (*gc*). The former denotes the individual's pure reasoning ability, and is assumed to be largely innate; the latter refers to the manifestation of this fluid ability as a result of the individual's environmental and cultural experience (*see* Kline, 1976). Thus Cattell's Culture-fair Test of Intelligence attempts to measure *gf* rather than *gc*.

Although Cattell's theory acknowledges the influence of the environment, it emphasizes the importance of innate ability. The relative importance of heredity and environment ('nature versus nurture') remains a contentious subject with political and social implications that transcend psychological theory. Eysenck and Kamin's (1981) book represents a debate between these two leading contemporary theorists, the former a proponent of the genetic, and the latter of the environmental, viewpoints. For the present purposes, a brief description of the type of evidence used to support these opposing viewpoints will suffice.

Findings that the IQ scores of identical twins are correlated more strongly than those of non-identical twins, and remain highly correlated even if the twins are separated and subjected to different environments, seem to support the genetic view. However, environmental factors have also been found to be important in many studies. For example, placing disadvantaged children in richer environments has been shown to increase their IQ scores, and it has also been demonstrated that the IQ of adopted children comes to resemble more closely that of their adoptive parents after a period of time. In summary, therefore, it seems likely that IQ is determined by a complex interaction between heredity and environment, and that the adoption of a polarized theoretical stance may ultimately prove unhelpful.

Aptitudes

In the previous section it was noted that intelligence tests are concerned primarily with the assessment of general ability. Although these tests have some usefulness in personnel selection, it is often necessary to obtain an indication of the individual's aptitude for a particular type of activity. Aptitude tests are much more specific in nature than intelligence tests; their content is determined by the requirements of the job.

It is important to distinguish between *aptitude* and *achievement* tests. The former predict the ability of an inexperienced individual to perform a particular task; the latter measure the individual's current capacity to perform that task. Thus aptitude testing typically occurs during selection, whereas achievement testing occurs during or after training.

Selection for many occupations may be achieved using published aptitude tests. For example, several tests exist for the measurement of mechanical aptitude. Among the best known of these are the Minnesota series (Spatial Relations Test, Mechanical Assembly Test, and Paper Form Board) originally published in 1930. Similarly, selection for clerical jobs is facilitated by the use of tests such as the General Clerical Test, which provides measures of clerical aptitude and of numerical and verbal ability.

Test batteries, giving scores on a range of aptitudes, are in some circumstances preferable to individual tests. For example, the Differential Aptitude Tests and the General Aptitude Test Battery are often used in vocational guidance and selection. The latter permits assessment of nine aptitudes found to be important in a wide variety of occupations. The subject's scores may be compared with occupational ability patterns published in conjunction with the battery.

Although published tests have wide applicability, it is sometimes necessary to produce custom-made aptitude tests. The Complex Co-ordination Test (Melton, 1947), for example, emerged from a major research effort on flying ability by the US Army Air Force during the 1940s. This test, which requires the subject to manipulate a rudder and control column, was found to be useful in pilot selection. More detailed consideration of the problem of selecting aircrew, both civil and military, will be given in a later chapter.

The validity of aptitude tests can be determined only in relation to their intended applications. Since they are used to provide an indication of future performance, high *predictive* validity is particularly important. Thus a test used in pilot selection must be shown to predict the outcome of a suitable criterion, such as success in flying training.

Motivation

Human performance cannot be predicted merely by measuring ability. It is important also to consider the forces that incite the individual to pursue particular goals. The study of motivation is concerned with the psychological and physiological needs that produce these forces, and investigates *why*, rather than *how*, actions are performed.

Maslow (1943) proposed a theory of motivation, based on a hierarchy of needs, that has been applied in occupational settings. At the lowest level in the hierarchy are physiological needs, and at the highest are needs for self-actualization (*Figure 27.4*). Maslow postulated that the individual strives to work upwards in the hierarchy, satisfying the needs at each level in turn. Thus the source of motivation in a particular context can be identified as the lowest need level currently unsatisfied. For example, the need for security will become a motivator only when the physiological needs have been satisfied.

Although Maslow's theory achieved great influence, its propositions have not gone unchallenged (Davies and Shackleton, 1975; Thierry and Koopman-Iwema, 1984). Some studies have failed to find categories of needs corresponding to those of Maslow, while others have presented evidence that certain needs may act as motivators even if more basic needs remain unsatisfied.

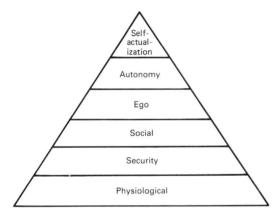

Figure 27.4 Maslow's hierarchy of needs. (After Maslow, 1943.)

The two-factor theory proposed by Herzberg (1966) represents another approach to the problem of motivation. Herzberg and his colleagues asked workers to describe job-related factors that produced positive or negative attitudes, and to indicate the effects of these factors. They found that positive attitudes were generated by factors such as achievement and promotion that were intrinsic to the job and fulfilled the need for self-actualization, whereas negative attitudes were associated with factors such as salary and company policy that constituted the context rather than the content of the job.

These findings suggested that job satisfaction and dissatisfaction do not form a continuum; rather, each has qualitatively different sources. In his two-factor theory, therefore, Herzberg referred to job-content factors as 'motivators', and suggested that only they could produce satisfaction and

influence productivity; the job-context ('hygiene') factors could merely prevent dissatisfaction.

Since Herzberg's theory refutes the notion that job satisfaction and productivity are influenced by changes in working conditions, attention has been directed towards redesigning the job to provide greater intrinsic motivation. Job enlargement, in which the individual is given further responsibilities, has been advocated as an effective means of achieving this goal. However, Davies and Shackleton (1975) in reviewing the evidence from various studies conclude that job enlargement does not necessarily improve both productivity and satisfaction. Indeed, it may lead individuals who reject established attitudes concerning the value of work to become less satisfied.

The importance of individual differences in motivation has been highlighted in the work of McClelland (e.g. 1961), who used the Thematic Apperception Test to assess the need for achievement, often abbreviated to nAch. High nAch has been shown to be associated with superior performance on laboratory tasks such as anagram solution, and with occupational success.

References

ALKOV, R.A. and BOROWSKY, M.S. (1980) A questionnaire study of psychological background factors in US Navy aircraft accidents. *Aviation Space and Environmental Medicine*, **51**, 860–863

ANASTASI, A. (1968) *Psychological Testing*. London: Macmillan

BARTRAM, D. and DALE, H.C.A. (1982) The Eysenck Personality Inventory as a selection test for military pilots. *Journal of Occupational Psychology*, **55**, 287–296

CATTELL, R.B. and WARBURTON, F.W. (1965) *Objective Personality and Motivation Tests*. Champaign: University of Illinois Press

DAVIES, D.R. and SHACKLETON, V.J. (1975) *Psychology and Work*. London: Methuen

EYSENCK, H.J. and EYSENCK, S.B.G. (1969) *Personality Structure and Measurement*. London: Routledge and Kegan Paul

EYSENCK, H.J. and EYSENCK, S.B.G. (1976) *Psychoticism as a Dimension of Personality*. London: Routledge and Kegan Paul

EYSENCK, H.J. and KAMIN, L. (1981) *Intelligence: The Battle for the Mind*. London: Pan

FARMER, E.W. (1984) Personality factors in aviation. *International Journal of Aviation Safety*, **2**, 175–179

FRANSELLA, F. (ed.) (1981) *Personality: Theory, Measurement and Research*. London: Methuen

FRY, G.E. and REINHARDT, R.F. (1969) Personality characteristics of jet pilots as measured by the Edwards Personal Preference Schedule. *Aerospace Medicine*, **40**, 484–486

GUILFORD, J.P. (1967) *The Nature of Human Intelligence*. New York: McGraw-Hill

HEIM, A.W. (1968) *Manual of AH5 Group Test of High Grade Intelligence*. Windsor: NFER Publishing Co.

HERZBERG, F. (1966) *Work and the Nature of Man*. London: Staples Press

HUNT, E. (1980) Intelligence as an information-processing concept. *British Journal of Psychology*, **71**, 449–474

KLINE, P. (1976) *Psychological Testing: The Measurement of Intelligence, Ability and Personality*. London: Malaby Press

KLINE, P. (1983) *Personality: Measurement and Theory*. London: Hutchinson

LEVINE, J.B., LEE, J.O., RYMAN, D.H. and RAE, R.H. (1976) Attitudes and accidents aboard an aircraft carrier. *Aviation Space and Environmental Medicine*, **47**, 82–85

MASLOW, A.H. (1943) A theory of human motivation. *Psychological Review*, **50**, 370–396

MCCLELLAND, D.C. (1961) *The Achieving Society*. New York: Van Nostrand

MELTON, A.W. (ed.) (1947) *Apparatus Tests*. AAF Aviation Psychology Program Research Report No. 4. Washington: Government Printing Office

NOVELLO, J.R. and YOUSSEF, Z.I. (1974a) Psycho-social studies in general aviation: 1. Personality profile of male pilots. *Aerospace Medicine*, **45**, 185–188

NOVELLO, J.B. and YOUSSEF, Z.I. (1974b) Psycho-social studies in general aviation: 2. Personality profile of female pilots. *Aerospace Medicine*, **45**, 630–633

SANDERS, M.G. and HOFMANN, M.A. (1975) Personality aspects of involvement in pilot-error accidents. *Aviation Space and Environmental Medicine*, **46**, 186–190

SANDERS, M.G., HOFMANN, M.A. and NEESE, T.A. (1976) Cross-validation study of the personality aspects of involvement in pilot-error accidents. *Aviation Space and Environmental Medicine*, **47**, 177–179

SHAW, L. and SICHEL, H.S. (1971) *Accident Proneness*. Oxford: Pergamon Press

SPEARMAN, C. (1904) 'General intelligence' objectively determined and measured. *American Journal of Psychology*, **15**, 201–293

SPEARMAN, C. (1927) *The Abilities of Man*. New York: Macmillan

THIERRY, H. and KOOPMAN-IWEMA, A.M. (1984) Motivation and satisfaction. In *Handbook of Work and Organizational Psychology, Volume 1*, edited by P.J.D. Drenth, H. Thierry, P.J. Willems and C.J. de Wolff, pp. 131–174. Chichester: Wiley

THURSTONE, L.L. (1938) Primary mental abilities. *Psychometric Monographs*, No. **1**. Chicago: University of Chicago Press

THURSTONE, L.L. and THURSTONE, T.G. (1941) Factorial studies of intelligence. *Psychometric Monographs*, No. **2**. Chicago: University of Chicago Press

VERNON, P.E. (1964) *Personality Assessment: A Critical Survey*. London: Methuen

28

Selection and training

J.W. Chappelow and M. Churchill

Selection

Introduction

When the Royal Flying Corps was established, it was generally believed that the best predictor of success in flying training was the ability to ride a horse. However, it soon became apparent that this was not an effective selection procedure; many individuals failed to acquire the complex skills of a pilot, with expensive and time-consuming consequences. In Britain, a selection procedure was introduced, based on a medical examination of the physiological systems most affected by altitude, and on simple tests of motor co-ordination; whereas the system adopted in the United States examined emotional stability, perception of tilt, and mental alertness (Koonce, 1984).

Although the psychology of selection developed during the inter-war years, there was little change in the procedures used by the Royal Air Force until 1941 (Vernon and Parry, 1949). However, the increased demand for pilots during the Second World War, and the serious consequences of poor selection, stimulated the development of more rigorous criteria.

There have been rapid developments in aircraft technology in recent years. Goodman *et al.* (1983) have suggested that:

'The successful tactical air mission of yesteryear depended predominantly upon a pilot's psycho-motor abilities in guiding his aircraft and its projectiles, success for the modern-day counterpart relies also upon his ability to process vast arrays of complex information, make rapid, highly-consequential decisions, *and* execute a large number of co-ordinated responses.'

(p.541, the authors' emphasis)

The techniques developed in the 1940s are still used, but new tests are continually being evaluated and introduced into modern selection schemes.

Principles of selection

Any selection test must satisfy two criteria of *reliability* and *validity*.

Reliability

The reliability of a test reflects the consistency of its scores. A test would be perfectly reliable if it yielded the same score on two separate occasions. In practice, however, such consistency is unlikely because error is introduced by extraneous factors, such as changes in emotional state or differences in environmental conditions. To minimize error, tests are administered under standardized conditions.

Test reliability can be estimated by several methods, all based upon the statistical technique of correlation. This procedure expresses the level of agreement between two sets of scores as a correlation coefficient. All coefficient values fall between -1 and $+1$. A correlation of $+1$ indicates perfect agreement; a correlation of 0 indicates independence; a correlation of -1 indicates an inverse relationship.

Methods of assessing reliability

1. *Test–retest reliability*—The same test is given to the same people on two occasions, either with no inter-test interval (immediate test–retest), or after a specific time interval (delayed test–retest). Not surprisingly, the immediate retest

method generally produces the higher estimate of reliability because virtually everything is held constant over the two test sessions. In fact, the level of reliability may be artificially high because testees are likely to remember and repeat their responses on the second occasion.

2. *Split-half reliability*—The internal consistency of a single test is assessed by examining the degree to which the different test items measure the attribute in question. Items are allocated to one of two groups (e.g., odd, versus even, numbered questions) and scores on the two halves are then correlated.

3. *Equivalent-forms reliability*—Sometimes it is desirable to develop more than one test. The correlation of results on these different versions is equivalent-forms reliability.

Validity

Test validity reflects the degree to which a test measures what it purports to measure. Although a psychological test cannot be valid unless it is reliable, it can be reliable without being valid if it measures behaviour that is irrelevant to the attribute being examined. Different forms of validity are recognized.

Types of validity

1. *Face validity*—A test has face validity if it appears to measure the particular attribute in question. A test that has face validity is not necessarily a good selection tool. Thus a test of the theoretical aspects of flight might appear to be relevant to pilot selection, although it would not necessarily provide any information about an individual's aptitude for flying. Face validity is usually adduced from the reaction of those sitting the test. If a test has little face validity, candidates may fail to take it seriously. This in turn can affect test reliability.

2. *Content validity*—When a test is designed to examine the ability to perform a complex task, all aspects of that task must be included in order for it to have content validity. Content validity is established through job analysis (a procedure that involves identifying a job's constituent parts) rather than by any statistical procedures.

3. *Predictive validity*—Predictive validity is concerned with a test's ability to predict the outcome on some independent criterion. In aircrew selection the criterion is usually the successful completion of training. Predictive validity can be assessed by allowing all candidates to proceed into the training programme regardless of performance on the selection test.

Success during training can then be correlated with selection test scores (*see* Koonce, 1981).

4. *Concurrent validity*—If a test can distinguish between different levels of performance attained by current incumbents (rather than applicants), it is said to have concurrent validity.

Practical aspects of selection

Typically, selection is based on the results from a battery of tests which measure a number of attributes including intelligence, ability and aptitude (*see* Chapter 27 for a discussion of individual differences). *Figure 28.1* represents a situation in which both the selection and training criteria have been established. The ellipse represents a positive correlation between selection and success in training. Had there been a perfect relationship between the two sets of results, the ellipse would be replaced by a straight line and all those who were selected would have satisfied the training criterion.

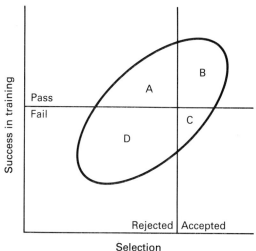

Figure 28.1 The relationship between selection and success in training.

Figure 28.1 demonstrates two major problems in selection. First, some of those who do well on the overall selection criterion do not satisfy a subsequent training criterion. These 'false positives' are in sector C in *Figure 28.1*. Second, some of those rejected as a result of their performance on the selection test would have succeeded had they been selected. These 'false negatives' appear in sector A in *Figure 28.1*.

The selection ratio is calculated by dividing the number who are selected (B+C) by the number of candidates (A+B+C+D). In *Figure 28.1* this ratio is approximately 33%. However, the *success* ratio

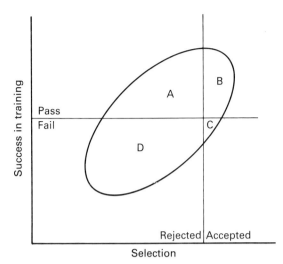

Figure 28.2 As a result of raising the selection criterion, fewer candidates enter training. A higher success ratio is thus achieved, but the proportion of false negatives (area A) is also increased.

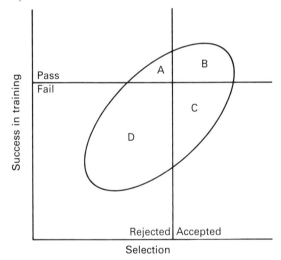

Figure 28.3 When the entry standard is lowered, the proportion of false negatives is reduced, but the success ratio is also negatively affected.

(calculated by comparing the number who succeed (B) to those who are selected (B+C)) is only 2:3. In other words, a third of the selected applicants fail to perform satisfactorily during training. When training costs are high, as in aviation, such a substantial proportion of 'failures' would be unacceptable. When a large number of applicants is available, the selection criterion can be set higher, thus reducing the number of training failures (*see Figure 28.2*). But when too few high-scoring candidates are available, a decision has to be taken either to accept fewer people into training, or to lower the entry standard. If the standard is lowered, fewer of the able candidates (sector A) will be ignored, but the

number of training failures will increase (to approximately 60% of those selected in *Figure 28.3*). The optimum selection ratio obviously depends upon cost of training and the number of suitable applicants.

If the validity of the selection criterion is increased, the proportion of individuals falling into sectors A and C is reduced. In other words, fewer acceptable candidates are lost, and fewer unsuitable candidates are passed into training. Selection tests must be continuously validated for this reason.

Content validity, once established, can be maintained by frequent job analysis, but the investigation of predictive validity poses a more difficult problem because of the cost and potential danger in allowing unselected candidates to go forward into pilot training. The predictive validity of a test, therefore, is generally evaluated by comparing its success ratio with that of existing tests. This ignores the problem of denying able candidates the opportunity for training, but represents the best practical solution to a difficult problem.

Pilot selection

General criteria

Pilot selection is not based on aptitude alone. Civilian and military organizations selecting *ab initio* pilots also try to satisfy criteria relating to mental and physical ability, and personality.

Civilian selection

In order to cope with the need to fly various aircraft during an airline career, the civilian candidate must be adaptable. Moreover, he or she must demonstrate both the level of ability and personality to attain the airline's ultimate goal, command of the flight deck. Selection is therefore complicated because attributes that make for an efficient and effective First Officer may not be those of a skilful Captain, and vice versa. Those who are willing to be led do not always make good leaders.

Since a review of jet transport accidents revealed the importance of crew co-ordination to flight safety (Cooper, White and Lauber, 1980), there has been increasing interest in social interaction on the flight deck (Helmreich *et al.*, 1986; Lauber, 1987; Wheale, 1984). 'Cockpit Resource Management' (CRM) has become a major concern both of commercial and of military organizations (Orlady and Foushee, 1987). Foushee (1983) provided an excellent summary of the flight-deck milieu:

'Since the cockpit crew is a highly structured small group, a number of socio-psychological, personality, and group process variables are relevant to crew effectiveness. The complexities of the operational environment, aircraft systems, and the sheer volume of information that must be processed (often in brief periods of time), mandate highly co-ordinated team performance.'

Military selection

Military selection often involves dual criteria. Frequently, those wishing to become pilots also have to be selected for officer training. In Britain today, all three military services select pilots. The Royal Air Force and Royal Navy have commissioned officer pilots, whereas Army pilots may be either commissioned or non-commissioned officers. In the United States a similar situation exists. Again, it is the Army who are the exception having accepted pilots with Warrant Officer status. Although Warrant Officers in the US Army are regarded as commissioned officers, they are employed as specialists and do not progress through the normal rank structure. A detailed explanation of these contrasting policies is beyond the scope of this chapter: but they can be partly explained in terms of different attitudes towards fixed-wing and rotary-wing aircraft (Brown, Dohme and Sanders, 1981).

Where the dual criteria of pilot and officer are employed, difficulties can arise because an individual with the appropriate aptitude, who is highly motivated to fly, may not be thought of as 'officer material'. The candidate may be rejected, either because he or she failed to display an interest in the additional duties and responsibilities usually assigned to commissioned officers, or simply because he or she failed to satisfy some personal or social criterion. So long as there is a plentiful supply of suitable applicants, the more discriminative criteria would not interfere with the Air Force or Navy's ability to meet their respective selection ratios. When such dual criteria are employed, however, a situation could arise in which the selection ratio was not being met because too few candidates were regarded as officer material. To ameliorate this situation, those responsible for selection would have to choose between three alternatives. First, they could fall short of the training quota; second, the overall criterion level could be lowered, thus decreasing the success ratio (*Figure 28.3*); or third, the selection criteria could be modified to allow for the training of non-commissioned pilots.

Specific criteria

Royal Air Force selection procedure

So far, the actual procedures employed by either civilian and military selectors have not been discussed in detail. However, a definitive selection procedure cannot be described here, because different organizations have developed their own systems. Therefore, the procedures employed at the Officer and Air Crew Selection Centre (OASC), RAF Biggin Hill, will be discussed in more detail to demonstrate the complex criteria by which applicants are judged.

Before an applicant arrives at OASC for his 3-day Selection Board, he will have completed an application form and had a preliminary interview with a serving RAF officer. At this initial interview the officer checks the applicant's eligibility (i.e. is between 17.5 and 24 years old and has a minimum of 5 'O' level passes at the General Certificate of Education Examination or equivalent qualification), and makes a preliminary assessment of his personality, i.e. does the candidate show 'officer potential', and motivation? On arriving at OASC candidates experience 5 hours of ability and aptitude tests. Together, these tests examine intelligence, psycho-motor co-ordination (e.g., candidates manipulate hand and foot controls in order to keep a moving spot over a target), and instrument comprehension. The score from each of the aptitude tests is multiplied by a factor, which reflects the individual test's predictive validity, to produce the Pilot Index score (p-index).

Those who achieve the criterion level in the aptitude tests must then pass a rigorous medical examination before going on to the Part 1 interview. This interview, conducted by two boarding officers, is used to assess personality, attitudes and motivation. In the first part of the interview the candidate is asked to give biographical information. Personality is assessed in terms of both presentation and content (i.e. can the candidate give a good account of himself, and has he made the most of his opportunities?). The second part of the interview examines the candidate's motivation and attitudes, in particular his grasp of current affairs. Following this interview the candidate's overall performance thus far is reviewed, and a decision made as to whether or not he should continue on to Part 2 which includes individual and group exercises. Candidates must demonstrate in these tests their ability both to command and to be a constructive member of a group. From the Part 2 tests, the boarding officers assess whether the candidate has the necessary maturity, and social skill, to pass initial officer training.

By grading candidates using a combination of objective tests (attainment, ability, and aptitude), a structured interview, and exercises, OASC has been able to meet its selection target. The tests currently in use are constantly validated against success in initial pilot training (IPT). In 1983, the 'P' score was introduced following one such validation which identified the following as the best predictors of success in training: previous flying experience; pilot aptitude score; age; and Part 1 Interview grading.

Other selection procedures

The aptitude tests used at OASC, designed for fixed-wing aircraft (i.e. 88% of the RAF's fleet), are used to select all military pilots. In 1980, because of perceived differences between fixed- and rotary-wing piloting skills, the Army Air Corps (AAC) commissioned a study to develop tests specifically for rotary-wing aircraft. The Micropat system which was produced (Bartram and Dale, 1985) was primarily designed to test cognitive load and risk perception although it also included personality questionnaires. A validation of these tests on 105 AAC candidates revealed higher levels of predictive validity for both Basic and Advanced training (0.52 and 0.57, respectively) compared with using the p-index (i.e. 0.23 and 0.16). Although these results appeared convincing, they were based on a relatively small and highly restricted sample (i.e. 105 candidates who had been selected on the basis of the p-index). Moreover, since 1980 the RAF has devised its own tests of cognitive workload, so the AAC has decided to continue using the OASC tests rather than introduce the Micropat system. However, in addition to these computerized aptitude tests the AAC employs a system of flying grading, assessed in terms of 15 hours on a Chipmunk.

This move towards tests that examine cognitive workload is vital in view of the new pilot role discussed above. Moreover, Gopher (1982) increased the predictive validity of the Israeli Air Force pilot selection procedure using a dichotic listening test. Those who graduated from the 2-year training programme had significantly lower error scores, compared with those who failed training. The selection ratio of the test battery would have been improved by including the results from the dichotic listening test, because the number below the selected criterion would have increased from 17.4% to 35.5%, although there was no similar improvement in the success ratio. Similarly, Damos and Smist's (1981) research, using a dual-task paradigm, revealed important individual differences in the ability to adopt the most efficient response strategy (i.e. simultaneous responding). When informed about the simultaneous strategy, those who naturally adopted an alternating response strategy performed at a similar level to those who adopted this strategy spontaneously, whereas those who originally adopted a massed strategy were unable to achieve a level of performance similar to the other two groups.

RAF selectors assess personality by interview and observation. Although other techniques are available (*see* Chapter 27 for a more detailed discussion), research has so far failed to identify more effective procedures. Nevertheless, personality questionnaires such as the 16PF may be used more appropriately to eliminate those with particularly unsuitable personality profiles (e.g., an individual whose profile suggested that he or she was extremely tense, apprehensive, and undisciplined).

Personality can also be assessed using projective tests (i.e. tests that demand responses to ambiguous stimuli). Although Swedish research suggested that accident-prone candidates could be identified using the Defence Mechanism Test (DMT), an evaluation by the RAF failed to produce comparable data. Although the theoretical basis underlying the DMT is open to question, the statistical and procedural shortcomings in the Swedish study undermine the original results (Chappelow, 1985). Moreover, there are serious doubts concerning the reliability and validity of projective assessment, because of the subjective nature of these tests (*see* Chapter 27).

Training

Introduction

Contemplation of the complexities of training necessarily requires some understanding of the learning process. What is learning? The answer to this question is not as straightforward as it at first appears. Clearly, objective evidence of learning can be obtained only if there is an observable change in behaviour. But it is obvious that other processes (e.g. maturation, fatigue, disease) can also change behaviour. Changes due to learning tend to be relatively permanent and to result from experience or practice. In general they are not likely to occur unless the student is motivated to learn. Several paradigms of learning have been explored experimentally; these may reflect different types of learning or different aspects of the same underlying processes.

Paradigms of learning

Classical conditioning

Pavlov (1849–1936) established many of the basic principles of conditioning in his work with dogs. He observed that some stimuli (such as the sight and smell of food) elicited simple responses (such as salivation). By repeatedly presenting the unconditioned stimulus (food) in conjunction with another stimulus (e.g. the sound of a bell, usually presented slightly before the food) he found that it was possible, eventually, to elicit the response by presenting the bell alone. Pavlov was able to show how the strength of the conditioned response (the amount of saliva produced at the sound of the bell) increased as training progressed. He demonstrated several other phenomena common to many learning situations:

1. *Extinction*—If, after training, the conditioned stimulus (the bell in the example above) is repeatedly presented without the unconditioned stimulus (i.e. without *reinforcement*), the strength of the conditioned response will decline and, eventually, disappear.
2. *Spontaneous recovery*—If, after a period of extinction, the subject is returned to the experimental situation, the conditioned response is often found to have recovered some of its former strength. This suggests that the extinction procedure does not simply weaken the original conditioning but either interferes with the response (the subject learns not to respond), or that the conditioned response is suppressed by a temporary inhibition.
3. *Stimulus generalization*—This is an important characteristic of all learning. Once a response has been conditioned to a stimulus, other similar stimuli also acquire the power to elicit the response in proportion to their similarity to the original conditioned stimulus.
4. *Higher order conditioning*—Once a conditioned response has been established, it may be used as the basis of further conditioning so that the conditioned response can be associated with other stimuli. In this type of experiment, the first conditioned stimulus provides *secondary reinforcement*, and no primary reinforcement is given.

Although Pavlov (and many others) illuminated some important characteristics of learning, the classical conditioning paradigm is not an adequate model for the rich variety of learned behaviours observed in man and other animals. An attempt to cope with this variety is embodied in the instrumental conditioning paradigm.

Instrumental conditioning

The responses learned in instrumental conditioning have one or both of two objectives: they may result in a positive reinforcement (food, water, sexual intercourse, etc.) or the avoidance of a negative reinforcer (pain, fear, etc.). In both instances the reinforcer may be a secondary one—a stimulus that has been associated with a primary positive or negative reinforcer. A typical instrumental response is that of pressing a lever to obtain food. An animal that is motivated (has been deprived of food) may, in the course of general exploratory activity, press the lever that causes a food pellet to be delivered. After a few such accidental responses the rate of responding increases; the animal has learned a response that is instrumental in the attainment of a

goal. The goal need not necessarily be linked to a physiological drive. Thus instrumental responses can be learned to satisfy curiosity. In this manner apparently incidental (or latent) learning can occur which only becomes apparent when a reward is provided to motivate performance. Long and complex sequences of responses can be established by careful training, as can discriminations between classes of stimuli or even concepts. Extinction, stimulus generalization and secondary reinforcement can be demonstrated in a manner similar to that for classical conditioning. Partial reinforcement has been found to be an important manipulation of the experimental conditions. By requiring several responses for each reinforcement, high rates of responding and a resistance to extinction can be established, particularly if a variable ratio of responses to reinforcements is used.

Insight

Although the paradigm of instrumental conditioning is relevant to many aspects of learning and training, there are some varieties of learning that require more complex formulations. Some animals, in particular humans, seem to be able to learn in a way that involves sudden solutions to a problem rather than blind trial and error and reinforcement of simple responses. Such solutions may be obtained by covert (i.e. conceptual) trial and error based on previously learned habits. The notions of motivation and reinforcement are by no means irrelevant in this context. It is worth noting, however, that humans (among others) will undertake such hypothesis testing out of sheer curiosity and that the only reinforcement they receive may be the knowledge of their success. The informative aspects of reinforcement may have an important function, perhaps the critical one, in apparently simpler forms of learning. It is certainly true that feedback of information on accuracy or speed of performance is essential to the development of skills of all types.

Verbal learning

The earliest systematic studies of learning were conducted by Ebbinghaus (1850–1909) using verbal materials such as poems, lists of words and nonsense syllables (meaningless, but pronounceable, combinations of letters). Although verbal material presents special problems in experimentation (e.g. covert rehearsal and interaction with experiences outside the experiment), it represents an important area of learning with wide relevance. Some of the more significant findings from this type of study are:

1. Forgetting is most marked immediately after training.

2. Forgetting is at least partly caused by interference from other learning activities.
3. The beginning and end of a list, or a lesson, are more easily learned than the middle.

Human learning

Examples of human learning may be found that are adequately described by the simplest instrumental or classical conditioning paradigm. And, although much human behaviour seems far removed from simple responses and basic drives, the differences appear to be of complexity rather than of kind. This applies even to complicated training objectives like learning to fly. A systematic analysis of the task can often simplify the trainee's—and the trainer's—job by identifying component skills that can be learned separately and by setting objective standards of performance to aim for. Crucial factors are the trainee's motivation and the reinforcement of correct responses (with the emphasis on the informing rather than rewarding role of reinforcement). Some generally important aspects of training are discussed below.

Massed versus distributed practice

Is it better to learn by practising for relatively long periods or to have frequent, short rests? This question was once of considerable theoretical interest in connection with the role (and varieties) of inhibition in learning. Many experiments gave results like those shown in *Figure 28.4*; Digman

(1959) trained two groups on a tracking task giving each group 18 trials of 30 seconds each day. One group had 90 second rests between practice trials (spaced or distributed practice); the other group had only 2 second breaks (massed practice). Several effects are apparent in the results:

1. The improvement shown by the massed-practice group on any one day was less than for the spaced-practice group.
2. The massed-practice group showed an overnight improvement on the first trial of each day—this effect (*reminiscence*) suggests that they had learned more than was evident in their previous day's performance.
3. The spaced-practice group needed some time to 'warm up' on each new day before attaining the level of performance of the previous day.
4. On the final day, both groups were given spaced practice, and the difference between them reduced markedly.

Some experiments seem to show a residual benefit of spaced practice. This may be due to a number of factors that are difficult to control. For example, the spaced-practice group may get more practice by rehearsing mentally during the rest periods. The massed-practice group may get less practice owing to lapses of concentration resulting from fatigue. Overall, it appears that the detrimental effects of massed practice are confined to immediate levels of performance, with little long-term effect on learning (Holding, 1965). However, from a practical point of view, if spacing practice has no drawbacks (such as disruption of the training programme), then there may be some advantages. The student's motivation

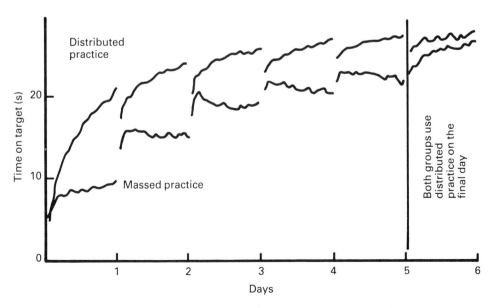

Figure 28.4 Effects of massed and distributed practice. (Adapted from Digman, 1959.)

may be enhanced if his performance shows obvious improvement. In complex tasks, an adequate performance on elements of the task allows the student to tackle more advanced procedures (e.g. positioning the aircraft in the circuit requires a certain minimum of skill in attitude flying). Finally, it is obvious that the effects of massed and spaced practice should be familiar to trainers so that they can make sensible assessments of a student's progress in comparison with others or with the required standard.

Whole versus part practice

Some activities are naturally divisible into component parts; map reading and basic attitude flying are both required for cross-country navigation, for example, but each could be further divided into simpler sub-tasks. To what extent is it advisable to decompose tasks into simple constituents for the purposes of training? There is no clear-cut answer to this question. Practising part tasks seems to be advantageous when the whole is too complex or too large for a novice to tackle conveniently (e.g. learning a long part in a play). It may also have the advantage of maintaining the trainee's interest as progress is more obvious when sub-tasks are being mastered. In general, however, whole-task practice is advantageous, especially when the whole forms a meaningful unit and when the trainee is capable of rapid progress. For practical purposes, it can only be stressed that a systematic task analysis may reveal ways in which the trainee's job could be simplified by separating components of the task, but that care must be taken not to destroy important interrelationships that also have to be learned.

Phases of learning

If a measure of performance in a complex skill is plotted against time in practice, some features commonly emerge. First, in the early stages there may be little improvement; later, performance may improve rapidly. In the final stages, the rate of improvement again slows down. For many skills, the trainee faces an initial conceptual task; he must learn to organize the requirements of the skill and the information to be used into easily understood units. Little change in performance may be evident until this task is completed. In the next phase, psychomotor co-ordination improves and the trainee becomes skilled in sub-tasks. In the final phase, the various components of the skill are integrated into a smooth operation and improvements in timing, speed and ease of performance become evident. Some skills, especially those with a strong hierarchical structure, tend to show rather discontinuous improvements in performance; for considerable periods the trainee may show little or no progress. Good examples are learning to play a musical instrument or to receive Morse code. In the latter case, having achieved a certain standard (speed) receiving letter by letter, the trainee will show no improvement for a while. Eventually, a further improvement occurs when the trainee learns to interpret whole words. A further increase in speed may eventually be apparent when whole phrases are received as a unit. Obviously, there is a risk of discouragement and loss of motivation for the trainee who has reached such a plateau in performance. However, many skills are not especially susceptible to this phenomenon, and erratic performance may be more of a problem.

Knowledge of results

One of the most important features of any training situation is the feedback provided to the student. The role of feedback can be viewed in two ways: it furnishes the information the trainee needs to adjust his actions to match those required of him, and it reinforces correct responses. The former is essential to the development of a skill but the style in which feedback is presented can also have important effects on the trainee's motivation. Feedback of one sort or another is intrinsic to many tasks; most vehicle-control tasks rely on visual feedback—the distance of a car from the kerb, the rate of closure on the vehicle in front, etc. Skilled movements in tasks requiring manual dexterity involve not only visual feedback but also internal, proprioceptive feedback. The trainee may be assisted in learning to use the feedback intrinsic to the task by additional, artificial feedback. Such knowledge of results can be manipulated in several ways that have an influence on learning and performance. One possible drawback is that it may distract attention away from intrinsic cues.

Goldstein and Rittenhouse (1954) provided artificial feedback in an air-to-air gunnery trainer in the form of a buzzer sounding when the target was correctly ranged and sighted. Although a group trained using this method appeared better than one trained without it, removing the buzzer caused a large drop in their performance. The trainees had used the artificial cue to guide their actions, not to evaluate their results. In this particular experiment, the artificial feedback was concurrent with the task. By delaying the feedback until the completion of an action (terminal feedback), better results can be obtained in training relatively uncomplicated tasks. Simply delaying the feedback even further (within reasonable limits) has little effect on learning. This is in contrast to the dramatic effects on performance induced by even small delays in intrinsic feedback.

There are advantages in elaborating feedback beyond the simple report of success or failure. Graphical presentation of, say, control movements could allow the trainee to compare his technique with that of an expert and to modify it accordingly (Holding, 1965). Similarly, the verbal feedback traditionally employed by instructors can, in the hands of a competent instructor, be both informative and highly motivating. In addition, by presenting feedback not only on current responses, but also on accumulated progress, the trainee's performance can be set in context—by comparison with long- or short-term goals, or with others' rates of progress. This feedback can influence the trainee's motivation and efforts to improve—particularly when combined with detailed analysis of his strengths and weaknesses.

Transfer of training

The fundamental purpose of training is to effect a change in the trainee's behaviour or capabilities in situations remote from that in which the training occurs. The assumption that skills once acquired will transfer to the real world, which may be very different from the classroom, is implicit in all training. Over what range of differences does such an assumption hold true? Early interest in this question centred on the notion of ability training; for example, is it possible to improve one's memory simply through practice in memorizing? In general, little transfer seems to occur between unrelated tasks (e.g. learning poems and learning lists of nonsense syllables) unless the trainee is also given instruction on, in this case, general techniques of memorization. In some circumstances the trainee may 'learn to learn' without special prompting (particularly if exposed to a variety of tasks) and, in this event, a degree of non-specific transfer of training may be evident, i.e. the trainee can learn other tasks in the same broad category faster. The saving in training time required to reach a criterion performance on one task produced by practice on another is the standard measure of training transfer. Variables with an important influence on transfer of training are:

1. *Stimulus similarity*—The phenomenon of stimulus generalization was mentioned in connection with simple conditioning. Many skills require the same response to a general class of stimuli. The definition of that class may require the trainee to learn to discriminate between what initially appear to be very similar stimuli (e.g. detecting the spin on a cricket ball). In general the greater the similarity between the stimulus elements of two tasks, the greater will be the transfer of training between them.

2. *Response similarity*—Obviously, when the responses required by two tasks are identical, or very similar, the transfer of training between the tasks can be very high. If the responses are not similar, little or no transfer would be expected (there may be some due to the learning of stimulus discriminations). A third possibility arises when the tasks require basically similar responses with small, but functionally significant, differences. In this case, previous training with one task may hinder progress on the second task—negative transfer. The use of a tiller in steering a boat seems 'unnatural' to many car drivers, and they may make many mistakes before adjusting to the apparent reversal of control sense. Typically, it is intrusions of the previously learned, and now inappropriate, control movements that cause problems early in training. Mastering the new skill may have a retroactive effect on previously learned skills. Although the control movements required by the two tasks may quickly become differentiated in the trainee's mind so that he can perform adequately on both tasks, there remains the possibility of intrusions of inappropriate behaviour in times of stress or inattention. This can be particularly hazardous in aviation where aircraft of the same class (fast jets, four-engined transports, etc.) have broadly similar cockpits; aircraft of the same type within a fleet or squadron may incorporate different modifications. Both states of affairs invite, and have caused, operation of controls in error, with costly consequences.

3. *Task difficulty*—Transfer of training between two tasks may be unequal because the tasks themselves demand different levels of skill. Two opposing principles seem to apply: first, the more difficult task may give better transfer to the easier task because it allows the trainee a greater breadth of experience and may even, in some sense, include the easier task; second, the easier task may permit more accurate learning and so show better transfer to the more difficult task.

Psychomotor skills

An important variety of learning is that used in the acquisition of psychomotor skills. Of particular significance in aviation is skill in tracking such as is necessary for control of an aircraft's flight path. Two major types of tracking task are:

1. *Pursuit tracking*—In this type of task, the operator has to match the position of a controlled element (e.g. a pointer on a display or the position of his own vehicle) with that of a target. Formation flying is an obvious example.

2. *Compensatory tracking*—In this type of task, the operator's display shows only an error signal which he should attempt to reduce to zero. Flying an instrument landing system approach using a zero reader type display uses this type of tracking.

Experimental studies of tracking usually include manipulation of the forcing function, that is the path that the target or error signal follows. The operator's control may work in several different ways; its position may be directly related to the position of the controlled element, or it may control its velocity. In some, generally more difficult, tasks control position affects acceleration of the controlled element. The relationship between the direction of movement of the control and that of the displayed response can have a strong influence on both the level of performance attainable on the task and on a typical operator's rate of learning. Incompatible control–display relationships (i.e. those that oppose previous learning) generally produce an initially poorer performance, but allow greater gains to be made in training. However, experimental studies indicate the persistence of a residual deficit due to incompatibility. Some psychomotor skills, particularly those including manual dexterity, have been studied over long periods of time. The indications are that performance goes on improving indefinitely with practice unless physically limited by the equipment.

Practical aspects

The variety of training undertaken in pursuit of aviation is immense. In addition to the basic psychomotor skills used in control of an aircraft, aircrew are trained in procedural, problem solving, social and managerial skills. Training continues throughout the career. Aircrew will occasionally receive conversion training for a new aircraft type, and at regular intervals will undergo continuation training and assessments. Any generalizations intended to cover this spectrum of activities must necessarily be broad. What follows obeys this dictum.

General principles

A primary requirement of successful training is adequate motivation on the part of the trainee. Maintaining such motivation should be an important concern of the trainer. Knowledge of results provides a significant source of motivation for most trainees. When the results are poor, there may be an immediate depression of performance; this need not do lasting damage if the trainee's overall motivation

is satisfactory and the feedback is both informative and relevant to the trainee's needs. In addition, feedback can be arranged in ways that make learning easier—by drawing the trainee's attention to subtle distinctions or cues; by allowing comparison with ideal responses, and so on. The analysis of the trainee's performance is as important as the practice itself.

Most tasks in aviation are relatively complex. It should, generally, be possible to make the novice's task easier by identifying sub-tasks that can be practised separately. Certainly the task should be analysed and the goals of training specified in objective terms. This not only standardizes the basis on which the trainee is assessed but permits another important form of feedback—assessment of the training system. Without such assessment, and systematic evaluation of changes in the training programme, there can be no rational basis for improvement of the training system. A formal analysis of the training task should also permit the balance between theory and practice to be optimized and appropriate training techniques to be selected (lecture, tutorial, group discussion, simulation, etc.) so as to maximize transfer to the real world.

Simulation

The widespread use of flight simulators brings many training issues, particularly the maximization of transfer, into sharp focus. Flight simulators could be regarded primarily as teaching machines but the impetus for their employment generally owes far more to economic and safety considerations than to a detailed analysis of training objectives. Nevertheless, simulators offer some important advantages over real aircraft:

1. The task can be simplified and the level of difficulty easily matched to the trainee's capabilities. For example, instrument landing procedures can be introduced without cross-winds, turbulence and other traffic to complicate the task and distract the trainee's attention from the essentials of the task.
2. Similarly, discrete components of the job can be taught in part-task trainers without unnecessary distractions.
3. Practice may be intensified on important aspects of the task by using the reset or reposition facilities available on modern simulators to eliminate, for example, flying the whole circuit in order to practice the approach and landing, or the preparatory manoeuvring necessary for air combat training.
4. Feedback can be optimized; some simulators allow the instructor not only to arrest the flight

for an immediate diagnosis of problems, but also to replay short periods so that the trainee can have a second opportunity to see what went wrong. In addition, graphical and numerical analysis of performance is readily provided.

It should be apparent that many of these training advantages are in direct opposition to the 'common-sense' requirement for maximum fidelity in a flight simulator. Obviously a degree of fidelity is required for transfer of training to the real aircraft, but there are two major ways in which total fidelity is a needless (and, in some cases, impossible) target.

First, there are many things to learn about the operation of a complex system; some of them do not require that the system be fully functional or be accompanied by all the incidental stimuli available in flight. For example, the positions of displays and controls and the order in which they are used during a drill can be learned from a static cardboard mock-up.

Second, even when an attempt is made to simulate important cues, only the psychologically important aspects need to be reproduced. Modern motion platforms now extend to the full six degrees of freedom (roll, pitch and yaw angular movements; and surge, heave and sway translations). Common devices for making the limited travel available on such a platform seem like the unlimited freedom available in the air include wash-out, wash-back and subthreshold movements. *Figure 28.5* compares the roll angles produced in an aircraft and in a simulator during a co-ordinated turn. The aircraft's initial acceleration in roll is matched fairly faithfully by the simulator; eventually, the simulator washes out the roll velocity to avoid reaching the end of its available travel. The cockpit is then washed back to a neutral position at an undetectable rate; as a result, the apparent normal acceleration vector rests where the pilot would expect it to be during the turn. Some of the sensations produced by longitudinal acceleration

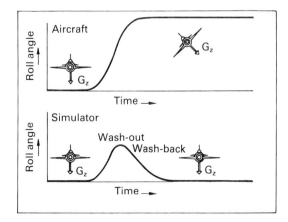

Figure 28.5 Simulation of roll motion.

(surge) can be suggested by pitching the simulator up at an undetectable rate; with the pilot's impression of attitude stabilized by the simulator visual system or instruments, the resulting rotation of the gravity vector is interpreted as a longitudinal acceleration.

Although motion platforms are a common feature of modern simulators, their training advantages seem to be limited. Most flying tasks are visually controlled. In the aircraft, kinaesthetic motion cues provide concurrent feedback on the response of the aircraft to control movements. Providing such cues in a simulator seems to allow experienced pilots to employ control movements more like those they would use in the aircraft and to fly more accurately than they would in a fixed-base simulator (Rolfe *et al.*, 1970). However, there appears to be little direct advantage in terms of training. Jacobs and Roscoe (1975) showed roughly equal transfer in three groups of *ab-initio* students trained in a simulator with normal motion, no motion or motion randomly reversed in bank. Nevertheless, motion simulation probably serves some useful training functions. It can provide alerting stimuli, e.g. yaw signalling failure of an outboard engine. It can support a level of performance that may be necessary to practise advanced tasks, or, at least, reduce the pilot's workload in producing that performance. There is some evidence that intensive, high-rate manoeuvring in a fixed-base simulator, particularly one with a wide-angle visual system, can provoke prolonged and unfortunate effects in pilots who adapt to this dynamically unrealistic regime (Kennedy *et al.*, 1986), though this is not a universal feature of using such simulators (Parfitt and Chappelow, 1986) and the necessary conditions have yet to be fully exposed.

Research into the features required in visual simulations has generally lagged behind the technical developments. Modern, computer-generated visual systems have now attained high levels of performance in terms of dynamic response, angle of view and fidelity of screen content. Their limitations include low levels of brightness, less than realistic texturing, and absence of stereoscopic information (the last may be significant in some specialized tasks such as air-to-air refuelling). The complexity of the tasks undertaken using visual references and the ability of experienced pilots to adapt to manipulations of the cues provided make research using realistic tasks difficult. There is some evidence that pilots learn to use idiosyncratic repertoires of cues selected from the totality of redundant cues normally available in the visual world (Chappelow and Smart, 1982). This finding would go some way to explaining why some experiments show little performance decrement when cues are selectively manipulated (Armstrong, 1970; Lewis and Krier, 1969) and, incidentally, why some pilots, but not others, have accidents when faced with extra-wide or sloping runways or a dearth of cues (e.g. approaching over the sea at night).

References

ARMSTRONG, B.D. (1970) *Flight Trials to Discover Whether Peripheral Vision is Needed for Landing.* RAE TR 70205. Bedford: Royal Aircraft Establishment

BARTRAM, D. and DALE, H.C.A. (1985) The prediction of success in helicopter pilot training. In *Proceedings of the Sixteenth Conference of the Western European Association for Aviation-Psychology*, edited by M. Sorsa, pp. 91–101. Helsinki: Finnair Training Centre

BROWN, W.R., DOHME, J.A. and SANDERS, M.G. (1981) Changes in the US Army aviator selection and training program. In *Proceedings of the First Symposium on Aviation Psychology*, edited by R.S. Jensen, pp. 267–278. Columbus, OH: Ohio State University

CHAPPELOW, J.W. (1985) *The Defence Mechanism Test and Pilot Selection.* RAF Institute of Aviation Medicine Divisional Record, F11, February, 1985

CHAPPELOW, J.W. and SMART, J. (1982) Putting texture in perspective. In *Proceedings of Symposium on Flight Simulation.* London: Royal Aeronautical Society

COOPER, G.E., WHITE, M.D. and LAUBER, J.K. (eds) (1980) Resource management on the flight deck. In *Proceedings of a NASA/Industry Workshop.* Washington, DC: NASA-CP-2120

DAMOS, D. and SMIST, T. (1981) Individual differences in multi-task response strategies. In *Proceedings of the First Symposium on Aviation Psychology*, edited by R.S. Jensen, pp. 279–288. Colubus, OH: Ohio State University

DIGMAN, J.M. (1959) Growth of a motor skill as a function of distribution of practice. *Journal of Experimental Psychology*, 57, 310–316

FOUSHEE, H.C. (1983) Dyads and triads at 35 000 feet: factors affecting group processes and aircrew performance. In *Flight Operations Symposium*, edited by N. Johnson. Dublin: Irish Airline Pilots' Association/Aer Lingus

GOLDSTEIN, M. and RITTENHOUSE, C.H. (1954) Knowledge of results in the acquisition and transfer of a gunnery skill. *Journal of Experimental Psychology*, 48, 187–196

GOODMAN, L., MCBRIDE, D.K., OWENS, J.M. and WHERRY, R.J. (1983) The identification of processes underlying the skilled aviator. In *Proceedings of the Second Symposium on Aviation Psychology*, edited by R.S. Jensen, pp. 541–546. Columbus, OH: Ohio State University

GOPHER, D. (1982) A selective attention test as a predictor of success in flight training. *Human Factors*, 24, 173–183

HELMREICH, R.L., FOUSHEE, H.C., BENSON, R. and RUSSINI, W. (1986) Cockpit resource management: Exploring the attitude–performance linkage. *Aviation Space and Environmental Medicine*, 57, 1198–1200

HOLDING, D.H. (1965) *Principles of Training.* Oxford: Pergamon Press

JACOBS, R.S. and ROSCOE, S.N. (1975) *Simulator Cockpit Motion and Transfer of Initial Flight Training.* ARL-75-18, Aviation Research Laboratory, Institute of Aviation, University of Illinois

KENNEDY, R.S., LILIENTHAL, M.G., BERBAUM, K.S. and DUNLAP, W.P. (1986) Issues in simulator sickness. In *Proceedings of International Conference: Advances in Flight Simulation Visual and Motion Systems.* London: Royal Aeronautical Society

KOONCE, J.M. (1981) Validation of a proposed pilot trainee selection system. In *Proceedings of the First Symposium on Aviation Psychology*, edited by R.S. Jensen, pp. 255–260. Columbus, OH: Ohio State University

KOONCE, J.M. (1984) A brief history of aviation psychology. *Human Factors*, 26, 499–508

LAUBER, J.K. (1987) Cockpit resource management: Background studies and rationale. In *Proceedings of the NASA/MAC Workshop: Cockpit Resource Management Training*, edited by H.W. Orlady and H.C. Foushee, pp. 5–13. Washington, DC: NASA

LEWIS, C.E. and KRIER, G.E. (1969) Flight research program: XIV. Landing performance in jet aircraft after loss of binocular vision. *Aerospace Medicine*, 40, 957–963

ORLADY, H.W. and FOUSHEE, H.C. (eds) (1987) *Proceedings of the NASA/MAC Workshop: Cockpit Resource Management Training*, (in press)

PARFITT, A. and CHAPPELOW, J.W. (1986) Results of the survey into simulator sickness in the RAF. In *Proceedings of International Conference: Advances in Flight Simulation Visual and Motion Systems.* London: Royal Aeronautical Society

ROLFE, J.M., HAMMERTON-FRASER, A.M., POULTER, R.F. and SMITH, E.M.B. (1970) Pilot response in flight and simulated flight. *Ergonomics*, 13, 761–768

VERNON, P.E. and PARRY, J.B. (1949) *Personnel Selection in The British Forces.* London: University Press

WHEALE, J.L. (1984) An analysis of crew co-ordination problems in commercial transport aircraft. *International Journal of Aviation Safety*, 2, 83–89

Further reading

ANASTASI, A. (1982) *Psychological Testing*, 5th edn. London: Macmillan

FITTS, P.M. and POSNER, M.I. (1973) *Human Performance.* London: Prentice-Hall

29

Stress and workload

E.W. Farmer

Psychological stress

In the physical sciences, the term *stress* denotes a force that acts to produce strain in a material. In other words, stress is considered a type of stimulus. Psychological stress, however, is generally defined as a reaction, or response, to adverse environmental conditions called stressors (Cox, 1978). Since the aviation environment is rich in potential stressors, and since stress-induced errors may have disastrous consequences, this topic is of particular interest to aviation psychologists.

The pioneering work of Hans Selye (1976) concentrated on the physiological response to stress. *Figure 29.1* depicts the General Adaptation Syndrome (GAS) that he proposed as a model of the stress response. The use of the term 'general' signifies Selye's belief that this was a stereotyped syndrome which did not depend upon the precise nature of the stressor.

The GAS comprises three stages. The first, the *alarm reaction*, incorporates a *shock* phase, involving immediate responses such as tachycardia, followed by a *counter-shock* phase in which the body marshals defensive mechanisms including the secretion of corticoid hormones. In the second stage, called *resistance*, successful adaptation occurs; this coping process, however, decreases resistance to other noxious stimuli. A particularly prolonged stressor may over-tax the body's ability to maintain resistance, leading to the re-emergence of the original stress symptoms, and eventually to collapse or even death (the stage of *exhaustion*). An individual attempting to cope with stress is, according to Selye, likely to experience illnesses ('diseases of adaptation') whose nature is determined by existing weaknesses in his physiological constitution.

The GAS approach is of limited relevance to aviation. The stress experienced by aircrew is generally less severe than that to which Selye exposed his laboratory animals, and does not present a direct threat to life; interest lies primarily in its effects upon aircrew performance, which may compromise flight safety. Moreover, since each stress state has its own 'cognitive patterning' (Hockey and Hamilton, 1983), the notion of a generalized physiological response cannot be extended to psychological analysis.

A distinction can be drawn between *life stress*, *environmental stress*, and *cognitive stress*. Life stress is produced by adverse occurrences in everyday life (such as divorce or family bereavement). Environmental and cognitive stress are more closely bound to the specific activities that the individual undertakes. The former includes the effects of factors such as heat, noise, and sleep disturbance associated with

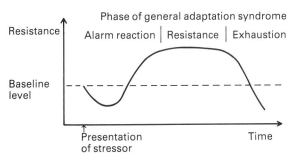

Figure 29.1 Selye's General Adaptation Syndrome.

the flying task; the latter refers to the cognitive demands of the task itself.

Life stress

Life stress is generated by major life changes to which the individual must re-adjust. Typically, it is assessed by the questionnaire method. Holmes and Rahe's study (1967) led to the development of the Schedule of Recent Experiences (SRE), comprising questions concerning the incidence of 42 life events (such as death of a spouse or changes in conditions of work) in the previous year of the individual's life. During the development of the SRE, each event was assigned a weighting based upon subjective ratings of the amount of adjustment it necessitated, relative to an 'anchor' point of marriage which was arbitrarily assigned a value of 500 points. The final values obtained were divided by 10 to produce 'life change units'. Using this method, death of a spouse was found to represent 100 life change units, marriage 50 units, and minor violations of the law 11 units. Scores on the SRE have been found to be correlated with incidence of depression, heart attacks, and other serious illnesses (*see* Johnson and Sarason, 1979).

Sarason, Johnson and Siegel (1978) noted several weaknesses in the SRE, such as its failure to distinguish between positive and negative life changes and to address individual differences in the perceived desirability of a given event. Their Life Experiences Survey (LES) obviated some of these difficulties by requiring subjects to indicate both the desirability and the impact of a particular event. Findings using the LES indicate that only negative life change, rather than any change, constitutes a source of stress (Johnson and Sarason, 1979).

There is evidence that life stress may contribute to aircraft accidents. Alkov and Borowsky (1980) and Alkov, Borowsky and Gaynor (1983) investigated individuals involved in US Navy accidents, and found that factors such as a recent major decision regarding their future, marital problems, or recent marriage, distinguished those whose errors contributed to the accident from those who were considered blameless.

Correlational methods, upon which life stress research is heavily dependent, do not permit conclusions concerning causality. As Johnson and Sarason (1979) note, some life events (such as change in sleeping habits) may be the consequence rather than the cause of illness. Moreover, external factors such as personality may underlie both major life changes and their apparent consequences. Nevertheless, the associations that have been established suggest that life change merits investigation by those wishing to enhance flight safety.

Environmental stress

Environmental stress is more amenable than life stress to direct experimental investigation. Thus for example, the effects of heat may be assessed by testing performance in the laboratory at different ambient temperatures, or by testing individuals working in tropical regions as they perform their normal duties.

The effects of environmental stressors are often explained by recourse to the notion of arousal change. Arousal is a continuum of wakefulness extending from deep sleep or coma to a state of frantic excitement. It can therefore be defined as the inverse probability of falling asleep (Corcoran, cited by Davies and Tune, 1970). The individual's level of arousal is controlled by the ascending reticular activating system (ARAS), part of the reticular formation that extends along the brainstem and midbrain. Thus a lesion in the cat's ARAS produces permanent sleep (Lindsley, 1952), whereas stimulation of this area produces wakefulness (Moruzzi and Magoun, 1949).

The relationship between arousal and performance is described by the Yerkes–Dodson Law, originally derived from work using laboratory rats (Yerkes and Dodson, 1908), which comprises the following postulates:

1. There is an optimal arousal level for the performance of any task, performance declining as arousal level increases or decreases (the *'inverted U'* relation).
2. The optimal arousal level is inversely related to task difficulty. Thus, easy tasks are performed best at a higher level of arousal than are difficult tasks.

The Yerkes–Dodson Law is illustrated in *Figure 29.2*. The inverted U hypothesis has obtained widespread support (Hebb, 1955; Duffy, 1962), although it has become the subject of increasing criticism (Hockey and Hamilton, 1983). Consideration of the strengths and weaknesses of this

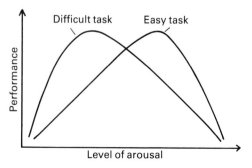

Figure 29.2 The Yerkes–Dodson Law.

approach will be deferred until the effects of various stressors encountered in aviation have been discussed.

Sleep loss

Civil aircrew frequently experience loss or disturbance of sleep. Transmeridian flight, irregular work–rest cycles, and a variety of other job-related factors contribute to this problem (Hawkins, 1978), which is cited in about 30% of reports submitted to the UK Confidential Human Factors Incident Reporting Programme (CHIRP). A few reports concern involuntary sleep during flight; more typically, an error is reported that appears to be a direct result of fatigue.

There has been some interest in the development of devices to prevent involuntary sleep. Such devices present an alarm if physiological measurement suggests that the onset of sleep is imminent (Kennedy, 1953; Farmer, Chappelow and Fletcher, 1985), or if the individual has failed to perform a particular action within a pre-determined time interval (Gardner-Medwin, 1986).

Since the incidence of involuntary sleep is relatively small, it is perhaps more appropriate to direct attention towards the behavioural changes induced by loss of sleep. One of the most commonly reported effects is the appearance of periodic 'blocks' or lapses in performance, during which slowing of the EEG is noted (Bjerner, 1949). These effects are revealed by performance tests that impose continuous demands to respond. A particularly sensitive test is that of continuous serial reaction, devised by Leonard (1959), in which a new stimulus is presented each time the subject makes a response (*Figure 29.3*). On this test, sleep deprivation greatly increases the frequency of abnormally long reaction times ('gaps'). On tasks in which the subject is permitted only a finite time interval in

which to respond, lapses are evident in the form of increased errors of omission.

Sleep loss also affects the subject's distribution of attention between task components. Greater difficulty is experienced in devoting particular attention to important aspects of the task (Hockey, 1970b). On the flight deck, one possible consequence of this reduced attentional selectivity is a less efficient instrument scan.

The Yerkes–Dodson Law predicts that the state of low arousal produced by sleep loss will be accompanied by a greater performance decrement on simple than on complex tasks. This has been confirmed in several studies. For example, Wilkinson, Edwards and Haines (1966) found that performance on an easy vigilance task was impaired if subjects had less than 5 hours' sleep, whereas impairment on a more difficult calculation task was observed only if subjects had less than 3 hours' sleep.

Farmer and Green (1985) reported the findings of a study designed specifically to address the effects of sleep loss on pilot performance. Sixteen civil pilots were subjected to loss of a single night's sleep (a relatively common occurrence in their professional life), and were required to fly a light aircraft and a simulator, and to perform laboratory tests. The EEG was recorded during flight.

The results indicated considerable performance decrement on various measures of flying performance. There was some evidence for a greater disruptive effect of sleep loss in the simulator than in the aircraft. The potentially more serious consequences of error during actual flight may therefore have induced subjects to expend greater effort, counteracting to some degree the effects of sleep loss.

Data from the laboratory tasks confirmed that simple activities are most vulnerable to disruption under sleep loss. Decreased performance was observed on tasks that required minimal storage of information (continuous serial reaction, and a tracking task performed whilst monitoring a peripheral display for the occurrence of signals); however, performance on a verbal reasoning task, which placed heavy demands upon working memory, was unaffected.

Power measures computed from the EEG records appeared to reflect the subject's level of arousal. For example, EEG power was negatively correlated with the frequency of gaps on the serial reaction time task.

Eventually, it may be possible to use relatively simple psychological or physiological measures to determine the fitness to fly of the sleep-deprived pilot. Meanwhile, the severity of this problem in civil aviation must be recognized, and every effort made to ensure that aircrew sleep disturbance is minimized.

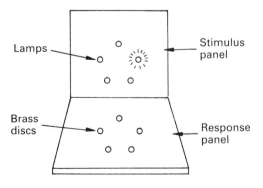

Figure 29.3 The continuous serial reaction task. (After Leonard, 1959.)

Heat

In some types of flying, heat represents a source of aircrew stress. The CHIRP scheme, for example, has received reports from helicopter pilots on North Sea operations concerning thermal discomfort associated with use of immersion suits and Mae Wests.

The effects of heat have been summarized by Poulton (1970) and Ramsey (1983). An excessive level of heat causes arousal to increase. As suggested by the Yerkes–Dodson Law, efficiency on difficult tasks is therefore particularly affected. However, even simple tasks exhibit performance decrement under very hot conditions. Pepler (1959), for example, demonstrated that both error rate and the frequency of gaps on a continuous reaction task increased when air temperature was 100°F (38°C). Increased errors are a common feature of performance in heat, and reflect a change of criterion towards fast but inaccurate responses.

Since heat and sleep loss have opposite effects on arousal level, their effects on attentional selectivity are not surprisingly also contradictory. Heat produces a focusing of attention on the important aspects of the task, an attentional 'tunnel vision' (Bursill, 1958). Such involuntary stress-induced changes in the distribution of attention are sometimes referred to as 'focused' attention, to distinguish them from the processes of 'selective' attention that are under the subject's control.

Noise

Noise is one of the most extensively studied stressors because of its predominance in industrial and military situations (*see* Poulton, 1970). This problem is more severe for the military than for the civil pilot, although some civil helicopters generate considerable noise levels.

Noise may obviously interfere directly with the reception of auditory signals. However, it also affects the processing of information received by other modalities. Noise increases the level of arousal, and its effects are in some respects similar to those of heat. It is more disruptive on difficult than on easy tasks (Hockey, 1979). Moreover, increased attentional selectivity (Hockey, 1970a; Smith, 1985) and decreased accuracy (Broadbent, 1971) are associated with noisy environments. However, noise and heat do not produce an identical pattern of performance change on the serial reaction task (Jones, 1983) and a decrement in short-term memory capacity is observed in noise but not in heat (Hockey and Hamilton, 1983).

The individual is often unaware of the progressive decline in his accuracy when working in a noisy environment (Davies and Shackleton, 1975). Further, his decisions are likely to be more extreme than is warranted by the available evidence (Broadbent, 1971; Jones, 1983). These effects, considered together with the tendency to focus attention on a restricted range of task components, suggest that noise will impair the ability of aircrew both to detect and to cope with unexpected events.

Particularly on relatively easy tasks, performance in noise may initially be better than that in quiet, the advantage gradually reversing; there may also be a further decrement in performance when the noise level is reduced (the 'after-effect of noise'). Poulton (1979) attempted to explain this pattern of results by a two-factor theory involving masking and arousal. He proposed that masking, both of inner speech and of auditory feedback from the operator's equipment, produced a constant performance decrement. During initial exposure to noise, this effect was outweighed by a sharp arousal increase; however, the arousal level gradually declined to normal as the subject became habituated to the noise, permitting masking effects to produce a net performance decrement. The after-effect of noise was attributed by Poulton to a drop in arousal level below the baseline when the noise level is reduced. Other explanations of the effects of noise are discussed by Jones (1983).

Threatening environments

Some studies of stress have exposed subjects to situations that they believe to represent real danger. For example, Yagi, Knox, and Capretta (1959) led army trainees to believe that the DC3 aircraft in which they were flying was about to crash Performance in completing an 'official emergency data form' distributed to the trainees was used to measure the effects of this apparent threat to personal safety.

Fear-inducing environments have also been studied under more ethically acceptable conditions, such as parachute jumping, in which no deception is necessary. This topic has been reviewed by Idzikowski and Baddeley (1983). The physiological correlates of the state of over-arousal induced by fear include tachycardia and increased secretion of adrenalin and growth hormone. The major effects on performance are disruption of manual dexterity and motor skill, and of secondary task performance in divided attention tasks. The latter effect is probably attributable to increased attentional selectivity.

Other stressors

It is beyond the scope of this discussion to consider each of the many environmental stressors to which aircrew may be exposed. The reader is referred to Poulton (1970) and Hockey (1983) for a more detailed treatment.

Personality and stress

Everyday observation suggests that individuals differ in their response to stress. This conclusion has been confirmed experimentally: both extraversion and neuroticism have been shown to influence the effects of particular environmental conditions.

Extreme introverts are chronically over-aroused, whereas extreme extraverts are chronically under-aroused (e.g. Corcoran, 1981). Exposure to a stressor that influences arousal level may therefore have profoundly different consequences for these individuals. For example, the stimulant caffeine was shown by Revelle, Amaral and Turriff (1976) to impair the performance of introverts but to improve the performance of extraverts, a finding entirely consistent with the Yerkes–Dodson Law (*Figure 29.4*). However, Eysenck (1982) discussed a number of complicating factors that argue against the notion that a single arousal mechanism mediates the performance differences between these groups. For example, he noted that introverts adopt a slower and more cautious approach than extraverts, but that the state of high arousal attributed to introverts is usually associated with rapid but inaccurate responses.

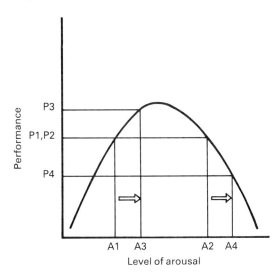

Figure 29.4 Differential effects of an arousing stressor on introverts and extraverts, explained by the Yerkes–Dodson Law. Normal low arousal level of extraverts (A1) is raised to A3, with consequent improvement in performance (P1 to P3); normal high arousal level of introverts (A2) is raised even further (A4), causing performance decrement (P2 to P4).

Individuals with a high level of trait anxiety (neuroticism) are more likely to experience increased state anxiety as a result of environmental stress. One of the major effects of state anxiety is to produce worry, which diverts some of the limited mental processing resources from the task in hand. Only when task demands are high does a difference emerge between the performance of subjects low and high in anxiety (*see* Eysenck, 1982, 1983).

Stress and the Yerkes–Dodson Law

The Yerkes–Dodson Law clearly has some success in accounting for the effects of the specific environmental stressors described above. For example, it correctly predicts the relative effects on easy and difficult tasks of stress-induced increases and decreases in arousal level. It must be noted, however, that the distinction between easy and difficult tasks appears to depend critically upon the degree to which memory storage is required. Thus manipulations that might be expected to increase task difficulty, such as increases in signal rate, may have little effect on performance under stress if memory requirements are unaffected.

The validity of the notion of an inverted-U relation between arousal and performance can be tested by applying two stressors simultaneously. If both stressors have a similar effect on arousal level, their combined effect on performance should be additive; if, however, they have conflicting effects on arousal level, then their effects should cancel. Several studies have supported these assumptions. For example, Wilkinson (1963) showed that incentive (a mild personal threat) further impaired performance in a noisy environment; on the other hand, Corcoran (1962) showed that noise decreased the number of gaps on a continuous serial reaction task in sleep-deprived subjects. This last finding illustrates why the drowsy driver is well advised to turn on his radio.

Despite the apparent validity of the Yerkes–Dodson Law, it is open to criticism. It has already been noted that the effects of noise and heat, although similar, are not identical. It is difficult to account for this discrepancy within a simple framework which suggests that high arousal, produced by whatever means, will have consistent effects upon performance. For a more detailed discussion of this problem, *see* Hockey (1979).

A further inadequacy of the Yerkes–Dodson Law is its suggestion that identical performance decrement will be observed in states of low and high arousal. As has already been shown, these states produce opposite effects on attentional selectivity.

The 'inverted-U' notion provides a superficial explanation of the reactions of introverts and extraverts to stress. However, as noted above, some aspects of the performance differences between these groups cannot be accommodated by this simple model.

A final characteristic of the Yerkes–Dodson Law, which may be considered either an advantage or a disadvantage, is its extreme flexibility, and its consequent failure to provide rigorous predictions concerning performance. By referring to *Figure 29.2*, the reader may easily confirm, for example, that either an increased or a decreased level of arousal may improve, impair, or have no effect upon performance of a given task, depending on the difficulty of the task, the subject's initial level of arousal and the magnitude of arousal change.

Mental workload

Central to any definition of mental workload is the assumption that the human operator has limited capacity to process information. Workload can be considered to be the total demand upon the operator associated with a particular level of output. Demand is determined by characteristics of the task, environmental conditions, and attributes specific to the individual, such as level of skill. Because of the complexity of this topic, some investigators have found it convenient to confine their interest to factors such as task requirements or level of performance (Gartner and Murphy, 1979).

In aviation, there is increasing awareness of the importance of workload measurement. In the United States, for example, the Federal Aviation Authority has specified that a formal workload assessment must be conducted as part of the certification procedure for all new aircraft. Paradoxically, interest in aircrew workload has expanded partly because of increased automation on the civil flight deck, which has created a trend towards reduction in crew complement. The additional workload imposed by the loss of the flight engineer from the traditional three-man crew is a matter of some current concern.

Workload measures

Measures of workload should be unobtrusive, reliable, sensitive to a wide range of workload variation, and diagnostic with respect to the sources of change in demand (Wickens, 1984). They should also be easy to implement and be accepted by the operator (O'Donnell and Eggemeier, 1986). Since no single measure is likely to satisfy all of these criteria, a battery of measures is typically employed.

Techniques for the assessment of workload can be divided into four major classes: task analysis, subjective reports, physiological measures, and performance indices. Each of these is considered briefly below. For a more detailed discussion, *see* Wickens (1984), O'Donnell and Eggemeier (1986) and Gopher and Donchin (1986).

Task analysis

A major example of this approach is time-line analysis, in which the duration of sub-tasks is plotted along a time axis, and workload is defined simply as the total time spent performing tasks in relation to the total time available.

Time-line analysis is used primarily as a predictive tool during the development of systems, and may help in the allocation of tasks to various team members. It does, however, have serious limitations. It fails, for example, to take account of the operator's level of skill, and it ignores the fact that some tasks may be performed simultaneously with little mutual interference; moreover, it is inappropriate for tasks in which operators have freedom to 'self-pace' their activities, deferring responses without loss of overall efficiency until a workload peak has passed (Wickens, 1984).

Subjective estimates of workload

It could be argued that the best way to assess workload is simply to ask the operator to estimate the demands produced by his activities. Subjective workload ratings are easy to obtain, and are relatively unobtrusive. Moreover, they have high face validity, an important consideration for any measure that addresses 'real-life' performance. Nevertheless, there are disadvantages associated with this type of procedure. Operators, for example, experience difficulty in comparing the workload imposed by qualitatively different tasks, and their estimates are typically correlated rather weakly with task performance (Gopher and Braune, 1983). It is therefore advisable that subjective estimates be used in conjunction with performance measures.

Some of the subjective workload assessment techniques that have been applied to the flying task are described in *Table 29.1*.

Table 29.1 Subjective workload assessment techniques

Technique	Description
Cooper–Harper rating scale	Originally developed for the assessment of aircraft handling qualities, this method uses a decision tree to arrive at a workload score between 1 and 10
Subjective workload assessment technique (SWAT)	This technique is based upon three dimensions of workload: time load, effort load, and psychological stress load. A scale development phase is followed by an event scoring phase in which workload estimates are obtained
Pro-SWAT	This technique is a projective application of the SWAT method, and is useful in assessing the workload of hypothetical systems. The event scoring phase of SWAT is replaced by a structured interview method in which operators, expert in the use of an existing system as similar as possible to that under investigation, provide workload estimates
NASA Task Load Index	This method assumes six dimensions of workload: mental demands, physical demands, temporal demands, own performance, effort, and frustration. Scores on these scales are weighted according to their subjective importance within a specific application

Table 29.2 Physiological workload assessment techniques

Measure	Relationship to workload
Heart rate variability	Decreases as workload increased
Pupil diameter	Increases as a function of workload
Brain activity	The P300 component of the evoked potential to a stimulus declines as load increases
Muscle tension	Tonic electromyographic activity increases as a function of mental load

Physiological measures of workload

The major advantages of physiological measures are that they do not disrupt the operator's performance, and that they permit a continuous record to be obtained. However, the recording equipment is often physically intrusive, and these measures provide only an indirect indication of performance change at different levels of workload (Wickens, 1984).

Some of the more commonly used physiological measures of workload are listed in *Table 29.2*.

Performance measures of workload

There are two major approaches to assessing workload by means of performance measurement.

The primary-task technique determines performance on the task whose workload is actually under investigation; the secondary task technique, on the other hand, attempts to measure the operator's spare capacity (the capacity not used by the primary task).

Measurement of primary task performance has high face validity, but is often an unsatisfactory workload indicator. The operator may maintain a relatively constant level of performance despite increases in mental load, but have less spare capacity to devote to other activities. Nevertheless, since primary task performance is clearly of importance in any workload assessment, its measurement is desirable in conjunction with other indices.

The notion of using secondary tasks to measure spare mental capacity is intuitively appealing,

Table 29.3 Secondary tasks used in workload assessment

Task	Description
Memory search	Subjects must decide whether a 'probe' item is contained in a memorized set of items. Performance on this task has been shown to be related to the demands of the primary task
Probe reaction time	Reaction time to an unpredictable stimulus is assumed to reflect the demands of the primary task
Time estimation	The extent to which an operator under-estimates a given time interval is related to workload
Interval generation	When an operator is required to tap at a constant rate, the variability of the intervals between taps tends to increase as a function of workload
Random number generation	The randomness of numbers generated by the operator is inversely related to workload. When the operator is busy, he is more likely to resort to repetition of well-learned number sequences

particularly within the framework of single-channel models (*see* Chapter 26). However, this method may produce interference with performance of the primary task under investigation. Moreover, the probable existence of specialized processing subsystems is a complicating factor. Consider, for example, the problem of assessing the workload imposed by a task that is predominantly spatial in nature. Although the operator may be quite unable to cope with additional demands for spatial processing, he may be able to perform an additional verbal task with ease. The use of a verbal secondary task under these circumstances would create a misleading impression that the total demand of the primary task is minimal. Thus the secondary task technique must be used in conjunction with careful analysis of the operator's primary task. *Table 29.3* describes a selection of secondary tasks that have been reported in the literature.

Comparison of workload assessment methods

Casali and Wierwille (1983) compared the sensitivity of 16 measures of communications-imposed workload during simulated flight. They found that subjective ratings, time estimation, pupil diameter and measures of communication performance were sensitive to workload variation, but that primary task (aircraft control) measures, tapping regularity, and physiological measures such as heart rate and respiration rate were not. Wierwille and O'Connor (1983), in a comparison of 20 workload measures, confirmed that subjective measures were particularly useful in the assessment of psychomotor load.

However, for activities such as flying, in which the efficiency of performance is of critical importance, it would be unwise to depend entirely upon subjective estimates, since these may in some circumstances be uncorrelated, or even negatively correlated, with operator efficiency (*see* Wickens, 1984).

The consequences of high workload

When workload is high, the skilled operator is particularly prone to action slips. As Reason (1981) notes, 'some motor programmes possess the power to lure us into unwitting action, particularly when the central processor is occupied with some parallel mental activity'. Even during largely automatic skilled performance, conscious attention is required at critical decision points. Thus a particularly 'strong' (well-learned) motor programme may be erroneously executed when attention is directed to other activities.

The increased level of arousal associated with high workload may lead to increased attentional selectivity, similar to that found in noise. Williams (1982) showed that the size of the functional field of view (the area of the visual field from which information is extracted) was inversely related to the cognitive load imposed by a task.

In most tasks, the operator can choose to trade off speed of responding against accuracy. At a high level of arousal, accuracy of responding is often sacrificed for increased speed. Thus the highly loaded operator is likely to perform task components rapidly but carelessly.

It has been seen that performance on the primary task may be relatively unaffected by changes in task demand. However, the operator may be unable to respond effectively to the additional load imposed by unexpected events. Thus high workload may present difficulties only when emergencies arise.

Reducing workload

The design of displays and controls according to sound ergonomic principles provides an important means of maintaining workload at a manageable level. Existing displays, for example, may be improved by the use of colour coding (Holmes, 1980). Moreover, new types of display, such as head-up displays, multi-function cathode ray tubes and the Peripheral Vision Device, may present information in a more accessible form, and hence reduce workload.

Workload may also be reduced by training. The development of a high level of skill has two important consequences: it permits delegation of the control of sub-tasks to motor programmes that require minimal mental processing capacity, and it produces increased economy of motor action. Thus for a given task, the skilled operator has a lower level of workload than his unskilled counterpart.

A further means of ensuring that task demands do not exceed operator capacity is by appropriate personnel selection. Anxiety, for example, reduces working memory capacity, and this may contribute to the low success of trait-anxious subjects during flying training (Jessup and Jessup, 1971).

References

ALKOV, R.A. and BOROWSKY, M.S. (1980) A questionnaire study of psychological background factors in US Navy aircraft accidents. *Aviation Space and Environmental Medicine*, **51**, 860–863

ALKOV, R.A., BOROWSKY, M.S. and GAYNOR, J.A. (1983) Pilot error and stress management (US Navy experience). In *Flight Operations Symposium*, edited by N. Johnson. Dublin: Irish Air Line Pilots' Association/Aer Lingus

BJERNER, B. (1949) Alpha depression and lowered pulse rate during delayed reactions in a serial reaction test. *Acta Physiologica Scandinavica (Supplementum)*, **19**, 65

BROADBENT, D.E. (1971) *Decision and Stress*. London: Academic Press

BURSILL, A.E. (1958) The restriction of peripheral vision during exposure to hot and humid conditions. *Quarterly Journal of Experimental Psychology*, **10**, 113–129

CASALI, J.G. and WIERWILLE, W.W. (1983) Communications-imposed pilot workload: A comparison of sixteen estimation techniques. In *Proceedings of the Second Symposium on Aviation Psychology*, edited by R.S. Jensen, pp. 223–235. Columbus: Ohio State University

CORCORAN, D.W.J. (1962) Noise and loss of sleep. *Quarterly Journal of Experimental Psychology*, **14**, 178–182

CORCORAN, D.W.J. (1981) Introversion–extraversion, stress and arousal. In *Dimensions of Personality: Papers in Honour of H.J. Eysenck*, edited by R. Lynn, pp. 111–127. Oxford: Pergamon Press

COX, T. (1978) *Stress*. London: Macmillan

DAVIES, D.R. and SHACKLETON, V.J. (1975) *Psychology and Work*. London: Methuen

DAVIES, D.R. and TUNE, G.S. (1970) *Human Vigilance Performance*. London: Staples Press

DUFFY, E. (1962) *Activation and Behaviour*. New York: Wiley

EYSENCK, M.W. (1982) *Attention and Arousal*. Berlin: Springer-Verlag

EYSENCK, M. (1983) Anxiety and individual differences. In *Stress and Fatigue in Human Performance*, edited by R. Hockey, pp. 273–298. Chichester: Wiley

FARMER, E.W., CHAPPELOW, J.W. and FLETCHER, Y.L. (1985) *Preliminary Evaluation of the 'Dormalert' Arousal-Monitoring Device*. RAF Institute of Aviation Medicine Divisional Record No F15

FARMER, E.W. and GREEN, R.G. (1985) The sleep-deprived pilot: Performance and EEG response. In *Report of the Sixteenth Conference of WEAAP*, edited by M. Sorsa, pp. 155–162. Helsinki: Finnair Training Centre

GARDNER-MEDWIN, A.R. (1986) Device to prevent vehicle drivers falling asleep. *Journal of Physiology*, **371**, 22P

GARTNER, W.B. and MURPHY, M.R. (1979) Concepts of workload. In *Survey of Methods to Assess Workload*, edited by B.O. Hartman and R.E. McKenzie, pp. 1–2 (AGARDograph No. 246). Neuilly-sur-Seine: AGARD

GOPHER, D. and BRAUNE, R. (1983) On the psychophysics of workload: Why bother with subjective measures? In *Proceedings of the Second Symposium on Aviation Psychology*, edited by R.S. Jensen, pp. 253–268. Columbus: Ohio State University

GOPHER, D. and DONCHIN, E. (1986) Workload—An examination of the concept. In *Handbook of Perception and Human Performance Volume II: Cognitive Processes and Performance*, edited by K.R. Boff, L. Kaufman and J.P. Thomas. New York: Wiley

HAWKINS, F.H. (1978) *Sleep and Body Rhythm Disturbance in Long Range Aviation: The Problem and a Search for Relief*. London: F.H. Hawkins

HEBB, D.O. (1955) Drives and the CNS (conceptual nervous system). *Psychological Review*, **62**, 243–254

HOCKEY, G.R.J. (1970a) Effect of loud noise on attentional selectivity. *Quarterly Journal of Experimental Psychology*, **22**, 28–36

HOCKEY, G.R.J. (1970b) Changes in attention allocation in a multi-component task under loss of sleep. *British Journal of Psychology*, **61**, 473–480

HOCKEY, R. (1979) Stress and the cognitive components of skilled performance. In *Human Stress and Cognition: An Information Processing Approach*, edited by V. Hamilton and D.M. Warburton, pp. 141–177. Chichester: Wiley

HOCKEY, R. (ed.) (1983) *Stress and Fatigue in Human Performance*. Chichester: Wiley

HOCKEY, R. and HAMILTON, P. (1983) The cognitive patterning of stress states. In *Stress and Fatigue in Human Performance*, edited by R. Hockey, pp. 331–362. Chichester: Wiley

HOLMES, R.H. (1980) The influence of the design of displays on cockpit workload. In *High-speed, Low-level Flight: Aircrew Factors*, edited by D.H. Glaister (AGARD Conference Proceedings No. 267). Neuilly-sur-Seine: AGARD

HOLMES, T.H. and RAHE, R.H. (1967) The social readjustment rating scale. *Journal of Psychosomatic Research*, **11**, 213–218

IDZIKOWSKI, C. and BADDELEY, A.D. (1983) Fear and dangerous environments. In *Stress and Fatigue in Human Performance*, edited by R. Hockey, pp. 123–144. Chichester: Wiley

JESSUP, G. and JESSUP, H. (1971) Validity of the Eysenck Personality Inventory in pilot selection. *Occupational Psychology*, **45**, 111–123

JOHNSON, J.H. and SARASON, I.G. (1979) Recent developments in research on life stress. In *Human Stress and Cognition: An Information Processing Approach*, edited by V. Hamilton and D.M. Warburton, pp. 205–233. Chichester: Wiley

JONES, D. (1983) Noise. In *Stress and Fatigue in Human Performance*, edited by R. Hockey, pp. 61–95. Chichester: Wiley

KENNEDY, J.L. (1953) Some practical problems of the alertness indicator. In *Fatigue*, edited by W.F. Floyd and A.T. Welford, pp. 149–153. London: Lewis

LEONARD, J.A. (1959) *Five Choice Serial Reaction Apparatus*. Medical Research Council Applied Psychology Unit Report No. 326/59

LINDSLEY, D.B. (1952) Psychological phenomena and the electroencephalogram. *Electroencephalography and Clinical Neurophysiology*, **4**, 443–456

MORUZZI, G. and MAGOUN, H.W. (1949) Brain stem reticular formation and activation of the EEG. *Electroencephalography and Clinical Neurophysiology*, **1**, 455–473

O'DONNELL, R.D. and EGGEMEIER, F.T. (1986) Workload assessment methodology. In *Handbook of Perception and Human Performance Volume II: Cognitive Processes and Performance*, edited by K.R. Boff, L. Kaufman and J.P. Thomas. New York: Wiley

PEPLER, R.D. (1959) Warmth and lack of sleep: Accuracy or activity reduced. *Journal of Comparative and Physiological Psychology*, **52**, 446–450

POULTON, E.C. (1970) *Environment and Human Efficiency*. Springfield: Thomas

POULTON, E.C. (1979) Composite model for human performance in continuous noise. *Psychological Review*, **86**, 361–375

RAMSEY, J. (1983) Heat and cold. In *Stress and Fatigue in Human Performance*, edited by R. Hockey, pp. 33–60. Chichester: Wiley

REASON, J. (1981) Actions not as planned: The price of automatization. In *Aspects of Consciousness*, edited by G. Underwood and R. Stevens, pp. 67–89. London: Academic Press

REVELLE, W., AMARAL, P. and TURRIFF, S. (1976) Introversion/extraversion, time stress, and caffeine: Effect on verbal performance. *Science*, **192**, 149–150

SARASON, I.G., JOHNSON, J.H. and SIEGEL, J.M. (1978) Assessing the impact of life changes: Development of the Life Experiences Survey. *Journal of Consulting and Clinical Psychology*, **46**, 932–946

SELYE, H. (1976) *The Stress of Life*, 2nd edn. New York: McGraw-Hill

SMITH, A.P. (1985) Noise, biased probability, and serial reaction. *British Journal of Psychology*, **76**, 89–95

WICKENS, C.D. (1984) *Engineering Psychology and Human Performance*. Columbus: Charles E. Merrill

WIERWILLE, W.W. and O'CONNOR, S.A. (1983) Evaluation of 20 workload measures using a psychomotor task in a moving-base aircraft simulator. *Human Factors*, **25**, 1–16

WILKINSON, R.T. (1963) Interaction of noise with knowledge of results and sleep deprivation. *Journal of Experimental Psychology*, **66**, 332–337

WILKINSON, R.T., EDWARDS, R.S. and HAINES, E. (1966) Performance following a night of reduced sleep. *Psychonomic Science*, **5**, 471–472

WILLIAMS, L.J. (1982) Cognitive load and the functional field of view. *Human Factors*, **24**, 683–692

YAGI, K., KNOX, R. and CAPRETTA, P. (1959) *Development of a Verbal Measure for Use in Stress Study*. Paper presented to Western Psychological Association, USA

YERKES, R.M. and DODSON, J.D. (1908) The relation of strength of stimulus to rapidity of habit formation. *Journal of Comparative and Neurological Psychology*, **18**, 459–482

30

Ergonomics

R.G. Green and E.W. Farmer

Introduction

The earliest objective studies of man in his working environment were concerned primarily with measurement of overall production time. In 1760, the Frenchman Perronet conducted a study of the time required to manufacture pins. At the turn of the twentieth century, F.W. Taylor developed in the United States his system of 'scientific management' that introduced an analytic approach to industrial tasks and formed the basis of time and motion study.

In Great Britain during the 1920s, the Industrial Fatigue Research Board and the National Institute of Industrial Psychology conducted vigorous investigations of human efficiency in the working environment. Research interest in this topic declined during the depression of the 1930s, to be reawakened in response to the increasing demands upon the human operator as a result of developments in military equipment during the course of World War II.

Interest in human aspects of work efficiency continued during the post-war years, and in 1949 the efforts of Hywel Murrell led to the adoption in Britain of the term 'ergonomics' for this emerging discipline which eroded the boundaries between psychology, physiology, engineering, and related sciences. Ergonomics is virtually synonymous with the American term 'human factors', since both are concerned largely with man–machine interaction.

In this chapter, consideration is given to the design of displays and controls, which represent the interfaces between man and machine. The optimal integration of these devices within the workspace is then discussed. It must be borne in mind, however, that the following sections are not intended to be a primer for aircraft designers, but simply an introduction to the problems and principles.

Displays

Flight-deck displays are devices for enabling information to pass from the aircraft to the human operator. They are necessary only because the operator is unable to sense directly all the information that is required for flight. It is of obvious importance that the information conveyed by these instruments should be presented clearly and unambiguously. To do so would not appear to be an insuperable intellectual challenge, yet the most cursory review of aircraft accidents shows how easily poorly designed displays can have catastrophic unforeseen consequences.

Altimeters

The most frequently quoted example of a misleading display is that of the three-pointer altimeter. In these instruments, an example being shown at *Figure 30.1*, a small pointer is used to indicate the tens of thousands of feet, one of medium size to show the thousands of feet, and a large pointer is used for the remaining information. As long ago as 1947, Grether pointed out that the probability of misreading such multiple pointer instruments is high, yet in 1958 two aircraft crashed into the ground within months of each other because the crews had misread such altimeters and thought that they were 10 000 feet higher than they were. Even more surprising is the fact that these instruments are still being fitted to aircraft. It is clear, therefore, that the capacity to generate good designs is of no consequence unless such designs are implemented.

The three-pointer altimeter suffers from a number of problems. The most important needle is the smallest, farthest from the scale, and consequently

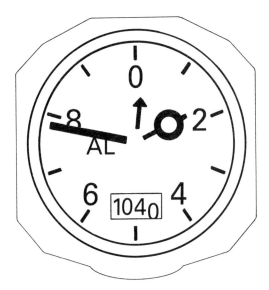

Figure 30.1 A three-pointer altimeter.

the easiest pointer to misread. It can also be easily occluded by the other pointers on the display. There is a further problem with such instruments, however, in that their interrogation is cumbersome. In order to extract information, the small pointer must first be fixated visually and the indicated value stored in memory. This must be followed by an eye movement to the medium pointer where the process is repeated, and then by a further iteration on the large pointer. The stored values are then combined to provide the pilot with the information required. Such a process creates unnecessary workload, and is both time consuming and error prone. If the reader compares the ease of extracting the value shown by the instrument in *Figure 30.1* with that of extracting the value shown by the digital indicator in *Figure 30.2*, the difference is striking.

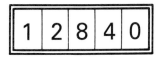

Figure 30.2 Digital representation of altitude.

It is, in fact, so striking that one wonders why three-pointer altimeters ever came to be designed. The answer lies largely in tradition. In mechanical, geared, devices it is convenient to make displays circular so that the pointer reflects the position of a driven shaft. Early altimeters were almost unmodified barometers with just one pointer. As aircraft flew to greater heights, two-pointer, and then three-pointer instruments were introduced. It is probably only because aircraft did not go on to fly at hundreds of thousands of feet that a four-pointer instrument has been avoided.

It seems, then, that a digital display is to be preferred if the pilot requires digital information. Digital displays are poor, however, at representing the rate of change of a value, the rate at which a pointer moves round a scale being much more effective. In order to combine the best qualities of both digital and analogue displays, 'counter-pointer' altimeters were developed. Unfortunately, some variants of these instruments could easily be misread. *Figure 30.3* illustrates a counter- or drum-pointer instrument in which a drum shows the tens of thousands and thousands of feet, and a pointer the remainder. It is easy to see that such an instrument may be read with a 1000 feet error because it succeeds in incorporating similar problems to those of the three-pointer device.

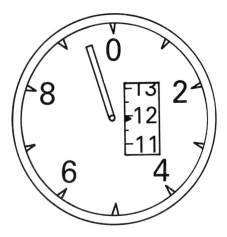

Figure 30.3 A counter-pointer altimeter.

In the types of altimeter so far described, the pilot is concerned with learning an absolute value, but there is a further form of altimeter—the radio altimeter—from which the pilot may be more concerned with gaining an analogue impression of his height above a surface, and his rate of closure with that surface. Since such altimeters are at their most useful when in close proximity to a surface, a long range of indication is not required and a single pointer is therefore sufficient. However, the importance of the height information provided by such an instrument becomes greater as the surface is approached, and *Figure 30.4* shows some ways in which designers have attempted to address this problem. Some instruments have logarithmic scales so that the scale divisions become progressively smaller as altitude increases, some have a scale divided at 200 or 500 feet with high resolution below this and low resolution above, and some function only for low altitudes and devote the whole scale to a limited range. The situation is complicated by the fact that in some radio altimeters the zero point of the scale is at the top of the instrument, whereas in others it is at the bottom.

It is easy to understand the thinking of the designers of these instruments, but less easy to predict which is best. If a logarithmic scale is used, reading may be made difficult by the inconsistency of scale divisions, and rate of closure with the surface may be misperceived because a constant rate of descent will not produce a constant rate of pointer movement. Similar problems beset the split-scale

instrument, and the limited-scale device may have its usefulness curtailed by the limited maximum altitude. It is not known which of these devices should be adopted as the standard, and it may not matter which. What is clear, however, is that there should be a standard. Pilots may well fly more than one type of aircraft type and examples abound in aviation of pilots who have committed errors because of 'negative transfer' of a skill (in this case the visual skill of reading an instrument) between one aircraft and the next.

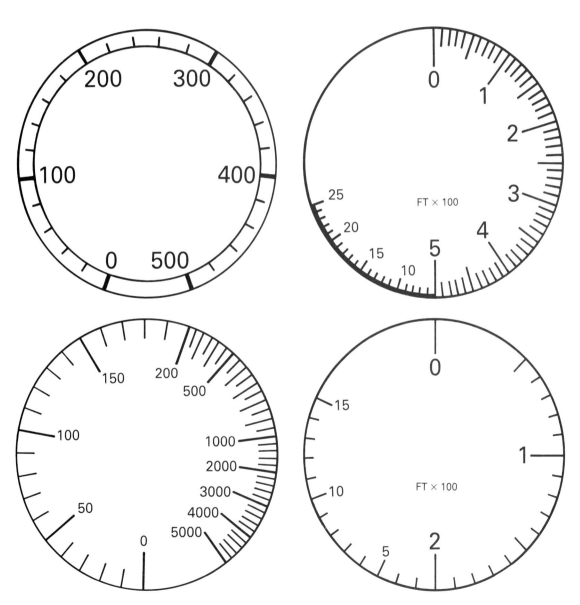

Figure 30.4 Examples of radio altimeter design.

Attitude indicators

Although it is obviously important for the pilot to maintain an awareness of his height, the most important cockpit display in instrument flight is the artificial horizon, attitude indicator or attitude director indicator. All members of this family of instrument provide the pilot with indications of earth-referenced roll angle (angle of bank), and pitch angle. Serendipitously, it is straightforward to provide mechanical linkages from a vertical gyro to produce a display that can be Earth-stabilized and mimic the behaviour of the real horizon.

It has not proved straightforward, however, to decide whether to design such displays so that the aircraft symbol on the display remains stationary with regard to the aircraft, with an Earth-stabilized horizon line (the 'inside-out' approach, illustrated in *Figure 30.5*), or whether to keep the horizon line on

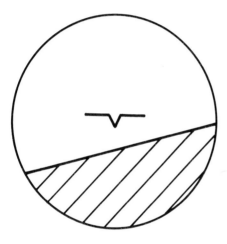

Figure 30.5 An 'inside-out' attitude indicator.

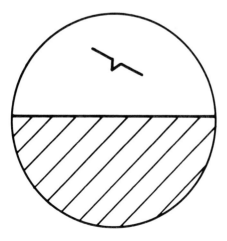

Figure 30.6 An 'outside-in' attitude indicator.

the instrument aircraft-stabilized and move the aircraft symbol in relation to the horizon line thus modelling the appearance of aircraft and horizon to a ground-based observer (the 'outside-in' approach, illustrated in *Figure 30.6*). Other configurations are possible, and some early attitude indicators were designed with an aircraft symbol that moved in relation to the airframe to indicate roll, and a horizon line that moved to indicate pitch. There have even been 'frequency-separated' instruments in which the aircraft symbol moved with regard to the airframe (i.e. outside-in) during angular accelerations, followed by the display assuming an 'inside-out' mode during any constant attitude. The object of such complex displays was to match the subjective perceptions of roll during angular change and of dynamic constancy during a co-ordinated turn (when the resultant force vector would be aligned with the pilot's own z-axis).

With practice, it is undoubtedly possible to use all such instruments, though the standard presentation is now 'inside-out'. However, practice is certainly required to make sense even of the standard inside-out device; the naïve observer is very unlikely to be able naturally to interpret a modern attitude indicator display and will often believe that a display indicating, for example, right bank is showing the opposite. Even if the observer is briefed that he should regard the instrument as a window in the instrument panel providing a limited view of the outside world, it is of little help, yet when the observer is able to see the real outside world, he will have no doubt about his orientation. This gulf, between the capacity for natural perception of orientation when the world may be seen and the capacity to interpret an attitude indicator, is so large that it is embodied in legislation. The pilot who has no 'instrument rating' (i.e. who has not demonstrated the skill of attitude indicator interpretation) is limited to flying only when good vision of the ground is available. Since the real world and the attitude indicator provide, apparently, the same information, it is puzzling that one should be so easy and natural to interpret and the other so difficult.

The difference lies in the fact that the real world fills the observer's vision, providing a powerful stimulus to the ambient visual system (*see* Chapter 26), yet the attitude indicator subtends a relatively small visual angle of perhaps 5 degrees, addressing only the focal visual system. Whereas the ambient visual system seems designed automatically to drive the sense of orientation, the focal visual system seems to be designed to provide information for conscious attention. It thus seems that the design of the conventional attitude indicator owes a great deal to the availability of vertical gyros and to the established technology of the watch and instrument maker, but owes fairly little to the provision of a device that best exploits the characteristics of the human visual system. Its design compels the operator to deal with the instrument as a conscious activity, rather than utilizing the information in a natural and unconscious way.

This realization has prompted the development of new types of ambient or peripheral attitude indicator in which a horizon line is projected across the whole instrument panel, or in which the canopy arch is used to represent horizon location and ground texture by covering the arch with small light sources and illuminating them in a way that provides an Earth-stabilized visual pattern. The object of both of these devices is to provide the ambient visual system with Earth-stabilized information and hence to provide a natural sense of orientation, making disorientation episodes less likely. Neither of these devices is yet in common usage, but they are included here as examples of attempts to match displays to the characteristics of the operator rather than simply to provide what is convenient.

The two displays already described provide extremely basic information to the pilot and have probably been the subject of more human factors research than any others. Both of them represent elements of the basic blind flying instrument array; the remaining instruments in this array being the airspeed indicator, the direction indicator, the vertical speed indicator, and the turn and slip indicator. Between them, these instruments provide the data from which the pilot may build a comprehensive model of the aircraft's static and dynamic state with relation to the Earth and the airflow. The attitude indicator and direction indicator may also incorporate information from radio navigational stations on the ground, and be linked to a flight directing computer in the aircraft. When enhanced in this way, these instruments are often referred to as the attitude director indicator and the horizontal situation indicator.

Aircraft status displays

In addition to those displays described above that inform the pilot of the aircraft's relationship with the world, there are many displays that are required to inform the crew of the state of the aircraft's own systems. Engines, fuel, hydraulics, cabin temperatures and pressures and aircraft avionics are all subject to comprehensive monitoring, the data from which must be displayed.

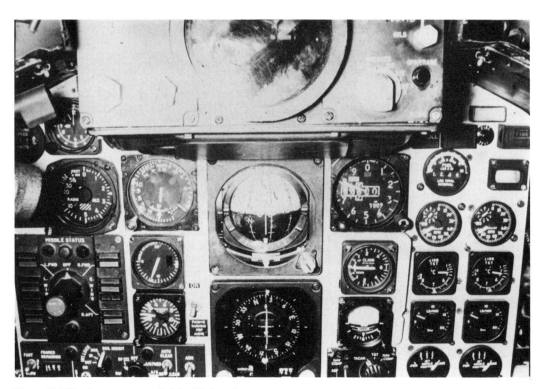

Figure 30.7 The instrument panel of the F4 aircraft.

The design of such displays, and their organization, is dealt with fully in texts listed under 'Further Reading' at the end of the chapter, but an example serves to illustrate the importance of good design.

In the F4 aircraft there are two engines, and consequently two sets of engine instruments. These engine instruments may be seen at the right in *Figure 30.7* in two columns of dials. This is obviously not only a convenient way of organizing these devices but is ergonomically sound, since if both engines are functioning correctly, the pointers on the instruments in each pair will be aligned. Furthermore, the scales on the instruments should be arranged such that when the pointers are in their normal operating position they will point, on all instruments in the array, to the same part of the scale, perhaps the top. Failure to do so reduces the number of instruments that may be checked in 0.5 seconds from 32 to as few as four (Senders, 1952).

The problem embodied in the design of the F4 arises not from the engine instruments, but from the two fire warning captions that may be seen above the engine instruments. Each of these captions is divided into three parts as shown in *Figure 30.8*. Ideally, these warning captions would have been

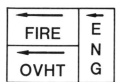 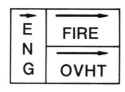

Figure 30.8 The fire warning captions used in the F4 aircraft.

located directly above the relevant set of engine instruments, but space constraints have resulted in their being located above and slightly to the right of their ideal location. There would still appear to be no doubt about the engine to which each of these fire warning blocks refers, until the night situation is considered. All of the instruments in the panel are internally illuminated, and the fire warning blocks are consequently totally invisible unless one of the captions is lit. If it should be the vertical ENG caption of the left engine that illuminates, the possibility exists that the pilot might misidentify it as the identical right ENG caption, since the left caption is located almost exactly on the mid-line of the two sets of engine instruments which act as visual landmarks. This confusion has resulted in the loss of an aircraft, but it was only after the loss that simulator records were examined and revealed an error rate of 15% in the responses of pilots to this particular caption.

Current display trends

The main change that has taken place in flight-deck displays has been in the replacement of pneumatic and electro-mechanical dedicated displays by multi-function, computer-driven cathode ray tubes (CRTs). Such electronic displays—popular with engineers because of their economy, maintainability and flexibility—also offer human factors advantages and pitfalls. Some of these are now discussed.

Flight-deck simplification

Traditional displays have tended to show only one flight parameter (they are 'dedicated' displays). Some integration of information has been provided even by electro-mechanical attitude directors and horizontal situation indicators, but to nothing like the extent that can be engineered if computer-driven CRTs are used. The result is the production of an uncluttered flight deck that contains a relatively small number of CRTs instead of many individual dials.

Graphic presentation

On a CRT, there is no mechanical limitation to the nature of the display, and symbols may thus be allowed to change shape, size, and their location on the screen. Thus a horizontal situation indicator may be made to give an essentially map-like representation of the world instead of the traditional compass-like representation. Furthermore, because of the integration facility referred to above, information from the aircraft's radar may be presented on the same display as information derived from the aircraft's internal inertial platform and information derived from ground-based radio navigational aids.

Use of colour

Colour has long been used on the face of displays to indicate, for example, areas of normal operation and areas of hazard. On CRTs, however, colour may be used more flexibly, in that text or graphics may be made to change colour without changing their screen location. The principal use to which colour may be put is in the categorization or grouping of information. Thus the use of different colours for electrical, hydraulic and fuel status displays may assist in their subjective categorization. Colours may also be used to indicate changes of state (e.g. a rise in engine temperature to a hazardous level), but care must be exercised in this practice since colours have no direct semantic content, though a very few do have strong associations with safety, caution, and danger. Such use of colour (analogous to the use of abstract audio warnings) should be most limited.

Information selection

In the traditional flight deck containing dedicated displays, the selection of information has been the task of the pilot, since it is largely true that all available information is continuously displayed. CRT displays may be multi-function in the sense that one screen may be used to present more than one type of information, the pilot or computer selecting the display 'page' that is appropriate to the phase of flight, or perhaps relevant to an engineering problem that has occurred. If the computer is to be required to monitor a large number of variables (that would previously have been scanned by, perhaps, a flight engineer), alerting the pilot only when a pre-programmed combination of events occurs, a large burden is clearly placed on the system designer to anticipate all possible problems, and decide the appropriate system response.

Location flexibility

Since electronic displays produce a luminous image, they are amenable to a considerable flexibility of presentation. The head-up display (HUD) in which the electronic image is collimated (brought to a focus at infinity) and projected on to an angled image glass before the pilot, is now a familiar part of the military cockpit. It enables flight and weapons information to be integrated into one display that may be viewed at the same apparent range as, and overlaid on, the real outside world. An attentional shift is required if the pilot wishes to interrogate the display rather than the world, but such an attentional shift is considerably preferable to the head movement and accommodational change that is demanded by the interrogation of a panel-mounted or head-down display (HDD). The symbology on current HUDs is restricted to lines and alphanumerics which impose limitations. For example, if the horizon is to be represented by a line it may appear very similar when presented inverted. Electronic displays may also be presented in a head-mounted form, in which some form of optical system is fastened to the pilot's helmet to produce a head-stabilized display. If such a display is coupled to a system that detects head orientation, the result can be used as a weapon aiming system. Although such devices are produced, their use in environments where there is vibration causing angular head movements at greater than 1.5 Hz may be limited, since the human vestibular and ocular systems are designed to stabilize retinal images of the outside world (i.e. to compensate for head movements), and if the image is already head-stabilized, these reflexes

will, paradoxically, result in retinal destabilization and blurring.

Perceptual distance

It was noted, at the beginning of this section on displays, that their purpose is to present the pilot with information that he is unable to sense directly. He must then use this information to construct a mental model of the external world. In early displays, the 'distance' between the aircraft sensor and the display was short—a card was directly mounted on a gyro, or air pressure produced a needle deflection—and readily understood by the pilot, but the display itself was abstract and bore little resemblance to the world. Today, the sensor–display distance is long, complex and incomprehensible, the information is heavily prioritized and processed before being given to the pilot, yet the display bears a much closer resemblance to the real world. This increased perceptual distance, or separation from the outside world, combined with a realistic and compelling display, may induce a pilot to regard manipulation of the display as his object and not to regard the display simply as a source of information to be used in the creation of a model of the real world. If so, then there may be consequences for the pilot's perception of risk: the avoidance of a green area on a display may seem less important than the avoidance of the mountain that it represents.

Display principles

When any new display is being contemplated, there are a number of factors that must be considered, and these include the following:

1. *Display type*—The designer must carefully consider the function of the display, and ask himself what information the observer needs. If the display is provided to inform the operator when some critical value is exceeded, then it is inappropriate to provide a continuous scale since doing so will provide the operator with a monitoring or vigilance task. In this instance, the operator should be provided with a labelled warning light or illuminated caption, perhaps with an attention-getting sound (an 'attenson'). If a quantitative reading is required, then consideration should be given to the provision of a digital display (perhaps augmented with a moving pointer if rate information is also required). If an analogue reading is required, such as some indication of magnitude of deviation from some optimal value, then a

linear (thermometer-type) or circular scale may be appropriate.

2. *Viewing distance*—There are many factors that will constrain viewing distance. For example, the display may be mounted on a panel that also contains controls that must be within easy reach. The critical consideration, however, is that individual symbols, such as letters or digits, on a display should subtend at least 5 minutes of arc when viewed from the normal range even if the viewer has 6/6 vision.

3. *Display orientation*—Ideally, the plane of the display should be normal to the line of sight.

4. *Illumination*—Some displays will depend on reflected light, and some may be internally illuminated. In either event, care must be taken that illumination is appropriate and free from glare or reflection.

5. *Array organization*—If the display is to be used as part of a panel, care must be taken that all displays in the panel contain scales which increase in value in the same direction, that displays that will be used in conjunction with one another are located together, and that each display is well identified.

6. *Interaction with other equipment*—Until recently, a protective visor was the only visual equipment that the pilot was likely to wear. Today, this is likely to be complicated by the provision of a transparency in the chemical protective respirator, and by the use of night vision goggles (NVGs). Although the problem of reflections that may be presented by viewing instruments through multiple transparencies must be considered, it is more transient than the problem of viewing cockpit displays with night vision, or light-intensifying, devices. The purpose of NVGs is to enable the pilot to view a distant, dimly lit, external world, but the pilot must also be able to view a close, relatively brightly lit, instrument panel. There are a number of ingenious solutions to this problem which involve illuminating the displays with narrow band light at wavelengths chosen carefully to complement those used by the goggles, but improved solutions to the difficulty are still being developed.

7. *Display–control compatibility*—Many displays are associated with a particular control. The problems of making displays and controls compatible with one another are discussed below.

Controls

Controls mediate the flow of information from man to machine. The importance of control design was illustrated in a classic study of 460 pilot errors by Fitts and Jones (1947). The most frequent cause of error was confusion of controls. Pilots were sometimes found, for example, to have changed the gasoline mixture when they had intended to pull the throttle. These errors could be considered examples of negative transfer between aircraft types: controls for the throttle, propellor, and gasoline mixture were arranged in a different sequence on each. This problem was exacerbated by the close proximity of many of the controls. A particular source of difficulty was the side-by-side positioning of controls for the flaps and landing gear, which required opposite movements during both take-off and landing. Errors due to control crowding could emerge either because the pilot selected the wrong control, or because he unintentionally altered the position of another control when attempting to operate the correct one.

'Reversal' errors (moving a control in the wrong direction) were also identified by Fitts and Jones (1947), and were clearly a result of poor control design. An even more fundamental design error was that in some instances the pilot simply could not reach the control that he wished to operate.

In the discussion that follows, many of the basic principles of control ergonomics will be seen to be directly related to the types of error described above. Modern aircraft design has benefited from increased awareness of these principles; however, although control-related errors feature less prominently in contemporary accident causation, they have not been eliminated. The CHIRP scheme has received several reports of civil aviation incidents attributed to control characteristics, and Chappelow (1984) reported that poor control ergonomics were the direct cause of about 3% of Royal Air Force accidents in the period 1972–82.

Types of control

Broadly, controls can be divided into two major categories: those that give continuous adjustment, and those that give discrete movement. Each may be in rotary or reciprocating form (*Table 30.1*). Note

Table 30.1 Examples of major types of control

Type of control	Type of adjustment required	
	Continuous	*Discrete*
Rotary	Knob	Knob
	Crank	Handwheel
	Handwheel	Handgrip
Reciprocating	Lever	Lever
	Joystick	Push-button
	Roller-ball	Toggle-switch

that the same type of control may be used to give either continuous or discrete adjustment. For example, a knob may be used on a radio for tuning (continuous) or for the selection of wavelength range (discrete). For a discussion of various types of control, and their suitability for particular applications, *see* Murrell (1965).

Compatibility

A compatible control is one whose operation 'naturally' produces the desired outcome. It seems natural, for example, that clockwise rotation of the steering wheel will move a car to the right. Such commonly held expectations are called population stereotypes. Some, such as the example above, are almost universal; others are clearly defined by past experience. The British visitor to the United States may find himself switching a light off rather than on, since he is accustomed to associating the down position with the on state.

Compatibility of controls is often considered in relation to their associated displays. The expected display changes for given movements of controls such as levers and dials have been well researched (Murrell, 1965); typical examples are illustrated in *Figure 30.9*.

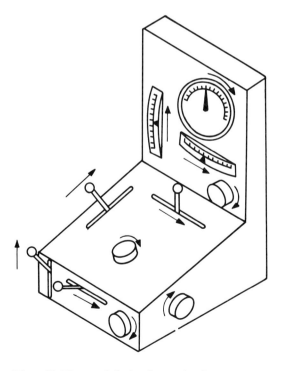

Figure 30.9 Expected display changes for given movements of controls.

Another aspect of compatibility is the ease with which a particular control may be associated with a particular display. Sometimes, controls may be located in close proximity to their respective displays. Often, however, they must be physically separated. Under such circumstances, spatial configuration is an important means of achieving compatibility. As a simple example, consider a cooker with four hobs arranged in a square. If the controls are arranged similarly, then their relationship to the hobs is obvious; if, however, the controls are arranged in a horizontal strip, then their assignment to the hobs must necessarily be more arbitrary.

Hartzell *et al.* (1982) identified a common source of low display–control compatibility in military helicopters: altitude is controlled by the left hand, but the altimeter is located on the right of the instrument panel; airspeed is controlled by the right hand, but indicated by a display on the left.

The amount of training required is inversely related to the compatibility of the controls incorporated in the equipment. Moreover, although incompatible control movements may eventually be learned successfully, individuals will tend to revert to the most natural response movement under stress. Murrell (1965) described an accident on board a ship that illustrates this point. A lubricating oil cooler was controlled by a valve whose rotation moved an indicator in the opposite direction. During an emergency, a sailor was instructed to select the bypass position. Since this position was on the right of the display, he turned the valve clockwise, unintentionally switching off the valve and causing considerable damage.

Control coding and confusability

In Fitts and Jones' (1947) survey, confusion of aircraft controls was found to be a common error. There are several ways in which the coding of controls—by means of physical characteristics such as location, size, shape, symbology, and colour—can be used to reduce confusability (Anastasi, 1979).

Standardization of coding is an obvious and powerful means of reducing confusion errors. A familiar example is the use of blue and red labels on cold and hot water taps, respectively. On the other hand, inconsistencies of location of controls can still be identified in many aspects of everyday life. Switching on the windscreen wipers instead of the direction indicator in an unfamiliar car is exactly analogous to the confusion of aircraft controls noted by Fitts and Jones.

The discriminability of controls can be improved, and hence the probability of confusion reduced, by appropriate selection of codes. Since it is often desirable that the operator be able to locate a particular control without diverting his gaze towards it, non-visual coding dimensions are likely to be particularly useful. Jenkins (1947) investigated the number and types of shapes that could be distinguished tactually. He arranged 22 control knobs, each a different shape, on a turntable. Subjects were blindfolded and permitted to feel one of the shapes for 1 second; the turntable was then rotated, and they were then required to locate the correct knob. Analysis of errors permitted the identification of eight shapes that were never confused with any other. To this basic set of shapes, developed for the US Army, three others were later added for Navy use, producing a negligible increase in confusion errors.

The use of meaningful codes may also enhance performance. When the coding dimension is visual, meaningful associations with function may easily be achieved by the use of verbal labels or images. However, such associations can also be achieved by non-visual means. The US Air Force, for example, developed a set of control knobs whose shapes were consistent with their functions, such as a wing-shaped flap control.

Dynamic control: tracking

A few of the control characteristics that influence human tracking efficiency will be considered briefly. For a comprehensive review of this topic, *see* Wickens (1986).

In dynamic systems, the relationships between the operator's input and the system's output are called transfer functions. One of the most important is the control/display ratio (the relationship between movement of a control and movement of a corresponding display element). When this ratio is low, i.e. when the gain of the system is high, large corrections can be made with little effort, but the probability of over-correction is increased. When the control/display ratio is high, more time is required to make the initial correction, but final adjustment can be made more quickly.

The optimal control/display ratio is dependent upon other transfer functions, such as system lag. The delay in a system may be pure, reproducing the input exactly after a given time period, or exponential, gradually attaining the demanded outcome. The former type of lag has a greater disruptive influence on tracking performance. Lags become increasingly detrimental when combined with a high control/display ratio, but may improve performance when the control/display ratio is low (Rockway, 1954).

The final transfer function to be considered here is system order. With zero-order or position control,

the system responds to a given control input with a proportional change in position; in a first-order or velocity control system, the response is a constant velocity of movement proportional to the input; and with second-order or acceleration control, a constant acceleration is produced whose magnitude is a function of the input. In general, zero- and first-order produce equivalent overall performance, since tracking requires control both of position and of velocity, and are greatly preferable to second- (or higher-) order control, which places excessive demands for prediction upon the operator (Wickens, 1984, 1986).

Current trends in control design

The principal controls in any aircraft remain the control column, joystick, or control wheel (used to effect changes in the pitch and roll attitudes of the aircraft), and the power control. The changes that have occurred in display technology have been paralleled in the development of modern controls, and this is perhaps most striking if the control column of large commercial aircraft is considered. Early commercial aircraft required a large control column since a direct connection, usually by control rods and wires, existed between it and the control surface on the aircraft. The control column had to be large in order to provide sufficient mechanical advantage for the pilot to be able to produce the forces required.

As hydraulic controls and powered flying controls were introduced, the requirement for the control column to be so large gradually disappeared, but convention prevented it from being redesigned. Today, the Boeing 757 still has a central, substantial control, but the designers of the European Airbus have taken the bold step of replacing this with a small joystick placed to the side of the pilot. In many modern aircraft a further change has taken place concerning the nature of the connection between control and control surface. Even in aircraft with sophisticated powered controls, control column input mapped directly onto control surface deflection. This is no longer so. The control is connected to the control surface via a computer which is programmed to produce a combination of changes in the control surfaces, the net result of which should be to produce the effect desired by the pilot. Thus the pilot is no longer controlling the aircraft directly but is using the control to indicate a desire to the computer, which then chooses the optimal method of expression for this desire.

The large human factors change produced by this technology is that the controls may be made 'carefree', in the sense that the computer may be programmed to produce only those changes in the flight regime that are safe. Thus the pilot who requires the maximum possible pitch rotation, on overshooting or when encountering wind shear, is free to pull the control column fully back, leaving the aircraft to provide the maximum safe pitch-up. Indeed it may, in future, not even be necessary for the pilot to touch the control column, since computers are already able to recognize a limited repertoire of spoken phrases, and the use of such direct voice input (DVI) may well enable the pilot simply to tell his aircraft what to do.

The technology underlying these control changes has been developed principally on fighter aircraft. Such machines are required to be as manoeuvrable as possible and are therefore built with extremely low levels of natural aerodynamic stability. In order to make them possible to fly, 'active' controls produce synthetic stability, and these controls have also enabled aircraft to be designed that could not otherwise have been controlled by the pilot. Interestingly, the sophistication of control over ailerons, spoilers, elevators and canards is now such that forces can be produced on the airframe (producing, for example, direct vertical translation without any change in pitch) for which no conventional aircraft control exists.

Arguably, these changes in technology add to the difficulty of the military pilot's task, in which performance is the overriding criterion, but simplify the civil pilot's task for which efficiency and safety are paramount. It might be predicted that the civil pilot would resist such change on two counts; because he may perceive the technology as de-skilling his task, and because he may not understand, and hence be inclined not to trust, the technology. These problems do not, in fact, seem to materialize. Pilots appear to accept empirical evidence that a system works. Autolandings and automatic terrain following were readily accepted once pilots gained practical experience that the systems were reliable. It also seems true that pilots are prepared to accept that their job is changing, to welcome technology that improves safety (even if it reduces the satisfaction associated with the execution of motor skills) and to accept that piloting a modern aircraft is principally a problem of system management. It is difficult to know how long this can remain true, however. The introduction of artificial intelligence into aircraft computers is rapidly making the pilot redundant even with regard to the high-level decisions that he is presently required to make, and, already, it is said that the most common remark made on current automated flight decks is 'Now why is it doing that?' It may be that a radical rethink of the pilot's task will have to be undertaken if he is to be provided with a role on the flight deck that is both sensible in system terms and acceptable in terms of job satisfaction.

Workspace

The essential characteristics of any workspace are that the displays should be visible and the controls within reach. However, in all workspaces there are compromises that must be made, and these compromises are probably best illustrated by consideration of the design of the workspace in a single-seat fighter aircraft.

In such aircraft, the overall amount of space available will be constrained by the fuselage dimensions, and aerodynamic considerations will force these to be minimized. The pilot will require the best possible external view, but providing a large canopy transparency will limit the panel space available for displays. Considerations of reach, and of the range of size of pilots, will limit the location of controls.

Figure 30.10 shows some of the more important geometric problems presented by the design of a fighter cockpit. The first point that must be fixed is the 'design eye position'. This immediately locates the height of the canopy (which must be at least 255 mm above the eye in order to provide adequate head mobility) and the top of the forward instrument panel (which must be at least 15 degrees or so below the horizontal vision line if the pilot is to have sufficient external, forward, downward vision for landing). The position of the eye will also determine the orientation of the instruments since they should, as far as possible, be normal to the pilot's line of sight when they are fixated.

The neutral seat reference point must be positioned below the eye at a distance designed to suit the pilot of mean size. Pilots vary in size, however, and it is customary to design for all pilots between, for example, the third and ninety-ninth size percentiles. Deciding on the appropriate size limits may not be straightforward but, once settled, enough seat adjustment must be provided to accommodate the decided range.

Seat position determines the location of the legs, which in turn constrains the lower extent of the space available for the forward panel. The maximum distance of the forward panel from the pilot will be limited by the reach of the pilot with the shortest acceptable arms, and the panel must also be located sufficiently distant from the pilot to enable a clear ejection path to be maintained. The requirement to maintain a clear path for ejection also prevents the provision of any protruding controls on this panel.

It is clear from the above discussion that the cockpit workspace is extremely tightly constrained, and that change in any one factor will have immediate repercussions on others. For example, it may be desirable to tilt the pilot's seat backwards to improve his G tolerance (*see* Chapter 11). Doing so, however, reduces the vertical distance between the

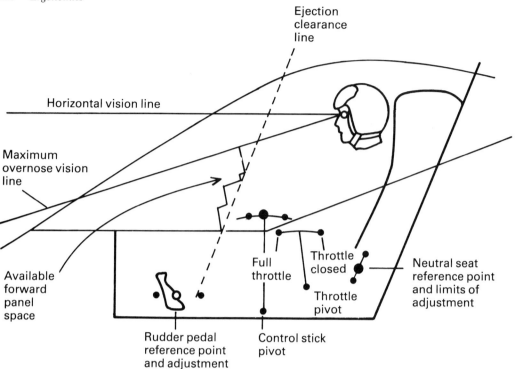

Figure 30.10 Geometric problems presented by the design of a fighter cockpit.

pilot's eye and his knees, and consequently the area available for forward panel space. It may also make it difficult for the pilot to use a central control column, compelling the provision of a side-arm controller which must be mounted on one of the side panels, consuming further panel space.

Once the areas available for displays and controls have been defined, their distribution within these areas must be carefully considered given their relative frequencies of use and importance. The precise nature of the displays in any aircraft will depend on the role of the aircraft, and the radar and weapons with which it is fitted. Generally speaking, the forward panel of fighter aircraft is reserved for the basic flight and navigational displays, the left side panel is used for throttles and secondary flight controls such as flaps, and the right panel for the displays and controls concerned with the aircraft's systems such as radios, oxygen, and autopilot. The weapons and systems of such aircraft are now so closely integrated that the controls for both are frequently mounted on a downward extension of the forward panel between the pilot's legs.

A great deal of effort is put into the workspace design of modern aircraft, but mistakes still occur. In one aircraft type, a set of weapons switches was located in a low position behind the control column, a location that was unsatisfactory for short pilots. Such pilots required the seat to be at its highest

position to maximize their external view, but they also tended to have short arms, and were thus unable to reach the low switches which consequently had to be relocated.

Relocation of controls always provides the potential for negative transfer of skill, but seldom as obviously as in an example provided by another fast jet. In this aircraft, the pilot was provided with an inconveniently located manual fuel control unit switch (the MFCU) which may have to be selected rapidly if automatic fuel control fails (and selection of which necessitates extremely careful throttle control). The aircraft's anti-skid unit was, however, selected by a conveniently located switch. Although the anti-skid switch is used frequently, its use is not time-critical in the way that the use of the MFCU is, and the decision was consequently made to exchange the position of the two switches. Such a change would have been sensible at the design stage, but conspicuously less so after pilots had gained experience with the aircraft. A number of inadvertent selections and, consequently, dangerously mishandled engines, were caused by this change, since it failed to take into account the learned behaviour or motor programmes of the aircraft's pilots.

It is beyond the scope of this brief résumé to present detailed recommendations for the design and location of the many types of controls and displays that may be used in aircraft. There are many excellent texts that provide data on these matters, and the interested reader is referred to Boff and Lincoln (1987) for an exhaustive discussion.

References

ANASTASI, A. (1979) *Fields of Applied Psychology*. Tokyo: McGraw-Hill Kogakusha

BOFF, K.R. and LINCOLN, J.E. (1987) *Engineering Data Compendium*. New York: Wiley

CHAPPELOW, J.W. (1984) *Human Error in Aircraft Accidents: A Review of Psychologists' Reports on Royal Air Force Accidents 1972–1982*. RAF Institute of Aviation Medicine Report No. 633. London: Ministry of Defence

FITTS, P.M. and JONES, R.E. (1947) *Analysis of Factors Contributing to 460 'Pilot-error' Experiences in Operating Aircraft Controls*. Report No. TSEAA-694-12. Dayton, Ohio: Engineering Division, Air Material Command

HARTZELL, E.S., DUNBAR, S., BEVERIDGE, R. and CORTILLA, R. (1982) Helicopter pilot response latency as a function of the spatial arrangement of instruments and controls. In *Proceedings of the 18th Annual Conference on Manual Control*. Ohio: Wright–Patterson Air Force Base

JENKINS, W.O. (1947) The tactual discrimination of shapes for coding aircraft-type controls. In *Psychological Research in Equipment Design*, edited by P.M. Fitts,

AAF Aviation Psychology Program Research Report No. 19. Washington: Government Printing Office

MURRELL, K.F.H. (1965) *Ergonomics*. London: Chapman and Hall

ROCKWAY, M.R. (1954) *The Effects of Variations in Control–Display Ratio and Exponential Time Delay on Tracking Performance*. USAF Wright Air Development Center Technical Report No. 54-618

SENDERS, V.L. (1952) *The Effect of Number of Dials on Qualitative Reading of a Multiple Dial Panel*. USAF Wright Development Center Report No. 52-182

WICKENS, C.D. (1984) *Engineering Psychology and Human Performance*. Columbus: Charles E. Merrill

WICKENS, C.D. (1986) The effects of control dynamics on performance. In *Handbook of Perception and Human Performance, Volume II: Cognitive Processes and Performance*, edited by K.R. Boff, L. Kaufman and J.P. Thomas. New York: Wiley

Further reading

KVALSETH, T.O. (ed.) (1983) *Ergonomics of Workstation Design*. London: Butterworths

MORGAN, C.T., COOK, J.S., CHAPANIS, A. and LUND, M.W. (eds) (1963) *Human Engineering Guide to Equipment Design*. New York: McGraw-Hill

Human Engineering Design Criteria for Military Systems, Equipment and Facilities (MIL-STD-1472C) (1981) Washington: US Government Printing Office

31

Social psychology

R.G. Green

Some animals lead solitary existences, but man is not one of them. All of us belong to groups of one sort or another, whether we wish to or not. We may lead one group and be led in another. We may wish to change the behaviour of our colleagues in a group or we may be happy to go along with the wishes of others. We may find ourselves to be uncomfortable with the direction in which our group seems to be going and have difficulty in deciding whether to go along with the trend. Social psychology is the study of how people behave in groups, and of how their judgements, attitudes and opinions are influenced by others.

Groups in aviation

In aviation there are many identifiable groups, the most obvious being the flight-deck crew of an aircraft. The number of people in a crew of large civil aircraft has decreased progressively from the early days of intercontinental travel (when a crew of seven was commonplace), to the current long-range jets which are capable of non-stop sectors in excess of 14 hours, but may be handled, technically, by just two crew. Many military aircraft in maritime reconnaissance and airborne early warning still carry large numbers of crew, but an immediate distinction presents itself between the flight-deck crew and the rear crew. A similar distinction may be made on civil aircraft between the flight-deck, or technical, crew and the cabin crew. These groups will have interests in common and interests that divide them even though they share the same aircraft. And there is, of course, another conspicuous group on civil and military transport aircraft—the passengers.

The group effects that probably have the most important safety repercussions for the largest

numbers of people are those that take place on the civil flight deck. At the time of writing, long-haul flights are approaching the end of an era in which they are manned by an engineer as well as two pilots, and the two-man cockpit is rapidly becoming the norm. These crew members may or may not know each other before the flight and they may or may not like each other. Their task, however, is to work together safely and effectively. This chapter begins by examining this group, the flight-deck team, and uses examples of team problems on the flight deck to introduce some of the concepts of social psychology.

The flight-deck group

On March 27 1977, a Boeing 747 lined up for take-off at Tenerife was given a route clearance but not a take-off clearance. Although the situation was probably accurately appreciated by the co-pilot (first officer), the captain thought he was cleared to roll. The co-pilot asked the captain whether they had had the right clearance, but did not insist on holding, as he might have, until he had personally checked. The aircraft accelerated down the runway and collided, in fog, with another 747 that was taxiing the other way. It was the worst aircraft accident ever, with 585 passengers and crew losing their lives.

Why would a competent pilot prefer to risk his life in fog rather than ensure that to proceed would be safe? It will occur to the reader that by asking the captain to hold until he had checked the clearance, the first officer would, at once, make himself look incompetent for missing the clearance, and suggest that the captain might be incompetent for believing that he had received a clearance that had not been given. The reader will probably have some added sympathy for the first officer if informed that the captain was a training captain. If the captain had had a very dominant personality, and the first officer had been rather submissive, then we would be even less surprised that he did not voice his doubts.

There was, however, a simple solution for the first officer. He could have said, 'I'm sorry Captain, I must have missed the clearance. Just hold for a second while I check with air traffic.' The captain would probably not have taken any umbrage, the first officer would have demonstrated his diligence, and this accident would not have happened.

Compliance, conformity, and obedience to authority

Social factors are obviously important, and we have already seen that there are a number of important variables; the role or job of the individuals, the status of the individuals, and their personalities. Clearly, a high-status training captain, in command and in control of the aircraft, perhaps with a dominant personality, is going to present difficulty to a junior, and perhaps submissive, first officer.

The first officer, in the example above, can be said to have been compliant or to have conformed to the behaviour of his group leader, but the terms COMPLIANCE and CONFORMITY have specific meanings within social psychology. Compliance is used to mean accession to the request or actions of another, and a good deal is known about the conditions that make compliance likely. For example, if a large and unreasonable request is made a compliant response is more likely if it has been preceded by a smaller, more reasonable, but similar request—the so-called foot-in-the-door technique. It is sometimes possible to see situations growing on flight decks where a co-pilot goes along with an unreasonable action on the part of another because it has been prefaced by a series of similar actions that were not as objectionable. Paradoxically, a compliant response is also more likely if the request or behaviour has been preceded by a request that is obviously outrageous, and which has not been complied with (the door-in-the-face-technique).

Conformity is a related term that is used to refer to those occasions on which an individual changes his behaviour towards a group norm. There are some remarkable experiments that demonstrate this effect, the best known being those of Solomon Asch (1955). He produced an experimental paradigm in which a group of subjects (all but one of whom were accomplices of the experimenter, or stooges) was shown a line drawn on a card and asked to match the length of the line with one of three test lines. The correct answer was obvious, and the experiment started with all subjects giving the correct response.

As matters progressed, however, the stooges began to give unanimous incorrect judgements, and on these occasions most of the test subjects agreed with the clearly wrong judgement on at least some occasions. The size of the opposing majority had a clear effect in these experiments, but interestingly the effect rapidly reached its maximum magnitude with an opposing group of just four individuals.

Other variables influencing the outcome of the experiment outlined above are the self-esteem of the test subject (low self-esteem subjects being more conforming), and the desirability or attractiveness of the group making the incorrect judgements. There are occasions on which a pilot may be called to resist the social pressure to conform exerted by another crew member, and experimental work strongly reinforces the common-sense notion that support by another individual has a powerful effect, particularly if that individual has obvious credibility. Although the debate over the three- versus two-crew aircraft has centred on issues of workload, it may be that there are good social reasons for keeping three crew. If a high-status and dominant captain behaves unreasonably in a two-crew aircraft he is much less likely to be challenged by his co-pilot than if there is a crew of three in which the co-pilot feels that he will receive support from the third pilot or engineer.

On the flight deck, the problems of compliance and conformity merge into the issue of obedience to authority, and the experiments of Milgram (1974) must be mentioned in this context. He used volunteers from the street in what was purported to be a memory experiment. One subject was assigned to be a learner, and the other to be a teacher. The learner was to memorize lists of words, and the teacher was to punish, by the administration of progressively more severe electric shocks, any errors. In fact, the learner was an actor and there were no shocks, but the teacher was not aware of this, and as he administered increasingly severe 'shocks' the learner cried out and complained of a heart condition. Milgram had asked psychiatrists how far they thought the teachers would go before refusing to administer more shocks, and they consistently underestimated by a large amount the degree of 'shock' that the teachers would be prepared to administer. Even though many of the teachers in this experiment overtly demonstrated acute anxiety about their actions they continued to administer shocks, under the encouragement of the experimenter, that they believed were not only painful but possibly dangerous.

Such controversial, and possibly unethical, experiments make a fairly sad commentary on humanity. They do, however, help to put into perspective the actions of all those who claim that they are simply doing their duty and do help to explain the behaviour of many pilots who believe that the actions they take are those that would be approved by their superiors. Obedience to the group leader seems to be a very basic human property, an attribute that may have had distinct survival value for a pack animal, and its power is not to be underestimated.

Group decision making

The function of having more than one pilot on a flight deck is, at least in some measure, to produce consensus decision making. Hopefully, a group decision about a given problem will be a better decision than might be made by any one of the individuals. There is, however, a group effect that is sometimes termed 'risky shift' which means that group decisions are not always more prudent than those of individuals. There are many laboratory examples of risky shift, and these generally involve presenting hypothetical problems to subjects about a man who is, for example, contemplating giving up a secure job for a better paid, but less secure position. Should he take the new job? Generally, a group that discusses the problem favours greater risk taking than a comparable set of individuals.

The following example of risky shift on a flight deck is taken directly from a report to the UK Confidential Human Factors Reporting System, and is in the pilot's own words:

'Venerable Captain, experienced P2 and P3. First approach made flying cat 1 automatic approach, at decision height (DH) of 220 feet, P2 initiated overshoot. During the overshoot the airfields lights were seen so we went round for another approach still on autopilot. The second approach was an action replay of the first, as was the overshoot.

'As we entered the hold to contemplate the situation, another aircraft landed. A suggestion was made that we should fly down 50 feet lower but as this was not legal, it was ruled out. We then managed to delude ourselves that flying level at the DH of 220 feet was a legal and reasonable way to achieve our landing. To do this the autopilot was disengaged for the last approach and the P2 flew a manual approach to 220 feet and levelled off. Within seconds the Captain shouted "I have control" and the aircraft continued to fly more or less level for several more seconds. From my position I studied the information on the flight instruments with a growing feeling of unease. The glideslope was fully fly down and had been for some time, we had no way of knowing how far we were beyond the threshold. The brightness of the runway lights convinced me that the Captain could see and knew what he was doing. I called out our radio height at the same time as the equally concerned P2 called the speed and rate of

descent (ROD). The next few seconds saw the cockpit filled with height, speed, and ROD.

'We touched heavily on the centre-line. Heavy braking followed what can only be considered a "max performance" stop. We cleared the runway well down. The pregnant silence which followed served to reinforce our feelings that we'd been party to an act of supreme folly and bravado and were lucky to escape with a few grey hairs and severely battered personal pride.'

Generally speaking, despite the effect of 'risky shift', it is true to say that the quality of a decision made by a group is better than that made by the average group member, but worse than that of the best group members (Shaw, 1971). This begs the question of whether, and if so how, members of the flight-deck group may be trained to get the best from one another. Since the management of the crew is the clear responsibility of the captain, this also becomes a question of leadership training.

Leadership styles

Prominent among those who have considered the qualities of leadership is Fiedler (1971). He has suggested that leaders may be either 'task oriented' or 'relationship oriented'. These terms are largely self-explanatory, and the concepts underlying them have been used in a number of training courses such as those used by United Airlines and Dan-Air Services. In these courses pilots and engineers are given a two-dimensional model of leadership styles such as that shown below (*Figure 31.1*).

Group duration

Another factor that must be taken into account when considering the behaviour of a group is the length of time for which that group remains in existence. In this respect a marked difference exists, within the UK, between military and civil flight-deck crews. Generally speaking, civil crews exist as a group only for the duration of the flight or, for long-range crews, for the duration of the trip (which may vary between just a night or two up to almost 3 weeks). Military crews, however, tend to be 'constituted', which is to say that a given crew will stay together, once formed, until circumstances, such as postings or promotion, necessitate change. The obvious difference between such groups is that the members of a military crew will be very familiar with the ways in which each other work, but the members of a civil crew may never have flown together or never even have met before they are required to function as a working unit.

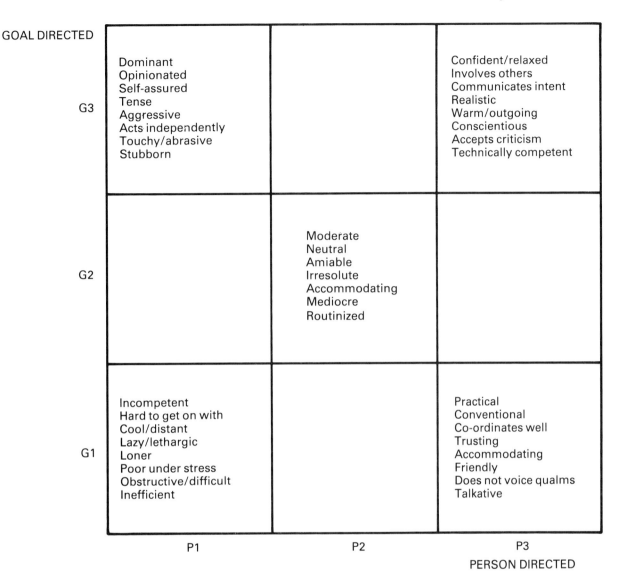

GOAL DIRECTED

G3

Dominant
Opinionated
Self-assured
Tense
Aggressive
Acts independently
Touchy/abrasive
Stubborn

Confident/relaxed
Involves others
Communicates intent
Realistic
Warm/outgoing
Conscientious
Accepts criticism
Technically competent

G2

Moderate
Neutral
Amiable
Irresolute
Accommodating
Mediocre
Routinized

G1

Incompetent
Hard to get on with
Cool/distant
Lazy/lethargic
Loner
Poor under stress
Obstructive/difficult
Inefficient

Practical
Conventional
Co-ordinates well
Trusting
Accommodating
Friendly
Does not voice qualms
Talkative

P1   P2   P3

PERSON DIRECTED

Figure 31.1 A two-dimensional model of leadership styles.

The first consequence of having a non-constituted crew is the importance that becomes attached to the roles (i.e. the functions) of each crew member. Obviously, these roles must be defined closely so that a given first officer can perform in exactly the same way regardless of the captain he finds himself with, and vice versa. There is little room in such crews for independence of action, and the close adherence to what are termed 'standard operating procedures' is of paramount importance.

The military crew can afford a somewhat more flexible approach since they should be more aware of each other's strengths and weaknesses: they may be able to tailor their mode of operation to take these factors into account to the best overall effect. There are, however, four main disadvantages to this 'constituted' approach. The first is that the crew members may become so familiar with each other's ways of working that they begin to depart from standard procedures and develop idiosyncratic work patterns with possible unforeseen implications. The second is that the crew members may begin to assume that another crew member has undertaken an action because he habitually does so, and consequently fail to carry out proper checks that critical items have been actioned. The third is that if a crew is constituted with a particularly difficult or argumentative member, the remainder of the crew is forced to tolerate the individual, possibly for a long time, and this may have implications for job-satisfaction or morale. The fourth is that the crew members are likely to grow to know their captain well, will be aware of his weaknesses, and this familiarity may engender contempt—it may be relatively difficult for a captain to be both a full social member of the crew and its leader.

The non-constituted crew also has disadvantages. If the crew members do not know one another, it is relatively easy for one crew member to upset another by remarking on a topic of special sensitivity. Although operating procedures may be standardized, it is very difficult to standardize the non-flying behaviour of the individuals in a crew, and the members of a non-constituted crew have no chance to grow to any sort of mutual understanding. This factor places extra emphasis on the requirement for the type of flight-deck management course described above.

There is a possible longer term disadvantage to the non-constituted approach. It prevents, to a large extent, the crew member from feeling that he belongs to an identifiable small group with which he has interests and problems in common, and from which he may draw support. Not all pilots are highly group dependent, and some will not need the security that such group membership may provide, but those who are may feel themselves rather isolated. A common complaint of pilots is that they are treated by airline managements as small cogs in a large machine, and are rostered for duty in exactly the same way as the aircraft is provided with fuel and catering supplies. Indeed, although modish terms such as 'human resources' have been introduced in place of 'personnel department' in an attempt to show concern for the workforce, they may actually reinforce this notion that the human is a resource available to management to be used like any other. This feeling may be strengthened further by the extremely automatic nature of modern flight decks, in which the pilot can see that tasks traditionally regarded as the skilled role of the controlling human are being carried out more effectively by the machine.

Such perceptions may create in pilots an effect that Festinger (1957) has termed 'cognitive dissonance', a state in which two incompatible perceptions, attitudes or opinions must be reconciled. In the present example, the pilot is encouraged to perceive himself as a highly trained, highly paid, professional, directly responsible for several hundred lives and many millions of pounds of machinery. Nevertheless, as noted above, he is expected to behave in a very constrained way, must spend a large portion of his time in the routine monitoring of automatic equipment, and has little or no say in the way he tackles his own task, let alone any wider responsibility for the management of his company.

Membership of a permanent group may help to provide the pilot with a route to the resolution of such dissonance. If such a group were required to meet occasionally, and if it were provided with responsibilities to be carried out as a team, it might provide the pilot with a better sense of group identity, and enable him to feel that he had a role that used intellectual judgement as well as the exercise of a trained skill. This philosophy of providing teams with responsibility has been used with effect in 'job enrichment' programmes in a number of industries.

Although operational reasons will preclude airlines from operating a constituted crew policy (and it is noted above that such a policy is, in any case, probably undesirable), it could be possible to roster crews from a group smaller than that comprising all pilots of that aircraft type. In one study (Wheale, 1983) civil pilots expressed a preference for being rostered from a group of about 60 members. The possible advantages of doing so are that such a group is large enough to avoid the constituted crew problems of over-familiarity, yet small enough for the pilots to know one another.

It may occur to the reader that something akin to the military squadron has just been described, and it may also be noted that such units are remarkable for the strength of group membership that they engender. Not only do members of most squadrons take pride in their belonging, but group membership becomes so valuable to them that they frequently seek to resurrect it by holding reunions long after functional membership has ceased. The ubiquity of such reunions stands as testimony to the importance of the squadron system in the emotional as well as the operational life of its members.

The cabin-crew group

Cabin crew are clearly different from flight-deck (technical crew) in a number of respects, the most obvious being the different sex ratio in each group. Today, technical crews are largely male, but cabin crews are more variable in their constitution. Qantas, the Australian flag-carrying airline, ran, for many years, a policy of employing all-male cabin crew. Dan-Air, a leading British independent carrier, was compelled by law to drop its policy of all-female cabin crews, and in most airlines today a roughly equal mix of sexes will be encountered.

The cabin crew are also likely to be less highly selected than the technical crew and to have a lower level of academic achievement. These factors, which tend to prevent these two sets of individuals from performing as a single group, are reinforced by a number of other influences, such as staying in different hotels during en-route stopovers. There is also an effect of physical location, which is sometimes commented upon by Boeing 747 crews, in that in most airliners, the flight deck is level with the cabin and easily accessible to cabin staff. On the 747, however, the removal of the flight deck to an upper level produces a physical distance between the flight-deck and cabin crews that also appears to increase the social distance between them.

Another social effect of the introduction of wide-bodied aircraft is that the reduction in the number of technical crew has been matched by an increase in the number of cabin crew—many large aircraft now carrying 14–16 flight attendants. This increase in number has generated not a wider and flatter hierarchy in the cabin crew, but been used as an opportunity to increase the responsibility of the senior cabin-crew members. A 707 might have carried four stewards and a purser, but a 747 might carry as many as 13 stewards, two pursers and a 'cabin service director'. This apparent increase in the status of the cabin crew may also serve as a source for division between the two groups.

The considerations above illustrate the factors, such as similarity of function and physical proximity, that enable individuals to form groups and perceive themselves as belonging to a particular group. The group to which an individual belongs is sometimes referred to as the 'in-group' (the 'we' group) and those groups that he may recognize but not belong to, as 'out-groups' (the 'they' groups). The nature of the in- and out-groups may, however, be changed by circumstance. For example, a flight attendant might clearly identify himself with a cabin crew in-group and see the technical crew as an out-group when the interests of the two groups conflict, but see himself as a member of the 'aircraft crew' in-group when dealing with a troublesome member of an out-group such as a passenger or hotel manager.

The passenger group

The third easily identifiable group in civil aviation comprises the passengers, but in some respects they do not operate as a group at all. They will probably have no common purpose or goal beyond the arrival at their destination, will not have to come to common decisions, will probably have no communication within the group, and have no functions assigned to them. The passengers may be defined as a group only by virtue of their physical proximity to one another—all are seated in the same aircraft.

Passengers are likely to function as a group, with the emergence of intra-group discussion and leaders, only if the group is subjected to some form of stress. For example, if their aircraft is delayed and a common feeling emerges that the operating company is not trying hard enough to correct the problem, strong group identity emerges. Furthermore, the group polarization effects referred to

above (under risky shift) become readily apparent. Those who, individually, feel that they have a grievance, will have the feeling reinforced and made more extreme by discussing the grievance with others in the same boat (or, in this instance, the same departure lounge).

The passengers in an aircraft have no real role beyond acting in a subordinate way. They are not expected to know anything about aircraft or aviation, and consequently must be told what to do and when to do it. Passengers readily accept such subordination, and behave in appropriate and socially acceptable ways. They queue to enter the aircraft, smoke only when and where permitted, keep their seat belts on while the signs are illuminated, and remain seated until the aircraft has come to a complete stop.

Such social order breaks down only in extreme circumstances, and notably during an emergency evacuation when a direct threat is perceived. The threat need not be real, so long as it is perceived as real. In 1986, a Boeing 707 was starting up in the Mediterranean when a fuel excess caused one of the engines to 'torch' (a spectacular but benign flame carried in the engine's exhaust gases). An alarmed passenger rose from his seat shouting 'Fire', causing other passengers to rush to the rear of the aircraft. The cabin crew inferred that the cabin was on fire and informed the captain. He then ordered a completely unnecessary evacuation of the aircraft.

Passenger behaviour in aircraft emergencies

A knowledge of passenger behaviour in emergencies is important for two reasons. The internal layout and design of aircraft must take the likely behaviour of passengers into account, and the evaluation of the evacuation acceptability of that layout (required for the aircraft's certification) should be carried out in a suitably enlightened manner.

The design of seats, aisles and exits in theatres and other public places has been influenced by the lessons learned from disasters, and the designers of aircraft must clearly take similar heed of experience. Sadly, the sort of descriptions given of aircraft evacuations today parallel closely those given of, for example, theatre fires earlier in the century. Roger Brown (1965), in discussing group behaviour, quotes an eye-witness account from Eddie Foy, a comedian, of a 1903 Chicago theatre fire. Foy describes the 'panic' of those closest to the flames, the shouted appeals for order, the way in which those with a clearly defined role (the musicians) stuck to their posts, the difficulty encountered in finding and opening exits, the way in which people piled up where there was the slightest impediment to their flow (e.g. a turn in a stairway), and the desperation of the escapees—'The heel prints on the dead faces mutely testified to the cruel fact that human animals stricken by terror are as mad and ruthless as stampeding cattle'.

Competition

Although experimental evidence is understandably hard to come by, it is not unreasonable to suggest that the behaviour described above does not derive from blind irrational responses to a threatening environment, but from a combination of responses to fear and to an obviously competitive situation. Brown points out the importance of the limited potential for escape in generating a group 'panic', noting that although there can be very high levels of fear generated in threatened submarines, the crew do not panic since escape is not possible. Conversely, where there is no fear, but limited access to a desirable resource (such as in the china department of Harrods at sale time), intensely competitive behaviour results that contains many of the elements of a group panic. Any form of competition is, however, conspicuously lacking in those evacuation demonstrations organized to show that an aircraft can comply with the well-known 90 second rule—a point returned to below.

The effect of competition for some limited resource has been studied in ways that produce results that effectively mimic real observed behaviour. The best known such experiments are those of Mintz (1951). He devised a task in which aluminium cones attached to long strings were put into a large, but narrow-necked, bottle. Only one cone at a time could be extracted from the bottle, but subjects (who were each assigned one string) were normally able to co-operate well in removing the cones in an orderly fashion. If, however, they were rewarded for the successful removal of their own cone but the bottle was filled, from the bottom, with water and the subjects fined if their cone was wetted, then blockages at the bottleneck always occurred even if the subjects were allowed to discuss a co-operative plan before the trial.

If the passengers' perception of limited potential for escape is crucial to the generation of panic, then it is clearly incumbent on aircraft designers and operators to consider whether there are any techniques that might be employed to reduce the feeling. Two possibilities come immediately to mind, and the first concerns the conspicuity of exits. It is reasonable to suppose that clear sight of an exit, and preferably sight of an exit being used effectively, will reduce the perceived threat of entrapment. However, the emergency exits in aircraft, and especially the smaller overwing exits, are generally designed to blend visually with the interior trim of

the aircraft rather than to be visually conspicuous. Such exits are, of course, placarded with illuminated signs, but these are generally small and readily lost in the visual clutter of the environment. There is no obvious reason why the emergency exit signs on aircraft should not be of the same dimensions as those that are obligatory in theatres, or why the door frame should not be illuminated in an emergency to provide the clearest visual target for escapees.

The problem of exit inconspicuity is exacerbated in many aircraft by the internal fit of galleys and bulkheads that can visually obscure the doors, and thus prevent those passengers who are queuing in the aisles from seeing that the exits are being used at all. If they were able to see that passengers ahead of them were leaving at the maximum possible rate, then they may be somewhat less likely to take precipitate individual action. Incidentally, this also provides an excellent reason for the cabin crew to use their loudest and most visible efforts to enjoin the passengers nearest to the exits to leave as quickly as possible. These passengers, who are possibly somewhat distanced from the immediate threat, may hesitate over their departure, and loud encouragement for them to leave will have not only the obvious effect of actually maximizing the utilization of the door, but also that of serving to increase the impression given to those behind them that the exit is being used, and hence their interest served, as well as possible.

The second way in which the perceived likelihood of escape may be increased is by the use of protective smoke hoods. Those who have worn such devices sometimes note the feeling of security that they provide, and the readiness with which people accept that the protection provided is effective. If this is so, then we may predict with some confidence that passengers who are able to breathe at least relatively freely, and who have their vision at least relatively conserved, will be significantly less likely to panic than those exposed directly to the frightening, choking, and blinding effects of smoke. The use of such hoods is generally advocated on the basis of the protection that they provide to the respiratory system, but it may be that they could save more lives by reducing the chances of a stampede than by their direct protective effects.

All of the foregoing has been predicated on the assumption that more passengers are likely to escape if the evacuation is orderly than disorderly. This is almost certainly true, and if the motivation of every passenger were to co-operate in getting as many people as possible out of the aircraft, then there would surely be orderly queues to leave. In fact, of course, every passenger is subject to the group pressure for orderliness, and the motivation for self-preservation that compels individual, possibly anti-social action. The threshold for taking individual action will doubtless depend to some extent on personality, to some extent on the threat to which the individual is exposed, and to some extent on the role of the individual. The last of these factors can have a powerful effect. It was noted above in the eye-witness testimony of the theatre fire that some of the musicians kept playing ('Some of the musicians were fleeing, but a few, and especially a fat little violinist, stuck nobly'), and there are many stories of the courage of cabin crew who have even died while carrying out their role.

This difference in motivation (individual *v.* group) provides an important differentiation between real and demonstration evacuations. In the demonstration, all the subjects are motivated to provide a low time for the group. There is no penalty in being the last to leave, and there may even be some kudos in being the one whose departure stops the watch. In evacuating from a burning aircraft, however, there are no points for being last, and the ignominy of queue-jumping may seem quite acceptable when balanced against the alternative. Such evacuation demonstrations, required for aircraft certification, are defended on the entirely justifiable grounds that they are not intended to show that, in emergency, an aircraft really can be emptied in 90 seconds, but that they represent the best method attainable for comparing the time required for an aircraft to be evacuated with a standard, and hence with other aircraft. There is just one point that is ignored by this argument, and this concerns the possibility that there will be a material interaction between the aircraft fit and the motivation of the passengers. An example that clarifies this point concerns egress from overwing exits. Manufacturers' demonstrations suggest that if a row of seats is placed below such an exit, its presence slows the egress of passengers forced to step on it by a possibly acceptable 10%. It may seem obvious to the reader, however, that although placing a row of seats beneath an exit may slow an orderly progress by only 10%, it may produce a dramatic increase in the probability that a member of a frightened crowd will trip and cause a catastrophic pile-up at that point.

There are, however, less obvious problems. At points where the cabin aisle passes through some form of bulkhead, is it preferable to make the aisle width as great as possible, or to limit it to that through which only one person at a time could obviously pass? Which is more likely to clog, given the press of a crowd? It is probably impossible to predict the answer to such questions, and some form of empirical approach is clearly called for. Such an approach may be possible if the distinction between the arousal state (i.e. the fear) and the motivational state (i.e. the competition) is maintained. Nobody can today contemplate frightening evacuation volunteers, but there is no reason why a suitable population of volunteers could not be motivated to compete with one another for the exits by manipulating the pay-offs they are given.

Fear

All of the above has concerned the behaviour of the group, but the fear associated with being inside a burning aircraft may act as a stressor to produce performance effects in the individual members of the group. Fear will undoubtedly heighten autonomic activity in that heart, respiration and sweat rates will all increase, but, as well as this, there is reasonably good evidence that attention will narrow so that only matters directly associated with physical escape are dealt with, and any intellectual activity—such as following the simplest instructions—will be materially impaired. Evidence for these suggestions is provided by some remarkable experiments conducted by Kan Yaki and Mitchell Berkun (reported in Watson, 1978) in which some soldiers were led to believe that they were in an aircraft that was about to crash, and others that they were inadvertently being shelled with live ordnance. These soldiers were required either to complete forms or to follow instructions to repair some equipment they believed they needed—both tasks actually being designed to measure the extent of the degradation in their performance.

There is an interesting and direct parallel between these experiments and the requirement that passengers follow simple instructions in order to don life jackets, operate oxygen masks, or open overwing exits in many aircraft. All of these acts are designed to be trivially straightforward, and they almost certainly are so on the second trial. If the first trial at, for example, door opening is considered, the naïve subject has to identify the handle, pull it in the correct direction, and then successfully manhandle the removed plug door. In one well-documented evacuation, two of these three phases of door removal went wrong. The young lady operating the door firstly misidentified the handle (believing it to be the armrest of her seat which was fixed to the door), and then proved unable to manhandle the door—probably partly because of its weight, and partly because of its awkward presentation and her lack of skill. Similar experiences have occurred with the use of oxygen masks.

The best solution to the door problem would be to provide the passenger seated next to the door with the elementary skill required to open it before departure. A dummy door in the departure lounge is all that would be required. A video of this door being opened would be the next best thing, but interestingly even the more modern safety videos now in use do not include any portrayal of how a passenger should open such doors. At the very least, the cabin crew should, before departure, call the attention of the person seated next to the door to the fact that it will be his or her responsibility to open it, indicate the handle to this person, explain how it works, and suggest how the door should be jettisoned or stowed after removal.

Carrying out any of these procedures would not only increase the probability of a passenger actually being able to remove the door but would also, by giving that particular passenger a role, increase the chance that the passenger will take prompt action. It is easy for those in the airline world, or for the regular passenger, to forget how unusual flying for the first time can be, and it has been noted above that passengers are required to act a subordinate role on aircraft. Yet in this environment the passenger must make his own decision about when to start interfering with the aircraft by opening a door and perhaps throwing it away. If the person is not explicitly provided with the role, some reluctance to adopt it may be expected.

Airlines might object to the last paragraph not just on the grounds of expense or impracticality, but because they are reluctant to give any passenger a particular responsibility for safety, feeling that it may cause unnecessary anxiety. There may be some justice in such concern, but if a fit passenger who is not showing any obvious signs of anxiety is invited to sit beside the door, then he will probably be pleased to be reassured that it will be appropriate for him to take action when required, and he will probably also interpret his selection as a status-enhancing rather than anxiety-provoking event.

In summary, then, it has been suggested that in an emergency evacuation we must expect passengers to be frightened, and that this fear will tend to produce both a degradation of performance in the individual and a breakdown in social order such that passengers will compete, rather than queue, for the exits. Evaluating aircraft evacuation demonstrations in a rather more realistic way, making exits more conspicuous, briefing more effectively the passengers seated next to emergency exits, and providing smoke protection hoods may all be ways of manipulating the social environment to the advantage of safety.

Hijack

The other extreme, but unlikely, form of stress to which the passengers and crew of an aircraft may be subject is hijacking. All airlines have established procedures for dealing with this problem, but one or two points are worth noting in the present context.

At the beginning of a hijack, the group structure is clear. The hijackers separate themselves from the other passengers, the passengers and flight crew form a group (though usually with the flight crew retaining a differentiated role from the passengers), and those inside the aircraft are likely to perceive a common external out-group of all those who are involved—rescue services, air traffic control, and security forces. The reason why it has traditionally been considered appropriate to maintain a gentle and unprovocative approach in such situations is because, as time passes, the hijackers will both gain a familiarity with their captives, and begin to gain an identity of purpose with them. The external out-group presents, constantly, the implicit threat that it may start violent action which could threaten the immediate safety of both groups on board the aircraft. These two groups may, consequently, begin to coalesce to some extent. The more strongly the hijackers identify with the crew and passengers aboard the aircraft, the less likely they are to harm them.

It is therefore in the interest of the passengers and crew to appear to reinforce the identity of purpose that they have with the hijackers, by indulging in such in-group activities as discussing families and other topics that are likely to establish common ground. The crew should, however, attempt to maintain a consciousness of what they are doing so that they do not themselves succumb to the technique that they are attempting to employ, and consequently fail to exploit any weakness that the hijackers may show. Unfortunately, modern hijackers are well aware of the social dangers they face and are schooled to maintain the maximum social distance between themselves and the passengers and crew.

Cultural effects

The cultural group to which flight crews belong probably has two main influences on their job. The first concerns the fact that both airlines and air forces have requirements of their employees that run counter to cultural norms. For example, the long-haul pilot or cabin-crew member may spend half of his time away from home and is consequently unable to fulfil the culturally accepted roles of husband and father. His wife must be capable of undertaking those everyday tasks that are normally carried out by the male member of the household. Male pilots and stewards frequently remark that they feel not to be required at home because their wives are compelled to know how to get the car or plumbing repaired. A review of the domestic and social stress to which pilots are exposed is provided by Sloan and Cooper (1986).

Military pilots may also find their lifestyle to be at variance with cultural norms. This probably mattered less during, say, the early post-war period than it does today, for the military pilot used to live a life with his family that was effectively cut off from the rest of society. He was likely to live on or near his flying station, his wife was unlikely to work, and his friends and social life were also likely to be exclusively service orientated. Today, however, financial pressures compel the pilot to buy his own house, his wife is likely to have her own career, and they will have civilian friends and neighbours. It requires an understanding wife to be consistently reasonable when her husband is sent on detachment at short notice or when she has to leave her job and find another at two yearly intervals on her husband's postings.

The cultural problems noted above are, perhaps, peculiar to the United Kingdom, or at least to a Western country, but there is a second type of cultural problem in aviation. This is that aircraft and flying procedures are designed, in large part, by industrialized Western societies but must be operated across many cultures. Assumptions that are made without question during the design may not be valid when the aircraft is operated in a different cultural context. For example, it is implicit in the operating procedures of all commercial aircraft that the first officer acts as a check on the behaviour of the captain. It has already been seen that in Western cultures it can be difficult for the first officer to act in this way, but in some Eastern cultures, in which the norm is to afford high levels of respect to age and status, the problem could clearly be exacerbated.

Social psychology is unquestionably less definitive than other areas of psychological endeavour, and this is likely to remain so. As the more transigent problems of aviation human factors are resolved, however, the importance of social problems will probably increase, and this is an area whose importance may confidently be predicted to grow.

References

ASCH, S. (1955) Opinions and social pressure. *Scientific American*, **193**, 31–35

BROWN, R. (1955) *Social Psychology*. Toronto: The Free Press

FESTINGER, L. (1957) *A Theory of Cognitive Dissonance*. Stanford: Stanford University Press

FIEDLER, F.E. (1971) Validation and extension of the contingency model of leadership effectiveness: a review of empirical findings. *Psychological Bulletin*, **76**, 128–148

MILGRAM, S. (1974) *Obedience to Authority*. London: Tavistock

MINTZ, A. (1951) Non-adaptive group behaviour. *Journal of Abnormal and Social Psychology*, **46**, 150–159

SHAW, M.E. (1971) *Group Dynamics: The Psychology of Small Group Behaviour*. New York: McGraw-Hill

SLOAN, S. and COOPER, C. (1986) *Pilots Under Stress*. London: Routledge and Kegan Paul

WATSON, P. (1978) *War on the Mind*. London: Hutchinson

WHEALE, J. (1983) Crew co-ordination on the flight deck of commercial transport aircraft. In *Flight Operations Symposium*, edited by N. Johnson. Dublin: Irish Air Line Pilots Association/Aer Lingus

Further reading

PENNINGTON, D.C. (1986) *Essential Social Psychology*. London: Edward Arnold

Part VI

Special Types of Flight

Medical aspects of special types of flight

R.M. Harding

with contributions by J.C.D. Turner and M. Bagshaw

Introduction

This chapter is concerned with the medical aspects of some of the less common, but no less important and perhaps more glamorous, forms of manned flight. Historically, the development of the helicopter is considerably more ancient than that of its fixed-wing counterpart. But, despite this venerability and its present-day ubiquity, the helicopter has remained until recently the Cinderella of the aviation medicine world: it is therefore entirely appropriate that the first section of the chapter should deal with the particular problems of helicopter aircrew. Since the late 1950s, however, helicopters have not been the only machines capable of taking off or landing vertically and, although commercial VTOL aircraft have not yet proved themselves, the outstanding combat success of the Royal Air Force Harrier and the Royal Navy Sea Harrier has assured that military V/STOL jet aircraft are here to stay; the second section addresses some of the problems peculiar to that operating environment. The 1960s saw a revolution in two further forms of manned flight: the first was the introduction of commercial supersonic transport (SST) aircraft, and this forms the subject of the third section; whilst the success of the manned spaceflight programmes brought to fruition the dreams of centuries and is the subject of the fourth and final section.

Helicopters

J.C.D. Turner

The helicopter is now an indispensable military tool. It has also earned the respect of the public as a form of aerial transport that is both practical and efficient in those areas, such as the North Sea, where conventional means of air transport cannot be used. However, despite the helicopter's frequent appearance in the media as a life-saving vehicle, following either an accident or a natural disaster, the stigmata of unreliability, expense and environmental pollution have not yet been completely removed. Furthermore, both civil and military budgets continue to favour fixed-wing development in preference to rotary wing, and this attitude, not surprisingly, is also reflected in the proportion of effort expended on the aviation medicine aspects of rotary wing flight.

There are few, if any, aspects of aviation medicine which are unique to this form of flight; usually there is just a shift in emphasis, and so a distillation of fixed-wing solutions to any problem has often been considered sufficient. This decade, however, has seen the development of a large number of airborne systems where rotary wing applications have led the field—e.g. night vision goggles—and this has resulted in a greater willingness to instigate dedicated rotary wing research effort.

The aviation medicine aspects of helicopter operations which are of particular concern include comfort and fatigue, thermal stress, crashworthiness and survivability, vibration, noise and disorientation.

Comfort and fatigue

The present generation of helicopters is easily capable of a 10-hour flying day: that is equivalent to an intercontinental jet transport flight in duration but very different in profile. These helicopter sorties almost always contain a large number of short legs, each often terminating in a difficult approach to an unprepared or exposed landing area such as an oil exploration rig. In such operational circumstances the comfort of the crew and passengers is of paramount importance.

The standard of crew seating is improving, but the prevalence and incidence of occupational back disorders in helicopter crews remains high; in the region of 70%. The size, contour and adjustment of the seat pan and seat back have all been optimized in many helicopter types, along with the provision in many civil variants of foldaway armrests. Many military aircrew have found the use of an individually moulded lumbar support beneficial in alleviating their symptoms. Nevertheless discomfort is still reported and most commonly attributed to the posture enforced by the control geometry of the helicopter, which predominantly requires 'hands on flying' (despite improvements to automatic flight control systems), and the harmonization of both cyclic and collective flying controls through a large range of movement. Even when provided with a wide range of seat adjustment in fore and aft travel, height and yaw pedal position, the pilot often has to adopt a hunched posture with loss of lumbar lordosis and a tendency to a scoliosis of the spine towards the collective. The resultant discomfort is aggravated by cockpit environmental factors and the need to wear immersion protective clothing and a life-preserver or, in the case of some military pilots, a load carrying jerkin with associated body armour.

A significant improvement in helicopter aircrew comfort is unlikely to occur until there is a radical departure in control geometry and design philosophy. The technology for seat-mounted, side-stick flying controls, which enable aircrew to adopt a considerably more comfortable posture, is available but the commercial incentive is not. In addition, the aviation regulatory bodies do not, as yet, have the experience to ensure the straightforward provision of a certificate of airworthiness for a helicopter fitted with side-arm controls.

To ensure maximum comfort, helicopter crew seats should have a good range of adjustment, sufficient for the desired anthropometric range of aircrew (including female); lumbar support adjustable both in thickness and in height; a seat back which can be raked through at least 10°, but ideally 15°; stowable arm-rests; and a rigid, contoured sitting platform with an adequate (but incompressible on impact) cushion covered in a durable material.

Passenger/troop seats in helicopters are rarely more than a tubular frame construction and are usually extremely uncomfortable. This form of seating is attributable to the requirement for it to be removed or stowed easily so that freight can be carried instead of passengers and also to the very limited amount of weight that a helicopter can carry.

Fatigue in helicopter crews remains a serious concern as improvements in endurance, reliability and capability result in longer sorties of an increasingly more complex nature; compounded in some military scenarios by a frequent requirement for single pilot operation. In these situations the aircrew will have to be considerably more dependent on automatic flight control systems to reduce the workload to acceptable levels and leave the major share of the tactical management to the mission specialist whether he be observer, navigator or air gunner.

Thermal stress

Even in Europe a helicopter may have to operate in ambient temperatures ranging from −30°C to +35°C. In the near future, it is unlikely that helicopter cabin conditioning systems will achieve a level of sophistication and performance that will prevent thermal stress in military helicopter crews or do more than ameliorate it in their civilian colleagues. Conditioning systems require considerable power if they are to be efficient and are relatively heavy so reducing the helicopter's payload. Their effectiveness is further reduced by the profile of helicopter transport operations which involves frequent opening of the cabin doors to emplane and deplane troops or passengers. Furthermore, during transport of troops in the Arctic the use of any form of cabin heating is forbidden because 'warming up' the troops results in perspiration and damp clothing, which can predipose to cold injury. Electrically heated gloves and socks are issued to aircrew who have to operate in such environments but, because of their bulky and cumbersome nature, they have never been popular.

Studies of pilot aircrew wearing immersion protection whilst operating in temperate climates revealed subjective signs of discomfort but did not demonstrate any definite evidence of physiological heat stress. However, it has been shown that helicopter aircrewmen, who have a high physical workload associated with their flying task, would be at risk from heat stress if required to wear the additional clothing for protection against biological and chemical warfare agents.

An effective personal conditioning system (*see* Chapter 18) for helicopter aircrew has yet to be demonstrated in an operational environment, but remains the most practical solution to the problem of thermal stress in helicopter aircrew.

Crashworthiness and survivability

Analysis of helicopter accident statistics during the 1950s and 1960s reveals a disastrous level of mortality and morbidity following impact forces *within* the levels of human tolerance. The incidence of helicopter accidents due to mechanical failure has reduced but will inevitably continue as there are still features of helicopter design where duplication of vital components or the provision of alternative loadpaths has not been achieved; hence failures can have catastrophic results. Accidents caused by human factors remain prevalent and may increase in incidence as the helicopter is required to operate at higher speed, at lower level and in poorer weather by both day and night. Some improvement is evident from analysis of British military helicopter accident statistics for the 1970s and early 1980s. There is nevertheless still a considerable amount of progress required. Similar shortcomings have been identified in civilian helicopters by a Helicopter Airworthiness Review Panel of the Airworthiness Requirements Board.

For most operational scenarios, assisted crew escape (although technically feasible) is not economically viable because of system complexity and the consequent weight penalty. Parachute escape following manual bale out is worthwhile in those missions, such as Airborne Early Warning and passive Anti-Submarine Warfare, where the helicopter frequently operates at altitudes greater than 2000 feet.

For the majority of helicopter accidents the survival of the crew and passengers will depend on good crashworthy design. The features of such design are well documented in the United States Army Crash Survival Design Guide and acknowledged in the UK Defence Standard 00-970, Aircraft Design, as being the ideal.

These design features can be summarized as follows:

1. The cabin and crew compartment should be sufficiently rigid to ensure the maintenance of the container space following impact and to resist intrusion from external structures and rotor blades.
2. The aircraft occupants must be well restrained, ideally by a five-point harness. The penalties of inadequate restraint have been known for many years. Even a four-point harness has unacceptable deficiencies. Torso movement on impact results in tension on the shoulder harness, which causes the quick-release fitting to rise up into the abdomen and is frequently followed by the occupant 'submarining' out of the harness under the lap straps. The quick-release fitting should be of a design that prevents inadvertent release due to rotation or inertial forces following contact with objects such as the cyclic control during the crash sequence. Helicopter loadmasters/ aircrewmen present a particularly difficult problem as their duties require mobility around the aircraft cabin. At present, the designs of despatcher harness provide limited protection against falling out of the helicopter, but do not provide any impact restraint whatsoever.
3. Sharp projections within the cockpit and cabin should be minimized and ample stowages and tie-down points for loose articles provided. Conflicts in design are bound to occur (for example, with sighting systems) and careful consideration must be given to the stowage and rigidity of such items during impact. Wherever possible, an energy absorbing material should cover all surfaces. None of the foregoing reduces the importance of helicopter occupants wearing adequate head protection; not only to survive the initial or subsequent impacts, but also to reduce the risk of even temporary incapacitation and thus enhance the occupants' chances of extracting themselves from possibly either a burning or sinking wreckage.
4. Methods whereby the energy of an impact and the change in velocity experienced by the occupants of a helicopter may be reduced during a crash are becoming more efficient. Incorporation of such technology has already shown a significant and cost effective improvement in survivability in the Sikorsky UH-60A (Black Hawk). Energy attenuation for land impacts begins with the undercarriage, which should be highly resistant to collapse, as an asymmetric failure usually results in the helicopter rolling over. The 'hull' of the fuselage structure should compress progressively and in such a manner as to discourage earth scooping and consequent somersaulting. The energy absorption mechanism of the crew seat or troop seat (e.g. invaginated tube, wire and bollard, rod and die, helical wire, crushable composite) should attenuate any remaining energy to within levels of human tolerance by 'stroking' through at least 30 cm.
5. The risk of post-crash fire must be reduced to an absolute minimum. Crash inertia switches to isolate the electrical system on impact and prevent electrical arcing; flexible, self-sealing coupling joints for the fuel system and the discharge of inert gas into the fuel tanks from either storage cylinders or on-board inert gas generation systems (OBIGS) are all effective.

Emergency exits should be as numerous as possible. The ideal is one per occupant. They must of course be of adequate size: intermediate size exits may encourage two occupants to attempt a physically impossible simultaneous egress. The exits must be easy to identify, well illuminated, jettisoned by a simple and standard action, and of a design unlikely to jam due to deformation from impact forces.

The hazards of a ditching are also considerably

reduced by incorporating in the design of the helicopter an adequate emergency flotation system which is capable of ensuring buoyancy in those sea states over which the helicopter routinely operates. An emergency flotation system also increases the likelihood of salvaging a ditched helicopter.

Vibration and noise

There has not yet been a helicopter introduced into British military service which shows a marked reduction in vibration levels over its predecessors and vibration remains a significant problem in helicopters. Although predominantly in the vertical axis (heave—a_z), helicopter vibration is typified by large linear and angular accelerations in all three orthogonal axes (shunt, a_x; sway, a_y). The multitude of moving parts in a helicopter all contribute to vibration of varying frequencies. It is the lower frequencies in the range of 1–20 Hz that have the most effect on helicopter aircrew and passengers and their dominance is a function of the 'blade passing frequency' for each particular helicopter type, e.g.:

The Sea King 1R vibration : 203 RRPM/60 = 3.38 Hz, where nR is the number of rotors and RRPM is the rotor revolutions per minute.

However, the Sea King is a five-bladed helicopter and the most significant frequency is therefore:

5R vibration : 203 RRPM × 5/60 = 16.9 Hz.

Resonant frequencies which are multiples of this, i.e. 10R, 15R etc. will all be present.

The vibration levels are usually greatest in heave, and levels of 6 m/s² rms (0.6 g) may be experienced; particularly during phases of flight such as the transition to and from the hover, in the hover, and during flight at the aircraft's maximum speed for a particular all-up weight and density altitude (V_{max}). The relationship between such levels of vibration and human performance, and attempts to quantify them by such means as the ISO Standard 2631, is complex and is dealt with in greater detail elsewhere (*see* Chapter 14).

The operational effectiveness of helicopter aircrew is impaired by vibration as a result of increased difficulty in interpreting the information required from instruments, maps, weapon-sighting systems and helmet-mounted devices, and of the reduction in the manual dexterity needed to operate controls, switches and keyboards. An increase in subjective discomfort and fatigue, as well as specific symptoms such as backache, teeth chatter, nasal itch and flutter of the facial muscles may all be caused by helicopter vibration.

Engineers now attach considerable importance to the control of helicopter vibration, both in the initial design and during in-service maintenance, because of its known detrimental effect on the operational availability and serviceability of the helicopter. Improved techniques for recording, analysing and storing a helicopter's vibration spectrum and its subsequent rectification, by such means as blade tracking, have resulted in significant reductions in vibration levels. Design features such as the so-called 'nodal beam' and 'self-tuning vibration absorbers' have helped in attenuating, absorbing and isolating the helicopter occupant from vibration but none has so far provided a complete answer.

The remarkable success of the British Experimental Blade Programme (BERP) in improving the aerodynamics of the rotor blade is usually associated with having enabled a British helicopter to regain the world speed record (Westland Helicopters Ltd. Lynx, 1986, 249.1 mph (400 kph)). However, one of its most practical consequences is a reduction in vibration imparted to the airframe. Further technological advances enabling the active control of helicopter vibration are imminent. Active Gearbox Interface Control (AGIC) uses electro-hydraulic actuators mounted at the gearbox attachment points to isolate the fuselage from the rotor forcing frequencies. Higher Harmonic Control (HHC) cancels rotor induced vibration at source by employing electronic actuators at the level of the rotor blade pitch control rods to introduce anticipatory, small amplitude, high-frequency blade pitch motions to redistribute blade air loads.

Like vibration, the ambient noise levels encountered within even the most recent types of helicopter accepted into military service have shown an undesirable increase in cockpit and cabin noise levels; a sound pressure level of 115 dB is quite common. Long-term exposure to noise is deleterious and its effects are described in detail elsewhere (*see* Chapter 24). The short-term insult results in reduced operational efficiency through distraction, interference with communication and masking of audio signals, both those designed to warn the aircrew and those of an operational nature such as sonar. A large external noise footprint is often unacceptable to the public for operations in urban areas, as well as increasing the detection and identification distance of a helicopter during military operations.

Sound-proofing material can be effective if sufficient is used but it is rarely adequate because of the concomitant weight penalty. Hitherto the only practical method of noise attenuation has been a headset or helmet. However, the ultimate efficiency of such passive protection, particularly for the lower frequencies prevalent in helicopter noise, is a function of the volume of the ear shell and is thus limited by what is practical or comfortable to wear. Technological developments such as Active

Noise Reduction (ANR), Adaptive Noise Cancelling (ANC), Voice Operated Switching (VOS), in conjunction with continued improvements to noise cancelling microphones (*see* Chapter 24) can, however, do much to improve the quality of communication in helicopters.

Disorientation

Illusory sensations of aircraft motion and attitude experienced by helicopter aircrew are similar to those reported by pilots of fixed-wing aircraft with 'the leans' being the most commonly reported phenomenon (*see* Chapter 21). The inherent lack of aerodynamic stability of the helicopter, its propensity for cross-controlled, out-of-balance flight and its ability to accelerate in all three orthogonal axes predispose to disorientation in its crew. These features also complicate any recovery action initiated by the pilot, which has to be prompt to be successful as the helicopter most commonly operates at low level.

In order to maintain a safe hover, in manual control, a helicopter pilot has to have adequate visual cues. Denial of these cues at night, in cloud, fog, mist, recirculating snow, sand, dust or smoke rapidly leads to disorientation unless a transition to forward flight on instruments is made or an automatic flight control system with an automatic hover capability (usually Doppler) is selected.

Illusory sensations of movement can be induced when hovering over water due to the outward motion of the waves caused by the rotor downdraught or by the downward movement imparted to any spray (or snow) drawn through the rotor disc.

Blade flicker from sunlight through the disc or at night from the reflection of the anti-collision beacon is most usually only a distraction although vertigo can occur. The frequency of blade flicker is, for many helicopter types, within the range that can induce an epileptiform attack, but fortunately this is extremely rare as potential aircrew are screened for susceptibility to this condition.

The accident rate for Army Air Corps helicopters where disorientation was a contributing factor has remained constant over the period 1965 to 1981 at 0.2 per 10 000 flying hours. The United States Army reported in 1987 an upward trend for accidents to helicopters where the aircrew were using night vision devices such as night vision goggles. The most frequently cited reason for these accidents was 'lack of contrast and visual cues' and 'that the 40° field of view of night vision goggles tends to promote disorientation'. The full significance of this trend is yet to be established. The effectiveness of devices, such as the Malcolm horizon which provide orientation information to the pilot's peripheral vision to reduce disorientation, is still under investigation.

The future

Experimental prototypes of novel and weird forms of rotary wing flying machines are not recent phenomena but the progress made during the last 15 years in the strength of new light-weight materials is extraordinary. It is this fact which has largely resulted in the apparent success of the present generation of prototype rotary wing aircraft. This generation includes the tilt rotor and the contra-rotating rotors of the advancing blade concept helicopter. Perhaps the most adventurous of all is the 'X' wing which will combine the versatility of rotor-borne low-speed flight with the efficiency of fixed-wing high-speed flight. These aircraft, and the systems they will carry, will mean that no aspect of aviation medicine will be irrelevant to rotary wing flight.

Vertical/short take-off and landing (V/STOL) aircraft

M. Bagshaw

Vertical take-off and landing (VTOL) is defined as the ability of an aircraft to take off and land vertically, and to transfer to or from forward motion at heights required to clear surrounding obstacles. Short take-off and landing (STOL) is the ability of an aircraft to clear a 50 foot (15 m) obstacle within 1500 feet (460 m) of commencing take-off or, on landing, to stop within 1500 feet after passing over a 50 foot obstacle. The capability of an aircraft to meet both VTOL and STOL requirements is defined as V/STOL.

To be able to carry passengers and freight to and from city centres, without the need for long and expensive runways, and to operate military aircraft away from vulnerable airfields or battle-damaged runways, has been an aspiration of fixed-wing aircraft designers for several decades. Today, both the civil and the military flying worlds are enjoying various aspects of V/STOL technology.

Commercial V/STOL aircraft

The first potentially viable commercial V/STOL aircraft was the Fairey Rotodyne, an aircraft with turbo-prop engines for forward propulsion and a large single rotor for vertical operation, capable of carrying up to seventy passengers in the production version which first flew in 1957. Successful development continued until 1962 when the project was abandoned on the grounds of high operating costs and excessive noise. The high power-to-weight ratio and large thrust requirements needed to lift a heavy payload inevitably generated much noise which was, and remains, unacceptable in an urban environment. Since the early 1960s, the development of efficient wing design, together with improvements in powerplant and propeller technology, has led to the evolution of quiet and economic STOL passenger-carrying aircraft such as the Buffalo and Dash-7 aircraft produced by the de Havilland Company of Canada. Fixed-wing VTOL aircraft for civilian commercial use are, however, unlikely to be developed in the foreseeable future.

Military V/STOL aircraft

The constraints of noise are less important in the case of military aircraft, and the world's first operational V/STOL fighter aircraft, the Hawker Siddeley Harrier, entered service with the Royal Air Force in 1969. The concept of a high-bypass-ratio, turbo-fan engine with ducted vectored thrust has proved highly successful, and variants of the Harrier are now in service with a number of Western air forces and navies. The Soviet Forger V/STOL aircraft utilizes small vertical lift engines in addition to the main propulsion unit; a concept which appears to be less successful than ducted vectored thrust.

In addition to the aeromedical problems associated with any high-performance military jet aircraft, and described in earlier chapters, there is a number of topics particularly associated with operation in the V/STOL mode. These topics include the requirement for an escape system which will allow abandonment both at high speed and high altitude, and at low level, especially when in vertical flight where engine failure is followed by a catastrophic rate of descent (high sink rate). Other areas of concern are those associated with vision in the VTOL mode, noise and communication, and the human factors and ergonomic aspects of cockpit and control system design. And, although not unique to V/STOL operations, the problems of aircrew and groundcrew fatigue take on another dimension when associated with the practicalities (such as facilities for rest, feeding and sanitation) of working in and from relatively unprepared landing sites in the forward edge of the battle area.

Escape systems

The requirement for a rapidly responding automatic escape system which will provide protection against hypoxia and extreme cold at high altitude and against windblast at high speed, and which will place the aircrewman within the envelope for successful parachute deployment, descent and landing is common to all high-performance combat aircraft. The additional problems of escape from V/STOL aircraft occur during the hover, and transition between the hover and forward flight, when there is little or no forward component of thrust available to assist the establishment of seat trajectory on ejection. The ejection seat must also be capable of overcoming the subtractive components of the high sink rate which rapidly develops in the event of an engine failure or loss of control when in the hover. These requirements are met by the use of an ejection seat employing an especially powerful gun (typically 24.5 m/s (80 ft/s)) and with a rocket motor designed to sustain acceleration away from the stricken aircraft, and which enable successful abandonment to take place at all but the extremes of the V/STOL aircraft flight envelope (*see* Chapter 15).

Visual problems

The successful landing of any aircraft is dependent upon the presence of good external reference and visual cues. In the case of a conventional landing, judgement of the final stages is based partly on a combination of the streaming effect seen in the peripheral vision and the change in the perceived subtended angle at the far end of the runway. During a vertical landing, although the apparent change in the angle subtended at a distance remains important, the streaming cues are replaced by changes in parallax between ground objects seen peripherally and it is necessary for the visual gaze to be shifted continually between a distant reference point, the ground area immediately ahead of the aircraft, and the aircraft instruments. Since a V/STOL aircraft is operating at the limits of its technical performance when in the hover, reference to attitude and engine performance instruments during the later stages of the landing is more important than is the case during a conventional landing. This task is usually eased by the provision of a head-up display (HUD) which allows external visual reference to be maintained while monitoring essential instruments. Another difficulty in V/STOL landing is sometimes encountered when operating onto semi-prepared or unprepared landing sites, or onto a wet runway, when the downward jet efflux creates a cloud of dust or spray which further compromises vision. This problem can be helped by adopting the technique of a rolling vertical landing, whereby the aircraft is allowed to land with some forward motion so that the pilot is kept ahead of the dust or spray.

Noise and communication

The high thrust-to-weight ratio necessary for V/STOL operation gives rise to high levels of engine noise, levels which are exacerbated by the downward vectoring of the jet efflux and its subsequent reflection from the ground. This noise is apparent in the cockpit but is even more of a problem for groundcrew operating in the confines of a forward site in close proximity to the aircraft. Carefully designed and compatible communication systems and well-fitted protective helmets or ear defenders are therefore essential for aircrew and groundcrew.

Cockpit ergonomics

During the preliminary design phase of the P1127 Kestrel, forerunner to the Harrier, it was planned to provide cockpit controls similar to those of a helicopter, with the equivalents of cyclic and collective levers. It was soon appreciated, however, that a military V/STOL aircraft is simply a fast jet with a V/STOL capability and the cockpit was then designed conventionally with the addition of a single lever to control the position of the jet efflux nozzles.

When learning to operate a V/STOL aircraft, a pilot first practises conventional and vertical flight as discrete accomplishments before tackling the more difficult aspects of transitions to and from these modes, short take-offs, and rolling vertical take-offs and landings. Take-off and landing in a conventional jet aircraft is achieved by moving the control column at the appropriate time; but, for V/STOL operations, take-off is accomplished by adding power or rotating the engine nozzles downward, while landing requires some reduction of power or backward rotation of the nozzles. The control column is thus almost redundant during these phases: a habitual control column movement at the wrong time may, at best, produce a poor take-off or landing but can be disastrous. Fortunately, confidence in the new and unusual operating techniques is soon gained, even in that of Viffing (vectoring in forward flight), and V/STOL handling has not proved to be as difficult as was at first predicted.

Problems of battle operations

The ability of the Harrier to operate from relatively unprepared landing sites enables it to be deployed at the forward edge of the battle area in support of land-based forces. Although of comparatively short duration, V/STOL sorties are usually at a high-generation rate with aircraft replenishment and aircrew re-briefing taking place during rapid turn-rounds, the pilot remaining in the cockpit. This high-intensity activity leads to fatigue, both for aircrew and groundcrew, particularly when wearing clothing for protection against biological and chemical warfare agents.

Finally, general medical and hygiene requirements may also be a problem when operating from tented encampments in primitive surroundings. And the toxic hazards from fuels and oils are always present although the difficulties associated with the transport and use of liquid oxygen will be alleviated by the introduction of molecular sieve oxygen concentrators for later variants of the Harrier.

Supersonic transport (SST) aircraft

Supersonic Transport (SST) Aircraft, for example the Anglo-French Concorde, cruise at altitudes of 50 000–65 000 feet, and at speeds above Mach 2. During the early development of this advanced aircraft, a joint Anglo-French Aeromedical Group was established to consider the potential problems presented by such extremes of operation. Clearly, the most important of these is related to the high cruising altitude: not only is control of cabin pressurization of vital importance, but so too is the influence of ionizing radiation and ozone. In addition, unusual heat loads are imposed by frictional skin heating at high indicated air speeds, while the noise created by supersonic flight is probably the most publicized problem.

Cabin pressurization and oxygen equipment

Concorde typically cruises at about 60 000 feet with its cabin pressurized to 5000–6000 feet (that is with a cabin differential of about $11 \, \text{lb/in}^2$ (75.8 kPa)). Significant loss of cabin pressurization will clearly place the occupants at considerable risk. An early decision taken during the design phase of the aircraft was therefore that the strength and integrity of the pressure hull, and the reliability of the cabin pressurization system, should be such as to ensure that a serious loss of cabin pressure would be a very remote possibility. Furthermore, it was decided that, should a decompression occur, then the final cabin altitude should at no time exceed a level at which the aircraft occupants could be protected by oxygen equipment such as provided in conventional subsonic passenger aircraft.

Accordingly, Concorde specifications are such that the cabin altitude shall not exceed 15 000 feet after a reasonably probable failure (1 in 10^3 to 1 in 10^5 flying hours), shall not exceed 25 000 feet after a remote failure (1 in 10^5 to 1 in 10^7 flying hours), and will only exceed 25 000 feet after an extremely remote failure (1 in 10^7 flying hours). Studies have shown that a serious loss of cabin pressure is indeed a remote possibility, while the aircraft design offers several features to minimize the effects of a decompression. Thus multiple supplies provide a considerable reserve capacity to deliver air to the cabin, the windows are small (less than 15 cm in diameter) so limiting the size of potential defects, and there are small multiple discharge valves. It has been calculated that, following a typical emergency such as the loss of a window at 65 000 feet with descent initiated within 30 seconds, the cabin altitude will reach a maximum of only 25 000 feet in about 3 minutes.

If decompression does occur, Concorde passengers and cabin staff are protected by conventional drop-down oxygen masks which are deployed automatically when the cabin altitude exceeds 14 000 feet. Additionally, the usual provisions for therapeutic and walk-around oxygen supplies are made. The flight-deck crew, however, require a more sophisticated system so that emergency situations can be recognized and analysed, and descent procedures carried out with minimum delay. To this end, a pressure demand oxygen mask and regulator assembly is provided which can be donned using one hand within 5 seconds. On removal of the mask from its stowage, oxygen delivery is initiated. The head harness is inflated into a rigid loop which can then easily be placed over the head. Release of levers on the mask then deflate the harness and draw the mask firmly onto the face. The system is capable of providing up to 30 mm Hg positive pressure breathing.

Ionizing radiation

In addition to the natural radiation derived from terrestrial sources, the Earth is continually bombarded by ionizing radiations from beyond our planet: so-called cosmic radiation, of which there are two main types.

Galactic cosmic radiation originates from outside the solar system and produces a steady (background), reasonably predictable, low-intensity flux of high-energy particles. This radiation is attenuated by the influence of the Earth's magnetic field which deflects the charged particles, and by absorption in the upper atmosphere. The magnetic field effect is clearly most evident at the equator and declines to virtually zero at the poles, while the effect of atmospheric reduction becomes less as altitude increases. Thus background radiation increases with latitude and altitude. At Concorde's cruising altitude the intensity of galactic radiation (6 milli-Sieverts (mSv)/h (0.6 mrems/h) at 45° latitude) is no more than about twice that encountered at the cruising altitudes of subsonic aircraft. Since flight times in the latter are approximately twice those of

Concorde, the total dose for a passenger is about the same in the two cases.

In the United Kingdom and France, the maximum permitted dose for radiation workers is that recommended by the International Commission on Radiological Protection: 50 mSv/year (5 rems/year). For members of the public the figure is 5 mSv/year (0.5 rems/year). Such a limit would permit many return trips across the North Atlantic and even the dose accumulated from this source by aircrew is unlikely to attain significant levels. For this reason, galactic cosmic radiation is not specifically monitored on board Concorde. On the other hand, solar cosmic radiation, the second type of importance, is potentially very dangerous. Solar radiation consists of low-energy particles but is occasionally produced with such high intensity that its rays can penetrate the upper layers of the atmosphere and reach Concorde's cruising altitude. A typical large Solar flare may produce a dose rate of over 1.0 mSv/h (100 mrems/h) at high latitudes. Since such flares are not easily predicted and the radiation therefrom is virtually unshieldable without massive and uneconomic structural penalties, Concorde is equipped with an in-flight radiation dosimeter mounted in the forward passenger cabin. This device provides a continuous display of the radiation dose rate. A preliminary warning is given to the crew if the rate exceeds 0.1 mSv/h (10 mrems/h) (the chances of this happening on a typical flight have been estimated at 10 000:1 shortening to 1000:1 in a year of high Solar activity), while a second warning is given when 0.5 mSv/h (50 mrems/h) is exceeded. A precautionary descent to a safer altitude would be the usual response to such an alert; but none such has yet been encountered during Concorde operations. A useful secondary function of the dosimeter is that it provides a measure of cumulative dose to the airframe, and so to the aircrew.

Ozone

As described in Chapter 1, atmospheric ozone (O_3) is formed in increasing amounts above 40 000 feet by the action of ultraviolet radiation on oxygen. It is a strong oxidizing agent and is toxic to man; its principal clinical effects being exerted on the respiratory system. Such effects depend upon the partial pressure of ozone and, in the concentration found at 50 000–60 000 feet (that is, perhaps as high as 4 parts per million by volume (ppmv)), ozone would produce respiratory distress within minutes when the air containing it was compressed to a cabin altitude of 5000 feet. The solution to this problem for the occupants of Concorde resides in the thermo-instability of ozone: dissociation and transformation to molecular oxygen is complete if it is exposed to 400°C for just 0.5 s. This happens to be the temperature to which gas in the air conditioning compressor circuit is brought during the climb and cruise phases of a Concorde flight. During descent, however, the compressor temperature falls to 300°C where dissociation is only 90% complete. Levels of 0.25 ppmv can be attained for as long as the aircraft remains at critical altitudes (normally about 3 minutes). It should be noted that, although for industrial ground-based workers a maximum allowable concentration has been set at 0.1 ppmv for a 5-day working week of 40 hours, such a regulation is clearly inappropriate for flight personnel, the population most at risk, who are only permitted a certain number of hours each month. Furthermore, ozone concentrations of 1.0 ppmv have been recorded in subsonic commerical aircraft flying at 40 000 feet without any evidence of distress in passengers or crew, and without there being any question of a need to take regulatory action.

Kinetic heating

At Mach 2, frictional skin heating of the external surfaces of Concorde can produce temperatures of 150°C. Clearly, it is of importance to ensure that unacceptable increases in temperature are not transmitted to the occupants of the cabin. As with many of its other components, the environmental control system of Concorde has considerable redundancy. Four separate units treat incoming air from the engines by passing it through a heat exchanger and compressing it in a cold air unit before delivering it to a second heat exchanger and then, somewhat unusually, to a countercurrent heat exchange cycle with its own (cold) fuel. The conditioned air is mixed with warm air if necessary before passing through a temperature control valve and a water separation unit. It is then passed between the double skin of the cabin wall before finally reaching the distribution outlets. The cabin conditioning system can maintain an internal temperature of 24°C (range 22–27°C) with all four compressors operating, while a temperature of 29°C can be maintained if one compressor fails. Even with a total system failure, cabin temperature would be unlikely to exceed 35°C: an uncomfortable but acceptable level in an emergency. A humidification unit incorporated within the conditioning system maintains relative humidity at about 30% throughout flight.

Noise

Although aerodynamically generated sound energy is a potential problem at supersonic speeds, the noise levels within the cabin of Concorde are similar to those of conventional subsonic aircraft because of the extensive use of sound insulating materials. Externally, also, sound levels during take-off and landing are similar to those produced by older subsonic aircraft such as the DC8: both generate noise levels of about 115 dB. Concorde is, however, considerably noisier than the modern generation of 'whisper' jets, such as the Airbus which has an approach noise level of just 102 dB, due largely to the use of high-bypass-ratio jet engines.

The emotive problems of sonic boom and 'super boom' have received much attention and aroused much ill feeling, but their medical consequences are poorly defined (*see* also Chapter 24). Notwithstanding this, however, Concorde does not fly supersonic over land, although a supersonic corridor was provided over the Middle East when Concorde flew to Bahrain.

Manned spacecraft

In the 27 years since Yuri Gagarin's epic flight in Vostok 1, over 200 men and women of 19 nations have spent a total of more than 6700 man-days in space. With some notable exceptions the physiological problems associated with space travel are simply extensions of those met in conventional aviation medicine. The success of the Russian and American manned spaceflight programmes provided clear evidence that the problems associated with existence in the ultimate hostile environment were not insuperable and that, apart from a few tragic exceptions, man can be sent into space and returned safely to Earth. Furthermore, the American Apollo flights demonstrated the ability to support manned activity on the surface of the moon, while many of the physiological problems associated with prolonged sojourns in space have been investigated throughout the Russian Soyuz/Salyut/Mir programme and during the American Skylab and Space Transportation System missions. This section discusses some physiological and psychological aspects of manned spaceflight with especial reference to established findings and their implications for the future. It is divided, somewhat artificially, into a consideration of the *immediate* problems which face any space traveller, followed by a consideration of those problems which confront a *prolonged* mission. The problems of principal concern may be summarized as follows:

1. *Immediate problems:*
   (a) Decreased pressure, with consequent risk of hypoxia, decompression sickness, ebullism, barotrauma, and thermal injury.
   (b) Accelerations of launch, re-entry and landing.

(c) Radiation
(d) Micrometeoroids.
(e) Nutrition, waste management, and personal hygiene.
2. *Long-term problems:*
  (a) Decreased accelerations (microgravity), with profound effects upon:
    (i) the neurovestibular system;
    (ii) the cardiovascular system;
    (iii) the musculo-skeletal system.
  (b) Behavioural aspects.

Immediate problems

Decreased pressure

The physiological consequences of an unprotected ascent to altitude have been extensively described in earlier chapters (hypoxia, decompression sickness and ebullism, barotrauma, and thermal injury in Chapters 5, 3, 2 and 16 respectively) and suffice to say that, except for their inevitable role in a very few tragic accidents, none of these risks has been a major problem for any of the 118 space missions so far flown. This is because all manned spacecraft are engineered with an Environmental Control System (ECS) capable of providing their occupants with adequate oxygen at adequate pressure in an environment at an appropriate temperature and with sufficient humidity. The environmental control system is also capable of removing carbon dioxide and other contaminants from the atmosphere.

Environmental control systems

At altitudes above about 100000 feet, cabin pressurization in the conventional manner is no longer effective since the reduced density of the air makes its compression inefficient and uneconomic. Craft destined to fly higher than this are therefore obliged to be hermetically sealed before flight either at a pressure equivalent to that at sea level or at another selected level. Thereafter, pressure within is maintained, despite losses through leaks from cabin to ambient and from oxygen consumption by the crew, by continual replenishment from stored or generated supplies.

The precise choice of atmospheric conditions is governed by both engineering and physiological considerations. The physiological ideal is clearly to provide an atmosphere at or near sea level pressure and with the gaseous composition of air. Despite the considerable engineering penalties which such a system incurs in terms of weight, bulk and complexity, all Russian spacecraft from Vostok onwards have indeed been so equipped. Although physiologically attractive for most spacecraft activities, pressurization to sea level equivalent provides

little protection against the risk of decompression sickness if the cosmonaut wishes to undertake extra-vehicular activity (EVA). Russian spacesuits are pressurized to 300 mm Hg and, since their pressure relationship is therefore close to the critical supersaturation ratio (CSR) (*see* Chapter 3), a period of up to 1 hour of pre-oxygenation with 100% oxygen at 760 mm Hg is required before venturing outside the spacecraft.

In American spacecraft before the Space Transportation System (Shuttle), a low-pressure single-gas cabin was proposed as the simplest engineering solution in terms of weight and control mechanisms (no inert gas was required and only one sensor system was needed to control both pressure and gas concentration). For Mercury, Gemini, Apollo and Skylab, an orbital pressure of 259 mm Hg was chosen with a gaseous composition of 100% oxygen. Furthermore, after adequate pre-oxygenation, the use of oxygen as the sole breathing gas eliminated the problem of decompression sickness. The disadvantages of such a system included the possible adverse long-term effects of exposure to reduced pressure (although 100% oxygen at 259 mm Hg is below any directly toxic threshold for oxygen), the reduced margin of safety in the event of loss of cabin pressurization, the additional heat load imposed on the cooling system by virtue of poor heat conduction in a low density gas, and of course the omnipresent risk of explosion and fire. Projects Mercury and Gemini were completed using just such a single gas system, but the tragic loss of the crew of Test Apollo 204 (later re-named Apollo 1 in their honour) in an oxygen-fuelled flash fire led to a redesign for later missions. In order to reduce the fire hazard during the critical launch period, a two-gas system was introduced. Thus, for all the Apollo and Skylab flights, a mixture of 36% oxygen and 64% nitrogen was used to pressurize the cabin at 760 mm Hg for launch. The pressure was reduced, again to 259 mm Hg, within a few hours of launch and nitrogen was purged from the cabin so that, by 3 days after launch, the cabin atmosphere was approximately 95% oxygen and 5% nitrogen for Apollo and 70% oxygen, 30% nitrogen for Skylab. Since the Apollo suit pressure was 191 mm Hg for these missions, the critical supersaturation ratio was not approached and no pre-oxygenation was required prior to either free space or lunar extra-vehicular activity.

The Space Transportation System is the first American spacecraft to utilize an atmosphere of sea level composition and pressure. Extra-vehicular activity from the Shuttle is therefore preceded by a period of pre-oxygenation. In order to reduce the time necessary for adequate pre-oxygenation, however, the whole pressure cabin undergoes an intermediate decompression to 527 mm Hg, the entire crew then breathes 27% oxygen for 12 hours before the two astronauts destined to leave the craft breathe 100% oxygen for 40 minutes. The Shuttle spacesuit is pressurized to a level of 222 mm Hg.

The concentration of carbon dioxide in inspired gas must be strictly controlled if serious disturbances of physiology and performance are to be avoided. Carbon dioxide control within spacecraft environments is achieved by chemical scrubbing (Russian craft), by a molecular sieve (Skylab), or by lithium hydroxide cannisters (all other American craft). An optimum mission design limit for the partial pressure of carbon dioxide both in Russian and in American spacecraft has been 3.8 mm Hg, rising to 5 mm Hg in Skylab, with a maximum limit for continuous exposure of 7.6 mm Hg. In practice, however, levels have usually been maintained near to just 1 mm Hg for long periods, although some did approach the critical value of 15 mm Hg during the ill-fated Apollo 13 mission.

Other cabin contaminants, both chemical and biological, such as those from the life support system itself, waste disposal systems, spacecraft materials and paints, and indeed crew members, must also be considered and removed. This has usually been accomplished by circulating the cabin air through activated charcoal filters. By this means even the 50 or so contaminants identified within the command module during one Apollo mission were kept at very low concentrations, but the reliability and effectiveness of such control will have especial importance when planning the long-duration missions of the future.

Other features of spacecraft environmental control systems include control of temperature and humidity. Within spacecraft and spacesuits, the principal problem of thermal control has always been that of heat dissipation from various engineering systems and from metabolism. Control, over ranges within the limits of 10–32°C, has been successfully achieved by a variety of conventional heat dissipation mechanisms including sublimation, evaporation, radiation, and liquid–air heat exchange. Likewise, control of cabin humidity has been successfully achieved by the use of sophisticated water extractors: once again, the main problem is that of water excess from metabolic production. Cabin relative humidity has been controlled over the ranges 40–70% (Russian) and 30–70% (American).

Spacesuits and portable life support systems

A spacesuit provides the means by which a space traveller can venture outside his craft either in free space or on the surface of another planet. It also provides a refuge within a spacecraft in the event of an on-board emergency. In its most simple form, a spacesuit consists of an inner rubber bladder to hold gas under pressure and an outer restraining layer which prevents ballooning and allows movement. Gas must clearly be delivered to or contained within the suit, as must other vital supplies such as a respirable atmosphere suitably cooled and humidified, and a supply of water. Waste products, both respired and excreted, must also be disposed of. Such facilities may be provided via an umbilical when the wearer remains dependent upon the mother ship. When the supporting facilities are self-contained, however, they are termed a Portable Life Support System (PLSS) and the user is entirely independent of his spacecraft: only the need for food may reasonably be omitted from such a system.

Spacesuits are thus designed and constructed in a similar way to, and have essentially the same function as, the full-pressure suits described in Chapter 7. Indeed, the Vostok cosmonauts and Mercury astronauts wore suits which were virtually identical with those of their colleagues flying high-altitude military aircraft. With later programmes came the need to venture beyond the confines of the spacecraft and so, while their basic function remained the same, several specialized features were introduced, including the extensive use of layering, the incorporation of special helmets, gloves and boots, and the evolution of sophisticated portable life support systems. For example, the layers and components of the Apollo Lunar extra-vehicular activity suit (from the skin outwards) were as follows:

1. Faecal containment system, essentially an adult nappy (diaper).
2. Liquid cooling garment (LCG), of the kind described in Chapter 18.
3. Multi-layered pressure garment assembly, comprising:
   (a) Comfort layer.
   (b) Pressure bladder.
   (c) Restraint layer.
   (d) Cover layer.
   (e) Pressure gloves and pressure helmet.
4. Multi-layered integrated thermal micrometeoroid garment, designed for thermal protection and to arrest micrometeoroid particles and comprising:
   (a) Nylon inner layer.
   (b) Five Mylar thermal layers with four Dacron spacer layers between.
   (c) Two laminate thermal layers.
   (d) Teflon abrasion layer with additional reinforcing Teflon patches.
5. Lunar extra-vehicular visor assembly, the visor itself being coated with gold to protect against solar glare and ultraviolet light penetration.
6. Layered glove shell and lunar overboots, designed to provide protection against temperature extremes.
7. Portable life support system.

A typical American portable life support system, as used for the Apollo Lunar landing missions, comprised five main systems, all housed in a back-pack and supplying the suit itself via a series of umbilicals. The primary oxygen system provided breathing gas from a gaseous store and also pressurized the suit and helmet to 191 mm Hg. Pressurization to a higher level, while physiologically more desirable, would have decreased mobility to an unacceptable degree. (Russian spacesuit technology, in this respect, appears to be more advanced since mobility is retained at a pressure of 300 mm Hg.) A ventilating system circulated and purified the oxygen by passing it through a carbon dioxide absorber, such as lithium hydroxide, and through a filter which removed trace contaminants. The gas was then cooled by a porous plate sublimator (a self-regulated heat-rejection device) and any excess water from respiration and perspiration was removed by a water separator. The third major system was a water transport loop which removed metabolic heat by circulating chilled water through the network of plastic pipes which made up the liquid cooling garment (*see* also Chapter 18). For the Lunar suit, the temperature of the cooling fluid could be controlled by the astronaut at one of three levels by means of a valve which diverted water either through or past the sublimator. Use of this system with the liquid cooling garment enabled very high metabolic rates ($278 \, kcal/m^2/h$; $1.2 \, MJ/m^2/h$) to be sustained for several hours while sweating at rates of $200 \, kcal/m^2/h$ ($840 \, kJ/m^2/h$) could be suppressed, and the average metabolic rate for all lunar activities ($130 \, kcal/m^2/h$; $550 \, kJ/m^2/h$) could be tolerated for 8 hours: the maximum duration of the portable life support system oxygen supply.

An independent and manually operated oxygen purge system provided an emergency breathing and pressurization supply for up to 40 minutes should the main supply be exhausted or in the event of loss of suit pressure. A final system provided communications and biotelemetry facilities. Two-way voice transmission was supplemented by physiological and spacesuit environmental data such as electrocardiograph, oxygen supply and suit pressures, and water inlet and outlet temperatures. Analysis of these data enabled the ground-based monitoring medical officer to derive a rough estimate of metabolic oxygen consumption and energy expenditure which, when compared with data obtained pre-flight, ensured that each astronaut was kept within the safety limits of his oxygen supply and heat removal systems.

Increased accelerations

To achieve Earth orbit, a velocity of about 8 km/s (28 800 km/h, 17 900 mph) depending upon the altitude of orbit required must be attained, while to leave the Earth's gravitational influence (Earth escape) the corresponding figures are 11.6 km/s (41 760 km/h, 25 950 mph). These velocities may be reached by any number of combinations of acceleration and time provided that their product is 828 G-seconds for Earth orbit and 1152 G-seconds for Earth escape. The magnitude of spacecraft acceleration is determined by constraints on rocket design and performance so that, in practice, a staged launch is used to achieve the final velocity required. Thus, for example, a Mercury–Atlas orbital launch comprised a two-stage acceleration profile of 6.0 G for 35 seconds followed by 6.4 G for 54 seconds with peaks of 8.0 G. Subsequent American and Russian launch profiles have been somewhat less severe with little time spent above 4.0 G even for the Apollo lunar missions. With the exception of the glide return of the Shuttle at 1.2 G, spacecraft re-entry accelerations have occasionally been considerably more severe with an average maximum G of up to 10.0 for Vostok, 8.9 for Mercury, and 5.9 for Apollo. Voskhod and Soyuz re-entry profiles have an average maximum of 4.0 G.

As described in Chapter 10, levels of acceleration such as these will have profound cardiovascular effects and be poorly tolerated unless applied transversely; that is, in the G_x axis. Consequently, body orientation during launch and re-entry has been in that axis, with the accelerative forces acting in the $+G_x$ direction. The exception is the $+G_z$ orientation of returning Shuttle crews who are exposed to just $+1.2 \, G_z$ during re-entry, although the duration of this applied force is seventeen minutes.

The final increased acceleration imparted to a returning crewman is that of landing shock. The Russian programme has consistently called for landings onto terra firma while the Americans chose water. In both cases, retardation of the capsule has been by means of parachutes deployed at an altitude of about 30 000 feet. The exceptions to this are the Shuttle with its runway return and Vostok from which the one-man crew was obliged to eject.

Radiation

Most electromagnetic radiation coming from space is either shielded by the Earth's atmospheric blanket or is deflected by its magnetic field. Spacecraft, by definition, venture beyond these protective layers and so they, and their occupants, are exposed to the full power of the electromagnetic spectrum and especially of ionizing radiations (IR).

Types of ionizing radiation

All of the forms of ionizing radiation which may affect supersonic transport aircraft and were described earlier will clearly also affect spacecraft, but do so to a much greater degree. Thus galactic radiation and, particularly, solar radiation provide a serious threat to the well-being of the space traveller. In space, however, there are two other sources of ionizing radiation. The first is trapped radiation, the energy found within the two bands of geomagnetically trapped particles which form the Van Allen belts. The inner belt lies at an altitude of 150–600 miles (241–965 km) depending upon latitude, while the outer belt begins at 4950 miles (7966 km) and may extend as high as 27 250 miles (43 853 km). Since most manned space activities now take place well below the inner belt, ionizing radiation from these sources presents no major problem, although it was of potential concern for the lunar missions and would be of concern for high Earth orbiting craft. Unfortunately, there is also a discontinuity in the Earth's magnetic field over the South Atlantic and here the high-energy particles of the inner Van Allen belt can be detected at altitudes as low as 80–160 miles (129–257 km). The implications for spacecraft such as Salyut, Mir and the Shuttle when operating in Low Earth Orbit in this region are clear and extra-vehicular activity is avoided during such passages.

The second additional type of ionizing radiation is the so-called energetic neutron. Such neutrons are probably formed within spacecraft as secondary radiation when internal components are bombarded by primary radiation from, for example, the Van Allen belts. Energetic neutrons are potentially most dangerous since they cause disruption of biological tissue when they collide with hydrogen nuclei.

Space radiation can therefore take many forms but should be regarded as a single threat; indeed it is considered by many to be the primary source of hazard for orbital and interplanetary space flight.

Biological effects of ionizing radiation

With remarkable speed, ionizing radiation disrupts all living tissue at the cellular level and devastates crucial cell components. For obvious reasons, the descriptions of the biological effects of ionizing radiation on man have largely been based upon clinical studies of acutely ill individuals and it is therefore unwise to extrapolate such findings to the healthy space traveller. Furthermore, some types of ionizing radiation experienced in space are unique to that environment. But Earth-based clinical experience does provide the best indication at present of the effects likely to be seen in space. *Table 32.1* lists the clinical effects of exposure to ionizing radiation and reflects the progressive influence radiation has on the most sensitive body tissues; that is, those that are most actively growing.

Using this sort of clinical classification, certain levels of radiation, above which astronauts and

Table 32.1 Clinical effects of acute exposure to ionizing radiation

Dose (Sv)*	Clinical effect
0.1–0.5	Minor blood changes
0.5–1.0	Vomiting and nausea for one day. Fatigue but no serious disability
1.0–2.0	Vomiting and nausea for one day. 50% reduction in circulating white blood cells within 3 days
2.0–3.5	Prolonged vomiting and nausea, loss of appetite, diarrhoea and minor bleeding within 4 days. Marked platelet (clotting) dysfunction within 6–9 days; 20% dead in 2–6 weeks
3.5–5.5	As for 2.0–3.5 exposure, but 50% dead in 30 days
5.5–7.5	All have vomiting and nausea within 4 hours. Nearly all dead within 1 week, but survivors ill for 6 months
10.0	All have vomiting and nausea within 1–2 hours. All dead within days
50.0	All incapacitated by nausea, vomiting and diarrhoea within minutes; followed by disorientation, uncoordinated movements (ataxia), shock and coma within minutes/hours. No survivors

*1 Sv = 100 rem.

cosmonauts should not be exposed, can be determined. Thus, for example, NASA has imposed a career limitation on astronauts of a cumulative long-term dose of 4.0 Sieverts (Sv) (400 rem) to the bone marrow, 6.0 Sv (600 rem) to the lens of the eye, and 12.0 Sv (1200 rem) to the skin. It is calculations of this sort which have determined that tours on board Space Station for a career astronaut will be a maximum of 90–120 days.

Radiation levels have been routinely monitored on board all Russian and American spacecraft, using passive dosimeters to assess cumulative exposure and active pocket dosimeters to assess immediate risks. Of course, both free-space and lunar extra-vehicular activities would have been avoided if there was any increase in Solar flare activity (for an astronaut to be caught outside his spacecraft during a Solar flare would have been rapidly fatal), and at no time so far have serious levels of ionizing radiation been encountered. Even on the longest Skylab mission (84 days) the cumulative dose to the skin was only 78.1 milli-Grays (mGy) (7.81 rad). Russian experience has been similar. Of course, the even longer missions planned for the future will pose a much increased risk and this is why radiation effects are regarded so seriously. So far, however, passive shielding against ionizing radiation by physical means has been effective. A limit exists, however, for the thickness of a physical barrier (a lead shield 1 m thick would be needed to provide protection in space equivalent to that of the Earth's atmosphere). And so for the future, active methods, perhaps by inducing a magnetic field around an individual spacecraft or perhaps by pharmacological means, may have to be considered.

Micrometeoroids

Micrometeoroids are the small bodies of solid matter, usually made of stone or iron, which comprise the so-called interplanetary dust. Vast quantities of such material are present throughout the galaxy: indeed over 10 000 tonnes of it survives the plunge through the atmosphere each day to fall on the Earth's surface! The particles are usually very small but may be of sufficient energy to form craters in, but not to penetrate, metal sheets. The conventional walls of spacecraft thus form an effective passive shield against impacts. Whilst undertaking extra-vehicular activity, however, those in spacesuits are at some risk, albeit low, and hence the need for suitable layers of protective material in the integrated thermal micrometeoroid garment described above.

Nutrition, waste management and personal hygiene

Food

Although the precise way in which food is presented to the space traveller has undergone considerable and necessary refinement throughout the manned spaceflight programmes, the metabolic and nutritional needs for that food were initially based upon values from Earth-bound studies of the energy cost of various activities. Confirmation of the requirements came from in-flight studies as the programmes progressed. Thus, for example, the early Soyuz cosmonauts were provided with a daily caloric intake of 2800 kcal (11.8 MJ) but this had risen to 3150 kcal (13.2 MJ) by the time of the Salyut 6 missions. Similarly, the American daily allowance has risen from 2500 kcal (10.5 MJ) to 3000 kcal (12.6 MJ) on board Skylab and the Shuttle, reflecting the intense physical activity scheduled for those flights. Female daily requirements are lower at 2700 kcal (11.3 MJ) and 2000 kcal (8.4 MJ) for Russian and American women respectively.

Early space food was provided as rather unappetizing purées and juices contained like toothpaste in soft metal tubes. Food technology has advanced considerably, however, and crews are now able to pre-select meals from a large menu of foodstuffs, both fresh and prepared in a variety of other ways such as freeze dried, thermostabilized, and rehydratable.

Finally, early fears with regard to difficulties of ingesting food in microgravity were ill-founded and incorrect: indeed, the ability to eat in space was conclusively demonstrated by Gagarin during the first manned spaceflight.

Water

For all Russian space missions, water has been carried as a potable store prepared on Earth. The recommended total daily intake for cosmonauts, as water and in food, has been about 2.5 l for the relatively benign missions within spacecraft, but double this amount if extra-vehicular activity was undertaken. Similarly, pre-loaded supplies have been sent aloft in American spacecraft but, since the introduction of electrical fuel cells as a power source and the ability to purify the water generated as a by-product in that process, pre-loaded supplies have been secondary to on-board generation. A daily consumption of about 3 l is recommended for astronauts.

Waste management

It is quite apparent that the adequate disposal of human waste products is a vital aspect of life support engineering in space. Carbon dioxide and water vapour are satisfactorily dealt with by the environmental control system, but the management of liquid and solid waste has presented considerable problems.

Russian spacecraft, from Vostok onwards, have been equipped with waste disposal ventilators, rather like vacuum cleaners, which are able to draw off urine and faeces simultaneously, and are capable of use even when a spacesuit is being worn. This level of sophistication was not achieved in the American programme until the flights of Skylab and the Shuttle. Prior to this, urine was initially collected by means of roll-on rubber cuffs and tubing for delivery either to a flexible plastic bag or to the overboard dumping system: a method which was relatively simple and effective, but regarded as unhygienic. For later missions, urine was voided into a hand-held receptacle, so removing the need for intimate contact, where it was held by a hydrophilic filter and then passed as before to the urine dump-line. Disposal of solid waste when on board the spacecraft was by means of the universally detested 'faecal mit'. This device consisted of a finger cot and plastic bag with a self-adhesive orifice which was applied to the anal area. After use, which was by no means easy within the confines of a small but public spacecraft, and took approximately 45 minutes, the bag was sealed and its contents mixed by hand with a bactericidal fluid before being stored for later analysis. Defaecation when inside a spacesuit was even more basic; and perhaps not surprisingly there is no record of the spacesuit faecal containment system, which was really an adult nappy, ever having been used.

Personal hygiene

Generally, human beings like both themselves and their surroundings to be clean and tidy; and this aspect of living in space is as important psychologically, in terms of maintenance of morale, as it is clinico-pathologically, in terms of maintenance of good health. Thus it is not surprising that the need for adequate facilities and materials for the maintenance of oral hygiene has always been recognized as vital. Similarly, the disposal of other less obvious forms of human waste such as epithelial debris, hairs and nails has been an important part of the ritual of life on board spacecraft; as has the provision of sufficient supplies of water and other skin cleansing materials.

Long-term problems

Decreased accelerations—microgravity

With the exception of very brief periods during violent and unnatural flight manoeuvres, microgravity is a phenomenon which affects man only in space. (The term microgravity is preferred to the more familiar weightlessness since the force of gravity decreases with the inverse square of the distance from the centre of the Earth. The Earth's gravitational attraction will always be present, therefore, although it's intensity may be very small, until the gravitational influence of another planetary body is entered. Thus, even in deep space, conditions of zero gravity do not exist; and the occupants of spacecraft are normally exposed to a microgravity of 1×10^{-4} to 1×10^{-5} G, rising to 1×10^{-3} G during spacecraft manoeuvres.) Although the absence of weight is implied, an appreciation of the *nature* of weight itself is helpful in understanding the full significance of the state.

Weight can be considered to be a constant for a particular body and so it is a characteristic physical property comparable with mass, geometric dimension, shape and density, etc. This only applies, however, when an object of specific mass is either resting on a supporting surface or moving at a constant velocity relative to the centre of the force of gravity. Thus man is made aware of his weight by virtue of the fact that there is a supporting or external medium (the Earth's surface) pushing back against his body with an inertial force equal to the gravitational force attracting it towards the centre of the Earth. If there is no external supporting influence, as in space, then the conceptual 'requirements' for weight are incomplete and the body is weight-less.

Once a spacecraft and its occupants are in orbit above the effective limits of the atmosphere, they are in a state of free-fall about the Earth because of the continuous accelerative force of gravity pulling towards the centre of the planet. The craft does not fall back to Earth, however, because if orbital velocity is maintained (*see* Increased Accelerations above) the resultant tangential and inertial forces exactly counterbalance the force of gravity. When this state of equilibrium is attained, the spacecraft and its crew are in microgravity.

Microgravity cannot be adequately simulated in a laboratory on the ground, although certain techniques have proved successful in providing partial models of that state. Such techniques include suspension in water at neutral buoyancy but, while this has been helpful in training in techniques of movement and equipment utilization, its use as a physiological tool is limited primarily because normo-gravitational proprioceptive function is retained. A similar criticism can be applied to prolonged bed-rest studies, and even to those involving head-down tilt which simulates microgravity well. Nevertheless, such terrestrially based experiments do provide at least some clues as to the physiological mechanisms invoked by exposure to microgravity.

The period of microgravity generated during Keplerian (parabolic) flight trajectories in large aircraft is too short (at 12–40 seconds) to provide any valuable physiological model, but again has been useful as familiarization training of personnel prior to space missions.

Thus the physiology of microgravity has relied of necessity upon spaceflight experience. Investigations were begun, initially purely in support of the operational requirements of the manned spaceflight programmes, during the Vostok, Voskhod, Mercury and Gemini missions, and continued throughout the Apollo programme. It was not until the dedicated scientific missions of Skylab, Salyut, Shuttle and Mir that detailed physiological studies could be undertaken. Even then, it must be emphasized that the total number of experiments remains small, the sample population is likewise small and highly selected, the potential benefit of any countermeasure has led to its use despite a lack of supporting evidence, and the operational constraints of a mission have always, correctly, held sway over the needs of scientists.

The physiological consequences of microgravity

The manned spaceflight programmes have conclusively demonstrated that man can work and live effectively in space for days, weeks and months despite conditions of microgravity. Not surprisingly, however, microgravity does produce considerable changes in all areas of physiology; changes that are of vital importance to the prolonged missions planned for the future since a safe return to Earth is predicated upon their successful reversal. The principal physiological effects of microgravity are

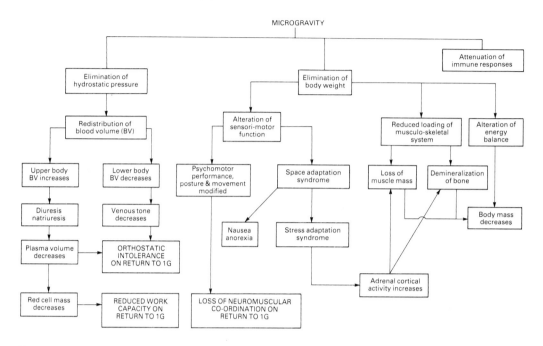

Figure 32.1 The physiological consequences of exposure to microgravity and their interrelationships.

wrought upon the neuro-vestibular system, the cardiovascular system, and the musculo-skeletal system (*Figure 32.1*).

The neuro-vestibular system

Space Motion Sickness is part of the so-called Space Adaptation Syndrome and is the most important vestibular consequence of spaceflight, affecting as it does over 45% of crew members in the current generation of large spacecraft. Cosmonaut Titov, the second Russian in space, was the first to report symptoms during his flight in Vostok 2, but American astronauts were unaffected until the Apollo programme because the ability to make body movements in the Mercury and Gemini capsules was limited. The aetiology, prediction, presentation, and management (prevention and treatment) of space motion sickness are described in Chapter 22. Similarly, the associated in-flight illusions of orientation, and the bizarre post-flight phenomena described by some returning astronauts, are described in Chapter 21.

The cardiovascular system

Microgravity neutralizes the hydrostatic pressure gradients within the circulation and the consequent uniformity of venous pressures, particularly, causes a headward shift of fluid which is complete within 24–48 hours. The magnitude of this cephalad shift may be as much as 2 litres in volume and manifests itself subjectively as persistent sensations of nasal stuffiness and feelings of fullness in the head. The veins of the head are visibly distended and remain so throughout flight.

The expansion of central fluid volume, with consequent distension of the left atrium and suppression of arginine vasopressin secretion, may be expected to stimulate a diuresis via the Gauer–Henry reflex. All cosmonauts and astronauts have indeed lost weight during spaceflight and the early phase of this weight loss has been attributed partially to a diuresis but mainly to suppression of thirst. When compared with pre-flight values, each Skylab astronaut excreted about 400 ml less urine daily over the first six days of flight, and drank an average of 700 ml less each day. Measurements of body mass, using a spring mass oscillator, on board Skylab reflected this fluid imbalance as a rapid loss in mass of 1–2 kg within 3 or 4 days followed by a steady but slower fall during the rest of the flight due to loss of muscle and fat: the results of atrophy (*see* below) and less than optimal caloric intake respectively.

The most important consequence of fluid redistribution is the development of orthostatic intolerance when blood pools in the legs on return to the 1G environment of Earth. Pre-syncopal symptoms are experienced and there is a reduction in exercise tolerance for several hours post-flight. The development and extent of orthostatic intolerance can be assessed by exposure to lower body negative pressure (LBNP). Such exposure results in a fall in systolic pressure, a narrowing of pulse pressure and an increase in heart rate; responses which were found to be exaggerated in returning Apollo astronauts. The large size of Skylab allowed in-flight lower body negative pressure measurements to be made for the first time, and these showed that, while intolerance improved slightly after 50 days in space, the test remained more stressful than before flight. Similar findings have been reported after the longer Russian missions and suggest that the orthostatic response to the challenge of lower body negative pressure, whilst still exaggerated, does not progress after 2–3 months in space. No countermeasures so far adopted by either the Russians or the Americans, including the use of G trousers inflated before re-entry to reduce peripheral pooling, and saline ingestion, have been entirely successful, and so the production of artificial gravity may be the only definitive solution to cardiovascular deconditioning in microgravity.

The musculo-skeletal system

Artificial gravity is also likely to be the only solution to the profound problems of muscular atrophy and bone demineralization seen as a consequence of prolonged exposure to microgravity.

Microgravity reduces the muscular effort required both for physical activities and for maintenance of posture. Thus, it is not surprising that there is atrophy of anti-gravity muscle groups, primarily in the legs but also in the buttocks and trunk. The arm muscles are least affected presumably because everyday tasks in space require the use of the arms considerably more than they do the legs. In confirmation of this, tests of limb strength have revealed that loss of strength in the arms is less than that in the legs. As would be expected, the atrophy is accompanied by increased urinary nitrogen and phosphorus excretion. Extensive and intensive exercise regimens have been shown to reduce the degree of atrophy, and such activity is now a mandatory part of life on board spacecraft. Nevertheless, skeletal muscle atrophy leads to a prolonged reduction in post-flight physical work capacity. Of recent concern, also, is the finding from animal studies on a Spacelab mission that cardiac muscle may also atrophy, although evidence from Skylab had suggested that there was no appreciable degradation of cardiac function despite reductions in ventricular end-diastolic volume, stroke volume, and left ventricular mass. Bone demineralization, similar to that seen in osteoporosis of the terrestrial elderly, undoubtedly represents the most serious consequence for man of exposure to microgravity.

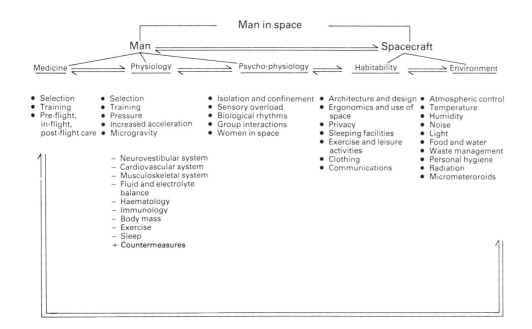

Figure 32.2 Space: interrelationships between man, his environment and his spacecraft.

There is an inexorable regional loss of bone, with greater losses from the trabecular form than from cortical.

The loss is reflected in a negative calcium balance which, in Skylab, was characterized by increased urinary and faecal losses in all nine crew members. Although similar states of hypercalciuria are seen in bed-rest and immobilization studies, the precise mechanisms operating during spaceflight are as yet unclear. It is vital that the condition is elucidated, and prophylaxis or treatment defined, so that future long-duration missions and subsequent return to Earth may be safely undertaken.

Figure 32.1 summarizes these physiological changes and suggests ways in which they, and others not discussed in detail, might interrelate.

Behavioural aspects of manned spaceflight

Until the advent of the Shuttle with its crews of pilot astronauts, mission specialists and payload specialists, manned spaceflight had been the almost exclusive preserve of military and civilian test pilots. The crews of early spacecraft were highly selected, highly motivated and highly trained individuals for whom spaceflight alone was the goal. With the inevitable progress of the manned spaceflight programmes, it is quite clear that the crews of future spacecraft will comprise individuals from disparate backgrounds and disciplines, with varying motivating drives, of different ethnic origins, and of both sexes. It is equally inevitable, therefore, that greater attention must be paid to the psycho-physiological or behavioural aspects of spaceflight. Furthermore, as flights become longer, both in duration and distance travelled away from Earth, the problems of spacecraft habitability will require further study and resolution. No longer will it be acceptable to consider manned spaceflight as a challenge to pure aeronautical engineering.

Figure 32.2 summarizes the interrelationships between man, his environment and his spacecraft including various psycho-physiological factors involved in present and future manned spaceflight, many of which have not been discussed in detail here.

Further reading

Helicopters

AGARD LECTURE SERIES NO 134 (1984) *Aeromedical Support in Military Helicopter Operations*. Neuilly sur Seine: AGARD/NATO.
ALLAN, J.R. and WARD, F.R.C. (1986) *Emergency Exits for Underwater Escape From Rotorcraft;* RAF IAM AEG Report No 528. London: Ministry of Defence.

BORRETT, W.G. (1977) *The Noise Discriminating Properties of Some First Order Pressure Differential Microphones:* RSRE Christchurch Test Report No 77/T4/2. London: Ministry of Defence.
BRAITHWAITE, M.G. (1985) Disorientation in army helicopter operations: a review. *Journal of the Royal Society of Medicine,* **78**, 856–859.
DESJARDINS, S.P., LAANANEN, D.H. and SINGLEY, G.T. (1980) *Aircraft Crash Survival Design Guide,* USARTL-TR-79-22A, Volumes I–V.
HARDING, R.M. and MILLS, F.J. (1983) Special forms of flight II: helicopters. *British Medical Journal,* **287**, 346–349.
Harp Report (1984) *Report of the Helicopter Review Panel (HARP) of the Airworthiness Requirements Board,* UK Civil Aviation Authority.
LOVESEY, E.J. et al. (1976) *Vibration and Other Measurements in RN Sea King Helicopters,* RAE Tech Memo FS 72. London: Ministry of Defence.
SKJENNA, O.W. (1981) *Cause Factor: Human, A Treatise on Rotary Wing Human Factors.*
VYRNEY-JONES, P. (1984) *A Review of Army Air Corps Helicopter Accidents 1971–1982,* RAF IAM Report No 632. London: Ministry of Defence.

V/STOL aircraft

GENTLE, R. (1980) *Aviation/Space Dictionary*, 6th edn. Fallbrook, Ca: Aero Publications.

Supersonic transport aircraft

BENNETT, G. (1962) Ozone contamination in high altitude aircraft cabins. *Aerospace Medicine,* **33**, 969–973.
LAVERNE, J., LAFONTAINE, E. and LAPLANE, R. (1978) The Concorde and cosmic rays. *Aviation, Space and Environmental Medicine,* **49**, 419–421.
Medical Aspects of Supersonic Flight. Medical Departments of British Airways and Air France.
MILLS, F.J. and HARDING, R.M. (1983) Special forms of flight III: supersonic transport. *British Medical Journal,* **287**, 411–412.
PRESTON, F.S. (1975) Medical aspects of supersonic travel. *Aviation, Space and Environmental Medicine,* **46**, 1074–1078.
WILSON, I.J. (1966) Radiation and supersonic flight. *Science Journal,* **66**, 31–37.

Manned spacecraft

CALVIN, M. and GAZENKO, O.G. (eds) (1975) *Foundations of Space Biology and Medicine.* Joint USA/USSR Publication in three volumes. Washington, DC: NASA SP-374. Vol. I—*Space As A Habitat.* Vol. II—*Ecological and Physiological Bases of Space Biology and Medicine* (2 books). Vol. III—*Space Medicine and Biotechnology.*
ENGLE, E. and LOTT, A. (1979) *Man In Flight: Biomedical Achievements In Aerospace.* Maryland: Leeward Publications.
HARDING, R.M. (1988) *Survival in Space: The Medical*

Problems of Manned Spaceflight. London: Routledge & Kegan Paul.

JOHNSTON, R.S. and DIETLEIN, L.F. (eds) (1977) *Biomedical Results From Skylab*. Washington, DC: NASA SP-377.

JOHNSTON, R.S., DIETLEIN, L.F. and BERRY, C.A. (eds) (1975) *Biomedical Results of Apollo*. Washington, DC: NASA SP-378.

MILLS, F.J. and HARDING, R.M. (1983) Special forms of flight IV: manned spacecraft. *British Medical Journal*, **287**, 478–482.

NICOGOSSIAN, A.E. (1985) Biomedical challenges of spaceflight. In *Fundamentals of Aerospace Medicine* (ed. DeHart, R.L.), pp. 839–861 Philadelphia: Lea & Febiger.

NICOGOSSIAN, A.E. and PARKER, J.F. (1982) *Space Physiology and Medicine*. Washington, DC: NASA SP-477.

Part VII

Commercial Aviation and Health

33

Commercial aviation and health—general aspects

F.S. Preston

Introduction

Civil aviation as we know it in the United Kingdom came into being during World War I: the first international airline company was formed in 1916. By 1919 there were flights from Hounslow Heath to Paris, Amsterdam, Brussels and Cologne and eventually to Copenhagen using converted World War I machines such as the de Havilland 4A, ill-suited for their role and flown by ex-RFC and RAF Pilots.

In the same year two young RAF officers, Alcock and Brown, made the first non-stop crossing of the North Atlantic in a converted Vickers Viking bomber from Newfoundland, crash-landing in a bog in Ireland to win Lord Northcliffe's offer of £10 000. The Minister of Air at the time, Sir Sefton Brancker, was preaching a global and Empire concept for civil aviation; but by a tragic turn of fate he was to die 11 years later in the airship R101 at Beauvais in Northern France bound, with many other notables, to India. This tragedy ended Britain's dalliance with ligher-than-air transport vehicles. The Germans continued with this form of transport, through the efforts of Count von Zeppelin, until the tragic end of their Hindenburg in 1937 when attempting to approach its mooring mast after a trans-Atlantic trip at New Jersey.

Despite the set-back for airships the years between the twenties and thirties saw the development of the British Empire routes using aircraft and the establishment of bases and refuelling stops. In 1926, Imperial Airways, which had been formed 2 years previously, re-equipped with modern aircraft fitted for passenger flying and for longer sea routes; flying boats were introduced, eventually reaching a

high level of comfort and performance in the Solent class operated by BOAC in 1949.

The Handley-Page HP 42s, very large four-engined biplanes, came into service in the early 1930s but they were slow, cumbersome and noisy, cruising at a reputed 105 mph with a critical range of 580 miles. They were, of course, unpressurized and had to fly at or below 10 000 feet. Nevertheless, they provided a high degree of passenger comfort, pre-cooked meals and drinks in flight, and special sound-proofing allowed passengers normal conversation in flight (Pudney, 1959).

Aviation medicine in civil aviation

Although aviation medicine started in the armed forces prior to World War I with the appointment of Captain E.R.G. Lithgow, RAMC, to the Royal Flying Corps, and Staff Surgeon H.V. Wells, RN, to the Naval Wing in 1912, it was the First World War that gave aviation medicine its great impetus.

H. Graeme Anderson, a naval surgeon who followed Wells, published *The Medical and Surgical Aspects of Aviation* in 1919 when he returned to civil practice after the war.

During this period, oxygen equipment, helmets, protective clothing, safety harnesses and parachutes were developed to protect military pilots in combat against the enemy, and the first medical tests for pilots were introduced by Lt. Col. Flack. With the entry of the United States into the war there was a great upsurge in the study of aviation medicine, and the first school for Flight Surgeons was set up in the USA in 1919. A Central Air Hospital devoted to the illnesses of naval and military flying officers was set up in 1918 at Hampstead. The same year saw the formation of the Royal Air Force, with its own medical service. Air Marshal Sir Harold Whittingham, later Director General of the RAF Medical Branch and Director Medical Services of BOAC from 1948 to 1956, was the first medical officer at the then RFC Hospital at Hampstead (Maycock, 1957).

It was not until 1937 that Imperial Airways appointed its first Chief Medical Officer. This was Col. Frederick P. Mackie, who had served for 29 years with the Indian Medical Service and was an expert on tropical diseases. In the 7 years he served Imperial Airways he built up an excellent medical department where previously there was none. He was the founding father of airline medical departments although most of the work of the new medical department was concerned with clinical rather than physiological problems.

After World War II, in which great strides had been made in every aspect of aviation medicine, airlines began to look for modern aircraft to supplant the converted military transports such as Yorks and Lancastrians which BOAC inherited from the RAF.

Although the Boeing Aircraft Company had produced the first pressurized cabin in their Stratocruiser in 1939 it was not until the late forties and early fifties that pressurized Hermes and Argonauts appeared in British airlines. Pressurized short-haul aircraft also appeared for the first time—the Airspeed Ambassador and the turbo-prop Vickers Viscount.

The advent of pressurization did much to improve passenger comfort and enabled aircraft to climb rapidly through and cruise above adverse weather conditions. The latter was further enhanced by the arrival of the Comet 1 in 1952, the first pure jet transport aircraft, followed later by the Boeing 707. Unfortunately, the Comet 1 had to be withdrawn from service in 1954 owing to a succession of pressure cabin failures. The investigation into the cause of the crashes involved the BOAC Medical Department and the RAF Institute of Aviation Medicine at Farnborough. Subsequently, later types of Comet aircraft were introduced and flown successfully in airline service for many years.

With the advent of supersonic travel much research work was carried out by the Anglo-French Aviation Sub-Group of the Concorde project involving many research establishments in France and the United Kingdom. The original group met first in April 1963 which was some 13 years before the aircraft entered airline service. Problems such as the protection of passengers and crew against the effects of high altitude exposure, cosmic radiation effects and the inhalation of high ozone levels were all carefully studied as well as problems of cosmic radiation at supersonic cruising levels. In many ways this aircraft has been the most researched ever to enter airline service (Preston, 1985).

Functions of an airline medical department

Commercial aviation is a rapidly expanding industry, working in a highly competitive and changing technological world. It is only some 80 years between the Wright Brothers and their flimsy machine rising a few faltering yards at Kitty Hawk, North Carolina and Concorde flashing across the Atlantic at twice the speed of sound. The doctor in civil aviation has therefore to keep abreast of events and be able to advise management, employees and unions of the particular environmental hazards facing the work-force of the airline and, for that matter, the passengers it carries.

Civil aviation medicine covers a very wide field in that the medical standards of aircrew demand a good working knowledge of clinical medicine and its application to aviation, the broader concepts of occupational and tropical medicine.

Unlike the military specialist the doctor in civil aviation medicine can rarely insist on things being done, but instead has to convince management and staff that his advice on the various environmental hazards are in the interests of the airline.

The medical department should be independent of management, preferably reporting to the highest level such as the Chief Executive or Managing Director, and as a result be able to advise employer, employee and trade union representative in a completely detached and professional way. The doctor, or for that matter the medical department, needs to win the necessary respect for independent and purely professional judgement.

Additionally, doctors in industry are frequently consulted by managers and employees on personal medical matters and, as a result, are required to maintain a strict doctor–patient relationship with these individuals which has to be respected at all times. This is frequently misunderstood by management who find difficulty in understanding the finer points of medical ethics.

To sum up, therefore, the doctor in civil aviation has to be a 'jack of all trades', in that he must know a great deal about aviation and occupational medicine, but also be competent in matters of food hygiene, tropical medicine, toxicology, ergonomics, physiology and psychology. The principal areas of responsibility are as follows (Harding *et al.*, 1983).

Flying staff

Because of the very high costs of training pilots and flight engineers, it is essential that an airline recruits only the highest quality of staff. Having trained these individuals it is equally essential that they are maintained in good health by adequate and regular medical supervision.

In some airlines the medical department is responsible for the conduct of licensing examinations, in others the licence medical examinations may be performed by independent examiners. Much can be said for either approach, but the essential matter is the broad medical supervision of the individual aircrew member and the factors that could influence his performance in the air.

Similarly, the medical department will be involved in the design and production of new aircraft types, aircraft equipment such as oxygen systems, survival equipment, protection against high altitude, problems of ozone, cosmic radiation, and so on. The medical department will also be concerned in the medical training of flight-deck and cabin staff, particularly the latter who necessarily require first-aid and survival training.

Such training should cover aviation physiology, food and tropical hygiene and the maintenance of good health on world-wide operations, sleep and exercise, etc. Particularly in the case of cabin crew emphasis must be given to passenger needs such as first-aid, resuscitation, food hygiene, emergency midwifery and survival problems, and on coping with time-zone and climatic changes.

To achieve this effectively requires a dedicated teaching group who are in close contact with flight-deck and cabin crew and are exposed occasionally to line flying.

Ground staff

These cover a wide variety of trades and professions from highly qualified airframe and power-plant engineers to catering staff employed in food production both at home and overseas. Additionally, engineering workshops employ modern methods of investigation and rectification, including the use of industrial radiography and processes such as synthetic paint spraying and chrome processing, microwave radiation and the stripping down of radioactive engine components, which have a high risk.

Tropical medicine and hygiene

World-wide flying exposes passengers, crew and personnel stationed on the ground overseas to endemic disease that is insect, food or water-borne. As a result suitable immunization has to be provided and employees and the travelling public educated in avoiding such conditions. The problem of protecting individuals against malaria is now very complex and there is no completely effective anti-malarial drug. Indeed, the situation changes rapidly from area to area so very recent information is necessary to provide protection.

Constant supervision of catering establishments, airport restaurants and staff canteens at home and abroad, plus the assurance of safe potable water and milk, are essential to safe airline operations. This involves regular and unannounced inspections of catering premises by properly trained hygiene advisers or by the aeromedical adviser himself. Fly-proofing, garbage disposal, disposal of aircraft toilet contents and disinfection of aircraft coming from tropical areas require regular supervision to ensure that they comply with international and national regulations.

Carriage of invalid and disabled passengers

Many airlines carry invalid and disabled passengers, and there has been a great increase in the carriage of these categories in recent years. Indeed, a number of pressure groups exist to compel airlines to carry such passengers 'without let or hindrance'. Among these is the 'Access to the Skies' organization and the Royal Association for the Disabled and Rehabilitation (RADAR) who have been in the forefront of campaigns to improve the lot of the disabled passenger.

Airlines belonging to the International Air Transport Association (IATA) have common standards of acceptance for sick and disabled passengers and a common medical form and acceptance procedure. On submission of the completed medical form to the airline booking office in any part of the world, the necessary details are transmitted by the most convenient route to the airline medical department for a decision to be made. The answer is transmitted rapidly back to the reservations office.

Special equipment such as high-lift vehicles, stretcher gear, wheelchairs, oxygen sets, suction apparatus, invalid and special diets can be provided given suitable notice, and the patient conveyed either in a stretcher or a wheelchair to his destination. Road ambulances can also be arranged to hospitals or elsewhere on request.

On the aircraft, special frames to support the stretcher, screens to protect the patient, and so on, can be provided. Obviously, cases of infectious disease cannot be accepted nor those cases who may deteriorate rapidly in flight resulting in a possible expensive diversion of the aircraft. Patients on a stretcher must be accompanied by a suitably qualified attendant who can administer to the patient's needs in flight, as cabin crew are essentially food-handlers and are not allowed to carry out nursing duties. In many instances the accompanying attendant could be a nurse, but in more serious cases a doctor may be required.

Applied research and development

While it is not a prime requisite of an airline medical department to carry out basic research, the very rapid advance in aviation technology means that the airline doctor must keep abreast of events in order to advise the various departments on the physiological and ergonomic aspects of new aircraft, ground equipment and systems.

For example, before Concorde entered airline service in 1976 the medical and physiological aspects of the aircraft had been very thoroughly researched by the Anglo-French Aviation Medical Sub-Committee which was set up in 1963. This Committee studied all the physiological and medical hazards connected with the project and these included the protection of crew and passengers against high altitude and ozone inhalation, the problems of cosmic radiation exposure and the monitoring of radiation levels, and so on.

In the passenger cabin there has been a great deal of medical input in seating design, particularly in sleeper seats, and in general toilet and galley design.

Medical involvement in helicopter design is considerable, particularly in pilot seat design, hearing protection and the provision and testing of immersion suits for use in long over-water flights, such as to oil rigs in the North Sea.

Frequently the medical department may be called in to adjudicate and give advice on workload problems affecting aircrew and cabin staff and undertake studies along the routes: these will normally include the day-to-day workload and sleep achieved en route.

Over the last few years some co-operative studies on aircrew sleep have been carried out in association with sleep laboratories in the USA, UK, Japan and Germany and have involved a number of international airlines.

On a completely different theme, recent work has been concerned with the possible introduction of food irradiation to prevent possible food poisoning of passengers and crew from contaminated airborne meals. Airlines have to pick up aircraft meals from not only their own catering departments but also from catering departments of other airlines at home and overseas and from private catering contractors in high-risk areas of the world. The legalisation by the UK and USA Governments of food treatment by Cobalt 60 or electron beam irradiation creates a new field in food safety. Airlines may well be the first to use this exciting new technology.

The International Health Regulations

The Twenty-Second World Health Assembly in 1969 produced a revised and consolidated version of the previous International Sanitary Regulations.

The purpose of these regulations is to prevent the international spread of diseases and, in the context of international travel, to do so with the minimum of inconvenience to the passenger (World Health Organisation, 1986).

In 1981 the 34th World Health Assembly amended the regulations to include smallpox among the diseases for which a vaccination certificate should no longer be required because its global eradication had been confirmed.

Nevertheless, there is still need for vaccination against yellow fever which still requires a valid certificate. Yellow fever is still endemic in Africa and South America, particularly in equatorial regions.

There is a constant need to protect aircrew and the traveller against endemic disease, particularly malaria and diseases such as cholera, typhoid and infective hepatitis. Airline medical departments are well situated to give practical advice to travellers regarding health risks and the need for immunization; and as they have to provide this for their own staff many can, and do, provide immunization services to the travelling public on a revenue-earning basis.

British Airways, for instance, have provided immunization facilities and advice to the travelling public for the last 35 years, which quite apart from the very useful revenue this produces, does help to project the caring image of the airline.

Summary

The aviation medical practitioner in the civil field is directly concerned with the health and fitness of airline staff and passengers and has to be aware of the world-wide implications of the hazards and endemic diseases that face the traveller. Additionally, in such a rapidly expanding and forward-looking industry he has to keep himself up to date on the new technologies as they develop and be able to advise management and employees on these matters as and when they arise.

References

HARDING, R.M., MILLS, J.F., GREEN, R. and CHAPMAN, P.J.C. (1983) *Aviation Medicine*. London: British Medical Association.
MAYCOCK, R. (1957) *Doctors in the Air*. London: Allen and Unwin.
PRESTON, F.S. (1985) Eight years experience of Concorde operations: medical aspects. *Journal of the Royal Society of Medicine*, **78**, 193–196
PUDNEY, J. (1959) *The Seven Skies*. London: Putnam.
World Health Organisation (1986) *Vaccination Certificate Requirements and Health Advice for International Travel*. Geneva: WHO.

34

Health and safety aspects of aircraft design

A.J. Palmer

Design concepts

The initial design concept of a new transport is usually produced by a small, far-sighted manufacturer's design team who are aware of market trends and likely airline requirements. Since the gestation period may be from 4 years upwards and the subsequent operational life about 20 years, it is essential—if the project is to be successful—for the aircraft to be designed to meet likely operational demands over a period of up to 25 years. The high non-recurring costs associated with an aircraft type are likely to require the sale of from 200 to 300 aircraft in order to break even financially. The technical, operational and commercial problems in sustaining an effort of this magnitude demand the participation of a large number of organizations: manufacturers, operators, regulatory authorities and other agencies.

In recent years, aircraft manufacturers have found it necessary to spread not only the financial risk but also some of the manufacture and design workload with other manufacturers. This trend in collaboration is now developing to the stage where most, if not all, new major transport aircraft will be built internationally. Such sharing widens the market for the aircraft. It is aided by the increasing airline grouping and airline co-operation in developing design requirements, together with increasing standardization of regulatory authority requirements. The airbus family of aircraft demonstrates this type of co-operation, produced by the combined efforts of British, French and German Aerospace Industry. A common design and certification standard in the form of the Joint Airworthiness Requirements (JARs) has been developed to control these joint ventures.

The initial design concept of the aircraft is developed into an initial design by a large design group. During this period considerable market research is necessary, and members of the design team visit the airline managements of potential customers to determine whether such a design is in accord with their requirements.

The airline will simultaneously be carrying out its own market research and it will make economic and route evaluations. In their selection of aircraft the airlines are influenced by the lineage of the aircraft and engines and by the fact that their major competitors may have already purchased a similar new type.

Once the project has reached a stage where airlines are likely to decide to purchase, a tremendous increase in activity occurs as the detail design and production programmes proceed. The manufacturer will be introducing new design and production features developed in his research department which may include the use of new materials, both metallic and non-metallic, new construction methods (particularly bonded and composite materials), and improvements in fabrication. Such developments have made major improvements in the strength-to-weight ratio and hence the ability to produce satisfactory large aircraft structures.

Large transport aircraft require the selection and development of a number of systems, including equipment for automatic flight controls, navigation, air conditioning, landing gear, electrical generation, instrumentation, etc. When these systems were comparatively simple, it was possible for individual airlines to specify their own selection of much of this equipment. This selection could frequently extend to the flight-deck layout and to the selection or positioning of equipment for maintenance purposes. However, the high costs of design and development, particularly where certification flying is required, have priced most of these options out of the market. It is therefore essential that the manufacturer meets the requirements of the widest selection of airline customers with a standard design. This is normally achieved by the manufacturer holding a Design Review Meeting at which he offers alternative designs for comment by the engineering, flight operations and other specialists of the potential customer airlines. Hence the detailed specifications are produced that form part of the aircraft purchase agreements and which enable the customer to select compatible commercial and electronic equipment.

Design requirements

British aircraft have until recently been designed to comply with British Civil Airworthiness Requirements (BCARs) published by the Civil Aviation Authority and also to carry equipment and operate in accordance with Air Navigation Orders. Joint European ventures such as the Airbus A300, A310 and A320 have demanded a common European standard and the controlling requirements are the Joint Airworthiness Requirements (JARs). Federal Aviation Regulations (FARs) are the corresponding regulations for aircraft of the United States of America.

In the design of structure and systems it is now generally assumed that the probability of failure can be determined by test, experience and analysis. Because of this certain vital structures or systems are duplicated, and some form of display is provided so that crew or maintenance staff may check that these duplicated systems are functioning satisfactorily.

This may be in the form of automatic self-monitoring of systems, and built-in test equipment (BITE) together with failure warnings.

This concept, of complex self-monitoring systems and multiple redundancy, is employed for automatic landing and other essential control systems.

Design features

Noise

Every aspect of aircraft noise is covered either by legal requirements, by airport rules or by agreement between manufacturer and airline.

A system of Noise Certification was introduced by ICAO and by the FAA in 1969, which specifies maximum noise levels at take-off, flyover and landing as a function of maximum take-off weight. A more stringent scheme was introduced in October 1977 for aircraft certificated after that date. The current certification limits reflect the adoption by aircraft manufacturers of new technology, high bypass ratio engines with low-noise design features such as acoustic nacelle linings.

While Noise Certification is the means by which aircraft have to be designed to technically feasible noise levels, a quiet environment will only be achieved as quiet aircraft displace noisy ones from the world's airlines. To this end, legislation has been introduced and is being developed, both nationally and internationally, that will stop the acquisition of noisier aircraft and limit the operational lives of those currently in service. Airline fleets should be almost entirely to Chapter 3/Stage 3 standards during the first decade of the twenty-first century. Local airport measures to reduce the impact of aircraft noise include noise monitoring systems, noise-related landing charges and night-time curfews or quotas.

Engine ground running can be a source of annoyance to communities, and special engine running facilities are a feature of most airports and airline maintenance bases. These facilities usually consist of detuners or tubes into which the engine exhaust efflux flows or, alternatively, an enclosure which protects surrounding areas by shielding. Airports usually impose tight restrictions in terms of power settings and night-time running.

Aircraft guarantees always include the specification of maximum noise levels in crew and passenger compartments to ensure that levels of comfort are not impaired. The almost universal adoption of on-board auxiliary power units (APUs) has made it necessary to specify maximum noise levels at cargo doors and servicing points to ensure that hearing conservation criteria are not exceeded during aircraft turnround.

Pollution

Early operations by jet aircraft (e.g. Boeing 707) were characterized by the emission of a large amount of visible pollution at take-off. Mixed with this smoke (or unburned carbon) were hydrocarbons, carbon monoxide and nitrogen oxides. As a result of retro-fitting the combustion in new technology engines, smoke is now rarely seen and pollution levels generally are much lower.

Emission standards have been introduced by ICAO internationally and the Environmental Protection Agency in the USA. The EPA regulations refer to hydrocarbons and smoke only and apply to engines manufactured since January 1984. The ICAO regulations include carbon monoxide and oxides of nitrogen and are effective for engines manufactured since January 1986.

In addition to the emission regulations, fuel may not be intentionally discharged into the atmosphere from engine manifolds.

Emergency escape

A new generation of large jet aircraft beginning with the Boeing 747 in 1966 has resulted in pressure on the designers to develop means of evacuating large numbers of passengers in the minimum possible time. The inflatable escape slide coupled with larger power assisted exits has largely satisfied this need. The manufacturers are required to demonstrate the evacuation capability of new aircraft—often referred to as the '90 second test'. In this test a full passenger load is evacuated given specific conditions and numbers of exits used.

Fire precautions

Following the Saudia Tristar accident at Riyadh in 1980 and the Air Canada DC9 accident at Cincinnati in 1983 the industry has never been under more pressure to improve the fireworthiness of civil aircraft.

Legislation has been issued both in the United States and in the United Kingdom stipulating significant improvements. Interior furnishings are being changed by the introduction of material with lower smoke and toxic gas emission. Polyurethane seat cushions are being replaced with cushions incorporating a 'fire blocking layer'. Emergency cabin lighting is now required in the form of underseat or carpet-mounted lights known as 'floor proximity emergency escape path markings'. These lights provide visual guidance for emergency evacuation when all sources of cabin lighting more than 4 feet above the floor are totally obscured by smoke. Cargo-hold liner materials have been improved often by the use of glass phenolics to prevent fire penetrating into the cabin. Finally, toilets are being equipped with smoke detectors and automatic waste bin extinguishers.

The future holds further changes. The new generation of aircraft should provide total fire and smoke protection for all passengers and crew in the form of self-contained protective breathing systems.

Water and waste

Historically the water and waste systems have always been 'afterthoughts' in terms of aircraft design. Leakage of water and toilet fluid have been a common problem and a source of corrosion and health problems. Cases of 'blue ice' striking the ground after falling from aircraft descending from cold to warm altitudes are all too frequent.

Toilet fluid leakage gives the most concern. Since the commencement of civil transport, toilet receptacles have consisted of a single holding tank to contain toilet waste. Perfume, dye and disinfectant are often added to mask offensive odours. The early turbojets benefitted from some improvements by the introduction of recirculating pumps which flushed the lavatory bowls with a mixture of toilet waste and dyes.

The Boeing 767 represented a significant landmark in toilet improvements. This aircraft is equipped with remote holding tanks located in the freight holds. During flight the pressure differential is used to suck waste material from the bowl into the tanks. These toilets are clean, odourless and reliable.

Water systems have remained unchanged for many years. Bacteria are controlled by regular hyperchlorination.

Oxygen

British Air Navigation Orders require aircraft capable of flying above flight level 100 (10 000 feet) to carry oxygen for continuous use by the flight crew and emergency oxygen for passengers during the descent and continuation of flight at a suitable lower altitude.

For aircraft operating above flight level 350 (35 000 feet) the requirement is sufficient oxygen for all passengers for 30 minutes during a descent to flight level 150, and, in addition, oxygen for 15 per cent of passengers for the remainder of the flight, when this is conducted above flight level 100. Oxygen is required in such aircraft for therapeutic use by at least two passengers simultaneously. Prudent operators specify larger oxygen capacities in order that normal system leakage and occasional crew usage and testing during several sectors will still leave an adequate supply to meet the minimal requirements. This reduces the need for topping up the system before each departure.

Usually gaseous oxygen is provided by charged cylinders which can either be changed or topped up from an external charging point. Considerable precautions are necessary in the system design and in servicing to prevent serious fires, for the ignition temperature of materials normally regarded as fire resistant is very much lowered in an oxygen-enriched atmosphere. Rapid pressure changes, producing high gas velocities, and rapid adiabatic compression are to be avoided as are any form of dirt, swarf and readily combustible materials, such as most greases and oil. Any sharp-edged orifices should be eliminated. Metal valve seats are preferable to plastic ones, particularly in high-pressure areas of the system. Metal brush-type heat sinks are frequently introduced into high gas velocity paths in the system to help dissipate locally generated heat. Isolation valves are essential so as to shut off oxygen in cases of local fire.

Chemically generated oxygen is becoming more popular and newer aircraft are fitted with generators installed above each seat row. These units are reliable and are cheap to maintain. Furthermore they are inherently safe in post-crash conditions and present a reduced hazard compared with gaseous oxygen in post-crash fires. Development is still required to produce units that will operate for longer periods of time.

Interestingly all flight crew oxygen masks now double as smoke protection equipment to protect the eyes, nose and mouth from the effects of smoke.

Protective paints

Paint finishes are used both for external decor, and in order to increase the life of the aircraft structure. Difficult areas to protect are the interior of fuel tanks, inside the fuselage, beneath toilets and galley, the bilge areas and, externally, the leading edges, steel fasteners and joints in the outside skin. The selection of paints is limited by the fact that they have to be resistant to phosphate-ester-based hydraulic fluids in many parts of the aircraft.

Epoxy-type paints were used in corrosion-prone areas for many years with Alkyd types for decorative finishes, but more recently the superior finish and resistance of polyurethane types has led to their widespread use by operators. To reduce the hazards to the painter of inhalation of isocyanate over-spray droplets, polyurethane paints are now usually applied with 'airless' type spray applicators. These devices, however, introduce other hazards to the operator since their high muzzle pressures can force misdirected paint into a wide area of tissue.

In order to avoid disrupting aircraft maintenance work whilst spray painting is in progress, some operators use latex, vinyl or acrylic finishes in decorative areas that are not exposed to attack by hydraulic fluids.

Airline pre-service planning

During a new aircraft procurement programme the operator will be preparing to introduce the aircraft into service. Where it has new features such as mechanized cargo handling devices, or where it is significantly different in size from previous aircraft, a wide range of new ground servicing equipment will be required.

When selecting these devices, considerable care is required to ensure that adequate personnel guards and safety devices are provided, particularly for those to be used in the open and at considerable heights from the ground. Many mechanical devices require noise attenuation.

New hangars and workshop facilities frequently take 2 or more years to construct so early decisions are required when these are necessary since the lead time for such facilities can actually exceed that for the delivery of the new aircraft. Multi-level docking structures are now commonly used for the major maintenance of large aircraft in order to provide adequate inspection and work access with satisfactory operator safety. They usually contain piped pneumatic and hydraulic services, and paint application and stripping facilities with effluent control.

During the pre-delivery phase, the operator assesses the requirements, purchases spares and test facilities, and trains air- and ground crews to standards to satisfy the certifying authorities.

The aircraft is operated in accordance with the requirements of the *Aircraft Flight Manual* which contains the mandatory operating instructions and operational limitations of the aircraft. The maintenance programme has to meet the minimum requirements of the aircraft *Approved Maintenance Schedule* which is prepared by the operator and approved by the Civil Aviation Authority. The requirements are determined on the basis of logical analysis of the design, and experience of similar equipment. Statistical analysis of failures and of the efficacy of remedial actions is frequently used to determine the details of maintenance in order to achieve the best reliability for systems and components.

Detailed operating information is provided in the form of *Flight Operations Manuals*; servicing is detailed in *Maintenance Manuals* and engine and component *Overhaul Manuals*. Owing to the size and number of manuals for servicing large aircraft, and the consequent difficulty of introducing frequent and extensive revisions, they are often provided in microfilm format.

35

Medical standards for civilian aircrew

D.W. Trump

Medical standard for commercial aircrew

Community expectations are for the highest standard of personal fitness and ability for operators of all forms of public transport. This is particularly so where an accident may have serious human and environmental consequences.

Medical supervision of aircrew has as its objective the maintenance and improvement of flight safety by attempting to answer two questions:

1. Does the candidate have the necessary mental and physical attributes, particularly in the special senses, to perform the tasks involved?
2. Is the candidate liable to become suddenly or subtly incapacitated while performing the task?

This objective is the basis for grading the strictness of medical standards and the timing of revalidation examinations for various categories of licences and age groups.

Pilot incapacitation and the resultant risk to flight safety has been of concern since the earliest days of flight. Incapacitation may occur in all age groups, at all phases of flight and take many forms. This risk cannot be eliminated by the imposition of even stricter medical standards.

The greatest change resulted from the mandatory introduction, from 1973, of specific incapacitation training drills for all pilots engaged in airline operations. Risks to operational safety imposed by all forms of incapacitation have subsequently been significantly reduced.

In 1984 Chapman reported an extensive evaluation of the impact of training, when incapacitation was introduced into routine simulator flight checks in conjunction with incapacitation training drills. Acute and subtle events were simulated at critical phases of flight, both as an isolated occurrence and in association with failure of another critical flight system. This study showed that in airline operations, the reported crash rate of 10^{-10} resulting from 'crew failure' was at least ten times better than the generally accepted airworthiness standards for failure of comparably vital aircraft systems.

However, it must be remembered that not all pilots operate in a multi-crew role and also that incapacitation drills so exceptionally effective in fixed wing aircraft are currently not demonstrably so in helicopter operations.

International civil aviation organization medical standards

The Convention on International Civil Aviation which was signed in Chicago on December 7th, 1944, called for the adoption of International Regulations in all fields where 'uniformity of practice would facilitate and improve air navigation'. The agreed Standards and Recommended Practices (SARPS) are promulgated in annexes to the Regulations.

The International Civil Aviation Organisation (ICAO) Medical Standards are contained in the ICAO publication *Personnel Licensing* (Annex 1, Chapter 6—Medical Requirements). Current standards were published in 1982, and will be referred to in this chapter as Annex 1 standards.

Most countries that are members of the United Nations have adopted and adhere to these standards, which cannot cover all eventualities but present in basic outline minimum requirements to be maintained for each class of licence. The medical examiner is asked to exercise clinical judgement, in the light of his knowledge of the particular privileges

501

granted by the licence and the specific flight environment involved, to determine whether the certificate may be issued or deferred. The *Manual of Civil Aviation Medicine* (1985), published by ICAO, gives extensive guidance to aid this decision and amplifies the standards in considerable detail.

In formulating recommendations for the grant and maintenance of a professional pilot's licence, ICAO has to take note of general standards of medical examination and facilities common throughout the contracting States. Care is taken that recommendations made are such as can be readily met by developing nations.

National Standards

National Standards set by individual nations amplify in detail those of Annex 1 and may be higher than those required by ICAO, leading inevitably to a minor degree of variation between one signatory country and another. There is, however, agreement on the basic ICAO standards. National variations in standards that are less stringent than those of Annex 1 must be notified by the country concerned to ICAO. The United Kingdom, for example, advised in 1985 of variations in the period of validity of medical certification for the younger age group of private pilots.

In the United Kingdom, statutory requirements detailing conditions of issue and renewal of all types of aircrew licences, including medical requirements, are contained in the *Air Navigation Order 1985* (Civil Aviation Authority, 1985). The Civil Aviation Authority gives details of the UK medical requirement for licensing in its *Guidance Notes for Authorised Medical Examiners* (1986). Similar published guidance is issued by other licensing authorities. National variations also arise in the requirement for, and periodicity of, such special investigations as chest radiography, audiometry and electrocardiography in various classes of licence.

The airline

The airline, as an employer, may impose medical standards that are more stringent than either ICAO or national standards. The financial cost to the employer of initial and continuation training is such that premature loss of aircrew through avoidable medical causes must be minimized. The airline and the candidate also expect a lifelong career prospect.

There is, therefore, a moral duty imposed on the aviation medical examiner—particularly at the initial examination—to advise the candidate meeting only the minimum ICAO standards permitting a licence, that acceptance by a major airline for training and employment may not be assured.

If, following medical examination, the two questions posed above are answered satisfactorily, a medical certificate is issued for a licence, valid for the period relevant to the specific class of licence. This certificate cannot be withheld even if it is clear that the applicant will become unfit at some time in the future beyond this period of validity. The candidate will be advised of any likely future problem, but may well decide to continue flying. It is, therefore, axiomatic that there can be no significant difference between the medical standards at initial selection and subsequent later medical supervision of experienced aircrew.

The airman

The airman also has a responsibility in respect of his own fitness. Annex 1 requires that the licence holder should not exercise the licence privileges at any time when aware of a significant decrease in medical fitness, which may affect flight safety. In the United Kingdom this is incorporated in the Air Navigation Order and a further statutory requirement added that any incapacitating injury, or illness in excess of 20 days' duration, must be notified to the Civil Aviation Authority. The licence is thereby deemed to be suspended and restoration of the privileges requires a satisfactory medical examination.

A female pilot is similarly required to advise the Authority when she has reason to believe that she is pregnant. Some licensing authorities allow flying (but not as pilot in sole charge) during the middle trimester, provided obstetric advice remains favourable.

Flexibility in the application of ICAO Annex 1 Standards

The wide range of individual variation must be considered whenever standards are being formulated or applied. If laid down too rigidly some individuals will be excluded who, while not meeting the standards in all respects, might well be competent and capable of performing the required tasks safely under all conditions of flight.

Annex 1, para. 1.2.4.8, recognizes the situation and provides for some flexibility to be applied in certain exceptional cases. Where, in the opinion of the Licencing Authority's medical advisers, flight safety will not be adversely affected when ability, skill and past experience are also taken into consideration, such flexibility may be recommended. Medical advisers may consult with specialists in the various fields of medicine who are also familiar with the flight environment; with flight managers; with flight operations and with other branches of the Licensing Authority before reaching a conclusion. Special flight tests or simulator details may also be used in reaching a final decision.

By these means the 'accredited medical conclusion' is achieved as required by Annex 1. The final licence decision may result in unrestricted licensing, or certain licence limitations may be applied. Such limitations may restrict the airman to fixed wing aircraft only; to acting as a pilot in multi-crew aircraft only; or require more frequent medical scrutiny to maintain the licence.

In certain medical conditions, the carefully considered application of operational limitations, notably that of restriction to a multi-crew role only, may permit the retention of older and experienced aircrew with their greater safety record in an active capacity.

The Authorized Medical Examiner

To be valid, all aircrew licences must contain a current certificate of medical fitness bearing the signature of a doctor specifically authorized by the Licensing Authority to conduct such examinations.

The Authorized Medical Examiner (AME) will have undergone specific training in aviation medicine and will subsequently be required to attend periodic seminars. Many will also be private pilots; some hold professional pilots' licences. All will be familiar with the flight environment and requirements of the various types of air operations. In the United Kingdom all AMEs conduct medical examinations for both the issue and renewal of the private pilot licence, but only a smaller proportion are authorized to undertake the periodic re-examination of professional aircrew. All medical examinations for the initial medical assessment of professional aircrew are conducted centrally. The geographical size of the United Kingdom, as in some other European countries, makes such a centralized arrangement possible.

Medical assessment standards

Three classes of medical assessment are specified by ICAO in Annex 1—each class details the physical and mental requirements, visual requirements and hearing standards applicable to the aircrew licence held or applied for.

Class 1 assessment standards

Class 1 assessment standards must be met by the following licence holder:

| Airline Transport Pilot | (ALTP) | both aeroplane and helicopter |

Senior Commercial Pilot	(SCPL)	aeroplane
Commercial Pilot	(CPL)	both aeroplane and helicopter
Flight Engineer	(FE)	

To hold a commercial licence the airman must be at least 18 years of age, the minimum age for other Class 1 licences being 21 years.

The period of validity of the medical certificate for each licence in the UK and in some other licensing authorities is as shown:

ALTP	6 months
SCPL	6 months
CPL (over 40)	6 months
CPL (under 40)	12 months
FE	12 months

However, Annex 1 recommends that the ALTP and SCPL medical certificates should have a period of validity not exceeding 1 year, this period reducing to 6 months only at the age of 40 years.

Class 2 assessment standards

Class 2 assessment standards must be met by the following licence holders:

| Private Pilot | (PPL) | both aeroplane and helicopter |
| Student Pilot | (SPL) | both aeroplane and helicopter |

A private pilot's licence cannot be held unless the applicant is 17 years of age or more and its recommended validity is for 2 years, this period reducing to 1 year after the age of 40.

Class 3 assessment standards

Class 3 assessment standards are to be met by air traffic controllers and are for all practical purposes identical with those for Class 1 assessments.

The final decision on a candidate's medical fitness for the issue, or continuation, of an aircrew licence is the responsibility of the licensing authority, through its medical advisers.

Decisions cannot always be made without additional specialized consultation and investigation. Ideally, the relevant specialist should be familiar with both medical requirements for licensing and the aviation environment. Thus a suitably informed opinion may be given both to the candidate and to the authority.

This ideal is not always attainable and conflict of opinion may arise between the specialist and the licensing authority. The comments following, which concern medical licence standards, should be read in conjunction with the relevant specialist chapters in this book, and also be amplified by reference to the *Manual of Civil Aviation Medicine* (ICAO, 1985).

Physical standards

The medical examination looks for freedom from disease or significant disorder which may impair flight safety. Ideally the examination should also contain a preventative element, identifying and modifying, where possible, risk factors for the development of future medical problems.

A personal and family history should be documented. A history of heart disease, particularly in association with early sudden death, and of hypertension, diabetes, epilepsy or atopic illness, can be significant. Familial hearing defects or visual problems, notably of myopia, glaucoma or colour vision defect, may indicate inherent problems in the special senses. Surgical procedures should be recorded and if necessary assessment deferred until full clinical details have been obtained.

Annex 1 standards require that:

'An applicant for any class of Medical Assessment shall be required to be free from:
  (a) any abnormality, congenital or acquired; or
  (b) any active, latent, acute or chronic disability; or
  (c) any wound, injury or sequelae from operation such as would entail a degree of functional incapacity which is likely to interfere with the safe operation of an aircraft or with the safe performance of his duties.'

The general appearance, particularly that of weight in relation to height, sex and age should be assessed. Obesity by itself is not a reason for denial of a licence, but if excessive can impair mobility and can have implications for future health problems.

All orthopaedic problems require special assessment. Abnormalities of, or loss of part of a limb may interfere with safe handling of aircraft controls. Loss of one or more digits with loss of dexterity and fine manipulative ability needs informed assessment. Loss of part of an upper or lower limb will be incompatible with a professional aviation career.

Cardiovascular standards

Cardiovascular supervision of aircrew remains essential because cardiovascular disease poses the most important medical threat to flight safety and the continuing medical fitness of pilots.

During the 10-year period from 1976 to 1985, professional licences were lost from medical causes in 236 United Kingdom aircrew. Of these, 123 (52%) were as a result of cardiovascular disease.

Annex 1, Class 1 medical assessment standards require that:

'The applicant shall not possess any abnormality of the heart, congenital or acquired, which is likely to interfere with the safe exercise of the applicant's licence and rating privileges. A history of proven myocardial infarction shall be disqualifying.'

and further requires that for Class 1 assessments:

'Electrocardiography shall form part of the heart examination for the first issue of a licence and shall be included in re-examinations of applicants between the ages of 30 and 40 no less frequently than every 2 years, and thereafter no less frequently than annually.'

A number of comprehensive reviews have been undertaken in the field of cardiology allied to aircrew licensing. That of the American College of Cardiology in 1975 and that of the Working Party of the Royal College of Physicians in the UK in 1978 both provided input on licensing decision making, but their recommendations were not adopted as presented by any licensing authority. More recently, the First United Kingdom Workshop in Aviation Cardiology was held in July 1982.* Its published conclusions (Joy *et al.*, 1984) have subsequently had a considerable influence on UK licensing decisions and have been quoted by many other National Licensing Authorities who, however, may not necessarily adopt the conclusions reached.

A history of, or physical findings suggestive of, congenital heart disease will, with few exceptions, lead to denial of licensing.

A history of myocardial infarction or electrocardiographic evidence suggestive of antecedent infarction will render the candidate unfit. However, some authorities will now reconsider such cases 12–24 months following infarction. Provided stringent criteria are satisfied, which will include an exercise ECG protocol and coronary angiography, a licence may possibly be restored although this may well not permit flight in sole command of an aircraft. A licence must be denied in all cases with symptoms suggestive of angina.

Valve disease—All murmurs and added sounds should be referred for informed cardiological assessment. Two-dimensional echocardiography has made accurate anatomical diagnosis possible in most

---

*A second UK Cardiological Workshop was held in 1987. Its proceedings will again be published as an Annexe to the *European Heart Journal*.

cases. The licensing decision will, in each case, be made by the licensing authority. Where fitness for licensing is agreed, detailed criteria for any periodic cardiological review required should be clarified to the candidate. A history of valve surgery or replacement will normally be disqualifying.

All ECG anomalies, changes in waveform, conduction disturbances, pre-excitation, rhythm disturbances (except for those of sinus arrhythmia or infrequent supra-ventricular extrasystoles) and changes in ST segment or T wave morphology require cardiological review and assessment.

Minor ST segment and T wave changes are common in all age groups and can present a diagnostic problem: symptomless coronary artery disease must always be considered. Such changes in the symptomless population have been extensively studied. In the United Kingdom, Joy and Trump (1981) studied the significance of such changes in the civil aviation population and Hampton (1984) the importance of these changes found in a wider population.

Exercise cardiography will resolve the diagnosis in many cases, but its use as a routine procedure in the initial or periodic examination of the pilot population has not been recommended by the CAA medical department, nor by its cardiological advisers, because of its known lack of specificity and sensitivity in a symptom-free population. The unacceptable number of false-positive results arising would necessitate the use of invasive studies to clarify the finding. The exercise test is, however, a powerful diagnostic tool when properly used. Ambulatory ECG monitoring, radionuclide studies and coronary angiography may be required in certain cases for a final diagnosis to be made securely.

Where coronary artery disease is found on investigation, its extent and distribution in the coronary arterial tree will need careful evaluation. Minimal non-critical disease may allow continued licensing in certain cases in a multi-crew role. Stringent follow-up criteria will be required.

Where coronary artery bypass surgery has been satisfactorily performed, some licensing authorities will reconsider the licence status 1 year after surgery. Each authority will have a protocol of investigative studies which must be satisfied if licensing is to be restored. Similarly, periodic follow-up studies will also be required. The licence may well bear an operational restriction to multi-crew aircraft only.

Hypertension

Hypertension is a common finding in the general population and the single most common cardiovascular problem found among aircrew. Because of the requirement for periodic re-examination it is usually detected in an early stage in this population.

Annex 1 requirements for all classes of licence are that: 'The systolic and diastolic blood pressures shall be within normal limits'.

Where systolic or diastolic levels consistently exceed the following levels, informed cardiological advice should be obtained:

Up to 39 years of age	145/90 mm Hg
40–49	155/95
50 and over	160/100

Risk factor analysis should be undertaken and freedom from 'target organ' damage ensured if the licence is to be maintained. The blood pressure must, however, remain at or below the following levels:

Up to 39 years of age	155/95 mm Hg
40–49	165/100
50 and over	170/100

Where readings are consistently above these levels, continuation of the licence will depend upon successful, acceptable treatment.

Certain drugs are unacceptable as therapeutic agents to the UK licensing authorities. These include methyldopa, hydralazine and ganglion blocking agents. Thiazide diuretics and spironolactone alone, or in combination, are compatible with unrestricted licensing. The United Kingdom currently limits aircrew being treated with beta-blockade to multi-crew roles only, removing the restriction after 3 years' stable control and in the absence of other risk factors. This also provides a period of satisfactory performance testing, assuring freedom from any covert physiological or performance decrement.

Annex 1 requirements for Class 2 standards have similar requirements in respect of hypertension, and the general clinical aspects of cardiology. The requirement for ECG examinations is, however, a recommendation only:

'Electrocardiography should form part of the heart examination for the first issue of a licence, at the first re-examination after the age of 40 and thereafter no less frequently than every 5 years, and in re-examination in all doubtful cases.'

Not all licensing authorities follow this recommendation, and international variations in this aspect of the physical examination arise.

The respiratory system

Respiratory disorders may be a cause of in-flight incapacitation, and functional assessment must always be considered in relation to the specific flight environments.

Annex 1 standards require for all classes of aircrew licences that:

'There shall be no acute disability of the lungs nor any active disease of the structures of the lungs, mediastinum or pleura. Radiography shall form a part of the medical examination in all doubtful clinical cases'

and it is recommended that:

'Radiography should form a part of the initial chest examination and should be repeated periodically thereafter'.

Licence decisions in candidates with traumatic or surgical deformities of the chest wall will be entirely dependent upon residual functional efficiency.

Active tuberculosis will not permit any licence to be held but following successful treatment, the licence status may be reconsidered. Quiescent or healed lesions may permit fit assessments. Restrictive or obstructive patterns of ventilatory impairment, found on spirometry, all merit investigation before any licence decision is made.

Three conditions require special consideration in the context of aircrew licensing:

1. Spontaneous pneumothorax.
2. Sarcoidosis.
3. Asthma.

The occurrence of a spontaneous pneumothorax demands the suspension of all classes of licence. Following resorption of the pneumothorax the established pilot may resume flying, but should not be permitted to fly as pilot in sole command for a period of 2 years. Recurrences are common. Should a second pneumothorax occur, the restoration of the licence must depend upon successful surgical pleurectomy, preferably bilateral.

A diagnosis of sarcoidosis, usually suspected on X-ray evidence of hilar gland enlargement, must lead to suspension of the licence and investigation. Other causes of lymphadenopathy must be excluded. In the UK, a confirmed diagnosis of sarcoidosis, deemed active, requires that the licence should remain suspended until the condition has resolved and no treatment is being given. When the condition is deemed inactive, respiratory and cardiological investigation must be undertaken before the licence may be restored. Subsequently, a limitation to a multi-crew role only is maintained for a 2-year period in all professional pilots. Sarcoid infiltration of the myocardium has been a postmortem finding in some instances of unexplained sudden death, and its relevance to aviation medicine was reviewed by Hill (1977).

Asthma or a history of antecedent asthma, in a candidate for aircrew licensing, produces considerable problems of assessment. A detailed history of the frequency and pattern of past attacks should be noted. Loss of schooling, periods of hospitalization and the use of steroids in treatment are relevant. Other atopic conditions in the candidate and a family history of atopy will also be of significance. Lung function, notably Peak flow rate, FVC/FEV^1 ratio and the effect of provocative exercise on these parameters should be studied.

Applicants with a history of recent attacks, particularly with the necessity for oral or inhalational steroids as therapy, will not be acceptable for any class of licence. Candidates with 'occasional' asthma and those using inhalational bronchodilators regularly will also be regarded with suspicion and will require the fullest possible investigation before any licensing decision can be made. Those with a past history of asthma, now 'cured', require careful assessment. In general terms there should have been freedom from attacks for at least 3–5 years, with no requirement for any form of medication, with the possible exception of sodium cromoglycate as prophylaxis. Lung function studies and consultant specialist advice should be obtained before a final decision is made. Residual functional capacity during an attack is difficult to quantify and the probability of such an occurrence needs careful consideration.

The licence status in these candidates, if agreed, will always be fragile. The applicant will be entering a demanding profession where the stresses imposed by the flight environment itself, particularly in difficult flight conditions, irregular working schedules, climatic changes and other factors, are all liable to trigger a recurrence of attacks in the vulnerable individual. The candidate should also be advised that a major employing airline may be cautious in accepting anyone with such a history for training and employment.

All assessments of potential professional aircrew should ideally include chest radiography and assessment of lung volumes and dynamics by spirometry. Smoking should be discussed and discouraged if necessary. However, respiratory pathology, in general, has a relatively small incidence as a cause of licensing problems.

Other significant medical conditions

Endocrine disorders

Thyroid disorders

Both hyperthyroidism and hypothyroidism are incompatible with continued licensing. Following appropriate treatment and a suitable interval to ensure that a stable euthyroid state exists, the licence may be reinstated. The licence will, however, be dependent upon continuing periodic specialist review throughout the flying career.

Diabetes

Glycosuria found at periodic medical examination requires that the licence is suspended until full investigation has been undertaken.

Should a diagnosis of diabetes be made, the licence must remain suspended until stable control is achieved.

Should control be obtained satisfactorily by modification of the diet alone, all classes of licence may be restored. Continued licensing will necessitate frequent medical monitoring to ensure that satisfactory blood sugar levels are maintained, the weight adequately controlled, freedom from ketonuria and glycosuria maintained and that the cardiovascular, neurological and ophthalmic status remain entirely normal.

Should control be obtained only by the use of oral hypoglycaemic agents, professional aircrew licences will be denied permanently.

Class 2 licences for private pilots may be reinstated, provided that satisfactory control is achieved by the use of biguanide hypoglycaemic agents only. Continued licensing will require monitoring as above.

Should control of the diabetic state require the use of insulin, no class of licence may be issued or reinstated.

Significant gastro-intestinal disorders

All aircrew with active peptic ulceration should be considered unfit until such time as healing has occurred, as proven by radiology or preferably endoscopy. Recurrent ulceration or evidence of occult bleeding must require suspension of the licence and possibly surgical treatment before restoration can be reconsidered. The complications of perforation or acute haemorrhage, if active ulceration continues, are such that flight safety might well be seriously jeopardized.

A diagnosis of active pancreatitis must result in denial of all classes of licence, until full and stable recovery has been assured. Alcohol as an aetiological factor must always be considered.

Candidates with active inflammatory bowel disease are usually unfit for all classes of licence. If medication is required, that in itself is usually a contra-indication to licensing despite absence of symptoms. Successful surgical treatment of ulcerative colitis or Crohn's disease may permit all classes of licence to be agreed.

Renal disorders significant in aviation

All candidates with albuminuria or haematuria on urinalysis should be referred for investigation into the cause. Those with orthostatic albuminuria are acceptable. The clinical findings in other cases will determine the licensing decision.

Urinary infections will entail temporary unfitness. Any underlying pathology found will require individual assessment.

Urinary calculi

Renal colic is a potential cause of acute in-flight incapacitation. The passage of an isolated calculus will permit continued licensing to be agreed provided radiological or ultrasound studies confirm the absence of further calculi.

If further calculi are demonstrated the medical certificate should be withheld until such time as they have been passed or removed.

Anaemias

Anaemias from any cause must be investigated and corrected. Other haematological disorders should be assessed individually.

Malignant disease

No return to flying can be considered for at least 6 months following surgical treatment or radiotherapy, and all chemotherapy must have been discontinued. The advice of the surgeon, radiotherapist and oncologist will all be essential before any licensing decision is made.

In all cases, return to flying must be in a dual role and increased specialist scrutiny will be required. Eventual return to solo flying will be dependent upon oncological advice.

Mental and behavioural disorders

About 80% of all accidents and 60% of fatal accidents are due to human failure—a high proportion through some error of judgement. In many cases inadequate information is provided or inadequate time is available to process the information and exercise judgement.

Information processing and the capacity to make decisions and initiate a suitable response may be disturbed by both psychiatric illness and organic mental illness resulting from brain injury or damage. Such disorders may be the cause of both subtle or acute in-flight incapacitation, and in the United Kingdom, remain the second most frequent cause for loss of licence in established aircrew. In the 10-year period from 1976 to 1985, of the 236 licences of all categories withdrawn, 57 (24%) were as a result of psychiatric disease.

Medical standards require that an individual presenting any such illness, or the potential for the occurrence of such disorders, should be excluded from licensing. This applies to all categories of flying licences.

Annex 1 requirements are that:

'The applicant shall have no established medical history or clinical diagnosis of:
(a) a psychosis,
(b) alcoholism,
(c) drug dependence,
(d) any personality disorder, particularly if severe enough to have repeatedly resulted in overt acts,
(e) a mental abnormality, or neurosis of significant degree, such as might render the applicant unable to safely exercise the privileges of the licence applied for or held, unless accredited medical conclusion indicates that in special circumstances, the applicant's failure to meet the requirement is such that the exercise of the privileges of the licence applied for is not likely to jeopardise flight safety.'

This is further amplified by the recommendation that:

'The applicant shall have no established medical history or clinical diagnosis of any mental abnormality, personality disorder or neurosis, which according to accredited medical conclusion makes it likely that within 2 years of the examination, the applicant will be unable to safely exercise the privileges of the licence or rating applied for or held.'

The AME is presented with a difficult decision in assessing those candidates vulnerable to psychiatric illness, the strongest evidence being a history of antecedent psychiatric illness. Some other indicators requiring careful assessment and possibly psychiatric advice include an inappropriate demeanour at examination, a poor academic record, sleep disturbances, frequent changes of employment without good reason, or a history of antisocial behaviour (particularly of alcohol or drug abuse or conflict with the law).

Answers to direct questioning may be avoided, deliberately falsified or coloured by the candidate, and overt signs of psychiatric illness or proneness may well not be evident. In the established pilot, considerable difficulty arises in assessing those showing uncharacteristic changes in mood, interpersonal relationships or behaviour. Such changes may be transient and a response to domestic or financial problems; they may be signs of early physical or mental illness, alcohol abuse, or a reaction to learning difficulties in the older pilot.

A history of, or the onset of, a major psychotic illness must result in the denial of all categories of licence. The manic–depressive psychoses, because of the known liability for unpredictable relapse, paranoid states and schizophrenic illnesses are all permanently disqualifying, even though stabilized by drug therapy.

An exception may be made in the case of an isolated episode of a reactive depressive illness, provided the previous personality was intact, the precipitating cause identifiable and unlikely to recur and all drug treatment discontinued for an 'appropriate' period of time. Reinstatement of the licence will be dependent upon informed psychiatric assessment and should include firm arrangements for periodic review. Flight in sole charge of an aircraft may well not be agreed.

The onset of a neurotic illness demands immediate withdrawal of the licence. The use of anxiolytic drugs is a bar to flying, and no consideration must be given to reinstatement of the licence unless the condition remits quickly and completely. Medication must have been discontinued for a suitable period. A prolonged neurotic illness or one that relapses is a strong indication for the permanent withdrawal of the licence.

Acute organic brain syndromes in association with severe systemic infections do not constitute a permanent bar to the restoration of a licence, provided the symptoms remit with recovery from illness and do not relapse. Psychiatric symptoms in association with organic brain disease should be evaluated individually, the underlying neurological disorder determining the licensing decision.

Neurological disorders

Annex 1 standards require for all classes of licence that:

'The applicant shall have no established medical history or clinical diagnosis of any of the following:
(a) a progressive or non-progressive disease of the central nervous system, the effects of which, according to accredited medical conclusion, are likely to interfere with the safe application of the applicant's licence or rating privileges;
(b) epilepsy;
(c) any disturbance of consciousness without satisfactory medical explanation of cause.'

and further:

'Cases of head injury, the effects of which, according to accredited medical conclusion, are likely to interfere with the safe exercise of the applicant's licence and rating privileges shall be assessed as unfit.'

This standard differentiates between the epilepsies, by definition characterized by multiple seizures, and the single disturbance of consciousness, which may result from a number of causes. The concern with either category is the risk of unexpected re-occurrence presenting an unacceptable threat to flight safety. The diagnosis of epilepsy—either focal, 'grand mal', or 'petit mal'—even though controlled by medication for a considerable time, is incompatible with any class of aircrew licence.

A single episode of disturbed consciousness must result in immediate suspension of the licence and investigation of the cause. Witness reports of the circumstances of the episode itself can be of significant value. Investigations may involve several medical disciplines and may require dynamic EEG and ECG monitoring, biochemical studies, drug screening, CAT scans and possibly cerebral angiography. If a cause cannot be established reliably, and shown to be non-recurrent, the licence must remain suspended.

Central nervous system disorders resulting from cerebro-vascular disease such as transient ischaemic attacks and cerebral or sub-arachnoid haemorrhage, will result in denial of a licence.

Migraine is a common complaint, characterized by incapaciting headache and preceded by an 'aura', often involving loss of central vision, hemianopia or diplopia. Mood changes, dysarthria, abdominal pain or limb dysfunction may also occur. Such symptoms are incompatible with any class of aircrew licence, but total freedom from symptoms for a continuous 2-year period may permit reconsideration. The degenerative CNS disorders, being progressive in nature, will normally be disqualifying, as will most demyelinating disease where episodic relapse and remission are a feature. Some cases of static neurological disorder or nerve lesions may be consistent with licensing.

All cases above will require informed neurological assessment. Closed head injuries may be allowed to return to flying on recovery, provided certain well-defined criteria are met, the duration of post-traumatic amnesia (PTA) being a reasonable indication of the degree of brain damage sustained.

However minimal any alteration of consciousness associated with trauma may be, no flying must be allowed for at least 1 week. Restoration and retention of the licence in other cases will depend upon the period of loss of consciousness and PTA, freedom from evidence of neurological deficit and from any risk of post-traumatic epilepsy.

Alcohol abuse

The airlines and licensing authorities have long recognized the adverse effect on judgement and performance of alcohol taken socially. A recom-mended minimum time of between 8 and 12 hours of abstention before flight is advised. Alcohol abuse, once diagnosed, must result in immediate withdraw-al of all classes of licence and referral for medical/psychiatric advice. If the prognosis for cure is considered good, the licence may be eventually reinstated. The applicant must demonstrate total abstinence for a period of at least 12 months. Abstinence must be substantiated by advice from the wife or family, the family doctor (who ideally should see the individual at fortnightly intervals) and psychiatric consultations at three monthly intervals are mandatory, before reinstatement is considered. After this period, continued licensing will be dependent upon abstinence and psychiatric review at three monthly intervals for a further 2-year period, with independent supportive evidence as before. Any relapse must result in permanent withdrawal of the licence. Alcohol may also be a significant factor in the maintenance of obesity, of hypertension, in the production of cardiac arrhyth-mias, peptic ulceration and changes in behaviour.

Drug abuse

The use of drugs for other than medical reasons must bring the individual's mental ability into question. Drugs impair judgement, alter perception, and affect the state of alertness. The unauthorized use of, or dependence on, any opiate, narcotic, hallucinogen, barbiturate or amphetamine must demand immediate and permanent withdrawal of the licence.

Although aviation has long attracted the eccentric and has reached its present state perhaps because of them, current airline operations demand both a stable personality and total freedom from behaviour problems among aircrew. There is always the difficulty of screening those whose unusual or eccentric behaviour represents a variation of the 'normal', from those with significantly disordered personalities. The ICAO concept of such disorder being 'manifested by repeated overt acts' is very useful in the context of aviation medicine.

The pilot with a physical disorder presents a serious risk to flight safety during a critical few minutes at the beginning and end of each flight. The pilot with a psychological disturbance presents a continuing threat throughout the whole flight.

Hearing requirements

Class 1 assessment standards required by Annex 1 are that:

'The applicant, tested on a pure-tone audiometer at first issue of licence, not less than once every 5 years up to the age of 40 years, and thereafter not less than once every 3 years, shall not have a hearing loss, in either ear separately, of more than 35 dB at any of the frequencies 500, 1000 or 2000 Hz, or more than 50 dB at 3000 Hz. However, an applicant with a hearing loss greater than the above may be declared fit provided that:

(a) the applicant has a hearing performance in each ear separately equivalent to that of a normal person, against a background noise that will simulate the masking properties of flight deck noise upon speech and beacon signals; and

(b) the applicant has the ability to hear an average conversational voice in a quiet room, using both ears, at a distance of 2 metres (6 feet) from the examiner, with the back turned to the examiner.

Annex 1 also details the reference standards for calibration of the pure tone audiometers, the background noise frequency range, and defines the 'quiet room'. Other methods providing equivalent results to those specified may also be used.

In contrast, the hearing requirement for *Class 2* candidates is that:

'The applicant shall be able to hear an average conversational voice in a quiet room, using both ears, at a distance of 2 metres (6 feet) from the examiner, with the back turned to the examiner.'

Audiometry is not a requirement unless the airman is to acquire an Instrument rating, when the permitted audiometric loss is that quoted above.

Nose, throat and ear examination

Nose, throat and ear examination must show a free nasal airway, any obstruction such as septal deviation or nasal polypi being referred for advice and treatment. Candidates with a history of frequent paranasal sinus infections or recurrent throat infections should also be referred for informed advice.

Eustachian tube patency must be confirmed at each periodic examination. The candidate with significant speech defects which degrade communication will be unfit for any class of licence. Most acute infections of the ear, nose and throat respond quickly to appropriate treatment.

Examination of the ear must demonstrate freedom from any acute or chronic disease of the middle and inner ear and the mastoid process. Chronic suppurative disease of the middle ear will be incompatible with any class of licence. A small dry perforation of the tympanic membrane, provided that hearing levels are maintained, will permit licensing.

Post-surgical assessment

The insertion of grommets for the treatment of secretory otitis media is compatible with continued flying, provided that eustachian tube function is normal. Successful tympanoplasty, where the graft is mobile, hearing levels satisfactory and there is freedom from vertigo, will allow the grant or restoration of all classes of licence. A simple mastoidectomy with the retention of adequate hearing is compatible with licensing.

Radical mastoid surgery, with resultant severe hearing loss and the potential for subsequent infection and vertigo will usually be incompatible with all classes of licence.

All cases of conductive and sensori-neural deafness should be referred for otological assessment before any licence decision is made.

Otosclerosis

Those with a minor blemish only on the audiogram may be licensed provided periodic specialist review is undertaken. Where surgical treatment (stapedectomy) is required to restore adequate hearing, no licence may be considered for 3 months after surgery. Evaluation will then be dependent upon the restoration of acceptable hearing, freedom from vertigo and upon the type of prosthesis introduced. With specialist concurrence, flying may be resumed in a multi-crew role for a suitable period of possibly up to 2 years, before solo flying is agreed.

The need for a hearing aid in flight is incompatible with a Class 1 licence although a Class 2 licence may be agreed in some cases.

Other hearing disorders

Sensori-neural deafness following childhood infectious fevers is usually unilateral and profound, and is the most common otological cause of rejection of initial candidates. A Class 2 licence may, however, be agreed following a suitable flight test. Deafness from other causes such as head injury, or following drug administration, will also be unacceptable for a Class 1 licence.

Meniere's disease is a disorder with serious implications for continuation of a flying career. The association of tinnitus, recurrent vertigo and sensori-neural deafness makes reinstatement of any class of licence doubtful. Informed specialist advice must always be taken.

Vertigo is a symptom of many middle- and inner-ear disorders and some neurological disorders and its occurrence requires immediate suspension of all licences, and investigation. Only where the cause is self-limiting and non-recurrent can a return to flying be considered.

Viral labyrinthitis is normally a short-lived infectious condition. Where this diagnosis can be made with complete confidence, a return to flying may be anticipated. Reinstatement of the licence will be dependent upon specialist advice and will require a suitable period of flight in a dual role before return to solo flying can be agreed.

Visual standards

Visual cues provide the pilot's most important sensory input, supplying approximately 80% of flight information. Good visual acuity over the entire field of view is essential for the safe operation of an aircraft.

Of younger candidates presenting for medical assessment for entry to a professional flying career, the greatest proportion of those rejected fail to meet the required visual acuity or colour vision standards. In the older age group of established aircrew, presbyopic changes affecting near and intermediate visual ranges present most commonly.

Annex 1 requires for all classes of licence that:

'The function of the eyes and their adnexae shall be normal. There shall be no active pathological condition, acute or chronic, of either· eye or adnexae which is likely to interfere with its proper function to an extent that would interfere with the safe exercise of the applicant's licence and rating privileges.'

Annex 1 standards for Class 1 assessment require that:

'The applicant shall be required to have a distant visual acuity of not less than 6/9 (20/30, 0.7) in each eye separately, with or without the use of correcting lenses. Where this standard of visual acuity can be obtained only with correcting lenses the applicant may be assessed as fit provided that:
(a) the applicant possesses a visual acuity without correction in each eye separately, not less than 6/60 (20/200, 0.1); or
(b) the refractive error falls within the range of ± 3 dioptres (equivalent spherical error); and
(c) such correcting lenses are worn when exercising the privileges of the licence or rating applied for or held;
(d) a spare set of suitable correcting lenses shall be readily available when exercising the privileges of the applicant's licence.'

and

'The applicant shall be required to have the ability to read the N5 chart or its equivalent at a distance selected by him in the range of 30–50 cm (12–20 inches) and the ability to read the N14 chart or its equivalent at a distance of 100 cm (40 inches). If this requirement is met only by the use of correcting lenses, the applicant may be assessed as fit provided that such lenses are available for intermediate use when exercising the privileges of the licence. No more than one pair of correcting lenses shall be used in demonstrating compliance with this visual requirement. Single vision near correction shall not be acceptable.'

Visual acuity

The young, healthy eye should achieve a visual acuity of 6/6 (20/20, 1.0) or better, either without correction or with any refractive error accurately corrected.

Those achieving only an acuity of 6/9, while meeting the minimum required visual fitness standard, should be examined carefully to exclude possible pathology. The specified limit of ± 3 dioptres equivalent spherical error (ESE) takes into account both the spherical correction and that of any cylindrical correction present.

The requirement for correcting lenses to be used must be endorsed on the medical certificate.

Candidates with sub-standard vision in one eye alone, when any refractive error is corrected, are unlikely to be accepted as *ab initio* professional aircrew, but those with minor errors may be acceptable for a private pilot licence by the application of the flexibility clause.

Contact lenses

Improvements in technology, materials and fitting techniques now permit most licensing authorities to allow aircrew to wear contact lenses.

The acuity must be accurately corrected, full-day tolerance achieved, and no adverse side effect present. Low cabin humidity may occasionally give rise to problems.

Near visual acuity and accommodation

This standard requires that professional aircrew have sufficient accommodative power to permit the Faculty of Ophthalmologists' Reading Chart N5 typeface, or its equivalent, to be read within the range of 30–50 cm, with each eye separately. This ensures that hand-held material may be accurately interpreted.

The further requirement to read accurately N14 typeface at 1 m ensures accurate interpretation of cockpit instrumentation. (The Federal Aviation Administration of the USA require the use of Sloane Letters, 20/40 equating with N5 and 20/80 equating with N14.)

With the onset of presbyopia, suitable correcting lenses will be required to achieve one or both of the requirements of this standard. Near visual acuity should be assessed with and without correcting lenses. It is important that the corrections prescribed are suited to the near working distances imposed on the aircrew by the flight deck of the aircraft. In the early stages of presbyopic changes this is not a critical problem, but becomes increasingly so as presbyopia progresses, with loss of residual accommodative power. The requirement for near vision correcting lenses to be available for use must be endorsed on the medical certificate.

Visual fields

All Annex 1 assessment standards require that: 'The application shall be required to have normal fields of vision.'

Perception of space is vital in the flight environment, and all classes of licence are required to have normal visual fields. One eye provides approximately 140° of vision in the horizontal plane and cannot be made to cover the field of both eyes simultaneously; thus in the uniocular individual, head movements cannot compensate for the visual field loss.

The visual fields are examined at each periodic medical examination. Any field defect discovered must be ophthalmologically assessed. The extent of the loss and its cause will determine the eventual licence decision. Loss of an eye from trauma or surgery will render an individual unfit for a Class 1 professional aircrew licence.

Monocularity

The Class 2 candidate with substandard central vision of such magnitude that, for practical and administrative purposes, a monocular state exists, may be considered for a licence. Here, however, where the loss of acuity is from amblyopia or a macular disorder affecting one eye, the peripheral visual field normally remains intact.

Glaucoma

All aircrew in whom ocular hypertension is found by tonometry must undergo increased ophthalmologic-

al scrutiny. Primary closed angle glaucoma requires immediate treatment. Ophthalmological review will be required before restoration of the licence can be considered.

Primary open angle glaucoma is insidious in onset and raised intraocular pressure may contribute to optic nerve damage and produce a characteristic field defect. A decrease in visual acuity is a very late manifestation. Control is normally medical and the medication used must be such that no unwanted side effects occur. Any field loss or cupping of the optic disc or rise in tension must be a reason for ophthalmological assessment.

Operative techniques may also be undertaken, and if successful will also permit relicensing to be agreed, provided fields are satisfactory.

Aphakia

The use of aphakic spectacles after cataract extraction produces such physiological disadvantages that restoration of any class of licence is unlikely to be agreed. The insertion of an intraocular lens implant and contact lens, or fitting of a contact lens alone may allow restoration of a licence in all classes.

Restoration of licence may be considered 6 months after surgery following ophthalmic advice. Periodic review must be maintained to ensure continuing fitness.

Ocular muscle balance

While standards are not specified in Annex 1, any degree of heterophoria should be assessed at the initial medical examination for all professional aircrew licences. After correction of any refractive error, a hyperphoria in excess of 1.5 prism dioptres or an esophoria or exophoria in excess of 6 prism dioptres should be referred for orthoptic and ophthalmological assessment. In practice, it is unlikely that a symptomless heterophoria would result in denial of a licence. However, the higher degrees of heterophoria may not be fully compensated if fusional reserves are weak.

A history of a childhood squint, treated surgically, requires careful ophthalmological assessment. The 'essential alternator' maintaining acceptable visual acuity in both eyes may be considered for licensing, provided ophthalmological assessment is favourable.

Acquired squints result from serious neurological or ophthalmological disease and produce diplopia; all classes of licence must be suspended.

The visual standards detailed in Annex 1 for *Class 2 licence assessments* permit a private pilot licence to be agreed, provided the distant visual acuity in each eye is at least 6/12 (20/40, 0.5) with or without correction. No limit is specified for unaided acuity. A refractive error of ± 5 dioptres ESE is permitted for licensing. Higher refractive errors may be acceptable, under the flexibility clause, provided ophthalmic opinion confirms that the eye is otherwise healthy. Near vision requirements are that N5 print can be read accurately within the range of 30–50 cm, with or without correcting lenses, this visual range being selected as meeting the visual requirements of the smaller cockpit of light aircraft.

Monocular candidates, as noted above, may be permitted to fly under defined training constraints, provided that the residual eye is normal and a suitable flight test confirms that flight safety will not be compromised.

Measurement of heterophoria is not a requirement.

Colour vision

Rapid and reliable perception of colour is an important factor in the acquisition of the total visual information necessary in all aviation duties and at all phases of flight.

Significant red/green defects occur in approximately 8% of the male population and constitute a major reason for denial of professional licensing at the initial medical examination.

Annex 1 standards require that for all classes of assessment:

'The applicant shall be required to demonstrate his ability to perceive readily those colours the perception of which is necessary for the safe performance of his duties.'

Colour vision is tested by means of a series of pseudo-isochromatic colour confusion plates, which must be accurately and quickly interpreted. The plates must be presented in daylight, or by means of artificial lighting 'of the same colour temperature as that provided by illuminant 'C' or 'D' as specified by the International Commission on Illumination.'

The Ishihara plates are standard in the United Kingdom; other test series include the Stilling chart; the Bostrom–Kugelberg set and the Dvorine test. Those candidates failing to identify the Ishihara plates correctly are referred for further ophthalmological assessment by means of a recognized colour vision lantern. Examples of suitable lanterns available are the Giles–Archer, the Martin, the Farmsworth and Holmes–Wright lantern. The Holmes–Wright lantern is that utilized as standard in the United Kingdom. Correct identification of colours presented, despite failure on the pseudo-isochromatic plates, allows all classes of licence to be agreed. Failure of identification of colours presented will result in denial of all professional licences.

A Class 2, private pilot's licence may be permitted under the flexibility clause, but will bear operational limitations confining the pilot to flight during daylight hours and operations into and out of airfields at which, if air traffic control is provided, it is by means of R/T communication and not by light signals.

The requirement for such an exacting medical standard has often been the subject of discussion. In the past, the standard has been related primarily to the requirement for a pilot to recognize coloured signal light codes, to avoid collision with ground obstacles or other aircraft at night. A new and complex colour environment has now been created by the introduction of colour-coded electronic flight instrument systems, increasing the reliance on accurate colour identification.

The 'X-Chrom' lens is a red-tinted lens, prescribed for the red/green colour defective to improve colour perception, and is normally fitted in the non-dominant eye. The lens may improve the interpretation of the pseudo-isochromatic plates but has little effect in improving interpretation of the colour vision lantern. The use of such lenses is not permissible in any class of aircrew. If it is suspected that such a lens is being used, the colour vision should be checked in each eye separately.

Precise assessment of the presence and sub-type of colour vision defect is possible by use of the anomaloscope but such precise assessment is not normally required. Practical testing by means of signal light guns, flares and medical flight tests have been used, but cannot possibly cover the reliability of colour perception under all conditions encountered in the flight environment. With scientific means available of measuring colour vision defects, such tests are not used by all licensing authorities.

Concluding remarks

The above discussions cover only the more important medical standards detailed in Annex 1. The many medical conditions not considered will require the AME to exercise careful clinical judgement in the light of his knowledge of the specific aviation environment.

The motivation for the airman to maintain optimum fitness is high. For those who earn their living by flying, fitness remains supremely important, not only for its impact on flight safety but also for future financial security.

Acknowledgement

I thank the Director of the Bureau of Administration and Services of ICAO for his permission to reproduce extracts from Annex 1, Chapter 6, Medical Provisions for Licensing.

References

American College of Cardiology (1975) Cardiovascular Problems Associated with Aviation Safety. Eighth Bethesda Conference of the American College of Cardiology. *American Journal of Cardiology*, **36**, 573–620

CHAPMAN, P.J.C. (1984) The consequences of in flight incapacitation in civil aviation medicine. *Journal of Aviation and Space Environmental Medicine*, **55**, 497–500

Civil Aviation Authority (1985) *The Air Navigation order 1985 (CAP 393)*. London: CAA

Civil Aviation Authority (1986) *Guidance Notes for Authorised Medical Examiners*. London: CAA

HAMPTON, J.R. (1984) The importance of minor changes in the resting electrocardiogram. *European Heart Journal*, **5** (Suppl. A), 61–63

HILL, I.R. (1977) Sarcoidosis: a review of some features of importance in aviation medicine. *Journal of Aviation and Space Environmental Medicine,* **48**, 953–954

International Civil Aviation Organisation (1982) *Personnel Licensing*, 7th edn. Montreal: ICAO

International Civil Aviation Organisation (1985) *Manual of Civil Aviation Medicine*, 2nd edn. Montreal: ICAO

JOY, M., BENNETT, G. and CAMPBELL, R.F.W. (eds) (1984) The First United Kingdom Workshop in Aviation Cardiology. *European Heart Journal*, **5** (Suppl. A)

JOY, M. and TRUMP, D.W. (1981) Significance of minor ST segment and T wave changes in the resting electrocardiogram of asymptomatic subjects. *British Heart Journal*, **45**, 48–55

Royal College of Physicians, London (1978) Cardiovascular Fitness of Airline Pilots. Report of the Working Party of the Cardiology Committee of the Royal College of Physicians of London. *British Heart Journal*, **40**, 335–350

Part VIII

Health and Hygiene

36

International health regulations

G.A. Faux and M.M. MacPherson

Introduction

International health control measures date back to 1340, when the City Fathers of Venice imposed 40 days' isolation on ships, passengers and goods arriving from other countries, presumably to allow infectious disease to manifest itself and allow primitive protective measures to be taken. From this the word 'quarantine' passed into everyday use.

The method was eventually abandoned as a health control procedure when the cholera pandemics of the nineteenth century swept unchecked into Europe, also because the accelerating pace of travel, together with the development of trade, made such restrictions impractical.

International co-operation in health protection began with the First International Sanitary Conference in Paris in 1851, and continued through the medium of international sanitary regulations updated as required for more than 100 years. In 1969, the World Health Organization (WHO) agreed a code of practice 'to ensure the maximum security against the international spread of diseases with minimum interference with world traffic'. This code was published as the International Health Regulations (IHRs) of 1969, which came into force in 1971.

Following the increasing emphasis on epidemiological surveillance for the recognition and control of communicable disease, the Regulations were designed for the following purposes:

1. To strengthen the use of epidemiological principles as applied internationally.
2. To detect, reduce or eliminate the sources from which infection spreads.
3. To improve sanitation in and around ports and airports.
4. To prevent the dissemination of vectors.

5. To encourage epidemiological activities on the national level so that there is little risk of outside infection establishing itself.

In 1973, the Regulations were amended, particularly as regards the provisions for cholera, and in 1981, in view of the global eradication of smallpox, the Regulations were amended in order to exclude smallpox.

The third annotated edition of the IHRs issued in 1983 (WHO, 1983a) is essentially the version adopted in 1969, with the subsequent amendments, and these are the Regulations currently in force. The IHRs are guidelines for participating countries to form their own legislations. Not all countries in the world are signatories to IHRs, and some have 'reservations', i.e. reserve the right to enforce their own additional requirements. Details of signatory countries and those with reservations are to be found in Annexes I and II in the IHRs.

In discussing the requirements of the IHRs in this chapter, only basic information can be given. For further details, reference can be made to the publication itself.

Entry of disease

Communicable disease and malaria can enter a country by means of an infected person, an infected vector, or through the medium of infected material, and provision is made in the IHRs to deal with all of these possibilities. Apart from recognizing persons suffering from infectious disease, health authorities have to recognize the possibility that incoming aircraft may carry mosquitoes infected with yellow fever or malaria, plague-infested rodents and their ectoparasites, or material contaminated with the organisms of cholera or plague.

There are now three diseases—cholera, plague and yellow fever—which are known as 'diseases subject to the Regulations' and the IHRs make special provisions for the control of them. The control of the three specified diseases is organized by WHO, and signatory members to IHRs are required to fulfil special obligations.

In 1969, the Twenty-Second World Health Authority, considering that epidemiological surveillance at the international level constituted the best weapon for preventing spread of infections from one country to another, felt it would be desirable to apply this not only to 'diseases subject to the Regulations' but also to five other diseases of international importance called 'diseases under surveillance'; these were louse-borne typhus, louse-borne relapsing fever, influenza, poliomyelitis and malaria. It is now agreed that the first two have not posed any threat in international travel for many years.

Diseases under surveillance can be added to as necessary, and since the Thirty-Third World Health Assembly in 1980 declared that smallpox eradication had been achieved throughout the world, WHO has maintained surveillance of suspected cases of smallpox which continue to be reported.

It should again be emphasized that although signatory countries to IHRs have formal obligations that must be fulfilled, these Regulations are also guidelines for the individual countries to form their own legislations. In the United Kingdom, for instance, the IHRs are applied at airports through the Public Health (Aircraft) Regulations of 1979. These concentrate on the 'diseases subject to the Regulations' to which are added lassa fever, Marburg disease, viral haemorrhagic fever and rabies as specific diseases, but extend to any other infection or infestation in a person or aircraft arriving or departing.

Health control measures for military aircraft are carried out by members of the armed forces at military airports.

Diseases subject to the Regulations

Thanks to preventive measures and improved therapy, the three diseases of cholera, plague and yellow fever no longer present the hazard that they have done in the past. A total of 28 893 cases of cholera, 908 cases of plague and 126 cases of yellow fever were reported to WHO in 1984 (WHO, 1985d).

In 1973, as a result of a WHO recommendation (WHO, 1973a), all reference to cholera vaccination was eliminated from the IHRs, as it was accepted that vaccination does not prevent transmission of the disease; however, some countries still make it a requirement. There will be no permanent radical change in numbers of cases until such time as an improved environmental situation, with provision of safe water and sewage disposal, makes it impossible for the disease to establish itself. In 1981, the Technical Advisory Group of the WHO Programme for Control of Diarrhoeal Diseases, after reviewing the current knowledge and experience in cholera control, concluded that since cholera generally creates problems in areas where other acute enteric infections are endemic, the development and implementation of national programmes for control of *all* diarrhoeal diseases was the best way to prevent and control cholera (WHO 1980).

The infectious agent in plague is the plague bacillus, *Yersinia pestis*. Wild rodents are the natural reservoirs. Bubonic plague is transmitted by the bite of an infective rodent flea, or by handling infected tissues or by contact with pus from an infected animal. Pneumonic plague is spread by the airborne route. Improved rodent control at airports is the best defence in prevention of international spread of plague.

Yellow fever is endemic in Africa and South America, and occasionally has extended into Central America and Trinidad. Two forms of yellow fever—urban and jungle—are epidemiologically distinguishable, although clinically and aetiologically they are identical. The causal agent is the yellow fever virus. In urban areas, the reservoir of infection is man and the *Aedes aegypti* mosquito, and the disease is transmitted by the bite of the mosquito. Preventive measures involve eradication of the *Aedes aegypti* mosquito and vaccination. Jungle yellow fever has as its reservoir vertebrates other than man, mainly monkeys, and forest mosquitoes and the best control here is vaccination of persons at risk. Control of the mosquito vector around airports and in aircraft is most important in prevention of international spread of yellow fever.

Smallpox

The eradication of smallpox from the world is of such significance in the field of international health control that a few words on the disease are appropriate here.

The smallpox eradication programme had its origins in 1958, when the Soviet Union proposed to the Eleventh World Health Assembly that the countries of the world co-operate in a co-ordinated effort to rid the world of smallpox. During 1958, 63 countries reported 280 000 cases to WHO, and because of the inadequate reporting at the time, it was agreed that this represented only a fraction of the cases occurring.

In 1959, the Assembly agreed that a global eradication programme should be undertaken as a matter of urgency, and it was thought that vaccination would achieve this within a period of 4–5 years. However, as this was not proceeding as rapidly as hoped for, in 1967 the programme was intensified with increasing emphasis on surveillance and containment measures as well as vaccination. The 1969 IHRs included smallpox as a 'disease subject to the Regulations'.

The last case of endemic smallpox in the world occurred in Somalia on 26 October 1977. In 1980, the Thirty-Third World Health Assembly in Geneva officially declared that smallpox had been eradicated world-wide.

In 1981, the IHRs were amended to exclude smallpox from the 'diseases subject to the Regulations' and they recommended that international certificates of smallpox vaccination should no longer be required of any traveller. International vaccination certificates for smallpox have not been in use since 1983.

The World Health Assembly in 1980 endorsed the post-eradication policy determined by the Global Commission for the Certification of Smallpox Eradication. A rumour register of suspected cases has been maintained, and about 20 cases per year have been reported. All have been investigated and found to be due either to misdiagnosis of chicken-pox, measles and skin conditions, or to errors in recording. WHO encourages the submission of reports of suspected cases in order to strengthen world confidence in the fact that smallpox has been eradicated.

The eradication of smallpox—the first disease ever defeated by man—is a triumph for international co-operation in preventive medicine.

Malaria

The Eighth World Health Assembly in 1955 formally endorsed a world-wide programme of malaria eradication, and in 1957, WHO took over the co-ordinating activities and the provision of technical assistance.

In 1969, the Twenty-Second World Health Assembly, noting the present and further increase in international travel, recommended to health administrations that they should report twice yearly to WHO on the malaria situation in the countries (Resolution 22.48) notifying areas where eradication is considered as completed, cases imported into these areas, areas with chloroquine-resistant parasites, and international ports and airports free of malaria. WHO would publish this information twice yearly and issue annual maps of areas at risk.

This information is presented in the WHO publications *Weekly Epidemiological Record* and the booklet *Ports Designated in the Application of the IHRs*.

There has been no real improvement in the world malaria situation over the 15 years 1970–85. While the number of cases reported in recent years to WHO has been about 5.5 million annually, the actual number of clinical cases is difficult to assess, owing to under-detection and/or under-reporting. According to estimates, the total incidence of malaria is in the order of 98 million cases annually (WHO, 1986).

Chloroquine-resistant *Plasmodium falciparum* malaria has been confirmed in more than 40 countries, including a few African ones. The situation is expected to deteriorate further, especially in Africa, as the use of drugs increases in the absence of large-scale vector control.

A WHO field test has been developed which denotes the response of the malaria parasites to chloroquine (WHO, 1973b). The degree of response varies from sensitivity (S) to resistance on a scale RI, RII, RIII, with RIII denoting high resistance. WHO now publishes data on chloroquine resistance referring to this scale.

Resistance to other antimalarial drugs is also beginning to be reported, and resistance to more than one insecticide now affects many anopheline species.

Of a total world population of 4751 million people, 48% live in areas where anti-malaria measures are carried out, and 8% inhabit areas where no specific measures are taken to control malaria transmission. The increase in international air traffic favours accidental dissemination of mosquitoes, a problem demanding great vigilance on the part of port authorities. Disinsection procedures on departure are very important as well as local control.

Application of International Health Regulations in disease control

The current edition (3rd annotated edition) lays down what organization, facilities, measures and procedures are required to maintain international health control in the most effective manner, while at the same time stating the maximum measures that may be applied.

The IHRs are divided into 94 Articles, four appendices and six annexes. Authority for various procedures is justified by reference to these divisions. Any updating required is published in the WHO publication, the *Weekly Epidemiological Record*.

Part I of IHRs gives definitions of terminology used—for instance references in IHRs to 'infected persons', 'infected or suspect aircraft' and 'infected area' all refer to the 'diseases subject to the Regulations'. An 'infected person' is a person suffering from the disease, and a 'suspect' is someone who has been exposed to infection and is considered capable of spreading it. 'Aircraft' means any aircraft making an international voyage, and 'airport' means any airport so designated by the State as an airport for international traffic, where formalities are carried out, which concern customs, immigration, public health, and animal and plant quarantine.

The various aspects of international health control for air travel can be considered under the following headings:

1. Notification and epidemiological information.
2. Health organization at airports.
3. Health measures and procedures at and between airports.
4. Provisions relating to diseases subject to the regulations.
5. Health documents.
6. Disinsection.

Notification and epidemiological information

This is covered under Articles 2–13 of the IHRs. When an outbreak of one of the three specified diseases occurs in a country which is a signatory to the IHRs, the Health Administration is required to take the following steps:

1. WHO is to be notified by telegram or telex within 24 hours of the first case of a disease subject to the Regulations occurring in the territory, other than an imported or transferred case.
2. The infected area is to be defined within the subsequent 24 hours, and as soon as possible, information on the source and type of the disease, incidence and mortality is to be provided; also the prophylactic measures taken, including, if indicated, those against insect vectors or rodents.
3. Follow-up information is to be supplied weekly, and incidence and mortality figures at least once weekly.
4. WHO is to be notified when the area is free from infection, i.e. when all prophylactic measures have been taken to prevent recurrence or spread to other areas.

Health administrations also have to notify when a case has been imported or transferred from another area within its jurisdiction into a non-infected area, or when an aircraft has arrived with a person on board who has one of the specified diseases—the notification here has to include the flight number of the aircraft, its previous and subsequent ports of call, and the health measures if any applied to the aircraft. A clinical diagnosis has to be confirmed as soon as possible by laboratory methods and the results notified to WHO immediately. Epidemiological information is reported until such time as an infected area becomes free from infection.

WHO disseminates information through its Automatic Telex Reply Service, the *Weekly Epidemiological Record*, and the annual publication *Vaccination Certificate Requirements and Health Advice for Overseas Travel*.

The Automatic Telex Reply Service was started to allow rapid dissemination of information of particular epidemiological interest. It is operational 24 hours a day. There is a daily relay of information from WHO headquarters to the six regional offices, and health administrations may receive information from these offices, or find out the latest on a situation by contacting the headquarters telex machine directly.

WHO's most useful organ of information is the *Weekly Epidemiological Record* (WER) which is published weekly in English and French and sent by air mail to subscribers. As well as enabling WHO to fulfil the obligations formally laid on it by the IHRs and various World Health Assembly recommendations, including updating the IHRs as required, it disseminates information on diseases subject to the Regulations as well as on any other internationally important disease. As required under Article 13 of the IHRs, it publishes an annual report on the functioning of the IHRs and their effect on international traffic. Data are published annually on epidemiological trends of diseases subject to the Regulations, illustrated with maps; information is also given about diseases subject to international surveillance. Information on malaria is published twice a year, and maps are issued annually showing areas at risk.

The booklet *Vaccination Certificate Requirements and Health Advice for Overseas Travel* is published annually by WHO, using information supplied by member countries. Unfortunately the requirements are not always adhered to, some countries making their own requirements in addition. The WER publishes any amendments, also any required for the other WHO publications *Ports Designated in Application of the IHRs* and *Yellow Fever Vaccination Centres*.

Health organization at airports

This is covered in Articles 14–22 in IHRs.

Each health administration is required to ensure that airports ('airports' as defined earlier) are adequately equipped and organized to meet the requirements of IHRs as follows:

1. Wholesome food and water from approved sources must be provided for local and in-flight

consumption; periodic checks on storage and handling practices are required, with analysis of food and water samples.

2. Each airport should provide for safe disposal of excrement and other waste material dangerous to health.
3. The airport and installations should be kept free from rodents.
4. The area within the airport perimeter is to be kept free of *Aedes aegypti* and other mosquito vectors of disease. This requires regular application of anti-mosquito measures over a distance of at least 400 m around its perimeter (defined as the line enclosing the buildings and the area used for parking of aircraft).
5. As many airports in a territory as practicable should have a medical and health service available with adequate staff, equipment and premises to provide facilities for isolation hospital care, bacteriological investigations, collection of food and water samples for analysis, disinsection, disinfection and deratting, and for the collection and examination of rodents for signs of plague infection.
6. Airports possessing a direct transit area have to be so designated. The direct transit area is a special area approved by the health authority and under its direct supervision for accommodating transit passengers and crews in segregation. Normally this is provided within the airport precincts. When the direct transit area is in a locality where mosquito vectors of disease are present, the accommodation for persons and for animals must be kept mosquito-proof.

Under Article 18 of IHRs, an adequate number of airports in a territory have to be designated as 'sanitary airports', which are required to have at their disposal the following:

1. An organized medical service and adequate staff, equipment and premises.
2. Facilities for the transport, isolation and care of persons infected with or suspected of having a disease subject to the Regulations.
3. Facilities for efficient disinfection and disinsection, for control of vectors and rodents, and for any other appropriate measures under IHRs.
4. A bacteriological laboratory, or facilities for despatching suspected material to such a laboratory.
5. Facilities within the airport or available to it for vaccination against yellow fever.

Each health administration is required to inform WHO of the airports and sanitary airports in its territory, together with the names of those having a direct transit area; changes must be notified as they occur. After appropriate investigations, WHO certifies that the airports fulfil the requirements of IHRs. Once a year each health administration must report on the success of disease vector control at its airports. The names of designated sanitary airports and airports with a direct transit area are published in *Ports Designated in Application of the IHRs*; this also indicates which airports are free from malaria.

Health measures at and between airports

This is covered by Articles 23–49 in the IHRs.

The health measures permitted by IHRs are the maximum measures which the State may apply to international traffic for protection of its territory against the diseases subject to the Regulations, and other diseases of significance in international travel. If a health administration introduces a measure believed to be excessive, WHO will draw attention to this during notification and will discuss the implications with the country concerned.

Travellers with diplomatic status are not exempt from compliance with the provisions of the IHRs.

Sanitary procedures such as disinfection, disinsection and deratting must be carried out without damage to persons, the aircraft or its contents and without creating any risk of fire. If particular procedures are recommended by WHO, these should be employed.

An airport health authority must issue free on request a certificate specifying the particular health measure carried out to an aircraft, together with the method employed and the reason for its application. This may be entered in the Health part of the Aircraft General Declaration. A health authority also issues on request certificates defining the health measures applied to freight and personal baggage, and when appropriate, the date of arrival or departure of a traveller.

A person under surveillance is allowed to move about freely. He may be required to report to the local authority at specified intervals for medical observation. If departing for another address in the same country or in another country, he must notify the health authority who informs the destination health authority; the person should report there on arrival.

All practical measures must be taken to prevent the departure of a person infected with a disease subject to the Regulations; if necessary, he may be medically examined before departure. A traveller under surveillance is allowed to depart, and the destination health authority is notified. Preventive measures must also be taken against the introduction on board of disease vectors, including disinsection as described in a later section.

No matter capable of causing any epidemic disease may be released from an aircraft in flight.

In-transit passengers and crew from a healthy aircraft may not be subjected to any health measures other than medical examination, provided they remain in a direct transit area of the airport; if they have to continue their voyage from another airport in the vicinity, the transfer must be made under the control of the health authority. 'Medical examination' refers to examination of persons or inspection of the aircraft for health reasons.

An aircraft may not normally be prevented, for health reasons, from landing at any airport. If that airport is not equipped for applying the required health measures, the aircraft may thereafter be ordered to proceed to the nearest sanitary airport. There are two exceptions to this regulation—they concern aircraft travelling from a yellow fever infected area and aircraft carrying pilgrims. Pilgrims may land only at an airport so designated for the purpose, and with regard to yellow fever, if an aircraft leaving an infected area has been disinsected, it may land at any sanitary airport; however, if it does not land at the sanitary airport, and the yellow fever vector is present in the area, it may only land at airports specified by the State.

On arrival, if no disease subject to the Regulations is on board, 'free pratique' is granted, i.e. permission for the aircraft to disembark and resume operation. Free pratique cannot be refused for diseases other than the three specified diseases except in case of an emergency constituting a grave danger to public health.

For aircraft arriving from an infected area, there are specific measures that will be described when provisions for the individual diseases are discussed. Provided that the health authority is taking appropriate precautions, these measures are limited to crew and passengers, and aircraft and contents, and 'free pratique' is issued on their completion.

Any aircraft and persons on board may be subjected to medical examination on arrival from an international flight. Further health measures may be applied to the aircraft after inspection, or because of in-flight occurrences that have given rise to concern. In the presence of a major threat to international health, a person may be required to give a destination address in writing. Apart from medical examination, any health measure applied at a previous airport may not be repeated subsequently, unless there is evidence that it was ineffective, or that another incident of epidemiological significance has occurred following departure.

An infected person on board may be removed and isolated, and the aircraft captain is entitled to insist on this. A suspect person coming from an infected area may be placed under surveillance, or even into isolation for a specified period if the risk of transmitting the disease is exceptionally serious.

An aircraft that has previously landed in an infected area, but only at a non-infected sanitary airport, is not regarded as coming from an infected area; neither are the crew and passengers, provided that they remained in a direct transit area as previously defined.

An aircraft captain who is unwilling to submit to health control procedures is allowed to take on fuel and stores and depart, but may not land at another airport in the same territory. Health control measures are obligatory, however, if an aircraft infected with yellow fever has landed at an airport in an area where the mosquito vector is present.

If for reasons beyond his control, an aircraft captain lands at an airport other than the scheduled one, he must notify this without delay to the nearest health authority, and without its permission nobody may leave the aircraft vicinity unless the captain decides it is necessary for health and safety reasons. Likewise, no cargo may be removed from the vicinity of the aircraft. After health control measures are completed, the aircraft may proceed to another airport.

Aircraft cargo and goods are subjected to approved health measures only if they have come from an infected area, and if there is a possibility of contamination or that they may serve as a vehicle for the spread of a disease subject to the Regulations. Goods, other than live animals, in transit without transhipment should not be subject to health measures or detained. Bilateral agreements between two countries may require a certificate of disinfection of merchandise to be issued. Disinsection and disinfection of baggage are necessary only if the owner is infected with or suspected of having one of the three specified diseases, or is carrying an insect vector or infectious material.

Containers used in international traffic must, in packing, be kept as free as possible of infectious material, disease vectors and rodents.

Mail, newspapers and other printed matter are not subjected to any health measure. Postal parcels may be subject to health measures only if they contain foodstuffs potentially infected with cholera, living insects or other animals capable of being vectors of human disease, infectious material, or soiled clothing etc. which may have been contaminated with the organisms of the specified diseases.

Infectious substances are carried by air subject to the requirements of the International Civil Aviation Organization publication *The Safe Transport of Dangerous Goods by Air* (ICAO, 1983). In this publication 'infectious substances' are defined as 'substances containing viable micro-organisms or their toxins'. They must be packed and labelled according to the ICAO publication *Technical Instructions for the Safe Transport of Dangerous Goods by Air* (ICAO, 1983). Infectious substances are acceptable in postal air mail packets subject to the provisions of the above instructions and those of the national postal authority.

Sealed coffins containing dead bodies are not subject to IHRs but are transported subject to IATA Regulations and the country's own requirements (ICAO, 1982).

Provisions relating to diseases under the Regulations

These are covered under Articles 50–75 of the IHRs.

Plague

For the purposes of the IHRs, the incubation period of plague is 6 days. Vaccination against plague is not a requirement associated with international travel. An aircraft is regarded as infected if there is a case of plague or a plague-infected rodent on board. Otherwise the aircraft is regarded as healthy.

The IHRs make the following requirements to prevent the spread of plague:

1. Every State is required to take all possible steps to prevent the spread of plague by rodents and their ectoparasites, and by regular collection of specimens to remain fully informed on the position.
2. At an airport infected with plague, special care is taken to prevent the introduction of rodents on board aircraft, and if rodents are suspected on board an aircraft may be subjected to deratting and disinsection procedures.
3. In an area where there is an epidemic of pulmonary plague, suspect persons must be kept in isolation for 6 days before being allowed to join an international flight.
4. Any suspect disembarking from an aircraft may be placed under surveillance for 6 days reckoned from the date the aircraft departed from the infected area.
5. On arrival of an infected aircraft, an infected person is removed to isolation care, and suspect persons are subject to disinsection, followed by surveillance for 6 days. If a case of pulmonary plague is on board, the crew and remaining passengers are liable to be placed in isolation for 6 days.
6. If a plague-infested rodent is found on board, the aircraft is disinsected and deratted, if necessary in an isolation area to prevent spread of disease.
7. The baggage of infected or suspect persons and anything else which may have been contaminated is disinsected and disinfected if necessary.

Once the health measures have been applied, the aircraft is given free pratique.

Cholera

For the purposes of the IHRs, the incubation period of cholera is 5 days. In 1973, the Regulations were amended so that cholera vaccination certificates were not required of travellers. However, a few countries still make it a requirement for entry, and the booklet *Vaccination Requirements for International Travel* gives details of these. Cholera certificates are valid for 6 months.

If a case of cholera is discovered on board an aircraft, the patient is removed to isolation care. The following measures are applied by the health authority:

1. Suspects among passengers and crew may be placed under surveillance or isolation for a period not exceeding 5 days reckoned from the date of disembarkation.
2. A person with symptoms who has come from an infected area within the incubation period of cholera may be required to submit to stool examination, but not to rectal swabbing.
3. Potentially contaminated aircraft water supplies must be disinfected before removal, and terminal disinfection of the aircraft water system must be carried out.
4. All human and other waste matter which is possibly contaminated must be disinfected before removal.
5. Samples of food and beverages on the aircraft (other than those in sealed packages and this includes cargo) may be removed for culture examination.

Once all the measures have been carried out, the aircraft is given free pratique.

Yellow fever

For the purposes of the IHRs, the incubation period of yellow fever is 6 days. A yellow fever certificate is now the only one that should be required in international travel.

The vaccine used must meet WHO requirements, and must be administered at an approved yellow fever vaccinating centre; WHO publish a booklet which lists all such designated centres, also the Institutes manufacturing approved yellow fever vaccines. The vaccination certificate is valid for a period of 10 years commencing 10 days after the date of vaccination; if revaccination is performed within the validity period of a certificate, the new certificate becomes valid immediately.

Vaccination against yellow fever may be required of any person leaving an infected area on an international voyage. If the certificate is not yet valid, he is allowed to depart, but may be subject to health control on arrival.

The following measures are applied by the health authority to persons:

1. Every person employed at an airport in a yellow fever infected area must hold a valid yellow fever vaccination certificate; the same applies to aircrew operating through the airport.
2. A person coming from an infected area without a valid vaccination certificate may be isolated on arrival if the yellow fever vector is present there—either until the certificate is valid, or 6 days have passed since the last possible exposure to infection. If the arrival airport does not have segregation facilities, the person may not be allowed to leave the departure area for the prescribed period. In the Indian sub-continent, as the insect vector, but not the virus, is present, the risk of importation of the disease is controlled by strict vaccination requirements for travellers from yellow fever endemic areas, even for those who have only been in transit through endemic areas, no matter from which country they departed.
3. In an area where the yellow fever vector is present, a suspect case on an arriving aircraft is isolated in mosquito-proof accommodation. Any person on board without a valid certificate is liable to be similarly isolated for the prescribed period.

An aircraft is regarded as infected if a case of yellow fever is on board. An aircraft is deemed 'suspected' if the health authority is not satisfied that disinsection was properly carried out, and has found live mosquitoes on board. Otherwise an aircraft is deemed 'healthy'.

The following measures are applied by health authorities to aircraft:

1. Aircraft leaving an infected area must be disinsected in accordance with Article 25 of the IHRs, using methods approved by WHO. Details of the disinsection are included in the Health part of the Aircraft General Declaration, unless this part is waived by the health authority of the arrival airport.
2. If a case of yellow fever is on board an aircraft arriving in an area where the vector is present, the aircraft is inspected and disinsected. Similar measures may be carried out if the aircraft is deemed 'suspected' as described above.
3. A healthy aircraft coming from a yellow fever infected area may be inspected and disinsected as necessary.
4. If an aircraft leaving an infected area has been disinsected, it may land at any sanitary airport, but otherwise only at airports specified by the State if the yellow fever vector is present in the area.

Health documentation

Personal documentation

Article 81 of the IHRs says that international travellers shall not be required to provide health certificates during international travel, apart from the current requirements for yellow fever, or as demanded by a few countries, cholera.

A model of a correctly completed vaccination certificate is reproduced in Appendix 2 of the IHRs. There are various requirements as follows from countries demanding personal documentation:

1. The certificate must be printed in English and French, and completed in either language.
2. The date must be recorded, for example as 5 January 1986, the medical practitioner must sign in his own handwriting, and the manufacturer and details of the vaccine are recorded. All certificates must bear the stamp of the approved yellow fever vaccination centre.
3. The certificate is rendered invalid by any amendment, erasure or inadequate completion.
4. Certificates are issued to the individual and must be signed by that person. A parent or guardian signs for a child who cannot write, and an illiterate appends his usual mark which is authenticated by another person.
5. A vaccination document issued by the armed forces to an active member of those forces is accepted *in lieu* of the exact format, if it substantially accords with the latter, and contains a statement in English or French that it is issued in accordance with the relevant article of the IHRs; the date and nature of the vaccination is also recorded.
6. If a medical practitioner considers a stipulated vaccination is contraindicated on medical grounds, he should give the traveller his reasons written in English or French, and health authorities are asked to take account of this document, which may refer to the clinical condition or age of the traveller. When the State agrees to waive the requirement for infants under a certain age, this is mentioned under the country's requirements in the WHO booklet *Vaccination Certificate Requirements for Overseas Travel*.

Aircraft documentation

The captain of an aircraft, on landing at the first airport in a territory, may be requested to deliver to the health authority a completed Health Part of the Aircraft General Declaration. This must conform to the model specified in Appendix 4 in the IHRs; he is also required to give any further information requested concerning health conditions on board during the flight. Details must be given of persons who have shown signs of illness on board other than motion sickness or the effects of accidents; details are also required of sick persons who disembarked earlier, and of any conditions on board that may lead to the spread of disease.

Any disinsecting or other sanitary procedure carried out during the flight must be noted, and the serial numbers of single-use aerosol insecticide dispensers expended during disinsection must be recorded. If no disinsection has been carried out during the flight, details must be given of the most recent disinsecting. Recent recommendations on disinsecting of aircraft include application of a residual insecticide film and a Certificate of Residual Disinsection is issued by the health authority. This certificate should be shown along with the Health Part of the Aircraft General Declaration. A health administration may decide to dispense with the requirement to submit the document, or may require it only if there is positive information to report or if the aircraft has come from certain specified areas.

Disinsection of aircraft

Article 83 of the IHRs describes the measures taken to prevent the transmission of insect-borne disease from one country to another. The aim of aircraft disinsecting procedures is to kill infected mosquitoes that have entered the aircraft, and also to destroy potential insect vectors which could become established in the destination area. The success of a major mosquito eradication project in an area could be seriously impaired by the importation of an insecticide-resistant species, or the re-introduction of a vector which had been eradicated from the area. Therefore, before departure on certain international flights, aircraft are treated with chemical insecticides, using an approved aerosol preparation. In passing, it should be mentioned that disinsection of aircraft flying on certain routes is also required to prevent the spread of agricultural pests from one country to another (but this is not under IHRs).

Under the IHRs, every aircraft leaving an area where transmission of malaria or other insect-borne disease occurs has to be disinsected using the methods approved by WHO. These methods have recently been updated (WHO, 1985a) and will be described in another chapter. Residual treatments with permethrin at regular intervals have recently been included in recommendations for disinsection, and a certificate is issued which becomes part of the documentation of the aircraft.

If a health authority is not satisfied that an arriving aircraft has been disinsected properly, or has other cause for concern, the aircraft may be disinsected on arrival. This is carried out before passengers disembark or luggage or freight are unloaded. All external and internal potential resting places receive insecticide spray treatment; the cabin doors, ventilators and other external apertures must be kept closed until spraying has been completed, and for at least 5 minutes thereafter. Details of the disinsecting procedure are entered in the health part of the Aircraft General Declaration.

Disease control into the future

Because of the success of co-ordinated programmes of disease control, notably the eradication of smallpox, the diseases formerly feared no longer constitute a major threat. Effective methods of immunization, vector control and improved therapy have minimized the need for port surveillance. Also the speed of air travel makes the importation of communicable disease in its presymptomatic period a very real possibility. It is possible to circumnavigate the world and keep within the incubation period of most diseases. Only staphylococcal food poisoning can be communicated, incubated and obvious before journey's end but this cannot menace the community.

However, because of the historical success of the international co-operation through application of the IHRs, it is generally agreed that the IHRs should be maintained as an instrument to guide member States for appropriate but flexible action when confronted by disease outbreaks elsewhere in the world.

A co-ordinated programme of disease control at entry to countries was put into action on a global basis during the outbreak of viral haemorrhagic fever in the Sudan and Zaire in 1976. The area was quickly defined and the disease contained, with international controls at airports being highly effective. On arrival, passengers were held on the aircraft until illness on board had been excluded. All passengers who had been in the infected area were identified and put under surveillance. As the disease and vector were unknown, there was some initial panic, but it was found that close and prolonged contact was necessary for secondary cases to occur.

The Committee on International Surveillance of Communicable Diseases in reviewing the outbreak decided against including viral haemorrhagic fever in a specified list as it was agreed that prompt reporting of outbreaks of communicable disease was the best foundation for their international control regardless of whether they are on any particular list.

The introduction of diseases through trade and travel is liable to continue, but with the eradication of smallpox from the world, the value of screening persons at entry to a country has diminished. In the United Kingdom, unless an aircraft captain as required under the Regulations notifies that a case of infectious disease is on board, it is not until the passenger reaches the Immigration desk that he may be referred to the Health Control Unit, as the United Kingdom 1971 Immigration Act permits Immigration Officers to refer certain categories of persons for medical examination.

All countries need to know if outbreaks of disease have occurred elsewhere. Unfortunately, first reports are often publicized in the media and grossly exaggerated before official confirmation. The *Weekly Epidemiological Record* remains the most reliable communication on the subject, and allows international requirements to be amended as necessary, either permanently or temporarily as disease patterns change.

Over the last few years there has been increasing emphasis in this journal on diseases such as hepatitis, tuberculosis, influenza, Legionnaire's disease, and the importance of food-borne disease is increasing all the time. Rabies and malaria remain a threat; and the importance of sexually transmitted diseases never diminishes, particularly with ever-increasing numbers of cases of acquired immunodeficiency syndrome (AIDS).

The acquired immunodeficiency syndrome was first identified in 1981 in the United States and has become a public health problem in a number of countries, with international implications.

An international conference on AIDS in Atlanta, USA was followed by a WHO consultation in April 1985 to review the information presented and assess its international implications. It was concluded that the information available was sufficient to permit health authorities to take action to reduce the incidence in certain risk groups. WHO were to establish a network of collaborating centres and co-ordinate the global surveillance of AIDS, disseminating all information on the disease as widely and rapidly as possible. Recommendations were also made that WHO should play an active role in developing an effective vaccine against the disease (WHO, 1985b).

Information on AIDS continues to be regularly updated in the *Weekly Epidemiological Record* and the numbers of reported cases are increasing all the time. Several countries were demanding certificates of freedom from AIDS at entry. In the *Weekly Epidemiological Record* of 4 October 1985, WHO stated that in accordance with Article 81 of the IHRs, 'no health document, other than those provided for in the Regulations, should be required in international traffic' and 'no country bound by the IHRs should refuse entry to a person who fails to provide a certificate stating he is not carrying the AIDS virus' (WHO, 1985c). However, the incidence of AIDS is increasing at such a rate that, at the present time, it is difficult to predict what controls may eventually be required.

There is no doubt that AIDS is the most important infectious disease of the present time.

The importance of food-borne disease is ever increasing. The Diarrhoeal Diseases Control Programme of WHO has estimated in 1983 that 500 million people travel as tourists every year, and as many as 20–50% get diarrhoea (WHO, 1983b). Vigilance must be kept on mass catering facilities.

International co-operation is essential for the control of infectious disease, and the main defences against the international spread of disease today are detection and elimination of sources of the disease, together with improvement in epidemiological and disease control activities on the national level; exchange of information and education of the travelling public also play a significant part.

No matter how the disease pattern in the world may change, the essential principles embodied in the original IHRs remain the same: namely, that travel should not spread disease, and that travellers should experience minimum inconvenience.

References

International Air Transport Association (1982) *Handling of Human Remains*. Airport Handling Manual 353 Section 3 Sheet 1.

International Civil Aviation Organisation (1983) *Technical Instructions for the Safe Transport of Dangerous Goods by Air*. Annex 18 to the Convention on International Civil Aviation, 1st edn. The Safe Transport of Dangerous Goods by Air. Montreal: ICAO

World Health Organisation (1969) *International Health Regulations*. Geneva: WHO

World Health Organisation (1973a) *WHO Official Records*, No. 209, p. 29 (Resolution WHA 26.55). Geneva: WHO

World Health Organisation (1973b) *Chemotherapy of Malaria and Resistance to Antimalarials*. Technical Report Series 529. Geneva: WHO

World Health Organisation (1980) *Guidelines for Cholera Control*. WHO/CDD/SER/80.4. Geneva: WHO

World Health Organisation (1983a) *International Health Regulations*, 3rd annotated edn. Geneva: WHO

World Health Organisation (1983b) Food safety: the role of food in the epidemiology of acute enteric infections and intoxications. *Weekly Epidemiological Record*, **58**, 241

World Health Organisation (1985a) Recommendations on the disinsecting of aircraft. *Weekly Epidemiological Record*, **45**, 45–47, 90, 345–346

World Health Organisation (1985b) Acquired immune deficiency syndrome (AIDS). WHO consultations. *Weekly Epidemiological Record*, **60**, 129–130

World Health Organisation (1985c) International health regulations. *Weekly Epidemiological Record*, **60**, 311

World Health Organisation (1985d) Functioning of the international health regulations for the period 1 January to 31 December 1984. *Weekly Epidemiological Record*, **60**, 387–388

World Health Organisation (1986) World Malaria Situation 1984. *World Health Statistics Quarterly*, **39**, 171–205

37

Epidemiological and immunological problems in international travel

J.M. Stewart

Introduction

In 1985–86 19.7 million passengers were carried by British Airways alone (British Airways, 1986). World-wide many hundred million passengers were transported at speeds that enabled them to complete their journey well within the incubation period of most infectious diseases. As a result of this, constant surveillance must be maintained at ports of entry and ultimate destinations in order to prevent outbreaks of disease, normally foreign to the area, from being imported into and possibly established in new locations. Maegraith (1963) in his classic treatise *Unde Venis* reminds us that 'eternal vigilance is essential if preventable tragedies are to be avoided.'

There are, of course, natural barriers—for example, climatic conditions prevent the establishment of diseases where the vectors cannot survive in the country of arrival. Thus although around 2000 cases of malaria are imported into Britain each year, each is an individual rather than a public health problem. Similarly, in countries with a high standard of hygiene it is unlikely that imported cases of cholera will become a serious threat. Outbreaks of typhoid and other faecal–oral spread diseases do occur but are normally quickly contained. However, in the absence of vigilance and the presence of civil or general war, natural disasters (earthquake, floods, etc.) or strikes by key workers in the water industry, serious outbreaks of disease in a non-immune community could arise.

A major triumph has occurred in recent years. The World Health Organisation (WHO) has been responsible for the successful eradication of smallpox. The last case of naturally transmitted disease occurred in Somalia in 1977. There were two laboratory acquired infections in the UK in 1978. No cases have occurred since, enabling the following declaration to be made in Geneva.

Declaration of global eradication of smallpox

The Thirty-Third World Health Assembly, on this 8th day of May 1980;
Having considered the development and results of the global programme on smallpox eradication initiated by WHO in 1958 and intensified since 1967:

1. Declared solemnly that the world and all its peoples have won freedom from smallpox, which was a most devastating disease, sweeping in epidemic form through many countries since earliest times, leaving death, blindness and disfigurement in its wake and which only a decade ago was rampant in Africa, Asia, and South America.
2. Expresses its deep gratitude to all nations and individuals who contributed to the success of this noble and historic endeavour.
3. Calls this unprecedented achievement in the history of public health to the attention of all nations, which by their collective action have freed mankind of this ancient scourge and, in so doing, have demonstrated how nations working together in a common cause may further human progress.

As a result of this, the *Weekly Epidemiological Record* of the WHO (WHO, 1986b) reporting the fourth meeting of the committee of orthopox virus infection stated:

'WHO has been informed that all of its Member States have discontinued routine vaccination. No country in the world now requires a certificate of smallpox vaccination from international travellers ....In 1984 seven countries produced smallpox vaccine totalling 3.8 million doses. Some of this production was for vaccination of military personnel.... WHO maintains reserve stocks of smallpox vaccine sufficient to protect 200 million people... more than 102 million doses of smallpox vaccine are held in 22 countries... the two laboratories which continue to hold stocks of variola virus, namely the Centers for Disease Control (CDC) Atlanta United States of America and the Research Institute for Viral Preparations, Moscow, USSR, were visited most recently by WHO inspection teams in November 1985 and January 1986 respectively. The inspection reports were satisfactory for both laboratories.'

Whilst the continuing vaccination of troops in some countries denies us complete peace of mind for the future, smallpox is at present no threat and smallpox vaccination is, by virtue of its distinct risks, contraindicated on medical grounds. It may in the future be possible to eliminate other diseases in a similar manner, for example measles and malaria— but the logistic and technical problems are immense.

More recently other diseases have caused public concern and much media coverage, notably the viral haemorrhagic fevers (Lassa fever, Marburg fever and Ebola virus disease). Public anxiety has probably been overstated but suspected cases should be managed using a high-security laboratory and strict isolation.

In the case of acquired immune deficiency syndrome the public, in the United Kingdom at least, is only now becoming aware of a disease which, if a means of controlling it is long delayed, will become as great a scourge as the Black Death or smallpox. In parts of Africa, this is already apparent. In the absence of a cure, the only hope of containing the epidemic would appear to be a radical change in the sexual behaviour of the majority of people. In the short term at least this may be an optimistic hope. Meanwhile education of all, not only the high-risk groups, screening of blood and treatment of blood products, a return to barrier methods of contraception for males, notification of cases and counselling of carriers as well as in some circumstances screening of individuals may slow down the spread of the disease.

International Health Regulations

'The International Health Regulations adopted by the Twenty Second World Health Assembly in 1969 represent a revised and consolidated version of the previous International Sanitary Regulations' (WHO, 1969). 'The purpose of the International Health Regulations is to help prevent the international spread of diseases and in the context of international travel to do so with the minimum inconvenience to the passenger' (WHO, 1987). To

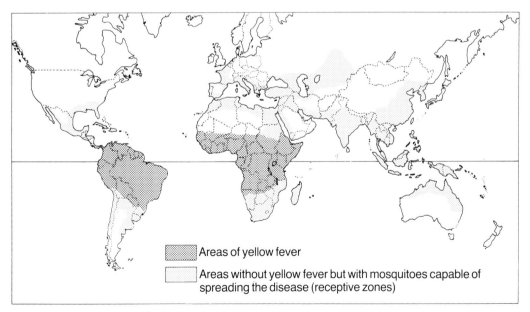

Areas of yellow fever

Areas without yellow fever but with mosquitoes capable of spreading the disease (receptive zones)

Figure 37.1 Geographical distribution of yellow fever and of mosquitoes capable of spreading yellow fever. (Reproduced from Dawood, R. (1986) *Travellers Health*, p. 114, Oxford University Press, with kind permission of author and publishers.)

this end, all countries are required to collaborate with each other through the WHO and to maintain national epidemiological services equipped to identify and control outbreaks of disease.

A looser, less legalistic approach than formerly to disease control led in 1973 to the Twenty Sixth World Health Assembly amending the Regulations with regard to cholera vaccination certificates. Vaccination does not prevent the spread of the disease across national boundaries. It was therefore logical to drop the requirement for an International Certificate. However, in 1986, 12 countries still required evidence of cholera vaccination if a traveller has come from an infected area and a further three require certification from travellers whose destination is a country which will require evidence of vaccination on leaving it.

In 1981, the Thirty Fourth World Health Assembly amended the Regulations to exclude the requirement of smallpox vaccination certificates. As previously stated this has finally been accepted world-wide.

Thus it will be seen that the only mandatory vaccination certificate should be for yellow fever. The disease is endemic in parts of Africa and South America (*Figure 37.1*).

Travellers to these areas should be vaccinated, though if only cities or unaffected areas are visited there is no epidemiological reason for it. Many countries do require evidence in the form of an International Certificate of Vaccination even if the traveller has only been in transit through an endemic zone. This is particularly rigidly enforced for persons travelling to the Indian sub-continent or Asia. It seems odd, though, that these potentially receptive areas with similar climate and the right vector for the disease have never experienced it. There must surely be some other factor, at present unknown, which prevents its establishment there.

Immunization requirements for international travel

From the above it will be clear that the number of mandatory immunizations required for international travel is small.

There are, however, a number that are strongly *recommended* both for the protection of the individual and for the control of disease in the community. These will be discussed individually later, together with a brief mention of the extremely important subject of malaria.

Exclusion of infectious disease

No airline will knowingly accept a case of infectious disease on any scheduled aircraft. Such exclusion

will even normally apply to the common childhood exanthemata during the infectious stage, because any aircraft complement may include expectant mothers, infants within either a few days or weeks of birth and elderly and infirm passengers—all of whom could be adversely affected by exposure to any infectious illness. Effective isolation is not possible in modern pressurized aircraft where there is a common ventilation system throughout.

Liberties of the individual

Irrespective of specific contraindications to any particular vaccine, enquiries may be received from prospective travellers who object to immunization on medical, religious, conscientious, or other grounds. Such individuals may be required to absolve the air carrier from any individual expenditure, difficulties or delays en route, and they should be advised that they may face isolation in quarantine in uncongenial surroundings for non-compliance with the conditions of entry into any country. Certainly, if time permits, passengers with irregular travel documents should obtain prior permission from the country of destination before ever embarking on their journey. Each case must be judged on its own merits. If there is no obvious risk of delays, fines or repatriation, most airlines will accept such passengers. Occasionally there are specific medical contraindications to immunizations:

1. Vaccines should not be administered to people suffering from acute infections.
2. Live vaccines should not be administered to those who are immunologically suppressed, i.e. the following:
   (a) patients taking steroids, or receiving radiotherapy or cytotoxic drugs.
   (b) Patients suffering from malignant disease.
   (c) Patients with gamma globulin deficiency.
   (d) Patients who are HIV positive.
3. Subjects with allergies to eggs or the various antibiotics that are constituents of the vaccines may react adversely to them, and all recipients should be questioned about this. Facilities for treatment of anaphylaxis should always be at hand. There should ideally be an interval of 3 weeks between the administration of live vaccines. Where this is not possible they may be administered on the same day at different sites.
4. Though all travel vaccines may be given to pregnant women if absolutely necessary, on theoretical grounds they are best avoided. Where an exemption certificate for yellow fever vaccination is acceptable and where no risk of the disease exists, this should be supplied. Killed (Salk) polio vaccine may be given if indicated instead of live Sabin. Of the killed vaccines,

typhoid in particular may produce a systemic reaction sufficient to induce abortion and should be avoided unless the risk of infection is great. Suitable advice regarding water purification and the hygienic preparation of food is essential. Occasionally it may be necessary to question the wisdom of travel.

Aircraft General Declaration of Health

The health administration of any territory may require the commander of an aircraft on an international journey to complete the Health Part of the Aircraft General Declaration, with notification of any persons on board suffering from illness, other than travel sickness. Particular reference is made to those with symptoms or signs suggestive of infectious disease such as rash or other skin manifestation, fever, chill, diarrhoea and vomiting. Most airline operators advise flying staff to report any such illness by means of air-to-ground communication prior to arrival, so that the local health authority may have advance notification of the possibility of an infectious disorder. Such air-to-ground communication may well prevent delays to service.

Specific vaccinations/immunizations

These are as follows:

1. Yellow fever.
2. Cholera.
3. Typhoid.
4. Poliomyelitis.
5. Tetanus.
6. Diphtheria.
7. Rabies.
8. Hepatitis A.
9. Hepatitis B.
10. Meningococcal meningitis.
11. Japanese encephalitis.
12. BCG.
13. Plague, tick encephalitis and pneumococcal pneumonia.

Yellow fever

Normally a zoonosis of monkeys in tropical rain forests, the disease is occasionally transmitted to man, who initiates the urban cycle. This is the only vaccination for which an international certificate should be required for travel into or between endemic areas and from endemic areas into receptive zones. The vaccine is a specially stabilized freeze-dried preparation of the living attenuated 17D strain of yellow fever virus which is avirulent

for man. It is propagated in chick embryos and contains neomycin sulphate and polymixin B sulphate. It is suitable for adults and children over the age of 9 months; reconstituted vaccine 0.5 ml is given subcutaneously and is the dose for all ages. Primary vaccination is valid for 10 years 10 days after vaccination and immediately following revaccination within 10 years of the last dose. An international certificate is valid only if the vaccine has been approved by the WHO and administered at a designated yellow fever vaccination centre.

Cholera

Cholera is a severe acute gastrointestinal infection caused by *Vibrio cholerae*. Classic cholera was responsible for devastating epidemics in India and the Far East. The recent pandemic began in 1961 and is caused by the biotype El Tor. Safe water and hygienic disposal of excreta prevents its spread in Europe but it is now endemic in the Near East and Africa as well as India and the Far East. Prevention is primarily by stringent hygiene and sanitary precautions in the preparation and handling of water and food. Now that air travel has replaced the caravan routes of earlier days the hygiene standards at each sector of a journey must be vigorously maintained.

Immunization against cholera does not prevent an individual from becoming a carrier, though it does confer up to 50% protection for the individual for up to 6 months (Wellcome Foundation, 1984). The vaccine contains *Vibrio cholerae*, serotypes Inaba and Ogawa with or without the El Tor biotype. Where the El Tor biotype is not included there is evidence of cross-immunity between the El Tor and classic cholera organisms. A primary course consists of two subcutaneous or intramuscular injections of vaccine preferably at least 1 month apart. This course need never be repeated as there will be a satisfactory anamnestic response to one booster at any time after the primary course. Second and subsequent doses may be given intradermally. As a single injection has been shown to induce a significant response and is enough for certification where required, and as the protection afforded is short lived (6 months), it may be felt that one injection is sufficient for most journeys, though for continued protection a primary course of two is recommended. The certificate becomes valid 6 days after the first dose, or immediately if boosted within 6 months of the previous dose.

Typhoid

Typhoid is endemic world-wide. It is a disease of poor hygiene and primitive sanitation which is spread by the faecal–oral route. In countries with good sanitation, the disease is normally spread by food handlers who are carriers. Immunization with monovalent typhoid vaccine is recommended for travel outside North Europe, North America, Australia and New Zealand, particularly for over-landers, trekkers, etc.—although a variable degree of risk exists anywhere where there may be a breakdown in the hygiene chain due to poor supervision or training of kitchen staff in endemic areas or to inadequate chlorination of water supplies.

As with cholera vaccination, one dose induces a significant response for several months (Wellcome Foundation, 1984) but for longer term protection two doses should be administered at an interval of 4–6 weeks. This course will protect for up to 3 years after which a booster should be given for further protection. If not, one injection on later travel is sufficient to produce immunity for a further 3 years.

The recommended dosage for primary immuniza-tion of adults is 0.5 ml given subcutaneously or intramuscularly though, in order to prevent reac-tions, the intradermal route (0.1 ml) may be preferred. This is generally accepted practice for the second and booster doses. Dick (1981) quoted studies which showed that the serum antibody response indicated no difference in efficacy whether the intradermal or subcutaneous routes were used even for first doses. Many centres use the in-tradermal method for all doses with a considerable lessening of unpleasant side effects.

An oral live attenuated vaccine, currently being used in Germany and Switzerland, which gives a high degree of protection, will become generally available in the near future.

Poliomyelitis

Before 1956 when the Salk poliomyelitis vaccine was first used, the disease was prevalent world-wide. In countries with a high rate of vaccination it occurs only sporadically so that in those countries the unvaccinated have little chance of acquiring 'natu-ral' immunity. For this reason it is most important that when travelling to areas where the disease is still prevalent, non-immune subjects should receive a full course of vaccine prior to travel. Others, who have had a full course, are advised to boost their protection after 10 years. People born much prior to 1956 may well have naturally acquired immunity to one or more strains but will still benefit from protection unless they are shown to be immune to all three polio viruses.

In the UK trivalent Sabin oral vaccine is generally used. Three doses at intervals of not less than 4 weeks constitute a primary course. In pregnancy or if there is a contraindication to a live vaccine the Salk inactivated vaccine may be given. Both types of vaccine contain very minute amounts of antibiotics including penicillin but this does not normally contraindicate their use except in extreme cases of hypersensitivity (Joint Committee on Vaccination and Immunisation, 1984).

Tetanus

It is wise for everyone to be protected against tetanus. Travel overseas is often an opportunity to initiate or bring up to date this protection. A primary course of adsorbed tetanus vaccine is two deep subcutaneous or intramuscular injections 0.5 ml at an interval of 6–12 weeks followed by a third 6–12 months later. Routine boosters are recommended every 10 years or *on injury* after 2–5 years if the wound appears to carry a high risk of tetanus. Too frequent dosage is apt to produce hypersensitivity reactions and should be avoided (Wellcome Foundation, 1984). In case of severe reactions to previous doses, tetanus vaccine in simple solution may be used in a dose of 0.1 ml intradermally. This preparation is not advised for primary immunization or for use in conjunction with antitetanus immunoglobulin.

Diphtheria

In many parts of the world diphtheria is still prevalent though in the developed countries, due to childhood immunization, the disease is rare and nearly all cases are imported. When the organism circulated freely most adults would have been immune but with routine immunization interrupting transmission of the organism, increasing numbers of adults are susceptible (Walker and Williams, 1985). Adults at high risk of infection should be immunized or receive booster injections. Schick testing is unnecessary if the low dose (2IU) preparation of the vaccine is used.

Rabies

Pre-exposure immunization against rabies is now frequently practised using human diploid cell rabies vaccine. This is particularly recommended for those travelling off the beaten track or to areas where vaccine may be hard to obtain. It should also be considered for expatriate families and others whose travel takes them to rabies endemic zones. Two doses of 0.1 ml intradermally (excellent technique is essential) or of 1 ml intramuscularly or by deep subcutaneous injection given at an interval of 4 weeks with a third after 6–12 months constitutes a primary course. This should be followed by boosters every 2 years if at continued risk or on later travel to endemic areas. The first two doses may be followed by an antibody test to confirm adequate seroconversion. The pre-exposure course does *not* obviate the need for treatment after a bite but booster doses only are needed and rabies immune globulin, often difficult to obtain overseas, is not required.

Hepatitis A

Until a suitable vaccine for hepatitis A is available human normal immunoglobulin should be offered for protection prior to travel in areas of dubious hygiene and primitive sanitation. In the older age groups or in those who have lived overseas as well as those giving a history of 'jaundice', it is wise to check for antibodies to the disease as a previous attack (either clinical or subclinical) will confer life-long immunity and remove the need for passive protection.

Hepatitis B

In certain areas of sub-Saharan Africa and the Far East up to 30% of the general population may be serum HBsAg positive (Fagan and Williams, 1986). Bearing in mind the mode of spread of the disease, some groups are recommended to be protected by vaccination. This applies particularly to health workers, and those exposed sexually or through drug abuse. For protection two 1 ml injections are given at a 4-week interval followed by a third 6 months after the first. Where possible it is wise to check anti-HBs levels 4 weeks after the last injection of the basic course of immunization. This gives an indication as to when it would be wise to give booster injections to those still at risk (Jilg *et al.*, 1984).

Meningococcal meningitis

Suitable polysaccharide vaccines against meningococcal meningitis A and/or C are available for travellers to highly endemic zones (e.g. the Sahel region of sub-Saharan Africa) or to areas where the disease is currently epidemic.

Japanese encephalitis

An arbovirus infection, Japanese encephalitis is endemic and occasionally epidemic in the Far East and Oceania, now spreading across the Indian sub-continent. A monovalent Japanese Encephalitis Vaccine (Biken) is available, for those at risk. Three 1 ml doses are recommended at 7–10 day intervals with annual boosters when at risk.

BCG (bacille Calmette Guérin)

This vaccine is recommended for all those who are tuberculin negative when travelling to areas of high prevalence of tuberculosis. A 3-week interval should be allowed to elapse between this and any other live vaccine. No further immunization should be given for at least 3 months on the arm used for BCG vaccination because of the risk of regional lymphadenitis (Walker and Williams, 1985).

Plague and tick-borne encephalitis

Vaccines against plague and tick-borne encephalitis are also available. These may be indicated for travellers in circumstances of particular risk. Polyvalent pneumococcal vaccine is indicated for patients with splenectomy who are at increased risk of this disease.

Malaria

This is not the place to discuss malaria at length but, sadly, it presents the other side of the coin to the successful campaign against smallpox. Insecticide resistance, lack of finance and less rigidly imposed disciplines in eradication campaigns together with ever-increasing drug resistance reflect a deteriorating situation world-wide in the control of malaria.

Whatever drug regimen is employed in prophylaxis, the principal aim must be to avoid bites by malarial mosquitoes by all means possible—nets, sprays, residual insecticides, repellants, coils, suitable clothing, etc. Proguanil 200 mg daily and/or chloroquine 300 mg base weekly remain the bastion of prophylaxis but in resistant areas this must be supplemented by other drugs (such as Maloprim—pyrimethamine 12.5 mg plus dapsone 100 mg). In the presence of resistant strains it is sensible, if travelling in areas remote from medical help, to carry additional *therapeutic* drugs in appropriate dosage in case of breakthrough—Fansidar (pyrimethamine 25 mg plus sulfadoxine 500 mg) or Mefloquine or a combination of the two (Fansimef). Aircrew are advised not to take chloroquine prophylactically because of the temporary effect it may have on visual accommodation.

Work is proceeding on the production of a vaccine that will be effective against malaria but at present this seems to be a dream for the future.

References

British Airways (1986) *Review of the Year—1985–86*. London: British Airways

DICK, G. (1981) *Mims Magazine*, 1 Feb.

FAGAN, E.A. and WILLIAMS, R. (1986) Hepatitis B vaccination and the traveller. *Travel Medicine International*, **4**, 2.59–68

JILG, W., SCHMIDT, M., RINEHARDT, F. and ZACHONAL, R. (1984) Hepatitis B vaccination; how long does it last? *Lancet*, **ii**, 458

Joint Committee on Vaccination and Immunisation (1984) *Immunisation Against Infectious Disease* (prepared by the Joint Committee on Vaccination and Immunisation for the Secretary of State for Social Services, the Secretary of State for Scotland and the Secretary of State for Wales). London: HMSO

MAEGRAITH, B. (1963) *Unde Venis. Lancet*, **i**, 403–404

WALKER, E. and WILLIAMS, G. (1985) *ABC of Healthy Travel—Articles from the British Medical Journal*, 2nd edn. London: British Medical Association

Wellcome Foundation Limited (1984) *Protection and Prevention*. London: The Wellcome Foundation

World Health Organisation (1969) *International Health Regulations*, 3rd Annotated edn. Geneva: World Health Organisation

World Health Organisation (1986) *Weekly Epid miological Record*, 19 Sep.

World Health Organisation (1987) *Vaccination Certificate Requirements and Health Advice for International Travel*. Geneva: World Health Organisation

38

Airline hygiene

P.J. Jerram

Introduction

International air travel has introduced its own special hygiene problems by bringing aircrews and passengers into rapid contact with new and varied situations before they have had time to acquire immunity or resistance to local diseases. Accustomed to safe water and food in their home countries, they have no choice but to accept what is offered either on the aircraft or at airports.

It is therefore vital that crews and passengers be safeguarded as far as possible from any health hazard. Some of the measures that should be taken to afford this protection are described in this chapter.

Aircraft catering

Since an airline is often assessed by the quality of the meals served on board, it is important to provide food of a high gastronomical quality, pleasing to the eye and acceptable to the taste. At the same time all food should be free from any bacteria or toxins that could cause discomfort or illness to the consumer and therefore precautions must be taken to prevent food poisoning on board.

Clearly, food poisoning that occurred during flight may in certain circumstances jeopardize the safety of the aircraft. One way to reduce the risk of its occurrence is by strict enforcement of the rule that the pilot and co-pilot must always eat completely different meals. Food hygiene in aircraft catering must be given a high priority which must not be lowered in the desire to satisfy operational and commercial targets.

While risks may be present in many countries, the uplift of meals from tropical countries demands extra vigilance to counteract the additional problems created by higher ambient temperatures, the prevalence of intestinal illnesses, the possibility of sub-standard premises and equipment, and often a lack of appreciation by food handlers of the possible causes and dangers of food-borne infections.

Since all food handlers, including cabin crew, ought to be free from any infection, it is advisable that they should satisfy a pre-employment medical examination which should include bacteriological and microscopic examination of stool specimens. They should also be medically cleared before returning to employment after absence due to sickness or after contact with any disease that could be transmitted by food. They should attend training classes and lectures on food hygiene and their personal hygiene should be frequently checked by, for example, the bacteriological examination of swabs taken from fingers.

Aircraft meals are supplied from the following categories of kitchens:

1. Those maintained by the airline and under its direct control.
2. Premises staffed and controlled by a catering contractor, but with surveillance by the airline.
3. Establishments of a catering contractor with no surveillance by the airline.

Whenever possible, category (1) is recommended, but economics are often the deciding factor. Category (3) should be employed only where the uplift is so small that any other system is impracticable.

In all cases the airline must retain the right of inspection, and it must be agreed that samples of food may be collected, as required, for bacteriological or other examination. Raw materials for aircraft meals must be of the highest quality as regards hygiene and, in particular, meat must be obtained only from fully inspected sources, the inspections being carried out by appropriately qualified local health inspectors or the caterer's own inspecting officials.

Certain foods present special risks, since they provide good media for the growth of bacteria. Examples are seafoods and cold meats (especially when excessively handled in preparation), fresh cream which has been inadequately heat-treated, or mayonnaise with a pH above 4.0. Wherever possible, menus should exclude such foods. Furthermore, oysters, clams, prawns and other shell-fish should not be used unless it is certain that they are fresh, that they are from non-infected sources, and that they are not likely to have been contaminated in handling, storage, transportation or preparation.

A modern trend in flight catering, particularly among charter companies, is to double-cater, that is, to provide meals for the return flight from the parent station. It is easy to see the potential danger in this practice, particularly where delays occur, and strict temperature control is therefore essential. Meals for the return flight must be held in refrigeration, i.e. below 10°C, during the outward flight. This can be achieved either by the use of solid carbon dioxide (dry ice) placed in the meal containers, or of specially insulated meal trays which hold the food at a near-constant temperature for several hours. The problem is not so acute on aircraft that have adequate in-built refrigeration.

Aircraft meals are often prepared many hours before they are eaten. During this time, if conditions are favourable to their growth, any potential food-poisoning organisms present could multiply. It is therefore vital to exercise strict temperature control. All cold meals must be stored at temperatures below 10°C, and all hot meals above 63°C. If an aircraft departure is delayed, and the meal cannot be served within the time limit for which it was prepared, it should be destroyed. Without refrigeration, this is usually a maximum of 4 hours. Because of the limited time available, bacteriological examination cannot be performed before the aircraft food is served. The avoidance of any contamination is therefore of added importance. However, frequent bacteriological examination of meals should be carried out where possible and appropriate remedial action taken when results are unsatisfactory. All large flight-catering establishments should have the necessary laboratory facilities for such examinations.

Deep-frozen meals, provided they are prepared hygienically, are by far the safest. They can be bacteriologically cleared before leaving the unit and, being transported in a frozen condition, can be used for second or third meals on long sectors or for supplying overseas stations.

All aircraft catering premises should be frequently inspected to ensure that any appropriate statutory regulations (e.g. the Food Hygiene (General) Regulations (1970) in the UK (HMSO, 1970)), the recommendations of the World Health Organisation (1960, 1977) and the requirements of the customer airline are being observed. Emphasis must always be placed on personal hygiene, and the provision of a bactericidal soap for hand-washing is strongly recommended. Cleaning and sterilization of equipment, and all surfaces with which food comes into contact, is essential. Where a temperature of at least 85°C for a hot water rinse cannot be guaranteed, an efficient chemical sterilizing agent should be used.

All salad items should be washed for 5 minutes in a solution of hypochlorite containing 50 parts per million (ppm) of available chlorine, and cabin crews should be instructed that the only ice they may place in passengers' or crew members' drinks must be made in ice-cube machines from chlorinated water, and supplied to the aircraft in sealed bags. Since milk and fresh cream are good media for the growth of organisms, only heat-treated products should be used.

The use of disposable catering articles such as piping bags, gloves, head covers, etc., is commended, while single-piece cutting boards made from synthetic rubber or other suitable composition are readily cleansed and sanitized and are generally much more hygienic than those made from wood, which often have open joints.

In the event of suspected food poisoning on an aircraft, every effort must be made to identify the cause. Samples of the suspected food should be obtained and sent for appropriate laboratory examination, so that the source may be traced if possible. It is also useful if cabin crew can record detailed information of the food and drink taken by the affected passengers or crew during the previous 24 hours, the times of consumption of the food and drink, and the onset of symptoms.

As passengers and crew may sometimes eat and drink at airports before or after flying, and while in transit, airport restaurants, bars, etc. should be frequently inspected to ensure that they operate only under the highest standards of hygiene. In addition, hotels where crew may be accommodated should be frequently inspected to ensure that any risks to crew members of contracting food poisoning or other associated infections (e.g. from the swimming pool or drinking water supply) are minimal.

Aircraft drinking water

International airlines operate through many countries in which water-borne diseases are endemic and where sanitation may be of a low standard. Aircraft do not carry sufficient water to last throughout an entire multi-sector flight, so that they are forced to uplift water from overseas sources. Consequently water-borne diseases can be spread through the medium of aircraft water supplies, and therefore water carried on aircraft for human consumption should be free from organisms or impurities that could cause illness.

All airports must have a pure water supply, and suitable equipment for loading water onto aircraft and for supplying the needs of passengers and crews on the ground. Samples for bacteriological examination should be collected frequently from different parts of the airport (e.g. the aircraft catering unit, the aircraft drinking water bowsers and the fill points used for the bowsers) to ensure that they meet the standards of purity laid down by the World Health Organisation (1984). Drinking water, in addition to being safe, must also be palatable, and free from turbidity, colour and odour.

During transit stops there is no time to drain, clean and refill aircraft water systems. Sufficient water is therefore pumped in to replace the water consumed during the previous stage of flight. As the flight proceeds, water on the aircraft thus becomes a mixture of various sources and quality.

Systems

The most basic system employs a special container, usually with a capacity of only a few gallons and designed to carry a sufficient supply for the drinking and culinary needs of passengers on a short flight. This is the only potable water on the aircraft, and should have been suitably treated with an appropriate sterilizing agent. Other supplies of water on the aircraft are designated 'unsuitable for drinking'. This system is not foolproof, since some passengers might still drink from or clean their teeth in supplies designated 'unsuitable for drinking' and subsequently develop water-borne infections if these supplies are polluted.

Most modern aircraft have large-capacity water storage tanks constructed of welded stainless steel or reinforced fibre glass. A single system supplies all the needs of the catering, drinking and hand-washing facilities throughout the aircraft, each point being fed either by gravity or through a pressurized system. This water must be suitably treated to make it wholesome. The advantage of this system is that only one quality of water is available, namely potable water. This is the normal standard on international services.

Because of the mixed supply of water resulting from the various points of uplift and the fact that the quality varies from country to country, it is necessary to carry out some form of treatment which will be a safeguard against possible contamination. This treatment is still required even when the purity of the mains water supply at an overseas airport can

be guaranteed, the reason being that at most airports, water that is uplifted may become polluted in unsterilized bowsers, hoses, hydrants or valves, or in the aircraft water tanks themselves, which can be sterilized only on return to base.

Treatment usually consists of adding chlorine in some easily handled form such as sodium hypochlorite to give at least 0.3 ppm residual chlorine or alternatively Chloramine T at a concentration of 16 ppm. Either substance will guarantee that the water remains pure in the aircraft tanks and pipes. Powder is preferable to tablets because it dissolves almost instantly.

There is less chance of contamination if the water is taken direct from a mains supply to the aircraft tanks, but it is still essential to introduce into the aircraft tanks a chlorinating substance which is usually metered in via an automatic injection unit. At present only a few airports enjoy the advantage of having mains water supply points available at aircraft parking bays, but this facility should be introduced wherever possible, since it eliminates the need for water bowsers, reduces the risk of contamination, and increases the palatability of the water.

It is essential that bowsers and delivery hoses, where still used, are regularly sterilized by hyper-chlorination. At all maintenance checks aircraft tanks must be sterilized. One method is by filling the entire water system with a solution of sodium hypochlorite to give 50 ppm available chlorine and leaving for 30 minutes before draining completely. The system is then thoroughly flushed with fresh water. By increasing the strength of the solution to 200 ppm available chlorine the contact time can be reduced to 5 minutes. At major checks the tanks should be removed for scouring and steaming. They should then be completely overhauled and after replacing, be sterilized by hyperchlorination.

Portable drinking water containers require cleaning and sterilization by hyperchlorination at each out-station, and on return to base. The delivery tap also should be cleaned and sterilized, and then protected with a polythene cover until delivered to the aircraft.

To test that the water contains the correct amount of free chlorine, some simple means of testing should be available. One such test is by the use of diethyl-p-phenylene diamine tablets, which indicate, by a colour change, correct or excessive chlorination. These water-testing tablets should be supplied where relevant to servicing engineers, catering officers and cabin crew.

To avoid complaints from passengers should the water become over-chlorinated, some form of on-board dechlorination is required and usually comprises tablets which are added to the water by the cabin crew.

In order to maintain a consistently high quality of

water, cabin crews and others responsible should be carefully instructed on the importance of their responsibilities in maintaining water tanks, water bowsers, portable flasks, etc. in a hygienic condition.

Samples of the water remaining in the tanks of aircraft arriving at base from abroad should be taken at regular intervals and submitted for bacteriological examination, the results being classified according to the WHO *Guidelines for Drinking-Water Quality* (1984). A system of constant supervision should be established, and there should always be close liaison with the Local Port Health and other relevant Health Authorities.

If water bowsers are employed, certain supply points at airports should be reserved exclusively for them. The tap should be protected and the end of the delivery hose immersed in a chlorine solution or covered in a plastic bag. In order to reduce accidental pollution, water filling points for toilet servicing units should be sited at least 30 m (100 feet) away from the water bowser filling points, and personnel engaged in operating drinking water bowsers must not also operate the toilet servicing units.

Aircraft toilets

Toilets in modern aircraft are basically chemical closets with retention tanks holding sewage until it can be conveniently discharged. They incorporate a complex mechanical flushing system, including a filtering arrangement to separate solids from liquids, and the latter are utilized in a recirculating cycle to clean the bowl.

The operation varies but is usually electrically operated. A solenoid energizes an electric timer and motor which simultaneously drive a pump and a mechanical self-cleaning filter. The pump draws liquid through the rotating filter and pumps it through a toilet bowl flush-ring into the bowl with a swirling action.

The bowl should be designed so as to produce an efficient cleansing action which will carry the deposits into the retention tank. The cycle takes about 15 seconds. When the circuit opens, the motor stops and the system is ready for the next operation.

An alternative method of operating the flushing system is by means of lowering or raising the toilet seat lid. When the lid is raised an air pump piston moves downward and air compressed in the bottom of the cylinder passes into the recirculatory piping, so forcing the water in the pipe out through the bowl flushing ring. As the piston moves downward, the upper part of the cylinder is charged with air ready for the reverse stroke. The emptying of the pipe causes a ball-valve to drop clear of its seating and admit filtered water from the tank for the next flushing operation. Lowering the seat lid moves the

air pump forward, closing the upper inlet valve and forcing the compressed air through to repeat the flushing cycle.

In both systems a minimum initial charge of liquid is required so that the flushing mechanism can operate immediately after the toilet is used. The minimum quantity of liquid should not be exceeded otherwise the tank capacity will be reduced. Construction of the system should be of stainless steel.

Aircraft toilets do not provide any treatment of excreta. To eliminate the possibility of disease transmission it is therefore essential to add a chemical to the water, and the chemical should possess the following essential qualities:

1. Be bactericidal against faecal-type organisms in the presence of faeces and urine within 15 minutes.
2. Be capable of preventing the development of any faecal, ammoniacal or other unpleasant odour, even at tropical temperatures.
3. Have detergent properties to facilitate the cleansing of the toilet.
4. Be consistent in performance and stable in storage for at least 12 months, at temperatures ranging from 1°C to 54°C.
5. Be non-corrosive to any of the metals or fabrics with which it may come into contact.
6. Be non-staining and non-irritating to human skin and membranes.
7. Have a flash point higher than 65°C.
8. Not produce gases at reduced cabin pressure when mixed with excreta.
9. Be non-detrimental to the correct biological working of sewage disposal plants.
10. Maintain when fully diluted a distinctive and aesthetically acceptable colour.
11. Remain bactericidal at its maximum dilution in a full toilet.

The chemical is usually purchased as a liquid or as a powder. Many different products are available. Unfortunately, some are little more than deodorants, while others (which usually contain quaternary ammonium compounds and/or formaldehyde) conform to the bactericidal requirement mentioned above. When the chemical is a liquid it is usually metered at the correct dosage rate into the fresh-water tank of the toilet servicing trolley (*see* next paragraph), and when a powder it is added in sachet form in water-soluble packages to each toilet after recharging with fresh water, following the emptying and flushing operations. Different-sized sachets are used according to the capacity of the toilet tanks.

All airports require adequate facilities for the hygienic removal and disposal of the contents of aircraft toilets, and they should be such that all hazards to health are eliminated. A special toilet servicing trolley, provided with a sewage tank and a fresh-water tank for flushing and recharging the toilets, and some means for ensuring that the chemical is added in correct concentration and quantity, are essential.

The ideal method of disposal is into a main sewer, or the airport sewage system. At all disposal points, adequate facilities for cleaning, washing and flushing must be provided, together with hand-washing arrangements for the operators. Toilet servicing operatives occasionally become contaminated accidentally by effluent, and such incidents emphasize the importance of using a bactericidal toilet chemical.

Aircraft pest control

Since some aircraft fly to all parts of the world, it is not surprising that various pests such as insects and rodents are sometimes found in cabins or freight holds. Insects can be a source of discomfort or annoyance to passengers, and a health hazard, since they can transmit diseases from one country to another. To prevent the transmission of such vectors, the International Health Regulations (WHO, 1983) consolidated by statutory rules and regulations issued by the governments of various countries stipulate the procedures that must be followed. In addition to the requirements of the Regulations, immediate action to destroy any other insects, whether harmful or not, is essential to the safety, well-being and comfort of the passengers and crew.

Many countries also require disinfestation of aircraft to prevent the entry of insects known to be agricultural pests. However, the insects most commonly found on aircraft—although they are not mentioned in the International Health Regulations—are cockroaches, and it is necessary to wage constant battle against them.

Pest control in aircraft is no simple matter because of the strict safety criteria. Pests must be eliminated because, apart from health considerations, they may be a threat to the safety of the aircraft. Rodents, for example, can damage control equipment and instrumentation. Moreover, no materials may be used in pest control that could affect aircraft structure or equipment. Hence the materials must be non-corrosive and non-flammable. Methods for controlling insect vectors of human disease, cockroaches and rodents on aircraft are given below.

Disinsection against insect vectors of human disease

'Disinsection' is defined in the International Health Regulations as the operation in which measures are taken to kill the insect vectors of human disease present in ships, aircraft, trains, road vehicles, other means of transport, and containers. The Regulations specify the measures that should be taken. They state essentially that every aircraft leaving an airport situated in an area where transmission of malaria or other mosquito-borne disease is occurring, or where insecticide-resistant mosquito vectors of disease are present, or where a vector species is present that has been eradicated in the area where the airport of destination of the aircraft is situated, shall be disinsected as near as possible to the time of departure, but so as not to cause delay in its departure. The Regulations permit the aircraft to be disinsected again if the Health Authority at the arrival airport is not satisfied with the work carried out at the port of departure, or if live insects are found on board. In addition, many countries have imposed their own laws and regulations upon airlines, and will not allow disembarkation of passengers unless satisfactory disinsection has been performed. The World Health Organisation's *Weekly Epidemiological Record* (1985a–c) gives specifications for aerosols and other relevant information which allow airlines a certain choice of materials and methods. The insecticidal action from any aerosol must not be biologically inferior to that of the 'Standard Reference Aerosol' which is also described.

The views expressed by the International Civil Aviation Organisation (brought to the notice of the World Health Assembly in 1970) and the requirements of some of the major airlines are as follows:

1. Any insecticide used must be harmless to humans and animals other than insects, both in long-term, repetitive exposure, and in the event of malfunctioning of the dispensing system.
2. Any insecticide used must not cause significant damage to aircraft materials, structural or otherwise (in particular, aluminium alloys and high strength alloy steel), it must not craze Perspex or Plexiglas and it must present no possibility of interference with aircraft systems or equipment (in particular, air conditioning system components and electronic and other instrumental equipment vital to the safety of flight).
3. Disinsection against insect vectors of human disease should be carried out as expeditiously as possible, only when necessary and with a minimum of discomfort to crews and passengers, and of delay in flight operations.

Methods

Three methods are currently in use:

1. Disinsecting before take-off.
2. Disinsecting on the ground on arrival.
3. Residual treatment of aircraft for disinsecting.

1. Disinsecting before take-off ('blocks away' disinsection)

This system was introduced in 1963 after many trials had been carried out and is still the most widely used method. Aerosols that contain enough insecticide to discharge 1 g/100 cubic feet (1 g/2.8 m³; the amount agreed necessary to disinsect effectively an aircraft) are used, and the containers must meet the IATA requirements relating to the carriage of restricted articles by air. They are single-use; that is, the contents are fully discharged (usually at the rate of 1 g/second) following one activation of the valve-operating button. The number of aerosol cans used is determined by the volume of the aircraft interior. Thus, two 140 g aerosols (i.e. 280 g) are used in a standard Boeing 747 aircraft with a cabin capacity of 28 000 cubic feet (790 m³). In this system, the procedure is not necessarily carried out at the port of departure but at the last airport prior to arrival in the country requiring disinsection, after embarkation of passengers, but before take-off. Since the object of disinsection is to kill any mosquitoes or other insect vectors of human disease harboured within an aircraft or its external recesses, it is necessary to carry out the procedure as near as possible to aircraft departure time. The 'blocks away' method comprises three separate phases of insecticidal treatment, as follows:

1. The flight deck (and, in the case of the Boeing 747, the upper deck) must be treated immediately before crew occupancy, and the access doors or curtains must thereafter be kept closed, except for the passage of crew members, until after take-off. The ventilation system and clear-vision panels and hatches must be closed during spraying and for at least 5 minutes thereafter.
2. External resting places such as wheel-bays and freight compartments are sprayed with insecticide as near as possible to 'start engines' time.
3. The aircraft cabin must then be treated during the period between closing the aircraft doors and take-off because the high rate of ventilation operating during flight would disperse the insecticide aerosol too rapidly for it to be effective. Using the single-use aerosol dispensers, the procedure is normally carried out by one member of the cabin crew who, on releasing the valve, walks the full length of the cabin, spraying the aerosol from side to side above seat level. In aircraft like the Boeing 747, the cabin size and seat configuration require that the task be carried out by several members of the cabin crew. During cabin spraying, all cupboards, compartments, and accessible cargo holds must remain open, and food and utensils must be kept covered. The serial numbers on the dispensers are then annotated on the Health Part of the Aircraft General Declaration and the empty containers kept as supporting evidence that disinsection has been carried out.

The 'blocks away' method of aircraft disinsection may be applied to most civil and military aircraft. Operating conditions and the very limited space in certain combat aircraft make it necessary to carry out a modified disinsecting procedure immediately before flight.

It would appear that because some airlines have been rather lax in their application of the 'blocks away' method, the system itself has been unjustly criticized as being unreliable, when the real fault has been failure to carry out the procedure correctly.

2. Disinsecting on the ground on arrival

This system has been in use ever since it was appreciated that some form of disinsection was required. However, it has a number of disadvantages:

1. Because a normal 'multishot' aerosol is used, the operator may discharge an insufficient quantity of insecticide to be effective.
2. Passengers are subjected, often at the end of a long and tiring flight, to unnecessary discomfort, more so as frequently the insecticide used is of doubtful effectiveness, yet pungent to the point of being obnoxious.
3. Live insect vectors of human disease might leave the aircraft at the same time as the disinsecting official boards and before spraying commences.
4. If disease-transmitting insects are on the aircraft, it is more logical to kill them at the start of the flight, rather than at the end when the health of passengers could already have been endangered.

3. Residual treatment of aircraft for disinsecting

Permethrin as a residual insecticide is sprayed on to all surfaces on which insect vectors might alight. A major advantage of this system is that the method of application decreases the risk of adverse effects in crew and passengers from inhalation of insecticidal aerosol components. However, the method is fairly new and has been accepted by relatively few airlines; spraying is required at intervals not exceeding 4 weeks (more frequently if cleaning or other operations remove a significant amount of the permethrin residue); and the treatment must be carried out to the satisfaction of an authorized officer of the appropriate government authority, who may then issue a certificate (valid for a maximum of 4 weeks) which becomes part of the documentation of the aircraft.

Disinfestation against cockroaches

Cockroaches gain entry to aircraft in many ways. They can be present in passengers' baggage, in cargo (particularly fruit and vegetables), or in food uplifted from countries where the insect is prolific. So long as there are cockroaches in the vicinity, it is impossible to stop their entry to an aircraft, and therefore regular treatment and preventive control measures are essential. Some airlines favour the use of insecticidal lacquer in the more vulnerable areas, for example, in cargo holds and galley areas, but this is often unsightly, especially in the galleys.

Routine spraying with a suitable insecticide is the best method of control. A procedure for treating all aircraft at regular intervals (on an average about every 6 weeks), regardless of whether insects have been reported, has been found to be most effective, particularly if two or more insecticides are used on a rotating basis to minimize the risk of resistance to the chemical being developed by the cockroaches. The corners, cracks and crevices of all cupboards, drawers and housings in all galley and bar areas are sprayed by means of a hand-held agricultural-type dispenser.

The fact that cockroaches are seldom found in treated aircraft indicates the success of the treatment, but it must always be remembered that even if spraying were carried out daily, cockroaches could still be found on aircraft. The important factor is that they should not be allowed to remain and breed.

Fumigation

'Fumigation' is used here as the term that describes the gaseous treatment for the destruction of rodents. Not only are rodents, particularly rats, found in aircraft a public health hazard—especially if the flight originated in a country where plague is still present—but they may also affect the safe operation of the aircraft. An airline must arrange for fumigation whenever rodents have been seen or reported on aircraft. It is permissible to use various fumigation agents provided they are of recognized effectiveness, but the one most commonly used is methyl bromide, which is normally used at a dosage rate of 8 ounces/1000 cubic feet ($8 \, g/m^3$) for a period of 4 hours.

Because methyl bromide is highly toxic, not only must it be handled by skilled and fully qualified persons, but the airline must also promulgate and enforce regulations to safeguard its own staff and prevent a public health hazard. A laid-down procedure should include:

1. Ascertaining that every part of the aircraft is clear of personnel before contractors start the fumigation.
2. Placing warning signs conspicuously around the aircraft.
3. Sealing all opening points into the fuselage.

4. Employing experts who will be fully responsible for complying with any relevant legislation, safety or guidelines (UK Health and Safety Executive, 1986).
5. Fully ventilating the aircraft after fumigation, and at this stage, guarding all entrances to prevent unauthorized entry.
6. Testing by contractors to determine that the aircraft is completely free from fumigating agents.
7. Certificate of clearance produced and signed by contractors.
8. Preventing entry by airline staff until the above certificate has been presented.

It is vital to adhere strictly to the above safety provisions.

Rats can be brought into aircraft freight holds with cargo, but they can and sometimes do enter the cabin via unattended passenger steps.

Keeping airports free from rodents will also greatly reduce the need to fumigate aircraft. Unfortunately, rodent control is often inefficient and sometimes non-existent at some international airports. It is a weakness of the International Health Regulations that failure to control rodents is not an offence, since a rat-infested airport is not only dangerous to ground personnel but also to aircraft.

Disinfection

On extremely rare occasions an airline receives a report that a passenger with a suspected or confirmed infectious disease has been carried on one of its flights. A decision must then be made as to what disinfection procedures, if any, need to be carried out on the aircraft. Advice should be sought from the local health authority, which may well have its own laid-down procedures that must be followed. The IATA Medical Manual (1979) provides some guidance on the selection of suitable disinfectants, but of paramount importance is the requirement that any disinfectant used will not harm the aircraft structure in any way.

Any disinfecting procedures necessary after the carriage of a passenger with a suspected or confirmed infectious disease will be kept to a minimum, provided that:

1. Appropriate chemicals are used routinely in the aircraft's water and toilet systems.
2. Toilet compartment surfaces and galley surfaces are always sanitized during routine cleaning operations.
3. All catering equipment is routinely sanitized before re-use.
4. All food waste and other garbage from the aircraft is disposed of hygienically as a routine.

Aircraft cabin cleanliness

When a passenger aircraft commences its flight the cabin interior should be sparklingly clean. During flight, conditions quickly deteriorate and therefore at each transit stop, or quick turn-rounds at terminal airports, it is necessary to perform a rapid cleaning operation. Special attention should be paid to the toilets and galleys. Litter must be removed and linen replaced.

The cabin must present an acceptable appearance to boarding passengers. A more thorough cleaning operation must be carried out when the aircraft is on the ground for a longer time or during a maintenance check. Cleaning staff must be provided with modern and adequate equipment and materials. A mobile vehicle fully equipped and with an abundant supply of hot water is a great asset. To lessen the risk of disease transmission, materials for cabin cleaning should include efficient bactericidal preparations which should be regularly used because, if a passenger has an infection, it is usually not discovered until after the aircraft has left on another flight.

Cabin interiors and furnishings, in addition to being attractive, should be designed with a view to easy cleaning. Galleys, in particular, can present cleaning difficulties which can be reduced considerably by the use of mobile fittings so that complete units can be exchanged for clean ones, all cleaning being done on the ground.

References

Her Majesty's Stationery Office (1970) *The Food Hygiene (General) Regulations*. London: HMSO

International Air Transport Association (1979) *IATA Medical Manual*. IATA Medical Advisory Committee. Montreal: IATA

UK Health and Safety Executive (1986) *Fumigation using Methyl Bromide (Bromomethane). UK Health and Safety Executive Guidance Note CS 12*. London: HMSO

World Health Organisation (1960) *Guide to Hygiene and Sanitation in Aviation*. Geneva: WHO

World Health Organisation (1977) *Guide to Hygiene and Sanitation in Aviation*, 2nd edn. Geneva: WHO

World Health Organisation (1983) *International Health Regulations*, 3rd edn. Geneva: WHO

World Health Organisation (1984) *Guidelines for Drinking-Water Quality*. Geneva: WHO

World Health Organisation (1985) (a) *Weekly Epidemiological Record*, No. 7. (b) *Weekly Epidemiological Record*, No. 12. (c) *Weekly Epidemiological Record*, No. 45

Further reading

Her Majesty's Stationery Office (1979) *The Public Health (Aircraft) Regulations*. London: HMSO

39

Health of airline ground staff

C.C.G. Rawll

Introduction

The prime function of an airline medical department is to provide a comprehensive occupational health service for the flying personnel. These are greatly outnumbered by those on the ground who support these operations in administration, sales and marketing, engineering and maintenance, catering, cargo handling etc., not only at the home base but also, often, in foreign countries. The occupational health team, therefore, must have expert knowledge of occupational medicine, public health, tropical medicine, aviation medicine and, of course, general clinical medicine. The occupational health team must be able not only to react to any problems that arise but also to give advice to management and to staff on how to control such problems; this preventive role is paramount.

To achieve this, the medical department must be kept up to date on all proposed changes over a very wide range: new building developments, new processes, new materials, and new equipment and facilities, so that the measures to deal with them may be established as early as possible—ideally at the planning stage. Additional sources of information are by inspection carried out periodically by members of the team, complaints from users, requests for advice, and feedback from formal or informal clinical consultations.

Clinical services
Work-related diseases

The clinical work of the occupational health service must obviously cope with accidents and illness occurring at work. By convention this also includes the classic occupational diseases, which, by definition, exclusively affect working people exposed to specific hazards and where there is a direct cause-and-effect relationship between the hazard and the disease.

It is now recognized that the work environment in all its facets can play a significant part, together with other risk factors, in the development of many diseases with a complex multi-factorial aetiology. These are the work-related diseases, e.g. hypertension, chronic respiratory disease, chronic locomotor system disorder, gastro-intestinal illness, and some behavioural or stress disorders.

Yet again, some diseases in the general population may be aggravated by occupational hazards, whereas other conditions may be a direct threat to safety at work. Thus the clinical practice of occupational medicine must provide for conditions occurring across a continuous spectrum of work association.

Treatment services

An efficient treatment service for illness and injury occurring at work is fundamental to good occupational health practice. These treatment services can be carried out by nursing staff who should have good general nursing experience as well as training in occupational health and aviation medicine and the relevant areas of public health and tropical medicine. In addition, it is desirable to standardize treatment and other nursing techniques in order to provide consistent guidelines for the handling of commonly occurring conditions, particularly where direct medical supervision is not available.

The treatment facilities must be located in areas where staff concentrations are highest or where the hazards are greatest; and they should be equipped to provide at least first-line response to any likely emergency. Emergency procedures should be established and rehearsed.

An efficient treatment service promotes trust in the medical department and can provide much information on the pattern of illness or occupational injury on which to base preventive action.

Consultation and advisory services

In addition to emergency and therapeutic services, the occupational health team must provide advice both to management and to staff on matters affecting health at work. In the clinical field this means, in the main, the provision of a consultation service, which should include the following.

Pre-employment medical examinations

Where deviation from normal health may affect the safety of an individual or his colleagues, some form of medical screening or assessment procedure is essential. This requirement is self-evident in the case of motor vehicle drivers, operators of machinery, workers in potentially hazardous processes and those who have to work at heights. A full medical examination is sometimes required to assess the candidate and additional investigations such as blood tests, chest radiographs and audiograms may be appropriate in certain circumstances. Food handlers should undergo microbiological tests for transmissible pathogens in the stools, and should be scrutinized for good personal hygiene and freedom from skin infection, otitis media and other conditions undesirable in those preparing food. Many groups of applicants may be screened using a medical questionnaire, examining only those with a relevant medical history. Questionnaires are best administered by an experienced occupational health nurse, who may also carry out vision, urine and blood pressure examinations, referring doubtful candidates for medical assessment or examination.

Selection procedures should include establishing medical guidelines or, sometimes, precise standards, often reviewing the requirements of jobs, either individually or in groups. These criteria should themselves be reviewed at intervals as job requirements change and medical knowledge grows.

National or other statutory standards obviously must be incorporated in company selection criteria, especially for drivers, as well as recommendations in recognized codes of practice, etc. This is particularly important for visual standards. Defective colour vision—as determined with Ishihara or other pseudo-isochromatic plates—is not an automatic bar to work in operational or engineering areas. Drivers in operational areas must pass a colour perception lantern test. Other applicants should be referred to line management for a practical or trade test.

Note that those with a history of atopy should not be accepted for apprenticeships in engineering as they run an unacceptable risk of skin breakdown. This is an example of a positive use of a medical examination to guide an individual into a less hazardous occupation.

Advice on working restrictions

It is often necessary, in the interests of the health of the employee, to restrict the range of his activities, either temporarily or permanently. Experience and knowledge of the tasks are essential to ensure that restrictions are adequate to meet the medical needs of the patient without incurring unnecessary social, operational or economic penalties either for the employee or employer. The restrictions, which commonly affect physical capacity, hours of work and environmental limitations, should be determined as precisely as possible and reviewed at regular intervals. Feedback from local management is valuable at such review.

Investigation of absence attributed to sickness

Employees with records of frequent or prolonged absence attributed to sickness should be assessed to exclude underlying unrecognized health problems; occupational causes; to arrange restriction of duties, if necessary, in the interests of safety or health; and to endeavour to remedy the underlying condition in the interests of employee and employer. Such consultations must include adequate information from local management about work performance and absence record.

Periodic examination or surveillance and screening

Employers are sometimes required by law to arrange periodic medical examinations for the protection of individuals in certain occupations; e.g. workers who are exposed to ionizing radiations, compressed air, lead and asbestos. Additionally, all instances of illness that might be attributable to work should be assessed by the occupational health team in order to protect the individual and to institute measures to protect the working group.

Regular medical surveillance, perhaps including biological monitoring, is recommended for those exposed to potentially hazardous agents, e.g. cadmium, beryllium, isocyanates. This surveillance is not a substitute for good engineering control or environmental monitoring. The results of such monitoring may indicate the nature and frequency of medical surveillance.

Any decision to introduce routine surveillance should only be made after careful review of the extent of the potential hazard and the results of monitoring. Surveillance is not an alternative to or substitute for adequate controls, including monitoring to assess the degree of success.

Routine 'executive' or 'health screening' examinations are a common feature of contemporary occupational health practice. While there is little doubt that examinations of the pre-symptomatic can have worthwhile results, the limitations as well as the advantages should be assessed with care, particularly the necessary resources for dealing with abnormal results. Such examinations do have value in establishing base lines and detecting abnormal trends in an individual and providing an opportunity for discussing work pressures and lifestyle in a neutral arena.

Problems peculiar to the industry may cause an emphasis to be placed on certain diseases; for example, in the aviation industry, an interest in noise-induced hearing loss and the risk of aerotitis and related problems focuses attention on ear, nose and sinuses, giving rise to frequent consultations in this field.

Open consultations

Anxiety about the effect of work on health or vice versa, together with a whole range of matters where work and health are interrelated—for example, the industry-wide opportunities for overseas travel—may give rise to requests for medical advice, and wide experience is required to ensure that this advice is appropriate and up to date.

Other components of the clinical services include special therapeutic activities such as physiotherapy, diagnostic procedures, immunization and health screening facilities. General preventive health measures such as cervical cytology services or health counselling are increasingly being promoted at the workplace. In addition, specific occupational health advice, such as instruction on the prevention of dermatitis, must be provided both to staff and to management. The medical problems on which advice will be sought and given are as diverse as the sphere of activities and range of occupations within the airline industry.

Many employers provide Employee Assistance Programmes to counsel staff, particularly those with alcohol or drug abuse problems. Occupational Health Departments may be directly involved in these or work in close but informal co-operation.

Ageing

The increased physical demands of working on larger aircraft weigh heavily on supervisory staff. They often have to cover several aircraft, whereas their tradesmen work in relatively small areas. These physical demands often reach their maximum as the supervisor's physical resources are declining. There is no easy solution but occupational health professionals should be alert to this.

Emergency facilities and procedures

The occupational health team will advise management on the location, facilities and training required for first aid services to all work areas. Specific training may be required for certain high-risk areas, i.e. cyanide tanks or for electricians. Basic emergency first aid training should be made as widely available as possible.

Airports and town offices are particularly vulnerable areas and the medical input to the emergency and evacuation procedures should be reviewed and rehearsed at regular intervals.

Environmental control

Control of the working environment is principally directed at avoiding and controlling hazards to the health and safety of airline employees, but there is an increasing awareness of the importance of comfortable working conditions in the interests of amenity and efficiency, even where there are no recognized specific medical hazards. In general, since effective environmental control depends on a flow of information, both in and out of the medical department, the organization of this flow is of paramount importance.

Particular care is needed to co-ordinate this interchange and the response when professional responsibility for health and safety is divided between different groups or individuals or there is no centrally directed health and safety team.

Hazards

The hazards to ground staff in the airline industry can be divided into those associated with physical, chemical and biological agents. The standard reference works deal with these in detail, but the following short review may be useful.

Physical hazards

The principal physical hazards encountered are as follows.

Ionizing radiation

Exposure to ionizing radiation may occur from the following sources.

Industrial radiography—Radiographic inspection techniques for airframes and engines are now commonplace using X-ray or gamma radiation from radioisotope sources.

Radioactive fall-out contamination of airframes, engines and aircraft components—Atmospheric testing of nuclear weapons led to the accumulation of radioactive materials in the stratosphere. This material concentrated on airframes, engines and ventilation system components during flights at high altitude. This has decreased to negligible proportions over the last decade but a short-lived 'peak' after the Chernobyl reactor incident in 1986 highlighted the need for awareness and preparation in dealing with contamination of staff and aircraft.

Radioactive cargo—Strict regulations govern the packaging and shipment of radioactive materials and risks should only arise if accidental serious damage occurs.

Depleted uranium balance weights—These are used on some aircraft for balancing purposes. The uranium is plated to contain the uranium, enabling the balance weights to be treated as sealed sources. Their location in the aircraft avoids hazards to passengers and crew. Care must be exercised in handling if the protective coating is damaged; advice should be obtained from a Radiological Protection Adviser. Advice should also be obtained about storage and disposal of these sources whether damaged or not.

Miscellaneous—These include radioactive gauges, sensors, luminescent aircraft instruments and radiographic security devices.

The handling of radioactive materials and exposure to ionizing radiation are internationally subject to legislation limiting exposures to internationally accepted standards, harmonized within the EEC countries. The principles of protection are based on reduction of exposure by time, distance and shielding. Additionally, in the case of unsealed sources, protection is conferred by practices designed to prevent absorption, inhalation and ingestion.

Non-ionizing electromagnetic radiation

The principal sources of such radiation are radar transmitters and microwave ovens.

Microwave energy—This can cause thermal damage to body tissues, the most vulnerable being those with a low blood supply since they do not benefit from the rapid heat dissipation produced by the blood circulation. The most vulnerable organ is the lens of the eye which is unable to dissipate microwave energy in excess of $10\,mW/cm^2$. Any thermal damage may cause the development of cataracts. Energy levels below $10\,mW/cm^2$ have generally been regarded as safe for continuous exposure. Protection is achieved by adequate shielding or controlling exposure.

Maximum field strengths for human exposure are now defined in terms of radiation frequency. A suggested schedule for whole body occupational exposure for total exposure not exceeding 2 hours per day is shown in *Table 39.1*.

Radar installations should not be tested on the ground where their emission can either cause harm to individuals or be a fire hazard (for example, by producing induction currents in flammable liquid tanks).

Ultraviolet light—Some techniques used to detect structural cracks in aircraft parts involve the use of ultra-violet light, generally in the least harmful range of wavelengths between 320 and 400 nm and at safe energy intensities, avoiding the need for personal protection. Ultraviolet emissions also arise from welding and certain other processes; shielding and appropriate eye protection must be provided for these.

Noise

Aero-engines and other industrial noise sources, such as machine shops, sheet metal working etc., are potential causes of noise-induced hearing loss. Ideally, noise should be reduced at its source, but where this is not possible and the noise is likely to exceed permissible levels, a hearing conservation programme should be instituted in which hearing protection is backed up by audiometric monitoring. Guidance for the United Kingdom on permissible noise levels, noise reduction and hearing protection is given in the Code of Practice for Reducing the Exposure to Noise of Employed Persons (Health and Safety Executive, 1972). Harmonization of

Table 39.1 Maximum field strengths for human exposure—now defined in terms of radiation frequency. Suggested schedule for whole-body occupational exposure for total exposure not exceeding 2 hours daily

Frequency (rms values)	Power density (W/m^2)	Electric field (V/m)	Magnetic field (A/m)
30–100 MHz	10	60	0.16
100–500 MHz	f/10	$6.0\sqrt{f}$	$0.16\sqrt{f}$
500 MHz–300 GHz	50	135	0.36

f = Frequency in megahertz (MHz).

noise control legislation is in progress in the EEC countries.

Employees with significantly impaired hearing should not be employed in operational areas where they are required to wear hearing protection. The combined effect of the attenuation of the hearing protection and of the pre-existing hearing loss may prevent them from hearing emergency signals or moving aircraft or vehicles.

Rules for the identification and labelling of noise hazard areas and the wearing of suitable hearing protection must be promulgated and enforced. When audiometry is undertaken records must be kept and appropriate advice given to those who are examined. Provision must be made for those who are advised to cease working in a noise area. EEC directives on hearing conservation will shortly require member states to introduce harmonized regulations, including audiometry and record maintenance.

Vibration

Vibration below 12 Hz may cause resonance of body organs and injury to skeletal tissues, notably the spine; of these the principal problem is repeated minor trauma of the spine from seat vibration in certain ground support vehicles such as tractors. There is little evidence of primary injury occurring as a result of lumbar stresses, but disc lesions and arthritic conditions of the spine may be aggravated. Ischaemic conditions of hands and arms can be caused by high-frequency vibrations from hand-held pneumatic tools such as hammers, drills and riveters; but most airline equipment operates outside the critical frequencies, and these conditions are uncommon in aircraft maintenance.

Barometric pressure

Pressure testing of aircraft hulls on the ground exposes some members of the staff to pressures in the order of 8–10 psi above atmospheric air pressure. On the other hand, test flying or normal passenger flying expose ground staff to a lowered barometric pressure. There is no risk of decompression sickness in either case, the only problems arising from the expansion of gases in normal and pathological body cavities.

Staff involved in aircraft pressurization tests should receive an initial medical examination, which in addition to establishing good general health, should be directed at permanently excluding those persons with conditions affecting the free ventilation of body cavities, or creating abnormal body cavities, e.g. blocked eustachian tubes, chronic sinusitis and lung cysts. Individuals suffering from acute respiratory infection should also be excluded for the period of the illness. Ideally, pressure changes employed in

the test procedure should be gradual: staff not actively involved in test procedures should be excluded from the aircraft.

General

Thermal injury may result from exposure to either high or low temperatures. Not only are there the climatic problems posed by world-wide airline operations that may expose staff to wide variations of ambient temperature, but also there are the problems encountered during maintenance using cold liquid gases or procedures performed at high temperatures. Adequate protective clothing must be provided and suitable handling procedures instituted. Repeated minor skin trauma may arise from the handling of fibrous materials such as fibreglass and carbon fabrics. Here again, appropriate protective measures must be instituted.

Chemical hazards

There is a wide range of chemical materials used in aircraft maintenance. The following simple non-comprehensive classification illustrates the nature and diversity of some common materials and discusses some basic principles of control. Routine medical surveillance may be required as well as engineering control and environmental monitoring:

1. *Metals and their salts*—Cadmium, mercury, chromium, nickel, beryllium, sodium and potassium cyanide.
2. *Acids and alkalis*—Ammonia, sodium and potassium hydroxide, nitric, sulphuric, hydrochloric, hydrofluoric and chromic acids.
3. *Gases*—Argon, carbon dioxide, carbon monoxide, oxygen and nitrogen (including liquid forms), refrigerant gases.
4. *Solvents and stripping agents*—White spirit, toluene, xylene, methylene chloride, chloroform, trichlorethylene, perchlorethylene, trichloroethane, ketones and phenols.
5. *Skin irritants*—Oils, degreasing agents, detergents.
6. *Aviation fuels*—Gasolene and kerosene.
7. *Hydraulic and de-icing fluids*.
8. *Plastic resins and surface coatings*—Epoxy compounds, isocyanates, primers and paints, polytetrafluoroethylene (PTFE).

The precise location and the method of use of each chemical should be recorded and be readily retrievable by reference and cross-reference. Each should be allotted a simple toxicity classification so that those who handle it are aware of the principal hazards, the necessary precautions and the emergency action in case of accident. Major processes using hazardous materials will normally involve the use of plant and equipment controlled by specified technical procedures and standards. Technical control documents should contain the specific precautions and first aid measures to be taken and should be available to all users. Records must be kept of significant individual exposures.

Records

Occupational health departments should maintain concise and accurate records of attendances, examinations, consultations, etc. together with details of accidents and significant occupational exposure.

The constraints of medical confidentiality apply to these records. Where they are maintained electronically consideration must also be given to the Data Protection Principles.

Occupational health records should be kept in such a way that extraction of epidemiological data is possible.

Safety and control procedures

The principles of control of hazardous material include:

1. The use of the least hazardous material compatible with technical requirements.
2. The use of plant and equipment for containment, extraction of hazardous vapours, dusts, gases, etc., or the avoidance of direct handling.
3. Good general standards of ventilation and housekeeping.
4. Safe methods of work.
5. The use, where necessary, of protective clothing and equipment.
6. Adequate initial and refresher training.

Control procedures should be based on the principle of achieving as low an exposure as reasonably achievable and not merely not to exceed any set limits (threshold limit value, maximum allowable concentration, etc.). These have their place, but caution is essential in their application. They are derived from experimental data of varying reliability and indicate exposure levels that are likely not to produce adverse effects in the majority of those exposed for 8 hours daily, 5 days a week, 50 weeks a year. Individual specific response is possible outside these limits and the effects of 'moonlighting' or unusual shift patterns must be remembered.

Chemical materials may exert injurious effects by surface contamination, inhalation or ingestion. These hazards may be controlled using the principles outlined above. Additional specific action may also be useful.

Skin contamination

1. Avoid contact.
2. Good personal hygiene with regular washing of exposed parts.
3. The use of protective clothing, especially gloves.
4. Barrier creams have some use, but the use of conditioning cream after washing is valuable.

Drench showers should be provided at sites where there is a risk of serious contamination by dangerous or irritant fluids, e.g. fuel, hydraulic fluids, solvents or toilet contents. Changes of clothing should also be available on loan.

Eye contamination

1. Avoid splashes.
2. Use of appropriate eye protection.

Eyewash facilities should be sited at potential hazard sites.

Inhalation

1. Avoid unnecessary inhalation of toxic substances.
2. The use of local or general extract ventilation.
3. Where necessary, the use of appropriate respiratory protection.

Respirators range from simple dust-filtering disposable masks to full-face air-fed equipment. All masks must be correctly fitted, regularly inspected and maintained in a serviceable condition. Where filters are used, they must be appropriate to the nature and degree of hazard and changed in accordance with established criteria for duration and/or intensity of exposure. Training is essential for those using any form of respiratory protection.

Ingestion

This is not a common hazard in normal airline maintenance operations but can occur during laboratory and testing procedures. A mechanical pipette should be used when hazardous substances need to be measured or aspirated.

Toxicology

An outline of the toxicological properties of the more important materials used in airline maintenance operations is as follows:

1. Many of the hydrocarbon solvents and detergents are a skin hazard because of their defatting action; the chlorohydrocarbon series are, furthermore, narcotic in high concentration and possibly carcinogenic in some instances.

2. Epoxy resins, isocyanate foam manufacturing reagents and polyurethane paints contain biologically active chemical groupings which can give rise to skin and lung sensitization.
3. Some metals, e.g. cadmium and mercury, have specific toxicological effects sometimes involving several end-organs. Metal spraying procedures and the use of polytetrafluoroethylene (PTFE) may give rise to so-called 'fume fevers'.
4. Some corrosive substances, for example, hydrofluoric acid and phenol, may have a singularly penetrating action if allowed to come into contact with surface tissues, as well as having systemic effects.
5. Some familiar substances, such as kerosene and hydraulic fluids, while not notably hazardous, may, because they are so widely used and involve frequent or prolonged contact, present a greater problem than hazardous materials, the use of which is strictly limited, contained or controlled.

The air transportation of hazardous cargo is governed by the IATA Restricted Articles Regulations. Nevertheless, spillages and breakages do occur and cause problems. Emergency procedures to deal with these should be prepared and rehearsed.

Biological hazards

World-wide travel may expose airline staff to a variety of communicable diseases and exotic infections; for example, cholera, polio and malaria. Potential risks also arise from passenger contact, and from human waste products encountered in aircraft cleaning and maintenance activities. Prophylactic immunization and advisory procedures must be established for all those involved at all stages of the chain—which will be found to be extensive! This is particularly important when an aircraft carries an unnotified or unrecognized passenger with a serious transmissible disease.

The carriage of animals by air requires consideration of diseases transmissible from animal to man. The IATA Live Animals Regulations list a number of precautions—*see* also Chapter 41. The prime objective is to avoid contact between these animals and employees by securely caging the animals and the use of protective clothing by airline staff. Prophylactic immunization against tetanus, and possibly rabies, should be offered to employees.

The IATA Dangerous Goods Regulations Section 3.6.6 defines infectious substances as those containing viable micro-organisms or their toxins which are known, or suspected to cause disease in animals or humans. There are relaxations in the carriage requirements for biological products or diagnostic specimens—as defined by IATA. For acceptance as

airfreight by an IATA carrier these materials must be declared by the shipper and packed in accordance with the Regulations. Nevertheless emergency procedures should be established for dealing with spillages or leakages at all stages of the airline's involvement.

General environmental considerations

Not only must the occupational health team play an active part in the control of the industrial working environment, it must also take an equally active part in the control of the general or office working environment in the interests of health, comfort and working efficiency. There is ample evidence that optimum working conditions improve accuracy and productivity and that sub-optimal conditions predispose to complaints such as fatigue—for example, where the temperature is too high or too low—or to eye-strain, where there is glare from lighting.

At least 50% of airline staff work in offices or similar non-industrial accommodation. In addition, therefore, to providing good working conditions for the industrial work-force, a concern in the environmental conditions for non-industrial staff is important in view of the increasing use of office machinery and semi-automated office procedures with their attendant ergonomic, visual, acoustic and psychological problems.

Office technology

Visual display units are in widespread use. The ergonomic criteria for their selection and installation are well established. There is no evidence to support the allegations that they are a cause of reproductive hazard, although research continues. Attention must be paid to the task and job design to ensure that psychological stress is minimized, it being clear that this area is where many problems are arising particularly for repetitive jobs. The effects of poor job design can easily cause physical health problems as well as psychological stress leading to occupational disease.

Ergonomics

While the term ergonomics covers a wide environmental field, its use here is limited to anthropometric factors. Seats, desks, machinery keyboards, etc. should be of such dimensions as to conform to the appropriate anthropometric requirements. Wherever possible, office furnishings should be capable of adjustment to meet individual variations in body size, and staff encouraged to use these facilities.

Examples of areas where anthropometric factors are particularly important are in the use of office machinery such as accounting machines, data processing equipment and visual display terminals; industrial bench work; and the handling of baggage and freight.

Temperature control

A dry bulb temperature of about 21°C (70°F) is suitable for sedentary occupations and a dry bulb temperature of 18.3°C (65°F) is satisfactory for active work. As the 'effective temperature' depends on the radiant heat component, air movement and relative humidity, clearly there are situations where the dry bulb reading is inadequate to define or assess thermal comfort. Maintenance of the working environment within the desirable thermal parameters depends on the capacity of the plant and the adequacy of the sensors and the controls.

Attention must be paid to providing adequate and controlled air movement and changes. Alterations in office layout can often lead to imbalance of the ventilation system and pockets of stagnation—or draughts. Provision for some degree of local control is valuable in terms of staff acceptance.

Building construction

Levels of noise and other atmospheric pollution often demand that airport buildings and town offices should be insulated against noise and be provided with air conditioning or other forms of mechanical ventilation. Care must be taken in siting intakes for systems and to ensure that cooling systems are regularly cleaned to prevent biological contamination.

Many older buildings may also contain asbestos for fire or noise insulation. This is unlikely to be a hazard if it is adequately and securely contained at all times. Any repair or removal work must be under strict and expert supervision.

Lighting

Lighting must be adequate both in quantity and quality to enable the visual task to be performed accurately, quickly and without discomfort. Recommended levels of illumination required for a range of visual tasks are given in the current edition of the IES (Illuminating Engineering Society) Code.

However, to achieve good quality lighting is more difficult, owing to problems of distribution, direction, glare, contrast, flicker, colour rendering and even aesthetics.

This subject is of particular importance in the airline industry with its large number of visual tasks, ranging from instrument fitting in the industrial sphere to the use of visual display terminals in offices.

Noise

The problems of damage to hearing have already been mentioned, but there are other important effects of noise. The principal problem is that of interference with communication and consequent irritation. At an airport, aircraft movements and engine-running produce high ambient noise levels, so at most airports it is essential to provide noise insulation for all accommodation where communication by speech is necessary.

The control of noise sources within buildings is also important, and the contribution of office machinery to noise levels in large open-plan offices often becomes evident when, as a result of noise insulation, the noise from external sources is reduced. One should not forget the major contribution of motor vehicle noise at an airport.

Wherever possible, noise must be reduced at source by the proper design of equipment. This is an important part of the specification which should be considered at an early stage of selection. Further reduction of noise from a particular source usually depends on interrupting the transmission pathways through the air, by acoustic enclosure, screening or distance; and through the building structure, by suitable mounting and location. Noise reflection from hard surfaces can accentuate problems, but it can be reduced by the use of noise-absorbent material such as acoustic ceiling tiles, drapes and carpets. Other effects of noise, such as fatigue and reduction in task performance, are commonly claimed even though they may be difficult to demonstrate either in the laboratory or in the workplace. Nevertheless, subjective complaints frequently merit attention.

Occupational stress

Much is heard today of stress in the workplace. Contrary to popular belief, adverse manifestations of stress are not confined to the top echelons of management but are equally prevalent in supervisory and other junior grades. The unpredictable nature of airline operations and their sensitivity to political and other external influences inevitably leads to a build-up of pressure on many in the operational areas, while the unrelenting demands made on those responsible for keeping an airline ahead of the market and its competitors are equally great. Domestic and social pressures may also combine with these.

The occupational health team has an important role in this situation. Informal and formal consultations may provide opportunities for discussion and advice on stress management. Employment Assistance Programmes and external courses may be useful. Formal medical and therapeutic intervention may be needed, including recommendations for modification of duties and discussions with members of the appropriate management team.

Stress reaction can also appear as group phenomena. An increase in short-term absence or of diffuse complaints about environmental conditions may be medical manifestations of organizational or occupational disease. Recognition of this by the occupational health team is important as resolution is more of a management than a medical exercise.

Overseas travel

Work in an airline often requires overseas travel on duty—as well as providing the opportunity for recreational travel.

Advice on health precautions, immunizations, malaria prophylaxis, etc. should be available, including specific advice on sexually transmitted diseases and other aspects of personal hygiene and behaviour.

Attention should be drawn to the problems associated with travel fatigue, especially with crossing more than five time zones without a break: advice should be offered on sensible schedules.

Staff consultation

The promotion of health and safety in any organization cannot take place as a medical activity in a vacuum. All proposals should be introduced after consultation with staff representatives in the appropriate forum—e.g. health and safety committees.

Results of individual examinations should be discussed with the individual, but pooled results of investigations should be made available to safety committees together with appropriate explanations.

Further reading

The standard textbooks of occupational medicine and occupational hygiene give detailed information on the topics outlined in this chapter. National sources should be consulted for local statutory requirements. Additional useful material will be found in the following.

BERGQVIST, U.O.V. (1984) Video display terminals and health. *Scandinavian Journal of Work and Environmental Health*, **10**, Suppl. 2

DAWOOD, R. (1986) *Traveller's Health*. Oxford University Press

Health and Safety Executive (1971) *Code of Practice for Reducing the Exposure to Noise of Employed Persons*. London: HMSO

International Air Transport Association (1986) *Live Animals Regulations*, 13th edn. Montreal: IATA

International Air Transport Association (1987) *Dangerous Goods Regulations*, 28th edn. Montreal: IATA

International Labour Organisation (1977) *Occupational Health and Safety in Civil Aviation*. Geneva: International Labour Organisation

Society of Occupational Medicine (1977) *Health Screening*. London: Society of Occupational Medicine

World Health Organisation (1985) *Identification and Control of Work-related Diseases*. Technical Report 714. Geneva: WHO

40

Carriage of invalid passengers by civil airlines

R.L. Green and S.E. Mooney

Introduction

The term 'Invalid Passenger' is used by airlines to denote those passengers who because of sickness or disability may require special assistance or consideration prior to or during an air journey. The modern airliner is in many ways a highly suitable vehicle for the transport of invalids but it also has some serious limitations. Invalid passengers may be considered under two headings.

By far the larger group consists of those travelling for business or pleasure whose incapacity or illness is incidental to their journey. In general these people present few difficulties since despite their disability they are usually capable of leading an independent life and their condition is unlikely to be affected by the flight. The second group comprises those whose disability is the reason for their journey; that is, those people who are travelling to obtain specialized treatment or advice. Passengers in this group may have problems, firstly because they are often too ill or too disabled to fend for themselves, and secondly because the flight environment may significantly affect their condition.

Invalid passengers may be refused carriage on normal scheduled flights if it is considered that their condition may deteriorate significantly, with the risk of possible diversion or delay of the aircraft. There are also certain practical considerations outside the control of the airline, such as the adequacy of ground handling and reception facilities at airports, and the attitude of Customs and Immigration departments to these special passengers. Most important of all, however, are the physiological and physical conditions faced by all air travellers, and these factors will be discussed with their relevance to specific medical conditions.

Physiological and physical factors

Physiological

Modern airliners operate mainly at altitudes between 25 000 and 45 000 feet and this high-altitude flight, which is above turbulence and adverse weather, is one of the features of air travel that makes it so suitable for the rapid transport of seriously ill patients. Cabin pressurization overcomes most of the physiological problems encountered at such high altitudes, but some reduction of cabin pressure has to be accepted, and most airliners operate with a cabin pressure range equivalent to altitudes of 5000–7000 feet, and rarely below an equivalent of 8000 feet. Although Concorde operates at a cruising altitude of 50 000–60 000 feet, its sophisticated engineering allows the cabin altitude to be maintained at around 6500 feet equivalent.

At 6000 feet the atmospheric pressure is 609 mm Hg (81.1 kPa) and under this reduced pressure gas in body cavities expands according to Boyle's law. Thus 100 ml of air at sea level will occupy about 130 ml at 6000 feet, and this may cause difficulties if it is unable to vent freely. The most common problems arise in the middle ear and occasionally the paranasal sinuses where acute catarrhal conditions prevent free air flow and pressure equalization. As described in Chapter 50 pressure damage (barotrauma) in these areas may be very painful but serious damage is rare.

The second and much more important physiological consequence of reduced atmospheric pressure is hypoxia. At sea level the alveolar partial pressure of oxygen ($P_{A_{O_2}}$) is 103 mm Hg whereas at 6000 feet it is about 75 mm Hg. Since the amount of oxygen taken up by haemoglobin is related to the $P_{A_{O_2}}$ this fall might be disastrous were it not for the sigmoid shape of the oxygen dissociation curve. Reference to Chapter 5 will show that a fall of the $P_{A_{O_2}}$ from sea level value to that at 6000 feet only reduces the oxygen content of the arterial blood by 3%. Until the $P_{A_{O_2}}$ begins to fall below 60 mm Hg (at approximately 10 000 feet) there is relatively little effect on the oxygen saturation of the blood, but below this partial pressure hypoxia becomes severe.

The fall in $P_{A_{O_2}}$ experienced in a modern airliner, with the consequent 3% desaturation of arterial blood, is not noticed by the healthy passenger at rest, although effects on night vision and on the learning of new tasks have been reported in experimental subjects (Denison *et al.*, 1966). However, it should not be forgotten that the effects of even mild hypoxia may be accentuated by such factors as smoking and alcohol in otherwise healthy passengers (Harding and Mills, 1983). For the unhealthy passenger, the sudden exposure to this mild hypoxia may be the final step over the threshold into significant tissue hypoxia. Conditions such as cardiac failure, any tissue ischaemia, severe anaemia and severe respiratory disease are among those that may cause severe adverse reaction to such hypoxia, and these will be discussed later.

The problems of hypoxia may be largely overcome by the use of supplementary oxygen in flight, and a portable set or the aircraft's main supply can be used to increase the $P_{A_{O_2}}$ in such cases. A relatively low flow rate will give adequate enrichment of the inspired air, but it must be remembered that continuous oxygen for a 10-hour journey, even at a low flow rate, may not be practical: it requires equipment that is both heavy and bulky in a situation where weight and space are expensive. Airlines will normally supply additional oxygen on request, but passengers' own oxygen cylinders are generally unacceptable as they may not comply with safety regulations.

Other physiological consequences of a long air journey may result from the very low cabin humidities encountered, and the disruption of circadian rhythms from the rapid crossing of several time zones.

Physical

Certain physical problems facing invalid passengers may be peculiar to air travel as are the physiological ones already outlined. Most, however, are more basic and common to travellers by any mode of transport. They must always be considered in the context of the journey to be undertaken as there are important differences between the flight on domestic routes in a narrow-bodied aircraft and that in a wide-bodied aircraft employed on long-haul operations. Not only is there a difference in the length of

journey but in the medical facilities that may be available at the destination or at transit stops.

The ergonomics of accommodating the incapacitated passenger give rise to most of the problems. There is not a great deal of space for the legs in an economy class seat and thus a passenger with an above-knee leg plaster, an ankylosed knee or hip, or a similar disability, may simply not fit in. Even if he can be accommodated with some effort, it must be remembered that he may have to maintain an uncomfortable position for many hours. In the first-class cabin there is altogether more room, but even here there are limits on available space. Certainly there are seats with a little more leg room than normal; for example, those in the emergency exit rows, but safety regulations prohibit the allocation of these to incapacitated passengers. This is to ensure that emergency exits allow free egress in the event of a rapid evacuation. It is often suggested that a passenger with, say, a plastered leg can be seated so that he can stretch his injured limb into the aisle of the cabin, but this too conflicts with safety regulations and would certainly inconvenience other passengers and crew. Space is also severely limited in the aircraft's toilets; also, passengers with mobility problems may have difficulty making their way from their seat to the toilet without assistance.

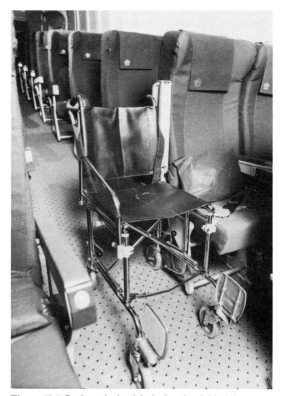

Figure 40.1 On-board wheelchair showing folded-down arm support and seat with lifting arm rest.

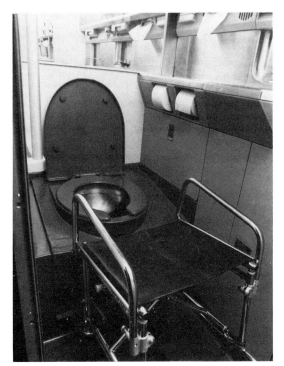

Figure 40.2 Aircraft toilet adapted for use by disabled passengers showing grab handle, low-level fitments and on-board wheelchair in position.

Some airlines have largely overcome these problems by the provision of a specialized wheelchair carried on board the aircraft (*Figure 40.1*), certain seats with lifting arm rests, and enlarged toilets equipped with aids for the disabled (*Figure 40.2*). However, sometimes the only solution for an immobile passenger is to travel on a stretcher.

Any long journey is tiring and air travel is no exception. Because of the speed of travel and consequent disturbance of circadian rhythm, sleep and appetite may be affected which will add to the feeling of fatigue. At the airport, passengers will encounter delays at Immigration, Security and Customs, as well as having to walk considerable distances between check-in and boarding. These factors make an air journey stressful or tiring for even the hardiest of travellers, but may prove intolerable or impossible for the incapacitated.

The International Air Transport Association recommends a maximum walking distance of 375 m from aircraft to kerbside, and similarly the United States Federal Aviation Administration recommends a maximum gradient for ramps at airports of 1 in 12. Many airports exceed these suggested maxima, which adds to the strain on the air traveller. An airline's medical department, with its passenger services section, can do much to relieve the elderly or invalid passenger of the physical and mental stresses that may occur. Baggage, ticket and passport formalities may be undertaken by passenger services staff and a wheelchair or even just a friendly arm to lean on may make the whole process less tiring. For those with mobility problems, special lifting arrangements are possible to overcome the problems of aircraft steps and where necessary arrangements can be made to lift the passenger to his seat.

An aircraft stretcher may be the only acceptable method of transporting a seriously ill or severely incapacitated passenger. In such cases an area is curtained off and a specially designed aircraft stretcher is fitted over the folded-down seats (*Figure 40.3*). The space available around the stretcher permits only the basic nursing functions, but it does allow a seriously ill patient to travel for treatment that otherwise may be unavailable to him. The stretcher passenger must be escorted by a trained person who can undertake any necessary treatment or nursing care in flight. In this context it must be remembered that airline cabin crew are trained only in first aid and are not qualified nurses. They cannot be expected to undertake nursing duties, administer injections or supervise treatment. Moreover, as food handlers it is not appropriate for them to provide bedpans or urinals in flight.

Air travel on a stretcher is naturally expensive, and the cost has to be borne by the passenger. The growth of air ambulance services has largely relieved the pressure on scheduled airlines to carry critically ill passengers or those requiring intensive nursing care in flight. Some passengers with terminal illness may wish to travel home to die and most airlines will consider such cases sympathetically on humanitarian grounds. Only if it seems likely that death will occur in flight will carriage be refused. This is because the practical and administrative problems that surround an in-flight death may be distressing and inconvenient to all concerned.

Clinical application

So far, the general principles affecting invalid passenger carriage have been discussed. The application of these to some common clinical conditions can now be examined.

Contraindications to air travel

There are no absolute contraindications to the carriage of patients by air, but most scheduled airlines would regard the following as unacceptable.

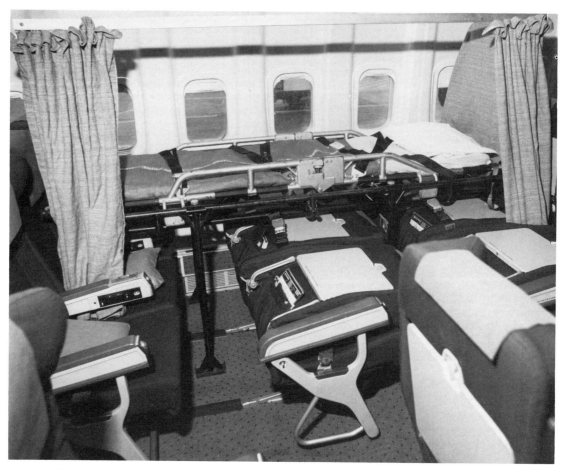

Figure 40.3 Stretcher in position.

Infectious disease

Passengers suffering from infectious disease will not be accepted until the period of infectivity has passed and they no longer constitute a risk to other passengers or crew.

Late pregnancy

Passengers near to term are not acceptable because of the risk of going into labour in flight, the aircraft cabin being less than ideal as a delivery suite. Airlines vary in their practice but most would be reluctant to accept a passenger in the last 4 weeks of her pregnancy.

The question often asked is how soon after delivery can a mother and baby safely fly? The mother can travel by air as soon as she feels able to make the journey, but the baby may present problems. In the first 48 hours of life the neonatal lung may still have small areas of atelectasis leading to ventilation–perfusion inequalities in the lung. As a general rule, therefore, it is prudent to wait at least 2 days and preferably 7 before flight unless the baby must travel for urgent treatment.

The moribund

The terminally ill passenger who is deemed unlikely to survive the flight will not be acceptable because of the distress and administrative difficulties caused by death on board.

Offensive conditions

These may include passengers whose behaviour is grossly disturbed, or those who may cause distress to others by their appearance or smell.

Conditions susceptible to hypoxia

It is recognized that the availability of oxygen to the tissues is dependent on the cardiac output, the haemoglobin level of the blood and its percentage saturation, which is in turn significantly affected by the $P_{A_{O_2}}$.

Slight reduction in any one of these three variables may be tolerable, but even a small reduction of two or more factors can lead to serious depletion of available oxygen.

Supplementary oxygen may overcome some of the problems by restoring the $P_{A_{O_2}}$ to sea level value, hence avoiding the reduction in haemoglobin saturation. However, considerations of weight and space may determine the quantity of oxygen available.

In assessing the patient's suitability to fly, the exercise tolerance is a useful practical guide. The ability to walk 50 m or climb one flight of stairs without undue distress suggests that the flight will be well tolerated.

Cardiovascular disease

Congestive cardiac failure, recent myocardial infarction, unstable angina and significant cardiac arrhythmia can all reduce cardiac output. In conditions where Pa_{O_2} is reduced, the associated reduction in the oxygen content of the blood may affect tissue oxygenation leading in turn to an exacerbation of the basic condition. Recent open-heart surgery is not in itself a contraindication to air travel unless the recovery has been complicated by any of the above conditions. After all, many post-surgical cases are far fitter when they fly home than when they flew in to their treatment centre!

Respiratory disease

Chronic bronchitis, emphysema, bronchiectasis and any conditions where respiratory exchange is compromised may be adversely affected by hypoxia. Although supplementary oxygen may be helpful for such passengers, in those bordering on respiratory failure this may be counterproductive by reducing the hypoxic drive to respiration. Once again, exercise tolerance is a good guide to fitness to fly. Dyspnoea at rest or the need for supplementary oxygen at sea level both suggest that the patient will be severely affected in the aircraft cabin and is unlikely to tolerate the physiological stresses of a long flight.

A pneumothorax will be complicated by the effects of gas expansion (*see* below).

Blood disorders

Severely anaemic patients may not tolerate the slight hypoxia and a haemoglobin level of 7.5 g/dl (1.2 mmol/litre) is generally regarded as the lowest acceptable. Much depends, however, on the cause of the anaemia, the chronicity of the condition and the length of flight; many chronically anaemic patients (e.g. those in renal failure) fly safely with haemoglobin levels of less than 7.5 g/dl. Sickle cell haemoglobinopathies may present special problems because of the known predisposition to sickling crises in hypoxic tissues, and once again supplementary oxygen may alleviate this (Green *et al.*, 1971, 1972).

Neurological disorders

Any condition where cerebral infarction is present—whether from thrombosis, embolism or haemorrhage—should be regarded cautiously until the acute stage is past. The elderly person whose cerebral oxygenation is just maintained at sea level despite arteriosclerosis may well become confused after some time at altitude, and this must be remembered when such a person wishes to travel alone on a long journey. Night-time confusion will indicate those who may be particularly susceptible to cerebral hypoxia in flight.

Epileptics may be slightly more liable to attacks during an air journey. Although hypoxia might theoretically lower the threshold to convulsions, this seems less important than the disruption of routine, the general stress and excitement of an air journey and the associated fatigue. Extra anticonvulsant medication around the time of the journey may be advisable for passengers whose epilepsy is poorly controlled.

Patients with closed head injuries and those with cerebral tumours tolerate air travel well, although they may, of course, require special nursing care during the journey.

Conditions susceptible to pressure changes

Ears and sinuses

Acute catarrhal conditions may prevent equalization of pressure in the middle ear by obstruction of the eustachian tube with resultant acute barotrauma. Similar effects may occur in the sinuses. It follows then that patients with acute otitis media, severe catarrhal obstruction of the eustachian tube, and acute sinusitis should be advised not to fly. A potentially more serious problem is that of recent middle ear surgery. Until the middle ear is dry and normally aerated it is unwise to fly and special care is necessary after stapedectomy. Some disasters have occurred when the prosthetic stapes has been disrupted by barotrauma, with serious consequences (King, unpublished observations).

Gastro-intestinal conditions

After recent gastro-intestinal surgery, expansion of gas in the gut will produce abnormal stress on suture lines, both in the gut itself and in the abdominal wall. Such cases should generally not fly until at least 10 days after surgery and if recovery has been complicated this period may need to be extended. Recent intestinal haemorrhage may be reawakened by gas expansion in the gut and in such cases adequate time should be allowed for healing to occur. Gas expansion may also lead to hyperactivity of a colostomy or ileostomy, and it is advisable for the passenger to take a good supply of bags and dressings in the hand luggage.

Chest conditions

The presence of a pneumothorax is a contraindication to air travel as the air trapped in the pleural cavity will expand and cause further respiratory embarrassment or even mediastinal shift. A pneumothorax secondary to trauma may be particularly dangerous as gas expansion may cause further distortion of the lung, leading to a tension pneumothorax. *Figure 40.4* demonstrates this problem in a patient who flew from the Caribbean to

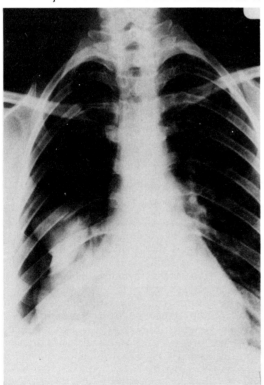

Figure 40.4 Large right-sided pneumothorax in patient who flew 7 days after closed chest injury.

London 7 days after a road accident in which some ribs were broken, there having been no evidence of a pneumothorax prior to flight. If such cases have to be moved before all the air has been reabsorbed then a chest drain of the Heimlich type should be *in situ*, or at least available to a suitably trained escort.

Emphysematous bullae do not appear particularly hazardous in flight, unless they are closed.

Other conditions

Other conditions that may be affected by gas expansion are fractures of the skull involving a sinus or the middle ear, penetrating eye injuries or recent intraocular surgery, and patients with a recently applied plaster of Paris whose limbs may be at risk from ischaemia owing to expansion of any air trapped beneath the cast.

Decompression sickness

Classic subatmospheric decompression sickness as experienced by aircrew does not occur below 18 000 feet and is extremely rare below 25 000 feet. However, this assumes that a subject is moving from normobaric to severe hypobaric conditions. A similar change of pressure can occur when moving from a hyperbaric to a mildly hypobaric environment. This situation faces the diver who boards an aircraft too soon after a dive. 'Bends' or more serious manifestations of decompression sickness have been reported in passengers who have flown too soon after a dive that normally requires stops during ascent (Diving Medical Advisory Committee, 1982).

Other conditions

Diabetes mellitus

Diabetic passengers often seek advice before travel. Most airlines can make a suitable diet available but the main problem is one of time zone changes with the risk of mistiming insulin dosage. With extensive time changes it is better for the passenger to remain on 'home base' time throughout the journey and only attempt readjustment when at his destination.

Fixed wiring of the jaws

Patients with wiring of the jaw, unless fitted with some quick release mechanism, will need to be accompanied by an escort carrying, and trained to use, wire cutters in case the patient vomits.

Tracheostomies

The very low humidity in many aircraft cabins (often less than 15% relative humidity) may cause excessive drying and crusting of secretions and this is a particular problem for infants. Nurses escorting such passengers need to be alert to this. Any such passenger who may require supplementary oxygen will need an appropriate stoma mask.

Psychiatric disorders

As passengers, the mentally ill may cause trouble in two ways. The obvious one, which is usually foreseen and relatively easily avoided, is when a potentially disturbed psychotic is travelling and may become a danger to himself or others, especially in the close confines of the aircraft cabin. A second group, less easily identified, comprises those psychotics or psychoneurotics for whom air travel may be particularly stressful and who may become bewildered, confused or lost during the journey. The atmosphere of an airport can appear unreal and bizarre: the lights, crowds and unfamiliar sounds and languages can at times have a nightmarish quality and be disorientating. Psychiatric patients who are well controlled in the sheltered environment of home or hospital, with regular routines of meals, rest and medication, are ill equipped to deal with the mental stress of a long journey, especially by air. A long intercontinental flight may involve several transit stops, perhaps a change of aircraft, considerable fatigue and some natural anxiety about personal safety. Unexpected delays or diversions due to weather or technical problems may add to the stress. These conditions, together with the busy atmosphere of a large airport, are enough to tax even the most placid person at times, and this is often overlooked by a doctor assessing his patient in the calm of a hospital or his consulting room.

Obviously the disturbed patient will require a suitably trained medical escort, and more than one may be needed if the condition is severe or the journey a long one. Passengers who may become disorientated, anxious or confused may simply need a responsible adult escort, as an airline cannot undertake to monitor their progress through the complexities and potential disruption of a long air journey.

Summary

The growth in air travel has been accompanied by an increasing awareness among airlines of the needs of incapacitated passengers. Most major airlines can provide specialist advice both to passengers and to their doctors, and full use should be made of such services.

Facilities for passengers with stable disabilities continue to be refined and improved, while the growth and availability of the air ambulance has relieved the scheduled airlines of the need to make provision for the passenger requiring intensive care or specialized treatment in flight.

For those between these two extremes, full consultation with the airline's medical department is important if inconvenience and even hazard to the patient or others is to be avoided. Cabin crew, although trained in first aid, are unable to offer a nursing service and if this is required then the passenger will need to be accompanied by a suitable attendant. Knowledge of the principles involved and the facilities available, combined with co-operation between the passenger, his physician and the airline's medical service should ensure that almost all invalid passengers travel safely and with minimum inconvenience.

References

DENNISON, D.M., LEDWITH, M.A. and POULTON, E.C. (1966) Complex reaction times at simulated cabin altitudes of 5000 ft and 8000 ft. *Aerospace Medicine*, **37**, 1010–1013

Diving Medical Advisory Committee (1982) *Recommendations for Flying after Diving*. London: DMAC

GREEN, R.L., HUNTSMAN, R.G. and SERJEANT, G.R. (1971) The sickle-cell and altitude. *British Medical Journal*, **iv**, 593–595

GREEN, R.L., HUNTSMAN, R.G. and SERJEANT, G.R. (1972) The sickle-cell and altitude. *British Medical Journal*, **i**, 803–804

HARDING, R.M. and MILLS, F.J. (1983) *Aviation Medicine*. London: British Medical Association

41

Airfreight—health and safety in the air transport of animals

G.E. Joss and T. Harris

Introduction

Airfreight companies may consider that their responsibilities for the shipment of animals by air are restricted to the time that the animal is in their possession. Even so, there are many factors that affect the health and safety of the animal not only during the time that it is in the possession of the airline but also from the time it leaves its natural environment, to the moment it is delivered into the hands of its ultimate owner. Any complaints with regard to the condition of the animal upon its receipt by the ultimate owner are likely to be directed at the airline operator. The final condition of the animal cargo at its ultimate destination is likely to be the criterion by which a customer judges the efficiency of the carrier.

This chapter deals with the non-domesticated animals which pose special problems. Attempts must be made to minimize stressful circumstances which, quite apart from the effects on the animal's temper, may turn a healthy animal into a sick one by the time it reaches its destination. The total journey that the animal undertakes—in which the flight plays only a small part—may impose such stress that the healthy animal becomes ill. Commensal bacteria and other infecting agents become pathogens, and silent infections become overt, so that the animal is not only a danger to others in the consignment, but possibly also to personnel or passengers. A wise carrier will therefore seek to influence the pre-flight and post-flight conditions, especially those of collection, distribution and packaging. In this way, he will play a positive part in the control of animal disease and zoonotic infections.

There are a number of quarantine and other importation regulations in force in many countries;

but as air transportation of animals increases, the regulations are likely to become more elaborate and more strictly enforced. In the past in air transport there has been some confusion arising from vague classification and description of animals, but in Great Britain this problem has been overcome by substituting zoological for domestic classification. The present classification (HMSO, 1974) lists most carefully those animals that are subject to quarantine in this country, and the possibility of such diseases as rabies being transmitted from animals imported by air was one of the reasons why stricter legislation has been imposed. Interestingly, prior to recent legislation it was possible to import many mammals (for example, skunks and bats) which may well have been carriers of the rabies virus.

Factors affecting the transported animal

There are three phases for an animal on its journey from the natural environment until arrival at the final destination.

Phase 1—collection and transport to airhead

It is undoubtedly regrettable that airlines have little or no direct control over the Phase 1 part of the total journey of the animal in which they have interest. The airline operator should certainly be aware of the problem and should perhaps consider accepting animal freight only from those shippers known to have a responsible attitude towards the acquisition of the animals that they are asking the airline to transport. Although the selection and methods of catching the animals may seem remote from Phase 2 of the total journey (*see* below) they often determine the success of the airlift. Ignorance of these factors may well negate any amount of care and attention lavished on the animals during the various stages of Phase 2.

Delay can be experienced by an animal during Phase 1, prior to its arrival at the airport. It may well be advisable for animals to be allowed to rest at the collecting centres and depots in Phase 1, during which time any overt disease could be noted, and the necessary action taken. In practice, such delays in Phase 1 may be only accidental since the collectors usually wish to export their animals as quickly as possible and present them at the airport before the weaker ones die.

The time an animal spends in a depot may be related to aircraft availability; therefore, close liaison here between the airline and the shipper is important. Short delays are generally not serious, and may indeed give the shipper the opportunity of removing ailing animals. Long delays, however, are a disadvantage both from the practical point of managing the animals in somewhat different circumstances, and because animals so delayed may acclimatize themselves to one location only to find themselves shipped on and having to readapt to the travel as well as to the new environment. It is probably advisable that, once the animals have left a collecting centre, their journey should be rapid and uncomplicated.

Since the importance of the stress of Phase I cannot be overstated it is advisable to consider some of the factors that contribute towards it:

1. The removal of the animal from its normal environment—its familiar territory, its intra- and extra-specific relationships—and the frustration of its normal behaviour must impose a great strain upon it.
2. There is the unfamiliar noise background to which the animal may be especially sensitive—perhaps to certain frequencies not noticed by man.
3. For the first time in the animal's life it will be in constant contact with man, normally regarded as an enemy.
4. Boxing and crating manoeuvres with their mixture of noise, the presence of man, and new circumstances, induce a high degree of fear and trepidation.
5. Nutritional factors may not be of great importance for short journeys, but there is bound to be some degree of change.
6. Unless proper care is taken, the animals may be exposed to unacceptable extremes of temperature and humidity.

Phase 2—airhead, flight and arrival at destination

In Phase 2, delays may be experienced by the animals at the airport holding centres, as well as during the actual loading or unloading of the aircraft. Of the various stages in Phase 2, the flying time itself is probably the least troublesome, since practical experience has shown that most animals adapt quite rapidly to flying. It should be remembered, however, that not all flights are direct, and that there may be periods of interchange on route. All airports should, therefore, have the benefit of veterinary consultant services, together with the appropriate accommodation for the animals that they may be holding. This should include facilities for the separation of incompatible species during any isolation period that may be required for local quarantine restrictions, together with any special requirements such as side-rooms for immediate laboratory work, and minor post-mortem facilities for immediate identification of the cause of death. There are those who feel that these facilities should be the responsibility of civil authorities; at the moment they are provided mainly by the airlines or by animal charities.

A factor that affects all phases of animal freight and that greatly influences not only the condition of the animal at its destination, but its ability to survive the journey is the condition in which it is packaged for transport. The techniques of packaging animals for flight are now fully laid down in *The IATA Live Animals Regulations* (IATA, 1986) which have been incorporated into the flight manuals of many airlines. Several countries have formally adopted the provisions of these Regulations as part of their legislation or through the issuance of a permit authorizing air carriers to carry live animals by air as defined in this IATA publication. These Regulations cover the factors that must be considered to ensure animals are carried without harm to themselves or to the handling personnel.

The crew of an aircraft carrying animals should be carefully instructed in their responsibilities. The pilots should be aware of the problems caused by height changes and sudden manoeuvres, and of the need to avoid turbulent air. The cabin crew should know how to look after the animals—if necessary a specialist handler should be on board.

Regulations are laid down for the protection of the crew against transmissible infection or from injury from animal freight. Aircraft must be disinfected after flights with animal freight, and only disinfectants that can dissolve fat and grease should be used and must not be corrosive to metals or plastics. Antiseptics are frequently not strong enough.

Phase 3—airport to final destination

Airlines should recognize the difficulties that animals may still have to face during their journey from the airport to their final destination; for example, they may have to go via a railhead or a road haulier, or be lodged with an animal agent, before they arrive at the destination.

Quarantine and import/export regulations vary internationally, but in the United Kingdom some of the most severe quarantine restrictions relate to rabies control. Airline operators must be familiar with all the relevant legislation current in those countries in which they have an interest. In Great Britain an order on rabies (HMSO, 1974) lists quite clearly those mammals that need quarantine facilities.

An airline should also be familiar with other infections of animals—particularly of primates—since these may cause disease in man. Correct handling facilities at airports and very careful documentation so as to make quite sure that animal batches can be identified rapidly should a disease problem arise are essential.

Rabies

The current spread of rabies across the continent of Europe towards the Channel ports highlights the risk that the disease may spread even more extensively. Since the domestic cat and dog in particular are potential carriers of the disease, regulations are being reinforced to ensure that no animals are landed in Great Britain either as accompanied passenger baggage or in the passenger cabin of an aircraft; they must be carried as freight and landed in a container of at least the appropriate IATA standard. The immunization of animal handlers is of course highly desirable, but here the distinction should be made between 'handlers' and 'loaders'. The former are seldom airline employees, but generally work for some other organization. On the other hand, loaders are airline employees, but the hazard to them is considered slight, since loading techniques and protective clothing and gloves are designed to keep the loader out of contact with the animal or its excretions. Should a person be accidentally scratched or bitten despite precautions, appropriate treatment should be given at once.

Hygiene problems in the carriage of animals

The IATA Live Animals Regulations (republished annually) (IATA, 1986) lists several hundred species, ranging from Aardvark to Zebu. Subsequent pages describe the problems associated with the air transport of most of the more exotic animals. Although airlines carry a wide variety of animals, many of them are very ordinary.

Larger animals, such as horses and cattle, are usually transported in charter freighter aircraft, but the bellies of modern wide-bodied scheduled aircraft may also be used for cattle, sheep, goats and pigs. On the other hand, animals such as cats and dogs are carried mostly in the cargo holds of passenger scheduled flights. Many airlines prohibit the carriage of domestic pets in passenger cabins; others may accept them under special circumstances as accompanied baggage.

The bulk of animals imported into the United Kingdom are primates and tropical fish, whereas domestic animals, particularly pedigree dogs and cats, are exported in large numbers.

The IATA Live Animals Regulations are informative and include the following sections:

1. General information.
2. Shipping procedures.
3. Carriage procedures.
4. Container requirements.
5. Government regulations.
6. Convention on international trade in endangered species (CITES).
7. Scientific names of animals.
8. Specific container and handling notes for each of the species listed.
9. Live animals acceptance check sheet.

Before any animal is accepted as cargo, the following main points should be satisfied:

1. The presence of the livestock will not cause discomfort to passengers or crew by reason of smell, noise or risk of escape.
2. Climatic conditions during the journey and stowage conditions on the aircraft will not adversely affect the health of the livestock.
3. The regulations regarding livestock are not infringed in the countries of transit and destination.
4. The animals are in a satisfactory physical condition to withstand the strain of the journey, for example, females should not be accepted when in an advanced state of pregnancy, so as not to give birth in transit.

Although hygiene problems may arise during flight, it is after the animals are off-loaded that the major sanitation problems occur. Odours emanating from either the animal itself or body waste products are usually present and are often penetrating and persistent. In addition there are waste products from animal feed stuffs and other types of rubbish. Fleas or other insects may have been carried, and surfaces might have been contaminated with harmful bacteria.

The contamination of the internal surfaces of the aircraft is reduced by placing plastic sheeting underneath cages and arranging it to extend 2 or 3 inches (50–75 mm) up the sides. Care must be taken not to block or impede ventilation holes.

To minimize odours during flight and handling, solid deodorant sachets are attached to each container, and, just before the hold doors are closed after loading, or when the hold is subsequently opened or closed, the interior is sprayed with a special animal deodorant.

The following hygiene precautions are recommended to protect staff involved in the handling of animals, and for cleaning aircraft after the animals have been off-loaded:

1. Only animals that are in good health should be accepted. Shippers should declare when animals are pregnant.
2. Different species should be isolated whenever possible.
3. Holding rooms or areas at airports should be cleaned and disinfected at least once every 24 hours.
4. Animal consignments should not be stowed near to foodstuffs.
5. Handlers must wear washable, impervious gauntlets of elbow length as well as face masks.
6. Gloves and hands should be washed with a germicidal soap after handling animals.
7. Physical contact with animals should be avoided as far as possible. People should not disturb the animals or bend down and peer into the containers.
8. Any person bitten or scratched by animals must report to a medical centre as soon as possible.
9. Handlers should be immunized against tetanus, and possibly rabies.
10. Clothing contaminated by blood or excreta from animals should be removed and sent for cleaning.

Cleaning procedures for aircraft

1. Cleaners must wear gloves and rubber boots which must be washed after use.

2. All polythene sheeting, netting, straps or other material used to cover or protect cages must be removed.
3. Waste foods or other debris from harbourage points must be removed with a vacuum cleaner.
4. Shelves and floors must be thoroughly washed or swabbed with a solution of approved fat solvent detergent/disinfectant that does not corrode metal or plastics.
5. The interior should be sprayed with an efficient odour counteractant, designed to neutralize the body odours from animals and their waste products. During the spraying all doors should be closed to obtain the maximum benefit.

The methods given are regarded as a minimum, and it may sometimes be necessary to insist upon more stringent cleaning procedures. However, if this system is operated after each cargo of animals, nuisance from smell etc. will be kept to an acceptable minimum, even if it is not completely eliminated. This will prevent a build-up which would obviously be much more difficult to remove at a later stage.

References

Her Majesty's Stationery Office (1974) *Rabies (Importation of Dogs, Cats and other Mammals)*. London: HMSO

International Air Transport Association (1986) *The IATA Live Animals Regulations (Republished annually)*. Geneva: IATA

Further reading

BISSERU, B. (1967) *Diseases of Man Acquired from his Pets*. London: Heinemann

Ministry of Agriculture, Food and Fisheries (1983) *Code of Practice for the Transportation by Air of Cattle, Sheep, Pigs, Goats and Horses*. London: MAFF

VAN DER HEODEN (1965) *Zoonoses*. Amsterdam: Elsevier Elsevier

Part IX

Clinical Aspects of Aviation Medicine

42

Sleep and wakefulness: clinical considerations

A.N. Nicholson

Introduction

Disturbed sleep is a frequent occurrence in aviation, and understanding sleep and wakefulness and the way in which they may both be disturbed are important facets to the work of the aeromedical practitioner. For this reason some knowledge of the sleep–wakefulness continuum and the circadian basis of the regular alternation of sleep and wakefulness is essential. However, though disturbance by the environment or by unusual patterns of work is likely to be of primary interest, sleep may also be impaired for other reasons, and so some familiarity with sleep disorders is desirable. Finally, every doctor concerned with the care of aircrew has been faced with the question of the use of hypnotics, and understanding their clinical pharmacology is necessary to ensure that they are prescribed effectively and that their use is free of adverse effects on subsequent performance. In this chapter we deal with these various aspects of sleep medicine as they may relate to aviation, and subsequently we deal with sleep disturbance in aircrew.

Sleep–wakefulness continuum

The electroencephalogram has contributed considerably to our present-day knowledge. The EEG together with the electro-oculogram and electromyogram (*Figure 42.1*) are used to define epochs of sleep usually of 30 seconds duration, and in this way the evolution of sleep over the night is described and disturbances are identified. The initial change from wakefulness is to drowsy (stage 1) sleep (*Figure 42.2*), and this involves a general slowing of the electrical activity of the brain with a decrease in the amount, amplitude and frequency of the alpha

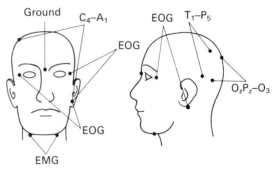

Figure 42.1 Electrode placements for recording the sleep EEG. The EEG can be recorded with three channels (C_4-A_1, T_1-P_5 and $O_zP_z-O_3$). The electro-oculogram (EOG) is recorded bilaterally, and the electromyogram (EMG) is recorded from the submental musculature.

rhythm (8–12 Hz). In the transition from wakefulness there are often slow eye movements, each of several seconds duration. Drowsy sleep is scored when alpha together with low-voltage activity amount to less than 50% of the record (*Figure 42.3*).

The onset of sleep (stage 2) is signalled by a K complex or by a spindle (*Figure 42.4*). K complexes can occur in response to sudden stimuli, but they also appear without any obvious reason. Stage 3 sleep is scored when at least 20%, and stage 4 sleep (*Figure 42.5*) is scored when more than 50% of each epoch consists of wages of 2 Hz or slower (delta waves) with amplitudes greater than 75 μV from peak-to-peak. Most stage 4 epochs have the appearance of continuous slow wave activity, although only slightly more than half the epoch may contain high-amplitude slow waves. Sleep spindles may or may not be present during slow wave sleep. Rapid eye movement (REM) sleep (*Figure 42.6*) is characterized by relatively low voltage, mixed

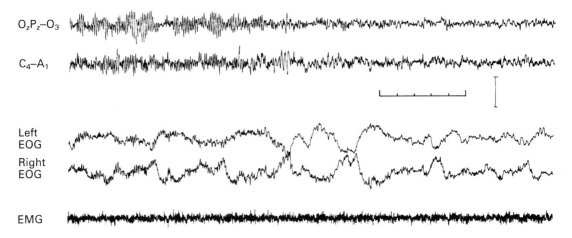

Figure 42.2 Change from wakefulness to drowsy (Stage 1) sleep with slow eye movements. Calibrations of 75 µV, and the time-base is 5 seconds with 1 second intervals.

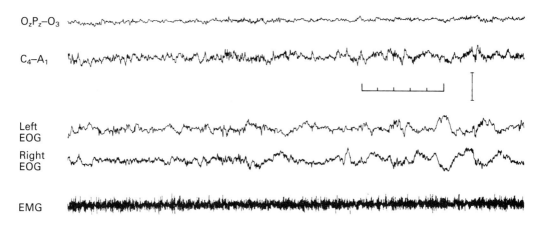

Figure 43.3 Epoch of drowsy sleep. Calibrations of 75 µV, and the time-base is 5 seconds with 1 second intervals.

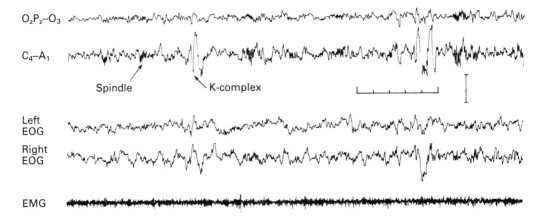

Figure 42.4 Epoch of stage 2 sleep with spindles and K-complexes. Calibrations of 75 µV, and the time-base is 5 seconds with 1 second intervals.

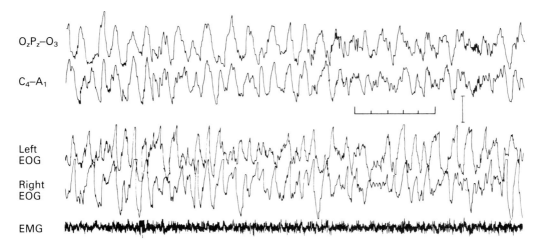

$O_zP_z–O_3$

$C_4–A_1$

Left
EOG

Right
EOG

EMG

Figure 42.5 Epoch of slow wave sleep (stage 4). Calibrations of 75 µV, and the time-base is 5 seconds with 1 second intervals.

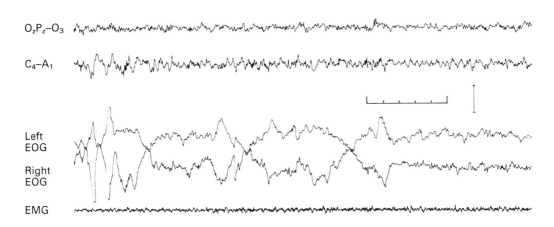

$O_zP_z–O_3$

$C_4–A_1$

Left
EOG

Right
EOG

EMG

Figure 42.6 Epoch of rapid eye movement sleep. Calibrations of 75 µV, and the time-base is 5 seconds with 1 second intervals.

frequency activity together with episodic rapid eye movements. The EEG has some resemblance to drowsy sleep, except that vertex sharp waves are never present, and the amplitude of myographic activity is low.

These various stages of sleep are used to describe a sleep period (*Figure 42.7*) Slow wave sleep predominates during the first third of the night, and the cyclical appearance of REM activity characterizes the latter two-thirds. The young healthy adult passes quickly from wakefulness into stage 2 and slow wave sleep, and about 70–90 minutes after the onset of sleep there is usually the first period of REM sleep which is fragile and may last only a few minutes. The first REM episode is followed by further non-REM activity which usually includes

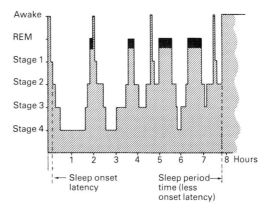

Figure 42.7 Nocturnal hypnogram of a young adult.

slow wave sleep, and then there is a further REM period of around 15 minutes duration. During the night the mean interval between REM periods is about 100 minutes, but it may vary between 70 and 120 minutes. In about 15% of sleeps the short first REM period may be absent, and then the subsequent REM periods appear somewhat earlier.

Sleep and age

Some individuals without complaints about their sleep or daytime function, and whose sleep is unbroken and normal, have substantially shorter or substantially longer sleep than the average amount for their age. Short sleepers have less than three-quarters of the norm, and some may even sleep less than 3 hours each night. Long sleepers have at least 9 hours, possibly between 12 and 14 hours. Long sleepers enjoy and protect their sleep, and may have difficulty in coping with restricted sleep schedules. There is no obvious psychopathology in these individuals, though it has been suggested that personality traits exist.

Total sleep time and the total nightly amounts of the various stages of sleep are related to age. Total sleep time is longest in infancy, and it stabilizes around 7 hours at about 20 years of age. It remains constant during adulthood, and changes little throughout old age. The most obvious change with age is the decrease in slow wave sleep. In young adults about 15% of nocturnal sleep is spent in slow wave activity, but in late middle age few have stage 4, although more women than men show it in their later years. Elderly men rarely show stage 4 sleep, but some may still be present in women. Rapid eye movement sleep has the longest duration in infancy and in childhood. There is a fall in the percentage of REM sleep from around 30% in young children to around 25% in adults, and there is another slight fall in the elderly.

Although the proportion of time spent awake during the night may change very little, the number of awakenings tends to increase with age. Awake time in adults is usually below 2% of the sleep period, but it tends to increase after 40 years in males and over 50 years in females. However, the number of arousals may be more than that suggested by an analysis of the usual 30 second epochs. An awake episode of just less than 30 seconds could be divided evenly across two epochs, and so would not be scored as wakefulness for either epoch. Such a disturbance of sleep can be important in middle age and in the aged.

Middle age is an important span of life, and this is equally so for aircrew. At this time of life many are coping with exacting day-to-day lives. Their occupations may involve irregularity of rest, and they may well have difficulty in achieving acceptable sleep.

Sleep is less restful as we grow older, and a significant contribution to this deterioration may be due to leg movements and changes in the usual pattern of breathing. Leg movements and apnoeas are usually seen during the sleep of middle-aged individuals even though they do not have any complaint related to their sleep. Indeed, about two-thirds of middle-aged males have leg movements and around 90% have apnoeas or hypopnoeas, and some have an unusually high number of these events. Both may lead to brief arousals and lightening of sleep, though leg movements tend to be associated with drowsy (stage 1) activity, and so with disturbed sleep.

Daytime sleep latencies

Recently the EEG has been used in the study of daytime alertness (multiple sleep latency test). The time taken to reach a particular stage of sleep is measured five or six times during the day (*Figure 42.8*). A low mean value over the day is found in patients with disorders of sleep associated with excessive daytime sleepiness. However, many healthy individuals have low values, and so short latencies during the day do not necessarily imply sleep pathology, but could indicate a relative ease of falling asleep.

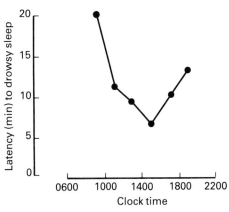

Figure 42.8 Multiple sleep latency test: the time taken to reach drowsy (stage 1) sleep is measured at intervals during the day.

Of particular interest to aviation medicine is the shape of the curve derived from sleep latencies during the day. During the early part of the day there is an increasing ease in falling asleep, and during the latter part latencies increase. The significance of the earlier and later parts of the curve remains to be fully established, but the progressive decrease in sleep latencies during the early part may be related to the interval since the last sleep period.

The increase in sleep latencies during the latter part of the day is related to the rising phase of the circadian rhythm of alertness, and can be used to measure the displacement of the circadian rhythm of the individual from the day–night cycle of a new time zone, and so to assess the rate of adaptation.

Neuroendocrinology

The secretion of many hormones is related to sleep and wakefulness, to the sleep cycle itself or to specific EEG activity. Circadian rhythmicity is an important variable, and other influences include the light–dark cycle and the episodic secretion of other hormones. For example, blood cortisol levels are lowest during the early hours of sleep and highest in the early morning hours, while secretion of the adrenocorticotrophic hormone (ACTH) is lowest in the few hours before and after sleep onset, and increases after 3–5 hours of sleep, reaching its maximum just before awakening. Individual episodes of ACTH secretion tend to occur about 10 minutes before an episode of cortisol secretion.

In most subjects the peak plasma level of growth hormone occurs during the first 90 minutes of sleep, and the episode lasts around 2–3 hours. About two-thirds of the total secretion occurs within 90 minutes of the onset of sleep. When sleep onset is delayed, the plasma peak of growth hormone is also delayed, and when subjects are awakened for 2–3 hours and sleep is resumed, there is another peak. Smaller peaks occur throughout the night, and these tend to be related to the appearance of slow wave sleep. After inversion of the sleep–wake cycle the pattern of secretion is also reversed. Growth hormone secretion may not be specifically associated with sleep onset, but rather to the onset of slow wave sleep.

The secretion of prolactin peaks about an hour after sleep onset, with subsequent peaks reaching maximum levels between 0700 and 0800 hours. During the hour after wakening the levels begin to fall, with the minimum before noon. When the hours of sleep are modified, there is an immediate shift. In this sense prolactin secretion resembles that of growth hormone. The individual secretory episodes of prolactin appear to be entrained to the NREM-REM sleep cycle, with nadirs of prolactin secretion occurring during REM sleep and peaks during non-REM sleep.

Melatonin is secreted principally by the pineal gland, although there is a secondary source in the retina. It is secreted at night, and is suppressed by light of sufficient intensity. It has been suggested that melatonin given at an appropriate time preceding the sleep period would advance the circadian cycle, and in this way alter the endogenous oscillator. Evidence is needed that melatonin has not merely distorted the observed rhythm, as this may be inadvertently interpreted as a phase shift. Published data are equivocal. There is, as yet, no convincing evidence that melatonin shifts the basic oscillatory function in man, and the situation is confused further as the drug would appear to have psychotropic activity such as sedation and mood elevation, and may even encourage sleep by lowering body temperature. The activity of melatonin in man has not yet been adequately explored, and the claim that it may be used to shift circadian rhythms after time-zone changes is premature (Anon, 1986).

Circadian rhythms

Human beings experience a regular alternation of sleep and wakefulness which has a constant relationship with the day–night cycle. The most important environmental influence on circadian rhythmicity is almost certainly the daily alternation of light and darkness, although social cues are also important. In the absence of the periodic time cues of the environment, as when living in caves, the rhythm is no longer entrained and is free-running. It then has a period of about 25 hours, and this is the intrinsic rhythmicity of man—an internal 'biological clock' which keeps time in the absence of environmental cues. It is important to realize that many factors can influence circadian rhythmicity, and that the observed rhythm may be easily modified by external events. Examples include the suppression of melatonin by bright light, the effect of posture on aldosterone secretion, and of sleep and exercise on body temperature. Such effects are transient modulations of the rhythm, and it is important that they are not interpreted as a fundamental change in the clock mechanism.

In many subjects living in the absence of external time cues the rest–activity cycle eventually splits apart from the body temperature cycle, and the two maintain different periods from each other. Rapid eye movement sleep, plasma cortisol release, urinary potassium excretion, sleepiness, and some aspects of performance are linked with body temperature; while slow wave sleep, growth hormone release, urinary calcium excretion and skin temperature are linked with rest and activity. The ability to sleep varies with the phase of the temperature cycle, and it is because the oscillator is slow to change that it is difficult to adjust sleep rapidly after a time-zone change or after a shift in the work–rest cycle.

Some disorders of sleep are believed to arise from modulations of circadian rhythmicity. In the delayed and advanced sleep phase syndromes sleep onset and wake time are later or earlier than desirable. Sleep occurs at the same clock time each day, and once it has begun there is no difficulty in maintaining sleep. The delayed sleep phase syndrome is usually seen in young people, and often presents with the complaint of difficulty in falling asleep at the conventional time. There may also be problems with getting up in the morning, and if sleep is curtailed there may be daytime sleepiness. The advanced sleep phase syndrome is much less common and does not interfere with daytime alertness. The complaint is that of an inability to stay awake in the evening, and to maintain sleep until the morning.

Other disorders may also be considered as modulations of circadian rhythmicity. The inherent circadian cycle of sleep and wakefulness may occur at a later clock time on successive days if entrainment to the light–dark cycle is weak. Further, complete loss of the entrained rhythm could lead to an irregular sleep–wakefulness pattern with frequent daytime naps and excessive bed rest. Sleep at night is not adequate even though the total amount of sleep may be within normal limits.

Disorders of sleep and arousal

As far as the aeromedical practitioner is concerned the most frequent problem with respect to sleep disturbance is likely to be irregularity of work. However, to assess adequately the problem it is necessary to be familiar with sleep disorders that arise for other reasons. Sleep disorders are part of the differential diagnosis, particularly in the middle aged if the primary complaint is that of persistent insomnia or excessive daytime sleepiness. The approach to the complaint of sleep disturbance must be logical; and in this sense it is convenient to consider, first of all, its duration. The chronic insomniac presents an unremitting history of disturbed sleep over months or even years, and careful assessment is paramount. On the other hand a history of a week or so (short-term insomnia) is usually related to a life crisis or to a medical illness, while transient insomnia, which is sleep disturbance over a day or two, arises when the circumstances that surround rest are not conducive to sleep or when rest occurs at unusual times.

The practitioner must always bear in mind that sleep disturbance in aircrew could be due to personal difficulties or to various forms of illness, and that the persistent complaint of insomnia or, perhaps even more important, excessive daytime sleepiness, may hide significant pathology. Possibly one-third to one-half of patients with chronic insomnia have an underlying personality disorder or psychiatric problem, such as depression. Some may have been prescribed hypnotics several years ago and have continued their use without an adequate reason, and some abuse alcohol or even drugs. However, in many cases there is no obvious cause,

and this is often referred to as primary chronic insomnia. Such individuals may complain of daytime sleepiness or loss of well-being without impaired daytime alertness, but on investigation show little evidence of sleep disturbance or of daytime sleepiness. They may have a neurotic attitude to sleep or may simply need more sleep than others; but some have a major and chronic dissatisfaction with their lives, and express this dissatisfaction in physical terms.

The sleep EEG of some patients with chronic insomnia shows brief arousals, and this finding raises the possibility that, perhaps, a more detailed understanding of sleep and the sleep of the chronic insomniac would reveal changes of clinical relevance. However, in some chronic insomniacs there are clear and multiple arousals during the night linked with somatic events such as apnoeas and leg movements. These events are of interest as they are related, at least in part, to the normal deterioration of sleep in middle age, and they may be an important finding in aircrew having difficulty in coping with unusual patterns of work.

Chronic difficulty with sleep may indicate more serious conditions than simply the usual deterioration with age, and the practitioner should bear in mind these clinical entities. In one series, the sleep apnoea syndrome accounted for over a half of patients who presented with the complaint of excessive daytime sleepiness, and about a fifth suffered from insufficient sleep, nocturnal myoclonus, or sleepiness associated with drugs and alcohol. It must also be remembered that narcolepsy does not only present itself in young adults. Indeed, in the same series narcolepsy accounts for a third of the patients. These sleep conditions can prejudice the ability to remain alert during the day, and for this reason narcolepsy and two of the commonest sleep conditions, sleep apnoea and the restless legs syndromes, are discussed below.

Narcolepsy

Excessive daytime somnolence always merits careful investigation. Narcolepsy is a prevalent cause, and though it is most frequently encountered between 15 and 25 years, the age of onset varies from childhood to the early fifties. The incidence is between 1 and 2 per 1000, and it is more common than many of the more familiar neurological diseases such as multiple sclerosis. The patient suffers from excessive daytime somnolence, and one or more of three other well-established features—cataplexy, sleep paralysis or hypnagogic hallucinations. There may also be disturbed nocturnal sleep. The features related to wakefulness are more frequent, but probably only 1 in 10 patients suffers from the complete tetrad.

Aetiology is unclear. A chronobiological basis is unlikely, but genetic influences are important, and there are associations with the HLA-DR2 antigen.

The primary and most disabling symptom is drowsiness which leads to short periods of daytime sleep, sometimes prevented by concentrating on staying awake. They occur at inappropriate times and last for 10–15 minutes, though if resting the patient may fall asleep for a couple of hours. They are usually, but not necessarily, refreshing. The attacks may occur with or without warning, and are common in situations that provoke drowsiness such as after lunch and during afternoon lectures, though they are not always related to monotonous activity. Patients not only feel sleepy, but also spend their days at a low level of alertness which may lead to poor work and memory lapses. A positive diagnosis requires one of the major features—either irresistible episodes of sleep or attacks of cataplexy—together with evidence of REM episodes immediately or within 10 minutes of sleep onset. Daytime sleeps are often used to establish sleep onset REM activity.

The most common symptom related to wakefulness is cataplexy. It occurs in some form or another in at least two-thirds of patients with narcolepsy. When fully conscious, patients suffer from a sudden decrease or abrupt loss of muscle tone which may be generalized or limited to certain muscle groups. There may be a transient weakness of the jaw, or in extreme cases, postural collapse. An attack may last for only a few seconds and is frequently triggered by exercise and emotion, such as laughing or crying, and it may terminate with REM sleep. Cataplexy may occur many times a day, or once a week or even less, and may disappear completely. Narcoleptics, particularly those in whom excessive daytime somnolence is accompanied by cataplexy, often have a REM period at sleep onset, and their sleep is often disturbed with awakenings and body movements, excessive drowsy and little slow wave sleep. Some patients may have excessive amounts of REM sleep.

Sleep paralysis and hypnagogic hallucinations occur while falling asleep or on waking, and recordings reveal REM sleep. In sleep paralysis patients feel they cannot move any muscles except those controlling the eyes, and this state is often accompanied by intense fear and by hypnagogic hallucinations. Respiration is not affected, and the paralysis can be terminated by vigorously moving the eyes or even by being touched. It lasts from a few seconds to several minutes. Hypnagogic hallucinations are vivid, frightening auditory or visual hallucinations experienced when fully conscious, and they often occur during an episode of sleep paralysis. Sleep paralysis and hypnagogic hallucinations are each present in about a quarter of patients with narcolepsy.

There is no consistent psychopathology associated with narcolepsy, though the patient may be considered as lacking motivation and having little interest in work. Often the history will include episodes of a disciplinary nature, and in about half of patients there is a history of an abrupt change in their sleep–wakefulness cycle, or recent personal distress. Narcolepsy can lead to driving accidents, a disrupted social life and depression. Treatment is somewhat uncertain though excessive daytime sleepiness may be alleviated by stimulants. If cataplexy is serious, drugs used as antidepressants but free of sedative activity may be helpful.

Idiopathic and recurring hypersomnias need to be distinguished from narcolepsy. In idiopathic hypersomnia sleep episodes are of longer duration and less irresistible without being refreshing; and hypnagogic hallucinations, cataplexy and sleep paralysis are absent. There are no sleep onset REM periods. Recurring hypersomnia is a manifestation of the Kleine–Levin syndrome and includes episodes of excessive somnolence, over-eating and abnormal behaviour, and may also feature depression.

Sleep apnoea syndrome

The sleep apnoea syndrome most commonly affects overweight males, especially between the ages of 40 and 60 years. There is excessive daytime sleepiness and frequent apnoeas during sleep. The syndrome can usually be recognized because of loud intermittent snoring, while respiratory recordings reveal apnoeic episodes. In these episodes there may be an absence of respiratory effort with cessation of diaphragmatic movement, but the upper airway remains open even though there is no airflow (central apnoea), or there may be obstruction to the airway with excessive respiratory effort (obstructive apnoea).

Because of the disturbed nocturnal sleep or hypoxaemia patients complain of excessive daytime sleepiness, and may take frequent though unrefreshing naps during the day—often at inappropriate times. The football fan may fall asleep at the match, and the teacher may fall asleep in front of the class. Obesity, in particular, and possibly depression may be associated with the condition. Nearly all are heavy snorers, and the diagnosis must always be considered in a patient who snores and complains either of excessive daytime sleepiness or insomnia.

The sleep apnoea syndrome develops gradually from heavy snoring with apnoeas and daytime somnolence to the complicated form with cyanosis, polycythaemia, right heart failure and oedema, enlargement of the liver, papilloedema and coma. Investigation should include both sleep studies and respiratory function during sleep. There may be mechanical abnormalities of the soft palate and jaw, laryngeal stenosis or even neurological disorders. However, some functional impairment such as decrease in the tone of the oropharyngeal musculature during sleep is necessary. In cases with either severe complications or excessive daytime sleepiness that compromises work a tracheostomy which is opened during sleep may be necessary. Alternative surgical measures may be more appropriate such as uvulopalatopharyngoplasty, though individual response varies and all do not benefit to the same degree. Weight reduction and sleeping on the side may help, and positive pressure breathing at night can be useful. Protriptyline 20 mg daily may lead to improvement possibly due to an effect on upper airway muscular tone.

Restless legs syndrome

Rapid, sporadic muscular movements occur during sleep, particularly during REM sleep, and sometimes there are massive jerks which may involve a limb or even the whole body. These are of little clinical importance, though frequent leg movements may lead to sleep disturbance. In nocturnal myoclonus leg twitches repeat themselves every 20–40 seconds during sleep, and recordings from the anterior tibialis show bursts of activity, with the episodes lasting from 5 minutes to 2 hours, and alternating with normal periods of sleep. In some individuals there are complaints of insomnia. In the restless legs syndrome there are similar jerks, but there are also uncomfortable and disagreeable sensations of cramp deep inside the calf muscles when at rest or in bed about to fall asleep. The sensations may be ameliorated by rubbing or movement of the legs. This condition can cause severe insomnia, though alterations in the sleep EEG are limited to arousals.

Hypnotics

The increasing awareness of the nature of sleep disturbance and the emergence of pharmacology as a clinical discipline have led to a greater understanding of the role that hypnotics should play in the management of insomnia. There has never been any doubt that hypnotics are effective in reducing wakefulness, but there has been less certainty concerning their place in the management of disturbed sleep. It is important that hypnotics are not prescribed for patients in whom they are contraindicated. It is now generally accepted that the approach to chronic insomnia is primarily that of assessment, and that hypnotics have a limited role in such patients. The most appropriate use of hypnotics is in those with a temporary problem, but with unequivocal evidence of disturbed sleep, and it is for

this reason that the aeromedical practitioner who inevitably deals with disturbed sleep must be familiar with their clinical pharmacology.

In the practice of aviation medicine the most relevant property of hypnotics is their duration of action, and this depends on absorption, distribution and elimination. The rate of absorption determines onset of action since hypnotics penetrate the blood–brain barrier with ease (*Figure 42.9*). Rapid absorption is associated with a quick onset of action whereas with slow absorption the desired effect may be attenuated or even absent. An adequate rate (peak plasma level around an hour after ingestion) is necessary if a drug is to be used as an hypnotic, whereas slower absorption may be more appropriate for the treatment of anxiety where a sustained effect with minimal initial drowsiness is sought.

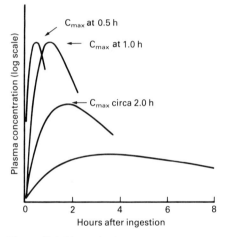

Figure 42.9 Absorption is an important feature of an hypnotic. Rapid absorption with peak plasma levels (C_{max}) about 0.5 hours after ingestion favour the use of small doses for sleep onset problems. An adequate rate of absorption has a peak plasma level around an hour after ingestion. Slower absorption may be more useful for sustaining sleep or for anxiety, though such drugs may lead to residual effects the next day.

After absorption an hypnotic is distributed to the blood and to highly vascular tissues such as the brain, heart, lung and liver, and peripherally to tissues of lesser vascularity such as voluntary muscle. The initial fall in the plasma concentration may be quite marked, and this relates primarily to the distribution of the drug. The latter part of the fall relates to elimination by metabolism and by excretion (*Figure 42.10*). In general, as hypnotics cross the blood–brain barrier with ease, a drug has a particular pharmacodynamic effect as long as its plasma concentration remains above a certain level. The duration of action will be short if this level is within the phase that predominantly represents distribution, but if the level is within the elimination

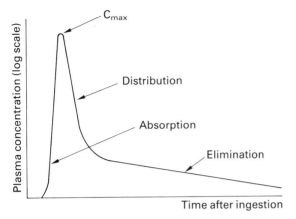

Figure 42.10 Plasma concentration after ingestion of an hypnotic. The slight delay before the drug can be detected in the plasma is related to the dissolution of the tablet, and the level then rises rapidly to the peak plasma concentration (C_{max}). The initial fall is related primarily to distribution, and the latter part primarily to elimination or metabolism.

phase, which is slower than the distribution phase, it may be much longer.

Distribution as well as elimination influence duration of activity, and so a relatively short duration of action may be attained with a single dose of a drug which is not rapidly eliminated (*Figure 42.11*). The influence of distribution on plasma concentration is important, and it follows that using the elimination half-life alone to indicate duration of action can be misleading. The elimination half-life provides a relative estimate of duration of action

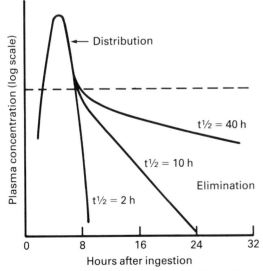

Figure 42.11 If the minimum concentration (dotted line) for a particular effect is related to the distribution phase the duration of the effect of a single dose will be independent of its elimination half-life ($t\frac{1}{2}$).

when the drugs in question have comparable absorption and distribution and the effect is related to the elimination phase, or, as with some rapidly eliminated drugs, when elimination is by far the dominant feature of the plasma decay—assuming again that they are absorbed in a similar manner.

Pharmacokinetic profile

Hypnotics that are currently available may be considered in two broad categories. Some have a pharmacokinetic profile with a clear biexponential decay (*see Figure 42.10*) in which the parts played by distribution and elimination in the decline in plasma concentration are clear, and some have an essentially monoexponential decay in which it is not possible to identify easily the separate phases of distribution and elimination. The duration of action of drugs which have a clear biexponential profile depends on distribution as well as elimination, and with some it can be relatively short because they have a marked distribution phase. Nevertheless, continued nightly ingestion may lead to accumulation if elimination is relatively slow, and the effect of repeated ingestion can be complicated further by accumulation of a slowly eliminated metabolite. It is for these reasons that a persistent effect may be avoided only when such drugs are used occasionally.

Clearly, slow elimination of parent compounds or of metabolites is disadvantageous if drugs are to be used on a nightly basis, and freedom from daytime effects is sought. However, a minor alteration in chemical structure may avoid this problem. For example, temazepam, a metabolite of diazepam, has a distribution phase similar to that of its parent compound but does not accumulate on daily ingestion as it is more rapidly eliminated and does not have a slowly eliminated metabolite. Thus daytime effects are highly unlikely unless inappropriately high doses are used. Diazepam and temazepam illustrate the parts played by distribution and elimination of parent compounds and their metabolites, and show that both factors must be borne in mind when the activity of any drug with a biexponential decay is under consideration.

Currently available hypnotics with an essentially monoexponential decay profile have a spectrum of elimination rates. The distribution phase does not play a significant part in the fall in plasma concentration for those drugs that are slowly eliminated, though it may contribute to the fall in plasma concentration for those that are rapidly eliminated. In each case the elimination phase is likely to be the dominant factor in determining the plasma decay.

Drugs that have a monoexponential profile can be divided clinically into two groups. Some are slowly eliminated and accumulation occurs on continued nightly ingestion, and some are rapidly or ultra-rapidly eliminated. The former group includes flurazepam and chlorazepate with their metabolites, desalkylflurazepam and desmethyldiazepam, respectively, and ingestion is likely to lead to a persistent effect. This may be useful as with chlorazepate in the treatment of insomnia with marked daytime anxiety, particularly as chlorazepate is free of impaired performance. However, tolerance, at least subjectively, may develop to all drugs that accumulate, and unwanted drowsiness may only be experienced early on in the course of therapy. Nevertheless, such subjective impressions of freedom from residual effects do not necessarily imply absence of impaired performance.

Nowadays, there is much interest in the rapidly and ultra-rapidly eliminated drugs, and several are available or may become available in the near future. Some are ultra-rapidly eliminated with half-lives of around 2–3 hours (midazolam, triazolam and zolpidem). Some, more usefully differentiated as rapidly eliminated hypnotics with a half-life of around 5 hours (brotizolam and zopiclone), are, in appropriate doses, free of residual effects the next day and of accumulation on continued nightly ingestion, and have the potential to sustain sleep. Single doses of compounds like brotizolam and zopiclone are not only more likely to sustain sleep than ultra-rapidly eliminated drugs, but are also more likely to sustain sleep than drugs which have a marked distribution phase.

Clinical pharmacology

An hypnotic may be used to shorten sleep onset when there is difficulty in falling asleep, to reduce nocturnal wakefulness, or to provide an anxiolytic effect during the next day. An hypnotic may help in one or more of these clinical problems, though a useful compound may meet only one criterion. There also arises the question of what improvement in sleep is required to constitute efficacy. This is uncertain, but the lowest dose that provides evidence of a beneficial effect on sleep in an appropriate group of healthy subjects would suggest what is likely to be the lower dose of the recommended dose range. With this approach, the use of unnecessarily high doses in some, if not many patients, will be avoided. Recommended doses and clinical use of currently available hypnotics and of those under development in various parts of the world are reviewed elsewhere (Nicholson, 1986a).

In general, hypnotics are adequately absorbed and so most are useful for difficulties in sleep onset. Some hypnotics are absorbed very rapidly, and an example is midazolam in which peak plasma concentrations may be reached in less than half an hour after ingestion. With very rapid absorption a very low dose may be quite adequate for difficulties with sleep onset. Some hypnotics are slowly absorbed (oxazepam and particularly loprazolam), and hypnotics are available in alternative formulations which may have different rates of absorption. An example of the latter is temazepam, and it is the soft gelatine capsule formulation (Normison) which is adequately absorbed with a mean delay to peak plasma concentrations of around an hour. This formulation in the dose range 10–20 mg is useful for difficulties with sleep onset. Other formulations of temazepam may be more slowly absorbed, and a higher dose may then be used in an attempt to produce an immediate effect, but this may lead to residual effects.

A reasonable duration of action is needed if frequent awakenings during the night are the main feature of the insomnia, and flurazepam and nitrazepam have been used for many years in this context. Low doses of these drugs should be used, but even if low doses avoid immediate residual effects on performance, accumulation will occur with repeated ingestion. Sustaining sleep without residual effects and without accumulation on nightly ingestion is more likely to be achieved with the newer generation of rapidly (as opposed to ultra-rapidly) eliminated hypnotics, such as brotizolam (0.125–0.25 mg) and zopiclone (5 mg)*. Their rates of elimination are still sufficiently fast for an appropriate dose to be free of residual sequelae.

It would appear that sustaining sleep without residual effects the next day with drugs in which the elimination phase is predominant requires a pharmacokinetic profile with a mean elimination half-life of around 5 hours. Ultra-rapidly eliminated hypnotics with mean elimination half-lives between 2 and 3 hours and hypnotics with a marked distribution phase are more appropriate when the only difficulty is falling asleep. With these drugs doses higher than those required to initiate sleep are needed to sustain sleep. Such high doses should be avoided as they may lead to high plasma concentrations during the early part of the night which could be accompanied by respiratory depression and alteration of sleep architecture, and lead to residual effects including anterograde amnesia and rebound insomnia on cessation of continued therapy.

The question of adverse effects of benzodiazepines arises frequently, but there is no convincing evidence that these are unavoidable. Unnecessarily high doses for unnecessarily long periods are the main causes, and essentially adverse effects imply

---

*At the time of writing brotizolam (Boehringer Ingelheim) is available in several European countries including Germany, the Netherlands, Belgium and Ireland. Zopiclone (May & Baker: Rhone-Poulenc) is still under development. Oxazepam (15–30 mg) is also useful for repeated nightly wakenings, but it is slowly absorbed.

misuse. Adverse effects include impaired perform-ance the next day and anterograde amnesia, and such sequelae are of considerable significance in certain occupations. A variety of tasks has been used to investigate residual sequelae, and there is now broad agreement on the nature and persistence of impaired performance the next day with the various hypnotics available. Impaired performance the next day is related largely to dose and pharmacokinetic profile, and so the correct dose of the appropriate drug is essential (Nicholson, 1986b).

Insomnia on cessation of treatment may also be a sequel to the misuse of hypnotics as rebound phenomena are a feature of many drugs if they are withdrawn suddenly. With rapidly eliminated hypnotics insomnia tends to occur during the first night or so after withdrawal, but with slowly eliminated drugs the fall in plasma concentration after withdrawal is relatively slow and sleep disturbance is unlikely to occur. Rebound insomnia occurs when relatively high doses of rapidly eliminated drugs are prescribed, and especially when they are used nightly for several weeks. It is not observed when these drugs are used in appropriate doses for a limited period. Dependency is also a possibility, but can be minimized by the intermittent use of low doses together with limited duration of ingestion, and gradual withdrawal in the event that continuous treatment has been given for more than a month. Dependency is unlikely to present as a problem with hypnotics if they are used judiciously.

References

Anon (1986) Jet lag and its pharmacology. *Lancet*, 30 August

NICHOLSON, A.N. (1986a) Hypnotics: their place in ther-apeutics. *Drugs*, **31**, 164–176

NICHOLSON, A.N. (1986b) Impaired performance. In *Iat-rogenic Diseases*, 3rd edn., edited by D'Arcy, P.F. and Griffin, J.P. Oxford University Press, pp. 671–679

43

Aircrew and their sleep

A.N. Nicholson

Introduction

The majority of healthy individuals who have a problem with their sleep complain of sleep disturbance lasting a few days. Disturbed sleep over a day or two may arise from a change in surroundings or from difficulty in coping with an unusual pattern of work, and it is in this way that we may consider the problem in aircrew. Indeed, changes in surroundings and rest at unusual times are for many aircrew part of their day-to-day life. Changed circumstances often lead to problems because preferences for sleep are usually well established, and even limited alterations disturb some individuals—particularly if they occur suddenly. Similarly, work by day and rest by night are in harmony with the normal pattern of sleep and wakefulness, and aircrew who work unusual hours and have to cope with time zone changes are likely to be out of phase with this natural rhythm.

Sleep disturbance due to adverse surroundings is characterized by an increase in wakefulness and drowsy sleep and by more frequent, and sometimes persistent, awakenings. Sleep onset and slow wave sleep may be little affected, presumably because they are related to the early part of the sleep, though REM sleep may be reduced during the early part of the night owing to the fragility of the first REM period. Disturbed sleep is also inevitable when resting during the day. The day does not favour sleep. There is more light and there is more noise. It is also warmer, and surrounding activity may disturb even the most tired sleeper. The individual may fall asleep quickly, but after a few hours sleep is broken and will be of short duration.

Sleeping at unusual times is inherent in most air operations. Even the duty hours of short-haul routes may encroach on the normal nocturnal sleep period,

and some sleep periods may be shortened. The mean duration of sleeps over several months may be similar to that observed in normal day-to-day activities, but the range is much greater (5 hours to more than 9 hours). This would appear to be the adaptation of the short-haul pilot to duty hours which encroach on early morning and, perhaps, late evening sleep. Naps are not usually a feature of the sleep of the short-haul pilot, and prolongation of some sleep periods is the essential compensation.

Disturbance of sleep related to overnight flights and to flights that include rapid and often large time-zone changes is of particular importance in aviation. Time-zone changes lead to complaints of tiredness, loss of appetite and a general feeling of loss of well-being, while sleep and wakefulness occur at unusual and often inconvenient times. Desynchronization of rhythms from those of the environment may lead to unusual levels of performance at certain times of the day, while the attempt to synchronize rhythms to a new time zone leads to sleep difficulties. Sleep disturbance that arises in this way is often encountered, and its management is an important aspect of the practice of aviation medicine.

Transmeridian flights

Sleep after transmeridian flights is influenced by a variety of factors including the timing of the flight and subsequent displacement of rest periods due to the direction of travel (Klein *et al.*, 1970; Klein, Wegmann and Hunt, 1973; Nicholson *et al.*, 1986a). After westward flights across the North Atlantic involving a delay of 5–6 hours to the first rest period, individuals tend to fall asleep quickly and sleep more deeply. There is some degree of sleep

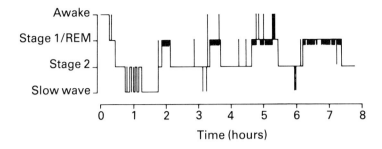

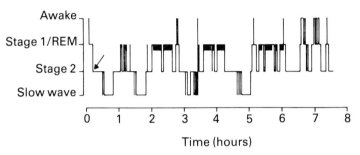

Figure 43.1 Control sleep recording (upper) and hypnogram of the first night after a westward flight with a 5-hour time-zone displacement (lower). The subject fell asleep quickly (arrow), but there was disturbed sleep during the latter half of the night.

deprivation, but falling asleep quickly may also be related to the lateness of going to bed which is well into the night of the natural rhythm for sleep and wakefulness. There tends to be less restful sleep during the latter part of the night as individuals try to sleep toward the local time of rising which is around midday in the home time zone (*Figure 43.1*).

A delayed rest period is also likely to modify the structure of sleep. There may be an increase in REM sleep as REM activity is likely to be greatest when individuals sleep later in their rhythm of sleep and wakefulness. However, by the third night after a westward flight normal sleep patterns are usually well established, and this indicates, together with the restoration of the rising phase of the circadian rhythm of alertness in the daytime sleep latencies, that the individual, at least as far as his sleep–wakefulness continuum is concerned, has adapted to the new time zone.

Sleep during the first night after an overnight eastward journey across the North Atlantic may be even better than before the flight if the subjects do not sleep on the aircraft or during the first day in the new time zone (*Figure 43.2*). However, in the new time zone with an advanced sleep period, sleep onset is delayed once the immediate effect of sleep loss is overcome. There is also likely to be a reduction in REM activity associated with the advance in the period of sleep. However, there is a significant development some days after an eastward flight. Slow wave sleep, total sleep time and sleep

efficiency are reduced and there are more awakenings. These changes, together with the slow realignment of the normal trend of increasing alertness in daytime sleep latencies, show that the sleep–wakefulness continuum may not relate to local time for several days after an eastward flight.

How are these differences in the rate of adaptation between eastward and westward flights interpreted? A reasonable explanation is that our innate circadian rhythmicity is longer than that of the day–night cycle, and that without the influence of the environment we have a natural desire to lengthen our day. This is the tendency after a westward flight with its delay to sleep; but after an eastward flight we have to shorten our day, and there may be an inherent resistance. Thus some individuals may even prefer to lengthen their day after eastward shifts. The extent to which this occurs is unknown, though it may lead to persistent sleep disturbance.

The main problem for aircrew with return transmeridian flights is coping with, rather than adapting to, a time-zone change (Nicholson *et al.*, 1986b; Wegmann *et al.*, 1986). After a westward flight crews usually sleep well, even though there may be somewhat less restful sleep in the latter half of the night. It is the timing of the return flight that would appear to be important, particularly if it is overnight. Although some shift of the circadian rhythm to the new local time will have taken place (*see* dotted lines in *Figure 43.3*) their period of

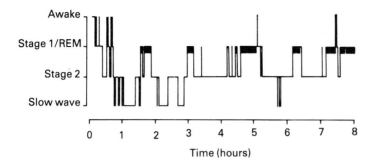

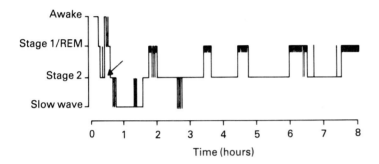

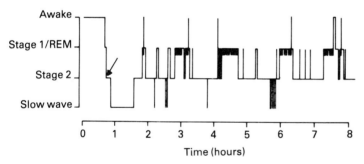

Figure 43.2 Control sleep recording (upper), hypnogram of the first (middle) and fifth (lower) nights after an eastward flight with a 5-hour time-zone displacement. The subject did not sleep during the overnight flight and so sleep onset during the first night in the new time zone (19-hour delay) was quick (arrow) and well sustained. During the fifth night sleep onset was slow (arrow), and there were many awakenings.

maximum alertness will still occur earlier than if the rhythm was fully synchronized. During the day of the return flight this may mean that they will be less alert than appropriate during the late afternoon and early evening, but a departure around 6 o'clock in the evening would allow the crews to take a nap in the afternoon. However, the advance of the phase of the alertness rhythm relative to the home time zone would ensure increasing alertness during the latter part of the flight terminating during the early morning (*Figure 43.3*). Although these observations

relate to a specific example it can be seen that correct timing of flights may have many advantages to the crew.

Irregularity of work

Aircrew are also likely to undertake repeated crossing of time zones, as in world-wide operations (Nicholson, 1970) or in repeated night flights during intercontinental north–south operations. In these

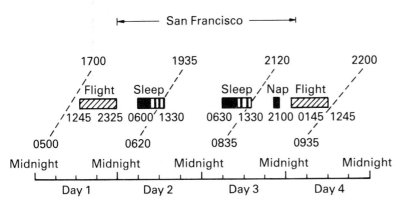

Figure 43.3 Importance of the timing of an eastward flight after a westward time-zone change of 8 hours. The scheduled departure time of the flight from London was 1245 (GMT) and it landed in San Francisco at 2325 (GMT) which was nearly 4 o'clock local time. The aircrew went to bed about 10 o'clock local time (0600 GMT the next day) and stayed in bed until nearly 6 o'clock the next morning (1330 GMT). They slept at about the same time the next night. Sleep may have been less restful than usual during the latter part of each local night, but it was nevertheless satisfactory. Arrangements preceding the return flight were of prime importance as the flight was overnight and followed several days of potential sleep disturbance. Departure time was nearly 6 o'clock (0145 GMT the next day), and the crews took a nap during the afternoon. The timing of the return flight was critical for another reason. The aircraft arrived in London at 1245 GMT, and though the rising phase of alertness during the day (dotted lines with minimum and maximum values at GMT times indicated) after the overnight return flight would have been somewhat later than usual owing to a shift of about 4 hours toward San Francisco time, it nevertheless would have increased alertness during the latter part of the flight.

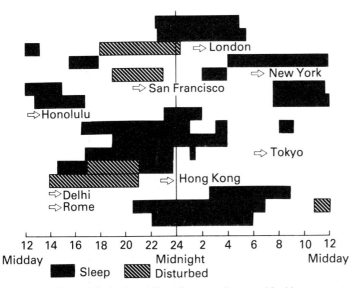

Figure 43.4 Sleep periods of an airline pilot operating a world-wide east–west schedule (Nicholson, 1970). The figure is read from the bottom line up, and each line is from midday of one day to midday the next, and each rectangle is a period of sleep. Hatched rectangles indicate subjectively poor sleep. Arrows indicate commencement of duty.

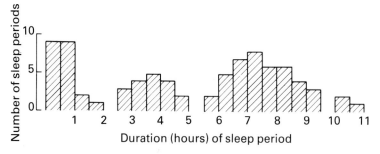

Figure 43.5 Frequency of sleeps of various durations over a month in a pilot operating world-wide routes. Sleep periods around 1 hour are naps whereas periods around 3–4 hours are often anticipatory sleeps.

circumstances their sleep patterns are irregular, and sleep disturbance may persist for several days after schedules including repeated transmeridian flights. The sleep of the pilot operating an eastward round-the-world schedule is illustrated in *Figure 43.4*. The irregularity of sleep both with respect to duration and time of day is evident. Indeed, the dominant feature of the sleep of aircrew who operate world-wide routes is irregularity both in terms of duration of sleep and of time of day when it occurs (*Figure 43.5*).

The adaptation of the sleep of pilots operating worldwide east–west routes has received much attention. With 24-hour rest periods a long sleep immediately after a flight could mean that the crew would not be in the most rested state possible during the next duty, and so, to avoid undue sleepiness during duty after a 24-hour rest, crews often split their sleep into two parts. The need for sleep immediately before duty (an anticipatory sleep) is created by restricting sleep immediately after the preceding flight. This often leads to sleep periods of 3–4 hours during long-haul schedules. During flights that extend wakefulness beyond 16 hours and flights that start during the early evening, naps of ½–1 hour duration are not uncommon, and they are clearly useful during westward flights when the day is lengthened (*Figure 43.5*).

Short periods of sleep are taken to maintain effectiveness during schedules that include irregularity of rest. However, though naps of about an hour decrease the tendency to sleep, it would appear they have a less beneficial effect on performance when an individual is impaired as when having worked overnight. On the other hand, periods of sleep of about 4 hours before overnight work may be very helpful. Levels of performance fall precipitously when the end of a long period of work coincides with the fall in performance associated with the circadian rhythm of the individual, but with a 4-hour period of sleep during the evening (anticipatory sleep) there can be a sustained improvement in performance over the night (Nicholson *et al.*, 1985). Performance overnight may be more easily sustained by a preceding sleep of several hours than by attempting to overcome the effects of sleep loss by a nap. Sleep preceding long duty periods may be the more appropriate strategy.

Careful attention to sleep is undoubtedly important in all air operations. Impaired performance follows sleep disturbance, even though the impairment is not easy to demonstrate. Sleep disturbance modifies circadian functions, impairs response to stress and upsets the normal sense of well-being. The measurement of performance is insufficiently sophisticated to detect change in many important aspects of behaviour; this has furthered the myth that disturbed sleep is of limited importance. This is not so. Performance is maintained by greater effort or by concentrating attention on limited aspects of the problem for a limited period of time, while interpersonal skills, judgement and decision making deteriorate even though such behaviour—and so impairments—is difficult to quantify.

Flight-time limitations

In 1944 the Convention on International Civil Aviation recommended limitations to the work of aircrew, and in the United Kingdom the requirement of the Air Navigation Order of 1950 was that the safety of operations should not be endangered by fatigue which may arise from excessive flying hours. The requirement was emphasized again by the Air Navigation Orders of 1957 and 1968, and in 1973 when the forerunner of the Civil Aviation Authority published the findings of a committee concerned with flight-time limitations. This led to the current recommendations (*Civil Air Publication 371—The Avoidance of Excessive Fatigue in Aircrew–Guide to Requirements* (1982), second edition). However, controversy concerning flight-time limitations has persisted world-wide, and at the time of writing there are fresh attempts to understand disturbed sleep in world-wide operations and its significance to the well-being of the airline pilot. The aim of such limitations must be to ensure safety and avoid unnecessary restrictions to the operation. It is the attempt to achieve this balance that raises difficulties.

Rate of working

Irregularity of work leads to disturbances of sleep, and it is widely accepted that duty hours must be arranged to ensure that aircrew can achieve acceptable sleep. There is a cumulative effect of irregular work, and a critical factor in achieving acceptable sleep is to limit total duty hours over any number of days (Nicholson, 1972; Wegmann, Conrad and Klein, 1983; Wegmann *et al.*, 1985). A small increase in duty hours may convert an acceptable to an unacceptable schedule, and so minor modifications in the overall number of duty hours may have particularly beneficial effects. Such modifications may provide an additional period of sleep within a schedule of many days or provide greater flexibility in the choice of time to sleep during a particular rest period. It is difficult to create ideal schedules with the complexities of present-day operations, but with care reasonably satisfactory

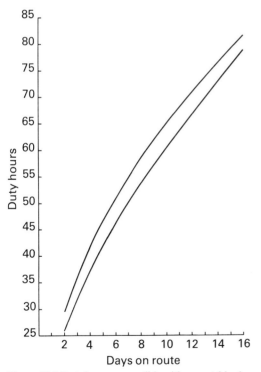

Figure 43.6 Duty hours compatible with acceptable sleep over a 16-day period. The lower curve indicates workload which is believed to be compatible with acceptable sleep, whereas the upper curve indicates a workload above which acceptable sleep is unlikely to be achieved (Nicholson, 1972).

schedules can be designed to include the facility to hasten operations, and to cope with the extra workload that minor changes in crew availability can create.

Duty hours that can be achieved by aircrew do not increase linearly with the number of days of the schedule (*Figure 43.6*), and this is due to the cumulative effect of the irregularity of sleep. In this sense aircrew operating world-wide routes are able to cope with 50–55 hours in the first 7 days of a world-wide schedule, but they can only manage about 75 hours duty by the end of 14 days. This reduction in the rate of working should be borne in mind in the scheduling of aircrew and must be one of the fundamental considerations of any system of flight-time limitations.

Continuously on task

Avoiding undue sleep disturbance is of prime importance to the safety of any operation, but a particular period of work could have characteristics that would adversely influence effectiveness. This is a possibility when individuals are expected to be continuously on task for long periods of time, and in these circumstances it is important that the durations and timing of duty periods should not adversely affect their ability to sustain vigilance. This is particularly relevant to the work of two-man crews. Workloads at any time of the flight may well be the same as, possibly less than, that of three-man-crew operations, but in two-man crews each is continuously on task. This is the important difference from three-crew operations in which it is highly unlikely that an individual would have to stay on task for more than a few hours.

Several factors influence continuous performance (Nicholson *et al.*, 1984; Minors *et al.*, 1986; Spencer, 1987):

1. The interval between the end of the previous sleep and the commencement of duty (time since sleep).
2. Duration of duty (time on duty).
3. The clock time of duty (time of day), assuming aircrew are adjusted to the local time zone.

If it is assumed that the individual is fully rested before the commencement of duty the effects of time since sleep and time on task are inseparable. In this circumstance performance rises during the first 5 hours. It then falls precipitously over the next few hours, and levels off around 16 hours. As far as time of day is concerned performance rises during the day and falls during the late evening and overnight to reach its nadir around 0500 in the morning (*Figure 43.7*). Clearly, very low levels of performance would be reached if the latter part of a prolonged duty period coincided with the nadir of the variation in

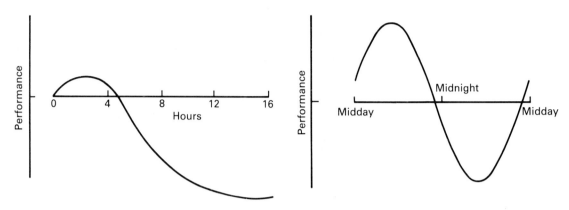

Figure 43.7 A model of change in performance with time on task (left-hand curve) and with time of day (right-hand curve) (Spencer, 1987).

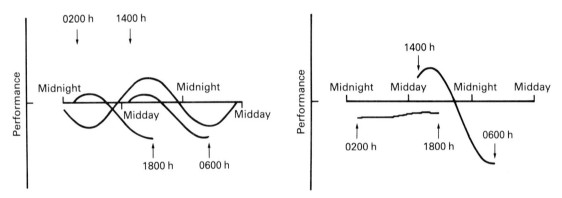

Figure 43.8 Time on task and time of day related to duty commencing at 0200 and 1400 (left-hand curves) and the resultant of the effects of time on task and time of day related to duty commencing at 0200 and 1400 (right-hand curves). If a 16-hour duty period commences around 0200 performance will probably be maintained as the fall in performance during the latter half of the work period will coincide with the rising phase during the day. On the other hand, if the duty period commences around 1400 the fall in performance during the latter part of the duty period would coincide with the lowest level during the night related to the circadian rhythmicity of the individual, and so very low levels of performance may be reached. Such adverse juxtapositions of time on task and time of day should be avoided if crews are expected to remain continuously on their task. For this reason careful attention must be given to the length of duty periods in such operations, and the length should be determined in relation to the time of day. These considerations assume that the aircrew are fully rested at the commencement of their duty (Spencer, 1987).

performance related to circadian rhythmicity (*Figure 43.8*).

There are, therefore, two overriding concerns in the design of schedules for aircrew who have to cope with world-wide operations. Over several days aircrew must be able to achieve acceptable sleep, and the arrangement of each duty period must avoid very low levels of performance due to the latter part of a prolonged duty period coinciding with low levels of performance related to circadian rhythmicity. Even so, as far as world-wide operations are concerned, we still need to know the pattern of alertness in relation to local time, and this is dependent on the number of time zones crossed and the speed of adaptations to the new time zone which

is different according to the direction of travel. More precise information on adaptation rates is needed before we can accurately predict performance at any time during world-wide operations. However, the general pattern of readaptation is known, so that reasonable predictions can be made in many cases.

Clinical considerations

The management of aircrew coping with irregularity of rest and activity is a complex matter (Nicholson, 1987), though the key is undoubtedly proper arrangements for duty. Long-haul operations incompatible with an acceptable sleep pattern and heavy short-haul schedules over many months could prejudice the safety of air operations, and so duty hours are of legitimate interest to the practice of aviation medicine. Workloads must allow crews to achieve acceptable sleep, and the scheduling of duty, particularly if the aircrew have to remain continuously on task, must avoid marked falls in performance due to the adverse juxtaposition of prolonged duty with the nadir of the circadian rhythm of performance. These are the primary considerations, and in this way flight-time limitations provide the foundation of effective management. However, even if flight-time limitations take into consideration these points, some aircrew may still find it difficult to cope with irregularity of rest, and this is particularly likely in middle age when sleep begins to deteriorate. Irregularity of rest superimposed upon poor sleep can be very troublesome, and a careful assessment should always be made if aircrew complain of persistent and unusual difficulty in coping with their work.

Persistent sleep disturbance could reflect illness. A history over many months would raise the question whether the individual is suffering from one of the many causes of chronic insomnia, and depression or unwise use of alcohol or drugs are possibilities. A more recent history in the absence of illness may suggest personal difficulties, either with the family or at work. Furthermore, the normal deterioration in sleep may be exaggerated with repeated arousals due to apnoeas and leg movements, and though such events in themselves may have limited or no clinical significance, they could herald a developing sleep apnoea syndrome or be a manifestation of the restless legs syndrome. Excessive daytime sleepiness as well as disturbance of sleep are often seen in these syndromes, and such sleep difficulties are unlikely to be compatible with arduous air operations.

When the practitioner is satisfied that there is no medical or psychological background to the complaint the initial approach is to counsel the individual to look after their sleep. Exercise and avoiding heavy meals as well as limiting the use of alcohol and caffeine will help. Less demanding routes should be considered. Persistence of the complaint after attention to sleep habits and to the nature of the work raises the question of the use of hypnotics to help the individual at specific parts of the schedule. Certainly, as it is a temporary problem and there is unequivocal evidence of disturbed sleep, the judicious use of hypnotics is warranted, but choice of hypnotic must relate to the nature of the insomnia and to the lifestyle of the individual. The prescribed hypnotic must be appropriate to the work of the airline pilot, and this means that normal sleep architecture both during ingestion and after withdrawal must be preserved, and that the drug must be free from unwanted effects on daytime function.

There are hypnotics that meet such requirements. Experience in the Royal Air Force (Baird, Coles and Nicholson, 1983) and in civil aviation (Nicholson, Roth and Stone, 1985) has led to temazepam (Normison, Wyeth) 10–20 mg as the drug of choice for aircrew, though it is important that this rapidly absorbed formulation is used (Nichoslon *et al.*, 1986). Temazepam has a relatively short duration of action due to its distribution phase, and its rate of elimination is such that accumulation does not occur, except possibly in the elderly, on daily ingestion. Its short duration of action provides an adequate margin of safety for use by aircrew during the schedule. However, if the problem is primarily that of disturbed sleep after returning home, a drug with a slightly longer duration of action with the potential to sustain sleep, but still free of residual effects, may be more appropriate. At the time of writing brotizolam 0.125–0.25 mg is the only one available (Nicholson, Welbers and Jady, 1983), and then only in some European countries (Federal Republic of Germany, Holland, Belgium and Ireland). However, oxazepam 15–30 mg, though slowly absorbed, can be useful.

An hypnotic with which the practitioner and the individual are familiar is appropriate, and it should be used 'on the ground' before it is prescribed during schedules. It should then be given at the lowest dose and as infrequently as possible. The practitioner should help to identify when its use is likely to be most beneficial. In general terms there should be an interval of 24 hours between ingestion and commencement of duty, though under supervision the interval may be reduced safely to 12 hours. Perhaps it is unnecessary to emphasize that if hypnotics are to be used in the management of sleep disturbance in aircrew the use of alcohol should be limited and preferably avoided.

In conclusion, there are now well-defined stages in the management of aircrew who have to cope with irregularity of work. Their pattern of work and of rest is largely determined by flight-time limitations, and so it is appropriate that expertise in aviation medicine is brought to bear on the formulation of these guidelines. However, the day-to-day care of aircrew is firmly in the hands of the aeromedical practitioner. The practitioner must be familiar with the work of the airline pilot, understand the rationale behind flight-time limitations and be conversant with disorders of sleep. It is important to remember that illness, both physical and psychological, may also lead to sleep difficulties, particularly in middle-aged aircrew. Finally, the practitioner must be aware of the clinical pharmacology of hypnotics as this, together with an understanding of the work of aircrew, will ensure that these drugs are used effectively. With such knowledge a confident approach will be presented to aircrew, and only in a few cases will it be necessary to use hypnotics, though these may be useful.

References

BAIRD, J.A., COLES, P.K.L. and NICHOLSON, A.N. (1983) Human factors and air operations in the South Atlantic Campaign. *Journal of the Royal Society of Medicine*, **76**, 933–937

KLEIN, K.E., BRUNER, H., HOLTMANN, H., REHME, H., STOLZE, H., STEINHOFF, W.D. and WEGMANN, H.M. (1970) Circadian rhythm of pilots' efficiency and effects of multiple time zone travel. *Aerospace Medicine*, **41**, 125–132

KLEIN, K.E., WEGMANN, H.M. and HUNT, J.B. (1973) Desynchronisation of body temperature and performance circadian rhythms as a result of outgoing and homecoming transmeridian flights. *Aerospace Medicine*, **43**, 119–132

MINORS, D.S., NICHOLSON, A.N., SPENCER, M.B., STONE, B.M. and WATERHOUSE, J.M. (1986) Irregularity of rest and activity: studies on circadian rhythmicity in man. *Journal of Physiology*, **381**, 279–295

NICHOLSON, A.N. (1970) Sleep patterns of an airline pilot operating world-wide east–west routes. *Aerospace Medicine*, **41**, 626–632

NICHOLSON, A.N. (1972) Duty hours and sleep patterns in aircrew operating world-wide routes. *Aerospace Medicine*, **43**, 138–141

NICHOLSON, A.N. (1987) Sleep and wakefulness of the airline pilot. *Aviation Space and Environmental Medicine*, **58**, 395–401

NICHOLSON, A.N., WELBERS, I.B. and JADY, K. (eds) (1983) Brotizolam: clinical and experimental studies. *British Journal of Clinical Pharmacology*, **16**, 1–440

NICHOLSON, A.N., ROTH, T. and STONE, B.M. (1985) Hypnotics and aircrew. *Aviation Space and Environmental Medicine*, **56**, 299–303

NICHOLSON, A.N., STONE, B.M., BORLAND, R.G. and SPENCER, M.B. (1984) Irregularity of rest and activity. *Aviation Space and Environmental Medicine*, **55**, 102–112

NICHOLSON, A.N., PASCOE, P.A., ROEHRS, T., ROTH, T., SPENCER, M.B., STONE, B.M. and ZORICK, F. (1985) Sustained performance with short evening and morning sleeps. *Aviation Space and Environmental Medicine*, **56**, 105–114

NICHOLSON, A.N., PASCOE, P.A., SPENCER, M.B., STONE, B.M., ROEHRS, T. and ROTH, T. (1986a) Sleep after transmeridian flights. *Lancet*, **ii**, 1205–1208

NICHOLSON, A.N., PASCOE, P.A., SPENCER, M.B., STONE, B.M. and GREEN, R.L. (1986b) Nocturnal sleep and daytime alertness of aircrew after transmeridian flights. *Aviation Space and Environmental Medicine*, **57**, B42–52

NICHOLSON, A.N., HIPPIUS, H., RUTHER, E. and DUNBAR, G.C. (eds) (1986c) Modern hypnotics and performance. *Acta Psychiatrica Scandinavica*, **74**, Suppl. 332

SPENCER, M.B. (1987) Influence of irregularity of rest and activity on performance: a model based on time since sleep and time of day. *Ergonomics*, In Press

WEGMANN, H.M., CONRAD, B. and KLEIN, K.E. (1983) Flight, flight duty and rest times: a comparison between the regulations of different countries. *Aviation Space and Environmental Medicine*, **54**, 212–217

WEGMANN, H.M., HASENCLEVER, S., MICHAEL, C. and TRUMBACH, S. (1985) Models to predict operational loads of flight schedules. *Aviation Space and Environmental Medicine*, **56**, 27–32

WEGMANN, H.M., GUNDEL, A., NAUMANN, M., SAMEL, A., SCHWARTZ, E. and VEJVODA, M. (1986) Sleep, sleepiness and circadian rhythmicity in aircrews operating trans-atlantic routes. *Aviation Space and Environmental Medicine*, **57**, B53–64

44

Cardiovascular diseases

J.N.C. Cooke

Introduction

The sudden incapacity of a pilot or other essential ground- or aircrew member is an obvious threat to flight safety and is the reason why cardiovascular disease forms the leading cause for loss of medical certification in civil aviation. The statistics for ICAO airline operations show that one or two such incapacitations occur every year; in recent times the risk of an accident has been avoided by the presence of another pilot and by his training in the management of such a situation. However, some risk clearly remains and is paramount in single-pilot operations, whether military or civil. The part played by medical examination in the reduction of this risk cannot be determined easily but must be considerable in general, even though it is constantly argued and reviewed in detail.

In the last 10 years the role of medical examination has resulted in a series of advisory reports especially from groups of cardiologists in the United States and United Kingdom; these have attempted to update the standards of medical validation in line with the rapid advances in cardiology, particularly in regard to the accuracy of diagnosis and prognosis. They include the Bethesda Conference (American College of Cardiology, 1975), the Royal College of Physicians Report (1978), the First United Kingdom Workshop in Aviation Cardiology (Joy and Bennett, 1984), and the American Medical Association's Review of Medical Standards for Civilian Airmen (Engelberg, Gibbons and Doege, 1986). The influence of these reports has been considerable, even though the natural conservatism of the various aviation authorities usually has not allowed the immediate implementation of all the recommendations. Nevertheless, the continuing progress of new diagnostic techniques and of new methods of treatment by drugs and by surgery, is improving prognosis but is also producing new problems in the decisions as to fitness for aircrew or for air traffic control duties. These can be resolved only by close co-operation between cardiologists and the aviation authorities. This has resulted in the formation of standing advisory committees in some countries, notably the United Kingdom. Over the same sort of period there has also been an increasing recognition by air forces and airlines of the need for preventive medicine and education, particularly with regard to the risk factors for ischaemic heart disease. These must also have an effect on morbidity. The whole picture, therefore, is one of active re-examination and change.

History and medical examination

Every national medical authority uses some type of questionnaire to act as a basis for the medical examination. The standard of excellence of such forms is variable, but all require that the examining doctor should use his initiative to pursue any aspect of the personal or family history of the candidate that appears to be significant, and particularly to seek any history of a possible cardiac event, past treatment, or reference for a consultant opinion. The clinical examination must be thorough, and note other factors besides the essential cardiological ones, such as evidence that may suggest premature ageing, hyperlipidaemia, or excessive consumption of alcohol. National civil and military medical authorities vary considerably in their requirements for ancillary examinations such as ECGs, chest radiographs and biochemical investigations; and there will be further variations in the requirements for the different standards of licence and the granting of waivers.

It has been argued that the ideal initial examination for professional licensing should consist of a more comprehensive survey, both to eliminate some cases of high risk, and to provide a baseline for future comparisons: but this would add to the costs of an already expensive procedure and alter the present philosophy of civil licensing, which is to validate medically an applicant for a limited period of licensing rather than form part of a preventive medicine programme. Such surveys are done at present by a number of air forces and major airlines who have to consider the cost of training and career implications for their candidates.

Ancillary examinations

Electrocardiography

12-lead electrocardiography is now virtually standardized as the format for aviation medical examination. However, despite the provisions of the ICAO Annex 1 (1982) the national requirements for the frequency and age relationship of the ECG are far from standardized, and are particularly variable for private pilots. The CAA in the UK stipulates that professional pilots should have ECGs at their initial examination, at every fifth year to age 30, then 2 yearly to 40, annually to 50, and thereafter every 6 months. The same pattern applies to other members of aircrew and air traffic controllers except that after the age of 40 the periodicity remains annual. Most other nations have similar regulations with differences of detail. Air forces also vary, but commonly have more frequent electrocardiography, with a younger age relationship, reflecting the greater frequency of single pilot operations and the greater physical stresses. With regard to private pilots, some nations do not insist on electrocardiography unless there is an indication in the history or physical findings. More commonly, there is a reduced requirement for these licences as compared with professional pilots. Thus in the UK the first tracing is required at the age of 40, and repeated 4 yearly to 50, 2 yearly to 60, annually to 70, and thereafter 6 monthly. All ECGs are valuable records, but their value depends upon a good quality copy produced by a machine of technical quality that has been properly standardized. The tracing must be free from artefact and be clearly labelled and identified. Long-term storage and an efficient retrieval system are essential if future comparisons are to be made; these are very important, since the pattern of an individual's ECG normally varies very little with the passage of years so that changes found on comparison may be very significant.

Information obtained from the ECG

A normal resting ECG does not exclude serious heart disease and, particularly, does not reveal a high proportion of cases of ischaemic heart disease (IHD) in the presymptomatic stage. Nevertheless, every year in the UK this routine examination shows up a number of cases of 'silent' myocardial infarction and larger numbers of cases of arrhythmia, conduction defects, and other myocardial disorders which might otherwise not have been detected. Computer programs for reading ECGs are now available with special and expensive recorders, but the reports still require scrutiny by consultants with special expertise on the wide range of normality and of the many borderline patterns. These consultants also interpret the vast majority of tracings that are produced by ordinary equipment. There are three main types of information obtained from the ECG:

1. Cardiac rate and rhythm.
2. Conduction of the cardiac impulse.
3. Evidences of myocardial abnormality.

Rate and rhythm

It is difficult to assess these factors with short strips of tracing of each lead derived from a single-channel recorder. Some authorities require an additional long (20 seconds) record from lead V2, while others advise a similar record only when a disturbance of rate or rhythm is noted in the ordinary tracing. Programmed three-channel machines usually produce a satisfactory length of recording for the purpose of interpreting most abnormalities of this kind, but the main method when a fuller assessment is needed is provided by the 24-hour ambulatory recording, which provides detailed information on the frequency and nature of arrhythmias.

Conduction

The standard resting ECG normally allows adequate measurement of the conduction times and pattern, though this may again be aided by a long strip in a single-channel recording. Holter monitoring is required when there are variations and intermittent changes in conduction, whether of delay or of pre-excitation. The effects of physical stress in showing up such abnormalities may occasionally require an exercise stress test.

Myocardial abnormalities

The suspicion of myocardial abnormality arising from the appearance of the ECG is a common problem for the interpreter. It may arise from a finding of an abnormal, or change in, axis or QRS form, but possible abnormalities of the ST segment form much the most frequent need for decision. Where there is doubt in a symptomless applicant the exercise stress ECG is the usual first additional investigation. This test has a very long history and many forms have been devised since the original step test of Master in the pursuit of a format with both high specificity and sensitivity for ischaemic heart disease (IHD). They all remain notorious for their liability to produce false-positive results in symptomless individuals as subsequently proved by normal coronary angiography (Froelicher *et al.*, 1976). Nevertheless, a properly conducted test continues to be the first stage of the necessary process of investigation until a better one is devised.

At the present time a standardized form of progressive workload such as the Bruce protocol performed on a treadmill with continuous ECG and blood pressure monitoring is generally favoured, with the exercise continued to an agreed endpoint, either to the limit of the individual's physical capability or to a calculated maximal heart rate related to his age. Other than the development of symptoms or a serious arrhythmia a 'positive' test is judged by the form and degree of changes that appear in the ST segment during exercise and the ensuing rest period. Once again, very considerable experience is needed to interpret such changes, the usual criteria requiring a minimum of 2 mm depression below the isoelectric level at a measured time interval after the J point. Unfortunately, these criteria themselves vary with the particular protocol in use, and their specificity is never good. Despite these shortcomings the test has been advocated for use as a regular examination for older aircrew and for those with apparent risk factors, but the high rate of false-positive results, quoted as over 50% in some series in symptomless pilots, have produced a very justified reluctance to introduce it as a routine in most countries. The test remains as an initial screening procedure where there are abnormalities of the resting ECG or other aspects of the cardiological examination.

Cardiac imaging

The chest radiograph remains the commonest form of cardiac imaging, as part of its other functions, and is carried out as a routine by most organizations at the initial medical examination and periodically at later stated intervals. It gives a useful measure of the size and shape of the heart, the aorta, and the pulmonary vessels. These measurements can be amplified by the rapidly developing science of echocardiography which is used to visualize and measure the myocardium and heart chambers, as well as providing an accurate assessment of the components and movements of the cusps of the heart valves. This harmless and non-invasive procedure is especially useful in aviation medicine to diagnose and monitor valvular lesions and myocardial hypertrophy, and has become a vital part of cardiac investigation.

Coronary angiography remains the ultimate method of studying the coronary circulation and is presently the only satisfactory procedure when a definite indication for it exists. Radionuclide scanning methods continue to be developed and can demonstrate areas of diminished myocardial perfusion and function. However, at the present time this technique more often acts as a confirmatory indication for angiography in an individual suspected of ischaemic heart disease than an accepted diagnostic criterion. Other methods of cardiac imaging are under intensive research and development and include nuclear magnetic resonance and advanced forms of computer assisted visualization.

Eventually, some method that allows competent non-invasive assessment of the coronary arteries will probably bring immense changes in our procedures and management.

Biochemical investigations

Some mention of these investigations is required because the trend to include biochemical 'profiles' in routine medical examinations has been increasing with the introduction of multichannel laboratory analyser equipment. The factors assessed usually include a full blood count, serum lipids, blood sugar, electrolytes, non-protein nitrogen, and tests of liver function. There have been repeated suggestions that such investigations should form part of the examination for licensing, initially and then at stated intervals, but there has been no general acceptance of this idea for a number of reasons. These include cost which is still significant despite modern equipment. Others are the dangers of inaccuracy due to sampling errors, and the difficulties of interpretation, particularly of abnormalities found in healthy symptomless subjects. Such tests are required by some air forces and airlines who use them to try to eliminate potentially high-risk individuals, such as those with hereditary hyperlipidaemia, before employment or training—and subsequently as part of the general preventive medicine effort. Biochemical tests are required as part of the investigations needed in the management of such conditions as hypertension.

Hypertension

The high incidence of hypertension among middle-aged men and women makes it the most common cardiovascular problem in aviation medical examinations. Despite the advances in control and management it remains a major risk factor for coronary, cerebral and renal vascular disease in the general population of advanced nations. The assessment of blood pressure at aviation medical examination therefore remains extremely important. There is general agreement that the recorded pressures should be 'casual', not those obtained after prolonged rest, and should be taken in the sitting position for standardization. Most authorities agree that the diastolic value is best taken as the 5th phase of the Korotkoff sounds (extinction), using the 4th phase only when there is no clear 5th phase. As regards acceptable levels, despite Pickering's (1972) assertion that there is no clear-cut level of blood pressure that separates health from disease it has been accepted that in aviation there has to be some pragmatic scale of limits. In many countries such a scale is age related, thus in the UK the Civil Aviation Authority defines maximal acceptable levels as follows:

Under 39 years of age	145/90 mm Hg
40–49 years of age	155/95 mm Hg
Over 50 years of age	160/100 mm Hg

Other authorities have different viewpoints. The three armed services in the UK have adopted a common policy that an initial candidate for aircrew must have a blood pressure below both levels of 130/90 mm Hg. But after flying training a different standard is applied, and the maximum acceptable level is set at 155/95 mm Hg regardless of age. This disregard of relationship to age has been followed in the most recent recommendations of the American Medical Association to the FAA (Engelberg *et al.*, 1986), where it is suggested that a single blood pressure standard of 150/95 mm Hg be used for all pilots, with an absolute maximum systolic level of 160 mm Hg regardless of the diastolic pressure.

All of these arbitrary figures still leave the problem of the nervous and reactive applicant in whom higher readings, particularly systolic levels, are claimed to be due to the stress of the examination. Such 'labile' cases whose levels vary between normal and abnormal on different occasions and with different examiners are more likely to develop persistent hypertension: about 10–25% will do so. As previously noted, there will be a definite difference of outlook for acceptance of such applicants between authorities involved in career prospects and those deciding fitness for a limited licensing period only.

Assessment of hypertension

Blood pressure varies in every individual with the time of day and the degree of physical activity and other stresses. When casual readings are consistently raised the increase in risk is related to the level and the presence or absence of other risk factors. In military aviation, where the physical stresses are high and the pilot is frequently flying without a co-pilot, the strictest standards will be applied to the initial applicant and close scrutiny to the trained

pilot. In civil aviation the arbitrary limits will tend to be more liberal and are often age related. Thus in the UK when special examinations show no evidence of other risk factors or target organ damage, an applicant may be accepted without restriction provided that the readings remain below the following higher levels:

Under 39 years of age	155/95 mm Hg
40–49 years of age	165/100 mm Hg
Over 50 years of age	170/100 mm Hg

Since these levels approximate to those at which many physicians would advise treatment it is clear that the applicant is being examined solely for a limited period of licensing, and not with a view to long-term preventive medicine. The assessment of risk factors is directed towards those known to be associated with the incidence of ischaemic heart disease and stroke. Inquiry will be made into lifestyle, smoking, previous and family history. Physical examination will be specially directed to detect any evidence of damage to the heart, retinal and peripheral vessels, and the kidneys. Ancillary examinations would include ECG, chest X-ray, and urine samples, together with a blood biochemical survey. Intravenous urography is not mandatory unless there are clear indications, but ultrasound scan of the kidneys is a very useful and harmless investigation.

Management of hypertension

When an aircrew member or an air traffic controller clearly does have significantly raised blood pressure, and the necessary preliminary examinations and investigations have been carried out, there needs to be a decision as to whether advice and treatment will reduce the risk to an acceptable degree to allow the individual to continue his flying career or private flying. Severe or accelerated hypertension is almost always disqualifying because by definition there is certainly going to be target organ damage. In cases of moderate and mild degrees of hypertension all authorities in aviation prefer that military aircrew and civilian licence holders should be managed without recourse to pharmaceutical drugs, so long as that management is effective. The correctable factors of excess weight and excessive consumption of alcohol are particularly important. Some physicians add reduction of salt intake to this list, and a reduction of heavy salt intake may be helpful and harmless. Smoking probably does not raise blood pressure directly, but its increase of the total risk demands its abandonment if the subject is to continue to fly. Such measures will often produce an aggregate fall in blood pressure to acceptable levels.

When these measures fail, the use of drugs is necessary to reduce the risk factor. The objectives of such treatment are to lower the blood pressure to values well within the accepted normal range without either any risk of excessive hypotension under the acceleration forces of flight, or any side effects that might prejudice the individual's performance of complex tasks. These requirements rule out a large number of hypotensive drugs, including those that act primarily through the central nervous system, or those that may cause drowsiness or produce significant orthostatic falls in blood pressure. Diuretics were the first compounds to be accepted as suitable for use in aviation and have been allowed by many national authorities without restriction of licensing. There has always been recognition that they can cause problems in the way of electrolyte disturbance, reduction of glucose tolerance, and raised serum uric acid levels; but recent emphasis has been on their capability to produce cardiac arrhythmias associated with potassium losses. This has led to a general recommendation that potassium sparing preparations should be used in preference to extra potassium intake, and for more frequent monitoring of the side effects of the drug.

Beta-receptor antagonists were soon recognized as a potentially suitable group of drugs for use in aviation, with the advantage that they oppose many of the catecholamine effects produced by stress. Glaister (1974) showed that they had no significant effect on G tolerance in human centrifuge experiments but the doubt remained that they might produce some decrement in human performance, especially as they are used in psychiatry to reduce somatic symptoms of anxiety. Research on these aspects is continuing, but the weight of extensive evidence of the side effects over many years does not suggest that the effects are significant. There does seem to be advantage in using beta-1 selective and hydrophilic drugs like atenolol, which are less likely to produce side effects than propanolol—and long-acting drugs are a convenience in the aviation environment. Many authorities now allow the use of these drugs either alone or combined with a diuretic. In the UK the CAA allows beta blockers for commercial pilots with an initial restriction 'as or with co-pilot' which may be lifted after a period of some years of satisfactory control. Private pilots and controllers are not usually restricted. Military aviation authorities normally impose restriction to roles with a co-pilot.

A number of more recently developed drugs remain under active consideration as possible acceptable therapies for hypertension in aircrew. They include the calcium antagonists, the angiotensin converting enzyme inhibitors and some alpha-receptor antagonists. Militating against their introduction is the great difficulty of showing that any drug is completely free of effects that might prejudice flight safety, and apart from special

research the main reliance must be upon a long experience of their use in the general population. Certain rules should apply to the use of any drug in aviation. The dose should be the smallest that is effective since many side effects are dose related. The drug should be given on the ground until the clinical objective is achieved without side effects; and in the case of drugs like beta blockers some authorities require simulator or flight testing before return to flying status, to check that there is no significant decrement of performance.

Follow-up of hypertension

The essential clinical points for follow-up are that blood pressure remains in an acceptable range and that there is no evidence of oncoming target organ damage. These observations will need to be supported by certain tests additional to the ordinary periodic medical examination and may include an ECG, chest radiography, biochemical tests, and occasionally such special procedures as a stress exercise ECG or echocardiography. The periodicity of examination may need to be more frequent than is routine, particularly for the younger pilot. If the regimen has to be altered, or drug treatment has to be changed or increased in dosage, the whole situation of the licence holder will need to be reviewed. The follow-up of drug therapy should include some specific questioning to uncover any possible side effects of the treatment.

Ischaemic heart disease
Risk factors

Ischaemic heart disease (IHD) in middle age remains predominantly a disease of men, with a risk of heart attack several times greater than in women of a similar age. The risk of incapacitation is also related to age with an exponential rise between 30 and 60. The likelihood of total incapacity or death as a first symptom cannot be accurately assessed but there is good evidence that 50% of those who die from an acute myocardial infarction (MI) do so in the first 2 hours after the onset. The accepted risk factors that have been identified in numerous population surveys (Kannel, McGee and Gordon, 1976) may be listed as follows:

1. Age.
2. Male sex.
3. Hypertension.
4. Cigarette smoking.
5. Hyperlipidaemia.
6. Family history of early IHD.
7. Diabetes.

Health education has had a considerable effect in relation to the correctable elements of this list, and the resulting changes in habits and lifestyle are regarded as the probable influence in the fall in mortality from IHD in some countries, notably the USA. Aircrew clearly have more than the normal motivation since their continuing flying status is dependent upon good health. Nevertheless, a significant proportion continue to smoke, especially in the armed forces, and there is certainly room for more preventive medicine. Other conclusions that might be drawn from consideration of this list are that more women should be employed in aircrew duties and that retiring ages should be adjusted so that the overall age distribution of professional pilots was younger. The former will depend upon social changes; the latter is not justified by accident statistics which show the advantage of the experience of older pilots.

Diagnosis of ischaemic heart disease

Symptomatic IHD is a differential diagnosis in many patterns of chest pain, which can lead to considerable anxiety both in the pilot and in his examiner. Typical angina and the classic pain of myocardial infarction are easily recognized, and the latter can usually be confirmed by a resting ECG, but musculoskeletal pains and the discomfort of oesophageal reflux can cause considerable problems. At the other end of the scale around 20% of survived myocardial infarcts are 'silent', causing no symptoms recognized as serious, and the first knowledge of the event by a licence holder is when a routine ECG shows typical changes. However, most cases of symptomatic IHD in aircrew and controllers will have been notified to the requisite medical authority as a result of a formal illness or a consultation resulting in the diagnosis. Where the diagnosis remains uncertain or suspect it is clearly necessary to ground the individual until investigation has clarified the situation.

The diagnosis of asymptomatic IHD remains an unsolved problem that constitutes a challenge for aviation medicine and for cardiology as a whole. Efforts to detect the condition are really quite recent in aviation medicine. Even routine electrocardiography has only been introduced in the last 25 years in most nations and is still not mandatory for Class 3 licences in the USA. The commonest clue that is pursued in present practice is an abnormality of the ECG, commonly an ST segment abnormality, but also QRS changes, arrhythmias, and conduction abnormalities. In addition, suspicion may arise from the physical findings on examination and can include:

1. Evidences of premature ageing.
2. Early arcus senilis, xanthelasmata.

3. Thickening of superficial arteries, poor pulses.
4. Hypertension.
5. Ectopic beats and arrhythmias.
6. Any new cardiac murmur or extra sound.

None of these physical findings are in any way diagnostic of IHD in a symptomless subject but may cause sufficient concern to warrant reference to a consultant for further evaluation. Resting ECG changes may be diagnostic, as for instance when they indicate unequivocal evidence of silent infarction, but beyond that the abnormal resting ECG is not a reliable indicator of asymptomatic coronary artery disease, though still requiring cardiological assessment.

When an applicant is referred for cardiac evaluation because of a suspicion of presymptomatic IHD, the important decision that needs to be made is the extent and depth of the investigation that should answer the query. This problem is far from simple since a number of autopsy surveys of airmen dead from other causes confirm that by middle age the question is more the extent of coronary disease than whether it is present. Since routine angiography still carries some small risk and would be quite unjustified in the majority of cases, that definitive investigation remains reserved as a final arbiter after a process of selection. This process requires some experience of dealing with asymptomatic individuals, which is not always available to cardiologists striving to cope with a heavy workload of overt cases of IHD. The management of an anxious and often resentful pilot who feels perfectly fit needs tact and repeated explanation of the detail and the reasons for each stage of the investigation. As a result, there has grown up in many countries a small group of specialists with a particular interest and experience of aviation cardiology and its problems.

The process begins in the usual way with an assessment of the personal and previous history, habits, and family history of the subject, with special regard to the established risk factors. The physical findings are checked, together with the resting ECG and chest radiograph, and the next stage is almost always a stress exercise ECG. Treadmill or bicycle ergometer exercise may be used, though the former is more favoured in the USA and UK, since hard cycling may be limited by fatigue of the thigh muscles in those unaccustomed to that exercise. A negative test result, judged by good exercise tolerance without symptoms, and without arrhythmia or 'positive' ST changes, will commonly be accepted as excluding serious coronary disease in the absence of other strong indicators, since false negative exercise ECGs are less common than false positive ones. A positive test result, though recognized as frequently misleading, demands further scrutiny. This often takes the form of a repeat of the exercise ECG after a short time interval, sometimes using preliminary betablockade to try to eliminate changes that may merely be the result of the effects of excessive catecholamine excretion. If the repeated test is still positive, or the first test was judged grossly abnormal, the continuing suspicion of liability to sudden incapacity remains and after explanation further tests are needed.

Radionuclide cardiac scanning may be helpful at this stage, performed after exercise and at rest, with gated studies that may allow an assessment both of the perfusion of the myocardium and ventricular motion as well as the ejection fraction. Despite claims, no complete reliance can be laid on the results, except that abnormalities shown by a thallium scan in a case with a positive exercise ECG greatly increase the likelihood that subsequent coronary angiography will show significant disease. A normal thallium scan in a dubious case with a positive exercise ECG but good exercise tolerance and no obvious risk factors may sometimes merit continuing observation with restriction of licensing rather than insistence on the need for angiography, though that investigation remains the final arbiter in those cases where suspicion of presymptomatic coronary artery disease cannot be eliminated. The cineangiogram films obtained are usually conclusive but can be reviewed by a panel of consultants when the findings require debate.

This section would not be complete without some mention of the changing attitudes towards the clues used to judge the need to investigate for asymptomatic disease other than those previously itemized. These attitudes relate to the import that should be placed upon obvious risk factors as indicators rather than relying upon ECG changes and physical findings alone. That would suggest, for instance, that a male smoker aged 50 with a blood pressure at the high limit for his age should be checked for blood lipid levels, and if they were also high, should at least be subject to an exercise ECG. Such suggestions have been made by advisory committees both in the USA and in the UK. Such surveillance would undoubtedly detect extra cases of latent IHD, but the acceptability and cost effectiveness of such measures are still being debated.

Management of coronary artery disease

A history, or the known presence, of coronary artery disease is the most certain predictor of subsequent coronary events. This fact dictated that for many years such a history or finding virtually always involved the permanent disqualification of aircrew or air traffic controllers. However, the increase in knowledge gained about the disease derived both from follow-up of infarction and of coronary bypass surgery, combined with modern methods of evaluation and monitoring, have

allowed some selected individuals to be returned to their occupations. These individuals are usually drawn from one of three groups:

1. Those recovered from a treated or silent MI.
2. Those diagnosed before infarction or symptoms.
3. Those treated by surgery or angioplasty.

In all cases there must be a time interval after the event during which the individual remains disqualified. The minimum period is usually 1 year during which the subject must be symptomless without need for treatment. Evaluation after that time has to be stringent and conducted by a specialist cardiologist. In the case of those with a history of infarction the necessary checks will include normal physical findings, a normal response to exercise stress ECG testing, and ambulatory ECG monitoring that shows no significant disturbance of rhythm. In the case of professional pilots angiography is usually demanded to assess the state of the coronary circulation; in others, radionuclide scanning may be acceptable. Those procedures must demonstrate that there are no other lesions likely to cause further coronary insufficiency and that ventricular function is normal.

If all these criteria are satisfied civilian licence holders may be relicensed on a restricted basis excluding single pilot operations. Such waivers are rarely offered to military pilots, because of the additional stresses they have to endure. Follow-up of these cases has also to be strict. Schemes vary between national authorities but most require repeated exercise ECGs, ambulatory monitoring, and thallium scans. Some lay down stated intervals for repeat of angiography. In the UK most decisions are referred to the Medical Advisory Panel to the CAA so that there is a frequent review of policies. Unrestricted licensing after a period of satisfactory follow-up is often requested but rarely allowed for professional pilots. Flight engineers and controllers may be so granted. Private pilots are the most frequent group to be fully relicensed despite the fact that they commonly fly in the single pilot role. This reflects the reality that private flying accidents are comparatively frequent and are related to bad weather and inadequate avionics and flying skills, rather than to medical causes.

Those individuals diagnosed as having coronary artery disease in the presymptomatic phase pose a difficult problem. Attempts have been made to quantify the extent of the disease as significant or not significant according to the anatomical site of the coronary narrowing and its degree as expressed in percentage terms. Thus narrowing equal to or greater than 50% in a major vessel might be regarded as disqualifying. While that sort of concept is always open to argument, there is also the uncomfortable fact that the progression of the lesion is initially difficult to predict. For practical purposes it seems reasonable to allow the milder cases to continue with restricted licences, subject to strict supervision, with angiographic review at an agreed time interval. More severe disease may well warrant bypass surgery or angioplasty as a prophylactic treatment in its own right, though it is an obvious fact that career consequences can easily affect the judgement of both the subject and his medical advisers when the only alternative to treatment is permanent disqualification.

Individuals who have undergone coronary artery bypass grafting (CABG) or angioplasty will undergo much the same examinations and investigations that are laid down for those that have had previous infarcts, except that coronary angiography is now essential in all cases both to demonstrate the patency of the grafts or of the vessels that have been dilated by balloon, and to check that there are no other significant narrowings left in the native circulation. In view of the known incidence of graft occlusions in the first few months after surgery, the check angiogram needs to be done at least 6 months or longer after the procedure. If these findings are satisfactory together with the rest of the exercise testing and monitoring, some professional pilots may again be returned to restricted licensing, subject to long-term follow-up. It appears that the number of CABGs required and performed at the original operation is less important to the prognosis than their continuing patency. Private pilots will also be allowed restricted licensing in countries where this waiver exists, and occasionally like those who have had previous infarcts they may be considered for full validation, depending upon continuing satisfactory follow-up. They should not, however, be allowed to undertake flying instructor responsibilities.

Cardiomyopathies

The incidence of cardiomyopathy varies considerably in different parts of the world and is a medical aviation risk because of its liability to produce incapacitation, whether its type is dilated or hypertrophic. The aetiology of the dilated form is very wide and includes alcoholism and virus infections as well as idiopathic and hereditary forms. The danger of arrhythmias, heart failure, or embolization, together with the unpredictable course of such dilated cardiomyopathies, makes disqualification on diagnosis the only safe course. Very occasionally apparent recovery to full normality may deserve a complete cardiological work-up to assess the possibility of some form of licensing.

Hypertrophic cardiomyopathy usually presents in aviation medicine as the result of an abnormal routine ECG indicating ventricular hypertrophy, rather than the characteristic symptoms of chest pain and dyspnoea. Definitive diagnosis requires echocardiography, and often cardiac catheterization and angiography. There may be little difference in prognosis between those with apparent degrees of obstruction to the outflow tract and those with none. There is no great problem in the decisions for proved cases. They should be denied any form of flying status because of the known high risks of sudden death from ventricular arrhythmia. However, there are some cases where the diagnosis is uncertain, with no conclusive echocardiogram and catheter findings. Their fitness for licensing may be considered provided that the close scrutiny and repeated investigation are acceptable. Some may belong to that group of athletes in whom excessive regular exercise is responsible for ECG changes and marked bradycardia.

Valvular heart disease

Abnormal conditions of the cardiac valves may be congenital in origin or acquired, but regardless of aetiology they may progress and cause haemodynamic effects of the greatest importance to aviation fitness. Their detection at the earliest possible stage of the lesion and of the individual's career is essential to allow proper initial assessment of the present fitness, future prognosis, and requirements for follow-up. Unfortunately, a proportion of these conditions are missed at the initial medical examination and at later stages so that the eventual diagnosis comes as an unexpected worry for airmen established in their flying career or occupation. Many of these problems are undoubtedly due to incomplete physical examination or misinterpretation of findings. A competent examination of the heart should include auscultation in three positions, namely supine, sitting, and left semi-decubital. It is particularly important that systolic murmurs and clicks should not be dismissed as 'functional' or insignificant without the concurrence of a specialist physician, or without an echocardiogram which can provide an objective method of evaluation. Diastolic murmurs do not occur in the normal heart. The risks of valvular disorders include arrhythmias, infective endocarditis, and embolization, as well as cardiac decompensation which may be rapid in onset under the physical stresses of flight.

Mitral valve disease

Mitral stenosis is virtually disqualifying for any form of certification of flying category because it carries all of the risks listed above. Even asymptomatic cases with mild stenosis can develop systemic emboli or even pulmonary oedema under special circumstances, such as the onset of atrial fibrillation. There are problems in refusing applicants with very mild stenosis and good exercise tolerance who have been told they do not require surgery; but the danger of complications remains, and the follow-up would have to be rigorous, frequent, and expensive. There may be a case for considering restricted licensing after successful surgery, but the results would have to be near perfect and there is still the risk of re-stenosis.

Mitral regurgitation has a large number of aetiologies with rather differing prognoses. The degree of regurgitation is itself very important in aviation, and all cases with severe, and most with a moderate degree are inevitably disqualified. Mild mitral regurgitation may be considered for civil licensing and exceptionally for restricted military standards, depending on the findings, aetiology, and the results of the investigations. The investigations would include echocardiography, exercise ECG, and ambulatory monitoring to show normal exercise tolerance and no arrhythmia. Left ventricular size and function should be normal, and there should be no more than slight left atrial enlargement. Echocardiography should also confirm that there is no associated mitral stenosis. The follow-up would require the repetition of these checks at intervals.

Mitral valve prolapse is now frequently diagnosed by the echocardiographic investigation of mid-systolic murmurs and clicks. The condition can vary in severity from slight redundancy of a mitral leaflet to severe prolapse with marked regurgitation. The severe cases are clearly unacceptable because of the risks of sudden incapacity and arrhythmias. Minor leaflet prolapse in asymptomatic applicants probably has a good prognosis providing they have the necessary prophylaxis against infective endocarditis and are followed up with echocardiography, Holter monitoring, and exercise ECGs at agreed intervals. Such reservations would probably bar them on initial examination from a military career, and may occasionally involve them in restriction of licensing for professional civil flying. The discovery of this abnormality at a later stage of career is at present quite common because of previous disregard or misinterpretation of the heart sounds at earlier examinations. Specialist assessment of the degree of the risk, and any necessary limitations that need to be imposed, is essential for a safe and a fair disposal of such cases, and the experience of their follow-up will provide valuable additional data for the future.

Aortic valve disease

Severe and moderate degrees of aortic stenosis carry such a risk of sudden incapacity that they are absolutely unacceptable for any form of licensing. The consideration of the mildest degrees would depend upon the results of complete cardiac assessment. The main criteria to be satisfied would require confirmation of a minimal degree of obstruction by both catheter studies and Doppler and two-dimensional echocardiography. These tests should also show normal left ventricular dimensions and function, and a stress exercise test should demonstrate normal exercise tolerance without ECG changes. Once again, full follow-up would be necessary and licensing would almost always be restricted.

Aortic regurgitation is recognized to be less likely to produce sudden incapacitation than stenosis, but the haemodynamic effects of severe degrees make them unacceptable in aviation. Mild aortic regurgitation would be disqualifying for initial air force selection but would be considered for some forms of civil licensing subject to a full evaluation of the cardiac state. Such a symptomless applicant would be one with the diastolic murmur of aortic reflux, but with a normal pulse pressure, normal resting and exercise ECG, and with echocardiographic findings that confirmed the absence of left ventricular enlargement. As always with valvular cardiac lesions follow-up would be mandatory at not less than annual intervals and would include all of the baseline investigations. The usual precautions would be needed to avoid infective endocarditis. A common problem that arises in these cases is the gradual increase in the amount of regurgitation with the passing of years. To some extent, such a deterioration can be allowed by the imposition of a restriction to flying only in a two-pilot role, but for the applicant who remains symptomless the judgement of a cut-off point at which licensing is no longer acceptable is a difficult one for the medical advisers. It will involve further investigations, probably including catheter studies, to gain objective data of the exact haemodynamic situation.

Valve replacement and valvuloplasty

The surgery of valvular heart disease continues to progress and presents new queries as to fitness for licensing. At the present time no mechanical valve can be acceptable because of the high risk of complications and the need for lifelong anticoagulation therapy. The First UK Workshop (Joy and Bennett, 1984) considered that there might be grounds for granting limited licensing of applicants who had a completely successful homograft replacement of the aortic valve, and that has now been allowed with the expected stringent follow-up criteria. Valvuloplastic procedures are being considered but so far no authority has adopted any firm recommendations.

Disturbances of rhythm and conduction

Disturbances of rhythm

These disturbances are frequently discovered at examination or by routine electrocardiography. Sometimes a suggestive history is obtained, but one of the problems affecting both diagnosis and follow-up is the fact that many individuals seem to be totally unaware of even major abnormalities or change in rhythm. Their importance in aviation medicine covers a wide spectrum. They can range in symptoms from the slight distraction that can result from unpleasant palpitations to the fatal disturbance of consciousness that may be produced by some ventricular arrhythmias. As previously noted, disturbances of rhythm may also be a clue to the existence of some underlying heart condition that requires further investigation. The physical finding of any disturbance of rhythm demands an immediate ECG, regardless of the normal periodicity of that procedure, so that the nature of the disturbance can be identified and analysed.

Sinus tachycardia and bradycardia

It is convenient to define these conditions as consisting of a resting heart rate of over a 100 beats per minute or under 50 respectively. Tachycardia may be a common response to the stress of medical examination but possible pathological causes should be considered when records for the individual show it to be a new finding. Important causes can include thyrotoxicosis and alcoholism as well as anxiety states. Bradycardia is an increasingly common finding as a result of the exercise regimens carried out by many candidates, including the middle aged, or may be due to the undeclared use of beta blocking drugs. It can also indicate the need for investigation. Electrocardiography should be done whenever there is any doubt.

Ectopic beats

This frequent finding causes a number of problems. Since the introduction of ambulatory monitoring there has been a considerable increase in knowledge of the frequency and forms of premature beats in the general population, and their prognostic significance. The results have been surveyed by Lown (1982) and suggest that isolated beats of supraventricular or unifocal ventricular origin occur in most individuals and are insignificant. Ventricular ectopics are more common than supraventricular, and over 50% of healthy people will show some degree of ectopic activity during a 24-hour recording. Simple and unifocal ventricular ectopic beats occurring at rest or during exercise are therefore

generally accepted as unlikely to be of any pathological significance so long as they occur singly. Ventricular ectopic beats that do demand consideration and further investigation include:

1. Ectopics of varying form and origin.
2. Two (doublet) or more successive ectopics in series.
3. R on T phenomenon.

Three or more successive ventricular ectopic beats are regarded technically as a burst of ventricular tachycardia (VT), which is definitely a disqualifying finding, but all the above forms of complex ectopic activity carry an increased risk of incapacity. The prescribed investigation would follow the expected form, and after repeated ambulatory recordings would include exercise ECG, followed by echo and thallium scans. Restricted licensing might be considered if these studies were satisfactory. Others might require complete evaluation including angiography.

Paroxysmal tachycardia

With rare exceptions an established history or finding of paroxysmal tachycardia is invariably disqualifying because of the possible dangerous consequences of the symptoms and haemodynamic consequences produced by the arrhythmia. Although supraventricular origins are clearly more benign than ventricular tachycardias, and may be more amenable to treatment, there are still problems related to unexpected recurrence or breakthrough, and the treatment itself gives rise to further consideration of side effects and control. In the most favourable cases restricted licensing may be considered after full investigation and a long period without recurrence.

Atrial fibrillation and flutter

Atrial fibrillation may be paroxysmal or chronic. It has a wide range of aetiological factors, of which rheumatic heart disease is now comparatively rare in aviation, whereas idiopathic or 'lone' fibrillation are diagnosed in about 50% of cases. Others turn out to have underlying heart disease, or different causes including viral infections, alcoholism, or a history of pericarditis.

The condition is found surprisingly often at routine ECG, and is more frequent in older subjects. Grounding is necessary because of the risk of embolism as well as the cardiac effects of uncontrolled ventricular rates. Some cases of paroxysmal fibrillation may be considered for restricted licensing provided that full investigation shows no evidence of an associated mitral valve lesion, coronary artery disease, or significant enlargement of the left atrium and ventricle, and particularly when there is a history of only a single attack. In others, there may be effective treatment for the underlying cause, such as thyrotoxicosis, when it may be reasonable to allow a return to duty after a sufficient time has shown no evidence of recurrence.

Follow-up of all paroxysmal cases must include ambulatory electrocardiography and be prolonged. The risk of embolization in chronic atrial fibrillation can sometimes be assessed as minimal when full investigation shows no valvular disease or progressive myocardial lesion, and there is good rate control and normal exercise tolerance. Such cases may be issued a limited licence or very occasionally an unrestricted private or controller's licence. Atrial flutter is less common than atrial fibrillation, but carries the risk that the atrioventricular conduction can suddenly change to allow very high ventricular rates. That fact, and the greater difficulty of effective control, makes atrial flutter normally unacceptable for licensing.

Disturbances of conduction

Sinus pauses

These may be noted on a routine ECG or ambulatory recording. Their significance may be difficult to determine especially in highly trained athletes, but any pause greater than 2 seconds should be regarded as requiring reference for investigation and opinion.

First degree A-V block

Defined as a P-R interval greater than 0.2 seconds, this finding is common in healthy young applicants. Provided that the block is reversible by exercise or the administration of atropine and the QRS complex is normal, the condition is acceptable.

Second degree A-V block

Mobitz type 1 with Wenckebach pattern may be acceptable for licensing subject to a very extensive cardiological assessment which may include invasive electrophysiological studies as well as exercise and ambulatory ECGs. Mobitz type 2 in which the A-V block occurs without prior lengthening of the P-R interval is disqualifying.

Third degree A-V block

Complete A-V dissociation even when symptomless is invariably unacceptable, and at present pacemakers are not allowable.

Right bundle branch block

When this condition is present as an incidental single finding in an otherwise normal applicant with a normal exercise tolerance, it is usually acceptable as conferring no increased risk. There is slightly more concern when it appears in middle age in an individual known previously to have had normal conduction, when full assessment and electrophysiological studies may be indicated and there may be a requirement for restriction of flying status.

Left bundle branch block

This conduction defect is more commonly associated with organic heart disease and is frequently unacceptable. Occasional cases may qualify for limited licensing when the fullest investigations have shown no evidence of disease that may progress.

Pre-excitation

Wolff–Parkinson–White and Lown–Ganong–Levine patterns are quite frequently found by routine electrocardiography with an incidence of around 2 per thousand. The patterns may only appear intermittently in the resting ECG and so some cases escape initial detection. Their importance in aviation lies in their association with tachyarrhythmias with high heart rates. Where there is no such history, opinion varies as to the risk of its occurrence later in life, so that after the fullest investigation no more than restricted licensing is usually offered. Surgery in suitable cases may greatly reduce the risk of tachycardia.

Peripheral vascular disease

Peripheral arterial disease may be identified in the history or by physical findings during the examination. To this end the palpation of the various arterial pulses should form part of the routine cardiovascular examination. Any history or finding that suggests occlusive arterial disease or aneurysm is important because of the close correlation with coronary artery disease, as well as consisting of a disability in its own right. Very few individuals with a history or symptoms of intermittent claudication will be considered for licensing. Where surgical treatment or angioplasty of the peripheral lesion has been effective, it will still be necessary to evaluate the coronary circulation by complete investigation before any form of licensing can be considered.

Venous thrombosis and thromboembolism

A recent history of thrombophlebitis or deep vein thrombosis is a cause for at least temporary denial of flying category until the condition has completely subsided and any anticoagulant therapy has been withdrawn without further symptoms. Recurrent venous thromboses will almost always require long-term therapy which will be unacceptable. Where pulmonary embolism has occurred there will need to be both a prolonged period of treatment and follow-up plus a cardiological assessment before any return to flight status.

Congenital heart disease

The assessment of individuals with congenital heart disease is likely to be a problem of selection at the initial medical examination. Excluding the more serious forms of congenital defects, decisions will be needed for the cases of mild disease who will fall into two groups; those who have had surgery, and those in whom it is not indicated. For the former at least 1 year will be needed after operation to allow evaluation of the results.

Atrial septal defect

Untreated cases will almost always be those with small defects of the ostium secundum and may be considered for licensing providing that investigations and catheter studies show that the left-to-right shunt is small and the pulmonary artery pressure is normal. Successful surgically treated cases may include both types of defect and the secundum group may again be suitable. Defects of the ostium primum carry a higher risk because of possible later problems with the mitral valve and conduction defects.

Ventricular septal defects

Very small defects may be considered for civil though not military flying. Repaired ventricular septal defects carry some risk of arrhythmia and careful follow-up and assessment will be required. Only restricted licensing is likely.

Pulmonary stenosis

Mild degrees of pulmonary stenosis carry no significant cardiac risk so long as there is evident stability. The results of surgery are also usually excellent and both treated and untreated mild cases may be fit for selection.

Persistent ductus arteriosus

Untreated cases should not be accepted. Individuals who have had successful surgical closure or excision may be entirely acceptable for civil licensing or a military flying category.

Coarctation of the aorta

Untreated subjects are not acceptable. The outlook for surgically treated cases depends somewhat on their age at the time of the operation for the repair. If it was done in early childhood, and there is no other congenital abnormality and the blood pressure is normal, the outlook is good enough for full certification. Where the operation took place after the age of 12, the prognostic doubt might involve restriction of licensing. At least 30% of cases of coarctation have other defects, notably bicuspid aortic valves.

References

American College of Cardiology (1975) Cardiovascular problems associated with aviation safety. Eighth Bethesda Conference of the American College of Cardiology. *American Journal of Cardiology*, **36**, 573–620

ENGELBERG, A.L., GIBBONS, H.L. and DOEGE, T.C. (1986) A review of the medical standards for civilian airmen. Synopsis of a two year study. *Journal of the American Medical Association*, **255**, 1589–1599

FROELICHER, V.F., THOMPSON, A.J., LONGO, M.R., TRIEBWASSER, J.H. and LANCASTER, M.C. (1976) Value of exercise testing for screening asymptomatic men for latent coronary heart disease. *Progress in Cardiovascular Disease*, **18**, 265

JOY, M. and BENNETT, G. (eds) (1984) The First United Kingdom Workshop in Aviation Cardiology. *European Heart Journal*, **5**, Suppl. A

KANNEL, W.B., McGEE, D. and GORDON, T. (1976) A general cardiovascular risk profile: The Framingham Study. *American Journal of Cardiology*, **38**, 46

PICKERING, G. (1972) Hypertension: Definitions, natural histories and consequences. *American Journal of Medicine*, **52**, 670

Royal College of Physicians, London (1978) Cardiovascular fitness of airline pilots. Report of the Working Party of the Cardiology Committee of the Royal College of Physicians of London. *British Heart Journal*, **40**, 335–350

45

Respiratory diseases

J.A.C. Hopkirk

Introduction

Respiratory disease is the commonest cause of morbidity and loss of time from work in the general community. Not surprisingly, therefore, it is of major importance in clinical aviation medicine and constitutes one of the major causes of loss of time from flying. To make a rational aeromedical decision it is necessary to be able to assess the effects that the disease process may have on the functional efficiency of that aircrew member. A detailed knowledge of the disease process is essential. This must encompass its short- and long-term pathological and physiological effects, the risk of possible complications, the prognosis in the short and the long term, and the requirements for and possible side effects of treatment.

The aeromedical problems will be described under three headings:

1. Sudden incapacitation: the risks of an aircrew member being affected to the extent that the safety of the aircraft would be jeopardized.
2. Operational efficiency: the effect of the disease on the individual's ability to perform his task regularly and efficiently over a period of time.
3. Treatment: the effects of drugs or surgical treatment on the aircrew member in the flying environment.

Asthma

Asthma is characterized by a wide variation in short periods of time in the resistance to flow in the intra-pulmonary airways. It has a wide clinical spectrum varying from a single mild episode not requiring treatment to constant disabling asthma.

The prevalence of asthma in the adult population in the United States and United Kingdom is about 2–5%. Asthma may be thought of as a state in which there is bronchial hyperreactivity. That is, the airways react to non-specific stimuli by excessive bronchoconstriction. This may be measured by a histamine challenge test in which increasing doses of histamine are inhaled until a measured variable, usually the forced expiratory volume in one second (FEV1), falls by 20%.

Natural history

There is a common belief that the prognosis of childhood asthma is excellent and that most children will grow out of their asthma by puberty never to be troubled again. Studies on the natural history of the disorder, however, do not bear this out (Hopkirk, 1984). Of childhood asthmatics about 50% will achieve a prolonged remission, 40% will continue with mild symptoms and 10% will have troublesome symptoms. If follow-up is prolonged about half of those who have had a prolonged remission will relapse, and having suffered such relapse have a smaller chance of obtaining a further remission; 10% of children will have continuing severe symptoms. So nearly 70% of children who have had asthma in childhood will have symptoms later in adult life, though these symptoms may be mild. In subjects with adult onset asthma the prognosis is less good. Of those with intermittent symptoms only 20–30% may expect prolonged remission, and approximately half of those who do remit will have a further relapse. Those with continuous symptoms have a small chance of a prolonged remission. The majority of those developing asthma after puberty will have either continuing symptoms or recurrent episodes of asthma throughout their adult life. In those with seasonal asthma there is a tendency for the season to extend as the years progress and many develop perennial asthma. Asthma caused by allergy to a single agent is rare.

Aeromedical problems

Sudden incapacitation

Sudden incapacitation is a potential hazard for aircrew members with asthma (Rayman, 1973) though its occurrence is uncommon. Unheralded life-threatening episodes of asthma can occur in brittle asthmatics with extremely hyperreactive airways. Exposure to smoke or fumes in the cockpit could provoke an asthmatic attack in a susceptible individual.

Operational efficiency

This is likely to be much more of a problem with asthmatics who may suffer exacerbations of their symptoms either spontaneously or in response to viral respiratory illnesses. These can cause prolonged periods of loss of time from flying. It is a disorder in which self-assessment is difficult because symptoms and impairment of lung function are often discordant. Aircrew may fly without realizing that they are unfit.

Treatment

Asthma may be treated with bronchodilators which reverse airway narrowing. These provide symptomatic relief but do nothing to affect the underlying condition. Recently asthma, even if mild, is being treated in the first instance with prophylactic drugs. With these the aim is to reduce bronchial hyperreactivity and therefore the susceptibility to develop airway narrowing. Commonly used bronchodilators are the beta-2 agonists, for example salbutamol or terbutaline. These drugs may have metabolic and cardiac effects when given intravenously or by mouth but these effects are not evident when they are given by the inhaled route. Muscle tremor, however, does occur. Prophylactic treatment is provided with inhaled cromoglycate or inhaled corticosteroids. In conventional doses these drugs do not have side effects that would be important in aviation medicine. Treatment with oral methylxanthines leads to a high incidence of side effects including central nervous system irritability. They are not suitable, therefore, for use in aircrew. There is a marked swing towards the use of prophylactic medication with cromoglycate or inhaled corticosteroids as a first-line treatment in asthma rather than regularly inhaled bronchodilators. This is an attractive concept for the management of asthma in

aircrew. Inhaled corticosteroids given twice daily may reduce bronchial hyperreactivity and therefore the risk of sudden bronchospasm in flight.

Disposition

Pilot training

Because of the uncertain prognosis of childhood asthma, and the enormous investment in time and money made in training aircrew, candidates with a history of childhood or adult asthma are unfit for entry into pilot or navigator training.

Trained aircrew

Trained aircrew who develop asthma need to be fully assessed. The pattern of asthma will determine the outcome. Those with extremely reactive airways are at risk for sudden incapacitation. Even though they may have infrequent attacks they are unfit for aircrew duties. Those with mild asthma requiring intermittent treatment are fit to fly but should probably be restricted from flying fast jets. This is because of the potentially adverse effect of pressure breathing and of G. Those with more continuous symptoms can be considered for restricted flying provided that their symptoms are well controlled with regular treatment with cromoglycate or inhaled corticosteroids. At present the restriction is that they are unfit for fast jet flying and must fly with or as a co-pilot.

There is a group of patients with mild but persistent asthma whose symptoms are extremely well controlled on treatment. Once it is established that an aircrew member falls into this group, that is their bronchial hyperreactivity is well controlled on regular medication and they have had no acute episodes for a prolonged period of time, consideration could be given to removing the restriction with or as co-pilot. Reasons for permanent grounding include persistent marked bronchial hyperreactivity, frequent exacerbations of asthma and inadequate control of hyperreactivity with drugs.

Sarcoidosis

Sarcoidosis is a systemic granulomatous disease of undetermined aetiology and pathogenesis. Mediastinal and peripheral nodes, lungs, liver, spleen, skin, eyes and parotid glands are most often involved but other organs may be affected. A Kveim reaction is often positive and tuberculin hypersensitivity frequently depressed. The characteristic histological appearances are of epithelioid tubercles with little or no necrosis. The diagnosis should be regarded as established clinically in patients who have consistent clinical features together with biopsy evidence of epithelioid tubercles or a positive Kveim test. Prevalence rates are variable depending on the detection methods used and are quoted as between 1 and 64 per 100 000.

Natural history

The most common presentation of thoracic sarcoidosis is with bilateral hilar lymphadenopathy which often occurs in asymptomatic individuals and is picked up on routine chest radiography. Most cases (80%) of bilateral hilar lymphadenopathy with or without erythema nodosum clear spontaneously within 2 years. However, some will progress to develop interstitial pulmonary shadowing. Again these patients are often asymptomatic and the shadowing may clear spontaneously. If the manifestations of the disease have cleared within 2 years this identifies a group who may be said to have acute/subacute sarcoidosis. If the disease is active for longer it is defined as chronic. If the shadowing persists for more than a year there is an increasing likelihood of irreversible pulmonary fibrosis. The occurrence of skin or bone sarcoidosis or posterior uveitis is associated with poorer prognosis. Cardiac sarcoidosis (Hill, 1977) is a major worry in aviation medicine. It is uncommon but not rare with an incidence *post mortem* in patients dying of sarcoidosis of between 13 and 20% (Longcope and Freiman, 1952). It occurs most frequently between the third and fifth decade. Most patients who present with cardiac symptoms rarely have symptoms of sarcoidosis in other organs. The prognosis is uniformly poor (Fleming, 1974). Sudden death occurs in about two-thirds, presumably due to arrhythmia, and congestive cardiac failure is the cause of death in about a quarter. It is not uncommon for sudden death to be the initial manifestation of sarcoid heart disease. ECG abnormalities include heart block and ventricular and supra-ventricular tachyarrhythmias. Widespread involvement leading to infiltrative cardiomyopathy is less common. Studies in the American literature (Kinney *et al.*, 1980) suggest that more than 30% of unselected patients with acute sarcoidosis have abnormal thallium myocardial scans suggesting granulomatous involvement of the heart. Unfortunately it appears that healed granulomas may lead to arrhythmias. Even patients whose disease is apparently in remission but who have had myocardial involvement remain at risk for sudden death.

Aeromedical problems

Sudden incapacitation

This is a major concern because of the possibility of occult myocardial sarcoidosis.

Operational efficiency

Chronic sarcoidosis is likely to be associated with symptoms seriously interfering with operational efficiency.

Treatment

The standard treatment for sarcoidosis is the use of corticosteroids and because of their widespread metabolic and central nervous system side effects subjects taking this treatment will be unfit for flying.

Disposition

Pilot training

Because of the anxiety about the development of myocardial sarcoidosis, candidates with a history of sarcoidosis are considered unfit for entry into pilot training.

Trained aircrew

Considerable controversy exists as to the fitness to fly of patients with sarcoidosis. There is little dispute that the following groups should be grounded:

1. Patients with acute symptomatic though mild disease, for example bilateral hilar lymphadenopathy.
2. Patients with chronic disease. It is likely that those with posterior uveitis, skin or bone sarcoid will fall into this group.
3. Patients requiring treatment.
4. Patients with persistent widespread pulmonary shadowing, particularly if associated with cyst or bulla formation or with abnormal gas transfer.
5. Those with evidence of myocardial sarcoidosis.

The difficulty exists in those with asymptomatic bilateral hilar lymphadenopathy with or without pulmonary shadowing unassociated with any measurable decrease in pulmonary function or with other organ involvement. The problems exist because of the possibility of occult myocardial sarcoidosis and the risk therefore of sudden incapacitation. Before returning aircrew to unrestricted military flying an attempt must be made to identify and ground those who are at highest risk for developing myocardial sarcoidosis. The way to do this is probably to investigate all aircrew with sarcoidosis with a full non-invasive cardiovascular work-up. This should include ECG, echocardiograms, exercise electrocardiography and cardiac scans. Where these are normal the risk of cardiac sarcoidosis is likely to be low. Because the risk of sudden death from myocardial sarcoidosis persists after the acute phase of the disease, those with any abnormality suggesting myocardial sarcoidosis should be grounded permanently. Those with a normal evaluation should be observed for a period of time following complete clinical and radiological resolution of their disease before being returned to unrestricted flying. In this way those of significant risk of sudden incapacity will be excluded from flying. As regards civilian flying, a more liberal approach may be appropriate.

Spontaneous pneumothorax

Spontaneous pneumothorax is a leak of air occurring from the lung into the pleural space with resulting collapse of the lung. It can be asymptomatic but often causes chest pain which may be severe. If the pneumothorax is large it may cause dyspnoea, and if a flap valve occurs then the pneumothorax may continue to enlarge with resulting compression of the contra-lateral lung. This is a tension pneumothorax, and it may cause cardiovascular collapse. There are two peaks of incidence of spontaneous pneumothorax. Those most commonly occurring in young adults are usually caused by rupture of sub-pleural blebs with usually no underlying lung pathology. Those occurring in middle age are usually associated with chronic airways obstruction and bullous lung disease and will be dealt with under those headings.

Natural history

A major problem with spontaneous pneumothorax is its tendency to recur. Most published series show a recurrence rate of about 30% after a first pneumothorax, 50% after a second, and 80% after a third (Cran and Rumball, 1967). When recurrence does occur it tends to occur early, usually within 12 months of the original episode. There is a risk of contra-lateral pneumothorax of about 10%.

Aeromedical problems

Sudden incapacitation

This could occur because of the sudden pain or dyspnoea associated with a pneumothorax. This is a theoretical problem because in-flight occurrence is rare (Cran and Rumball, 1967). If a pneumothorax occurs during flight and there is a reduction in ambient pressure the pneumothorax will increase in size, perhaps leading to a tension pneumothorax. If aircrew fly with a pneumothorax that occurs on the ground but is unrecognized it may become symptomatic as the ambient pressure falls.

The symptoms usually resolve on return to ground level.

Operational efficiency

This is likely to be compromised as an aircrew member who has suffered a spontaneous pneumothorax is at high risk for developing another, especially within the first 12 months. This may occur in flight or on the route with resulting complications. To avoid this risk aircrew need to be grounded for at least 12 months after the episode.

Treatment

Because of the high risk of recurrence definitive treatment is recommended for all aircrew with spontaneous pneumothorax. Chemical pleurodesis is not without morbidity and has a significant failure rate (Hopkirk, Pullen and Fraser, 1983). Current Royal Air Force policy is to recommend thoracotomy and pleurectomy. Recurrence post-pleurectomy in pneumothorax not associated with bullous lung disease is very rare (Askew, 1976). Three months after pleurectomy most subjects will be symptom free with normal lung function and fit to return to flying duty.

Disposition

Because of the risk of recurrence, a history of spontaneous pneumothorax in the past 2 years should be a bar to entry to pilot training unless definitive treatment has taken place. If the pneumothorax occurred more than 2 years before, the risk of recurrence is sufficiently small to be acceptable. In trained aircrew, unless a period of prolonged grounding is acceptable, definitive treatment (pleurectomy) should be offered with the expectation of return to flying duty in 3 months.

Traumatic pneumothorax

Traumatic pneumothorax is caused by a penetrating lung injury, often a fractured rib. Once it has resolved the risk of recurrence is extremely small and so no further treatment is required. Once the initial episode is over, aircrew may return to unrestricted flying duty.

Chronic airways obstruction

Chronic bronchitis is a disorder characterized by over-production of bronchial secretions, often associated with irreversible airflow limitation. It is caused by cigarette smoking. Emphysema is a pathological diagnosis defined as an increase in the size of the air spaces distal to the terminal bronchioles. It too is caused by cigarette smoking but may be associated with other abnormalities particularly, alpha-1 antitrypsin deficiency. In both bronchitis and emphysema there is an accelerated decline in lung function, the excess loss in FEV1 being about 500 ml/decade.

Natural history

By the time these disorders present they are usually well advanced in their natural history. If smoking continues the disease tends to progress with increasing symptoms of cough, sputum production, breathlessness and decreasing lung function. Slow, but nevertheless significant, deterioration will continue even if cigarette smoking ceases. Recurrent exacerbations lasting several weeks, with loss of time from work, can be expected usually associated with respiratory infections.

Aeromedical problems

Sudden incapacitation

In the absence of bullae which can be associated with spontaneous pneumothorax, sudden incapacitation is not likely to be a problem.

Operational efficiency

With increasing dyspnoea and recurrent episodes of acute on chronic bronchitis, functional efficiency is likely to be severely compromised in patients with anything less than extremely mild disease.

Treatment

Bronchodilator therapy with beta-2 agonists and anticholinergics is the only treatment available. Aircrew requiring regular bronchodilator treatment are unlikely to be fit for flying. Beta-2 agonists are acceptable provided they are not taken within 4 hours of flying. Methyl xanthine derivatives, because of their central nervous stimulatory effect, are unacceptable.

Disposition

In those subjects whose disease is uncomplicated by radiological evidence of bullae and who have no or only very mild impairment of lung function, unrestricted flying can be allowed. With moderate airways obstruction subjects should be restricted from flying high-performance aircraft. More severe disturbance of lung function or abnormal blood gas measurements, or frequent acute exacerbations of chronic bronchitis, will be incompatible with flying. Bullae in the presence of chronic airways obstruction should be disqualifying.

Tuberculosis

Pulmonary tuberculosis is a pneumonic infection with *Mycobacterium tuberculosis*. This may be associated with cavitation due to lung destruction.

Natural history

Adolescent tuberculous pleural effusion usually resolves spontaneously but in 30–40% classic pulmonary tuberculosis will occur later. Uncomplicated pulmonary tuberculosis can be cured with a negligible relapse rate with standard quadruple chemotherapy in 6 months (British Thoracic Society, 1984).

Patients with substantial lung damage may have bronchiectasis and will be susceptible to recurrent episodes of chest infection. In some countries where BCG vaccination is not routine, monitoring of subjects' Mantoux status is part of regular flight medical examinations. Mantoux conversion is a potent risk factor in these circumstances for the development of pulmonary tuberculosis, and isoniazid prophylaxis is warranted.

Aeromedical problems

Sudden incapacitation

This is unlikely to be a problem.

Operational efficiency

During the acute phase patients will be systemically unwell and unfit for flying duty.

Treatment

Standard quadruple chemotherapy consists of isoniazid, ethambutol, rifampicin and pyrazinamide. Isoniazid may cause hepatitis and may be associated rarely with convulsions and psychosis. In high doses peripheral neuropathy may be a problem. Ethambutol 15 mg/kg rarely causes optic neuritis but this is reported. Rifampicin may cause hepatitis and hypersensitivity reactions. These side effects also occur with pyrazinamide.

Disposition

Pilot training

Candidates with a history of tuberculosis in the past who have had adequate chemotherapy, and who show no significant underlying lung damage on chest radiography, are acceptable for entry into pilot training.

Trained aircrew

Those with active disease or who are taking therapy are unfit for flying duty. As soon as treatment is complete, provided that there is minimal residual lung damage, aircrew may be considered fit for unlimited flying. Those with substantial lung damage will need to be assessed individually. Aircrew members with persistent cavities will need to be carefully assessed. Tuberculous cavities are thick walled and will have a bronchial communication. The risk of significant problems with these is not great provided that they are not colonized by Aspergillus. Large cavities are likely to be associated with a moderate or severe degree of lung damage, and individuals with such cavities are probably not fit to fly. Patients with adolescent pleural effusions should receive treatment, and will be fit to return to flying duty once this is complete. Mantoux converters taking prophylactic isoniazid are probably fit to return to flying duty following a period of observation (Shub, Salmonsen and Jordan, 1971).

Bullae

Bullae are airspaces of greater than 1 cm in size occurring within the lung substance. They have very thin walls composed of connective tissue and compress surrounding lung tissue. Bullae may occur singly in young individuals who have no underlying lung disease, but more frequently they occur associated with chronic airways obstruction and emphysema. They may also occur in association with scars, sarcoidosis and pneumoconiosis.

Natural history

Bullae in young adults tend to be fairly stable or only slowly increase in size. There is a risk of rupture and spontaneous pneumothorax. Bullae in those with underlying emphysema tend to be progressive.

Aeromedical problems

Sudden incapacitation

There is a slight risk of spontaneous rupture of a bulla with the development of a spontaneous pneumothorax. Bullae do not have communication with the airways and therefore during decompression, particularly sudden decompression, there is a significant risk of rupture with spontaneous pneumothorax or even air embolus resulting.

Disposition

Pilot training

The presence of bullae makes a candidate unfit for entry into pilot training.

Trained aircrew

Aircrew with bullae associated with underlying emphysema are unlikely to be fit for flying. Younger aircrew with bullae, unassociated with underlying lung disease, should not be put at risk of sudden decompression. In military flying this usually means grounding until the lesion has been resected surgically. In civil aviation, in situations where the risk of sudden decompression is small, it may be reasonable for such aircrew to be considered fit for limited flying. In this circumstance regular follow-up is required and it is probably desirable to have altitude chamber assessment with decompression to 5000 feet. This must not be associated with symptoms or with significant increase in size of the bulla.

Lung cancer

Natural history

The outlook in lung cancer remains unfavourable. The 5-year survival for patients unselected for operability and cell type is about 3%. In cases of squamous cell or adenocarcinoma, however successful the resection, the 5-year survival is approximately 25%. The prognosis of small cell carcinoma is even worse with a 2-year survival of less than 5% (Rossing and Rossing, 1982). Metastatic disease, including intra-cerebral metastasis, is common in all forms of bronchial carcinoma. Recurrent or metastatic disease may occur years after apparently successful resection.

Aeromedical problems

Sudden incapacitation

There is a possibility of sudden incapacitation due to intra-cranial metastatic disease.

Operational efficiency

This is likely to be severely compromised. An initial period of prolonged convalescence would be required followed by indefinite follow-up because of the risk of late recurrence or metastatic disease.

Treatment

It is unlikely that anyone having had a pneumonectomy for carcinoma would be fit to return to flying because of the severely reduced pulmonary capacity. Lobectomy would not necessarily be a contraindication to a return to flying provided that residual lung function was adequate.

Disposition

Pilot training

No individual with a history of lung cancer is acceptable for entry into pilot training.

Trained aircrew

Because of the poor prognosis, prolonged follow-up and risk of sudden incapacitation, patients with bronchial carcinoma are unfit for all forms of military flying. Patients who have had a successful lobectomy for squamous cell carcinoma or adenocarcinoma and have been followed up for at least 5 years might be considered fit for very limited civilian flying.

References

SKEW, A.R. (1976) Parietal pleurectomy for recurrent pneumothorax. *British Journal of Surgery*, **63**, 203–205

British Thoracic Society (1984) A controlled trial of 6 months' chemotherapy in pulmonary tuberculosis. Final report: results during the 36 months after the end of chemotherapy and beyond. *British Journal of Diseases of the Chest*, **78**, 330

CRAN, I.R. and RUMBALL, C.A. (1967) Survey of spontaneous pneumothoraces in the Royal Air Force. *Thorax*, **22**, 462–465

FLEMING, H.A. (1974) Myocardial sarcoidosis. *British Heart Journal*, **36**, 54

HILL, I.R. (1977) Sarcoidosis: A review of some features of importance in aviation medicine. *Aviation, Space and Environmental Medicine*, **48**, 953

HOPKIRK, J.A.C. (1984) The natural history of asthma: aeromedical implications. *Aviation, Space and Environmental Medicine*, **55**, 419–421

HOPKIRK, J.A.C., PULLEN, M.J. and FRASER, J.R. (1983) Pleurodesis: the results of treatment of spontaneous pneumothorax in the Royal Air Force. *Aviation, Space and Environmental Medicine*, **54**, 158–160

KINNEY, E.L., JACKSON, G.L., REEVES, W.C. and ZEUS, R. (1980) Thallium scan myocardial defects and echocardiographic abnormalities in patients with sarcoidosis without clinical cardiac dysfunction. *American Journal of Medicine*, **68**, 497–503

LONGCOPE, W. and FREIMAN, D. (1952) A small study of sarcoidosis based on combined investigations of 160 cases including 30 autopsies from Johns Hopkins Hospital and Massachusetts General Hospital. *Medicine*, **31**, 1

RAYMAN, R.B. (1973) Sudden incapacitation in flight 1 Jan 1966–30 Nov 1971. *Aerospace Medicine*, **44**, 953–955

ROSSING, T.H. and ROSSING, R.G. (1982) Survival in lung cancer, an analysis of the effects of age, sex, resectability, and histopathologic type. *American Review Respiratory Disease*, **126**, 771–777

SHUB, C., SALMONSEN, P.C. and JORDAN, J.E. (1971) Safety of INH chemoprophylaxis in aviation personnel. *Aerospace Medicine*, **42**, 1325–1335

46

Renal disease

D.J. Rainford

Introduction

The aims of this chapter are to acquaint the reader with some aspects of renal physiology and pathology and to discuss the ways in which they may be influenced by flight.

No attempts are made to cover the whole field of renal medicine, but some emphasis is laid upon the implications of abnormal findings in urine testing at routine medical or licensing examinations (Rainford and Arm, 1984) and the problem of renal stone disease.

The problems of renal medicine and aviation are considered under six main headings:

1. Renal responses to the flying environment.
2. Haematuria.
3. Proteinuria.
4. Renal stone disease.
5. Chronic renal failure and transplantation.
6. Other renal disorders.

Renal responses to the flying environment

The important renal responses to the flying environment are mediated predominantly through changes in renal blood flow. These include changes in sodium handling and the excretion of protein. Positive radial acceleration ($+G_z$) causes a reduction in renal blood flow and consequent fall in glomerular filtration rate (GFR). There is a significant antinatriuresis which also appears to be medicated by a decrease in filtered sodium load and enhanced tubular reabsorbtion (Epstein *et al.*, 1974). With an anti-G suit, enhanced tubular reabsorption seems to be the dominant factor (Shubrooks, Epstein and Duncan, 1974). It has been postulated that the increased tubular sodium reabsorption is due to stimulation of intrathoracic volume receptors in response to a decrease in central blood volume during $+G_z$ stress. It is tempting to consider whether this may be mediated through the inhibition of atrial natriuretic peptide release.

In manned spaceflight a significant reduction in plasma volume is well documented (Fischer, Johnson and Berry, 1967). This follows a diuresis though the mechanism for this remains obscure. The work of Epstein and Saruta (1973) showed that the hyperoxic hypobaric environment of spaceflight did not contribute to the diuresis either by a primary suppression of the renin–aldosterone mechanism or by impairing the aldosterone adaptive response to the diuresis.

Changes in protein excretion during flight in response to $+G_z$ were first documented by Cromarty (1984) in an elegant study of urinalysis in fast-jet aircrew. Out of 39 pilots studied, one-third (13) showed at least a trace of protein in the urine after flight. It is likely that this is due to an increase of venous pressure within the kidney during $+G$ acceleration. Interestingly, Noddeland and his colleagues (1986) found significant amounts of protein and hyaline casts in the urine of 17 of 20 pilots after centrifugation without anti-G suits. This was, however, not seen in a further group of 19 fighter pilots after air combat manoeuvre training with anti-G suits.

A limited study of 39 fast-jet aircrew during fast low level flight showed the appearance of microscopic haematuria in 3 after flight. This is certainly benign but follow-up studies have yet to be done (Cromarty, 1984).

Haematuria

The complaint of frank haematuria by the airman leaves the medical officer in no doubt about management. The patient must be properly investigated and referred for specialist opinion.

The finding of so-called 'dipstick haematuria' at routine medical examination, however, raises a lot of questions. One thing is certain, it cannot be ignored. The modern dipstick test for haematuria is a reliable guide to the presence of abnormal numbers of red cells in the urine (Arm, Peile and Rainford, 1986; Arm *et al.*, 1986) and correlates very well with population studies with regard to defining an upper limit of normality of 8 RBC/μl (8 × 10^9/litre) (Fairley and Birch, 1982; Kincaid-Smith, 1982).

Investigation should be full and include competent cystourethroscopy. Some cases will be found to be due to asymptomatic posterior urethritis/prostatitis and are easily treated. Carcinoma of the bladder, though uncommon below the age of 40 years, must be excluded. Most adults in whom the cause of the haematuria remains undiagnosed after full urological assessment have glomerular disease at renal biopsy. The decision as to whether it is justified to proceed to renal biopsy can only be taken by an experienced nephrologist who is aware of the special needs of the aircrew.

In examining fast-jet aircrew, it should be remembered that microscopic haematuria may occur following the application of G forces. Therefore, to avoid unnecessary investigation, it is probably wise to avoid urine testing within 24 hours of this kind of flying.

Patients with continuing macroscopic haematuria should be grounded. Carcinoma of the bladder that is entirely localized to the bladder mucosa with no spread, and controlled easily by endoscopic means, is entirely compatible with a continuing flying category. In general terms this should be as or with co-pilot, but after a suitable period of total absence of recurrence on endoscopic examination (e.g. 18 months) solo flying may be permitted. The presence of microscopic haematuria presents the examiner with a more complex set of decisions. After the exclusion of urological disease, the majority of these cases will be found to have chronic glomerular disease. The discovery of chronic glomerular nephritis precludes entry to Royal Air Force flying training. However, the discovery of glomerular disease in a trained pilot must be viewed differently. The commonest form of glomerular disease in patients presenting with microscopic haematuria is mesangial proliferative nephritis, usually of the IgA type. In the presence of normal renal function, a normal blood pressure and the absence of proteinuria, this usually carries a good prognosis. A category of 'as or with co-pilot qualified on type' is appropriate. Occasionally this category will also remain appropriate with an elevated blood pressure, providing it is well controlled on allowed drugs.

Commercial pilots should be under the same stringent constraints and regular follow-up by a nephrologist at a minimum of six-monthly intervals should be mandatory. Mild mesangial proliferative nephritis with no adverse features should not preclude the holding of a private pilot's licence. Decisions on other categories of glomerular disease can be made only after very full clinical and laboratory investigation and must be made only in consultation with a nephrologist.

Proteinuria

Normal man may pass between 30 and 130 mg protein per day in the urine. Present information is that reagent strips (Albustix) will detect the presence of 50–200 mg/litre and so a trace result must be interpreted with some caution. A trace of protein in a dilute urine is clearly more significant in terms of abnormal excretion than a trace of protein in a concentrated specimen. None the less, persistent positivity at any level requires quantification of urinary protein excretion. A 24 hour urine should be collected and assayed for protein excretion. If this exceeds 0.1 g/litre then the patient should be referred for full evaluation by a renal physician. Proteinuria is nearly always a portent of underlying renal disease and this is usually due to chronic glomerular nephritis. It may also be a sign of systemic disease affecting the kidney or of underlying malignancy of bowel or lung. A full history and clinical examination is therefore vital.

Orthostatic proteinuria is present when protein is entirely absent from the urine in the recumbent position but appears in the upright posture. In general terms this carries an excellent prognosis. The tendency of true orthostatic proteinuria is to resolution, with up to 50% of patients remaining free from proteinuria in 10 years (Robinson, 1980). However occasionally, early glomerular nephritis may have a postural element to protein excretion. Caution is therefore advised in making this diagnosis.

Certainly benign is the development of proteinuria in response to +G_z in some aircrew, and this can be ignored. Urine testing should not be carried out within 24 hours of flight involving manoeuvres which subject the crew to repeated +G_z stress. In general terms, proteinuria of less than 1 g daily in the presence of normal blood pressure, normal renal function and the absence of haematuria or systemic disease carries an excellent long-term prognosis. After full evaluation, these patients may be allowed to return to full flying duties provided that they are carefully followed up at a minimum of six-monthly intervals.

Patients with greater than 1 g per day have a greater potential for the development of complications such as the nephrotic syndrome, hypertension or a decline in renal function. Solo flying should not be allowed and at the best a category of as or with co-pilot qualified on type should be awarded. Follow-up should be rigorously enforced and carried out by a renal specialist.

Renal stone disease

Over the last few years there have been many changes, both medical and surgical, in the management of renal stone disease. These changes have revolutionized the way in which renal stones are regarded in the context of aviation.

The concern about renal stones is, of course, their ability to produce sudden incapacity in flight by the development of acute renal colic. All aircrew interviewed who have experienced acute renal colic have testified to the author that they would have been unable to carry out their duties safely during the phase of acute pain. Renal stone disease is common, affecting some 2% of the adult population of the UK. This incidence is growing, chiefly because of changes in dietary habits.

The majority of stones contain calcium and oxalate, and the most prevalent form of calcium urolithiasis is the so-called 'idiopathic group'. This is defined as stone formation occurring when known causes have been excluded (e.g. renal tubular acidosis, medullary sponge kidney, hypercalcaemia, hyperoxaluria and infection). Unfortunately, the natural history of untreated renal stone disease is one of recurrence. Roughly half of the patients with a single stone episode will have suffered recurrence by 5 years, two-thirds by 9 years and beyond 25 years there is a 100% rate of recurrence. Clearly, therefore, the passage of even one stone in an airman cannot be ignored. It is important not only to investigate these patients thoroughly but also to institute effective measures to prevent recurrence and establish close follow-up procedures.

Investigation is directed towards excluding known causes of stone formation and should be carried out in a unit practised in the art of metabolic medicine. Equally important is assessment of the urinary tract by radiological and ultrasonographic techniques to identify any residual stones.

The single most effective form of therapy for prevention of further stone formation is thiazide diuretics. Following investigation, providing no more specific therapy is indicated then all aircrew at risk should be given the benefit of thiazide administration. Yendt and Cohanim (1978) described a 15-year follow-up of 346 patients with stone disease treated with hydrochlorothiazide. In those who took hydrochlorothiazide 50 mg twice

daily on a regular basis, stone progression ceased in greater than 90%. Side effects necessitated cessation of treatment in only 7% of patients and were minimized in all patients by starting treatment with a small dose and increasing gradually. No other treatment is equally effective, though general advice about maintaining a good fluid intake and avoiding high oxalate intake should be given to all patients.

The following is now accepted as the protocol for management of renal stone disease in aircrew in the Royal Air Force (Director General Medical Services (RAF), 1984):

1. At initial medical examination, a history of renal colic or the known presence of stones in the renal tract will render a candidate unfit for aircrew service.
2. All aircrew are grounded at the first attack of renal colic or with the discovery of renal calculi. They are then referred immediately for intravenous urography to exclude further stones and to ascertain urinary tract normality. A biochemical screen is performed to exclude renal dysfunction, hypercalcaemia and hyperuricaemia. In the absence of any continuing abnormality the patient may return to flying pending metabolic investigations at 6 weeks post stone passage. In the presence of residual stones, the patient remains grounded until they have either passed naturally or been removed.
3. Following metabolic assessment, all patients with no residual calculi are commenced on hydrochlorothiazide 25 mg twice daily. They remain unfit flying for 2 months whilst ensuring that they remain free from side effects of the thiazides. After 1 month, they are interviewed with reference to side effects and have a biochemical screen for blood glucose, uric acid, potassium and calcium levels. The dose is then increased to 50 mg twice daily and the patient returns after a further 1 month for repeat interview and biochemical screen. If all remains well then he returns to full flying duties.
4. Patients with residual stones are commenced on thiazides in the same way, but arrangements are made for stone removal. It has been our recent experience that the majority of these can be dealt with by extracorporeal shock-wave lithotripsy. This involves the minimum of trauma and the minimum of time on the ground.
5. Six monthly follow-up is continued indefinitely both from the metabolic point of view and to ensure that the small group who will continue to form stones while taking thiazides can be identified early. Most of these respond to the addition of allopurinol to their regimen.

In civil aviation the more advanced age of the pilots may allow occasionally a relaxation of the rules. The tendency for idiopathic stone formation declines gradually after the age of 40 and therefore it may not be so important in the first-time stone producer over 45 years to institute prophylaxis. This decision should be made only by an experienced aviation physician and in these circumstances follow-up with radiological confirmation of the absence of any new stones becomes even more vital. No aircrew member performing an important role should be allowed to fly in the knowledge that he has a stone in the urinary tract.

Chronic renal failure and transplantation

Chronic renal failure is usually a progressive disorder due to a variety of renal disorders. The rate of decline of renal function is often predictable and follows a steady downhill course to end-stage renal failure. If a plot is made of the reciprocal of creatinine excretion versus time then a very reasonable prognosis can often be given. There are several factors that will accelerate the rate of decline, but uncontrolled hypertension is probably the most important.

Chronic renal failure shows little in the way of symptoms or major biochemical change except for nitrogen retention until the creatinine clearance falls below 20 ml/min. In these patients fitness to fly will be related to the factors governing licensing as described above in the sections on haematuria and proteinuria, as most will have chronic glomerular or renal interstitial disease. Flying duties, however, should only be sanctioned where the patient is normotensive, or if on hypotensive therapy is being controlled with drugs that are acceptable for flying. All flying duties should be proscribed when creatinine clearance is below 20 ml/min.

Occasionally, patients have stable renal failure due to previous obstructive atrophy. These patients have an excellent prognosis (Gower, 1976) and as long as they are followed up to exclude the development of hypertension, renal functional decline is not to be expected and a full flying category is appropriate.

The requirement for dialysis therapy for chronic renal failure should preclude any flying duties and these patients should not hold private pilot's licences. They tend to be anaemic with labile cardiovascular systems and unstable biochemistry and although often appearing very well are more prone to sudden incapacity.

The return of 'normal' renal function in a patient following renal transplantation provides a difficult problem in terms of deciding on fitness to fly. The first year after renal transplantation is the most unstable and in my opinion no patient with a renal transplant should be allowed to undertake aircrew duties during this period. After this time return to flying duties may be considered provided that there is good renal function and the patient has a normal blood pressure. The use of modern immunosuppressive regimens to prevent rejection of the graft occasionally means that transplant recipients do not require steroids. In this situation a return to flying duties in the capacity of as or with co-pilot is acceptable providing that follow-up for assessment of graft function and blood pressure is at a minimum of every 6 weeks. The administration of steroids is not compatible with a flying career and so all other transplant recipients should remain grounded.

Other renal disorders
Renal anomalies

Unilateral renal agenesis occurs in about 1 in 500 of the normal population. This may therefore be discovered from time to time as an incidental finding. It is of no clinical importance and after documentation may be ignored. Horseshoe kidney occurs with about the same incidence as unilateral renal agenesis. These patients may be allowed normal flying categories, but must be followed up with annual radiographic studies as there is an increased tendency to renal stone formation.

Polycystic kidneys

Polycystic kidneys occur in about 1 in 350 of the population and they are therefore one of the commonest of the congenital renal disorders. Inheritance is autosomal dominant in the adult type with which we are concerned and so a family history is usually obtained. Associated problems are cysts in other organs, and between 5 and 16% of cases will have cerebral or abdominal arterial aneurysms.

The discovery of polycystic disease at initial medical examination should preclude aircrew training. The discovery of polycystic kidneys in trained aircrew requires a full renal assessment before decisions are made on fitness to continue flying. Complications include bleeding, urinary infections, renal calculi, hypertension and the development of chronic renal failure. Any decisions must therefore be made in the light of the presence or absence of these findings. The relatively high incidence of cerebral arterial aneurysms and the potential for sub-arachnoid haemorrhage should preclude any category better than as or with co-pilot.

Pelvi-ureteric junction obstruction

Pelvi-ureteric junction obstruction (PUJ) is a not uncommon cause of loin pain, often of a colicky nature following a fluid load such as a few pints of beer. Radiologically the renal pelvis is seen to be distended on intravenous urography, and the ureter below is not easily seen. Isotope studies will confirm either partial or complete blockage. Treatment is surgical, either by open pyeloplasty or by percutaneous techniques. Following repair, the patient is fit to return to full flying duties with no restrictions. Follow-up with isotope renography is essential as occasionally the disorder is bilateral and both sides do not always manifest themselves simultaneously.

Conclusions

This chapter has sought to discuss some of the more common renal disorders and the way in which they may affect the activities of the airman. The efficient prophylaxis for stone disease and innovations in stone removal have modified attitudes to urolithiasis and flying. Changes in treatment of chronic renal disease and transplantation are having slower but well-defined effects. The major problems for the physician remain the interpretation and management of asymptomatic urinary abnormalities and anomalies which present in increasing numbers with modern screening techniques.

References

ARM, J.P., PEILE, E.B. and RAINFORD, D.J. (1986) Significance of dipstick haematuria. 2. Correlation with pathology. *British Journal of Urology*, **58**, 218–223

ARM, J.P., PEILE, E.B., RAINFORD, D.J., STRIKE, P.W. and TETTMAR, R.E. (1986) Significance of dipstick haematuria. 1. Correlation with microscopy of the urine. *British Journal of Urology*, **58**, 211–217

CROMARTY, I.J. (1984) *Microscopic Haematuria in Fast Jet Aircrew*. MRCC project 042. Unpublished data. London: Ministry of Defence

Director General Medical Services (RAF) (1985) *Recommendations for Management of RAF Aircrew with Renal Stones*. EMR Clinical Memorandum 1/85. London: Ministry of Defence

EPSTEIN, M. and SARUTA, T. (1973) Effects of an hyperoxic hypobaric environment on renin-aldosterone in normal man. *Journal of Applied Physiology*, **34**, 49–52

EPSTEIN, M., SHUBROOKS, S.J., FISHMAN, L.M. and DUNCAN, D.C. (1974) Effects of positive acceleration (+G_z) on renal function and plasma renin in normal man. *Journal of Applied Physiology*, **36**, 340–344

FAIRLEY, K.F. and BIRCH, D.F. (1982) Haematuria: a simple method for identifying glomerular bleeding. *Kidney International*, **21**, 105–108

FISCHER, C.L., JOHNSON, P.C. and BERRY, C.A. (1967) Red blood cell and plasma volume changes in manned space flight. *Journal of the American Medical Association*, **200**, 579–583

GOWER, P. (1976) A prospective study of patients with radiological pyelonephritis, papillary necrosis and obstructive atrophy. *Quarterly Journal of Medicine*, **45**, 315–349

KINCAID-SMITH, P. (1982) Haematuria and exercise related haematuria. *British Medical Journal*, **285**, 1595–1596

NODDELAND, H., MYHRE, K., BALLDIN, U. and ANDERSEN, H. (1986) Proteinuria in fighter pilots after high +G_z exposure. *Aviation, Space and Environmental Medicine*, **57**, 122–125

ROBINSON, R.R. (1980) Isolated proteinuria in asymptomatic patients. *Kidney International*, **18**, 395–406

RAINFORD, D.J. and ARM, J.P. (1984) Urinalysis in routine medical examinations. *British Journal of Aviation Medicine*, **2**, 16–22

SHUBROOKS, S.J., EPSTEIN, M. and DUNCAN, D.C. (1974) Effects of an anti-G suit on the haemodynamic and renal responses to positive (+G_z) acceleration. *Journal of Applied Physiology*, **36**, 345–349

YENDT, E.R. and COHANIM, M. (1978) Prevention of calcium stones with thiazides. *Kidney International*, **13**, 397–410

47

Other important medical conditions:

Diabetes; obesity; thyrotoxicosis; gastrointestinal disorders; sickling; anaemia; malignancy

David H. Hull

Introduction

This chapter deals with several disorders which are commonly seen by flight medical officers amongst civil and military aircrew. Only those aspects that are of aeromedical importance are discussed. Standard texts should be consulted for complete accounts.

The standards of fitness proposed are in general those required for unrestricted flying in single-seat high-performance aircraft. Similar though not identical standards apply to pilots holding Class 1 (Airline Transport Pilot) licences. Slightly less stringent standards will apply to two-pilot operations, military or civil, and to holders of commercial or private pilots' licences. Standards are further relaxed for other flight-deck crew and for cabin crew. Leniency must be tempered by the consideration that incapacity of any crew member will at least prejudice the success of the flying task, and may even be a hazard to flight safety.

Differing requirements for military and civilian aircrew arise in part from the severe physical stresses inherent in combat flying, the risk of injury, and the potential need for ejection, survival, escape and evasion in military operations. There is also a difference in time perspective. The medical examiner for a civil licensing authority assesses fitness for flying duties for a restricted period—say, 6 or 12 months. The air force medical officer is part of a full-time occupational medical service, and must decide the implications of any condition, however apparently trivial, for flying fitness over a full career. The question of possible attributability of deterioration in health to conditions of service has also to be considered. The great cost of fast-jet training is an additional reason for the inflexible application of standards for air force flying, especially at initial examination.

Standards for air traffic controllers (ATCOs) are closely similar to those for aircrew; in the RAF they are identical. Standards for civilian ATCOs, or at least their application, seem less stringent. The restriction 'unfit solo control of aircraft', sometimes imposed where the risk of incapacitation is appreciable, is rarely compatible with long-term career requirements.

Interpretation of aircrew medical standards has become overall somewhat more lenient in the past decade. Reasons include better aircrew health, medical advances including safer drug and other treatments, investigational methods allowing improved assessment and follow-up, and awareness of a better prognosis than was formerly believed, e.g. in mild hypertension. Aircrew are now often well informed on many medical matters and their professional associations will dispute unfavourable medical recommendations, often successfully. There is an increasing requirement to supply numerical estimates of relative and absolute risks for any medical condition; ultimately, the acceptance of any level of risk is the responsibility of the employer and licensing authority rather than the medical adviser. Waivers, usually for restricted flying or ATC duties, are quite often awarded; usually to individuals with mild forms of otherwise disqualifying disorders, where the prognosis seems relatively favourable. Specialist evaluation and follow-up are usually required.

In relation to other hazards, the contribution of medical disorders to aviation accidents is extremely small, so that some liberalization is justified; this will, however, invite greater vigilance from flight medical officers who must supervise aircrew flying with disorders that, in earlier years, would have resulted in grounding.

Medical standards for women aircrew are similar to those for men. Their generally higher percentage of body fat suggests that weight standards may require some modification. Use of oral contraceptives is generally permissible despite adverse cardiovascular effects. Overall, pre-menopausal women experience much less ischaemic heart disease than men, and sustain any level of hypertension with fewer complications. Despite notable efforts, women have not as yet established careers as high-performance jet pilots; physiological limitations may have been less important than cultural, political and financial considerations. Women aircrew fly some USAF fast jets, including instructional duties, but remain restricted from combat duties.

Certain types of sport flying (gliding, hanggliders, microlight aircraft) require no formal licence, but their pilots or others may ask for medical advice. In the absence of regulations, it seems reasonable to insist on standards no lower than those for a driving licence. Unusual and difficult cases should be referred for specialist opinion.

Medical ethics and aviation

Most practitioners will become aware of ethical problems in the practice of clinical aviation medicine. Confidentiality can never be absolute; documents are often duplicated for transmission to a central authority or records department, and the employer is likely to have *de facto* access to diagnoses. In air forces, non-medical authorities may have a prescriptive right to examine medical records.

No occupational health service can conceal medical data that may be crucial to public safety, and the flight medical officer may be obliged to alert the employer or licensing authority to medical, including psychiatric, disorders that necessitate executive action. Aircrew are aware of this situation and may feel that the doctor is serving the interests of the employing authority rather than their own. Not surprisingly, evasion and concealment of disability and even covert consumption of drugs (e.g. antihypertensives or hypoglycaemics) may occur. The risks are obvious. All doctors practising clinical aviation medicine have an important duty to minimize such abuses by doing all in their power to obtain and retain the confidence of their aircrew patients. High standards of clinical practice, flexibility in the interpretation of restrictions where that is compatible with safety, and readiness to obtain further opinions before hard decisions are made are likely to assist this objective. Willingness to discuss medical problems with aircrew organizations is helpful. Unfortunately, the flight medical officer's findings and opinions may sometimes end a career,

and this knowledge inevitably colours the doctor–patient relationship.

Healthy aircrew are subject to regular statutory medical examinations which may include X-rays and blood tests. Their right to refuse such examinations is in practice, if they are to be employed, quite hypothetical. Actual or suspected abnormalities will lead to specialist referral and to further investigations, some (e.g. coronary angiography) being potentially hazardous. The propriety of submitting asymptomatic individuals to such procedures for the sake of their employment appears dubious. Sometimes the results of the investigations may clearly benefit the individual, perhaps disclosing a condition that may be corrected or controlled by timely treatment. Quite often, however, this argument looks very thin. Aircrew may resist or refuse certain investigations, and the doctor may be tempted to exert unusual persuasive pressure or point out the likelihood of suspension if adequate investigation is not completed. Sometimes, however, the aircrewman is uncritical in his willingness to undergo any test that may promote his return to flying, however remote the possibility, and the doctor must be prepared to counsel restraint where the likely benefit to risk ratio appears low. No test should be undertaken, in the absence of a clear clinical indication, when it has no chance of influencing a decision in favour of return to flying. This often means careful 'sequencing' of investigations so that any test whose results may be disqualifying is completed and assessed before proceeding to other potentially hazardous tests. In this connection the necessarily inflexible machinery of research protocols requires the closest monitoring.

Many conditions detected on routine screening may be insidiously progressive—examples include arterial hypertension, mild aortic valve disease, and glucose intolerance. A decision on when to initiate appropriate treatment is often extremely difficult. Particularly when drug treatment may itself be a cause of temporary or even permanent grounding, there is a tendency to defer a decision to treat until well after it is clinically indicated, with obvious risks to patient and public. The converse error—initiation of treatment to enable a pilot to meet the requirements of flying standards when clinical indications are inadequate—must also be resisted.

Compromise and accommodation are essential in aviation practice; but unfortunately disagreeable, even harsh decisions are commonplace. Irreproachable ethical standards are difficult to sustain in such an environment. Nevertheless the welfare of the patient must remain the first even if not the exclusive consideration. The closer that aviation medical methods can be kept to standard clinical practice, the less likely it is that serious harm will be done. Free use of consultant services is often a safeguard, as is use of specialist panels and medical boards. Nevertheless, there is a clear individual responsibility incumbent on all practitioners to be vigilant in avoiding the potential abuses inherent in the exceptional powers and responsibilities vested in the flight medical officer.

Obesity

There is no universally accepted definition of obesity, which is commonly diagnosed by clinical inspection. Obesity usually means severe overweight, incompatible with good health, but there is no medical or other basis for such a definition; overweight and its hazards are continuous variables. Obesity is a term carrying derogatory, even insulting overtones, and for this reason its use is unhelpful, or worse, in clinical consultation. 'Adiposity' is more acceptable; and few will object to 'overweight', qualified by degree (mild, moderate, etc.). Definitions of obesity based on some arbitrary excess of weight over the 'ideal' for a given age and height involve a decision on what is 'ideal', and cannot allow for variations in body build. Many weight tables recognize the undoubted tendency to weight gain during adult life by increments for each year or two of age. For example, Royal Air Force tables give the average weight of a man 178 cm (70 inches) tall as 69 kg (151 lb) at age 24 and 78 kg (172 lb) at age 55.* There is little physiological justification for such an age allowance, as the weight of muscle and bone decline with age and any weight increase is normally due to fat. However, overweight contributes a proportionately much smaller independent risk to health as age increases, its effect being slight by the sixth decade, so that some increase in weight with age may be acceptable even though not ideal.

By contrast, weight tables for the Metropolitan Life Insurance Company (Metropolitan Life Insurance Company, 1960) give different 'desirable' weights for adults depending on small, medium or large frames, making no allowance for age. Rather often, unfortunately, frame size is difficult to assess. The Body Mass Index (BMI, Quetelet index) defined as weight in kg divided by height in metres squared, is increasingly used. A BMI exceeding 30 defines obesity, but a more stringent standard of 27–28 has been proposed recently (Foster and Burton, 1985). The BMI makes no allowance for variations in body build. More accurate methods of measuring body fat (body composition, immersion studies) are impracticable for routine clinical use. Measurement of skinfold thickness (DHSS, Medical Research Council, 1976) is reasonably reproducible, fairly well correlated with percentage body fat, and

is acceptable to patients. Arbitrary standards for the subscapular skinfold range from 1.5 cm or below for lean to over 2.5 cm for severe overweight. Multiple skinfold measurements (biceps, triceps, subscapular, suprailiac) may be summed; up to 4 cm for lean, over 8 cm for obese. In practice, a combination of weight, including records from early adult life, visual assessment and skinfold measurements is likely to give a reasonable clinical assessment of the degree of overweight.

Mild or moderate overweight may confer some advantages on the military aviator, during cold climate operations, escape and survival, malnutrition in captivity, and above all during immersion in cold water. Men of heavy, stocky build resist G-forces better than asthenic individuals, but this is probably due to physical strength and shorter heart to brain blood column rather than to fatness. Overweight aircrew are said to be vulnerable to decompression sickness; there are difficulties of fit with clothing and other flying equipment, mobility and physical fitness are harder to maintain, accidents and injuries may be more common, and a smart military appearance and self-respect may be prejudiced. In general, there are health disadvantages to any degree of overweight; indeed, if diseased individuals are excluded, the underweight person suffers less illness than those of normal weight.

Multivariate risk factor analyses of cardiovascular disease usually find overweight to be a fairly minor risk, much below that of hyperlipidaemia, hypertension or cigarette smoking. Such analyses tend, however, to exaggerate the importance of major factors at the expense of minor. Overweight is related in so many ways to more important risk factors for coronary disease and stroke that it deserves serious assessment and determined treatment.

The risks of developing diabetes mellitus and arterial hypertension are much increased by overweight, and both disorders are common causes of loss of licence. Their treatment often involves drugs which themselves constitute a potential hazard to flying safety. Weight reduction almost certainly reduces the chances of developing these disorders.

Overweight aircrew are commonly referred for exclusion of any endocrine or neurological abnormality, e.g. Cushing's syndrome, hypothyroidism or brain tumour. Such an aetiology is excessively rare and can usually be excluded by clinical examination. Assessment should include other risk factors, notably adverse family history, blood pressure, glucose intolerance, cigarette smoking and hyperlipidaemia; the risks of overweight appear increased in the presence of such risk factors, and weight reduction becomes even more desirable. Weight loss should improve glucose tolerance, blood fats and blood pressure.

---

*Obesity is defined as 15% or more above 'the accepted ideal for height and age' in aircrew, and 25% or more in others.

Table 47.1 shows the hazards of being 25% overweight, estimated as relative risk for various disorders (Royal College of Physicians, 1983). Often the size of the risk is unknown (*Table 47.2*). Risk varies directly with degree of overweight, possibly accelerating with more extreme degrees of obesity.

Table 47.1 The hazards of overweight

Condition	Risk factor
Mortality:	
Overall	+ 20–25%
Age 20–29	+ 60%
Age 50 +	Nil
Coronary mortality:	
In overweight cigarette smokers	+ 40–50%
In overweight female 40–49	+ 171%
In overweight male 70–79	+ 20%
Gall-bladder disease	+ 50% (?)
Malignancy	+ 20%
Blood pressure	+ 15/10 mm Hg
Hypertension needing treatment	× 5
Diabetes mellitus	× 3–4
Varicose veins (deep vein thrombosis)	× 2

Table 47.2 Conditions in which the influence of overweight is not known or of uncertain magnitude

Level of blood lipids
Hiatus hernia
Oesophageal reflux
Post-operative chest infections
Gout
Osteo-arthritis
Accidents
Psychiatric disorders
Heat stroke
Decompression sickness

Correction of overweight in aircrew is therefore almost always worthwhile. Drug treatment is at best of partial and temporary efficacy, at worst dangerous and ineffectual; it should be avoided. Overweight results from imbalance between energy intake and output, and its correction requires reversal of this trend. A sustained effect can be obtained only by permanent modification of personal habits; most people find this inconvenient and uncomfortable and will require motivation, repeated encouragement and support. Explanation in terms of the threat to the flying career, e.g. from blood pressure or glucose intolerance, is often effective especially when other risk factors have been found.

A calorie-restricted diet (e.g. 1500 kcal/24 hours, 6.3 mJ/24 h) is essential and should result in a loss of 0.5–1.0 kg weekly. Hazards (e.g. hypoglycaemia) are negligible but discomfort and constipation are likely. A high-fibre diet low in refined carbohydrate and animal fat is suitable. Few people can lose weight without abstaining from alcohol. A gradu-

ated exercise programme will improve fitness and morale and benefit blood lipids and metabolism generally, but is a disappointing calorie expender (e.g. 7–11 kcal/minute for jogging). However, regular exercisers are leaner than sedentary people and have a lower expectation of heart disease (Morris *et al.*, 1980). As most aircrew tasks are sedentary, frequent (four or five times weekly) recreational exercise, such as swimming, cycling or jogging, is to be encouraged.

Despite these measures, weight reduction is often incomplete, patients becoming 'stuck' at some particular weight still appreciably above the ideal. They often lose heart, feel unable to sustain the discipline of dieting, and insidiously regain some or all of the earlier loss. In practice this situation may have to be accepted. Loss of licence is exceptional unless obesity is severe, or complications are present. A restricted category may be awarded, especially for military flying. Special investigations (e.g. blood lipids, glucose tolerance test, or exercise test) may be appropriate. Discovery of weight-related abnormalities, e.g. of blood pressure or glucose tolerance, will justify renewed efforts at weight reduction and will often lead to flying restrictions.

Severe progressive (morbid) obesity is rare in aircrew. It usually originates in childhood or adolescence, and is notably resistant to all treatment. For this reason, substantially overweight applicants for flying training should be rejected. A few will re-apply after a period of drastic dieting; if they meet the weight standards, they may be accepted. However, the lost weight is then almost invariably regained, often rapidly, with further progression to unacceptable levels. Permanent disqualification of seriously overweight applicants would therefore be rational; though such a draconian regulation would be hard to enforce. Deferment for some arbitrary period, to test the individual's ability to remain slim, is a reasonable compromise.

Diabetes mellitus

Diabetes mellitus (DM) commonly leads to permanent grounding, mainly because of the risks of ketoacidosis, of hypoglycaemia or other drug effects, and of cardiovascular, renal, neurological or ocular complications. Because of the serious career implications, precision in diagnosis is essential. This is rarely a problem with symptomatic diabetes, which will be managed by standard measures. Difficulties are much more likely to arise with asymptomatic diabetes or with aircrew showing asymptomatic abnormalities of glucose tolerance.

Insulin-dependent diabetes (Type I or juvenile DM) is a bar to flight-deck duties and, despite advances in insulin types and modes of delivery, is likely to remain so. Reluctance to recognize the inevitability of this outcome may lead to mismanagement, such as attempts to persist with dietary or tablet treatment in the presence of ketonuria and weight loss, or even the withholding of any treatment despite persistent glycosuria and hyperglycaemia. These well-intentioned but misguided endeavours are dangerous; the airman should be treated precisely as any other diabetic and must be reconciled to grounding. The common apparent 'remission' in Type I DM which may enable insulin to be withdrawn for a few weeks or months early in the course of the disease is invariably followed by relapse and should not lead to resumption of flying.

Mild, usually asymptomatic non-ketotic (Type II) DM may respond to non-drug treatment, clearly an attractive option for flying personnel. A high-fibre diet low in refined carbohydrates, restricted in calories and possibly supplemented with gums (e.g. guar) will improve glucose tolerance and help with the weight reduction that is usually necessary. Some patients regain apparently normal glucose tolerance on such a regimen and can be considered for return to aircrew duties. Prior exclusion of detectable complications is essential, with lifelong follow-up. Practical problems include difficulties over obtaining or adhering to a suitable diet world-wide, tendency to regain weight, for the disease to progress, or for complications to develop insidiously or abruptly. Flying may continue for a few more years but a lengthy career is unlikely.

When hyperglycaemia cannot be controlled by diet and weight reduction, oral hypoglycaemic drugs must be considered. Diguanides (metformin) rarely if ever cause hypoglycaemia, and if control is good a waiver for restricted Class 1 or for air force flying (as or with co-pilot) may be suggested. The sulphonylureas (e.g. tolbutamide, chlorpropamide, glibenclamide) may all cause hypoglycaemia and are therefore unacceptable for most types of military flying and for Class 1 licensing. However, the likelihood of hypoglycaemia in otherwise healthy aircrew is claimed to be very small, and there is increasing pressure for waivers for Class 2 and Class 3 flying for pilots well stabilized on sulphonylureas. Instructor pilots should not be licensed. Non-pilot aircrew are likely to receive waivers for most duties.

Indefinite specialist follow-up is essential. Hypoglycaemia or loss of diabetic control necessitate grounding and reassessment. Review of asymptomatic diabetics must include search for complications (proteinuria, neuropathy, retinopathy, cataracts) whose development will attract further restrictions, often permanent grounding.

Glycosuria found at a routine aircrew medical examination must always be investigated by a formal glucose tolerance test (GTT); a diagnosis of 'renal glycosuria' entails the demonstration of glycosuria at the time of a normal GTT. Renal glycosuria is accepted as benign, though occasionally a marker of other renal tubular defects. There is no predisposition to later development of diabetes, but of course diabetes may later develop independently, so that the GTT may have to be repeated if glycosuria increases and particularly if symptoms develop. Renal glycosuria tends to decrease with age.

A few people have an abnormally high renal threshold for glucose and urine test results may be normal with frankly diabetic blood sugar levels. Diagnosis and follow-up must depend on blood sugar measurements.

Modern aircrew medical examinations usually involve blood biochemistry, which includes blood glucose. A fasting specimen is needed; a level above 6 mmol/litre (108 mg/100 ml) necessitates further appraisal, by GTT if the initial specimen was truly fasting (12 hours without oral calories). Interpretation is easy if the test result is obviously normal or abnormal. Intermediate values cause problems. The World Health Organisation (WHO) identify 'impaired glucose tolerance' in symptomatic patients when the fasting blood glucose is between 6 and 8 mmol/litre (108–144 mg/100 ml) and the blood glucose 2 hours after a 75 g oral glucose load is between 8 and 11 mmol/litre (144–200 mg/100 ml). Asymptomatic patients require an additional intermediate abnormal value, e.g. a 1-hour figure of 11 mmol/litre or more. Lower values constitute normality, and higher figures definite diabetes (*British Medical Journal*, 1980). Because so much turns on the diagnosis, neither impaired glucose tolerance nor definite diabetes should be diagnosed in an asymptomatic airman without a second GTT being carried out a week later. Great care should be taken to ensure standard conditions for the tests, as over-indulgence, sleep-deprivation and 'jet lag' may affect results. Some have practised admission to hospital, use of a high-carbohydrate diet for 72 hours before the test, intravenous GTTs and even steroid provocation. The prognostic validity of such measures is uncertain.

The importance of impaired glucose tolerance rests in its propensity to progress to DM and a probable increased risk of arterial (including coronary) disease. Recruitment to flying training is inadvisable. Established aircrew should be investigated for lipid and vascular disorders, and other risk factors (especially overweight and tobacco smoking) corrected. Diet and weight control as previously described, and vigorous daily exercise, should further reduce the risk. Provided they remain asymptomatic, regular follow-up including specialist review and GTTs should enable many, perhaps most aircrew with impaired glucose tolerance to continue flying, at least for a few years.

The chances of progression from impaired glucose tolerance to frank diabetes is said to be about 3%

per annum (*British Medical Journal*, 1980) but is probably higher in young people. Correction of risk factors, notably overweight, may reduce the risk substantially.

Measurement of serum glycosylated haemoglobin (Hb A_{1c}) is helpful in follow-up of aircrew with impaired glucose tolerance or mild diabetes. Measurements reflect the prevailing blood glucose levels over several previous weeks. A normal (< 8%) or unchanging mildly elevated level of Hb A_{1c} is reassuring; progressively rising levels strongly suggest deterioration. This test is not universally available and serum fructosamine assay has been proposed (Baker, Reid and Holdaway, 1985) as a cheaper and simpler equivalent.

Impaired glucose tolerance rarely may be due to drugs (diuretics, steroids) or to endocrine disorders (hyperthyroidism, Cushing's disease or acromegaly). Withdrawal of drugs or appropriate treatment of the disease will often restore normal glucose metabolism.

Candidates for flying training with two or more diabetic first-degree family members have a greatly increased risk of developing the disease themselves. A normal GTT is required before acceptance for RAF training; absence of glycosuria suffices for civil licensing.

Thyroid disease

Both hyper- and hypothyroidism are much more common in women than in men. However, because of the need for lifelong follow-up, thyroid disease is quite common in clinical aviation practice. Aircrew should not fly with untreated thyroid dysfunction; successful suppressive or replacement therapy is compatible with return to full flying duties, under medical supervision.

Hyperthyroidism in men is easy to miss because of an atypical presentation, e.g. predominantly psychiatric, musculoskeletal (proximal myopathy), cardiac (atrial fibrillation) or lacking usual features such as exophthalmos, weight loss, goitre and tachycardia. Thyroid function tests should be done on least suspicion and repeated if there is doubt. Blood tests have been progressively improved, and new methods make it likely that estimates of thyroid stimulating hormone (TSH) alone will suffice to diagnose both hyper- and hypothyroidism. Reliance on T4 (thyroxine) measurements alone is unsafe; T4 may be normal in the rare T3 toxicosis.

Surgical treatment of hyperthyroidism is in decline, and will rarely be appropriate for aircrew in whom some complications (e.g. recurrent laryngeal nerve damage) may end a career. Radio-iodine treatment has many attractions; unfortunately the modern smaller doses may result in delay in control,

and eventual development of hypothyroidism still remains the rule. A large, ablative, dose with acceptance of lifelong L-thyroxine replacement treatment has been advocated; follow-up is somewhat simplified but the inevitability of lifelong tablet taking, with insidious disability if compliance lapses, makes this option unattractive for aircrew. Radio-iodine is unsuitable for women in their reproductive years.

Drug treatment (carbimazole in divided doses, initially 45–60 mg daily by mouth, maintenance 5–20 mg daily) is usually successful, and rarely harmful in the form of rashes or agranulocytosis. Follow-up every 2 or 3 weeks until control is established, thereafter every 3–6 months, involves clinical assessment and serial TSH. A 2-year course is followed by early or late relapse in almost half of cases, so that lifelong follow-up is needed. The treatment can be repeated; ultimately radio-iodine is a likely choice for repeated recurrence. A few authorities treat all hyperthyroid patients with large (e.g. 45 mg daily) doses of carbimazole throughout the course of treatment, the resultant complete thyroid suppression being corrected by full replacement doses of L-thyroxine.

The onset of hypothyroidism is usually insidious and routine blood tests including thyroid function, the ECG, chest film (cardiomegaly), slowing of performance or minor clinical features may lead to diagnosis. Treatment with L-thyroxine, starting with a low dose (e.g. 25 µg daily) if there are cardiac features, ultimately about 100 µg twice daily by mouth, is readily monitored clinically and by serial TSH (6 U or below). Indefinite annual follow-up is advised, mainly to verify continued drug compliance.

Gastrointestinal disease
Acute conditions

Acute gastroenteritis is a common cause of incapacity in aircrew, who are usually well aware of the hazard and will postpone a flight if they notice even slight warning symptoms. Fortunately most attacks are self-limiting and normal flying duties may be resumed as soon as symptoms have resolved and the patient feels well again. Specific antimicrobial treatment is rarely required, even when a susceptible pathogen is identified; antibiotic treatment may even prolong symptoms. Symptomatic treatment for nausea or diarrhoea may be required. Ideally, aircrew should not fly if they need medication. Certain drugs, e.g. Lomotil (diphenoxylate and atropine), and most opiates are unsuitable. Loperamide (Imodium) or codeine phosphate may be safer, but only for those who have taken the drug before and experienced no side effects.

In two-pilot operations, aircraft safety should be ensured if captain and co-pilot invariably choose different meals, a common airline rule. Many if not most acute infections can be avoided by observing preventive health measures and using common sense. Selection, regulation and supervision of caterers is clearly very important.

Peptic ulcer (PU)

Duodenal ulcer (DU) is much more common than gastric ulcer (GU) in most Western communities, especially in young men. The major hazard to flying safety is from haemorrhage or perforation; but uncomplicated dyspepsia is distracting and may be disabling if severe. An airman with unhealed peptic ulcer should not fly.

Aircrew with dyspepsia require prompt investigation; endoscopy, though not infallible, is probably preferable to contrast radiography, which has particular problems in determining DU activity. Negative tests invite review of the differential diagnosis especially pancreatic, gall-bladder and heart disease. However, most aircrew with normal investigative findings have a benign or functional disorder, e.g. irritable bowel syndrome, requiring simple measures but no flying restrictions.

Both duodenal and gastric ulcers respond well to H2 receptor blockers (cimetidine, ranitidine); other medical regimens, some just as effective, are rarely needed. Endoscopy-proven healing rates of 80–90% at 2–3 months are commonplace. Unfortunately relapse is the rule, especially with duodenal ulcer, where rates approach 100% by 1 year. About 30% of relapses are asymptomatic; short of repeated routine endoscopies, an unacceptable measure, many relapses are undiagnosable. Unfortunately, there is no evidence that a painless DU is less prone to perforate or bleed. One bleed is predictive of others; fortunately, few perforations recur.

These facts have led to early surgery for peptic ulcer in aircrew; vagotomy, especially highly selective vagotomy (HSV) with drainage, has superseded gastrectomy for peptic ulcer; but though less disabling, it is not free of complications such as dumping syndrome and diarrhoea. Relapse of duodenal ulcer is more common after HSV than after gastrectomy, and HSV is a difficult operation requiring much experience for best results. Aircrew with a good operative result, conventionally supported by normal endoscopy at 3–6 months, can be returned to unrestricted flying duties. Unsatisfactory results create very difficult problems of aeromedical disposal.

Reluctance to resort to surgery for patients with short histories, often asymptomatic for much of that time, has prompted search for other strategies. Stopping all tobacco smoking promotes healing and probably reduces likelihood of relapse. No other non-drug intervention has been effective. As a result of research (Nicholson, 1985) into ulcer-healing drugs, maintenance H2 receptor blockade, particularly with ranitidine which is notably free of side effects in a single 150 mg dose on retiring to bed, is likely to gain increasing acceptance to allow flying in a two-pilot role.

At present, candidates for flying training with a dyspeptic history are usually rejected. Acceptance may be proposed following a negative endoscopy but the author's experience of this course is adverse. History of a proved peptic ulcer should be a bar to flying training.

Inflammatory bowel disease

Though varying enormously in severity, both ulcerative colitis and Crohn's disease are prone to complications, some acute and disabling. Inflammatory bowel disease is a bar to entry to flying duties and commonly ends a flying career. Drugs (systemic steroids, sulphasalazine, immunosuppressives) essential in treatment have potential side effects and should not be prescribed for general use in aircrew. Occasionally an aircrewman has mild or moderate disease apparently completely controlled on sulphasalazine or possibly immunosuppressives and may be considered for restricted licensing. Normal colonoscopy, haematology and biochemistry will be prerequisites. A very few aircrew have flown after colectomies, with permanent ileostomies—but this course would rarely be authorized today.

Disease, in the form of proctitis, strictly limited to the rectum often presents with bright blood flecks on stool or paper, with minor diarrhoea or sometimes constipation. There is no systemic, haematological, biochemical or other upset, barium enema (double contrast) is negative and colonoscopy confirms normality of the rest of the bowel. Appropriate tests exclude infective and other causes, rectal biopsy shows only non-specific inflammatory changes, and spontaneous long remissions are common; response to topical steroids (suppository, foam) is good. Disability is minimal and maintenance on full flying status is usually possible, though indefinite clinical follow-up is needed. Rarely, the disease extends proximally. However, a mild onset most commonly predicts a benign course.

Biliary tract disease

Biliary stone disease is becoming more common in men. Most will require surgery and can expect return to full flying duties on recovery. Endoscopic or (rarely) medical treatment may be appropriate. Aircrew who have had symptoms should not fly with stones *in situ*.

Pancreatitis

This is also becoming more common. Recovery from a single acute attack, without persisting sequelae, is compatible with return to flying. Recurrent acute episodes, or chronic pancreatitis, will rarely allow return to flying duties. Alcohol-related disease requires permanent abstinence as a condition for consideration of re-licensing.

Anaemia

Anaemia in a candidate for flying training is an absolute reason for rejection, whether temporary or permanent depending on the outcome of investigation and treatment. Symptomatic anaemia in aircrew is extremely rare. Immediate grounding is essential and ultimate return to flying depends on complete correction of the anaemia following discovery of a curable cause.

Lesser degrees of anaemia (Hb below 130 g/litre (2 mmol/litre) in men, 120 g/litre (1.86 mmol/litre) in women) may be discovered on haematology at a routine medical examination. Immediate investigation is invariably required prior to return to flying. Specialist help from physician and haematologist is advised.

Primary iron deficiency is much more common in women; a few adolescent men (e.g. recruits), usually with bad dietary habits, have iron deficiency but the diagnosis requires exhaustive exclusion of causes of blood loss, usually intestinal, or malabsorption. Response to oral iron should allow resumption of flying duties. The similar anaemia due to blood loss is rarely due to a permanently correctable cause; tropical infestation (hookworm, schistosomiasis) and certain surgically cured conditions (e.g. Meckel's diverticulum, bleeding polyp) being exceptions.

Mild anaemia due to heterozygous haemoglobinopathies (e.g. beta-thalassaemia) requires individual assessment. Sickle-cell trait is usually a bar to recruitment, certainly for military flying, for fear of sickling crises with hypoxia and other stresses. The magnitude of the risk is uncertain but is probably not great. Where rejection would involve a substantial proportion of aircrew candidates, a decision to accept the risk may be taken by licensing authorities or government departments.

Macrocytosis, usually mild (MCV 95–105 fl) is a common 'routine' finding; alcohol, drugs, vitamin B_{12} or folate deficiency and hypothyroidism are possible causes that should be considered. Rarely, occult malabsorption (adult coeliac disease) may present with macrocytosis.

Candidates with a 'perfect' result of childhood splenectomy for congenital spherocytosis (acholuric jaundice) have a normal Hb and minimal haematological features. Although fulminating fatal infections (pneumococcal, malarial) may occur, acceptance for flying duties is common.

Gout

Acute gout, often recurrent, usually of the metatarso-phalangeal joint of a great toe, is not uncommon in aircrew. Familial or constitutional factors are more important than overweight and alcohol, but combinations of predisposing and precipitating factors are usual. Acute gout and its immediate drug treatment should preclude flying duties, which may be resumed 24 hours after conclusion of treatment. The inconvenience of this restriction often leads to maintenance treatment with allopurinol (Zyloric) 300 mg daily by mouth, earlier rather than later. Allopurinol may precipitate acute gout early in the course of treatment, so prophylactic treatment with an anti-inflammatory drug such as indomethacin is usually prescribed simultaneously for the first few weeks of treatment. Allopurinol may disturb liver function and rarely causes more serious side effects, usually early in treatment. In practice, it is generally well tolerated, normalizing the serum uric acid, preventing attacks of gout and development of complications, and it can, and usually should, be continued indefinitely. Periodic follow-up is usual. Most aircrew can remain on unrestricted flying status.

Asymptomatic hyperuricaemia is common, especially in overweight and hypertensive men, who may be taking diuretics. Only a minority will progress to clinical gout. Asymptomatic hyperuricaemia carries a small risk of urate stone or nephropathy, potentially preventable by prophylactic treatment with allopurinol; but in practice the inconvenience and other disadvantages of indefinite drug treatment outweigh any benefits. Low purine diets are rarely practicable. General health measures such as weight reduction, alcohol restriction, and a review of need for diuretic treatment should be attempted. 'Crash diets' are apt to precipitate clinical gout.

Theoretically, serious diseases such as blood dyscrasias might underlie the appearance of asymptomatic hyperuricaemia. The chances of this are very small, and otherwise negative results from the haematology and biochemical tests of the modern aircrew medical examination should exclude the possibility.

Hyperlipidaemia

Abnormal blood fats are a common finding on routine biochemical tests. Constitutional and environmental factors are often evident. Causes of secondary hyperlipidaemia (diabetes mellitus, hypothyroidism, chronic renal or liver disease) should be excluded before a diagnosis of a primary hyperlipidaemia is accepted.

Referral to a lipid expert will be needed for the assessment of serious elevation, especially of cholesterol. Heterozygous familial hypercholesterolaemia is suggested by a family history of premature coronary disease or hyperlipidaemia, or the presence of tendon xanthomas at the extremities, especially Achilles tendons, tibial tuberosities, hand tendons, and elbows. Eyelid xanthelasmas and arcus lipoides are less specific. Familial combined hyperlipidaemia is distinct in that blood triglycerides as well as cholesterol are elevated, xanthomas usually absent, but premature coronary disease is prevalent in close relatives. Either type of familial disorder greatly increases the risk of arterial and particularly coronary disease (e.g. 50% of men with familial hypercholesterolaemia have developed symptomatic coronary disease by age 50); they are a bar to recruitment for flying training, and their discovery in trained aircrew necessitates detailed evaluation including exercise stress testing, drug treatment and long-term follow-up by a cardiologist and lipid specialist. Unrestricted flying is unlikely to be possible, and premature grounding the rule.

Most aircrew with hyperlipidaemia will not, however, have a familial disorder, but so-called 'common' or 'polygenic' hyperlipidaemia often aggravated by dietary factors including alcohol, overweight, physical inactivity or drugs such as beta-blockers and diuretics. Classification into the Fredrickson grouping is usually possible but rarely of practical usefulness. There is moderate elevation of either cholesterol (6.5–9.0 mmol/litre, 250–375 mg/100 ml) or triglycerides, or both. Triglycerides will vary due to such factors as covert eating, overweight, alcohol and physical inactivity; fortunately triglycerides are weak factors compared with cholesterol, which is one of the strongest risk factors for vascular and particularly for coronary disease. The advantages to the individual of intervention to reduce moderate elevations of blood cholesterol are at present uncertain, though there is some evidence that prognosis may be improved. Unfortunately, drug treatment is potentially hazardous, is expensive and sometimes unpleasant, and will generally be inappropriate for aircrew. Dietary treatment using vegetable oil and polyunsaturated fats as substitutes for dairy and meat products, and weight reduction often improve the blood fats, sometimes to normal.

Fractionation of cholesterol into high density lipoprotein (HDL) and low density lipoprotein (LDL) may be helpful prognostically. The higher the ratio of HDL to LDL or to total cholesterol, the better; though this has been disputed recently. Certain drugs such as beta-blockers and diuretics,

cigarette smoking, overweight and physical inactivity adversely affect the ratio, whereas weight reduction, stopping smoking, regular vigorous exercise and small amounts (e.g. two drinks daily) of alcohol increase HDL cholesterol at the expense of LDL cholesterol. Resulting benefits are uncertain, but the measures suggested appear unexceptionable on general health grounds.

Aircrew with common hyperlipidaemia should be assessed by a cardiologist who will probably carry out echocardiography, exercise and possibly isotope studies. If the cardiovascular system is normal, most aircrew may be returned to unrestricted flying, but require indefinite follow-up, with periodic repetition of specialized studies.

Malignant disease

The annual physical examination and other routine screening methods will occasionally disclose the first evidence of malignancy. More commonly, aircrew will present with symptoms of the disease. Any suspicion of neoplastic growth should lead to immediate grounding and full investigation. Treatment will be in accordance with normal practice.

The question of return to flying duties after treatment is extremely difficult. Traditionally, permanent grounding has been commonplace. This is probably still appropriate for tumours with the most adverse prognosis (e.g. most bronchial and gastric cancers), certainly for single seat flying duties. Return to unrestricted flying is unlikely in the presence of metastatic disease, or where remission in response to chemo- or radiotherapy is incomplete.

The greatly improved results of modern treatment for some solid tumours (e.g. Hodgkin's disease, testicular tumours) and some blood dyscrasias mean that many patients enjoy an apparently complete remission; a substantial proportion are cured, though unfortunately time alone can confirm which individuals are so fortunate. Re-licensing of aircrew in apparent full remission requires considerable caution, because of the risks of insidious relapse with subtle disability, or of sudden incapacitation such as may occur with neurological or bony metastases. In every case the opinion of an oncologist with experience of aviation medicine should be obtained. Regular expert follow-up with modern diagnostic equipment such as computerized imaging is essential in all cases.

References

BAKER, J., REID, I. and HOLDAWAY, I. (1985) Serum fructosamine in patients with diabetes mellitus. *New Zealand Medical Journal*, **98**, 532–535

British Medical Journal (1980) Impaired glucose tolerance and diabetes—WHO criteria. *British Medical Journal*, **281**, 1512–1513

Department of Health and Social Security. Medical Research Council (1976) *Research on Obesity*. ISBN 0 11 450034 7, pp. 5–6. London: HMSO

FOSTER, W.R. and BURTON, B.T. (eds) (1985) Health implications of obesity; NIH concensus development conference. *Annals of Internal Medicine*, **103**, 977–1077

Metropolitan Life Insurance Company, New York (1960) *Mortality Amongst Overweight Men and Women.* Statistical Bulletin 41. New York: Metropolitan Life Insurance Company

MORRIS, J.N., EVERITT, M.G., POLLARD, R. *et al.* (1980) Vigorous exercise in leisure-time; protection against coronary heart disease. *Lancet*, **ii**, 1207–1210

NICHOLSON, A.N. (1985) Central effects of H1 and H2 antihistamines. *Aviation, Space and Environmental Medicine*, **56**, 293–298

Royal College of Physicians (1983) Obesity—a report. *Journal of the Royal College of Physicians of London*, **17**, 6–65

48

Psychiatry

E. Anthony

Introduction

This chapter contains a description of the psychiatric problems most likely to be met by doctors in their clinical contacts with aircrew and an outline of their treatment. In presenting the subject in this way it has been assumed throughout that the reader possesses some knowledge of psychiatry and no attempt has been made to present a complete review of psychiatric disorders and their treatment.

Much of the subject matter presented in this chapter may appear to be no more than the common sense of good medical practice, and that is what it is. There is, however, good evidence that 'obvious' emotional problems are often overlooked, particularly in patients who present with somatic symptoms, and a significant proportion of patients with conditions that have been accepted by general practitioners as bona fide physical illnesses are exhibiting significant symptoms of psychiatric disturbance. Some surveys have put the figure as high as 50%. There is also good evidence that in routine clinical practice up to half of such disturbances remain unidentified. Aircrew are likely to be over-represented among such patients.

Personality characteristics in aircrew

To understand the attitudes of the majority of aircrew to emotional disorders it is necessary to have some model of the 'typical' airman. Many attempts have been made to describe him (and more recently her), particularly in the American literature. What emerges is, of necessity, a stereotype which is useful only as a means of summarizing some of the personality characteristics found frequently in aircrew. Typical of the profiles that have been produced was that by Fine and Hartman (1968) who described the 'modal' military pilot as psychiatrically normal, matter-of-fact, terse, utilizing direct ways of coping, having strong needs for personal achievement and high regard for the responsibilities of family life. Complexity is added to the picture by the airman's postulated need to keep emotional distance in interpersonal relationships, particularly those with women. They often have excessive unconscious aggressive hostility, and internal tensions appear to be related to this hostility as well as to frustrated achievement, distance in relationships and feelings of responsibility inconsistent with their need for novelty. According to Fine and Hartman inner tensions are reflected in particular areas of personality vulnerability:

1. The potential to 'act-out' when frustrated.
2. Reductions in efficiency in important areas (to the individual) such as productivity, contentment, and self-acceptance.

British authors are less expansive, confining themselves to pointing out that many aircrew exhibit moderate or pronounced obsessional traits, are very aware of the need to have few psychological failings in order to achieve respect and that virtually all of them experience anxiety when exposed to constant threat of danger. In a minority this anxiety becomes incapacitating and this is more likely to happen following an incident where threat of danger has been converted into reality, for example incidents resulting in ejection. There are reports that from 30 to 70% of aircrew who have ejected subsequently experience significant emotional consequences and that only a minority successfully resolve these although the majority continue to fly despite their significant fears, apprehension, resentment and anger (Fowlie and Aveline, 1985).

Among commercial aircrew psychiatric disorders are second only to cardiovascular disease as a cause of loss of flying licence and, as among military aircrew, anxiety is more common than depression. The final 'wastage' rate is low, 34/1000 at risk but, as Bennett (1985) points out, this is unlikely to represent the true incidence of psychiatric disorder in professional commercial pilots as it is certain that some continue to fly while suffering psychological disturbances, sometimes shielded by colleagues in the mistaken belief it is in the sufferer's best interests.

The consequences of ejection are an example of the result of interaction between an individual and a particularly stressful event. The links between such interactions and disease are not straightforward. The particular event is important but its interaction with predisposing factors, including the personality, is vital. Surviving sudden emergencies and disasters can precipitate neurotic symptoms even in the absence of apparent constitutional vulnerability.

The re-discovery in World War II that individuals not predisposed to emotional disorders manifested disabling anxiety and its autonomic concomitants when subjected to very stressful experiences stimulated interest in the prevalence of such symptoms in the general population. The discovery that they are widespread has prompted much discussion of what constitutes a 'psychiatric case' and encouraged the development of instruments such as the General Health Questionnaire (GHQ) by Goldberg and the Present State Examination (PSE) by Wing and his colleagues in an attempt to introduce some consistent criteria as a basis for determining when the manifestation of psychiatric symptoms justifies categorizing an individual, should he or she seek medical advice, as having a psychiatric or psychosomatic disorder. Goldberg and Huxley (1980) present a very balanced account of the evidence of undeclared psychiatric symptoms in the community in their review of the subject.

It has been suggested that as aircrew are volunteers who have been rigorously selected and trained for their profession, different criteria should be used when assessing them, particularly for fear of flying, than would be appropriate for assessing the general public. Whilst one may assume it is normal for non-aircrew to be afraid of flying low-level missions, or at night in bad weather, or air combat manoeuvres, or mid-air refuelling, or low altitude parachute extraction, for those trained to carry them out it is not. According to this argument manifestation of fear in a trained flier who was previously unafraid represents a serial change, a loss of adaptation in one previously able to cope with the realities of operational flying.

Systems of classification

No predisposing or protective factor is predominant in determining the occurrence of psychiatric illness nor can one compile a comprehensive list of such factors. Where predisposing personality traits are prominent relatively minor stress will precipitate illness, but overwhelming stress will precipitate illness in the most resilient. It was pointed out above that a large proportion of the population exhibits symptoms of emotional disturbance at some time in their lives. The relevant question is, when do such symptoms constitute a significant psychiatric illness? In many circumstances that point is reached when an individual seeks help from a medical or paramedical agency. In the case of aircrew, because undetected emotional disturbance, however minor, may represent a hazard to themselves and others it is not acceptable to wait until an individual recognizes or is prepared to acknowledge such a disturbance.

The major mental disorders should not present serious problems of discrimination from normal mental health because the sufferers exhibit symptoms such as delusions, hallucinations and severe abnormalities of mood, which are not experienced by those in normal mental health. Patients with such disorders comprise a minority of those who require help from caring professions, however, and because aircrew are, when initially selected, young and apparently in normal mental health they subsequently produce fewer major mental illnesses than a random sample of the general population.

The majority of mental disorders encountered in aircrew will be minor; and since the symptoms exhibited by those with such disorders, for example anxiety and its physical and autonomic concomitants and relatively mild dysphoria, are experienced in some degree, at some time, by everyone, what reliably discriminates the 'neurotic' patient from his normal neighbour? The answer is nothing apart from the intensity and persistence with which the patient experiences his symptoms and the extent to which they disrupt his life, particularly his ability to make interpersonal relationships and his ability to function efficiently. The morbid phenomena of the minor mental disorders are quantitative deviations from the phenomena of normal living. The diverse, individual and unique patterns of psychological functioning presented in them can be understood only by a systematic approach to the assessment of the sufferers' personalities in terms of traits, dimensions, categories, or dynamics.

Two systems of classification are in common use, the 9th revision of the *International Classification of Diseases* (World Health Organisation, 1978), and DSM III which was published by the American Psychiatric Association in 1980. The difference in the nomenclature used in the two systems highlights their arbitrariness when applied to minor mental disorders since the ICD 9 denotes arguably its largest grouping as neurosis while the DSM III has done away with the term on the grounds that it groups together conditions that are better classified in other ways and introduces unsubstantiated ideas about aetiology. In addition it is claimed that neurosis is too general a grouping and its boundaries with normality and with personality disorder are difficult to draw. The most powerful argument for retaining the overall category of neurosis is that not all the conditions that would generally be thought of as neuroses fit neatly within the diagnostic criteria for particular syndromes such as anxiety disorder, obsessional disorder or hysteria. There are many intermediate cases which are characterized by a mixture of anxiety, depressive, obsessional and hypochondriacal symptoms, which have in recent years been called 'minor affective disorders'. Such conditions, together with psychophysiological disorders (somatization of anxiety), are the most prevalent among aircrew, and whereas they might be of relatively little consequence in those practising in many occupations, in aircrew they can be lethal. When added to the many physiological stresses involved in flying, even minimal mental disorder becomes disabling.

The majority of aircraft accidents are attributed to human error, approaching 60% between 1967 and 1971 according to an estimate by the Civil Aviation Authority. It surveyed accidents occurring on public transport, commercial, executive, club, private and training flights, and all but 4% of those involving human error were attributed to pilot error. It is therefore of paramount importance that any remediable contributor to such error is identified and dealt with effectively, and minor affective disorders clearly fall into this category. More major psychiatric disorders are, of course, equally important to identify although they may not be remediable to the point where the patient can return to flying.

Psychiatric disorders and grounding

Attempts to determine the proportion of aircrew grounded on medical recommendations where the responsible disorders have been psychiatric have produced widely different figures. A study, over 10 years, of United Kingdom military aircrew categorized as medically unfit to fly indicated 41% were grounded for 'psychiatric reasons', and comparable figures have been reported in some studies on United States military aircrews. In a review of all such studies in America between 1975 and 1979, however, Ursano and Holloway (1985) quoted a figure of 13% of whom approximately half were later returned to flying duties in some, but not necessarily their original capacity. A study of United Kingdom commercial airline personnel stated 67%

of 'medical groundings' were psychiatric, but figures derived from data collected by companies insuring professional civilian aircrew indicated that the figure was 13.4%. There would be little purpose in debating which of the figures is most accurate since they were collected in different ways, for different purposes and using different criteria. The only useful conclusion that can be drawn is that a substantial number of highly and expensively trained aircrew have their careers wrecked or curtailed because they become disabled, as far as flying is concerned, by psychiatric illness. What can also be said, with some certainty, is that the prospect of being diagnosed as psychiatrically ill is for many, if not most, aircrew more unacceptable than being given a diagnosis of physical illness. This is a factor that must always be considered when evaluating somatic symptoms presented by aircrew for which no appropriate organic pathology can be discovered, since to some the idea that they might have a 'mental illness' is unthinkable and this may significantly influence their presentation.

The management of anxiety in aircrew is facilitated, as it is in other patients, by early recognition and this is most difficult when it is something of which the individual is not consciously aware or which he does not wish to acknowledge. In such circumstances, and they are frequent, the initial presentation is with somatic symptoms, leaving the doctor to determine at what point, for example, the perpetually hyper-alert posture in the cockpit caused the physical changes in the head and neck that are being experienced and presented as a headache. Any doctor presented with such a symptom complex must include an evaluation of the possible underlying psychological correlates, particularly the patient's true motivation to continue flying, if a satisfactory formulation of the problem is to be made. Jones (1986) suggested that the most notable characteristic in successful fliers is their absolute faith in themselves. Anything that shakes or destroys this, that casts doubt on their self-control, may lead to disproportionate anxiety about flying. It may occur following hyperventilation and vertigo which are interpreted as, and may momentarily be, an unexplained loss of self-control. Unable to predict when it might recur and feeling helpless to control it if it did they find the attendant anxiety intolerable, and such anxiety may become associated with all flying situations.

Accounts of attempts to identify and define psychological mechanisms and their relationship to somatic manifestations imply a causal connection between the two. The significance of such a connection in the aetiology of 'psychosomatic disorders' has been discussed at length by many authors over the years with strong views expressed both for and against. Mitchell (1984), in an evaluation of the current position, after admitting that he had been until recently a 'don't know' on the question, pointed out that the beta blocker heart attack trial has shown that psychological stress must now be included as a factor when considering the aetiology of heart attacks and their prognosis. Earlier studies, summarized by Brandon (1983), indicated a causal relationship between stressful events and both emotional disturbance and increased mortality in stable people. Therefore, it can now be said with confidence that however difficult it may be to identify, much less quantify, there is a causal relationship, mediated through many intermediate variables, between 'stress' and both physical and mental illness.

'Stress', personality and disease

Whenever the relationship between stressful environmental circumstances and disease, whether psychiatric or psychosomatic, is discussed the role of personality as an intermediate variable is invariably emphasized. Attempts to evaluate personality, both clinically and psychometrically, in a way that permits accurate prediction of the influence particular traits have on determining the probability of an illness occurring, or the form of an illness when it does occur, have largely proved fruitless. However, personality is undoubtedly a vital component of the interactions that result in illness. It has long been known there is no personality type that is a necessary precondition for mental disorders to occur. The appropriate question to ask is whether particular sorts of personality are at greater risk of developing physical illness, as the research into Type A personalities has suggested, or whether particular personality traits increase the risk of psychiatric disorder. When calculating such a risk it is important to remember that only a small proportion of psychiatric illnesses are treated by the psychiatric services. Thus the idea that abnormal personalities are at a greater risk of psychiatric illness, as investigators like Hurry, Tennant and Babbington (1980) have suggested, may simply reflect the greater likelihood of those with such abnormalities being referred for a psychiatric opinion. Most of the research published is based upon patients who have been referred to the psychiatric services, whereas the present discussion is concerned with minor affective disorders which are often treated exclusively by general practitioners. In addition the reader must bear in mind the impossibility of drawing sharp lines of demarcation between predispositions to, for example, depressive illnesses of varying grades of severity.

A further complication is introduced into the consideration of the effect disorders of personality have on psychiatric disorders by the fact that the two are not discrete entities. Usually, for convenience, they are separately classified but they are not sharply differentiated. An argument can be made for not making the distinction between abnormal personality and minor neurotic illness which is familiar in Anglo-Saxon psychiatry. The term 'neurosis' has been removed from the American Psychiatric Association's DSM III. This was anticipated by 30 years when Schneider described neurosis in 1950 as 'out of date, discredited by facts and therapeutically harmful since it gives the patient a false picture of himself and his condition'. Schneider felt it was important that the patient saw himself as a neurotic not as someone who has a neurosis, the practical implication being that as a neurotic he must take some responsibility for himself whereas if he had a neurosis, that is an illness, the responsibility for curing him rested with the doctor (Schneider, 1950). This is an important practical distinction when considering the therapeutic approach most appropriate for aircrew. Although Schneider's approach does have certain disadvantages these are largely theoretical and of importance mainly to research investigators. For the clinician the appropriate stance is that advocated by Cawley (1983), that 'classifications are necessarily arbitrary: definitions are incomplete, nomenclature tends to be confused and distinctions remain blurred. The best nosology is likely to be the one that achieves the greatest reliability while attaining the greatest validity in terms of clinical usefulness and predictions concerning the course of treatment and outcome'.

The Type A personality

Intensive study in recent years has produced some potentially useful results by defining Type A personality and a putative relationship between it and psychosomatic illness, particularly coronary heart disease. Type A personalities have many of the characteristics itemized by Fine and Hartman in their stereotype of the aggressive military airman. They are aggressive, ambitious and competitive, and along with their hard-driving competitive behaviours they tend to express hostility and irritation in response to challenge or threat. The importance of the role of environmental milieu in either inducing or interacting with such observed behaviour has been stressed in the more recent research and has indicated that although Type A persons are in a chronic struggle to achieve more and consequently in habitual conflict, they tend to ignore, suppress or deny physical or psychological symptoms while working under pressure, reporting them when work is over. Although it is generally believed Type A behaviour (TAB) occurs usually when environmental challenges are added to personality attributes in predisposed individuals some research workers have placed so much importance on the role of challenges in evoking TAB that they have claimed that, when these are severe enough and of a chronic nature, almost any individual may respond with TAB regardless of basic personality.

The sense of threat that a situation may present is related not only to the individual's personality characteristics but its impact is also dependent on the amount of available interpersonal and social support. An event or situation may pose a threat because of uncertainty of outcome, risk of physical or psychological harm, or the need for continued vigilance, and the effect any event or situation will have on a particular individual will depend on how he or she perceives it. Johnson and Sarason (1979) found that negative life change was significantly correlated with measures of trait anxiety and depression in subjects who believed they were not in control of their environment. Work is itself a potential source of stress, as Cooper (1985) has pointed out. Having set out sources of stress at work he suggested that one or some combination of these, together with certain personality traits, may be predictive of a variety of consequences including mental ill health, excessive alcohol or drug taking, coronary heart disease and marital disharmony.

Heightened affective arousal is associated with physiological cardiovascular changes such as increase in heart rate, blood pressure, cardiac output and peripheral resistance. A true psychosomatic pathogenesis has been hypothesized by Brandt et al. (1976) where Type A behaviour together with frequent affective and autonomic arousal due to environmental demands leads to atheromatous deposits in coronary arteries and, in turn, to ischaemic heart disease.

The airman's environment is designed to provide the type of challenges shown by research to increase the evocation of TAB; this is a lifestyle associated with hyper-alertness, muscular tension and a chronic sense of time urgency that underlies habitual acceleration of the pace of most activities and thought. A prominent outcome of this orientation is frustration and associated irritability that is manifested by enhanced hostility, although this is often covert. Similar findings have been regularly quoted by researchers into the effects of stress on aircrew.

Air traffic controllers have frequently been studied as a group in whom stress-induced illnesses directly attributable to working conditions occur. Among the findings in different studies have been an increased prevalence of hypertension, diabetes and peptic ulcers. Some of the specifically stressful aspects of an air traffic controller's job, identified by different investigators, have been shift work, fatigue (as a reflection of work overload) and too little work leading to periods of boredom interspersed with sudden upsurges of physical and mental activity during emergencies which lead to very high arousal.

This responsibility for people's safety has been repeatedly identified as a major long-term stressor which may lead to physical and/or mental ill health.

This is an appropriate point at which to attempt to summarize some of the factors common to different aspects of research into possible causal factors in the precipitation of non-psychotic psychiatric disorders and psychosomatic disorders. We can say with some confidence:

1. That personality is an important variable helping to determine an individual's vulnerability to such disorders and in determining whether distress is exhibited through psychological or somatic symptoms.
2. That 'stress' interacting with personality is an important variable helping to determine the occurrence of such disorders.
3. That 'stress' in any individual is determined not simply by the objective content of the stressful event but how the event is perceived by the individual, and that this perception is determined to some extent by the individual's personality. 'Negative' life-events are more stressful than 'positive' life-events.
4. The environmental milieu is important in determining whether an individual responds to stress with psychological or somatic symptoms. Some investigators believe that the environmental milieu is as important, or even in some cases more important, than personality in determining an individual's response to 'stress'.

Measurement of personality

While it is true that personality is important, interacting with environmental factors impinging on an individual and so determining his ability to cope with any particular experience, this is a platitude, more comforting than helpful in predicting vulnerability to the development of psychiatric illness or prognosis when such an illness has occurred, unless both components of the statement can be described in such a way that they can be used reliably in the prevention and management of somatic or psychiatric disorders. Many inventories are used to measure various aspects of psychological functioning. Rating scales and similar devices such as symptom inventories attempt to increase the precision with which psychopathology, abnormal behaviour and personality variables are recorded. Symptoms or aspects of personality can be evaluated more precisely than by global, general assessments so that sophisticated statistical techniques can be used in their development and analysis. High reliability is possible when the scale is expertly constructed and refined when it is used by properly trained personnel. The most important attribute of the rating scale, however, is its validity. Does it really measure what it purports to measure? Scales are most useful when they transcend cultural boundaries. To some extent they can be regarded as verbal surrogates for behaviour samples and in this respect their usefulness depends on how reliably and faithfully they correlate with the type of behaviour or condition in which the investigator is interested. In practice the results have been disappointing and in recent years there has been a marked decline in the use of inventories that measure personality traits. This has stemmed both from practical considerations such as the cost of training testers and doubts about the validity of the inferences frequently drawn from test findings and consequent reservations about their usefulness.

The Minnesota Multiphasic Personality Inventory (MMPI) is probably the most widely used of all inventories, especially in North America where it has been extensively used in the assessment of aircrew in an attempt to identify those most likely to be disabled by psychiatric symptoms, particularly anxiety which is the most common symptom experienced and the greatest contributor to poor flight performance. Investigators in the United Kingdom (Goorney, 1970; Aitken, Lister and Main, 1981) have not found it particularly useful in this respect. Other inventories have been widely used including Cattell's 16 PF questionnaire and, particularly in the United Kingdom, the Eysenck Personality Inventory (EPI), but these have shown no improvement on the MMPI. The EPI poses questions which have to be answered 'yes' or 'no'. The answers when analysed are expressed in terms of extraversion–introversion and neuroticism (emotional lability) scores which it is claimed represent fundamental dimensions of personality. Individuals are arrayed along two continua which are claimed to be orthogonal and Eysenck found that patients with anxiety states scored highly on neuroticism and introversion, as did obsessive-compulsives and those with reactive depression. He classified all such individuals as 'dysthymic'. Studies searching for the 'accident-prone', an issue of primary importance to anyone caring for aircrew, have shown that 'neurotic extraverts' are more accident-prone than 'stable-introverts' and that those identified in questionnaire studies as 'adventurous' have a much greater probability of being involved in a flying accident (Green, 1983).

Despite its popularity and the claims that have been made for it the EPI, and its predecessor the MPI, have come in for considerable criticism. Among the most cogent when normal personality functions are being assessed is that they were originally derived from assessment of psychiatric patients who were vaguely labelled as 'neurotic' or 'psychotic'. The use of such criterion groups is highly suspect as they are invariably heterogeneous. Aitken found no significant difference between the

EPI scores for aircrew with phobic anxiety when he compared them with those of normal operational aircrew, while Goorney found that aircrew with phobic anxiety who were 'dysthymic' on Eysenck's criteria before treatment reverted to the normal range for both neuroticism and extraversion–introversion after treatment. Instability of scores measured under different conditions is an obvious further limitation on the usefulness of a personality inventory as a predictive instrument and must raise doubts whether what is being measured are, as Eysenck claimed, 'fundamental dimensions of personality'.

The term 'asthenia' was introduced into psychiatry more than a 100 years ago to describe individuals with an 'irritable weakness', easily fatigued, who respond readily to minor stress by experiencing discomforts and pains. Although widely used clinically and considered to predispose to affective disorders it was not placed on a sound theoretical basis until 1966 when Hagneil carried out the research which demonstrated, apparently conclusively, that asthenic personality traits are important in increasing vulnerability to psychiatric illness. A total population of 2550 inhabitants of an area in Sweden were screened for 'asthenia', that is complaints of habitual tension, fatigue and nervousness. Ten years later those who had been initially assessed as exhibiting asthenia whose onset was in adult life had a significantly increased risk of developing mental disorder during this follow-up period. His study supports the view that those who develop minor 'asthenic' symptoms in early adult life are thereafter at greater risk of developing psychiatric illness, and this finding is independent of the tendency of the individual to seek medical care for his symptoms.

The fact that introverted–neurotic individuals (after Eysenck) have been highlighted as being predisposed to affective disorders has tended to distract attention away from the fact that extraverted–neurotics are also liable to develop such disorders in appropriate circumstances. It is clinically commonplace that depression tends to accentuate 'acting-out' by individuals with such personalities so that they appear more histrionic and manipulative than when they are well. Remembering that it has been shown earlier that many aircrew are extraverted, this emphasizes the need for flight medical officers to consider the possibility that aircrew are depressed or hypomanic when they are observed acting-out exaggeratedly and this constitutes a significant change from their normal behaviour pattern.

Having established that certain personality traits can be identified reliably premorbidly and that they interact, to some extent predictably, with environmental stresses in causing psychiatric or psychosomatic illness, what else can be said with any confidence about factors that influence predisposition to psychiatric disorders? Life events and the difficulty in evaluating their 'stress potential' has already been discussed. Early childhood experience is another topic about which much has been written since Bowlby stimulated interest with his publications in the effect of attachment, separation and loss of parents to children (Bowlby, 1969, 1973, 1980). Subsequently some of Bowlby's conclusions were challenged and Rutter (1985) has recently exhaustively reviewed the evidence about factors that influence 'Resilience in the face of Adversity'. His conclusions confirm the importance of a person's appraisal of a situation and his ability to process the experience, attach meaning to it and incorporate it into his belief-system in determining his response to it. He emphasized the importance of people dealing with adversities and life stresses and not simply reacting to them; the fact that they do act is more important than the particular strategy they adopt and this ability to act positively is a function of their self-esteem and feelings of self-efficacy as much as of their problem-solving skills. He opines that such a 'cognitive act' is fostered by secure, stable affectional relationships and success, achievement and positive experiences as well as by personality characteristics. Such personal qualities seem to be operative as much in their effects on interactions with and responses from other people as in their role in regulating individual responses to life events. Coping successfully with stressful situations is strengthening since it is normal throughout life to have to meet challenges and overcome difficulties. The promotion of resilience does not lie in an avoidance of stress but in encountering it at a time and in a way that allows self-confidence and social competence to increase through coping successfully and accepting appropriate responsibility.

Lastly, Rutter emphasizes that all the evidence points to the importance of developmental links, pointing out that protection does not primarily lie in the buffering effect of some supportive factor operating at one point in time, or even over a prolonged period of time. Early life experiences, happenings during later childhood and adolescence, and circumstances in adult life all contribute to the buffering effect. No one experience is in itself determinative of later outcomes but in combination they may serve to create a chain of indirect linkages that foster escape from adversity. We don't have a clear or adequate understanding of how this development takes place but it is undoubtedly a 'final common path' that can be arrived at by a variety of different routes.

If we now attempt to summarize, it can be seen that despite all the research in various areas no comprehensive picture has emerged of the factors which, in combination, result in psychiatric disorders or their avoidance. We have, however, progressed some way beyond re-stating the obvious, that both personality and environmental factors contribute and interact in determining their outcome, and can identify some of the threads of information which when woven together comprise the material of these disorders:

1. Certain personality configurations when subjected to stress present, with a high degree of probability, with predictable symptomatic pictures. Asthenic personality traits, which can be reliably identified before psychiatric symptoms are declared, predispose to 'minor' affective disorders. In contrast, Type A personalities are likely to respond to stress by developing psychosomatic disorders, particularly coronary heart disease.
2. Some definition of stress can be attempted by cataloguing 'significant life-events' which, if they impinge on an individual may precipitate psychiatric illness. 'Negative' life-events can be discriminated from 'positive' life-events and have a higher stress loading. The stress-loading of an life event for a particular individual is determined not simply by its 'objective' characteristics but also by the way he perceives it.
3. The way in which situations are perceived is influenced by prior experiences in which opportunities to develop positive emotional relationships with significant 'role-models', usually parents, in a supportive environment are important. Such relationships enable individuals to develop realistic 'self-concepts' and appropriate self-esteem. In their absence negative self-concepts develop resulting in low self-esteem and a fundamental lack of confidence in their own value—a belief that they are worthless.
4. Negative self-concepts may remain latent during periods of healthy adjustment but are activated by adversity (negative life-events).

The neuroses

When discussing more formal psychiatric disorders in aircrew, where symptomatic presentations leave less room for argument about whether they constitute deviations from the norm, it is appropriate to concentrate on the 'neuroses'—anxiety states and minor affective disorders (depressive reactions) in particular, since these comprise the large majority of conditions presented by aircrew to the flight medical officer.

For simplicity and clarity anxiety states and depressive reactions are dealt with in this chapter as if they are separate entities, but the reader should keep in mind that this is no more than a matter of convenience since attempts to discriminate reliably between the two in diagnostic practice have been largely unsuccessful.

Anxiety neurosis (states)

The syndrome of anxiety neurosis is a relatively recent nosological entity. In the First World War the majority of patients who would now be regarded as presenting with cardiac and respiratory symptoms of anxiety neurosis were diagnosed as suffering from 'irritable heart'. Today the diagnosis 'anxiety neurosis' is used imprecisely and too often to include patients whose anxiety is associated with prominent phobias, obsessions or depression. Such patients are better categorized as *mixed neurotic disorders*. Where phobic symptoms appear as virtually the only manifestation of anxiety the diagnosis *phobic anxiety state* should be made. More recently it has been suggested that panic attacks should be differentiated from anxiety neurosis because they respond differently to the antidepressant drug imipramine. Although this grouping has been included in the American Psychiatric Association's DSM III its validity as an independent diagnostic entity has not been firmly established.

The phenomena of anxiety neurosis fall into three groups:

1. The patient complains of *feeling anxious* with fearful anticipation and apprehension.
2. The patient has *other psychological disturbances* in addition to feeling anxious. He may complain of irritability, poor concentration, overreaction to noise, and restlessness. Memory is not impaired but inability to concentrate may lead to complaints that relate to impaired recall. A group of psychological symptoms that have been neglected until recently are apprehensive thoughts which are associated with and seem to be initiated by somatic symptoms. For example, a patient who feels his heart beating rapidly whenever he is anxious may think repeatedly that he is about to have a heart attack. Such thoughts amplify the original anxiety because they lead to further anxiety which, in turn, increases the somatic symptoms that set the thoughts in train initially. Other thoughts that are common in anxiety states are ruminations about life problems and personal inadequacy. These add to the sum of anxiety the patient experiences.
3. *Somatic symptoms* in anxiety neurosis are very variable. Many stem from over-activity of the autonomic nervous system and common complaints are palpitations, dry mouth, nausea, abdominal discomfort, diarrhoea, frequency or urgency of micturition and sweating. Men often complain of impotence. Other somatic symptoms relate to the somatic musculature: patients often describe headaches and these usually indicate increased tension in the neck and scalp muscles. Dyspnoea is also common and overbreathing can at times lead to faintness, dizziness, pins and needles in the hands and feet and occasionally to hyperventilation–tetany. A variety of other muscular tensions may be experienced; undue fatigue is commonly described and so is tremor of the hands. Patients often describe difficulty in falling asleep (as opposed to the early waking experience in depression) and say they feel tense and cannot stop ruminating about the events of the day or worrying about the future. Many report frightening dreams.

Any of the somatic symptoms described above may be the presenting complaint and it must be remembered that any one can be the first evidence of organic disorder rather than anxiety.

Many aircrew patients presenting with symptoms attributable to anxiety will be experiencing short-lived reactions through being subjected to unusual but short-lived stress. Such patients are properly diagnosed, according to ICD 9, as *adjustment reactions* and comprise mild or transient disorders which occur in individuals without apparent pre-existing mental disorder. They are relatively circumscribed, situation specific, generally reversible and last a few months at most. Where very acute and occurring in response to exceptional physical or mental stress the diagnosis of *acute stress reaction* is appropriate. Such reactions usually subside within hours or days and *combat–stress reaction* is an example with which flight medical officers are likely to be familiar. Symptoms persist when the stress lasts longer or when there is an underlying disorder of personality, and it is such patients who are usually referred for a psychiatrist's opinion. It appears that about 75% of patients with anxiety managed by general practitioners recover within 6–12 months and that most of those who are unwell at the end of a year will still have symptoms 2 years later.

Owing to their careful selection one might expect the prognosis in aircrew to be better than that for the population as a whole although the more stringent criteria applied in assessing recovery might modify this expectation. The prospect of aircrew referred for specialist psychiatric opinion returning to unrestricted flying was discussed earlier and found to be poor. Patients with anxiety neuroses referred to hospital have a worse long-term prognosis than those with depressive disorders. Fortunately, most anxiety neuroses can be managed on an outpatient basis provided the appropriate therapeutic resources are available.

Treatment

The allocation of treatment should be preceded by a thorough assessment of the relative importance of psychological and social stresses and personality factors. The success of treatment depends on the accuracy of such assessment. This should make possible a judgement about the chances of spontaneous recovery. A reaction is likely to pass quickly if it is recent, a response to temporary stress and occurs in a stable personality. In such cases the essential steps are to reduce the anxiety symptoms by simple means—encouraging the expression of emotion about stressful events and giving advice, explanation and reassurance. Where absolutely necessary an anxiolytic—a benzodiazepine—may be given on a short-term basis but it is to be avoided wherever possible in aircrew since it must be associated with grounding them for the duration of the treatment. An alternative is provided by relaxation exercises or the somewhat more elaborate procedures known as *anxiety management training* which will be described in detail later. This may be carried out in conjunction with the prescription of beta-blockade medication where somatic and autonomic concomitants of anxiety are troublesome.

As soon as the patient is sufficiently composed he should be encouraged to consider his problems constructively and take any practical steps he can to resolve them, and to come to terms with any difficulties he cannot influence. Psychotherapeutic treatment is important at several levels. It is at its simplest above. In more complicated situations it is not limited to resolution of the immediate problems but concerned also with helping a patient acquire insight into the ways in which he habitually attempts to cope with stress and how he might do so more appropriately. It is also concerned in an important way with the patient's perception of himself and his relationships with other people. If these are important aetiological factors more intensive psychotherapy may be required in either an individual or a group setting, but it is fair to say that in such cases there is little likelihood that a patient will be able to return to flying in anything but the most restricted capacity.

Phobic anxiety states

Although the idea of a separate phobic syndrome was first raised over 100 years ago the development of behavioural methods of treatment in the last two decades has focused attention on the aspects of situational anxiety and the avoidance of feared situations, and confirmed the practical value of recognizing phobic disorders as a group of distinct syndromes. Such an approach is particularly apposite in the management of 'fear of flying' in aircrew.

The definitive characteristics of phobic anxiety are:

1. Anxiety is a central component; not free floating as in panic disorder but attached to a specific object, activity or situation.
2. The anxiety is not justified by the stimulus that invokes it or is out of proportion to the real situation.
3. The sufferers are completely aware that their reactions are irrational.

It is easy to state the features that define a phobic disorder but it can, at times, be difficult to decide whether the response to the external situation is, in fact, justifiable. At one extreme it is obviously reasonable to experience fear in the face of an enemy charging with a loaded gun and at the other unreasonable to experience panic when venturing into one's own peaceful garden. In between these two ends of the spectrum lie many situations, of which fear of flying by aircrew can be one, in which the absence of a quantitative measure of the degree of the external danger and of the level of anxiety makes the assessment of the reasonableness of the response a matter of imprecise clinical judgement. When making such a judgement it is essential to exclude irrelevant extraneous considerations such as the pressures of operational commitments on military pilots. Such considerations have to be taken into account when considering management strategy but not when making a diagnosis.

It was pointed out earlier that some have suggested that different criteria have to be adopted when considering 'flying phobias' in aircrew because what would be understandable fear in a member of the general public represents a serial change in someone with training and experience which have enabled them to cope previously and adequately with the situation. When assessing such a situation the relationships built up by medical officers with special responsibility for the health and welfare of aircrew are invaluable. The shared experience of having flown with aircrew is irreplaceable when making such assessments. His acceptance as 'one of the squadron' enables the flight medical officer to become a confidant of the squadron commander and is a powerful argument in favour of air force psychiatrists making themselves known personally to squadron commanders and aircrew personnel, who are more likely to accept recommendations and advice from someone they know and in whose competence they have confidence.

There is little sound evidence on which to judge the prognosis of anxiety neuroses, of which phobic anxiety of flying is one presentation. Specific phobias, uncomplicated by more generalized 'free floating' anxiety, are particularly accessible to a behavioural treatment approach, but those who are immediately involved in the treatment of 'phobic aircrew' usually become convinced that the true incidence of such disorders is low. On closer examination such specific phobias are often found to be complicated by general anxiety, usually unrelated to flying. A frequent precipitant of such anxiety is marital disharmony which may stem from the irregular lifestyle and family disruption associated with being a professional military or civilian aviator. Depending on the particular role of the aviator his wife may fear more or less for his safety and this may, in turn, have a corrosive effect on the relationship, not least because declaring such fears openly is often regarded as unacceptable.

Aircrews' motivation for flying stems from different sources. Young fliers may be truly fearless because they do not understand the dangers of flying, but as the realities impinge on them they must find the courage and confidence in their own abilities, which come from adequate training, to cope, using a range of mechanisms which include denial, humour, suppression, intellectualization and rationalization. The investigation of any presentation of fear of flying must include inquiry into the patient's expectations and aspirations at the time he reached his decision to become an airman, and an attempt to trace and explore any subsequent changes in these. The issues have been sensitively explored by Jones (1986).

Treatment

Whatever the admixture of specific phobic anxiety and free-floating anxiety revealed by enquiry, treatment can be approached in only three ways:

1. *Behaviourally* which now usually comprises a combination of the 'exposure' form of behaviour therapy and anxiety management. Before embarking on this form of treatment it is important to look for evidence of a depressive disorder. When such a disorder is detected its effective treatment makes the anxiety more accessible to treatment and improves the prognosis.
2. *Anxiolytic drug therapy*. In practice this means a benzodiazepine or a beta blocker.
3. A combination of (1) and (2).

Rational treatment must be preceded by a thorough assessment of the relative importance of psychological and social stressors, personality factors and real motivation (as opposed to declared motivation) to fly, along lines already discussed. This should allow some judgement about prognosis. In practice, in aircrew, the behavioural approach, where possible not combined with benzodiazepine medication except in the very short term, is favoured since introduction of psychotropic medication involves grounding for the time the drug is administered. Where somatic (autonomic) concomitants of anxiety are making a significant contribution to the clinical picture the judicious employment of a beta blocker is advisable and this can be achieved without the patient being grounded. The question whether the patient should be grounded while treatment is carried out is one that must be dealt with at the outset, and it may involve the therapist in a dilemma. To prevent the phobia becoming 'fixed' it is advantageous not to ground the airman. Such a decision inevitably leads to role conflicts and places a heavy responsibility on the therapist who must consider any threat this may impose on his patient and any of his patient's colleagues whose safety may be jeopardized by it. It can be contemplated only with the consent of the patient and the informed support of his squadron commander. A therapeutic programme initiated while the patient continues to fly is easier to organize and more likely to be successful if it is to be carried out in the patient's own unit with the active co-operation of his flight medical officer—who may ideally be the therapist—and squadron commander rather than in a hospital setting.

The severity of anxiety experienced by aircrew when they present is one of the criteria that determines whether they will be grounded during treatment and whether, if they are sufficiently motivated, treatment is aimed at returning them to a flying role in some capacity, not necessarily that in which they were employed at the time of their referral for assessment. Those accepted for treatment with the intention they will eventually return to flying have, until recently, usually undergone relaxation/desensitization associated with 'anxiety management'. The addition of anxiety management, which the patient must learn to use both when he is in situations that provoke anxiety and also immediately before he goes into them since anxious anticipation is an important component of most phobic states, has been shown to reduce the risk of relapse following successful treatment, presumably by changing the way in which the patient responds to the onset of symptoms when he encounters new stressful situations. In particular, anxiety management can be expected to break the vicious circle in which symptoms cause worry and worry leads to more symptoms.

When Wolpe developed desensitization it was the first practical behaviour therapy technique and a landmark in the development of the subject (Wolpe, 1958). The patient is first questioned carefully to determine the full range of stimuli which invoke anxiety. These are then arranged in ascending order of severity and patients are encouraged to encounter them in a carefully graded sequence, or to create them in imagination. In either case anxiety is inhibited, usually by relaxation exercises but occasionally with anxiolytic drugs. Treatment begins with the stimuli which produce least anxiety and progress up the hierarchy one step at a time. The method is still widely used but is gradually being replaced by *exposure treatment*. This, in addition to attempting to modify stimulus–response relations, pays considerable attention to the consequences of abnormal behaviour. It differs from desensitization, where the subject encounters stimuli only briefly in a context of minimal anxiety, by exposing the phobic subject to anxiety-provoking stimuli for long periods—an hour or more, while anxiety is kept at a moderate level. The essential features of treatment are simple. The patient must enter the situations that provoke his fears and learn not to leave them until fear has subsided. It has become apparent that it is generally more effective to enter the real situation than to imagine it, and that moderate anxiety levels are better than very high ones, as in flooding, or very low ones such as are used in desensitization. This is probably because patients need to master their feelings of anxiety and they cannot do this when levels are too high or too low. The 'reality' element in the flying situation can be achieved at the onset of treatment by using the appropriate simulator and the level of anxiety controlled by modifying the simulator programme, maintaining the presence of the therapist or, in the last resort, an anxiolytic drug such as a benzodiazepine. These supports should be discontinued at the earliest opportunity to encourage self-reliance on the patient's part.

The therapist should act more as a teacher than in his usual role and make it clear to the patient that improvement depends largely on the effort he makes to overcome the fear in his daily life between treatment sessions. Strenuous efforts are made to increase the patient's motivation to carry out a programme that is inevitably repetitive, sometimes frightening and frequently monotonous. If a close friend who is also a professional colleague can be enlisted to take a close interest in the treatment it is often of significant help. Once again the most crucial factor in the patient's prognosis is his true motivation to continuing flying. This largely determines how conscientious he is in applying himself in the therapeutic programme. Regular practice of simple measures is more important in the outcome than the introduction of procedures such as interpretive psychotherapy or marriage counselling which usually only complicate treatment. The outcome is also significantly influenced by the attitudes adopted towards him by members of his immediate family and close professional colleagues.

Somatic anxiety

The use of medication in the treatment of states of anxiety in aircrew is limited by the necessity to ground them if they have been prescribed psychotropic drugs, including benzodiazepines. In recent years consideration has been given increasingly to the use of beta-blockade medication in controlling the somatic symptoms of anxiety. Tyrer (1976) distinguished patients with somatic anxiety, which he suggested would be better termed *somatosthenic anxiety*, from those with psychic anxiety and emphasized it was not simply a matter of somatic symptoms playing a more important part in the former's presentation. Such patients regard their major problems as somatic in nature, sometimes denying anxiety altogether.

In such patients beta-blockers have been reported as being as effective as the benzodiazepines in controlling symptoms whereas in patients experiencing overt anxiety they are ineffective. The somatic symptoms most favourably influenced by beta-blockers are tremor and those associated with the cardiorespiratory system. Sweating, nausea, dizziness and bowel disturbances are largely unaffected.

In morbidly anxious subjects who complain primarily of somatic symptoms bodily feelings are increased and correlate highly with physiological changes. When the physiological effects are altered by peripheral pharmacological blockade there is a corresponding reduction in bodily symptoms accompanied by an improvement in subjective anxiety. In morbidly anxious subjects who complain primarily of psychological symptoms, however, although bodily feelings are increased these correlate poorly with physiological changes and are unaffected by pharmacological blockade.

The action of beta-blockers in the doses used in patients with somatic anxiety, that is propranolol 40–120 mg daily or the equivalent in other drugs, is entirely peripheral. It has been postulated that beta-blockers alleviate anxiety by interrupting the feedback loop between the perception of autonomic and somatic symptoms of anxiety and the central awareness of anxiety which these otherwise reinforce.

In view of the large proportion of anxious aircrew patients who present with predominantly somatic symptoms and the relative acceptability of beta-blockers, because under certain circumstances aircrew can continue to fly while taking them, their use as an adjunct to behavioural methods in the management of anxiety states in such patients would repay further exploration.

Obsessional disorder

Obsessional disorder, more properly described as obsessive–compulsive disorder, exemplifies the difficulty, discussed earlier, in determining whether neurosis and personality disorder should be regarded as part of a continuum or as separate although related conditions.

The essential features of an obsessional symptom are:

1. It is an idea, thought or impulse which comes repeatedly into a patient's consciousness against his will.
2. It is always recognized by the patient as his own idea or impulse.
3. It cannot be accepted by the patient as harmless. He tries therefore to push it from his mind and resist its implications. His failure to do so generates anxiety and tension.

The content of an obsession is usually, but not necessarily, unpleasant, abhorrent or frightening.

The status of true obsessional disorder as a neurosis is uncertain. It rests on the understanding that obsessional patients retain insight, but in severe cases insight may be very limited and incapacity virtually complete. Minor variants of morbid obsessional symptoms can, however, be recognized frequently in persons not regarded as ill by themselves or others. Such traits are over-conscientiousness, tidiness, regularity and a tendency to rigidity and inflexibility. When such traits are present to a striking but not troublesome extent the individual can be regarded as an *obsessional personality type*. This is consistent with great ability and achievement and such ability may enable an individual to perform creditably even when obsessional traits are so marked that they dominate other aspects of the personality and it is legitimate to categorize him as an *obsessional personality disorder*. The presence of more than a minimum of obsessionality constitutes a handicap to aircrew because of the associated tendency to doubt and indecisiveness. Where highly motivated they may conceal this more or less successfully unless promoted to command where critical decisions have to be made under highly stressful conditions. Unless faced with such overwhelming stress obsessional individuals may hide their symptoms for years, often by employing extensive behavioural rituals to allay their anxiety. When they are eventually identified, close relatives or colleagues often report behavioural changes towards reticence and withdrawal associated with vague aches and pains, irritability and even frank hypochondriacal worries about serious illness. This information is often available to the flight medical officer but, unless he is alert to its significance, he may not recognize it as a manifestation of an obsessional disorder. Findings from a number of studies have indicated that about 50% of the patients studied have had some fairly obvious recent stress or life change linked with the onset of their illness, and illness or death of someone with whom they have had a close relationship has been particularly identified in this respect by some investigators. Identification of precipitating causes is made more uncertain by difficulty in identifying the onset of obsessional illnesses.

There is a strong clinical impression that people with marked obsessional personality traits are particularly prone to develop major depressive illnesses in which agitation is prominent and that they are usually recognized when they are depressed. When such individuals present clinically it sometimes seems that they have been precipitated into their illnesses by changes of status at work, particularly if these involve increased responsibility. While mixtures of obsessional and depressive symptoms are most common, mixtures of obsession-

al and schizophrenic symptoms also occur. In both instances the clinical skill is in assessing the significance of each group of symptoms and determining the primary diagnosis. This is important because of its implications with regard to treatment. If the illness is primarily depressive and it is treated effectively the obsessional symptoms will usually remit. If the illness is basically obsessional the mistaken use of ECT may exacerbate the patient's difficulties whereas treatment with a tricyclic antidepressant such as clomipramine often facilitates a behavioural approach to the obsessional symptoms and rituals.

Most obsessional patients have some sort of sexual problem but no common theme appears to exist. They have excessive and turbulent sexual drive and complain of a poor level of satisfaction. This is frequently a contributing cause to the high incidence of problems among those who are married, although it is reported that the rate of marriage, about 50%, is well below that for other categories of neurotic patients and the general population.

It is important to distinguish obsessional disorder from 'impulse disorders' in which the subjects claim they are subject to powerful impulses to carry out acts which when carried out are, at the time, intensely pleasurable, for example gambling, drinking, and some sexual activities. Obsessional thoughts hardly ever give rise directly to acts, except rituals to ward off harm which are not themselves pleasurable but at most successful in temporarily and partially allaying anxiety and tension.

It was mentioned earlier that somatic symptoms, manifest apparently as part of the presenting symptomatic picture of a neurotic disorder, can be the first evidence of an organic disorder. *The role of organic influences* runs a considerable risk of being overlooked when the aetiology of neuroses and personality disorders is considered. The association is rare in relative terms and organic psychiatric disorders usually carry distinctive hallmarks such as clouding of consciousness or cognitive impairments so that when these are absent there is less likelihood that the diagnostician will search for brain malfunction. Yet both neurotic and personality disorders can owe much to organic factors—either intrinsic brain disease or somatic pathologies which serve to compromise brain function. The relationship may be of so direct a nature that the organic influences on the mental state largely transcend differences in constitution and background, leading to similar forms of disturbance in widely dissimilar persons. The characteristic changes in personality which follow frontal lobe lesions are an obvious example. In other examples interaction is seen, the organic contribution serving to accentuate or liberate pre-formed tendencies in the individual. The patient who presents with depression while harbouring a cerebral tumour or who becomes seclusive in the early stages of dementia is likely to be illustrating multifactorial causation. He may be reacting to a subjective awareness of cognitive decline. Such reactions may not always be accompanied by detectable cognitive changes, and may antedate other clear clinical evidence of the organic nexus of the problem.

Cerebral tumours

Cerebral tumours may sometimes present with neurotic symptoms or change of disposition. Depression and anxiety are not uncommon. More elaborate developments with obsessional and hysterical features may emerge before focal signs are apparent. Slow-growing tumours in the frontal or temporal lobes may declare themselves by an insidious alteration in the personality. Thus when the tumour is in neurologically silent parts of the brain the true diagnosis may be considerably delayed. A special source of error is readiness to attribute such symptoms to current stresses in the life situation. Sometimes the patient's attempts to cope with such stresses eventually unmask his reduced adaptability.

Post-traumatic neuroses

Post-traumatic neuroses are the most frequent of the psychiatric sequelae of head injury. The degree to which brain damage can be held responsible is much debated. In the early post-traumatic phase many quasi-neurotic manifestations are often much in evidence—anxiety, depression and irritability, often coupled with headache and dizziness. Their frequency and stereotyped nature would alone suggest that they owe much to disturbed brain function. However, where they become long lasting and floridly elaborated, other sets of factors such as pre-morbid constitution, current stresses, or problems inherent in litigation are usually principally responsible. Lishman (1973) comprehensively reviewed such issues. Some head-injured patients will fall into the 'borderland' with both organic and non-organic aetiological influences operating together and reinforcing one another. Clinical appraisal must attempt to apportion such causative influences in the individual case so that treatment and prognosis can be correctly formulated.

The importance of head injury as a cause of personality disorder is well appreciated even in cases where intellectual competence is unaffected. Frontal lobe damage is again the classic example. Diminished control over aggression may sometimes be traceable to factors such as alcohol abuse, but in other examples disturbed cerebral function may emerge as the only reasonable explanation.

The appearance of 'neurasthenic' symptoms as a sequal to viral infections is a topic discussed in detail by Crow (1978). The mechanisms behind such associations remain unclear, though in the case of herpes simplex infections it has been hypothesized that the link may lie in disturbance of brain monoamine synthesis.

Epilepsy

Epilepsy has been closely studied in relation to personality disorder. Though still disputed, the balance of evidence supports the view that epilepsy arising within the temporal lobes is unusually prone to be associated with personality difficulties, especially aggressive tendencies of an explosive, immature kind.

Metabolic and endocrine disorders

These show how readily disturbances of the 'milieu interieur' can lead to emotional symptoms. Uraemia, electrolyte disturbances and liver disorder are quite regularly associated with states of depression and anergia. Anxiety states may accompany thyrotoxicosis and lethargic depression occur in myxoedema. In both hypo- and hyperparathyroidism affective disorder can be the presenting feature, the serum calcium level having a decisive influence on mood.

Of toxic disorders alcoholism is the best known in relation to change of personality. This may depend on minor degrees of brain damage more often than is commonly supposed. A relationship between chronic cannabis intoxication and personality alteration is a great deal more controversial.

Dietary insufficiencies

Dietary insufficiencies can cause neurotic symptoms. Lack of B vitamins is clearly incriminated as a principal cause. Thiamin deficiency can lead over several weeks to depression, weakness and insomnia, later to forgetfulness and impaired concentration. Less severe but more prolonged deprivation produces emotional lability, moodiness and depression. Nicotinic acid deficiency often shows a long prodromal period of neurotic manifestations which can respond promptly to replacement therapy. Folic acid deficiency may be related to depression and, at least in epileptics, to lethargy, irritability and personality difficulties.

Covert brain disease and brain damage

In addition to the foregoing, where disease processes or deficiencies are ultimately identifiable, it seems likely that a proportion of neurotic and personality-disordered patients may harbour some degree of covert brain pathology, and the possibility must exist that this has altered the patients' reaction to life stresses and facilitated the development of the neurosis. Hysterical conversion symptoms may also be facilitated by brain damage. Whitlock (1967) found evidence of preceding or co-existing brain disorder much more commonly in such patients than in controls with other forms of neurotic illness. Some cases diagnosed as 'hysteria' subsequently proved to have multiple sclerosis. All in all the wise clinician steers clear of diagnosing hysteria. With regard to personality disorder the principal evidence comes from electroencephalography. A high proportion of patients with disturbed personality, particularly those with aggressive antisocial behaviour, were found to have abnormal EEGs.

The management of combat-stress reactions in aircrew

The principles of proximity, immediacy and expectancy in the management of combat-stress reactions in aircrew are as valid as they have proved in every other context. Because aircrew operate in a uniquely stressful milieu, however, in some cases without the immediate support of any colleague, the principles have to be interpreted and applied to them by someone with insight into their special circumstances if optimal results are to be obtained. That 'someone' is the flight medical officer and his role in the management of combat-stress reactions is a logical extension of his role in managing stress-precipitated neurotic or adjustment reactions in peacetime, and his ability to carry it out effectively will depend to a large extent on how successful he has been previously in establishing his professional credibility with the squadron executive and aircrew.

Similar symptoms, both psychological and somatic, are precipitated by combat stress as by the more familiar stressful situations encountered in peacetime. They will, however, be more acute and florid, the circumstances under which they have to be evaluated will be less favourable, they may be exhibited by a number of aircrew simultaneously rather than by single individuals as in peacetime, and the source of the precipitating stress will be obvious. The same difficulty will be experienced in determining the point at which 'normal' anxiety shades into psychopathology which requires formal psychotherapeutic or chemotherapeutic intervention (rather than general support and reassurance). The same predisposing personality traits influence the prognosis of combat reactions, and positive motivation to continue flying is perhaps even more influential in determining their outcome than when similar symptomatic reactions occur in peacetime.

The flight medical officer who has got to know the individual members of his squadron well and gained their trust and confidence will find this invaluable in supporting them in their attempts to cope with their operational commitments in wartime. His knowledge of their individual strengths and weaknesses will enable him to recommend short-term and temporary withdrawal from duty of an airman in danger of exceeding his stress-tolerance, and to do so in a way that does not humiliate him and so diminish his chance of returning to operational flying within a few days. The understanding of, and relationship with, individual aircrew which enables such decisions to be made appropriately has to be gained before war is declared. Squadron personnel have to be fully briefed about what to expect by way of psychological and physical symptoms of fear when in combat, and warned that these will be experienced by everyone. They must accept that the tremulousness, dry mouth, sweaty palms, palpitations, rapid heartbeats, breathlessness, 'stomach-churning'—and on occasions even nausea, vomiting, urinary frequency and diarrhoea—are normal physiological responses. Unless aircrew are totally incapacitated by such symptoms they must continue to fly operationally.

Squadron executives must be instructed to look out for warning signs in an individual such as insomnia, nightmares, unremitting restlessness, decreased appetite, irritability, increased startle reflex, increased smoking or drinking, loss of sense of humour and changes in normal temperament beyond those taking place among his colleagues. At this stage a good night's sleep and being stood down for 24–48 hours with an opportunity to ventilate his feelings to his flight medical officer, secure in the knowledge he is not going to be criticized or judged, may rescue an individual from progressive loss of efficacy which will otherwise lead to permanent removal from the operational role. The medical officer's response must be understanding and supportive, and he must express optimism amounting to a conviction that recovery from this understandable 'exhaustion' will be swift and associated with a return to operational flying duties.

It may be appropriate to prescribe a benzodiazepine for some individuals as part of the management of combat-stress reactions. Their appropriate use in this context is dealt with in detail elsewhere.

The affective disorders

The classification of affective disorders in both the ICD 9 and DSM III is essentially into major and minor disorders. In the ICD 9 these are called *affective psychoses* and *depressive neuroses* (depressive reactions) respectively. In the DSM III they are called respectively the *major affective disorders* and *other specific affective disorders*. The latter include cyclothymic and dysthymic disorders but do not attain the severity or duration of the major disorders.

To avoid confusion the ICD 9 classification will be used in this account although in some ways the classification in DSM III conforms more closely to the common clinical presentations.

In ICD 9 major affective disorders are categorized mainly as *manic–depressive psychoses*, although in many cases a patient will only manifest either the depressive phase or the manic phase of the illness. The depressive phase occurs much more frequently than the manic phase and usually does not attain psychotic intensity. Where hypomania or mania occurs it is usually either succeeded or preceded in the total history of the patient's illness by an episode of depression.

Provision is also made in the classification for a depressive psychosis described as 'similar in symptoms to manic–depressive psychosis (depressed type) but apparently provoked by saddening stress such as bereavement or a severe disappointment or frustration'. This also usually fails to fulfil the criteria for a psychosis.

To complete the picture of conditions dominated by alterations of mood, affective (cyclothymic) disorders of personality should be included. They are characterized by a lifelong predominance of a pronounced mood, which may be depressive or elated or alternatively one and the other, which does not attain the status of an affective illness.

Depressive reactions

Definitions of depressive reactions are unsatisfactory but in practice they are depressive states which fall short of the diagnostic requirements for 'affective psychosis' or 'major depressive illness'. They must be persistent and include pathological depression—an intense, exaggerated form of sadness accompanied by symptoms such as anorexia, fatigue, insomnia, loss of sexual drive, loss of motivation, anhedonia (loss of the ability to derive pleasure from life), indecisiveness and a negative self-concept. The diagnosis should only be made when there is a reason to suspect a disorder of psychobiological equilibrium which goes well beyond a mood swing and is accompanied by other phenomena. There is no evidence that genetic factors make a specific contribution to the aetiology of depressive reactions. Research has shown, however, that traits variously described as 'self-confident', 'active', 'vigorous' and 'surgency' are strongly determined by genetic factors. Such traits are the obverse of the neurasthenic traits which, as was stated earlier, put those exhibiting them at a higher risk of becoming psychiatrically ill. Minor affective disorders are more likely to occur among

those with a general susceptibility to anxious and neurasthenic traits. Three groups of factors need to be considered in relation to the aetiology of a particular depressive disorder. They are, *loss events*, *physical illness* and *stressful social circumstances*. These various factors typically occur in combination with one another, with symptoms gradually developing in response to each factor until the individual reaches a state of depression which is unresponsive to homeostatic mechanisms. Physical illness—often but not exclusively infectious such as influenza, glandular fever and infectious hepatitis—is often followed by depression.

Bereavement

Bereavement on its own is often succeeded by a fairly clear-cut clinical syndrome which is in many ways a good example of a depressive reaction, as defined by the World Health Organisation, in that it follows a psychic trauma. The depression typically proceeds through a series of stages. The most frequent immediate reaction is a state of numbness, sometimes preceded by a brief period of distress during which panic attacks may occur. About 5–7 days after the death there is a sharp increase in affective symptoms and preoccupation with thoughts of the deceased (Parkes, 1970). The latter are a central and pathognomonic feature of grief and without them it cannot truly be said to have occurred. There are wide variations between individuals in the time course of events. Some are severely disturbed in the first week and thereafter gradually improve over the subsequent 3 months. Others express little or no distress in the first 2 weeks but a steady increase thereafter. Most are depressed by the end of the third month. There is no overall increase in the use of psychiatric services following bereavement, perhaps because the depression is understandable. There is an increase in the rate of visits to general practitioners, often with headaches, backaches or other pains. The physical symptoms may so distract the doctor that the depressive syndrome of which they are a part may pass unrecognized.

The reluctance of aircrew to acknowledge emotional distress that may be interpreted as evidence of psychiatric illness must be kept in mind when assessing a patient who presents with unsubstantiated physical symptoms following the death or serious injury of a close relative, friend or colleague, particularly if the latter was in the same squadron. A typical presentation is with 'gastritis' caused by heavy drinking to relieve the symptoms of depression. Evidence of excessive eating or smoking, as well as of drinking, or all three combined may be picked up incidentally, for example at the periodical medical examination, and associated symptoms of affective disturbance should always be inquired after in such cases. It is important when seeing such a patient to inquire whether his perspectives have changed recently. Is he dwelling inordinately on problems, particularly those for which he feels responsible, and inflating their importance? Does the future seem unrealistically bleak and does the patient entertain a feeling of hopelessness about it? Does he blame himself for the way he feels and is he comparing himself more unfavourably with others than is usual for him? Is he having increased difficulty in making decisions, either because of a lack of confidence in his ability to make the right decisions or because of subjective difficulty thinking through the consequences of alternative plans of action? The physical presentation is important. Depressed mood will influence the way a patient speaks, walks and sits. In making such assessments the knowledge the flight surgeon or medical officer has of the patient's normal presentation is invaluable. In minor depressive illnesses an increased appetite and weight gain is almost as common as anorexia and weight loss. There is diminution in sexual interest and general energy. Sleep is hard to come by, light and unrefreshing.

The concept of a 'depressive reaction' caused by a particular psychic trauma carries with it the implication that after a time homeostasis will occur and the patient will recover whether or not he has treatment. In practice he often does not and minor depressive states are frequently chronic and associated with disadvantageous life situations rather than isolated traumatic events. The more closely the illness does follow a single trama, such as bereavement, the more likely it is it will resolve completely; in the case of bereavement the majority will have done so within a year. In many patients who suffer recurrent episodes of illness, investigation reveals an underlying disorder of personality. In one study 79% of such patients had an unfavourable outcome compared with 11% of those with no such component. This supports the view that patients diagnosed as depressive reactions are a heterogeneous group, a view supported by the fact that some patients change from 'neurotic illness' to 'psychotic illness' during follow-up.

The major affective disorders

The major depressive disorders aircrew present to their flight medical officers are likely to be distinguished from depressive reactions by the intensity of the dysphoria and relative absence of obvious precipitating events. If the selection process has been successful candidates for aircrew status with identifiable pre-disposing factors in either their personal or first-degree family histories will have been selected out, but no such process is completely successful and occasionally typical manic–depressive illnesses are seen in their depressive phase.

Just as the characteristic mood in depression is intense sadness, so that characteristic of mania is elation. Difficulty is often experienced in the milder examples of hypomania in distinguishing the appropriate cut-off point between extreme normal high energy and drive and the pathological elation often associated with expansive euphoria seen in hypomania, but it is important that the two are not confused. Most energetic people do not have a manic disorder and most manic individuals expend considerable energy but accomplish very little. Observations made by close colleagues or relatives of such frenetic but ill-directed expenditure of energy, especially when it is associated with irritability and consequent fraying of interpersonal relationships, should always alert the doctor to the possibility of a pathological elevation of mood. Other symptoms characteristic of the disorder are hyperactivity, pressure of speech, flight of ideas, diminished need for sleep, increased self-esteem to the point of grandiosity, extreme distractability and extraordinarily poor judgement in the interpersonal and social areas. The patient is invariably resistant to acknowledging that he is ill, insisting that he is well and functioning at the top of his form. He claims he has boundless energy and ideas, is working much faster and more efficiently than normally, and that any problems stem from the inability of his colleagues to keep pace with him. Attempts to reason with him are likely to be met with anger and even rage if the doctor persists in suggesting he is ill and needs treatment. Once the diagnosis has been made it is a time for firm action and admission of the patient to hospital for further assessment and treatment, on an involuntary basis if necessary.

Serious difficulties can arise where the clinical presentation amounts to an exaggeration of the normal forceful presentation in a senior airman with a cyclothymic personality. In such cases the flight medical officer may be uncertain of his diagnosis. The danger of allowing someone with a hypomanic illness to fly makes it essential to ground the patient in such circumstances until a second opinion has been sought.

Management and treatment

The most irrevocable consequence of depression is suicide and it is appropriate therefore when considering management to assess this risk first. It is not true that those who talk about suicide never carry it out. The majority of those who kill themselves have communicated their intentions to others beforehand, and approximately 10% of those who attempt suicide eventually complete it. The risk of suicide increases with advancing age, where there is a history of attempted suicide previously or a family history of suicide, and where there is associated alcoholism or other drug addiction. The risk is greater in men. Social isolation, unemployment or the threat of unemployment and sudden financial difficulties all increase the risk. It is important to make a thorough assessment of the severity of the patient's depression. The presence of psychotic phenomena greatly increase the risk, particularly where the phenomena present as delusional ideas about serious physical ill-health. If the patient admits to entertaining ideas of suicide, these should be explored to discover whether specific ways and means have been considered. There is no evidence to suggest that asking the patient about suicidal intentions increases the risk. In most instances the flight medical officer can adequately assess the risk. Only where he is in doubt or judges it to be real need the patient be referred.

Aspects of treatment can be divided into those that are non-specific and those that are specific. The doctor's confidence that he can help his patient is a very potent example of the former, particularly where he is a trusted colleague with responsibility for the patient's general medical care. The doctor also has the power to temporarily remove professional and social obligations, allowing the patient to rest without a sense of failure. Where medication is prescribed, by setting the regimen and its timescale—'improvement in 10–14 days'—the doctor promotes the strong expectancy that improvement will indeed occur and the side effects the patient will experience from the outset, which must be discussed with him, provide a constant reminder he is on 'real treatment'.

It is usual to discover that reactive depression is in an understandable relationship to the patient's life situation or the way in which he handles his interpersonal relationships. The opportunity exists to attempt improvements in these areas. Such attempts have been formalized by Klerman as 'Interpersonal Psychotherapy', consisting of approximately 12 weekly sessions for ambulatory depressed patients (Klerman et al., 1979). Efforts are focused on improving the quality of current interpersonal functioning. Constructive improvements the patient might make to his life are discussed and modifications he might make in the way he habitually responds to other people are suggested. Expression of affect is encouraged and, where appropriate, directive techniques, role-playing and the making of a therapeutic contract can be utilized.

In contrast to the more general techniques utilized in interpersonal psychotherapy, Beck's 'cognitive therapy' for depression is based on an assault on some of the self-defeating strategies and unflattering self-concepts typically seen among depressed patients (Beck, 1976). The negative thoughts the patient holds about (1) himself, (2) his world and (3) his future are described as a 'cognitive triad'.

The cognitive therapist has four tasks:

1. To help the patient appreciate the connections between thoughts, feelings and behaviour.
2. To encourage the patient to monitor his negative thoughts.
3. To examine the evidence for and against his negative thoughts.
4. To substitute more reality-orientated interpretations for his negative thoughts.

It has been claimed that cognitive therapy is equally as effective as anti-depressant medication in the short-term treatment of depressed outpatients and improvement is better maintained at 6-month follow-up.

Choice of treatment

An important principle in rational therapeutics is to *know* what is being treated. Unfortunately in the treatment of affective disorders, where many deviations of normal mood are indiscriminately treated with antidepressant drugs, this basic axiom is often forgotten. As we have seen, the point at which 'normal' dysphoria and euphoria become psychopathological is problematic. When considering the use of mood enhancing or controlling drugs, however, some criteria must be applied to ensure they are used appropriately. There is a considerable consensus that this means restricting them to the major disorders whose symptom profile includes pervasive loss of interest and pleasure (anhedonia), qualitative depressive mood changes, lack of reactivity to external stimuli, middle and late insomnia, psychomotor disturbances, anorexia and weight loss. In the absence of such features or the presence of a high neuroticism level, marked anxiety and/or agitation, and associated real life events, the response to tricyclic or tetracyclic antidepressants will be poor. It has recently been suggested that 'dysthymic' patients displaying anhedonia, guilt and hypersomnia respond favourably to such medication.

The choice of treatment is also determined to some extent by the severity of the depression. Mildly depressed patients often respond to psychotherapy alone and if consideration is being given to aircrew continuing to fly while undergoing treatment, medication which necessitates grounding should not be prescribed for them. Where the severity of the depression would in itself ensure grounding this obstacle to medication is removed.

When introducing a tricyclic or tetracyclic antidepressant into the treatment regimen it is essential to explain the following to the patient:

1. The side effects immediately on starting treatment, what these are and how he can ameliorate them.

sychiatry

2. There will be a latent period of about 14 days before any therapeutic effects are experienced.
3. Treatment in full dosage must be maintained for 6 months even though the patient may become asymptomatic before that, after which medication will be reduced gradually while the patient's progress is carefully monitored.

A second group of antidepressant drugs, the *monoamine oxidase inhibitors*, are probably best avoided in general practice because of their propensity to provoke hypertensive crises if taken in conjunction with tyramine-containing foods. Members of this group should never be taken in conjunction with tri- or tetracyclic antidepressants for the same reason. If they are considered it is the responsibility of the doctor to select and educate suitable patients regarding potential toxicity and to ensure the patient has a thorough understanding of the potential interactions of the drugs.

Non-compliance

Non-compliance is a frequent cause of failure of treatment with anti-depressants. It can be minimized by creating a strong therapeutic alliance and the flight medical officer is in an ideal position to do so by using his status as professional colleague as well as medical adviser.

Lithium is the accepted treatment for established hypomania/mania. Neuroleptics (phenothiazines and butyrophenones) may still be used to control the acute presentation of symptoms where these are severely disruptive. Both treatment regimens are better initiated on an inpatient basis.

Side effects and toxic effects of tricyclic antidepressants

Tricyclic antidepressants (TCA) can be divided into those with marked sedative effects, of which *amitriptyline* is the most commonly prescribed, which are preferred in the treatment of patients with prominent anxiety or agitation; and those drugs such as *imipramine* which are less sedating and a suitable alternative for patients who are retarded. *Clomipramine*, which is chemically related to imipramine, has been claimed to have a specific effect on obsessional symptoms in addition to its antidepressant properties, but this has not been unequivocally substantiated.

Antidepressants are rapidly absorbed, long-acting and need to be given only once daily, usually at night because of their sedative effects. Patients can show a 10–20-fold variation in plasma levels at the same oral dose and this is reflected in response to treatment. Dosage therefore has to be adjusted using careful monitoring of clinical progress as a guide. Once started on antidepressants patients

should be encouraged to persevere on full therapeutic dosage, which averages amitriptyline 150 mg or its equivalent daily in healthy young adults, for at least 4–6 weeks before discontinuing the drug if a satisfactory response has not been obtained.

Most TCA side effects are benign and transient, fading in about 2 weeks in young otherwise healthy adults. The most common potentially dangerous side effect is orthostatic hypotension because it may induce falls and consequent injuries. Significant hypotension is experienced by about 20% of patients and is not dose related. Palpitations and tachycardia have been reported with most TCAs but at therapeutic levels TCAs have a negligible effect on the healthy heart although in overdose they can be lethal.

Anticholinergic side effects are troublesome and can precipitate serious medical problems. Dry mouth, constipation and blurred vision occur most frequently whereas more serious side effects such as urinary retention, paralytic ileus or precipitate narrow-angle glaucoma are usually confined to older age-group patients. Combination of a TCA and a phenothiazine increases the risk. The toxic syndrome is characterized by confusion, disorientation, delirium, auditory and visual hallucinations, agitation, hyperpyrexia (often attributed to infection) and concomitant anticholinergic symptoms. The second-generation 'tetracyclic' antidepressants such as *mianserin* hydrochloride have fewer adverse side effects, particularly anticholinergic manifestations. Mianserin hydrochloride has been found, however, occasionally to depress bone marrow function, patients usually presenting with agranulocytosis which is reversible by stopping the drug. Central nervous effects are rare but do occur in concentrations above the therapeutic and range from a parkinsonian picture to tardive dyskinesia and seizures which are particularly likely to occur in alcoholics. Hypomania may be precipitated by TCA and not recognized for some time if the patient's progress is not carefully monitored.

Lithium treatment monitoring

Monitoring of lithium treatment is carried out by regular estimations of serum lithium value. Initially a level of 0.9–1.0 mmol/litre is aimed for to control the acute manic or hypomanic episode but a serum level of 0.7 mmol/litre is usually adequate for maintaining a patient in remission. Serum estimations should initially be carried out at weekly intervals, increasing progressively as the patient stabilizes on the drug so that eventually estimations every 3 months are adequate.

The psychotic patient

The definitive characteristic of the psychotic patient is loss of the insight which is present in members of the general population including those with neurotic disorders. This renders the patient impervious to reason and obviously disqualifies him from flying. When recognizing the psychotic patient the flight surgeon or medical officer should always consider the possibility that the underlying cause may be an as yet unidentified organic illness rather than the more likely functional illness (schizophrenia, depressive, manic or paranoid).

Drug abuse and dependence

From the point of view of their pharmacological action, drugs of dependence are classified as narcotic analgesics, central nervous system (CNS) depressants, stimulants and hallucinogens. *Drug abuse* is defined as persistent or excessive drug use unrelated to or inconsistent with acceptable medical practice. *Drug dependence* is defined as a state, psychic and sometimes also physical, characterized by behaviour and other responses which always include a compulsion to take the drug on a continuous or periodic basis in order to experience its psychic effects, and sometimes to avoid the discomforts of its absence.

In morphine, alcohol, barbiturate and amphetamine dependence, physical dependence may occur and is characterized by a specific withdrawal syndrome when consumption is abruptly stopped or substantially reduced. Other drugs produce only psychological dependence.

Drug dependence is essentially a psychic rather than a physiological phenomenon and the drugs used reduce anxiety or alter mood in a way which is experienced as pleasurable or desirable. The psychological motives initiating and continuing drug use include self-medication for anxiety and depression, recreational hedonistic use, and the desire to experience altered states of consciousness. The pharmacological action of drugs is modified by psychological factors and there is considerable individual variation in response to psychoactive drugs. Drug effects are also influenced by the social setting in which they are taken and smoking cannabis or drinking alcohol when alone may have little euphoriant effect, whereas when taken with friends they may produce a pleasant experience. Similarly, adverse reactions to LSD are less likely to occur in the presence of a companion who is an experienced user. Social influences are especially significant in initiating drug use in a non-medical context, the commonest examples being smoking and drinking. Social reinforcement through acquisition of companionship or status, or pharmacological reinforcement through euphoriant or anxiolytic effects help to establish a pattern of repetitive drug use. It may then become a generalized conditioned response to unpleasant psychic states of tension,

anxiety or boredom. Relapse after prolonged abstinence can be precipitated by environmental cues and all flight medical officers are familiar with such consequences when alcohol-dependent patients succumb during a squadron celebration.

Patients suffering from drug dependence show an interesting interaction between the personality features and the problems of social adjustment which render them vulnerable, neurotic symptoms such as anxiety or depression which may lead them to drug use, the psychological effect of the drugs themselves and finally the consequences of the drug dependence on their mental health.

Alcoholism

Aetiology

The pattern of a population's alcohol consumption strongly suggests a multi-factorial explanation for drinking, not that there is one explanation for 'normal' drinking and another for 'abnormal' drinking or alcohol abuse. It is convenient to examine the multiple determinants of drinking under separate personal and environmental headings although in practice one is always dealing with the interactive effects. Aircrew are exposed to many of the environmental influences that encourage drinking. They are relatively well paid and can afford to drink; they spend a lot of time away from home, much of it in premises that sell alcohol and in circumstances of considerable boredom; they are in a stressful occupation and alcohol provides immediate if temporary relief from tension and anxiety; and they are part of a culture that sets great store by team spirit and camaraderie, much of it fostered by alcohol-facilitated social gatherings, either formal or informal. Among the personal factors alcohol is a social facilitator for those who are anxious, uneasy or under-confident, helping to substitute for confidence they naturally lack.

Although abnormal personality development and neurotic symptoms may render patients vulnerable to dependence on alcohol there is no 'addiction-prone' personality and a variety of social and psychological factors contribute to the development of dependence. When a drug is widely used and socially acceptable, as is alcohol, many individuals without serious psychopathology may become dependent on it. Among the factors that increase the likelihood of dependence occurring are exposure, availability, group pressure and the social context of drinking. In a carefully selected group such as aircrew these features are likely to be more influential in determining the pattern of inappropriate use of alcohol than the abnormal personality characteristics which have been postulated as antecedents of dependence. Such characteristics have not been shown to predict reliably subsequent dependence on alcohol but young alcoholics more often display marked personality disturbance and more anti-social behaviour than those with later onset. Most aircrew with an alcohol problem fall into this group with later onset.

Attempts to 'place' alcoholism in categories have been largely unsuccessful. An alternative formulation suggests that rather than there being a multiplicity of true sub-types of alcoholics, drinking behaviour is moulded by a range of factors (personal, cultural, and social), to give rise to a wide variety of possible presentations. A recent World Health Organisation formulation (Edwards *et al.*, 1977) suggests that a core syndrome of alcohol dependence can be identified which exists in degrees not as an all-or-none phenomenon, and with a presentation which will be influenced by the factors mentioned above. The meaning currently being given to the concept of dependence is subtler than older 'addiction' formulations. There is growing evidence that the repeated experience of alcohol withdrawal symptoms and repeated engagement in withdrawal-relief drinking may constitute a crucially important learning process during which the individual graduates from 'drinking too much' to 'alcohol dependence'. It is also possible for someone to experience serious alcohol-related problems without being dependent, and in practice the term 'alcoholic' is appropriate for any severe problem with alcohol whether or not dependence is involved. Abuse of alcohol not associated with gross psychopathology is particularly apposite to aircrew and such abuse frequently raises the question whether alcoholics can return to safe drinking. The answer must rest on what is meant by 'alcoholics'. In such a heterogeneous population there will be some who could succeed in returning to controlled drinking but in the very demanding circumstances in which aircrew work it is not appropriate to accept the risk inherent in the attempt to do so. Any attempt to restore to flying an airman who has experienced a significant alcohol problem must be associated with a condition of total abstinence, and the regulations are written so that they give formal expression to this. One lapse from total abstinence following symptomatic recovery from diagnosed alcoholism, especially where associated with further professional, personal or social difficulties, results in permanent loss of flying licence.

When assessing a patient with an alcohol problem the clinical skill lies not only in knowing what questions to ask but how to ask them in a way likely to obtain an honest response which can form the basis for subsequent co-operation between patient and doctor in management of the problem. The threat to his livelihood perceived by the patient must be recognized and appreciated by the doctor who must be able to convince the patient he has more to gain by being frank than by being devious.

Corroborative information against which to assess the patient's account should always be sought from a close relative—his wife where available—and the employer.

The most effective way to obtain an accurate account of the patient's alcohol consumption is to get him to reconstruct a typical heavy-drinking day, taking a specific day, for example yesterday; when does he take the first drink? Reconstruct, hour by hour, the day's drinking and the circumstances of each drink. The summated picture is likely to be very different from what usually emerges from casual questioning along the lines 'how much do you drink in a day?'

When determining whether an individual is alcohol-dependent enquire for *withdrawal symptoms*, including tremor, sweating, nausea and mood disturbance. Skilled questioning has to be directed at discovering the intensity, frequency and duration of the problem. It is important that the patient recognizes that alcohol relieves his withdrawal symptoms. Subjective awareness of dependence may be difficult for the patient to verbalize. At its most severe his drinking and the next drink will preoccupy him and he will describe classic *'loss of control'*. *Narrowing of the repertoire* implies that the patient is becoming more severely dependent and his drinking pattern stereotyped. *Heightened tolerance* is associated with regular drinking but is lost in the later stages of dependence.

The overall coherence of the story is important. If the severity of the different symptoms that the patient describes are not consistent he is probably being less than frank. Alternatively the questioner may have confused him and so obtained a distorted picture.

When questioned about his attitude to drinking the patient is invariably ambivalent. He wants both to continue drinking and ameliorate the consequences. The assessment therefore involves drawing up a profit and loss account. The doctor should start by emphasizing that he will not accept that the patient believes drinking is a totally bad experience and emphasizing that he wants to hear what is enjoyable about it. He may then hear about alcohol relieving apprehension, producing an agreeable euphoria, making him more social and self-assertive. It may become clear that a major attraction is the social setting and companionship of the bar. Exploration of the debit side involves persuading the patient to consider the consequences of his drinking, including the possibility of losing his livelihood. Other potent threats may be loss of health or break-up of marriage.

Management

The so-called 'minimal approach to treatment', which is now gaining popularity, is particularly appropriate to the management of patients with alcohol problems recognized at a relatively early stage. It is based on the belief that what was previously considered the non-specific element in the treatment is the very essence of the therapeutic process. This is combined with a determination that the patient should not be over-treated with the attendant dangers of iatrogenic learned helplessness. Treatment starts with patient and doctor considering the nature of his predicament in an attempt to persuade him to surrender the denials and defences with which he has sustained his drinking. Particular attention must be paid to discussion of the degree of the patient's dependence, the criteria on which the diagnosis has been made and its personal implications. The patient's negative feelings towards a life without alcohol have to be explored empathetically and dealt with rationally. The doctor's success will depend on his credibility with the patient and here the flight medical officer should have a marked advantage. Once the patient has reached broad decisions about what he is going to do about his drinking he can be helped to interpret these in terms of short-term and long-term goals in a number of areas, including marital, parental and professional. Establishing the drinking goal is vital and it must be clearly formulated as total abstinence if return to flying is the objective. Coexistence of other psychopathology, for example a depressive illness requiring active treatment, reinforces the need for abstinence while this is dealt with.

It is easy for a patient with a drinking problem to leave the consultation bemused. At worst he may accidentally have got the message that he is a sick alcoholic whose sickness excuses his behaviour, when what he needs is to accept responsibility for it. It is not a matter to be handled negatively or pessimistically. The message to be conveyed is confidence that the patient can help himself which, if effectively transmitted, can help to restore his self-esteem. Progress of treatment must be carefully and conscientiously reviewed with no issues fudged and a clear recognition of the consequences of failing to maintain total abstinence in the forefront of both the patient's and the doctor's minds.

Where the extent of the problem requires specialist referral, with the likelihood of detoxication, immediate grounding is inevitable and although, on the whole, there has been loss of faith in the intensive intervention and prolonged inpatient treatment which used to be the norm, there is still a place for such regimens for carefully selected patients. It can apply to aircrew who cannot continue to practise their profession unless and until their alcohol problem is resolved, and is particularly appropriate where this is associated with an affective disorder or significant organic pathology. Excessive drinking frequently coexists with other psychiatric problems, and admission simply for diagnosis where this is suspected may be indicated. The treatment of the coexisting condition may be vital for dealing with the drinking, while a confused therapeutic approach with no clear priorities and too much prescribing of drugs to a patient who is still drinking is a recipe for wasted time and can lead to disaster.

One is frequently faced with the alcoholic patient who is miserable and may be threatening suicide, and suicide is common among alcoholics. Depression is, however, over-diagnosed in alcoholics because labile disturbance of mood is a common feature of intoxication. The typical biological features of a major depression are often confused by the drinking and a clear history is of paramount importance to indicate whether there is purposive self-medication with alcohol. Antidepressants should not be given as a therapeutic trial to the alcoholic who is still drinking. It is worthwhile trying on an outpatient basis to get the patient to stop drinking, so that the depression can be properly assessed; but if the flight medical officer is in any serious doubt it is wise to admit the patient for detoxication and assessment. Patients with hypomanic illness may drink excessively, either as a consequence of a general disinhibition or because of an unpleasant element of anxiety in the mood disturbance which is relieved by drinking. Brain damage is widely recognized as a potential consequence of excessive drinking but it is less well recognized that a cerebral tumour may present as 'alcoholism'. The airman suffering from a phobia of flying may be drinking to cope with his anxiety and may view alcohol as an indispensible medicine. In such circumstances admission for detoxication is an essential preliminary to assessment of the phobia. Social phobia may also be a contributory cause of excessive drinking and detoxication followed by assessment is similarly indicated. Anxiolytic medication is contra-indicated in such cases because of the risk of dependence on such drugs being substituted for dependence on alcohol. A common-sense emphasis on 'learning to live with it' by finding other strategies such as relaxation training is the best approach. Where autonomic or somatic concomitants are severe, a beta blocker such as propranolol is indicated. Pathological jealousy is classically described as a consequence of excessive drinking with speculation that it may be associated with alcohol-induced impotence. Although adequate studies are lacking it seems likely that in many instances the jealousy has been a long-standing problem with alcohol used to relieve the associated anxiety. If the patient can be helped to give up drinking in such cases, although the jealousy will remain its more anti-social manifestations may be brought under control.

Other drugs

With the exception of alcohol there is little information about possible long-term adverse effects of most drugs of abuse on mental functioning, and what there is is largely circumstantial. *Barbiturates* are the most commonly abused sedative drugs apart from alcohol. Addiction is associated with increasing tolerance so that, ultimately, enormous quantities may be consumed. States of fluctuating confusion follow ingestion or injection, with slurred speech, ataxia and tell-tale nystagmus. The usual mood is towards euphoria though irritability and uninhibited behaviour may be marked. Withdrawal effects are similar to those with alcohol, with epileptic fits and delirium among the more severe. Analogous withdrawal effects may be seen with glutethimide, meprobamate, and other sedative drugs.

The *specific central anxiolytics* (ataractic drugs), of which meprobamate is probably the most prescribed especially when combined with analgesics (for example Equagesic—with aspirin, ethoheptazine and calcium carbonate), were the forerunners of the benzodiazepines and have been largely superseded by them. They induce drowsiness and commonly tolerance and dependence, withdrawal symptoms developing if the drug is suddenly stopped in a patient on a high dosage. The *benzodiazepines* differ from the general and other specific central anxiolytics by reducing anxiety without significant impairment of consciousness. They have selective effects in the limbic system where high concentrations of benzodiazepine receptors have been demonstrated as well as in the cerebral cortex and cerebellum (the latter possibly explaining their anticonvulsant effects and tendency to produce ataxia). The usual calming effect of benzodiazepines can sometimes be reversed in individuals in whom they appear to release aggression. The explanation for this is that the drug has a disinhibiting effect on the individual who has previously been suppressing aggression. Usually hostility occurring as a consequence of anxiety (a common association) is improved by benzodiazepines. Skeletal muscle relaxation is a property of the benzodiazepines independent of their anxiolytic effect and the use of 'muscle relaxants' should always be enquired after in aircrew in case benzodiazepines are unwittingly being used for this purpose.

Although the benzodiazepines are remarkably free from toxic effects they may produce drowsiness even in normal therapeutic doses and they always increase reaction-time and adversely affect performance. Although the risk is much less than with barbiturates or meprobamate true pharmacological dependence does occur with benzodiazepines, and tolerance and active drug-seeking behaviour after high dosage may be associated with severe withdrawal reactions after stopping the drug. There is evidence that withdrawal reactions are more severe after stopping a short-acting benzodiazepine such as lorazepam than a long-acting one such as diazepam. There may be difficulties in distinguishing withdrawal effects from a return of pre-existing anxiety, and in the minor manifestations of the syndrome such a distinction may be impossible. Insomnia, muscle tension, headaches and panic attacks come into this category.

Chlormethiazole has similar properties pharmacologically to the benzodiazepines. It is markedly anti-convulsant and an effective anxiolytic and hypnotic with relatively few toxic effects, of which drowsiness, conjunctival and nasal irritation are the most common. There is an additive effect with other central depressant drugs, including alcohol, and patients should be warned of this since chlormethiazole is frequently used to ameliorate the symptoms of alcohol withdrawal. The major criticism of the drug is its capacity to produce pharmacological dependence and when using it in alcohol withdrawal its use should be completed within 10 days, rapid step-wise reduction of dose being employed during that time.

Bromide intoxication may still be seen occasionally in patients who consume large quantities of proprietary 'cough cures' or 'nerve tonics'.

Amphetamine use (and that of related stimulants) leads to hyper-arousal and restless overactivity. The most remarkable effect on the mental state is the not infrequent development of an acute paranoid psychosis which at initial presentation can be hard to distinguish from acute schizophrenia. Distinguishing features are acuteness of onset, brisk and predominantly fearful affective response and the presence of visual as well as auditory hallucinations. Persistence of the paranoid features for more than a week after the urine is free from amphetamines makes it likely one is dealing with an endogenous schizophrenia.

Hallucinogens such as LSD-25 or mescalin produce perceptual distortions—vivid hallucinations in many modalities. They carry the special hazard that they can be administered without the subject's knowledge. Striking alterations of body image occur, typically without clouding of consciousness, and in this respect differ from those associated with most other agents. Occasionally, even in habitual users, acute panic reactions or explosive outbursts of anger or paranoia occur. Acting-out of impulses can lead to dangerous situations, for example leaping from heights. Both brief and long-lasting schizophrenia-like psychosis may be precipitated and probably owes much to premorbid vulnerability. 'Flashback' phenomena may occur in which abnormal experiences induced during acute ingestion— vivid images or perceptual distortions—recur intermittently for several weeks or months thereafter.

Marijuana intoxication leads usually to a mildly euphoric state, often with slight impairment of consciousness and distortion of time sense. Fragmentation of thinking and hallucinations may occur but the latter lack the profusion and vividness of those following LSD ingestion. With more severe intoxication, waves of ecstasy, perplexity and terror may be experienced plus depersonalization and derealization. Spontaneous recurrences of marijuana effects can apparently occur after discontinuation of the drug, as with LSD. It remains controversial how commonly serious adverse affects can ensue with marijuana. Acute disturbances include episodes of panic or hysterical dissociation lasting from minutes to hours. Chronic effects associated with long-term abuse, ascribed to possible CNS damage, include an insidious change of personality ('amotivational syndrome') and progressive social and intellectual decline. With all such syndromes definitive evidence of the role of marijuana has been hard to obtain and matters of special selection and vulnerability have probably been operative in most cases.

Narcotic drugs such as heroin and morphine are usually without the florid psychiatric effects of the drugs described above. A state of drowsy euphoria is the usual aftermath of their administration.

Airline passengers may experience overdose or withdrawal from drugs in flight and create an emergency.

Toxic levels of an *opiate* result in the triad of decreased level of consciousness (ultimately coma), depressed respiration and myosis, as well as hypotension, hypothermia and pulmonary oedema. Initial treatment is basic life-support and, where it is available, administration of an opiate antagonist parenterally. High doses of such an antagonist may precipitate withdrawal symptoms. These, while dramatic, are not usually life-threatening but can be extremely disruptive and the patient needs to be restrained from injuring himself and others. The symptoms can be rapidly terminated by administering an opiate, preferably parenterally.

The signs and symptoms of *stimulant toxicity* from amphetamines and cocaine are not dissimilar and may be considered together. The presenting symptoms are extreme restlessness and agitation which may progress to panic state and frank psychosis. Management in the air depends on the degree of life-threat and disruption and ranges from reassurance and restraint, to protect the sufferer from injuring himself or others, to basic life support following cardiovascular collapse, hypertensive crisis or fits. Alpha-adrenergic blocking agents are useful in the management of hypertensive crises and fits are best treated with intravenous diazepam.

Toxicity from *central nervous system depressants*, including alcohol, may, ultimately, present with coma, apnoea, hypotension and cardiovascular collapse. There are no specific antagonists for this group and so treatment must be supportive while the drug is being eliminated. Withdrawal symptoms in those dependent on CNS depressants may be life threatening and must be viewed as a medical emergency. The appropriate immediate in-flight response is administration of the drug on which the individual is dependent as soon as the early symptoms of anxiety, irritability and tremulousness are manifest. If this is not done the patient may progress to status epilepticus, hyper-pyrexia, hallucinosis and delirium tremens.

Inappropriate medication

Whenever the flight medical officer is faced by an aircrew patient exhibiting atypical behaviour or symptoms for which no ready explanation is available he should consider the possibility that the inappropriate use of drugs is responsible. Such a high index of suspicion is necessary and is perhaps particularly apposite when clinically assessing aircrew because they have ample opportunities when 'down route' or on exercises or detachment outside the United Kingdom to obtain drugs 'across the counter' which are available in this country only on prescription. In addition the knowledge that taking any form of medication may jeopardize their flying may persuade aircrew to seek medical advice from independent medical practitioners who may prescribe without realizing the implications. When more than one doctor is prescribing, albeit unknowingly, for one patient, or individuals are self-medicating, the potential for drug interactions is increased. Atropine, scopolamine, belladonna and antihistamines are commonly the active ingredients in over-the-counter sleeping pills available without prescription. An overdose or an individual drug sensitivity to these so-called anti-cholinergic substances may produce similar effects, i.e. what is in effect an atropine psychosis, through their anticholinergic side effects.

One of the most common drug effects results from the additive side effects of sedative hypnotics (including alcohol) and tricyclic antidepressants. Patients with severe hepatocellular disease are particularly sensitive to the sedative properties of a variety of psychotropic drugs. In patients with liver disease such as alcoholic cirrhosis the half-life of the drugs is increased, the volume of distribution increased, plasma-binding reduced and clearance is decreased.

Barbiturate and non-barbiturate sedatives and alcohol speed the metabolism of the phenothiazines and tricyclic antidepressants. Disulfiram (antabuse) can prolong the half-life of benzodiazepines.

The most effective way to limit the unwanted secondary and interactive effects of prescribed drugs is for medical officers to look critically at the need for such prescriptions, ensure that they enquire about other medications (prescribed or otherwise) which the patient is taking and familiarize themselves with the likelihood of interactions occurring between the drugs they prescribe. They should encourage aircrew to ask themselves the following questions:

1. 'Do I need this medication, even if it has been prescribed for me?' They should be urged, however, not to discontinue medication without informing their doctor.
2. 'Have I given the medication a thorough trial on the ground before taking it when I am due to fly?'
3. 'Do I feel fit to fly when taking this medication?'

A negative response to questions (2) or (3) should be regarded by the medical officer as sufficient grounds for ensuring that the patient does not fly again until any doubt has been resolved.

Sexual problems

Sexual relationships like many other aspects of peoples' lives vary from the highly successful to complete failure and there are probably few couples who do not experience at least temporary difficulties at some stage in their sex lives. It was pointed out earlier that aircrew's lifestyle, with its frequent separations and high level of stress, is likely to precipitate difficulties in those whose sexual adjustment is not wholly secure. Dissatisfaction with sexual relationships is more closely associated with other types of difficulty—for example poor communication, inability to relax and low sexual interest—than with sexual dysfunction *per se*. Experience of the kind of difficulties most frequently reported by aircrew supports this view. Moreover, only a small proportion of the large numbers of individuals who are dissatisfied sexually seek help. Men presenting a sexual problem predominantly complain of erectile or ejaculatory problems and relatively rarely of low sexual interest which may, however, be one of the presenting features of a depressive illness. Psychological factors influence reactions to erotic stimuli and although it is far from clear that sexual dysfunction is a direct consequence of these emotional states it is reasonable to assume that treatment aimed at alleviating the emotional disturbance is likely to improve the sexual response. Psychological and physical factors frequently interact in creating difficulties. Side effects of drugs are an important cause of sexual dysfunction, though in most instances the pharmacology is not understood, in particular whether the effects are peripheral or central. Drugs involved in lowering blood pressure are commonly implicated. Cerebral pathology has a very unpredictable association with

sexual dysfunction, though temporal lobe epilepsy is associated with a loss of sexual interest and arousability. Interference with normal erectile mechanisms may be the only obvious manifestation of the disease. Erection normally becomes less efficient with advancing age and this is liable to be regarded by older aircrew as an indication of more general waning of their capabilities. The resultant anxiety is likely to reinforce the difficulty and set up a vicious circle. Low self-esteem is also liable to have sexual repercussions.

It is surprising how often couples fail to recognize the link between long-standing resentment between them and problems in their sexual relationship. Communication in general is of fundamental importance and problems that should otherwise be transient become chronic because of poor communication. The flight medical officer with his first-hand professional and social contact with the airman and his wife, and his privileged position of being able to discuss matters in complete confidence, is in a uniquely advantageous position to offer help in such situations.

Sexual deviations and disorders

These are described in the ICD 9 as sexual inclinations and behaviours which do not serve approved social and biological purposes. If such behaviour becomes manifest during mental illness it should be dealt with as part of the management of that illness. Where it occurs in isolation it is not likely to bear directly on an individual's capability as an aviator but certainly in the case of military aviators it is likely to be incompatible with membership of the armed forces.

References

AITKEN, R.C.B., LISTER, J.A. and MAIN, G.J. (1981) Identification of features associated with flying phobia in aircrew. *British Journal of Psychiatry*, **139**, 38–42

BECK, A.T. (1976) *Cognitive Therapy and the Emotional Disorders*. New York: International Universities Press

BENNETT, G. (1985) Aviation safety, physical and mental incapacitation. In *Occupational Health in Aviation and Space Work*: 4th UOEH International Symposium vol. 7; Supplement March Journal of UOEH: 45–42

BOWLBY, J. (1969) *Attachment and Loss: I. Attachment*. London: Hogarth Press

BOWLBY, J. (1973) *Attachment and Loss: II. Separation, Anxiety and Anger*. London: Hogarth Press

BOWLBY, J. (1980) *Attachment and Loss: III. Loss Sadness and Depression*. New York: Basic Books

BRANDON, S. (1983) Chest pain in patients with normal coronary arteriograms. *British Medical Journal*, **287**, 1491–1492

BRANDT, D.J., ROSENMAN, R.H., SHOLTZ, R.I. and FRIEDMAN, M. (1976) Multivariant prediction of coronary heart disease in the Western Collaborative Study compared to the findings of the Framingham Study. *Circulation*, **53**, 348–355

CAWLEY, R.H. (1983) The neuroses and personality disorders: concepts in classification. In Russell, G.F.M. and Hersov, L.A. (eds). *Handbook of Psychiatry*, vol. 4. Cambridge University Press

COOPER, C.L. (1985) The stress of work: An overview. *Aviation, Space and Environmental Medicine*, **56**, 627–632

CROW, T.J. (1978) Viral causes of psychiatric disease. *Acta Psychiatrica Scandinavica*, **43**, 144–162

EDWARDS, G., GROSS, M.M., KELLER, M., MOSER, J. and ROOM, R. (1977) *Alcohol-Related Disabilities*. WHO Offset Publication No. 32. Geneva: WHO

FINE, P.M. and HARTMAN, B.O. (1968) *Psychiatric Strengths and Weaknesses of Typical Air Force Pilots*. Technical Report 68-121, USAF School of Aerospace Medicine, Brooks AFB, TX

FOWLIE, D.G. and AVELINE, M.O. (1985) The emotional consequences of ejection, rescue and rehabilitation in Royal Air Force aircrew. *British Journal of Psychiatry*, **146**, 609–613

GOLDBERG, D. and HUXLEY, P. (1980) *Mental Illness in the Community: The Pathway to Psychiatric Care*. London and New York: Tavistock Publications

GOORNEY, A.B. (1970) Treatment of aviation phobias by behaviour therapy. *British Journal of Psychiatry*, **117**, 535–544

GREEN, R. (1983) Aviation psychology: Assessing workload and selecting pilots. *British Medical Journal*, **286**, 1947–1949

HAGNELL, O. (1966) *A Prospective Study of the Incidence of Mental Disorder*. Norstedts: Svenska Boleforlagets

HURRY, J., TENNANT, C. and BEBBINGTON, P. (1980) The selective factors leading to psychiatric referral. *Acta Psychiatrica Scandinavica*, **62**, Suppl. **285**, 315–323

JOHNSON, J.H. and SARSON, I.G. (1979) Recent developments in research on life stress. In Hamilton, V. and Warburton, D.M. (eds) *Human Stress and Cognition*, pp. 205–233. Chichester and New York: John Wiley and Sons

JONES, D.R. (1986) Flying and danger, joy and fear. *Aviation, Space and Environmental Medicine*, **57**, 131–136

KLERMAN, G.L., ROUNSAVILLE, B., CHEVRON, E., NEU, C. and WEISSMAN, M.W. (1979) *Manual for Short-term Interpersonal Psychotherapy (IPT) of Depression*. New Haven: Boston Collaborative Depression Project

LISHMAN, W.A. (1973) The psychiatric sequelae of head injury: a review. *Psychological Medicine*, **3**, 304–318

MITCHELL, J.R.A. (1984) Hearts and Minds. *British Medical Journal*, **289**, 1557–1558

PARKES, C. (1979) The first year of bereavement. *Psychiatry*, **33**, 444–467

RUTTER, M. (1985) Resilience in the face of adversity: protective factors and resistance to psychiatric disorder. *British Journal of Psychiatry*, **147**, 598–611

SCHNEIDER, K. (1950) *Psychopathic Personalities* (translated by M.W. Hamilton). London: Cassell

TYRER, P. (1976) *The Role of Bodily Feelings in Anxiety*, Institute of Psychiatry Maudsley Monograph number 23, Oxford University Press

URSANO, R.J. and HOLLOWAY, H.C. (1985) Aerospace operations. In Kaplan, H.I. and Sadock, B.J. (eds) *Comprehensive Textbook of Psychiatry*, vol. 2, 4th edn., pp. 1906–1907. Baltimore/London: Williams and Wilkins

WHITLOCK, F.A. (1967) The aetiology of hysteria. *Acta Psychiatrica Scandinavica*, **43**, 144–162

WOLPE, J. (1958) *Psychotherapy by Reciprocal Inhibition*. Berkeley, Cali.: Stanford University Press

49

Neurology

R.T.G. Merry

Introduction

Neurological disease is one of the commonest medical causes of aircrew or air traffic controllers becoming unfit to continue their duties. When considering the effect neurological disorders might have on flight safety we must take into account not only those diseases that cause permanent disability, either static or progressive, but also whether an individual harbours a predisposition to an intermittent disorder of neural function which, if it occurred during flight, might lead to a temporary safety hazard. Epilepsy or other causes of sudden loss of consciousness, migraine, periodic paroxysmal vertigo and the neuralgias can all be so disabling temporarily, that what may in other circumstances be purely socially inconvenient, becomes a potential hazard to survival of the person affected and often many others, not to mention the possibility of considerable material loss due to an accident. Many of these conditions occur commonly, tend to recur and are unpredictable in their natural history. As a result a history of these conditions or symptoms suggestive of a predisposition in a recruit for aircrew or air traffic control will often result in rejection.

The final decision on whether a person is fit to fly must always be based on the particular clinical circumstances pertaining to that individual, his or her role, and the possible natural history of the particular disease. While there are some neurological diseases that would be an automatic bar to a person flying, most decisions cannot be made by laying down rigid rules without considerable wastage of trained personnel, and must be based on informed common sense.

Permanent disability

Static disorders

Those diseases of the nervous system that cause permanent disability can be divided into static and progressive groups. The static disorders mainly include injuries, though occasionally other conditions such as an evolved stroke require consideration (*see* below). Injuries to the peripheral nervous system or spinal cord can be assessed entirely on the degree of disability, and the effect that this disability has on the individual's particular role. It must be emphasized that recovery of function after injury to the nervous system can be very slow, and may occur over a few years. Only after an appropriate time can a final prognosis be given, and then it may be possible to return a person to limited flying duties even though there may be a significant residual permanent disability. In this situation a medical officer pilot or flight medical officer can usefully employ his expertise in assessing how a particular disability would limit the patient in various aircrew roles, and sometimes a return to flying in a limited way may be possible.

Certain permanent disabilities of a static nature, but due to other underlying pathology, must be judged on the likely natural history of that particular disease and the residual neurological deficit. For example, an intracerebral haemorrhage in a young person due to a minute arteriovenous malformation which has been obliterated by the haemorrhage may carry a very low risk of rebleeding, but a residual neurological deficit such as a visual field deficit, or an increased risk of epilepsy, may render that person unfit to return to certain flying duties. Alternatively a transient cerebral ischaemic attack, or a completed stroke but with little residual deficit, may still be a poor risk for return to flying because the underlying pathological disorder is likely to remain, and the risk of recurrence consequently increased. For this reason cerebrovascular disease due to arteriosclerosis—whether causing ischaemic attacks, cerebral infarction or intracerebral haemorrhage—is usually considered incompatible with return to most flying duties. Subarachnoid haemorrhage due to a solitary ruptured berry aneurysm, which is subsequently clipped, or where angiography does not show an aneurysm, carries no increased risk of rebleeding.

However, there is a considerable risk of the development of epilepsy, even in those cases where craniotomy was not performed, and for some time the patient should be judged unfit to return to flying. If after 3 years epilepsy has not developed a return to a limited flying role may be possible, but not as a solo pilot of high-performance aircraft. Similarly, the risk of epilepsy is significantly increased after craniotomy, intracranial haemorrhage including subdural haematoma, cerebral abscess or severe head injury, and in these circumstances the patient should be grounded for a minimum of 2 years before return to flying is considered. Disorders of certain cranial nerves, such as the olfactory, optic, facial or auditory nerves, may cause problems with flight safety, or the wearing of equipment which would exclude a person from some aircrew roles. A permanent visual field defect will normally exclude the person from aircrew or traffic control duties.

Progressive disorders

Most permanent neurological disorders which are progressive are generally incompatible with normal flying duties. This is particularly so when the disease affects higher cognitive functions or the easy performance of motor skills. Parkinson's disease, Alzheimer's disease and other dementing or organic brain diseases and the demyelinating diseases are usually therefore a cause for permanent grounding as soon as the diagnosis is established. An occasional exception occurs in a progressive disease such as multiple sclerosis where if, for example, there has been an episode of demyelination in the spinal cord followed by complete clinical recovery, and without evidence of involvement of other areas of the central nervous system, an individual may be allowed to return to full flying duties. However, normal clinical examination is a relatively crude measure of function, and other covert plaques, particularly in cerebral white matter, may affect a person's judgement and higher cognitive function to a significant degree in the performance of his duties.

A member of aircrew who develops, or is suspected of having, multiple sclerosis and who makes an apparent full recovery may be allowed to return to flying, but he must be kept under regular review. In patients with multiple sclerosis who show even minor permanent deficits a flying restriction or permanent grounding is necessary.

The possibility of a return to flying in those with an intracranial tumour is dependent on type, site and the result of treatment. All intracerebral tumours, whether primary or secondary, are incompatible with continuation of flying duties. Extracerebral benign tumours, for example a meningioma, carry a better prognosis if complete removal has been achieved and no cerebral damage has resulted from tumour or surgery. However, the risk of development of epilepsy must be taken into account, this risk remaining high after removal of tumours such as a meningioma, and for a time after any supratentorial craniotomy. However, provided that the individual has made a full recovery and not developed epilepsy after 3 years, a return to flying in a full or restricted role is sometimes possible.

Head injury

Finally in the consideration of permanent disability we must consider head injuries. The earlier remarks concerning injury to the spinal cord or peripheral nervous system, that return to flying duties is entirely dependent on the degree of final recovery, still apply; but because of the involvement of the brain, with the possibility of psychological and intellectual disorders, as well as motor or sensory deficits and the risk of traumatic epilepsy, the assessment of recovery is inevitably more difficult. Again it may take several years for full recovery to occur, and certainly an adverse prognosis should be guarded if given before at least 2 years have elapsed since the injury. In penetrating head injuries irreversible damage to cerebral tissue always occurs, and the very high risk of neurological, cognitive or psychiatric disorders and epilepsy means that these injuries are usually incompatible with a return to flying. Any closed head injury sufficiently severe to cause disturbance of consciousness is inevitably associated with some degree of brain contusion, with a risk of permanent brain injury, and clearly the more severe the head injury the greater the risk of permanent brain injury. Even a minor contusion in aircrew can have profound effects on efficiency, particularly intellectually, and it is wise to ground an individual to a period of convalescence. Neurological complications of head injury include intracranial or intracerebral haemorrhage, focal neurological disorders, infection, epilepsy, intellectual difficulties and cranial nerve damage, either temporary or permanent.

The incidence of psychiatric disorder is increased after a head injury, the risk correlating with severity and site of the brain injury (Lushman, 1978). Most of the neuroses and psychoses show an increased incidence, and in any individual the risk depends not only on the above-mentioned factors but also on genetic susceptibility and premorbid personality, age, and motivation for return to flying. The incidence of prolonged neurosis in this population is less than in the general population, a finding which is in accordance with other groups who have a high motivation for return to a desired activity. There is an increased incidence of intracranial haemorrhage if there is a fracture of the skull, and an increased risk of intracranial infection with skull fractures involving the middle ear cavity or sinuses.

In assessing the severity of a past closed head injury, and so risk of residual brain damage, the symptom of most use is the duration of post-traumatic amnesia (PTA). This is defined as the interval between the moment of injury and the recovery of sequential memory. There is a good clinical correlation between the duration of PTA and risk of brain injury in closed head injuries and thus the incidence of neuropsychiatric complications and time taken to recovery. The duration of PTA is a record which is permanently held by the individual. Although the duration of unconsciousness would also show a correlation with the degree of brain injury, it is difficult to measure, is frequently not accurately recorded in hospital notes, and the patient often cannot recall for how long he was unconscious. The period of retrograde amnesia is often of short duration and less variable, even after more severe head injuries. For these reasons these two latter measures are of less use clinically. The period off flying, provided a full recovery has occurred, can be judged in relationship to the duration of PTA (*Table 49.1*). Where the PTA is more than 24 hours, not only is the individual at greater risk of more severe brain damage, but the risk of traumatic epilepsy is increased. For these reasons a minimum period of 6 months off flying is recommended, but in most cases where the risk of traumatic epilepsy is considered higher than 15% it is advisable for the period off flying to be between 1

and 3 years. Clearly these recommended periods of grounding are only rough guidelines and will always depend on a full clinical recovery, the patient's individual details of injury and aircrew role.

In deciding whether a person has fully recovered, apart from a complete clinical neurological examination, a detailed assessment of the mental state including intellectual function, should be made. This can be reinforced by a number of investigations, such as EEG or CT brain scan, where necessary as further measures of structure and function of the brain. However, many more subtle intellectual deficits may not be readily apparent on even a detailed clinical examination, and in those persons who are at high risk for enduring brain dysfunction it is wise to ask a skilled clinical psychologist to perform a neuropsychological assessment of cognitive function. The parts of the brain most vulnerable to damage are the frontal and temporal lobes, and it is those cognitive tasks of memory, higher abstract reasoning, judgement and mental flexibility which are largely mediated by these parts of the brain. Changes in these functions may be difficult to detect but may cause serious disability in the performance of the patient's duties as aircrew. Occasionally even a good neuropsychological assessment may not identify a serious disability, which may become apparent only after reports from the patient's close family or acquaintances. It is wise whenever possible to obtain a report from a perceptive relative or friend. If there is any doubt about recovery of higher brain function, a longer period off flying in a ground job will usually clarify whether there is any serious permanent disability.

Traumatic epilepsy

The overall risk of traumatic epilepsy after a closed head injury is 1–5%, and this risk is increased if one or more of certain complications occur (*Table 49.2*),

Table 49.2 Factors causing an increased risk of traumatic epilepsy (based on Jennett, 1975)

	Increase in risk (%)
Penetrating brain injury	40
Depressed fracture of skull vault	15
Intracranial haematoma	35
Intracerebral haemorrhage	35
PTA 24 hours	4
Early seizure	25

this risk being cumulative and rising to as high as 70%. If seizures do occur, 27% do so within the first 3 months, 56% within the first year, and 75% after 2 years (Jennett, 1975). An early seizure is one occurring within the first week after head injury, and is associated with a 25% risk of recurrence of seizures. However, this is significantly less than the risk of epilepsy developing after a late seizure (one

Table 49.1 Relation of the minimum period off flying to the duration of post-traumatic amnesia (PTA)

Duration PTA	*Minimum period recommended off flying*
Momentary	2–6 weeks
1 Hour	6 weeks
2+ Hours	8 weeks
12 Hours	4 months
24 Hours	6 months–1 year
1 Week 2 Weeks 3 Weeks	9 months–Indefinitely

occurring 1 week or more after the head injury) when the risk of recurrence is 80%. Although the risk of traumatic epilepsy is substantially reduced if 2 years have elapsed after the head injury without onset of seizures, it should be noted that in 25%, traumatic epilepsy develops many years after a head injury. Although it would be reasonable to allow certain aircrew who were initially estimated to have a high risk of traumatic epilepsy to return to flying after 2 years if seizures have not occurred, and even some pilots to return to certain flying duties, it is wise not to authorize a return to solo pilot duties in those considered to have a very high risk of developing traumatic epilepsy, even when no seizures have occurred within the first 2 years. An early seizure, even when not followed by recurrence within 2 years, is incompatible with a return to pilot or indeed any aircrew duties, except in very exceptional circumstances.

Finally, while a member of aircrew is taking a prophylactic anticonvulsant, he will be ineligible to return to flying until this has been withdrawn and he has been free of seizures for at least 6 months.

Transient disability

If for the purpose of our discussion normal physiological or psychological disorders such as depersonalization, or disorientation associated with flying, are excluded, the common disorders likely to cause a transient disturbance of consciousness or loss of control are epilepsy, migraine, paroxysmal vertigo and the neuralgias. Loss of consciousness from causes other than epilepsy should not be forgotten. Paroxysmal vertigo is incompatible with most flying duties except where it is due to a transient illness which is unlikely to recur and where vertigo has not recurred for some time despite discontinuation of vestibular sedatives.

Neuralgia can be so painful that it may be temporarily totally distracting and prevent the patient from performing his job. While the neuralgia persists, or while treatment is continuing, flying is not permitted. If, however, the condition has been in remission for at least 6 months without treatment, either due to a spontaneous remission or the success of surgical treatment, it is often possible for the patient to return to flying duties.

Epilepsy

In the population with whom we are concerned, the majority of episodes of spontaneous disturbance of consciousness are due either to an epileptic seizure or to a disturbance of circulation leading to transient cerebral hypoperfusion. This differentiation can be extremely difficult clinically, but must be attempted

as accurately as possible because of the prognosis for recurrence and the effect this might have on flight safety in the future. The history, including a good eye witness account, is all important, and the clinical diagnosis hinges largely on this. There is no investigation that will distinguish between epilepsy and syncope, though the EEG may show paroxysmal spike-wave complexes which correlate closely with a predisposition to epilepsy. Other investigations, including ambulatory ECG recording, may identify a cardiac dysrhythmia or other disorder which would predispose the patient to syncope. Clonic jerking of limbs or incontinence are not particularly useful symptoms in the differentiation between syncope and seizure, and indeed syncope with profound or prolonged hypoperfusion of the brain can lead to a generalized seizure. However, the tongue being badly bitten during an attack is indicative of a marked generalized tonic spasm and is very common with a generalized tonic–clonic seizure, but is very uncommon with syncope even with a secondary hypoxic seizure. A prolonged period of unconsciousness or marked confusion on recovery are also suggestive of an epileptic seizure, whereas a short episode of unconsciousness, little confusion on recovery, and marked pallor or clamminess are suggestive of syncope.

In aircrew, a clear syncopal attack in appropriate circumstances does not necessitate any medical intervention. If, however, the attack of disturbance of consciousness is of uncertain aetiology, a period of grounding and observation is advised. This period should be between 6 and 24 months, as we know that the majority of epileptic seizures will recur within 2 years from the first seizure. Because of the risk of recurrence, even a solitary definite epileptic seizure always results in permanent grounding of aircrew.

When selecting candidates for training, it must be remembered that epilepsy is one of the commonest medical disorders associated with accidents due to physical incapacity (Taylor, 1983; Raffle, 1983). In addition it has been shown that trainee pilots with paroxysmal/abnormal EEGs had a threefold increased crash rate compared with those pilots with normal EEGs (Lennox-Buchtal, Buchtal and Rosenfalck, 1959). Epilepsy is a common disease with a prevalence of 0.5–0.8% in the population. A predisposition to epilepsy is usually persistent, so the risk of a seizure over the professional lifespan of aircrew is cumulative. Any incident in a patient's history that indicates an increased risk of epilepsy, for example seizures occurring after the age of 5 years, a severe head injury, or other illness with a very high risk of epilepsy, should exclude that person from selection. In addition the occurrence of generalized or focal spike–wave paroxysms on an EEG suggest a predisposition to epilepsy, and it is recommended that an EEG should be an integral part of the initial medical examination, and that those with the above abnormalities (usually 0.5–0.7%) are considered unfit for training.

Migraine

Migraine is a disorder, probably of genetic origin, causing a predisposition to recurrent attacks of headache, often associated with vomiting and transient focal neurological dysfunction. It is a very common disorder and surveys have shown a prevalence of up to 19% (Walters and O'Connor, 1971). As the predisposition is inherited it is permanent, and can occur either spontaneously or be triggered by a large and varied number of precipitants. The diagnosis is clinical, there being no investigation that provides objective confirmation.

An attack may consist of headache with gastro-intestinal upset (common migraine) or be associated with focal neurological disturbance (classic migraine), but these syndromes are not clinically distinct, and a person who has had only attacks of common migraine may have an attack of classic migraine at any time. The commonest neurological disturbances include various visual obscurations, many of which cause serious temporary impairment of visual acuity, dysphasia, or loss of use or feeling of a limb. Because of the severity of the headache or associated vomiting, photophobia, or the occurrence of one of these focal neurological disturbances, what usually is a common benign disorder can become an extreme flight safety hazard for aircrew

or air traffic controllers. A recruit for training in either of these branches who gives a past history of migraine should be found unfit for training. In trained personnel the development of migraine must result in the imposition of limitations on their employability in those fields, and recurrent attacks are incompatible with continuing as aircrew or air traffic controllers.

References

JENNETT, B. (1975) *Epilepsy after Non-missile Head Injuries*, 2nd edn. London: Heinemann

LENNOX-BUCHTAL, M., BUCHTAL, F. and ROSENFALCK, P. (1959) Correlation of electroencephalographic findings with crash rate of military jet pilots. *Epilepsia*, **1**, 366–372

LISHMAN, W.A. (1978) *Organic Psychiatry*, Chapter 5, pp. 191–261. London: Blackwell Scientific Publications

RAFFLE, P.A.B. (1983) The HGV/PSV driver and loss or impairment of consciousness. In Godwin-Austen and Espir, M.L.E. (eds). *Driving and Epilepsy—and Other Causes of Impaired Consciousness*. Royal Society of Medicine International Congress and Symposium Series No. 60, pp. 35–39. London: Royal Society of Medicine

TAYLOR, J.F. (1983) Epilepsy and other causes of collapse at the wheel. In Godwin-Austen and Espir, M.L.E. (eds). *Driving and Epilepsy—and Other Causes of Impaired Consciousness*. Royal Society of Medicine International Congress and Symposium Series No. 60, pp. 5–8. London: Royal Society of Medicine

WALTERS, W.E. and O'CONNOR, P.J. (1971) Epidemiology of headache and migraine in women. *Journal of Neurology, Neurosurgery and Psychiatry*, **34**, 148–153

50

Otorhinolaryngology

P.F. King

Otic barotrauma or aerotitis media

Introduction

Otic barotrauma results from a failure to equate the pressure in the middle ear cavity with that of the external environment. It can occur in flight, in the decompression chamber or during sea-diving, and is characterized by pain in the affected ear, deafness and occasionally vertigo.

As described in Chapter 2, and as shown in *Figures 50.1* and *50.2*, two primary factors are involved in the production of otic barotrauma:

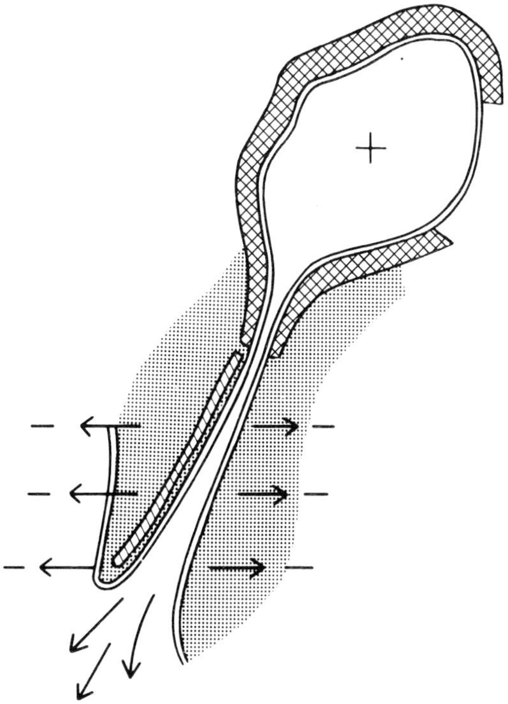

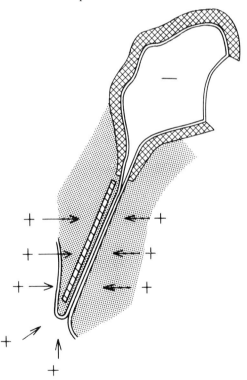

Figure 50.1 Diagrammatic representation of middle ear and eustachian tube during ascent. With reducing environmental pressure, the air in the middle ear expands, bulges the tympanic membrane and passively opens the eustachian tube.

Figure 50.2 Diagrammatic representation of the middle ear and eustachian tube during descent. With increasing environmental pressure the tympanic membrane is forced inwards and unless there is pressure equalization through the eustachian tube, barotrauma will occur if the descent is continued.

1. The expansion and contraction of gases under alteration of atmospheric pressure.
2. The collapsible nature of the proximal two-thirds of the eustachian tube.

The signs and symptoms occur in descent and follow the rapid reduction in volume of the gas in the middle ear, and the effect of increasing external pressure on the tympanic membrane, the ossicles and the lining membrane. The severity of the lesions sustained depends on the rate of descent and therefore on the rate of pressure change.

Aetiology

Under flight conditions barotrauma can occur in the presence of a normal eustachian tube when the subject is pre-occupied, asleep, ignorant of the technique of opening the eustachian tube by swallowing or by Valsalva's or Frenzel's manoeuvre, or when he is heavily sedated. Otic barotrauma is relatively common in invalids travelling by air under heavy sedation.

The rate of gaseous exchange along the tube will be reduced when the lumen of the tube is narrowed by mucosal oedema secondary to the common cold, sinusitis or allergy. Old nasal and facial fractures, deflection and spurs of the nasal septum, nasal polyposis, chronically infected tonsils and enlarged adenoids are also possible aetiological factors.

Symptoms and signs

One or both ears may be affected. The symptoms are pain, deafness, tinnitus and occasionally vertigo. If the tympanic membrane ruptures there will be bleeding from the ear.

Pain

Pain may be gradual or sudden in onset. It may be excruciating to the extent of causing fainting or it may be merely a sensation of dullness in the ear which, as the descent continues, gives way to pain resembling that of acute otitis media. It can radiate to the temple and the parotid area. In about 5% of ears the drumhead will rupture from the increase in external pressure; the pain will then go, and bleeding from the ear may be apparent.

Deafness

Deafness that arises during or after flight is usually conductive in nature due to effusion in the middle ear. Conductive deafness will resolve except in the occasional case where there are adhesions in the middle ear, ossicular dislocation, or unhealed perforation.

Deafness may also, though rarely, be perceptive, when it is likely to be due to rupture of the oval or round window. In such a case deafness is marked, and associated frequently with vertigo. Such sensori-neural deafness may be lasting if the window fistula remains open, so that surgical closure may be necessary.

Tinnitus

Tinnitus may accompany the hearing loss.

Vertigo

Vertigo is luckily rare, but if it occurs in a pilot especially during a fast descent, it may, of course, prove a hazard. In most cases, spontaneous nystagmus will be apparent.

When the ear is examined, a variable degree of invagination of the drumhead will be seen together with a fan-shaped congestion, extending from the tip of the malleus to the attic. Single or multiple interstitial haemorrhages occur and, with rapid rates of descent, large plum-coloured blisters may distort the surface of the drumhead and extend on to the adjacent meatal skin.

Effusion into the middle ear, which commonly occurs at any time from onset until 12 hours later, is characterized by an amber appearance of the drumhead. If the middle ear is not completely filled with fluid, a thin, blue or black hair-line meniscus may be seen, which will move when the head is flexed or extended on the neck. Occasionally, collections of bubbles will be seen in the fluid. If bleeding occurs in the middle ear (haemotympanum) there is a typical blue-black appearance.

Rupture of the tympanic membrane occurs in the pars tensa. The classic site of a tear is at the anterior inferior quadrant adjacent to the opening of the eustachian tube, but any area of scarring or weakness will tear in these circumstances.

Chronic otic barotrauma

Every incident of barotrauma sustained in flight is acute in itself, whether it is mild or severe. There are cases, however, in which resolution is not complete at the time when a return to flying is permitted. Such individuals are likely to suffer further episodes of barotrauma, which is then termed chronic otic barotrauma.

Delayed otic barotrauma

In this instance the subject starts to suffer from pain in the ear and hearing loss several hours after a trouble-free flight. This form of barotrauma occurs after long flights in which 100% oxygen is breathed. With partial occlusion of the tube the rapid absorption of oxygen via the middle ear mucosa results in a significant change in the pressure differential. Signs are minimal.

'Reversed ear'—barotrauma of the external auditory meatus

This will occur in descent if an obstruction at the meatal entrance prevents an increase in pressure in the external canal, with ambient atmospheric pressure in the middle ear via an open eustachian tube. In flight it is caused by a tight ear plug. The tympanic membrane bulges *outwards*, and may tear. Blood blisters may form in the external canal with possible bleeding.

Management

Prevention

In general, all those with any likely predisposition to the condition should be excluded from flying duties but careful judgement needs to be exercised in deciding which, if any, of marginal cases are fit for flying. In some cases recourse may be made to preliminary decompression chamber testing, and the use of tympanometry can give helpful information confirming tubal obstruction in a doubtful case.

It is essential that aircrew should be taught the causes of otic barotrauma, and how to prevent it, at a very early stage of their flying training. The Valsalva manoeuvre becomes much easier with practice, while some prefer Frenzel's method (1950).

The temporary grounding of aircrew personnel with upper respiratory infection is a wise precaution.

Immediate treatment

Treatment should be started as soon as possible, and should aim at:

1. Relieving the pain.
2. Reventilating the middle ear to relieve the pressure.

Pain rarely persists after landing and the administration of analgesics is not often required. If pain persists, it is likely that otitis media has supervened.

Ventilation of the middle ear presents some problems. Inflation will succeed only when the barotrauma has been sustained at a relatively slow rate of descent. Eustachian catheterization in unpractised hands can be uncomfortable at the least, and at worst potentially dangerous, and in a severe barotrauma it is unlikely to help even in skilled hands.

In the USAF, myringotomy is practised in the consulting room. This has the advantage of immediate relief of symptoms, and the disadvantage of possible transmission of infection to the middle ear and of some danger in inexperienced hands; a patent perforation may also persist.

The safest and most satisfactory early treatment is to give nasal decongestants, and this could include antihistaminics by mouth if nasal allergy is suspected. Where infection in the nose is present, the use of wide-spectrum antibiotics is justified. In general, treatment along these lines will reduce all signs of a tubal block in 7–10 days or less. There should be evidence of movement of the drumhead during self-inflation before a return to normal flying is permitted, and a preliminary flight or decompression chamber test may be helpful.

Delayed treatment

If there is no resolution by the end of a fortnight a search must be made for one or more of the aetiological factors noted above. If such a lesion is found it should be treated, often surgically, and this will generally bring a speedy resolution of the tubal obstruction.

Sometimes where no predisposing cause can be found, a course of eustachian inflation may be helpful. In recent years the problem has been overcome by fitting a Teflon or silicone grommet into the drumhead of the affected ear. This permits easy ventilation of the ear and, with the grommet in place, flying can be resumed. Ultimately the grommet will be shed, or it can be removed, when the ear will heal. This technique has replaced the use of irradiation to the nasopharynx and eustachian tube.

If the tympanic membrane has ruptured, there is the possibility of infection; so interference with the ear should be minimal and limited to inspection and the application of cotton wool at the entrance to the meatus. If infection supervenes, or is feared, systemic antibiotics should be given. In most cases, spontaneous healing occurs and a return to flying can be permitted. If a perforation persists, it may be closed by one of the simpler forms of tympanoplasty.

When fluid persists in the middle ear it can be drained easily by simple myringotomy and suction, or needle aspiration.

Prognosis

In the average case the likelihood of returning to flying is good. Fifteen per cent of those attending hospital will be grounded, and a further 15% will be suitable for flying in a restricted capacity, which will be determined by decompression chamber testing.

Sinus barotrauma or aerosinusitis

Introduction

The paranasal sinuses also contain air and symptoms can arise when communication between the interior of a sinus and the external atmosphere fails to cope with a change in the ambient barometric pressure. The incidence of aerosinusitis is one-third of that otic barotrauma, but some subjects may suffer simultaneous lesions.

The frontal sinus is involved more frequently than any other, either alone or in combination with the maxillary antrum. Barotrauma of the antrum alone is not uncommon, though involvement of the ethmoid sinus(es) is unusual. Barotrauma of the sphenoidal sinuses has not been recorded.

Aetiology

Any condition that causes narrowing of the ostium of a nasal sinus will predispose to sinus barotrauma. One should therefore consider nasal allergy, nasal polyposis, chronic nasal infection, deflection of the nasal septum and old fractures of the nasal and facial skeleton as being likely aetiological factors.

Delayed sinus barotrauma

This can occur after long flights in which 100% oxygen is breathed. Occlusion of the sinus ostium at the end of the flight is then followed by a rapid absorption of oxygen through the mucosa, with a consequent fall of pressure within the sinus.

Symptoms and signs

Pain, the predominant symptom, may be localized over the sinus involved, be more diffuse, or even referred to an unaffected area. It may start above or around the eyes, spreading to the vertex and the temples. Pain in the cheek is not uncommon.

In most cases pain occurs in descent. It is of sudden onset and severe in character, this feature being directly related to the rate of descent and hence the rate of pressure change. It may be sufficiently severe to cause fainting. Generally the pain eases and disappears on return to ground level although it may persist for several days until relieved. Pain occurring in ascent is slower of onset and progress and is not usually severe. Other

symptoms in sinus barotrauma are lacrymation and sometimes epistaxis. Occasionally patients describe a 'sucking noise' high in the nose before the onset of pain.

Signs are few, and include evidence of bleeding from the nose. The front wall and the floor of the frontal sinus may be tender on pressure, as may be the front wall of the antrum.

Radiological examination gives information both as to the location and extent of the submucosal haemorrhage, which classically is found in the upper outer angle of a frontal or maxillary sinus. Mucosal swelling of effusion into one or more sinus cavities may also be seen (*Figure 50.3*).

Differential diagnosis

One is unlikely to be misled in diagnosis although occasionally the apparent predisposing cause, for example, a subacute sinusitis, may, in fact, be the only cause of headache. As barotrauma is a condition which lends itself to hysterical mimicry, in doubtful cases this should be considered, and radiological examination will help to establish the diagnosis.

Management

Prevention

Acute and chronic upper respiratory infections are the most frequent causes of trouble, and aircrew suffering from these infections should not be permitted to fly.

Those with nasal allergy and chronic nasal infection should not be selected for flying training; when aircrew change from aircraft of lower performance to those of higher performance, a run in the decompression chamber may help to establish individual tolerance.

Treatment

Treatment should be directed to equalizing the intra-sinus and ambient pressures and to the relief of pain. Thus decongestants to the nose will relieve the congestion resulting from the original aetiological factor and hence will help to aerate the sinus involved. If infection is suspected, systemic antibiotics may help to control infection and reduce oedema.

Many cases are relatively mild and can be rapidly improved symptomatically. Others may need surgical intervention to resolve the immediate difficulty and to prevent recurrence.

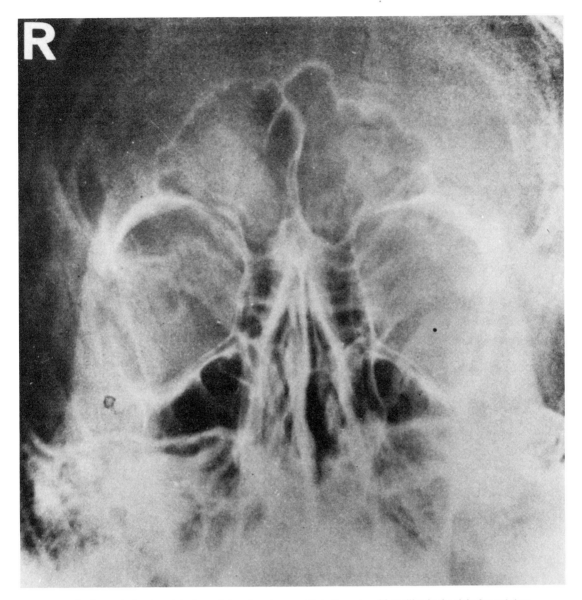

Figure 50.3 Radiograph showing right frontal sinus barotrauma. Note the polypoid swelling in the right frontal sinus which is the result of submucosal haemorrhage.

The progress of the barotrauma may be followed by serial X-ray examination. In many cases the submucosal swelling settles, and, with the completion of treatment, a return to flying can be permitted. If despite treatment a haematoma persists for 2 months it is reasonable to assume that the change is permanent and to recommend a decompression chamber or flight test before a resumption of flying duties is allowed. In recurrent cases, intranasal antrostomy may be necessary to ensure adequate ventilation of an affected antrum.

Prognosis

A large proportion of those who have suffered from the syndrome return to full flying; a small proportion are fit only for flying in a limited category, and about 15% of those coming to hospital for treatment have to be grounded.

Pressure cabins may have reduced, but they have not abolished, the tendency to develop either sinus or otic barotrauma which are still a frequent cause of loss of flying fitness in aircrew.

Conductive hearing loss in flying personnel

Introduction

Aircrew need good hearing both in the air and on the ground. The required range is from ½ to 3 kHz, for the reception of speech and audio signals. Most ear telephones have no appreciable response beyond 3072 Hz.

In general, the appearance of losses beyond a recognized normal level in either ear should be taken as a warning sign but this does not necessarily indicate the need for immediate withdrawal from flying.

Conductive losses are often associated with paracusis willisii, in which the subject hears better in a background of noise; improvement of the hearing can often be attained by amplification, so that subjects with conductive deafness often hear well in the air. However, the need to hear accurately on the ground (particularly unaided), the uncertain effects of fatigue, and the degree of progression of the hearing loss must all be borne in mind when making an assessment. Certainly, hearing loss in candidates for initial flying training should be viewed unfavourably, on both social and economic grounds.

The measurement of hearing

Hearing standards—national and international, military and civil—are usually based on pure tone audiometry.

The first step for the examiner is to take a careful history, noting particularly the occurrence of any acute infectious fever in the past, any head injury and history of previous trouble with the ears, together with any familiar history of deafness. Undue exposure to noise or any adverse response to medication should also be noted. This is followed by a full otological examination: the tympanic membrane, the middle ear and its adnexae, the patency of the eustachian tube and the range of hearing. Weber's and Rinne's tests are also important.

It is helpful to check the ability of each ear to hear a whispered voice, the other ear being masked. If responses are deficient, then this test is given at conversational levels. Opinions vary as to their usefulness, but provided one realises their limitations, such tests do give useful information, and so have a practical value.

Audiometry

Pure tone air conduction audiometry is the most satisfactory method of checking the hearing. These tests can be carried out on individual subjects or on groups.

Equipment must be calibrated to a recognized standard and the tests must be carried out by properly trained operators in an ambient noise level of low intensity. If testing conditions are standardized, initial and follow-up examinations of the hearing are comparable.

Within the Royal Air Force, pure tone audiometers constructed to the specification of British Standard 2980 (British Standards Institution, 1958) are employed, while the standard reference zero for the scale of hearing is that specified by British Standard 2497 (British Standards Institution, 1954). Each ear is tested separately in an ambient noise no greater than 25 dB overall relative to 0.0002 dynes/cm². In clinical practice, the hearing is considered to be within normal limits if there is no loss greater than 20 dB relative to the standard reference zero at ¼, ½, 1, 2, 3, 4 and 8 kHz. In doubtful cases, the estimation of a threshold by bone conduction may be helpful, as may speech audiometry.

Tests to measure the efficiency of the subject in discriminating speech in a background of noise have been devised, and several varieties exist. They are of particular value in determining the fitness of trained aircrew with hearing losses, though it should be remembered that ability to discriminate speech signals in noise will depreciate as a perceptive loss advances. In conductive deafness, however, the ability to discriminate speech in these conditions will be maintained, and may be better than normal.

Conductive deafness

The hearing loss results from an impairment of the transmission system in the middle ear. In the established case certain fundamental signs are recognized; Weber's test will be referred to the deafer ear, while Rinne's test will be negative in the affected ear(s). The ability to discriminate speech in ambient noise will be retained. With pure tone air conduction audiometry, in the uncomplicated case the greatest loss will be apparent in the low and middle frequencies; while testing by pure tone bone conduction audiometry will demonstrate near normal thresholds of hearing. There will be a relatively wide difference between air and bone conduction thresholds—the so-called air–bone gap.

There are several basic causes of this type of deafness, as follows:

1. Failure of sound to reach the tympanic membrane. A history and examination will quickly reveal such causes as impacted wax and otitis externa.
2. Failure of the tympanic membrane to act as a tambour and to collect sound. The commonest cause is perforation of the drumhead, but undue scarring or chalk deposits may also be the cause.

3. Impaired mobility of the middle ear ossicles which may stem from tubal block, interossicular arthritis, otosclerosis, ossicular disruption or dislocation, or adhesions from previous inflammation. (*Figures 50.4–50.7*).

4. Altered transmissibility of the middle ear space. This may be due to a reduced volume of gas resulting from chronic tubal block, or delayed otic barotrauma resulting from absorption of oxygen. A collection of fluid for example from secretory otitis media, blood following trauma, barotrauma, pus or seropus from otitis media may likewise cause deafness.

The significance of such a hearing loss in aircrew depends on the cause.

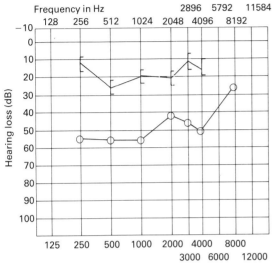

Figure 50.4 Pure-tone air (○—○) and bone ([–[) conduction audiogram (right ear) for a typical case of otosclerosis. Note the difference between the air and bone conduction thresholds—'the air–bone gap'.

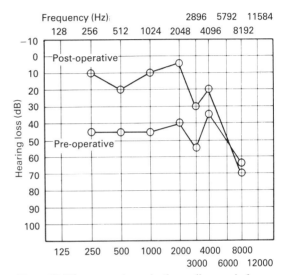

Figure 50.6 Pure-tone air conduction audiogram, before and after operation, in a case of incudostapedial dislocation treated by tympanotomy and repositioning of the ossicles.

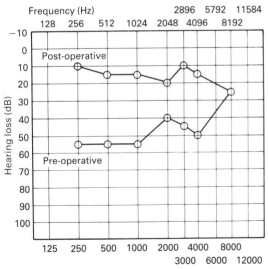

Figure 50.5 Pure-tone air conduction audiogram from the same case of otosclerosis as in *Figure 50.4* treated by stapedectomy showing the pre-operative and post-operative hearing levels. Note that the new hearing level by air conduction is the same as the hearing level by bone conduction in *Figure 50.4*, indicating closure of the air–bone gap.

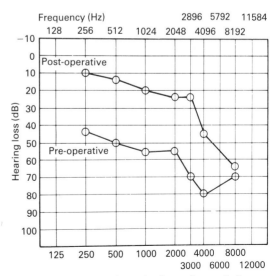

Figure 50.7 Pure-tone air-conduction audiogram before and after operation in a case of adhesive deafness, treated by tympanotomy and division of adhesions.

Secretory otitis media

In this condition, the secretion in the middle ear results from an upper respiratory infection, sometimes viral in origin, and often subchronic. It should therefore not be confused with otic barotrauma. With the deafness there may be a sensation of fluid swirling in the ear on movement of the head. The tympanic membrane is a little bulged out and is amber coloured owing to the presence of fluid in the middle ear. Mucus in the ear gives a dull, blue-grey appearance, whereas blood in the middle ear (haemotympanum) gives a blue-black appearance. Occasionally, a fluid level may be seen which moves as the head is flexed or extended, and sometimes bubbles may be seen in the fluid.

Treatment is by decongestion of the nose with attention to any infection. The fluid in the middle ear may be removed by myringotomy and suction, or by aspiration, and the fitting of a grommet. Flying should not be permitted while the condition is active.

Otosclerosis

While generally affecting females, otosclerosis is also common in the male. The hearing loss starts in the early twenties and slowly worsens, until the perceptive mechanism of hearing is involved. The loss is often bilateral. There is frequently a family history of similar deafness. The cause of otosclerosis is not known. Foci of otosclerotic bone form in the capsule of the inner ear, with some predilection for sites at or close to the oval window. As the process continues, the footplate of the stapes is trapped by the encroaching otosclerotic bone and hence an impedance type of deafness results.

Apart from the classic signs of conductive deafness, in some cases a pink suffusion may be seen through the tympanic membrane—the so-called 'flamingo flare'. Untreated, the otosclerosis will progress until a hearing aid is required. There is no medical treatment, but surgical treatment can be very successful in relieving the hearing loss.

The present-day practice is to remove the stapes (stapedectomy) replacing it with a prosthesis while closing the open oval window with a tissue graft. In carefully selected cases, this can give a good result.

So far as aircrew are concerned, there is a risk to the inner ear from violent movement of the prosthesis during sudden or marked pressure changes, with resultant vertigo and cochlear failure. Where military pilots are concerned, it is safer to advise withdrawal from flying duties if this operation has been performed. Depending on their roles, other crewmen can be given restricted flying categories, though they should be aware of the risk to the ear. There is evidence to support the view that

a wire prosthesis, securely anchored to the incus and combined with a fat graft, is free of hazard.

The operation of partial stapedectomy has been developed in recent years, with preservation of the incudostapedial joint, the stapedius muscle, one leg of the stapes and a small piece of footplate. The open window is covered by a tissue graft. This procedure gives a good hearing gain and risk to the inner ear in flight is reduced considerably.

Additionally, the stapedial bypass procedure in which the fixed stapes is retained, and a prosthesis fitted to the long process of incus and thence to a drill hole in the footplate of the stapes, can be regarded as effective and hazard free.

In practical terms, a member of aircrew with otosclerosis can often hear better than average in flight. There comes a time, however, when he will begin to have difficulty. One would then normally weigh the pros and cons of surgical treatment or of fitting a suitable hearing aid. The latter will not inspire confidence in crews or passengers; and some forms of stapedectomy, while providing a good hearing gain, may spell the end of flying. In practice good results in the short term can be produced by stapes mobilization which will permit flying for perhaps as much as a further 5 years. If the hearing then starts to fail, stapedectomy can be undertaken in the uncomplicated case, and while this will generally mean grounding or limitation in a military pilot, the subject is by that time well prepared for it. In civilian pilots the type of operation performed will need to be weighed carefully before a decision is made to permit flying.

Sequelae of otitis media and tympanoplasty

Perforation of the tympanic membrane, with or without hearing loss occurs as a result of infection in the middle ear, from trauma, and as a result of pressure changes acting on the tympanic membrane.

Two types of perforation of the tympanic membrane should be recognized:

1. Those involving the pars tensa and which generally result from acute otitis media.
2. Perforations in the pars flaccida. Perforations in this second group occur commonly as a result of chronic, often intermittent, negative pressure in the middle ear as a result of tubal obstruction. The thin membrane in the pars flaccida becomes sucked in and eventually atrophies, and perforates. Squamous epithelium invades the ear in an attempt to heal the defect, and cholesteatoma results from the accumulation of squamous debris that follows. This, in turn, initiates a chronic inflammatory response, so that apart from the cholesteatoma in the attic there may also be pus, granulations and polypi.

While perforations of the drumhead are uncommon in aircrew, they do occur; the site of the perforation, the presence or absence of infection, and the state of the hearing all influence the type of treatment which is undertaken.

Simple perforations in ears with good hearing require simple procedures; if there is advanced disease with marked hearing loss, a major excisive and reparative procedure is called for.

Aircrew with the simpler type of tympanoplasty are considered fit to fly, provided that the new tympanic membrane is sufficiently supple to permit easy adjustment to the pressure in flight. In such cases, some degree of conductive hearing loss is permissible. Cases with a well-encapsulated cholesteatoma which after excision and repair show a functioning middle ear should present no difficulty either; but where there has been an invasive cholesteatoma, and when the hearing loss is more advanced, it is doubtful if one is justified in permitting an unrestricted return to flying.

Sensori-neural loss in flying personnel

Introduction

The hearing of aircrew may be damaged by two conditions which are related to flying—otic barotrauma and noise. The first is not a common cause of perceptive or sensori-neural deafness, whereas the latter is decidedly common.

Damage to the hearing by noise (noise-induced hearing loss—NIHL) and the pathology of the condition have been described earlier. Suffice it to say that the degree of hazard to aircrew from excessive noise bears a direct relationship to the power, the number and the type of engines used in aircraft.

Noise-induced hearing loss may be acute or chronic. If acute, it is generally recoverable, and the hearing will return in hours or days. This condition is called auditory fatigue. The change in hearing from its original level is known as temporary threshold shift (TTS). With further, repeated, exposures to high noise levels, there is an increasing degree of temporary hearing loss, which slowly becomes permanent; the now permanently depressed level of the hearing is called the permanent threshold shift (PTS), and patients in this group have a chronic hearing loss.

It is known that the organ of Corti is damaged or destroyed by the buffeting of the basilar membrane which is induced by high intensity noise. In early cases of noise-induced hearing loss, the losses appear at 4 kHz and above, and these produce the characteristic dip or notch seen on the pure tone air conduction audiogram.

Hearing loss may pass unnoticed in the early stages because the loss is at a frequency above the speech range. This will improve, only to deteriorate again after the next flight. The process is a slow one and may take a long time before the subject is aware of any social disability or of any difficulty with hearing on the radio-telephone. Tinnitus may occur, but this more often follows exposure to impulsive noise, such as from firearms. In many cases the loss is noted on a routine medical examination.

Ultimately, the hearing loss will begin to involve the speech frequencies, with resultant social as well as occupational handicap. At this stage, the airman will himself be aware that he is having difficulty in receiving speech signals. This is to be expected from the nature of the condition—one of the features is the inability to discriminate speech in ambient noise.

Diagnosis

The need to assess the degree of hearing loss and its effect on the efficiency of the individual is a constantly recurring problem. In order to give the most suitable advice it is essential to take a careful history and to make a full clinical and audiometric examination.

There are many causes of perceptive hearing loss, but those of congenital origin can generally be excluded in aircrew as such a condition will have been detected at the initial medical examination. In taking the history and in the examination, one should therefore consider the following possible aetiological factors:

1. Injury to the skull, either with fracture of the temporal bone or by concussion.
2. The effect of chemical toxins, for example, alcohol, nicotine, quinine; dihydrostreptomycin and other aminoglycoside antibiotics.
3. The effect of bacterial toxins, for example, diphtheria, scarlet fever or syphilis.
4. The effect of viral toxins, for example, mumps, measles and herpes.
5. Meniere's disease.
6. Blood disease.
7. Arteriosclerosis.
8. The effects of noise from engines, workshops or weapons.

The clinical examination, which should take these factors into account, establishes a positive Rinne's test in the affected ear, while Weber's test is referred to the better ear. In the more severe cases, absolute bone conduction, elicited with a tuning fork, will be diminished when a comparison is made with a normal ear. By pure tone air conduction audiometry, losses will be demonstrable at 4 kHz and above. As the condition worsens, losses will extend down to 3 kHz and then to 2 kHz while

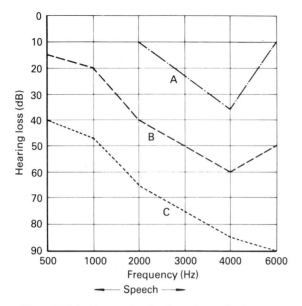

Figure 50.8 Audiogram showing three stages of noise-induced hearing loss. The hearing can be considered as being within limits of normal up to and including a hearing loss of 20 dB at any or all frequencies. (A) Early signs of noise-induced hearing loss. (B) After further exposure to noise the loss spreads to involve the speech frequencies. (C) In the late stage, the hearing loss is advanced and disability severe.

becoming more marked at the higher frequencies (*Figure 50.8*). Hearing levels when measured by pure tone bone conduction audiometry will show a similar pattern to and have the same levels as those measured by air conduction.

Initially, the power of discriminating speech in noise is not lost, but later this faculty deteriorates, and can prove a handicap. In the established case there is recruitment of hearing, which is a characteristic of deafness of cochlear origin. This is shown by diminution in hearing loss with increasing signal loudness. Thus if the acuity of one ear is demonstrably less than the other under normal conditions, the difference will be found to diminish as the loudness of the signal is increased, until a stage is reached when the acuity in each is the same.

Management

For the purpose of this discussion we can assume that all possible causes of the perceptive hearing loss have been enquired into, and that the hearing loss present is attributable to noise.

If the hearing loss involves only 4–8 kHz in one or both ears there is no indication to ground the subject, though regular examination by an otologist should be carried out to determine the subsequent

course of the hearing loss. In those with more extensive hearing loss a rest from flying may bring about a significant degree of recovery. If no recovery occurs, a return to flying may be permitted, provided that there is evidence of good speech discrimination in noise, that suitable ear protection is worn, and that a regular follow-up of the hearing is made.

Generally, despite adequate protection in these cases, as the subject reaches the age of about 45 years the hearing will eventually show some deterioration, which will be due to the physiological changes of early ageing.

In reaching a decision regarding fitness to fly, the examiner should bear several factors in mind:

1. The age of the subject.
2. The extent of the hearing loss and the rate of deterioration of the hearing.
3. The continued ability to discriminate speech signals in noise.
4. The crew role of the subject.

The extent of the hearing loss and the rate of deterioration of the hearing are obviously closely related. For example, a subject with a slowly progressing noise-induced hearing loss with good speech discrimination can be kept flying for years until the speech frequencies begin to show involvement. If further flying is then permitted there is a risk of further deterioration leading to social deafness. Should there be rapid deterioration of the hearing at any age, but particularly in a young subject, grounding is the only course. This is to protect the hearing from further damage and also because the effect of auditory fatigue, superimposed on waning hearing, may produce a degree of hearing loss in flight which can no longer be regarded as safe.

It is impossible to lay down hard and fast rules for those whose hearing fails to reach a given audiometric standard. Each case must be judged on its merits; it is easy to work to absolute standards, but the rigid application of these standards could be wasteful in terms of trained aircrew.

Sometimes, aircrew with apparently normal hearing for speech under test conditions and normal hearing for pure tones, none the less state that they cannot hear accurately in noise. This is quickly noted by other crew members who may lose confidence in the individual affected. It will be found that he does not discriminate speech well in noise when formally tested, and can therefore be considered to be suffering from a loss of faculty for discriminative listening. The cause of this is not known, but it may be psychogenic in origin. If the subject continues to fly, it is likely that he will suffer increasing anxiety, possibly leading to breakdown. The best course is to advise grounding.

Hearing and air traffic control

Air traffic controllers have an important role in aviation. The safety of aircrews and passengers depends on their ability to hear accurately. In general, evidence of hearing loss found at preliminary examination is grounds for unfitness for entry. If hearing loss develops during the course of a career, the type of deafness, and its management will have an influence in deciding fitness to continue. Successful surgical treatment of otosclerosis, or of the effects of trauma or infection in the middle ear, is not necessarily a bar, provided there is no residual vertigo or recurrent discharge.

One should also consider carefully the conditions under which the air traffic controller works and the techniques employed, bearing in mind that much information can come to him in the form of a visual display. Nevertheless, the attendant effects of both fatigue and low-grade ambient noise in depreciating the hearing in sensori-neural hearing loss should be remembered. Where the hearing is well below the hearing standard required, removal from active controlling duties is necessary in the interests of safety, and most controllers are the first to recognize this.

Vestibular disease in aircrew

Introduction

In this chapter we are not concerned with the problem of disorientation, which is dealt with elsewhere, but with the peripheral forms of vertigo, which can be defined as 'a sensation of disturbed equilibrium when the accustomed sense of orientation within one's environment is temporarily disturbed'.

A person experiencing an attack of giddiness generally has a sensation of movement, which may often, but not necessarily, be one of turning. He may stagger or fall: pallor, sweating, nausea and vomiting, and in severe cases even diarrhoea, may occur, and the patient may be prostrate and virtually helpless.

There are several broad groups of conditions that give rise to vertigo either solely or as part of a pattern of other symptoms and signs; these are as follows.

Trauma

This is a well-known cause of vertigo, following fracture of the temporal bone, head injury with concussion of the labyrinth, blast injury or possibly a surgical operation.

Specific infections

Conditions such as syphilis and tuberculous meningitis may also provoke vertigo, but these are rare. The condition may occasionally be caused by focal sepsis in the teeth or nasal sinuses.

The specific fevers

Mumps and measles, for example, may be responsible for producing vertigo—as may viral infections. One of these, vestibular neuronitis, will be discussed more fully.

Acoustic neuroma

Unsteadiness may be late in making its appearance, but can be the presenting symptom. The condition should be excluded in anyone with a unilateral progressive sensori-neural hearing loss.

Local conditions in the middle ear

Otitis media, cholesteatoma, and possible otosclerosis, may provoke vertigo. The diagnosis may be made quickly on the characteristic symptoms and signs of each condition.

Oto-toxic drugs

Alcohol, nicotine, streptomycin and other aminoglycosides such as kanamycin and gentamycin may also be the cause of vertigo.

Blood dyscrasias

Leukaemia may be accompanied by vertigo, and simple anaemia should not be forgotten.

Vertigo

Unless momentary and not repeated (as in that which occasionally accompanies the Valsalva manoeuvre) vertigo is an indication for withdrawal of the patient from flying, until the symptoms are no longer expected to recur. The cockpit is not the place to be incapacitated by an attack of severe vertigo.

It is important that each case should be thoroughly investigated so that the diagnosis and prognosis can be established. Before he is allowed to return to unrestricted flying, a pilot whose symptoms have subsided on the ground may be allowed a period of 'probation', flying with a co-pilot with the later introduction of aerobatics and the application of high G-forces.

Apart from these broad groups, the principal conditions with which one is likely to be concerned are:

1. Meniere's disease.
2. Vestibular neuronitis.
3. Positional (or postural) vertigo.

Meniere's disease

This is a disease of the pressure-regulating mechanism of the endolymphatic system. The cause is not yet known. The process leads to obstructive distention of the membranous portion of the inner ear. Vertigo, deafness and tinnitus comprise the classic syndrome, but a feeling of fullness in the affected ear is also noted and may sometimes be a premonitory symptom. The patient has a perceptive deafness which may be slight, or, in the later stages, almost absolute. While the hearing is deficient during and just after an attack, in the early stages it seems to recover, though a pure tone audiogram may contain evidence of high tone hearing loss. During the attack, speech reception is distorted. There is also sensitivity to sounds of high pitch.

Vertigo is the predominant and disabling symptom. The attack can occur at any time: stress and fatigue are often precipitating factors. The severity may vary. The duration of the attack may be a few minutes or days. Vertigo is almost always accompanied by nausea and sometimes by vomiting, and the symptoms are aggravated by movement. The vagal disturbance is followed by pallor, sweating and an unsteady pulse.

A feature of the disease is its tendency to return. There may be a history of attacks going back for years. In the long term the possibility of recurrence of vertigo undermines the self-confidence of the patient, to the extent that he may fear to cross the road, or have an alcoholic drink, in case an attack should put him in an embarrassing situation. The condition is more common in males than in females, and characteristically occurs in the age-group 30–50 years.

Signs

These include sensori-neural deafness demonstrated by tuning forks, pure tone audiometry, and in the advanced case by speech audiometry. Loudness recruitment is also present. During the attack there is spontaneous nystagmus which may be recorded by electro-oculography. Between attacks, caloric testing shows that labyrinthine responses are absent or abnormal in as many as 90% of cases.

Treatment

Initially, treatment should be direc[ted to] the vertigo and the attendant nause[a. In a] mild case the patient should be put t[o bed; in a] severe attack with vomiting, intramus[cular] mazine may be necessary. Any of [the following] drugs will be found useful, singly or i[n combination:] promethazine theoclate (Avomine, M&B) 25 mg three times daily by mouth; perphenazine (Fentazine A&H) 15 mg three times daily by mouth; or chlorpromazine hydrochloride (Largactil, M&B) 25 mg twice daily or 25 mg intramuscularly.

Vertigo can be controlled also by the use of such agents as dimenhydrinate (Dramamine, Searle), prochlorperazine (Stemetil, M&B) and hyoscine in the acute attacks. Cinnarizine (Stugeron, Janssen) 15–30 mg three times daily is helpful as a vestibular sedative, as is betahistine dihydrochloride (Serc, Duphar) 8 mg twice or three times daily.

Where there is a known history of allergy, antihistaminics may be used with good effect: and for those in the older age-group, vasodilators, such as nicotinic acid.

There are surgical measures available for treating the condition in the long term, the simplest of these being the fitting of a grommet to overcome possible negative pressure effects in the middle ear acting on the inner ear. Other surgical techniques are available to improve the vascular supply to the inner ear, to destroy, sometimes selectively, the end-organ of balance, or to drain off the excessive endolymphatic fluid.

Cases of Meniere's disease, in which surgical treatment has been carried out, sometimes come for assessment of fitness to return to flying, generally on the grounds that the individual is free of vertigo. Any opinion should be guarded, as Meniere's disease tends to affect both ears, and freedom from symptoms in one ear does not guarantee freedom from attack in the other. The diagnosis of Meniere's disease in aircrew effectively means the end of active flying, because no one can predict when the next attack of vertigo will come. If one adds to this the likelihood of increasing perceptive deafness, there is little justification for any disposal other than grounding.

Vestibular neuronitis

In this condition, the vertigo due to vestibular involvement is not associated with any cochlear upset. It is thought to be a selective lesion of the vestibular neurones—perhaps of viral origin. The onset of vertigo is often related to an upper respiratory infection, and while cases may be isolated, they also tend to occur in groups within a community—hence the name 'epidemic labyrinthitis'. Any age-group may be attacked but the 20–50 year age-group is particularly vulnerable. Males and females are equally affected.

Vertigo is accompanied by nausea and sometimes vomiting. During the acute phase vertigo may be frequent: it may be continuous, though varying in severity, for a day or two. Ultimate recovery is the general rule, although the patient may get slightly giddy on sudden movement of the head or body for a period of months, or even occasionally for years. The vertigo has no relationship to the position of the head, and cochlear symptoms and signs are absent. Abnormal caloric vestibular responses are present in nearly every case.

Treatment consists of bed-rest during the early phases, but rapid restoration to full mobility once the symptoms pass. Sedatives and drugs such as dimenhydrinate, prochlorperazine or hyoscine may reduce the nausea.

While the disorder is incapacitating at the time, it tends to be self-limiting, so that return to full flying can be expected. But the patient must be grounded until the symptoms have entirely passed—2–6 months, according to the severity of the symptoms and the rate of recovery. Thereafter, a graduated return to flying may be permitted, first with a co-pilot until the confidence of both patient and doctor is fully established; other members of aircrew may fly once the symptoms and signs of the acute phase have abated.

Finally, it should be remembered that an episode of this nature may be the start of a wider disease process—so that the patient should be kept under review for at least 2 years.

Positional nystagmus of benign paroxysmal type

In this condition, short-lived episodes of vertigo occur directly in relation to a change in position of the head. Each patient has a specific position of the head which induces a short-lived nystagmus and vertigo. If the situation is repeated immediately, each subsequent response is reduced until it finally disappears. The responses to caloric stimulation of the labyrinth are often normal. In addition, cochlear signs and symptoms are absent, though some abnormal hearing responses may be obtained if the condition is associated with middle-ear disease. The condition is believed to follow a degeneration of the maculae of the otolith organs. It requires no treatment, and the patient soon learns to avoid the critical head position. It is uncommon in aircrew though a similar condition may appear after head injury and persist. Provided that the critical head position is one that is uncommon during flight, it is safe to permit flying for most aircrew, though pilots should be advised to avoid high G-forces.

Hearing conversation in ground technicians

Noise seems to be inseparable from aviation. It most affects those who service and handle aircraft on the ground. These men (and women) for part or all of their working life are exposed to noise levels which are hazardous to hearing. To conserve their hearing certain measures are required; these are as follows:

1. A knowledge of the characteristics of the noise, and the duration of exposure, and hence the daily noise dose.
2. Control of exposure.
3. The provision of any necessary protective devices.
4. The measurement of each person's hearing before employment, and at regular intervals during employment.

Opinions vary as to what constitutes a hazardous noise and at what levels hearing conservation programmes should begin; but there is general agreement that noise exposure should be related to an 8-hour working day in terms of a man's working life. Some authorities advocate that a conservation programme should begin if 95 dB SPL (sound pressure level) is attained for 8 hours daily in either of two octaves 300–600 Hz and 600–1200 Hz; others put the figure lower. For military aviation the starting point is taken as 90 dB(A), indicated by a portable sound-level meter.

Measurement of the noise and assessment of risk

The first step in the examination of a potential noise hazard is a full octave band analysis. This requires a wide range of suitable instruments, and the measurement and subsequent analysis is a specialized task. Any variation of level or characteristics with time are of great importance. Details of noise measurement and analysis are contained in Chapter 24.

Finally, one must know the duration of the total daily exposure. With a knowledge of the SPL of the noise in question, its frequency distribution, and the duration and extent of the individual's exposure to it, we are in a position to assess the noise as a risk to hearing. This is done by comparing the spectral analysis of the noise against a chosen damage risk criterion; several versions have been computed but all rely on extrapolations of observed phenomena, and all are designed to define the maximum sound pressure level of a noise to which persons may be exposed if the risk of significant hearing loss is to be avoided. The permitted levels vary according to the frequency. The criteria employed within the Royal Air Force are as follows:

97 dB SPL at   63 Hz
91 dB SPL at   125 Hz
87 dB SPL at   250 Hz
84 dB SPL at   500 Hz
82 dB SPL at 1000 Hz
80 dB SPL at 2000 Hz
79 dB SPL at 4000 Hz
78 dB SPL at 8000 Hz

The frequency spectrum should be analysed and the components compared with the damage risk criteria. If the SPLs exceed the criteria, then protective measures must be taken.

Some factors in the character of the noise and in the type of exposure may alter the significance of such a comparison; for example, the criteria above should not be used for exposure to impulsive noise, such as that associated with riveting, hammering or small-arms firing.

L_{eq} and assessment of risk: the equal-energy principle

It has been shown that for steady-state noise, a relationship exists between A-weighted sound energy and persistent hearing loss—the 'equal-energy principle'—and this can be extended to include impact and weapon noise. This is expressed as equivalent continuous sound, L_{eq}, which is defined as the level of continuous noise in dB(A) which in the course of a working day would cause the same sound energy to be received as that from the actual noise in the same period. For convenience a working day is considered to be of 8 hours duration. The maximum permitted noise level is now regarded generally as being 90 dB(A) over 8 hours. *Table 50.1* shows a range of sound levels in dB(A), with permissible exposure times per day, each represent-

Table 50.1 Permissible equivalent continuous sound level (L_{eq}) for an 8 hour working day for the unprotected ear

Sound level dB(A)	Permissible duration of exposure per day
90	8 hours
93	4 hours
96	2 hours
99	1 hour
102	30 minutes
105	15 minutes
108	7½ minutes
111	225 seconds
114	112 seconds
117	56 seconds
120	28 seconds
123	14 seconds
126	7 seconds
129	3½ seconds
132	1¾ seconds
135	Under 1 second

From: Department of Employment (1972).

ing an L_{eq} of 90 dB(A) for 8 hours. These levels are advocated as the maximum permissible levels for noise exposure for the unprotected ear.

In order to measure equivalent continuous noise level, both sound level and time must be measured. This is achieved with a sound level meter which conforms to a recognized specification set to the A-weighting network, and a timepiece to measure exposure time.

Where there is wide fluctuation in the noise levels and the time scale, a work-study investigation may be required. In terms of individuals it may be necessary to measure their noise exposure, during a working day, by means of a noise *dosimeter*. While a static dosimeter may be employed the portable variation is that which is favoured. Such a monitor measures both A-weighted sound level and duration at the same time and provides a direct measure of L_{eq}.

Protection of the hearing

There are three ways to reduce the noise reaching an individual: diminishing at source the energy radiated; attenuating the energy; or removing the source to a distance. Sound-reducing devices may adversely affect the performance of aircraft, though some improvement can be attained. The residual noise when the aircraft is on the ground can be tackled by siting run-up areas at a distance, by employing engine detuners, earth walls, corrugated sloping fences and concrete walls; and by the attenuation provided by appropriate building techniques—insulation of walls, roofs and windows of buildings in which people work or live.

A combination of building techniques, sound-proofing and an engine detuner has resulted in the 'hush house', an engine-running cell which provides hazard-free observation by engineers, and a reduction in outside environmental noise of the order of 55 dB(A).

Protection of the individual hearing may be achieved by reduction of the noise reaching the hearing organ, and by reduction of the duration of exposure. The effectiveness of both measures can be monitored by pure tone audiometry conducted at intervals throughout the man's working life. Noise entering the ear can be reduced by wearing plugs in the external ear canal, or by protecting the ear and surrounding bone by a muff or helmet. Where noise levels, though harmful, are not excessively high, there may be difficulty in getting a man to wear protection, though this is not the case where the levels are so high that exposure is painful.

Ear plugs

Absorbent material may be used to plug the meatus. Cotton wool is the commonest, though its protective powers are slight. Glass down is frequently recommended, particularly for short-term exposure, and has an average attenuation of the order of 20 dB. It is cheap, disposable and comfortable, and irritation of the skin does not occur. When ground crew travel in noisy transport aircraft, those who have no personal ear plugs or ear defenders can be made more comfortable by glass down.

Personal insert ear plugs are made in a variety of designs, of which the most widely accepted is that made of soft synthetic rubber in five sizes. It is comfortable, and its attenuation ranges from 18 to 25 dB, being least at the low frequencies and best at 4 kHz (32 dB) (*Table 50.2*). Such plugs are effective

Table 50.2 Hearing conservation in ground technicians. Attenuation provided by glass down, the synthetic rubber ear plug and fluid-seal ear muffs

Octave band centre-frequency (Hz)	Attenuation value (dB)		
	Glass down	Synthetic rubber ear plug	Fluid-seal muff
63		11	17
125		13	18
250	11	15	20
500	13	18	30
1000	16	22	38
2000	26	27	40
4000	33	32	43
8000		29	35

From: Burns (1965).

only if they fit properly, and the size should be decided not just by the individual but by someone with fitting experience. If a plug is too tight it will be uncomfortable, though without some sensation of pressure in the external ear there is unlikely to be good attenuation. Plugs should be washed regularly in warm soapy water, being dried carefully before they are used again. If the wearer does not look after them he will contaminate the meatal skin and this can lead to otitis externa. Likewise, the onset of otitis externa will preclude the wearing of ear plugs, and may necessitate withdrawal of the individual from a noise-exposed working site.

Ear muffs

There are many variations in the design of ear muff but the basic pattern incorporates a pair of ear cups, generally made of plastic material, which fit over the ears and are secured in place by a tensile head band. The inside hollow of the cup is filled with synthetic sponge rubber, and may be occupied by an ear microphone. The edge of the cup is fitted with a fluid or foam seal of plastic or rubber, which provides a close fit to the head and gives good attenuation. The

attenuation provided by a muff is better than any other ear protection worn alone, being about 17 dB at the low frequencies, and improving to 40 dB or more at 2 and 4 kHz.

If ear muffs are used on a communal basis, particularly in hot humid climates, care must be exercised to prevent transmission of otitis externa from person to person. This can be controlled by washing the muff weekly with a solution of carbolic soap 5 g in 1 litre warm water, with separate washing of the foam pads, followed by drying in the sun and fresh air.

If adequate protection cannot be provided by a single ear muff or ear plug, both types may be worn together to provide better attenuation.

Helmets

The original patterns of helmet, designed principally for aircrew, were made of cloth, canvas or leather with varying sizes of the circumaural 'bun' of padded leather which provided a slight degree of attenuation against noise. This basic head cover has been utilized to support an ear muff, generally of fluid-seal pattern, with or without a telephone attachment. With the helmet secured by a chin strap, the ear protection is held firmly in place, so that this type of design is very suitable in exposed and very noisy situations such as the flight deck of an aircraft carrier. Suitable colouring or marking of the helmet also provides an indication of the wearer's role.

Aircrew in military aircraft usually wear a rigid protective helmet. It is designed to provide buffet and crash protection for the head, as well as a suitable mounting for an anti-glare visor and an oxygen and communications mask. The inside of the helmet is padded, and this, with the fibreglass which forms the shell of the helmet, provides sound attenuation which is further increased by seals around the ears. The level of attenuation of such a helmet when worn with an oxygen mask can be up to 40–41 dB. (*See* Chapter 24.)

Jerkins

If exposure to noise levels of 145 dB or more is undertaken, even for a short time, the body requires protection by a garment designed to break up the sound falling on the body and so prevent the visceral effects of noise, and reduce the volume of sound reaching the skull via the vertebral column. Since such garments cut down mobility, are heavy and hot, the cover is normally restricted to the trunk. It is doubtful if any of the known designs of jerkin could or would be worn for long in hot, humid climates. (*See* Chapter 14.)

Advice on protection

A decision regarding the correct form of protective equipment to employ may be reached by subtracting the attenuation values of the ear defender from the SPL of the noise, measured at the same octave bands. The resultant figure may then be compared with the chosen damage risk criterion, which will show which device will be adequate.

Whatever protective device is used, it should be remembered that, in actual use, the attenuation may drop by as much as 5 dB because the defender will work loose when the wearer moves about, and because head springs of ear muffs may be eased to make them more comfortable in wear.

In aviation it is unusual for ground personnel to be exposed to continuous noise during their working day. There are, of course, exceptions such as marshallers at busy airports and those employed on test beds and engine running. For these groups, if the overall level of noise falling on the unprotected ear during a full working day is greater than the permissible level, safety can be achieved by reducing the duration of exposure.

Where noise is continuous, the problem of protection and possible reduction in exposure are straightforward but where noise levels are variable in intensity and pattern, and the interval between each exposure short, with possibly little chance of recovery, the problem is more complex. In any instance where men are working in hazardous conditions with noise continuously or intermittently above a 'protected' criteria, advice should be sought of a specialist in this field regarding limitation of exposure.

Audiometric checking

The principles of audiometric measurement of the hearing have been discussed. If the data obtained are to be useful and reproducible, the hearing measurements should be carried out in standard circumstances using standardized equipment operated by properly trained technicians. The ears should be checked by a physician before audiometry to determine the presence of wax or discharge. A full clinical history should be obtained including that of any previous exposure to noise.

On entry into a noise-exposed job, a person's hearing should be measured by some form of pure tone audiometry. This will form a baseline for comparison and will also detect those who show any existing high tone loss which may predispose to noise damage. Those susceptible can be excluded from noise-hazardous trades, or else steps can be taken to ensure that such people have a full understanding of the damaging effect of noise and its consequences and that they are adequately protected and supervised. Follow-up audiometric examination should be repeated at routine intervals during the individual's working life, while he remains exposed to noise. An annual check is both practical and convenient.

The greatest change in the hearing in those susceptible to noise or those working in very high noise levels occurs early during exposure. This loss is, in a sense, protective. When susceptibility is known, an audiometric check should be repeated 6 months after starting in employment, and again after a further 6 months.

Management of those with hearing loss

If an audiogram shows evidence of noise-induced hearing loss, it will be necessary to decide whether the individual should continue in a noise-exposed occupation. The age, the extent of the hearing loss, and the type and frequency of exposure should all be considered.

When early signs of hearing loss appear at 4 kHz and above, it is probably sufficient to draw the attention of the individual to the loss, to warn him of its nature and the possible consequence. He should be provided with properly fitting ear protection and given instruction in its use and how to care for it. It is often advantageous to check the hearing by audiometry in 3 months and again 3 months later. If the result is unchanged the man can continue at work, properly protected, and audiometric and clinical checks can be made at yearly intervals. Sometimes a change from one type of defender to another may be indicated. Misleading results can be obtained if the hearing is measured too soon after a noise exposure, when there can be a temporary raising of the hearing threshold. If possible the hearing should always be tested when the man has been away from noise for at least 24, and preferably 48, hours.

Sometimes the hearing loss may be apparent early in a person's career and then remain unaltered for years. From the age of 40 years onwards additional change starts, and this is probably the sum of two factors at work—the cumulative effect of noise and the early changes of physiological ageing. The two combined can produce a sudden and dramatic deterioration in the hearing.

Individuals with this sort of hearing loss and those in whom a loss is first detected in middle age need careful management. Such a man will be both experienced and skilled, and premature withdrawal from his chosen work may have serious personal consequences. If he continues in the same way, however, he may become unable to discriminate speech, particularly in ambient noise. He will, in a word, be deaf. Tinnitus may be present, and this with the deafness may combine to make him irritable and withdrawn. The air conduction audiogram will show a loss extending down to 2 kHz and possibly involving 1 kHz, or lower in the frequency range.

If there is no cause other than noise for the hearing loss, it is essential to remove the individual from his noisy working environment and recheck the hearing in 2 or 3 months. Any improvement after this period will indicate the capacity for recovery. Ear protectors should be checked, as well as the noise pattern at his working site. Another 2 or 3 months away from noise will achieve as much recovery as is possible, when a return to work in noise, fully protected and not over-exposed, and under routine supervision, should be permitted.

If no improvement appears in the audiogram, and if none is forthcoming after a rest from noise of 2 or 3 months, what should be done? In some circumstances a man can continue in his trade in a supervisory or instructional capacity but unexposed to hazardous noise. This is the preferable course, but if it is not possible a return to work fully protected—with three-monthly checking of the hearing—may be permitted. Any subsequent deterioration of the hearing would require complete removal from a noise-exposed job, to save the man from disabling deafness. Beyond the age of 50 years, any deterioration in the hearing in the protected ear is probably due to early presbycusis. Removal from noise in such a case will not necessarily abate the hearing loss, which may worsen as age increases until a severe disability is present.

In addition, two further facets must be mentioned; pre-existent sensori-neural deafness from any cause should make an individual unfit for entry to a noise-exposed trade: and if sensori-neural deafness develops from any cause other than noise in a man in a noise-exposed trade, one should take the greatest care before deciding to allow him to continue.

Established deafness

In the established case of noise-induced hearing loss with a marked permanent threshold shift no medication is likely to be helpful.

It is worth trying a hearing aid if the patient has difficulty in discriminating speech, either at work or socially. Commonly, an aid worn at ear level will be both convenient and suitable. For this type of deafness performance can be improved by techniques such as 'peak clipping' which eliminates sound distortion due to overloading of the sound amplifying system and automatic volume control. It should be remembered that no aid can remove the difficulty, inherent in the damaged cochlea, in interpreting speech signals in ambient noise, so that in these conditions the wearer may face disappointment. Finally, for the severely deafened, lip reading

instruction will help. This, combined with an aid, will do much to reduce the disability.

The control of tinnitus may prove difficult. In some, tinnitus is disproportionately greater than the hearing loss, and in these some form of masking device may help if other treatment fails.

Stapedectomy

Ground engineers who have had the operation of stapedectomy for otosclerosis are particularly vulnerable to noise on return to work. This is principally because the protective stapedial reflex is lost in most of them. Every effort should be made to ensure that these patients understand the significance of the operation in relation to their job, and the importance of wearing ear protection whenever they are exposed to noise.

Bibliography

ARMSTRONG, H.G. and HEIM, J.W. (1937) The effect of flight on the middle ear. *Journal of the American Medical Association*, **109**, 417–421

British Standards Institution (1954) *British Standard 2497. The Threshold of Hearing for Pure Tones by Earphone Listening*. London: BSI

British Standards Institution (1958) *British Standard 2480. Pure Tone Audiometry*. London: BSI

BURNS, W. (1965) Noise as an environmental factor in industry. *Transactions of the Association of Industrial Medical Officers*, **15**, 2

Department of Employment (1972) *The Code of Practice for Reducing the Exposure of Employed Persons to Noise*. Industrial Health Advisory Committee Sub-Committee on Noise. London: HMSO

DICKSON, E.D.D., MCGIBBON, J.E.G. and CAMPBELL, A.C.P. (1947) Acute otitic barotrauma—clinical findings, mechanism, and relationship to the pathological changes produced experimentally in the middle ears of cats by variations of pressure. In Dickson, E.D.D. (ed.) *Contributions to Aviation Otolaryngology*, pp. 60–83. London: Headley Brothers

FRENZEL, H. (1950) Otorhinolaryngology. In *German Aviation Medicine World War II*. Vol. 2, pp. 977–984. Washington: Government Printing Office

GOODHILL, V. (1971) Sudden deafness and round window rupture. *Laryngoscope*, **81**, 1462–1474

International Organisation for Standardisation (1971) *Assessment of Occupational Noise Exposure for Hearing Conservation Purposes*. Recommendation R 1999. International Organisation for Standardisation

KING, P.F. (1965) Sinus barotrauma. In Gillies, J.A. (ed.) *A Textbook of Aviation Physiology*, pp. 112–121. London: Pergamon Press

MCGIBBON, J.E.G. (1947) Nasal sinus pain caused by flying. In Dickson, E.D.D. (ed.) *Contributions to Aviation Otolaryngology*, pp. 134–155. London: Headley Brothers

RAYMAN, R.B. (1972) Stapedectomy: a threat to flying safety? *Aerospace Medicine*, **43**, 454–550

51

Ophthalmological conditions and the examination of the eye

J. Cloherty

Fundamental principles

Introduction

Without vision man cannot fly, and since the earliest days of aviation the possession of a high standard of vision has therefore been a positive requirement as 80% of flight information is visually acquired (Stringer, 1978). In the past, in aircraft with open cockpits and with the pilot wearing a relatively ill-fitting helmet and goggles, this high standard had to be achieved without the use of spectacles or other aids. Today, with closed cockpits and with aircrew wearing well-fitting helmets or headsets, correction of defective vision in trained aircrew is generally accepted, and in some roles the training of new recruits who need spectacles is permitted although this may cause problems with the integration with advanced optical equipment.

In aviation the basic requirements are that the subject shall possess two eyes which see clearly distant and near objects; that the ocular muscle balance shall be within the normally accepted limits; that there shall be no significant restriction of the fields of vision; that colour perception shall be safe for the performance of flying duties and that neither the eyes nor their adnexa shall contain an anomaly likely to prejudice the safety of the individual or the aircraft and its contents.

Vision outside the aircraft is of great importance even with the development of radar and other devices. With the increase in number and complexity of instruments, vision inside the aircraft has also become a greater problem, particularly in the case of ageing aircrew who need spectacles to read hand-held material and overhead instruments.

In this chapter these functions and their anomalies will be described and their significance in aviation

will be discussed. As separate items a suggested form of examination will be given and recommendations made on the assessment of clinical findings.

Other attributes of vision such as dynamic visual acuity, speed of perception and/or interpretation, particularly in the high-speed low-level role, are considered in Chapter 23.

Visual acuity

Visual acuity may be defined as the ability of the eye to perceive form and is normally measured by reference to the visual angle subtended at the eye by a target; normal distant vision being assumed if a letter composed of lines subtending 1 minute of arc at the eye (the whole letter subtending 5 minutes of arc) can be correctly read (*Table 51.1*).

Near vision is normally measured by the ability to read standard printer's type of various sizes, the

Table 51.1 Equivalences of United Kingdom, United States and decimal visual acuities. Common values are in bold type

UK	USA	Decimal
6/3	20/10	2.0
6/4	20/13	**1.5**
6/4.6	**20/15**	1.3
6/5	20/16	1.25
6/6	**20/20**	**1.0**
6/9	**20/30**	0.7
6/12	**20/40**	**0.5**
6/15	**20/50**	**0.4**
6/18	20/60	0.3
6/21	**20/70**	0.28
6/24	20/80	0.25
6/30	**20/100**	**0.2**
6/36	20/120	0.16
6/60	**20/200**	**0.1**

666

present ICAO recommended type being the Times Roman N series, normal vision being assumed when the N5 size type can be read at a distance which, in the normal eye, is dependent on age (*see* Chapter 23—form vision).

Accommodation

The refracting structures of the eye—cornea, aqueous, lens and vitreous—together act as a lens of approximately 58 dioptres power which, in the normal eye, converges parallel rays of light to a focus on the retina according to the normal rules of geometrical optics.

If the object of regard is brought closer to the eye the place of image formation will fall behind the retina (*Figure 51.1*).

In order to maintain clear vision the process of accommodation occurs, whereby the lens becomes

more spherical, thus increasing its converging power, bringing the image to a focus upon the retina (*Figure 51.2*).

When the stimulus for near vision has been received, action of the third cranial nerve results in a convergence of the optic axes to maintain the position of the images on the foveae. Constriction of the pupils follows this and diminishes the spherical aberration produced by the periphery of the lens and increases the depth of field.

In each eye, contraction of the ciliary muscle draws the ciliary body forward around the circumference of the globe allowing the ciliary processes, to which are attached the zonular ligaments of the lens, to approach the centre of the eye. This relaxation of the zonule reduces the tension of the lens capsule which, due to its elasticity, moulds the soft lens cortex into a lens of greater power which moves forward towards the anterior chamber. On relaxation of accommodation,

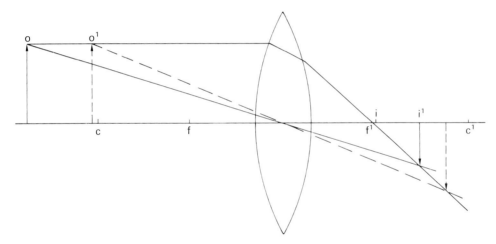

Figure 51.1 The geometrical formation of images.

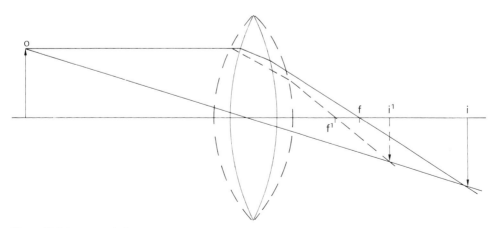

Figure 51.2 Accommodation.

the elasticity of the choroid draws the ciliary body backwards, thus restoring tension to the zonule, flattening the lens, and therefore reducing its power.

Accommodation is synchronous and equal in both eyes. Its amplitude represents the dynamic refracting power of the eye, and is the difference between the refracting power of the eye at rest when focused at its far point and the refractive power when maximum accommodation is exerted and the eye is focused at its near point. The amplitude of accommodation may be measured in dioptres or by measurement of the near point, the closest distance in centimetres from the eye at which small type can be read clearly.

The dioptre (D) is a unit representing the converging power of a lens and is defined as the reciprocal of the focal length of the lens expressed in metres. A lens with a focal length of 0.5 m therefore has a power of 1/0.50 = 2D.

The conversion of the near point in metres to amplitude of accommodation in dioptres or vice versa may be achieved by calculating the reciprocal of the unit available; for example, a near point of 0.25 m gives an amplitude of 1/0.25 = 4D. An amplitude of 5D gives a near point of 1/5 = 0.2 m.

The change of accommodation with age

Owing to progressive sclerosis and loss of elasticity of the lens the amplitude of accommodation diminishes with age, as is shown by a recession of the near point. This change commences in childhood, and when it has progressed to the stage when the individual can no longer see clearly at a practicable reading or near-working distance, the state of presbyopia is reached. This generally occurs at about the age of 46.

If normal distant or near vision cannot be achieved a refractive error may be present.

Refractive conditions

Production

Emmetropia results when growth of the eye proceeds in a perfectly co-ordinated manner so that optical perfection is obtained. Such a state is rare and some degree of refractive error is found in the majority of eyes. Most of these errors are simple and are due to a slight lack of co-ordination of development of the various parts of the refractive system and therefore only represent a biological variation from the norm and must not in any way be regarded as pathological.

Pathological refractive errors are relatively uncommon. They are due often to a gross abnormality of development and may often be hereditary and often show racial characteristics. The degree of error is usually high and the visual acuity is often not

fully correctable while, particularly in myopia, the eye may show visible degenerative changes.

Age variation

At birth the majority of children are hypermetropic; between birth and the age of 8 years this hypermetropia is seen to increase. After this age the refraction changes to being less hypermetropic or more myopic until approximately the age of 25–30 years when relative stability is reached. With the onset of middle age a slight increase in hypermetropia is seen, and at approximately the age of 65 years increasing sclerosis of the lens produces a final change towards myopia (*Figure 51.3*).

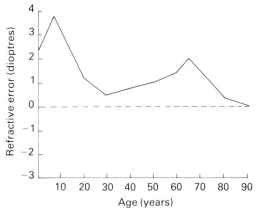

Figure 51.3 The age norms of refraction.

If, therefore, a child starts life with less than the average degree of hypermetropia, the natural reduction in hypermetropia or the increase in myopia can result in the development of overt myopia, a development that is likely to progress until the age of 25–30 years, when some degree of stability should be attained.

The variables, however, are such that it is most difficult to give an accurate prognosis of the progress of refractive errors since individual cases do not necessarily follow the population norm, and it is frequently seen in those who develop frank myopia that the progression is more rapid than for those who remain hypermetropic.

Care should therefore be taken in assessing young candidates for aviation training, particularly those in whom there is a recent history of low myopia, because in these there is a significant chance that they may need flying spectacles at an early age. Some organizations are unwilling to retain aircrew who require spectacles in flight.

Hypermetropia (Hm)

The hypermetropic eye may be considered as one in which either the axial length of the globe is less than normal or one in which the refracting media are less efficient. Parallel rays of light are thus brought to a focus 'behind' the retina. This defect is capable of correction to a greater or lesser degree by the exercise of accommodation.

The total amount of Hm present may be subdivided as follows:

Total		
Latent	Manifest	
	Facultative	Absolute

Latent Hm

The amount corrected by the normal physiological tone of the ciliary muscle. This amount is usually considered to be of the order of 1 dioptre and is normally demonstrable only under cycloplegia.

Manifest Hm

The amount uncorrected by the normal physiological tone of the ciliary muscle. This is subdivided into:

1. *Facultative Hm*—The amount correctable by an effort of accommodation.
2. *Absolute Hm*—The remainder unable to be corrected by an effort of accommodation.

With increasing age the amount of facultative Hm falls and absolute Hm increases, until all manifest Hm becomes absolute.

Total Hm: Latent + Manifest

In youth, when accommodation is active and the refractive error lies within the facultative range, an effort of accommodation will produce clear vision for far and near without symptoms; but with increasing age a decreased amplitude of accommodation leads to ocular fatigue, recession of the near point and, when the facultative Hm becomes absolute, to a decrease of unaided visual acuity.

For example (*Figure 51.4, curve B*), at the age of 12 years, a child with 4D of Hm has an accommodation of 13D available: 4D of the 13D will be used to overcome the refractive error, leaving 9D in reserve. Normal distant vision will be produced and the near point will be 11 cm.

At the age of 36 years, only 7D of accommodation are available: 4D will be used to overcome the error, leaving 3D in reserve. Clear distant vision will be possible, but symptoms of ocular fatigue are likely to be present and the near point will have receded to 33 cm (0.33 m).

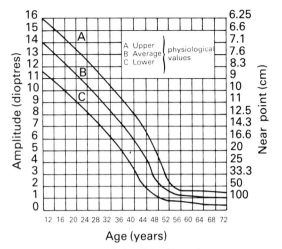

Figure 51.4 Accommodation (after Duane).

At the age of 44 years, 4D of accommodation are available. All the facultative Hm will be overcome by a maximum accommodative effort to see clearly at infinity and there will be none in reserve for close work. Distant vision may be clear but uncomfortable, but will probably be defective owing to accommodative fatigue preventing continued maximum effort.

At the age of 46 years, 3D of accommodation are available. This is insufficient to overcome the refractive error and the residual 1D of absolute hypermetropia leads to a fall of distant acuity to approximately 6/12 (*Figure 51.5*). Reading without the aid of spectacles will be impossible.

With increasing age more of the facultative Hm becomes absolute and the unaided distant acuity falls further, due not to an increase in the hypermetropia, but to a physiological failure of accommodation.

Myopia

Myopia is that optical condition in which parallel rays of light come to a focus in front of the retina. The condition occurs because the refractive power is too great for the length of the eye or because the eye is too long for the refractive power present. The condition is corrected by a concave or negative power lens, which diverges the light rays to bring them to a retinal focus.

Simple myopia, being a variant of normal growth, may show itself in childhood as a low degree of hypermetropia which decreases, or as emmetropia which becomes myopia. This tendency may progress through puberty and adolescence until stability is reached at maturity.

Whether or not progress occurs the simple myopic eye remains healthy, and must in no way be regarded as abnormal or diseased.

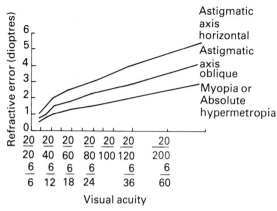

Figure 51.5 Approximate visual acuity and refractive errors.

As accommodation cannot correct myopia, the effect of the refractive error on the unaided acuity is marked (*Figure 51.5*), but it is frequently seen that young myopes can resolve small targets with remarkable ease.

With increasing age the unaided visual acuity of the myopic eye may be seen to fall. This may be because of a deterioration at the perceptual level and not necessarily to an increase in refractive error.

As the far point is at a finite distance from the eye, near vision is good and failure of accommodation does not lead to the onset of presbyopia at an early age.

Astigmatism

Astigmatism is an optical condition in which the refracting power of the eye is unequal in different meridians. Thus if the refracting power of the eye is 58 dioptres in the vertical and 60 dioptres in the horizontal meridian, two dioptres of astigmatism would be present. Astigmatism may be myopic where both meridians are focused in front of the retina, or hypermetropic where both meridians are intercepted by the retina before reaching a focus, or mixed where one meridian is focused in front of the retina and the other behind the retina. Lines at 90° with respect to each other cannot be brought to a common focus. For example, vertical lines may be brought to a focus in the 60D meridian whereas horizontal lines in the 58D meridian are blurred. The converse applies to the 58D meridian; when horizontal lines are sharp the vertical lines are blurred.

Ninety-five per cent of eyes show at least 0.5D astigmatism, and an error of over 6D is normally found in a pathological eye (that is, one affected by corneal trauma, conical cornea, dislocated lens, and so on) the 'Rule' being that the axis of astigmatism is horizontal in negative errors and vertical in positive

errors; astigmatic errors 'Against the Rule' being seen when the axis is at right-angles to these directions. It is generally accepted that such errors produce ocular symptoms.

Astigmatic errors may vary greatly in a random fashion with increasing age, and frequently the axis changes through a right-angle in old age.

Presbyopia

Accommodation increases the refractive power of the anterior segment by causing an increased curvature and thickness of the lens. This change in the shape of the lens occurs because of its inherent elasticity. The contraction of the ciliary muscle causes relaxation of the zonule and allows the lens to become more spherical. The lens loses its elasticity with age, the loss of accommodation being progressive with each year of life. Generally, there are about 14D of accommodation at the age of 10 years and by the age of 50 years this has fallen to 2D. The decrease occurs gradually, but when only 2D of accommodation remains, the near point is extended to 0.5 m from the eye. This results in difficulties in reading or other close work (*see Figure 51.4*).

In a hypermetrope, whose near point is further away than that of an emmetrope, presbyopia occurs earlier.

In a myope, who has a closer near point, the onset is later, or may not occur.

Treatment

Hypermetropia

In the absence of ocular symptoms, defective vision, heterophoria or squint, treatment is not required; but when any of these anomalies are present, convex lenses are required to reduce the need for accommodation.

Myopia

Concave lenses of sufficient power to produce comfortable and adequate vision are needed. Over-correction must be avoided as this will lead to over-accommodation.

Astigmatism

Cylindrical lenses are needed which have maximum power in one meridian and are a focal in the meridian at right-angles, this latter meridian being the axis of the lens. Spherical and cylindrical lenses of equal or opposite sign can be combined into a sphero-cylindrical lens. The type of astigmatism for which such lenses are needed is described according to the combined powers required; for example, hypermetropic astigmatism, myopic astigmatism or mixed astigmatism.

Astigmatic refractive errors are sometimes referred to by the term equivalent spherical error (ESE). This represents the sum of the spherical component of the error plus half the cylindrical component.

For example:

Spherical +3.00D with cylindrical +2.00D = (+3)+(+1) = ESE 4.00
Spherical −2.00D with cylindrical +1.00D = (−2)+(+0.50) = ESE −1.50

Lens prescriptions can be transposed. In transposition the algebraic powers of the sphere and cylinder are added to arrive at the new spherical power. The sign plus or minus on the cylinder is reversed and the axis of the cylinder is rotated through 90 degrees.

For example,

$$\frac{-2.00D \text{ sphere}}{+3.00D \text{ cylinder}} \text{axis } 90°$$

can be expressed also as:

$$\frac{+1.0D \text{ sphere}}{-3.00D \text{ cylinder}} \text{axis } 180°$$

A recent amendment to Annex 1 (Personnel Licencing) to the Convention on International Civil Aviation recommends the use of the equivalent spherical error notation in determining the fitness of initial applicants for professional and private pilots' licences.

Presbyopia

Convex lenses of gradually increasing power are required after the age of 40 years until the age of 65 years is reached, when further increase ceases. There are wide personal, familial and racial variations to this rule.

As changes of refraction or an increase of presbyopia are among the most common reasons for the referral of aircrew for specialist ophthalmic examination, their cause and natural history should be understood. It should seldom be necessary to recommend the removal of a trained member of aircrew from active flying due to the onset, or change, of a simple refractive error, provided both uncorrected and corrected vision are likely to remain at a safe level.

Spectacles

The examination for and the prescription of a spectacle correction should, whenever possible, be carried out by an examiner with some knowledge of the problems of vision in aviation, so that lenses and frames compatible with the aircrew task and equipment assemblies can be supplied. Also, presbyopic examinees should be advised to provide the examiner with a measure of the near working distance and field of vision required so that appropriate half-eye or multifocal lenses can be prescribed. Reading lenses must not be too strong, lest they significantly reduce visual acuity at the instrument panel distance.

The spectacle frame prescribed should be thin and light (preferably of metal) in order to reduce obstruction of the field of vision, and should completely surround the lens. The nylon thread or rimless type of spectacle are a flight hazard and should be avoided. The spectacle side-pieces should also be thin to avoid breaking the noise seal of the headset and to avoid painful pressure on the ears by a close-fitting helmet.

Concern is naturally felt, and often expressed, by aircrew and aviation organizations, that loss or breakage of spectacles in the air may constitute a flight hazard. It is difficult to convince an occasional or non-spectacle wearer that correctly chosen spectacles are rarely broken whilst on the face and aviation ophthalmologists agree that such incidents are most uncommon.

Over the years, however, there have been few instances reported in the Royal Air Force of lenses falling from their frames because of loose retaining screws. There are also cases on record of pilots ejecting from their aircraft without loss of spectacles.

In order to reduce ocular and facial injury in accidents, e.g. from birdstrike, spectacle lenses should preferably be of a synthetic material such as CR39 resin or polycarbonate and should not be made of glass. Polycarbonate lenses possess the maximum impact resistance but in higher powers their low 'V' factor or prismatic effect causes the dispersion of light into its spectral components. The resulting colour fringes reduce the wearer's acuity, and the use of polycarbonate lenses by aircrew is restricted to the lower powered lenses. Lenses may be of single vision or multifocal type, but lenses of continuous or variable focus are inadvisable owing to the distortion produced in their periphery.

Tinted lenses, either plano or corrective, may be prescribed where necessary, but these should be of good optical quality as the cheaper blown lenses, which are not optically worked, often distort vision. The polarizing type of tinted lens is also inadvisable owing to the bi-refringent patterns produced when worn in aircraft or cars fitted with toughened transparencies. With certain treated transparencies which also polarize light, the use of such lenses seriously reduces vision outside the aircraft, and some aircrew complain of distracting scintillation at high altitude.

In the RAF all aircrew wearing helmets with visors, one of which is tinted, are forbidden to wear tinted spectacles in flight. The combination of tinted spectacles and tinted visor could be hazardous under certain environmental conditions.

The use of corrective photochromic lenses may cause problems in flight owing to the dynamics of the photochromic chemicals, which darken rapidly but recover to a high transmittance slowly. This may cause difficulties when descending below clouds from bright ambient conditions above.

Contact lenses

Contact lenses should, in theory, produce excellent visual correction but they have not yet received full approval for use in aviation. In a well-motivated patient who has achieved a full working day's tolerance, visual results with the hard micro-corneal lenses are excellent; visual acuity is good, there is no obstruction of the visual field and there are no problems of integration with the helmet and oxygen mask. However, difficulties can be encountered with dust or other small foreign bodies passing between the lens and the cornea, and in cases such as this, and also in the presence of low flight-deck humidity, which leads to drying of the surface of the eyeball allowing the contact lens to adhere to the corneal epithelium, painful corneal abrasions may result which require removal of the wearer from flying for some days until healing is complete. The long duration of some civil and military flights may also lead to similar disabilities.

Since 1950 contact lenses have become an acceptable optical aid in the functional replacement of spectacles, although their use is not permitted by some air forces.

There are various types of contact lenses available and a few are suitable for pilots (Cloherty, 1985):

1. *The scleral or haptic contact lens* covers the anterior surface of the globe. It is large and uncomfortable, visual acuity is variable and air bubbles beneath the lens on decompression are commonplace. It is unsuitable for pilots, though such lenses may have a role in ocular therapy.
2. *The micro-corneal hard contact lens*—This lens is composed of either a polymethylmethacrylate (PMMA) material or an oxygen-permeable polymer mixture. The majority of such PMMA lenses have an overall diameter of 8–10 mm and rest on a thin tear film on the cornea. A well-fitted lens can move 3–4 mm on blinking without any loss of visual acuity or discomfort to the subject. Such lenses are only suitable for daily wear and cannot be worn for longer than 1 day without the onset of blurred vision and a painful red eye owing to corneal hypoxia.

   A new range of oxygen-permeable hard lenses is becoming available and these have an extended wear capacity. They are thinner and more delicate than the original daily wear PMMA lens. Hard lenses are not used by military pilots because they can readily become dislodged due to vibration or G forces, and are too great a hazard. A foreign body under a hard lens is also a hazard.
3. *The 38% water content soft contact lens*—The majority of soft contact lenses are of this type. This lens is oxygen permeable, and the diameter is between 12.5 and 13.5 mm. It is comfortable and gives good visual acuity in most people. A well-fitted lens moves 1–2 mm on blinking, floating on the fine tear film layer between the lens and the cornea. They are also daily-wear lenses and should not be worn longer or the wearer will develop the symptoms and signs of corneal hypoxia. These lenses are not used by RAF aircrew because of the limitation of daily wear. In the operational environment the airman may not be able to sterilize his lenses, and hostilities may not permit adequate rest periods when the lenses can be removed.
4. *The high water content soft contact lens*—A high water content contact lens (70–80%) possesses a high oxygen permeability; the diameter is between 13.5 and 14.5 mm. It is comfortable and a good visual acuity is normally achieved. A well-fitted lens also floats on a fine tear film, and moves 1–2 mm on blinking. Such lenses can usually be worn constantly for periods extending from weeks to months.
5. *The silicone lens*—This lens has the highest oxygen transmissability factor of all contact lenses. However, its surface is hydrophobic and the surfaces have to be specially treated to make it hydrophilic and thus wettable, this reduces its life. Its other attributes are similar to the high water content lenses.

A civil pilot may wear either a hard or a soft contact lens as he will have daily access to maintenance equipment and be assured of adequate rest periods. It is advisable that he flies with another pilot so that in the unlikely event of him suffering a foreign body in his eye he can remove his lens. A contact lens wearer should always carry spectacles to use in an emergency, although it must be realized that particularly with hard lenses he may suffer 'spectacle blur'. This can last from days to weeks and varies considerably in extent from individual to individual. The hard contact lens, worn regularly, slightly flattens the curvature of the cornea and this changes the refraction of the eye. The spectacle prescription is then incorrect. It may take from days to weeks for the cornea to return to its 'normal contour' and refractive state thus permitting clear vision when wearing spectacles, though in some individuals it may only take hours. Aircrew should be advised of the visual consequences of changing from hard contact lenses to spectacles. The blur suffered after removing 38% water content lenses and donning spectacles is less dramatic but good visual acuity must not be expected immediately. The change from high-water content lenses to spectacles can normally be accomplished without any loss in visual acuity.

If a pilot is flying solo missions, commercial or private, he should wear soft contact lenses preferably of a high water content. Licensing authorities should insist that contact lens wearers should always carry corrective flying spectacles with them at all times when they are exercising the privilege of their licences. Their prescription should be such as to give the best possible correction immediately after the contact lenses have been removed.

Finally, decompression to over approximately 23 000 feet can lead to gas-bubble formation between a hard lens and the cornea. If the pressure of these bubbles on the cornea cannot be relieved, erosion of the corneal epithelium may result. This has not been seen with high water content (75%) soft contact lenses.

Ocular muscle balance

Introduction

Ocular movements are mediated by six extra-ocular muscles which are inserted into the sclera of each eye. Their primary actions are shown in *Figure 51.6*; for simplicity, secondary or torsional actions have been ignored.

Acting with their contralateral synergists these muscles produce the following ocular movements:

Dextro-version	R. lateral rectus	L. medial rectus
Laevo-version	R. medial rectus	L. lateral rectus
Dextro-elevation	R. superior rectus	L. inferior oblique
Laevo-elevation	R. inferior oblique	L. superior rectus
Dextro-depression	R. inferior rectus	L. superior oblique
Laevo-depression	R. superior oblique	L. inferior rectus

Normally, these muscles are co-ordinated by a complex neuromuscular mechanism which results in the visual axis of each eye being directed towards an object which is at the time the point of regard: the image formed by each eye is fused centrally to give binocular single vision with stereopsis.

If such co-ordination is perfect both visual axes remain directed towards the object when binocular vision is interrupted by occlusion of one eye or by means of one of the dissociation tests used in clinical practice.

Anomalies

Such a state of orthophoria is rare and it is generally found that, when binocular vision is interrupted, the state of heterophoria (defective ocular muscle balance) is present, in which the non-fixing eye may deviate inwards (esophoria), outwards (exophoria) or vertically upwards (hyperphoria). By convention, vertical deviation downwards (hypophoria) is not considered separately, a downward deviation of, say, the right eye being considered as an upwards deviation of the left eye.

If, when the interruption to binocular vision is removed, the deviating eye resumes its original direction, this 'recovery' indicates the certain presence of heterophoria, the type of recovery indicating to a fair degree the quality of binocular vision present. If, however, the eye does not resume its original direction, heterotropia (manifest strabismus or squint) is present.

Slight degrees of heterophoria, except hyperphoria, usually produce no symptoms of headache, 'eye strain', blurring of vision or diplopia, particularly under conditions of fatigue, stress, hypoxia, anxiety, high G-forces, alcohol or drugs.

In the early days of aviation very small degrees of heterophoria, which today would be accepted as being within normal physiological limits, disqualified an applicant for piloting duties, since it was believed that this state of ocular muscle imbalance would lead to difficulty in learning to fly and, in particular, in landing an aircraft. The general belief was that esophorics tended to fly into the ground while exophorics judged the ground to be nearer than was actually so and tended to land high.

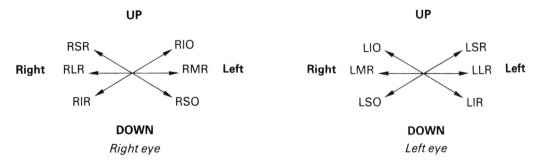

Figure 51.6 Ocular movements (simplified) and responsible extra-ocular muscles.

The reasoning behind this belief was that heterophoria was considered to be associated with defective fusion of the two ocular images; as a result stereoscopic vision and therefore judgement of the distance of objects and their relative positions were both defective.

This reasoning breaks down on two counts. First, heterophoria, particularly of moderate degree, is not necessarily associated with defective fusion, for if defective fusion were present the heterophoria would break down into a manifest strabismus. Secondly, defective stereopsis does not necessarily lead to defective distance judgement, as it is only one of the nine visual cues used in this estimation. The others are the binocular cue of convergence and the monocular cues of aerial perspective, linear perspective, light and shade, overlapping contours, motion parallax, angular subtense and association with other cues. Although the 'range finder base' between the two eyes is short, the depth cue of stereopsis is of great value in military aviation, although its necessity in the military transport role, or in civilian, professional and private aviation may be less important (*see* Chapter 23). Within the UK the desirability of normal stereopsis in aircrew is becoming accepted.

Small or moderate degrees of asymptomatic well-compensated horizontal heterophoria probably have little influence on an individual's ability to fly well and safely; and it seems somewhat anomalous that such an individual who, in the early stages of flying training, finds himself consistently landing high or low should take no steps to correct this fault. Conversely, it is of interest to note that over the years a number of 'bad landers' referred for ophthalmic examination have shown no significant ocular muscle defect.

What is more likely is that the stresses of flying, particularly fatigue and hypoxia, produce decompensation of a barely controlled heterophoria and thus lead to the appearance of symptoms.

The literature on this condition in association with aviation is vast and the exact interrelationship is in doubt, many investigators finding that flying stress produces an increase of exophoria and a decrease of esophoria. Other workers, however, have found the reverse.

The presence of heterophoria in a candidate for flying need not necessarily entail automatic rejection, and each case if otherwise suitable, should be assessed following specialist opinion, which may first require a detailed orthoptic examination with estimation of the fusional reserves, and possibly also a 'stress test' such as the production of mild hypoxia with measurement of any change of the degree of heterophoria.

If a pre-existing heterophoria should break down and produce symptoms, treatment is usually simple and involves only a short absence from duty. Orthoptic or ocular muscle training is of limited value and merely produces a short-term improvement; but well-planned and executed surgery to the appropriate extra-ocular muscles generally produces a permanent cure.

Convergence

The disjunctive extra-ocular movement of convergence is generally included under the heading of ocular muscle balance, and although it is of no direct importance in aviation a measurement of its near point should be made.

When an object approaches the eyes to within reading distance, both eyes should converge so that the image in each eye falls on each fovea. If this convergence does not occur, diplopia will result.

If the power of convergence is defective the individual—because of the accommodation convergence synkinesis—will not only be exerting an effort of accommodation to achieve near vision but may be exerting a maximum effort of convergence in an effort to maintain binocular single vision. This maximum effort may produce symptoms of asthenopia, so that reading for even short periods becomes uncomfortable.

If such a convergence insufficiency is found, a course of orthoptic training will almost invariably effect a cure, and rejection from aviation training should not be considered until such a course has been completed and its results assessed.

The visual fields

Although good central vision for distance and near is of major importance, the value of a full peripheral field of vision should not be neglected, for although its numerical value in terms of visual acuity is low (*Figure 51.7*), its use in the detection of objects in the vicinity of the observer is an important factor in flight safety and in some aspects of survival in a hostile military environment. Although the peripheral field can only perceive a target as an ill-defined blur or as a flash of light reflected from the wing or canopy of an approaching aircraft, such a stimulus, particularly if moving in relation to the observer, reaches consciousness and draws attention to itself, then by eye and head movement the observer can acquire the image of the target upon his two foveae.

The extent of the normal, static, uniocular field of vision depends on the size, brightness and colour of the target used, and also on the contrast between the target and its background; but when examined by normal clinical perimetric methods, the field for form may be expected to extend to more than 90 degrees temporally, 50 degrees superiorly, 60 degrees nasally and 65 degrees inferiorly, the

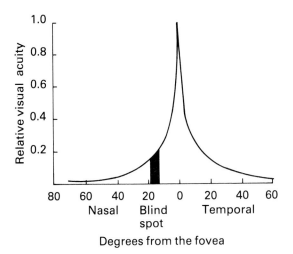

Figure 51.7 The regional variation of visual acuity (after Wertheim, 1894).

superior and nasal field being variable, depending on the cut-off produced by the eyebrow, cheek and nose. The fields for colour are smaller, that for red being larger than that for green.

Binocularly, part of each field overlaps that of the fellow eye (*Figure 51.8*); and if maximum head and eye movements are used the maximum field for form available is extended to approximately 240 degrees in the horizontal meridian and 130 degrees superiorly.

The normal blind spot occupies an area of about 5 × 7 degrees and is approximately centred on the horizontal meridian 16 degrees from the fixation point in the temporal field. As this area is overlapped by a seeing area in the field of the opposite eye, its presence, unless pathologically enlarged, may be ignored as with the normal scanning movements of the eye a target would not remain on this small blind area for a significant time should vision from the opposite eye be obstructed.

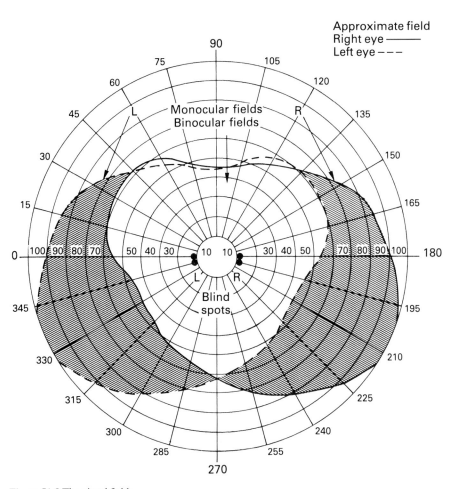

Figure 51.8 The visual fields.

Significant, or progressive, loss of either visual field should be a bar to flying, particularly if the loss is in the temporal field, because the temporal or 'outboard' field is the most valuable in aviation.

Small, stationary scotomata not affecting vision may be treated more leniently, as may peripheral losses of the inferior field not obscuring instrument warning lights.

Colour vision

See Chapter 23.

Examination

Method

Visual defects and medical ophthalmic conditions are among the major causes of rejection for flying duties, and a thorough and accurate eye examination is therefore of great importance in selecting flying personnel. It is important to know whether the subject wears glasses or contact lenses; if glasses are normally worn, the candidate should attend for his first examination wearing them, and bring the written prescription. If contact lenses (hard or soft) are normally worn, the candidate should attend wearing glasses. Contact lenses should not be worn for 2 weeks prior to assessment.

In order to reduce observer error and to ensure maximum test/retest reliability, certain standard examination techniques are recommended:

1. Adequate illumination and magnification is required for external examination.
2. A set pattern of examination should be followed. The following sequence is only one such pattern which follows a satisfactory instrumental sequence, and which reduces possible learning by the candidate.
   Colour perception.
   Personal and family history.
   External examination.
   Ocular movements and nystagmus.
   Cover test, distance and near.
   Trial frame on:
   Distant visual acuity.
   Near visual acuity (accommodation).
   Convergence.
   Manifest hypermetropia and/or refraction.
   Maddox Rod—distance and near.
   Trial frame off:
   Maddox wing test (if done).
   Stereoscopic vision (if done).
   Visual fields.
   Media and fundi.
   Intra-ocular tension (if done).

In the following paragraphs, the precise techniques will be described not necessarily in the order listed above—which is a practical examination sequence—but rather in the usual functional groups.

Colour perception

Two tests are in general use for the estimation of colour perception; *see* Chapter 23.

Pseudoisochromatic plates

Broadly speaking, these plates differentiate between colour normals and colour abnormals, but their use in the differentiation of minor degrees of colour anomaly is uncertain, particularly as various editions of plates differ so that validation data for one edition does not necessarily apply to another.

The most important source of error in the use of these plates is to administer the test in the wrong type of illuminant. These charts are balanced for a colour temperature of approximately 6500K, standard north daylight, so their administration in direct sunlight, in rooms with strongly coloured walls and in light with a reddish colour cast, that is, daylight in early morning or late afternoon, will prejudice the accuracy of the test. Testing under normal tungsten lighting is likely to give an increased pass rate for green defectives of approximately 4%.

The test should be presented orthogonal to the candidate at a distance of 3 feet (0.9 m), with spectacles, if worn, being used, in good diffused daylight, or its artificial equivalent of appropriate quality.

Approximately 5 seconds should be allowed the candidate to read each plate, and he should not be allowed to trace or otherwise handle the plate. It is normally not necessary to use the illiterate winding-line plates.

If all plates are read correctly, the colour perception is assessed as normal. If any mistake is made a lantern test should be carried out.

Lantern tests

These tests are of the nature of a 'trade test', used solely for the practical purpose of determining a candidate's safety in the recognition of signal lights under all conditions.

Their interpretation requires training and experience, and is generally carried out in specialist departments. The subject is, initially, required to identify the numbers on the Ishihara pseudo-isochromatic plates. Should he fail to read the plates correctly he may be classed as colour safe following a lantern test. The current lantern used in the RAF is the Holmes–Wright. The test is applied in a darkened room; two colours, one above the other, are shown to the subject at a distance of 6 metres, with the subject seated, and wearing spectacles if necessary. He is required to identify the colours naming the top colour first. The test is repeated with various colour combinations. If a mistake is made the subject remains in the darkened room for a further 15 minutes to become further dark adapted, when the test is repeated. If a mistake is made on the second examination he is classed as colour defective unsafe and would be unfit for military flying.

With the increasing use of multi-coloured CRT displays both in civil and in military aircraft it is necessary to review the testing of colour vision. Current tests only monitor red/green deficits (Brennan, 1985).

History

Personal

A personal history should always be taken, particular attention being paid to: the wearing of glasses; disease or inflammation of the eye or its adnexa; visual disorders associated with headache, eye-strain or diplopia; and difficulty seeing in the dark.

Family

Any history of squint, cataract, glaucoma or degenerative disease of the eye should be noted.

External examination

Eyelids, eyelashes and lacrimal apparatus

Ptosis, blepharitis, or any abnormal condition of the lacrimal apparatus should be noted.

Conjunctivae

The bulbar and palpebral conjunctivae, including the fornices, should be examined for signs of hyperaemia, infection or growths.

Corneae

The presence of corneal opacities or vascularization should be recorded.

Iris

Any abnormality of colour or configuration of the iris, or signs of past iritis should be noted.

Pupils

Any inequality of the pupils should be noted, for example, mydriasis, miosis or irregularity due to posterior synechiae, or any abnormal reaction to light or accommodation/convergence.

Ocular movements

Movement

Normally the eyes should move fully and equally in all directions, and no diplopia should be elicited in any quadrant. Particular attention should be paid to a candidate exhibiting a torticollis, as this sign is commonly present in cases of paresis of a vertically acting extra-ocular muscle.

Nystagmus (*Table 51.2*)

In testing for nystagmus, particular care should be taken to keep the fixation object inside the normal binocular field of vision. Physiological nystagmus can almost invariably be elicited in extreme positions of gaze, or if the fixation object passes from view of one eye behind the nose.

Distant visual acuity

This function is tested by means of Snellen test types, or similar optotypes, illuminated to an approved level and viewed at a measured distance which, in Great Britain, is normally 6 m. This may be obtained by either direct vision or mirror reversal.

Each eye should be tested separately, first without and then with spectacles, if worn; each letter should be read aloud and the eyelids should be open normally. The smallest line of type which is read completely and accurately determines the fraction used in recording visual acuity.

When spectacles are habitually worn, the prescription and corrected acuity of each eye should be recorded. When the unaided vision does not reach 6/6, or when the spectacles worn do not correct the vision to 6/6, the refraction and the corrected vision should be determined and the required prescription recorded.

Common errors

1. The chart not being at 6 m (20 feet) from the candidate. This completely invalidates the test unless the testing distance is recorded; for example, if at 7 m the 6/6 line is read, visual acuity is recorded as 7/6; if at 5 m, 5/6, and so on.
2. Too much light. This reduces visual acuity, particularly if glare is reflected from the surface

Table 51.2 Types of nystagmus

Type	Vision	Slow and quick component	Occurrence		Accompanied by vertigo, past pointing nausea
			Extreme positions	Any position	
Physiological	Not diagnostic	No	Yes	No	No
Ocular	Poor	No	No	When attempting to fix	No
Extra-ocular paresis	Not diagnostic	Usually	In direction of action of paralysed muscle	No	No
Central	Not diagnostic	Usually	No	Yes	Unusual
Labyrinthine	Not diagnostic	Yes	No	Yes	Yes

of the test type, or if extraneous light enters the candidate's eye.

3. The candidate viewing the chart with both eyes open, or memorizing letters before the test starts.
4. The candidate being allowed to read the chart with glasses on before the unaided visual acuity is determined.
5. The candidate or examiner pressing upon the occluded eye.
6. The candidate being allowed to cover his own eye and peeping from behind the occluder.
7. The candidate being allowed to 'screw up' his eye or adopt an unusual head posture.
8. Inaccurate recording. No reading errors are permitted, and it should be noted that errors with letters C, G and D sometimes indicate some degree of astigmatism.

Manifest hypermetropia

Some aviation organizations reject candidates for a licence or training if the manifest hypermetropia in either eye exceeds +2.25D.

This manifest hypermetropia can be measured with some degree of accuracy by recording the level of distant visual acuity obtained by each eye separately with the candidate viewing the test type through a convex lens.

There are two methods of conducting the test:

1. A +2.50D spherical lens is placed before the eye under test and the examinee is instructed to read all the letters on the test type. The lowest line of

letters read quickly and correctly is recorded, and if the 6/6 line is read correctly the examinee is rejected as having more than +2.25D manifest hypermetropia.
2. The highest power of convex lens through which the 6/6 line of letters can be read quickly and correctly is recorded.

A +2.50D spherical lens is placed before the eye under test and the examinee instructed to read the whole of the test type.

If the 6/6 line cannot be read, the power of the lens is progressively reduced with negative lenses until this line can be read correctly.

Common errors

1. The test being carried out immediately after the testing of distant visual acuity as the candidate may remember the 6/6 line.
2. Insufficient time allowed for the candidate to relax his accommodation and too low a level of manifest hypermetropia is recorded. The time taken to read the whole of the test type is usually sufficient to permit this relaxation.
3. Lack of appreciation that the candidate is guessing or memorizing the letters. If the test type cannot be changed, the lines of letters should occasionally be read backwards.
4. These tests for manifest hypermetropia are not sufficiently accurate when precise facts are required and, where possible, an objective refraction should be carried out, preferably under cycloplegia on first examination.

Ocular muscle balance

The tests used for the estimation of heterophoria are based on the principle that when dissimilar images are presented to each eye, fusional control of the extra-ocular muscles is prevented, and the eyes take up an abnormal position of rest.

Cover test

The purpose of this objective test is to determine whether manifest strabismus is present, or whether there is any tendency for the eyes to deviate when the two eyes are dissociated.

The candidate sits with his head in the 'Primary Position', fixing on the distant 6/60 letter with both eyes open, and is instructed to remain so. The examiner stands on the candidate's right and facing him, holding an occluder card in his right hand, so that when he covers one eye he can observe any movement of the occluded eye.

Orthophoria

The examiner observes the two eyes fixing on the distant object, and they appear straight (*Figure 51.9*). He covers the left eye, observing any movement of the right eye when the left is covered. He then observes the left eye behind the cover to see

Figure 51.9 Cover test: orthophoria.

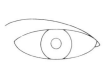

Figure 51.10 Cover test: orthophoria.

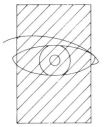

Figure 51.11 Cover test: orthophoria.

whether any movement occurs (*Figure 51.10*). In the case shown there is none. The occluder is removed to cover the right eye (*Figure 51.11*), and no movement is detected. In such a case the subject is orthophoric for distance.

Esophoria

In this instance the same sequence is followed, but movement inwards of the left eye, esophoria, is observed behind the cover (*Figure 51.12*). With the

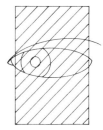

Figure 51.12 Cover test: esophoria for distance.

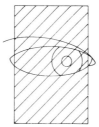

Figure 51.13 Cover test: esophoria for distance.

occluder removed, the eyes become straight. Occlusion of the right eye would cause the right eye to turn in (*Figure 51.13*)—the eyes again becoming straight after removal of the cover.

Exophoria

The reverse situation applies should the candidate be exophoric. In this instance the eye, under cover, will turn outwards (*Figures 51.14* and *51.15*), and when the cover is removed the eyes will again become straight.

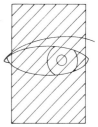

Figure 51.14 Cover test: exophoria for distance.

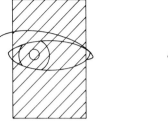

Figure 51.15 Cover test: exophoria for distance.

Convergent strabismus

In this case (*Figure 51.16*) there is a small right convergent strabismus. If the angle is small it may be difficult to detect. Occlude the left eye (*Figure 51.17*) and the right eye will be seen to straighten and take up fixation; the left eye will turn inwards behind the occluder. If the cover is removed, or the right eye covered, the right eye will turn inwards, and the left eye will again take up fixation (*Figure 51.18*).

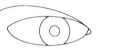
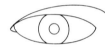

Figure 51.16 Cover test: right convergent strabismus.

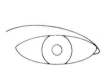
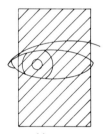

Figure 51.17 Cover test: right convergent strabismus.

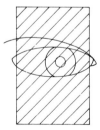
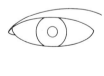

Figure 51.18 Cover test: right convergent strabismus.

Alternating convergent strabismus

In this instance examination shows a small right convergent strabismus (*Figure 51.16*). With the left eye occluded the left eye turns in behind the cover

and the right eye becomes straight on fixation (*Figure 51.19*). Remove the occluder from the left eye and the left eye remains turning in as a left convergent strabismus (*Figure 51.20*). If the right eye is occluded, the right eye turns in behind the cover and the left eye straightens on fixation (*Figure 51.21*). With the occlusion removed from the right eye, the right convergent strabismus remains (*Figure 51.22*).

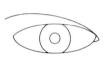
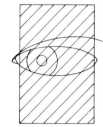

Figure 51.19 Cover test: alternating convergent strabismus.

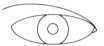
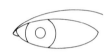

Figure 51.20 Cover test: alternating convergent strabismus.

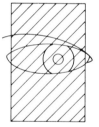
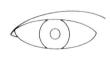

Figure 51.21 Cover test: alternating convergent strabismus.

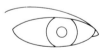
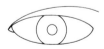

Figure 51.22 Cover test: alternating convergent strabismus.

The same procedure can be used to demonstrate a right or left divergent strabismus or an alternating divergent strabismus. The same procedure is repeated with subject fixing a near object at 33 cm distance in order to record the findings of the cover test for near vision.

In military flying no case of manifest strabismus is accepted for pilot training, though in civilian flying some cases may be accepted. Those candidates with phorias must have their phorias measured to determine whether they are within the acceptable limits. This measurement is performed using the Maddox Rod Test.

Maddox rod test

With this test heterophoria can be detected and its degree estimated both for distant and near vision.

The Maddox rod is a disc of red glass in the surface of which are moulded a number of grooves. If a spotlight is viewed through the disc the light is seen as a red line, the direction of which is at right-angles to the direction of the grooves. As the line and spotlight are dissimilar images the stimulus for fusion is absent and the covered eye takes up its position of rest.

Distance

With the candidate looking, with both eyes open, at a small light source at an equivalent distance of 6 m, the Maddox rod is placed in a trial frame before the right eye with the grooves horizontal. If binocular vision is present, a vertical red line is seen by the right eye and the spotlight by the left eye and both are seen simultaneously. If either the line or the light is not seen, binocular vision is absent, the vision of one eye being suppressed.

If orthophoria is present the red line appears to pass through the spotlight. If the red line does not pass through the spotlight the candidate is asked to which side of the spotlight the red line lies.

As the eye reverses and inverts images, in heterophoria the red line appears to go in the opposite direction to the movement of the eye. Therefore, with the Maddox rod before the right eye, if the red line is:

1. To the patient's right of the light = esophoria (*Plate 3(a)*, opposite page 345).
2. To the patient's left of the light = exophoria (*Plate 3(a)*).

Increasing powers of prisms are placed before the right eye, with the base of the prism towards the side on which the red line lies, until the red line appears to pass through the spotlight. The power of the prism, in prism dioptres, and the type of horizontal heterophoria it has corrected, are recorded.

The test is repeated in a similar manner with the Maddox rod placed in front of the right eye with the grooves vertical, producing a horizontal red line, and the degree of hyperphoria is recorded:

1. If the red line is above the light = Left hyperphoria (*Plate 3(b)*).
2. If the red line is below the light = Right hyperphoria (*Plate 3(b)*).

Near

The test is repeated in a similar manner using a torch bulb, at a distance of ⅓ metre, as the fixation target.

Whether testing for distance or near, in cases of incomitance—that is, when the degree of deviation differs according to which eye is fixing as may be demonstrated by the cover test—these tests must be repeated using the left eye for fixation. Any difference in the findings should be recorded, and assessment should usually be made in terms of the greater degree of deviation.

Heterophoria may also be measured by means of a Maddox hand frame. There are various types of this instrument, one being shaped like a lorgnette holding a Maddox rod in one eyepiece and a rotating prism in the other. To measure any deviation, the prism is rotated until the candidate sees the red line coinciding with the spotlight. The strength of the prism required is indicated on the scale engraved on the frame.

Common errors

1. The candidate shutting one eye.
2. The candidate not relaxing his accommodation in order to focus the distant spotlight. This results in a degree of esophoria which is too high and which does not match the deviation detected by the cover test.
3. Multiple red lines being seen, due to aberrant light sources. If the examination room cannot be blacked out, the proper red line should be indicated by flashing the spotlight on and off a few times.
4. Falsification by the candidate. Heterophoric candidates who know the test may claim that the line passes through the light. If, following the cover test, orthophoria appears unlikely, a prism should be placed in an appropriate direction before the Maddox rod. If orthophoria is still claimed, a closer check of the candidate's responses is indicated.

Maddox wing test

This test may be used for testing the muscle balance at reading distance. On looking through the eyepieces an arrow is seen with the right eye and figures with the left, white for horizontal and red for vertical heterophoria. The degree of heterophoria is indicated in degrees or prism dioptres by the figure to which the arrow finally points.

Owing to accommodative effects, this test cannot be correlated accurately with the Maddox rod test at ⅓ m, and it should be noted that, as 1 degree is approximately equivalent to 2 prism dioptres, the Maddox wing reading recorded in degrees should be doubled to compare it findings with those with the Maddox rod.

Accommodation (near vision)

Accommodation may be measured uniocularly and binocularly without and with spectacles with the RAF Near Point or similar rule. The examiner draws the drum containing the test types towards the handle, turns the N types towards the candidate, and places the shaped facepiece below the candidate's infra-orbital margins.

The candidate is instructed to read out the smallest print he can and, as the drum is moved at a steady slow speed towards his eyes, he is instructed to say when the print first becomes blurred. This distance, shown by the rear edge of the slide carrying the drum, is recorded in centimetres.

Doubtful cases may be checked by sliding the drum away from the candidate until the print becomes perfectly clear.

The accommodation of each eye should be measured separately as well as together since apart from differences in refraction, a weakness of convergence will cause the binocular reading to be greater than the uniocular.

The near vision standards for the issue and retention of a civilian aviation licence do not normally stipulate the exact measurement of the near point, the present requirement being that the examinee should be able, with or without spectacles, to read N5 type at a distance to be chosen by himself of between 30 and 50 cm with each eye separately. In order to ensure that the individual can read aircraft instruments, an additional standard requires the ability to read N8 typeface at a distance of 1 m.

Convergence

This test is carried out binocularly with the RAF Near Point or similar rule, using the test card bearing the line and dot. This target is moved towards the candidate, and he is instructed to say when the line becomes, not blurred, but double. This is the subjective convergence, and this distance is recorded in centimetres.

At some point on the scale, one eye may be seen to hesitate in its convergence and then, suddenly to diverge. This is the point of objective convergence, and its distance is recorded in centimetres.

These two measurements may or may not coincide and doubling of the line may or may not be noticeable by the candidate.

Stereoscopic vision

The requirement for testing stereopsis is, regrettably, not yet universal although its value is not doubted.

If such a test is required use may be made of the Howard–Dolman, Verhoeff, Titmus stereotest, standard orthoptic techniques or the TNO test.

The TNO (Toatepast Natuurwetenschap Onderzoek) test is a random-dot stereogram devised by Julesz (1961). The subject wears a pair of red–green spectacles, to view the test plates, which when viewed binocularly by a normal subject will elicit perception of an image in depth. The TNO test is graded to provide retinal disparities ranging from 15 to 480 seconds of arc.

The USAF requirement for stereopsis, using the Howard–Dolman or Verhoeff techniques, demands a minimum standard of 25 seconds of arc for military aviators (Tredici, 1985).

Visual fields

The visual function of the retinal periphery may be assessed by a measurement of the peripheral field of vision. It may be measured accurately by means of instruments such as a perimeter or it may be estimated by means of the confrontation test. The confrontation test is a gross test which is significant only when abnormal. If the peripheral vision appears normal with confrontation, a defect may still be detected by more sensitive methods of examination. The confrontation test is carried out as follows:

The examiner sits facing the subject at a distance of 1 m in an area with good illumination. The subject is asked to close one eye (e.g. right) using one finger. The examiner closes his own eye (left) which is directly opposite the closed eye of the subject. The examiner then places his hand midway between the subject and himself, bringing his hand slowly in from the periphery with one, two or three fingers extended. The subject is instructed to tell the examiner when he can see and count the number of fingers in his field of vision while continuing to fix the examiner's eye. As well as counting the fingers, the subject is asked to note if the examiner's fingers are still or moving. When the subject and the examiner have normal fields, each should see the fingers at the same time. The temporal and nasal fields and the upper and lower fields of each eye are tested in turn.

Media

The presence of any opacities in the corneae or other media should be noted and their effect on vision assessed.

Fundi

No active pathological condition is acceptable. The presence of retinal pigmentation, even if considered of no significance should be recorded, as should the appearance of deep physiological cupping of the discs.

Intra-ocular tension

An abnormality of the intra-ocular tension is unusual before approximately the age of 40 years, but if, in older aircrew, there is a family history of glaucoma, or if there is a suspicion that cupping of the optic discs is non-physiological, or there is a significant loss of visual field, the intra-ocular tensions should be measured by applanation tonometry.

Ocular disease

Introduction

The presence of any active ocular disease should be a bar to entry to flying training, and assessment should be deferred until it can be shown that the condition has been cured and is unlikely to recur.

Although vibration, acceleration and decompression sickness may produce a temporary effect on vision, and anoxia produces a number of visual effects, including decompensation of ocular muscle imbalance, failure of accommodation and convergence, depression of higher visual functions and (particularly in hypertensive subjects) retinal haemorrhage, flying does not cause ocular disease. Trained aircrew are, however, as liable to acquire ocular disease as other members of the population, and if it does arise it should receive prompt specialist care because any condition affecting vision or the integrity of the visual apparatus can result in a permanent loss of flying status, a penalty for delay which occurs in few other professions.

Fitness to return to flying after eye disease or injury should be carefully assessed because an eye that is irritable can be a flight hazard. In particular, no flying, especially as pilot in sole charge of an aircraft, should be permitted until all effects of hydriatic, miotic or steroid treatment have disappeared.

Owing to the strict pre-training medical examination given and the fact that professional aircrew retire from flying at a relatively early age, degenerative ocular disease is not commonly seen.

A few common ocular conditions will now be mentioned in slightly more detail.

Dry eyes

Owing to badly sited heating vents or low flight-deck humidity aircrew frequently complain of red, irritable or 'dry' eyes without discharge, but sometimes with reflex excess lacrimation. This condition usually responds to treatment during flight with eye drops of 0.5% methyl cellulose, which provides an emollient film over the surface of the eyes and eyelids.

Cataract

A small stationary lens opacity, congenital or acquired in origin, which does not interfere with vision need not impose any restriction on flying.

A cataract which interferes with vision may be due to ageing (senile cataract) or trauma (traumatic cataract) or inflammation (secondary cataract), or a combination of causes. In pilots the condition is often uni-ocular, and vision in that eye will be reduced.

Management

In military flying the uni-ocular cataract is managed on the following broad lines but each case is assessed individually.

In the 20–30 year age group a lensectomy and anterior vitrectomy is performed and thereafter the subject is fitted with an extended-wear soft contact lens. In the 30–45-year-old group an intra-capsular cryo cataract extraction is performed and thereafter the subject is fitted with an extended-wear soft contact lens. This enables the pilot to continue flying in fast jets or helicopters.

A posterior chamber intra-ocular implant after an extra-capsular cataract extraction is not used for the following reasons:

1. The possible long-term adverse effect on the endothelium of the cornea.
2. The loops of the posterior chamber implant are inserted into the capsular bag during surgery, but under high G forces or severe vibration they could impinge on the vessels in the ciliary body (Irvine, 1981; McDonell *et al.*, 1983). The capsule of the lens is a thin structure, particularly at the anterior and posterior poles where it is approximately 2.5–4.0 μm thick. The average mass of an intra-ocular implant is 2.5 mg. At 5G this implant weighs 12.5 mg; should the specific gravity of the implant and the surrounding aqueous differ significantly there would be differential movement inside the capsular bag, with the possible loss of lens retentivity. If the posterior capsule becomes opaque, a hole could be made in the capsule with a Yag laser in the

OBSOLETE & NOT ACCURATE

visual axis, which would restore good visual acuity, but the remaining opaque capsule would reduce the visual field.

In the age group above 45 years the normal surgical procedure is an extra-capsular cataract extraction with a posterior chamber implant. Following this treatment the pilot will be unfit for duties in fast jets and helicopter aircraft, but is fit to fly on other types. In civil aviation each pilot, with a cataract, will be treated and assessed taking all circumstances into account.

Glaucoma

An acute angle closure glaucoma is a surgical emergency which must be managed by an ophthalmic surgeon. The patient normally suffers prodromal episodes before a severe attack. These episodes may include eye ache, blurred vision and 'haloes' around lights particularly when daylight fades and night falls causing the pupils to dilate. Suspected prodromal attacks of angle closure glaucoma require that the patient be referred for investigation.

An attack of acute angle closure glaucoma is a surgical emergency and as narrow filtration angles are frequently bilateral there is a good case for a peripheral iridectomy to be carried out on the apparently unaffected eye following successful treatment of the affected eye. Such cases are uncommon, but the provision of an adequate passage between the posterior and anterior chambers of both eyes would probably enable the individual to return to flying, in a less demanding role.

Chronic simple glaucoma is more common and with closely supervised treatment may be compatible with continued flying. The silent, insidious, chronic simple glaucoma is usually diagnosed because of a family history or incidentally because of 'cupped discs' or raised intra-ocular pressure discovered during a routine examination. It must be remembered that the old treatment for this condition was miotic eye drops. These drops produced a spasm of accommodation for a time after instillation and the intense constriction of the pupil led to a serious reduction of night vision. The modern treatment is to use a beta blocker, such as timolol (Timoptol) drops. With these drops the intra-ocular pressure and field loss can be controlled and the pilot can continue flying, providing he remains under careful ophthalmic supervision. Drainage surgery such as trabeculectomy may be advised. Following surgery and providing the intra-ocular pressure and field loss are controlled, the pilot may return to flying but should not fly in fast jets or be subjected to high G forces. If any miotic is needed, grounding should be permanent unless the condition

can be completely relieved or controlled by surgery alone.

Although no accidents to the conjunctival bleb produced by external fistulizing operations have been reported, it is probably wise permanently to ban aerobatics, unnecessary exposure to the risk of rapid decompression and 'eyeballs out' G manoeuvres.

Glaucoma is a bilateral condition and can only be controlled, not cured. Specialist supervision should therefore be life-long as loss of control may result in serious visual loss without the patient necessarily being aware of its onset.

However, although pressure breathing may cause a rise in intra-ocular tension (*see* Chapter 7), this rise is transient and does not permanently affect the tension in either normal or glaucomatous individuals.

Amaurosis fugax

This is a term given to a sudden temporary failure of vision in one eye lasting several minutes. It may be due to a physiological or pathological reduction in blood flow through the internal carotid and basilar arteries.

Grey out of vision may occur under high G loads even if the subject is wearing anti-G clothing. It is due to the gravitational deprivation of oxygenated blood to the globe via the ophthalmic artery and to the occipital cortex via the posterior cerebral artery at the horizontal plane of the circle of Willis.

Should a pilot present with symptoms of amaurosis fugax, narrowing or pathology of the internal carotid artery on the affected side must be considered and investigations including ultrasound scanning and possible carotid angiography should be initiated.

Central serous retinopathy

This may cause distortions and reduced image sizes (micropsia) in the affected eye, together with macular oedema. The subject may not be aware of the condition unless he incidentally covers or closes his good eye.

This condition is one of unknown aetiology and is characterized by a comparatively sudden loss of central vision which may be recurrent. It occurs in healthy, young and early middle-aged people, predominantly males, the patient experiencing a central scotoma which may be of green or yellowish appearance. If the scotoma does not affect the master eye, the defect may not be noticeable until a routine eye examination takes place, and it is stated that myopes often do not notice the defect as early as hypermetropes and emmetropes.

The initial fall of visual acuity may be profound, but recovery, at least from the first attack, is common.

When the fundus is examined, one sees macular oedema, the swollen area exhibiting a circular light reflex at its periphery. General treatment has no effect on the course of the condition, some recovery of vision and loss of the scotoma occurring spontaneously with the passage of time. In some cases it is worth performing fluorescent fundus angiography: if leakage of dye occurs over a small area, provided the leak is a sufficient distance from the macula, it is often possible to seal the area by means of a light or laser coagulator.

The condition normally clears in time without treatment, though the vision does not fully return to normal. Initially the pilot should cease flying duties until the condition has resolved, and his vision has improved.

Uniocular vision

An individual can undoubtedly fly an aircraft safely with only one eye, or with only one seeing eye, and evidence produced by the Federal Aviation Administration of the USA shows little significant difference between the accident rates in one-eyed and two-eyed private pilots. However, the effect of complete loss of vision of one eye is seriously to restrict the field of vision on that side, and to produce a complete loss of stereoscopic vision. Although judgement of distance may still be possible by means of motion parallax these losses must constitute a flight hazard and, although acceptable in the past for certain experienced private pilots, they should probably be no longer permitted unless a satisfactory flight test has been performed and a safety look-out pilot is regularly carried.

The case of the 'administrative' one-eyed pilot, that is, an individual who has one amblyopic eye in which central vision is lost, or who has a central scotoma due to a retinal lesion, is slightly different. In this case, although the eye cannot see fine detail, the peripheral field of vision is full. This individual is therefore far more safe; and if he is experienced and by flight testing he can be shown to have adequate awareness he may often be retained in a limited capacity.

A trained pilot who has lost the sight in one eye because of disease or who has lost his eye through injury or enucleation may be permitted to continue in military flying with the limitation that he must fly as or with a co-pilot current on type, subject to expert approval.

Hypertensive and diabetic retinopathy

In both conditions small haemorrhages, exudates and oedema can occur at the macula. These can reduce the visual acuity and may be noted when the posterior pole of the fundi are examined. When fundal evidence is seen other signs should be apparent on a general medical examination.

Pilot applicants with a history of previous ocular surgery

Applicants for military flying may have had surgical treatment for a variety of conditions, and those in the following categories are unacceptable for entry:

1. Keratotomy for myopia.
2. Intraocular implant surgery following removal of a cataract.
3. Penetrating injuries or severe blunt trauma.
4. Surgery for retinal detachment.

A new type of refractive surgery, photoablative refractive keratectomy which uses a computer controlled excimer laser to recontour the cornea, has yet to be assessed.

Assessment of ophthalmic clinical findings

Assessment should be made in accordance with instructions issued by the licensing or employing organization, but it should be noted that differences exist between the acceptance standards for initial training, and those for continuation by trained aircrew.

Squint and the need for spectacles for other reasons are frequently hereditary, and a family history may give valuable information on the degree of deterioration to be anticipated in the candidate. The unaided visual acuity of the young myope is variable, and the hypermetrope may need spectacles only for reading, so the occasional use of spectacles may indicate the possibility of progressive deterioration of unaided vision, with or without increase of spectacle power, and therefore the candidate's unsuitability for a long-term engagement.

Ptosis interfering with vision is a cause for rejection unless surgical correction is successful.

Candidates with uncontrollable blepharitis, particularly with loss of eyelashes, are generally unsuitable for tropical service, and should be rejected. Less severe cases of blepharitis and chronic conjunctivitis should be assessed as temporarily unfit until the response to treatment can be assessed.

Naso-lacrimal occlusion producing epiphora, or a

mucocele, entails rejection unless surgery produces relief lasting a minimum of 6 months.

Uveitis (iritis, cyclitis, choroiditis) is frequently recurrent, and candidates giving a history of, or exhibiting, this condition should be carefully assessed.

Even if a corneal affection does not interfere with vision it should be carefully assessed, as many conditions are hereditary, degenerative or recurrent.

Visual disturbances associated with headaches of a migrainous type are not a strictly ocular problem and should be assessed in accordance with current regulations. Convergence insufficiency; diplopia due to heterophoria; concomitant, or paretic strabismus need not necessarily entail immediate rejection but will require specialist, including orthoptic, examination, evaluation and opinion.

In many instances the cause of apparent 'night blindness' is due to lack of adequate training, but persons suffering from certain progressive, genetically determined, incurable diseases of the eye—e.g. retinitis pigmentosa—exhibit this defect as an early symptom, and electro-diagnosis may be necessary to establish the true cause.

Visual acuity

The visual acuity requirements for the various categories of flying personnel are detailed in the appropriate publications.

Myopia

If there is a strong family history of myopia, particularly if the history of the candidate's visual defect is recent, if he is still growing, or if the fundus appearance indicates progress, assessment should be deferred, even if the visual acuity is within the limits prescribed.

Astigmatism

Many organizations limit the amount of astigmatism permitted, even if the visual acuity is within the prescribed limits. Current instructions should be consulted. Particular attention should be paid to astigmatism 'against the rule'. Astigmatism of ±0.50D cyl may be considered to be physiological.

Manifest hypermetropia

Organizations requiring this examination usually limit the permitted amount to 2.25 dioptres without the use of a mydriatic. Uncorrected hypermetropia above this level may possibly be associated with disturbances of accommodation and visual judgement, especially in conditions causing fatigue, anoxia or during tropical service, and with the deterioration of unaided visual acuity which is due to increasing age. In borderline cases with +2.00 or +2.25 dioptres of manifest hypermetropia using the present test, a full estimation of the refraction should be carried out.

Ocular muscle balance

Candidates with manifest squints are unsuitable for piloting, even after the objective deviation is corrected, unless good binocular function with a good range of fusion and stereopsis can be demonstrated before operation, and full normal binocular single vision is achieved after operation. The standards for heterophoria and the power of convergence, and for accommodation in relation to age are detailed in current instructions. The results of these tests must be considered together and re-assessment after treatment may be permitted.

The presence of a manifest squint in other flight personnel may be permitted, provided it is cosmetically acceptable, that there is no diplopia and that the visual acuity is not affected. Symptomless heterophoria also need not be a bar.

Visual fields

A defect of the visual field, particularly of the temporal fields, unless produced by a small, inactive lesion, entails rejection.

Media

An opacity of the cornea, lens or vitreous interfering with vision entails rejection, as does a small progressive lens opacity or pathological condition in the vitreous.

Fundus

The presence of an active pathological condition of the fundus or one interfering with vision or the visual field entails rejection. In cases of low myopia, careful consideration must be given to the appearance of the fundi. If there is any pigmentary disturbance which appears to be active or progressive, or which shows any indication of stretching or thinning of the retina or any degenerative changes in the retinal periphery, the candidate should be rejected.

[handwritten margin note, rotated: Much of this page seems to apply to military selection. Must is magically occurate.]

References

BRENNAN, D. (1985) Entry visual standards and ocular examination technique for future fighter aircrew. In AGARD Conference Proceedings No. 396. *Medical Selection and Physiological Training of Future Fighter Aircrew*. Neuilly-sur-Seine: AGARD

CLOHERTY, J.K. (1985) Contact lenses for pilots and aircrew in the services. In AGARD Conference Proceedings No. 379. *Visual Protection and Enhancement*. Neuilly-sur-Seine: AGARD

EGGERS, H. (1945) Estimation of uncorrected visual acuity in malingerers. *Archives of Ophthalmology*, **33**, 26

IRVINE, A.R. (1981) Extracapsular cataract extraction and pseudophakos implantation in primates: a clinico-pathological study. *Ophthalmic Surgery*, **12**, 17–37

JULESZ, B. (1961) Binocular depth perception without familiarity cues. *Science*, **145**, 356–362

MCDONNELL, P.J. *et al.* (1983) Pathology of intra-ocular lenses in 33 eyes examined post-mortem. *Ophthalmology*, **90**, 386–403

SLATAPER, F.J. (1970) Age norms of refraction and vision. *Archives of Ophthalmology*, **43**, 466

STRINGER, F.S. (1978) In AGARD Report No. 118, *Optimisation of Pilot Capability and Avionic System Design*. Neuilly-sur-Seine, AGARD

TREDICI, T.J. (1985) Ophthalmology in aerospace medicine. In de Hart, R.C. (ed.) *Fundamentals of Aerospace Medicine*. Philadelphia: Lea and Febiger

WERTHEIM, T. (1894) Über die indirecte Sehschärfe. *Zeitschrift für Psychologie und Physiologie des Sinnesorg, Hamburg und Leipzig*, **7**, 172

52

Orthopaedics

H.J.K. Vieyra and D.J. Anton

Introduction

The development of high-performance jet aircraft has led to considerable fresh thinking in terms of orthopaedic requirements for aircrew.

The standards described below are those expected of high-performance jet aircrew. The same standards should be applied to aircrew flying transport aircraft, helicopters and commercial aircraft. It might be thought that in the case of the latter categories, a slightly lower standard may apply in some respects. In fact, this is not necessarily so, owing to the heavier control forces in larger aircraft, particularly in asymmetric flight, and the multiplicity of controls situated on overhead panels and side controls which may be difficult to reach.

The musculo-skeletal system will be taken systematically, from the lower extremity upwards. The final section will deal with the spine, with a special discussion on the vitally important and vulnerable cervical spine.

Lower extremity

Ankle and foot

It is essential for the safe management and control of aircraft to have a good range of painless movement at the ankle and subtalar joints. There are a variety of conditions that could impair this faculty, e.g. painful trauma and infection. Certainly the presence of a fused or painful ankle or subtalar joint would raise the question as to a candidate's fitness to fly. In this, as in similar situations, the final decision would rest either on testing in a simulator, or on flying with a qualified flying instructor or

medical officer pilot in a dual control aircraft. In these days of widespread sporting activities, the incidence of foot and ankle injuries is on the increase. It is fortunate, therefore, that modern methods of internal fixation have improved the long-term outlook after injuries in this region and the facilities for rehabilitation are such that a rapid return to full function often can be assured.

The knee

Of all the joints in the body, the knee is probably the most prone to injury, particularly in contact sports. During recent years there has been a vast increase in our knowledge and understanding of the complexities of the joint, and the development of the arthroscope and of arthroscopic surgery have brought great improvements in diagnosis, and enabled relatively minor surgery to take care of what used to be major problems, e.g. torn meniscus, or a loose body. Recovery after arthroscopic surgery is remarkably quick, and when this is coupled with the rapid improvements that are being made in the field of ligamentous reconstruction, using either natural or artificial fibres, the long-term outlook for damaged knees is much enhanced. The minimum requirement for functioning capability at the knee is a range of movement from 0 to 90 degrees, and this must be painless and the joint must be stable. Arthrodesis of the knee or a total knee replacement would preclude any form of flying.

The hip

A pain-free range of at least 90 degrees of flexion from the neutral (extended) position is the minimum essential for hip joint function for safety in flight. A traumatic dislocation or a fracture–dislocation of the hip requires prolonged non-weight bearing after traction treatment in bed because of the danger of avascular necrosis, and the minimum period before return to flying is 3 months. Fortunately, in the young adult, hip joint pathology is rare unless it is of a congenital nature. Congenital dislocation of the hip, Perthes' disease, or slipped upper femoral epiphysis occurs in children, and one would expect an accurate diagnosis of a situation such as this to be made before entry into aircrew training.

Lower limb nerve injuries

A neurological deficit in the lower extremity, be it central or peripheral, should not cause difficulty in determining fitness. Careful clinical evaluation will establish the nature and the cause of the deficit, be it motor, sensory, proprioceptive, thermal or reflex. Further management will depend on the extent of the problem; a minor sensory loss is of little import, a drop foot is a potential disaster.

Upper extremity

The shoulder

The shoulder is also prone to injuries in contact sport, among the commonest being a traumatic dislocation of the shoulder joint itself or of the acromio-clavicular joint, a fracture of the clavicle, or damage to the supraspinatus and rotator cuff mechanisms. These injuries are easily diagnosed and treated, and in the main, the results are excellent after either conservative or surgical management. A good range of shoulder movement is essential for operating those controls which are positioned to the side of, behind, and above the seated crew member. In transport aircraft the standard cannot be reduced; here too controls are located in overhead panels and side consoles.

The elbow

A certain amount of loss of function in the elbow is acceptable, because its movements are complementary to those of the shoulder, and some impairment can be compensated for by shoulder movement. Trauma is the most common cause of elbow problems, but again, with modern surgical techniques and rehabilitation, restoration of adequate function should usually be possible.

Hand and wrist

The hand is probably the most vital part of the musculoskeletal system. The three basic types of function carried out by the hand, as described by Schlesinger (1983) are:

1. To grasp round or cylindrical objects.
2. To pinch by tip pressure, by pulp pressure or by lateral pressure.
3. To hook.

Any assessment of a hand's capability must be made with the realization that these three movements are essential. It would therefore require to be well nigh perfect, with complete intact sensibility and good finger and thumb movements on both sides, if aircraft control manipulations are to be carried out safely. Fortunately, major disabilities in this region are easy to identify. Arthrodesis of a finger in isolation need not necessarily preclude aircraft handling, but the hand would have to be assessed carefully as to overall function before flying was permitted. Painful conditions such as arthritis and unreduced dislocations or fractures would be a bar to safe flying. The presence of a plaster cast for, say, a Colles' fracture or even a scaphoid fracture should not be a problem. In the upper extremity two more important factors need to be considered.

1. *Peripheral nerve injuries*—These are usually the result of trauma, be it blunt or sharp. A careful history will elucidate all but the most complex. A working knowledge of how to examine the upper extremity is essential. The reader is referred to the Medical Research Council's War Memorandum No. 7 (1943) on aids to the diagnosis of peripheral nerve injuries for further information.
2. *Dupuytren's contracture*—This relatively uncommon condition of palmar subcuticular fibrosis, which usually involves the ulnar side of the hand, is fortunately rare among younger adults. Its presence in minor form is of little concern as it is slow to progress, and all that will be required is annual assessment. In its more aggressive form with fixed flexion contractures of the ulnar side fingers, surgical correction will be required before flying is permitted.

The back

Thoraco-lumbar spine and backache

During the transition of *Homo sapiens* from the quadruped to the biped position, the human spine has adapted itself to taking heavy loads. The spine itself is a complex of what Schmorl (1932) described as 'vertebral motor units'. These consist of a column of vertebral bodies with intervening intervertebral discs, with the facet joints posteriorly, the whole complex joined by anterior and posterior longitudinal ligaments in continuity with the annulus fibrosus. More posteriorly is a complex of ligaments supported by a muscle mass which helps to maintain the erect posture. In addition to supporting the erect posture this system also affords protection to the spinal cord and cauda equina.

In 1959 Karl Hirsch demonstrated that injection of saline into a disc produced low back pain, which could subsequently be relieved by an injection of local anaesthetic solution. An injection of saline into the superficial ligaments gave rise to local pain, whereas an injection into a posterior facet joint caused pain radiating to the buttock. This experimental work did much to explain the various modalities of back pain experienced by the human sufferer.

The complexity and the variety of causes of low backache are such that when it occurs in aircrew it becomes of particular importance to make a correct diagnosis so that the proper treatment may be applied. The work of Fitzgerald and Crotty (1972) on back pain in aircrew has been valuable, and the individually moulded lumbar supports that they advocated are widely used for the relief of intractable backache in aircrew. Fitzgerald (1972) in a further survey reported a 13% incidence of backache in RAF pilots between the ages of 20 and 50. This backache only occured at the actual time of flying. This incidence is even higher in helicopter pilots, though their symptoms are usually in the thoracic spine, due to the uncomfortable forward flexed position they have to adopt when flying the aircraft. Much work has been done to improve the positions of the seats in more recent aircraft, but further work is still required.

Every case of backache among aircrew before, during, or after training must be carefully evaluated, with particular reference to the history and the possibility of previous injury. Low back pain from mechanical factors must be distinguished from back pain associated with sciatica. The latter is most commonly due to the herniation of the nucleus pulposus in the lower lumbar region. X-rays are mandatory, and the advice of an orthopaedic surgeon or rheumatologist may be required. One must also keep in mind the various specific problems that may be responsible for low back pain, such as ankylosing spondylitis; rheumatoid arthritis and infection; and structural defects, including transitional vertebrae, spondylolysis, spondylolisthesis and other rare abnormalities. Functional defects of lateral imbalance—like leg length discrepancy, scoliosis or posture at work—are much easier to evaluate. Finally, the rare but ever-present possibility of a neoplastic process must also be borne in mind; this may be a primary tumour, an intradural space-occupying lesion, or a metastasis from a distant site.

The management of aircrew with backache will depend upon the underlying cause. Happily, the majority of patients appear to respond to simple conservative measures such as bed rest, certain forms of exercises, or physical treatment in the form of short-wave diathermy, ultrasound, or interferential or transcutaneous nerve stimulation. The provision of a temporary surgical corset can be helpful, and the empirical use of an epidural or caudal injection of local anaesthetic and steroid may be beneficial.

Unfortunately, surgical removal of a herniated intervertebral disc, even in a proven case, does not always lead to the impressive result that it was once thought to do. Despite the use of diagnostic and localizing aids such as radiculography, discography, computerized axial tomography and magnetic resonance imaging, the overall results leave much to be desired, and most orthopaedic surgeons now consider carefully before subjecting a patient to such an operation.

The common condition of lumbosacral strain can occur both in acute and in chronic forms. The former by a sudden movement or blow, moving the spine into an abnormal range of movement, or a sudden effort to prevent an injury, putting the muscles into spasm. Chronic strain may follow on acute strain that has not been treated adequately—when the back musculature has been allowed to deteriorate—or when a patient is overweight.

A discussion on the problem of low backache is not complete without mention of manipulative treatment for those cases with no overt organic cause for their symptoms. The help of a trained physiotherapist is often sought by aircrew in an effort to speed up their recovery. Fortunately, most physiotherapists and osteopaths are well aware of the potential damage that can be inflicted on a back if it is manipulated without proper assessment and radiography, and the likelihood of damage from injudicious treatment is now small. Finally, it is important not to ignore the possibility of psychological factors playing a part in backache, particularly in a patient who may have developed a hidden fear of flying.

The cervical spine

With the advent of highly manoeuvrable aircraft and the introduction of various helmet-mounted devices, considerable interest has been focused on the cervical spine. This interest arises partly because of the need to determine spinal structural strength in response to suddenly applied loads, and partly to ascertain whether long-term degenerative changes are seen in the necks of aircrew as a result of trauma consequent upon head movement in a high-G environment.

No evidence has yet emerged that the incidence of cervical spondylotic change is higher in aircrew than in any other group, with the sole exception of MacKenzie Crook's (1970) positive finding of a significant increase in the condition, as diagnosed radiologically, in aircrew who had ejected. Limited studies in Holland of F16 pilots have shown that they have eight times more cervical symptoms than F104 pilots and that 67% of them experienced cervical symptoms during the duration of the study (Aghina, 1985). No evidence emerged of an increased incidence of spondylotic change in this series of pilots, although a number of candidate pilots for the F16 were rejected because of degenerative disc conditions with osteophyte formation.

Despite considerable research effort, there is little data available in the literature that will provide detailed guidance as to what are the maximum loads that the cervical spine will resist. The fact that soft-tissue neck injury is a not uncommon sequel of ejection and that cervical fracture is a feature, albeit rare, of assisted escape suggests that current helmet weights and forces imposed by escape systems are close to the maximum allowable.

Anatomically the cervical spine is different from the thoraco-lumbar spine in that the former is subjected to far greater strains as the result of its mobility rather than from weight bearing. Degenerative changes occur commonly in the third decade at the C5 to C7 levels, and it is not uncommon to find changes as an incidental finding in people over the age of 40 years. Care must be taken to identify brachalgia, or referred pain down one or other arm, as this may result in muscle weakness and impairment of function while at the controls. Cervical disc prolapse may also occur, but it is uncommon in the younger subjects under discussion. Of greater importance are the neurocentral joints of Luschka which, as the result of loss of disc height, develop secondary arthritic changes, osteophyte formation and encroachment on the foraminal canals where the cervical nerve roots emerge to form the brachial plexus. Clinical examination will reveal any motor, sensory, or deep tendon reflex changes in the arms, and these should be searched for with great care. Investigations must include routine antero-posterior and lateral radiographs of the cervical spine with oblique projections if indicated. The more sophisticated investigations of tomography, discography, radiculography or computerized axial tomography are not normally indicated. Each case must be considered on its own merit, and it is indeed fortunate that most patients with acute stiff neck, or torticollis, respond to simple conservative measures such as rest, the wearing of a collar, traction, physiotherapy and a non-steroidal anti-inflammatory drug. Pre-existing radiographic changes if advanced and accompanied by a neurological deficit, be it episodic or permanent, should preclude aircrew training.

The possible existence of the rare forms of neck lesion be they metabolic, neoplastic, infective or traumatic must always be remembered.

Ejection injury

Cervical injury

There has been concern in recent years that improvements in the design of escape systems were being achieved at the cost of an increased incidence of neck injury. This problem was addressed by an AGARD Working Group (Anton, 1984) which failed to find any evidence in support of this hypothesis. What was noted, however, was that neck injuries did occur on 'within envelope' ejections with a reported incidence of between 1 and 2%.

The commonest type of injury noted was anterior compression fracture of the fifth cervical vertebra. Such a fracture is stable and does not affect the cord. More extreme forms of flexion injury with avulsion of spinal processes were also noted. Such damage may be associated with dislocation of the vertebral bodies with respect to each other leading to the risk of cord damage. More exotic neck injuries are extremely rare on 'within envelope' escapes; but it is prudent to check that no neck injury is present, and it is vital that the cervical spine is included in the standard post-ejection vertebral screen.

More recently it has been noted that a number of cervical fractures occur in-flight. The mechanism appears to be the sudden application of G forces catching the second crewman unawares at a time when the head is rotated to the side to obtain lateral vision. Whilst not an ejection injury, the mechanism should be remembered when analysing data relating to cervical injury in ejection, since ejection may follow a sudden, violent, flight manoeuvre.

Thoraco-lumbar injury

The loads applied to the spine during assisted escape from aircraft, parachute landing and in some aircraft—particularly helicopter—accidents may be sufficient to produce vertebral fractures. The injuries seen may be grouped into six different categories (King, 1984). These are:

1. Anterior wedge fractures.
2. Burst fracture.
3. Dislocations and fracture–dislocations.
4. Chance fractures.
5. Rotational injuries.
6. Hyperextension injuries.

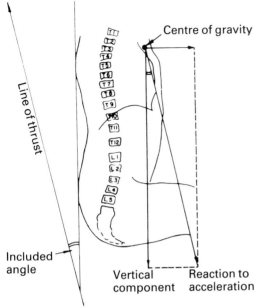

Figure 52.1 The relationship of the line of thrust of an ejection seat to the spine and to the centre of gravity of the upper torso (portion of body above T12) with the hands grasping the seat pan firing handle.

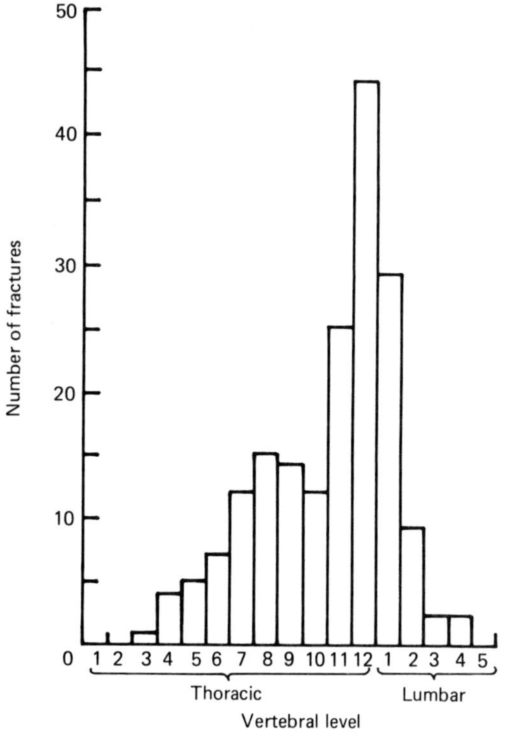

Of these six groups anterior wedge fractures are by far the most common. The mechanism of injury is the combination of axial compressive force and spinal flexion.

The flexion occurs because the centre of gravity of the upper torso lies in front of the spine. A bending movement is thus produced whenever loads are applied along the spinal axis, this bending movement being increased if there is any significant disparity between the line of application of force and the long axis of the spine (*Figure 52.1*).

Typically injuries occur at the thoracolumbar hinge (T12-L1) although a significant proportion of injuries also occur at the mid-thoracic level. The distribution of fractures seen in ejectees from RAF aircraft between 1968 and 1983 is shown in *Figure 52.2*. All of these fractures were of the anterior wedge type of which *Figure 52.3* is a typical example.

Anterior wedge fractures resulting from ejection are usually stable with no damage to the longitudinal ligaments or spinal cord involvement. This is not always so in the more uncontrolled environment of aircraft impact and ditching and under such circumstances, with higher energy input, burst fractures may be seen. These fractures are unstable

Figure 52.2 The distribution of 184 vertebral fractures in a group of 105 aircrew who sustained vertebral injury on ejection from Royal Air Force aircraft between 1968 and 1983.

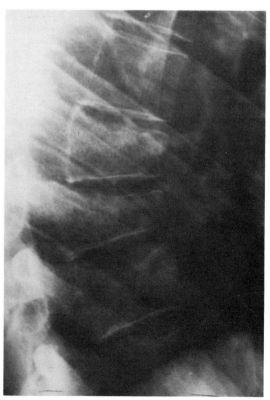

Figure 52.3 Lateral radiograph of a typical vertebral anterior wedge fracture, occurring at the 11th thoracic vertebra.

and neurological involvement is a very real possibility. With the exception of hyperextension injuries all of the other fracture categories mentioned are associated with varying degrees of extreme spinal flexion and/or rotation and are rarely encountered.

Diagnosis

Following successful ejection an airman should be assessed by the medical officer. If other injuries do not preclude it, he should then be admitted to hospital under orthopaedic care. A full spinal radiographic screen from C1 to the sacrum should be carried out. In the event that the screen is negative, that the patient is symptomatic, or there is an urgent requirement for him to return to the flying role, a bone scan should be ordered. A bone-seeking radiopharmaceutical, oxidronate labelled with technetium 99m, is injected intravenously for this purpose. No adverse effects have been noted and the radiation dose to the spine is less than 1 rad, which is regarded as safe for clinical radiodiagnostic procedures. Technetium 99m is taken up by active metabolizing bone thus highlighting fresh fractures and infractions. A gamma-camera study of the whole skeletal system will show a fresh bony injury as a 'hot spot' even in the absence of findings on a plain radiograph.

Treatment

The presence of a fresh fracture following an ejection demands 3 weeks total bed rest in hospital. Its purpose is to remove the load on the fracture until the cortical bone has regained some of its intrinsic strength. During this period as soon as the back has become pain free (7–10 days) extension exercises are carried out, first in the supine and then in the prone position. Gradual mobilization can then be resumed, but all forms of flying are barred (except as a passenger) for a period of 3 months. In the event of slow muscle recovery, a rehabilitation centre should be utilized.

Recovery

The majority of aircrew (90%) with simple, stable crush fractures go on to make a full recovery, and after a further orthopaedic check at the end of the 3-month period, return to flying, to include the use of ejection seats.

References

AGHINA, J.C.F.M. (1985) Systematic radiographic examination of the spine for selection of F16 pilots: a preliminary report. In van Dalen, A. and van den Biggelaar, N.H.M. (eds) *Medical Selection and Physiological Training of Future Fighter Aircrew*. AGARD Conference Proceedings No. 396, pp. 41–1. Neuilly-sur-Seine: AGARD/NATO

ANTON, D.J. (ed.) (1984) *Report of the Working Group on the Clinical and Biomedical Evaluation of Trauma and Fatalities Associated with Aircrew Ejection and Crash*. AGARD Advisory Report No. 194. Neuilly-sur-Seine: AGARD/NATO

FITZGERALD, J.F. and CROTTY, J. (1972) *The Incidence of Backache Among Aircrew and Ground Crew in the Royal Air Force*. RAF Institute of Aviation Medicine Report No 505, London: Ministry of Defence

HIRSCH, C. (1959) Studies on the pathology of low back pain. *Journal of Bone and Joint Surgery*, **41b**, 237–243

KING, I.A. (1984) The spine, its anatomy, kinematics, injury mechanisms and tolerance in impact. In Aldman, B. and Chapon, A. (eds) *The Biomechanics of Impact Trauma*. Amsterdam: Elsevier Science Publishers

MACKENZIE CROOKS L. (1970) Long term effects of ejecting from aircraft. *Aerospace Medicine*, **41**, 803–804

Medical Research Council (1943) *Aids to the Investigation of Peripheral Nerve Injuries*, revised 2nd edn. War Memorandum No. 7. London: HMSO

SCHLESINGER (1983) In Duthie, R.B. and Bentley, G. (eds) *Mercer's Orthopaedic Surgery*, 8th edn. p. 921. London: Edward Arnold

SCHMORL, G. (1932) Uber Verlagerung von Bandscheibengewebe und ihre Folgen. *Archiv fur Klinische Chirurgie*, **172**, 240

Part X

Accident Investigation

53

Accident investigation and its management

A.J.C. Balfour

The medical investigation of fatal aircraft accidents

The first thing to be done after an aircraft accident is to find and look after the survivors. This may prove more difficult than it sounds, because those who can are likely to run away and may be difficult to find, and others may be trapped within the wreckage where they cannot be seen; and fire or some other hazard may make it difficult or temporarily impossible to search the wreckage. Only about 25% of accidents happen in mid-flight, and over 50% on the approach or landing, so that most accidents happen close to an airfield, where there will be emergency services which should be organized so that they can reach the accident site quickly to set about finding and treating the survivors as rapidly as possible. It is likely that many of those who have survived the impact but are seriously injured will die in the 20 minutes or so following the accident, so that speed is important if lives are to be saved; and the need for haste may make it necessary to damage or destroy part of the aircraft in order to find survivors or possible survivors.

However, in an accident where there are no survivors or where all of the survivors have been treated already the situation is completely different, and there is no need for haste. What is needed then is a patient search to find and record all the evidence, so that the investigators may have the best possible chance of finding the cause of the accident; because only when the cause is known can measures be devised to prevent a recurrence. Both in cases where there are survivors and in those where there are none, the aim is to save lives.

Medical investigation is of the greatest importance in fatal aircraft accidents because there may be no witnesses as to what was going on in the aircraft before the accident, or to what the crew thought was going on; so that it is necessary to try to build up a picture of the situation by other means. The medical services played only a small part in accident investigation between the two world wars, possibly because aircraft usually crashed at relatively slow speeds so that it was usual to have a survivor who could give an eye-witness account; but the German Air Force developed a scientific approach to aircraft accidents, and studies of aviation injuries were made in USA. In the United Kingdom it was not until after the war that the report of a classic investigation by a forensic pathologist (Teare, 1951) correlated the safety equipment with the post-mortem findings. Four years later the medical investigation of the Comet aircraft accidents (Armstrong et al., 1955) led to a reconstruction of the sequence of events in the accident, and focused attention on the value of the pathology findings in fatal accidents. The Department of Aviation and Forensic Pathology at the RAF Institute of Pathology and Tropical Medicine (IPTM) was founded as a direct result of these investigations (Stamm, 1968), as was the Aerospace Pathology department at the Armed Forces Institute of Pathology (AFIP) in Washington.

Great interest was also shown in Canada (Mason and Reals, 1973), and the three countries joined to form the Joint Committee on Aviation Pathology in November 1955, whose objectives were:

1. Collection of information regarding the correlation between pathological evidence and causative factors of aircraft accidents.
2. Initiation of detailed pathological investigations which may yield information relating to the cause of hitherto unexplained aircraft accidents.
3. Improvement of flight safety records as a result of pathological correlation data.

4. Investigation of possible insidious changes induced by repeated and long duration exposure to environmental factors and forces present during flight.
5. Establishment of a long-range programme involving the accumulation of pathological data from a large series of cases.
6. Investigation of psychological and physiological factors which may produce pathological changes as a result of flight stresses.

Originally the Aviation Pathology Departments were concerned with Service accidents only, but energetic flight safety campaigns led to a fall in the number of fatal military accidents and allowed assistance with civil accidents also. In Great Britain distances are relatively small, so that it made good sense to establish a centralized Aviation Pathology Department to deal with all the fatal aircraft accidents within UK, on average between 40 and 50 each year. In other countries where the distances are larger and the legal system less homogeneous there are greater difficulties, and various systems have been tried depending upon local conditions.

International organization

The International Civil Aviation Organisation (ICAO) has published in the series of International Standards and Recommended Practices of the Convention on International Civil Aviation an Annex 13 on Aircraft Accident Investigation, which has been accepted by many States (International Civil Aviation Organisation, 1981). Annex 13 gives various definitions for aircraft accident investigation purposes; briefly, an event is considered to be an accident when between the time any person boards an aircraft with the intention of flight and the time before such persons have disembarked, somebody is fatally or seriously injured, or the aircraft sustains damage or structural failure requiring major repair, or the aircraft is missing or inaccessible. The State in whose territory the accident occurs undertakes to preserve the evidence and arrange for an investigation, to which the State on whose register the aircraft is entered may send an accredited representative, as may the State responsible for the certification of the airworthiness of the aircraft. The international co-operation resulting from these agreements has done much to make the investigation of accidents easier and more effective; there may still be complications when an aircraft crashes in international waters, and the accident is investigated by the State where the aircraft was registered, but the autopsies and the inquests are held in the State where the bodies of the casualties come ashore.

In the UK the coroner has very wide powers and is responsible for holding an inquest on unnatural deaths, normally in co-operation with the official accident investigators, either civil or service, from the same or another country. Strictly, HM Coroners officiate in England and Wales, and in other countries there will be legal officials with similar objectives but different procedures, such as the Procurator Fiscal in Scotland, while in the USA the word coroner has a different meaning. In England the coroner commonly opens his inquest a day or two after the accident and takes sufficient evidence to give the family a burial or cremation certificate, and then adjourns the inquest until such time as the investigation has been completed; he then reopens the inquest with all the relevant witnesses, and gives the family a death certificate after a verdict has been reached. The coroner usually has a jury, and may ask one of the official investigators to sit beside him as an assessor. The pathologist who has carried out the autopsies is expected to assist the court as an expert witness and give not only his observations but his opinions based upon his findings and his experience of past aircraft accidents; until the inquest is finally concluded all the evidence belongs to the coroner and must not be divulged to anybody else without his permission.

Accident investigators

In the UK the Chief Inspector of Accidents of the Accidents Investigation Branch (AIB) is directly responsible to the Secretary of State for Transport, and has the right to decide whether to order a formal investigation into a civil accident. If there are fatalities, it is likely that AIB Inspectors will make enquiries, whether or not a formal Inspector's Investigation is decided upon later; but if the accident is to a large public transport aircraft with many fatalities then the Secretary of State may order a public enquiry (Accidents Investigation Branch, 1984). The AIB inspectors have powers to require evidence to be produced and to retain it; the police assist them as appropriate, usually working in conjunction with the Coroner's Officer. The investigation of accidents involving gliders, hot air balloons or hang-gliders are usually delegated to the appropriate national association, but the Chief Inspector of Accidents retains the right to investigate any accident where he considers it necessary to do so. The purpose of enquiring into an aircraft accident is to establish the probable cause, so that appropriate steps may be taken to prevent a recurrence, and the assessment of blame or responsibility is not amongst the duties of the AIB. The Department of Aviation and Forensic Pathology at IPTM was established in 1955 to investigate Service accidents, but since the early 1960s has routinely assisted the AIB with the medical investigation of civil fatal accidents.

The pathologist must always act only upon the order of the coroner, who may ask the aviation pathologist to carry out the autopsies, or who may decide that some other pathologist should carry out the autopsies but that the aviation pathologist may attend as an official observer. Home Office Circular number 90 of 1971 suggests that whenever a coroner is called upon to investigate a death or deaths following an aircraft accident he may wish to consider asking an RAF pathologist to carry out any necessary post-mortem examination, and over the years the Department has had much help and co-operation from HM Coroners. In other countries the procedures will differ in accordance with local law, but the overall effects are generally similar; in the USA the National Transport Safety Board (NTSB) investigate major accidents, and call upon the assistance of the Aerospace Pathology Department of the AFIP to assist them with the medical investigation of major civil aircraft accidents, in addition to that department's ordinary task of investigating military accidents.

Military aircraft accidents are normally investigated by the Service concerned, the Board of Inquiry always working with HM Coroner, or the corresponding legal official, and with the police. Aircraft accidents cause a great deal of extra work for the police, and it is helpful to them if arrangements can be made for tasks such as guarding the accident site to be handed over to the Service concerned. It is for HM Coroner to decide who shall carry out the autopsy, but it is especially appropriate that it should be done by an RAF Aviation Pathologist because of the specialized nature of the aircraft, its task and the equipment of the aircrew. The Aviation Pathology team from IPTM try to attend all fatal aircraft accidents within the UK on behalf of all three Services or of the AIB, although in about 20% of accidents this proves impossible because the body of the pilot has not been recovered from the sea or for some other reason. They also assist the AIB at civil aircraft accidents overseas when requested by the Chief Inspector of Accidents, depending upon the circumstances. Under the Visiting Forces Act fatal accidents to military aircraft of friendly powers are normally investigated by the teams from their own country; so that the Aerospace Pathology team from Washington would normally attend a USAF accident in the UK. Similarly, the IPTM team may attend accidents to UK Service aircraft overseas. Whatever the circumstances of the accident, and whoever is carrying out the medical investigation, it is important that all the investigators should work together as a team and share the evidence they obtain so as to arrive at the truth.

The police are likely to be first on the scene, and to be responsible for co-ordinating the emergency services if there are survivors; and, after the survivors have been dealt with, for guarding the accident site and preserving the evidence. They will also co-ordinate the efforts and assistance of the civil or military investigation teams with the authority and requirements of the coroner; in each area the police will have disaster plans prepared, and will help the visiting team. All airfields will have their own disaster plans, prepared in conjunction with the police, the ambulance and fire services, which will all be standing by whenever aircraft are operating. The AIB have prepared a Memorandum on the Investigation of Civil air accidents, which outlines the essential procedures. Security of the accident site is one of the most important considerations, and once the rescue and fire fighting teams have completed their tasks only police, AIB personnel and Customs or Excise officers are allowed on site; it is all too easy for valuable evidence to be destroyed by the public, quite apart from evidence that may be removed by souvenir hunters. The AIB engineers complete their on-site investigation as soon as they can, so that the police do not have to guard the site any longer than is essential; and may then release the wreckage to the owner, or remove it for more detailed examination. It is also essential that the accident site should be mapped accurately, the positions of the pieces of wreckage and of the casualties recorded, and a complete photographic record made, starting with distant photographs so that the relationship of the wreckage and the casualties is shown, working up to middle-distance views and then close-ups showing the details.

Some pathologists prefer to see the accident site first and then go to the mortuary, while others like to make a rapid external examination of corpses and then go and examine the accident site before carrying out the autopsy in detail; often circumstances will dictate what the pathologist must do first, but the important thing is that he should examine both the wreckage and the bodies and then go to and fro between the accident site and the mortuary until he has correlated all the information available. If it is at all possible the pathologist should see the bodies in position at the accident site; there is usually no difficulty about this if the pathologist can reach the site reasonably quickly, and the site itself is such that reasonable privacy can be assured. No harm is done by keeping a body in a cool field for a few hours, and much irreplaceable evidence may be lost if the body is moved before it has been examined by a doctor on site and notes made and photographs taken. Sometimes a body may have been taken away to hospital if the rescue services thought that there was a chance of resuscitation, or it may be that the Incident Officer in charge considers it necessary to remove the body because of special risks; there may be hazards from fire, or chemicals such as pesticides in crop-spraying air-craft, which may threaten to destroy the evidence or put the rescue workers at risk. It is also a consideration that post-mortem changes will set in rapidly if a body is left in a warm place, so that if the pathologist cannot arrive at once a judgement has to be made as to whether keeping the body on site will lose more evidence than it will gain. It is important to preserve the bodies both as evidence and for the sake of human dignity if it is possible, but if this can only be done by putting the lives of rescue workers at risk then the living must come first and it may be necessary to abandon the bodies of the dead.

Mortuary organization

The next problem is where to put a large number of dead bodies, and how to get them there. A temporary mortuary is usually the best solution, perhaps an empty hangar on the other side of the airfield or any other large building where all the bodies can be stored together; tents have been used successfully, as have trailer trucks. The only essential requirement for a mortuary is security, so that no unauthorized person can interfere with the evidence, that is to say the bodies, or with the workers who are attending to them. It is very desirable to have space and light, perhaps heating, ventilation and running water; but even quite rudimentary facilities are adequate if privacy can be guaranteed, especially if some sort of refrigeration can be provided for the bodies. Freezing of bodies is not allowable; it is dangerous because the presence of ice may cause a knife to slip at autopsy, because it takes time for the body to thaw out, and because the appearance of the tissues may be altered by freezing. Refrigeration at about 4°C will keep the body in good condition until such time as the pathologists can perform an unhurried and careful autopsy, after which the undertakers can carry out embalming.

The great advantage of refrigeration is that it removes the need for haste in the investigation, which too often leads to evidence being overlooked or destroyed inadvertently. The amount of cooling that will be needed obviously depends on the local climate, but often some sort of cold storage may be available; if not, portable refrigeration or the use of freezer trucks with the thermostat suitably adjusted may be the answer. No other form of preservation is permissible before the autopsy, as embalming or even putting cotton wool in the orifices may alter the physical or chemical findings significantly, and embalming would obviously prevent any attempt at toxicology. Bagging the hands and head in separate small plastic bags is a useful refinement, but in an aviation accident rather than a criminal case the benefits might not justify the extra effort, and in a mass disaster it would probably overstrain the resources available.

Logical and orderly organization is necessary in the mortuary if a large number of bodies are to be dealt with carefully in a reasonable time. It will take many assistants dressed in suitable protective clothing to move them about as required; this work is often undertaken by the police, who also commonly cope with the paperwork and who may have computer facilities to assist the identification procedure. This will fall naturally into three stages; firstly, the examination and photographing of the clothed bodies and their possessions, which may often lead to a provisional identification, followed by careful undressing and the recording of the nature and state of all the clothing, equipment and possessions. The pathologist should see all the bodies clothed before the autopsy, and should witness the undressing of the aircrew. If the aircrew have flying equipment this must be removed by somebody who is familiar with it, both so that he can assess any damage and also so that he can deal with any pyrotechnics or other dangerous items. Secondly the unclothed body should be carefully examined by the pathologist and photographed, with close-ups of any injuries or identifying marks considered important, and at this stage the body should be X-rayed if this is practicable. The pathologist then carries out the autopsy, using whatever procedure his experience suggests for that individual, and taking specimens for histology and toxicology as a routine.

It is an advantage to take the whole heart for examination rather than just a few blocks, as it is then possible to make a detailed examination of blocks from the whole organ if it is found to be required later. Blocks are taken from each organ and from each lobe of the lungs, together with anything else that appears to be of interest or importance. The toxicology specimens taken will depend upon what is available, but if possible clean limb blood is taken in fluoride for alcohol estimations and in heparin for carboxyhaemoglobin, urine in fluoride and in a plain container for alcohol and drug screens; bile or CSF may also be taken. The most reliable specimen for alcohol estimation is vitreous humour from each eye taken separately into fluoride, and it is also important to take at least 200 g liver tissue preserved by deep freezing for drug analysis.

Photography of the internal findings and injuries is often unrewarding, but the facility should be available. Measurements of height and weight of the unclothed body and records of any tattoos or other identifying marks may confirm identification, and the injuries visible on the unclothed body can also be correlated with the flying equipment and clothing examined previously. Forensic odontologists will also be examining the dentition at this stage, working with the pathologist just before or just after the main autopsy, depending on the degree of injury to the head and jaws; if the jaws are intact the teeth may be charted early, but if there are severe facial injuries and the jaws are fragmented then the pathologist and dentist will have to work together. After the autopsy has been completed and specimens taken, the bodies are passed to the undertakers for embalming and restoration of their appearance to make them as acceptable as is possible to their relatives.

Identification

Identification is the responsibility of the police, but under the circumstances of a fatal accident it is likely that medical and dental evidence will be important in the identification process, and in practice it is properly a team effort.

Identification is important for medico-legal purposes for the coroner, for the family who naturally want to have the right body back for the funeral, and for the investigation of the accident; if it is suspected that the Captain of an airliner has had a heart attack and that this has led to the accident, then the next question is which of the several hundred bodies is the Captain. In ordinary civil life bodies are usually identified visually by relatives or friends, but after a large aircraft accident this is often unreliable because of the overwhelming emotional effects of a mass disaster, and also because many or all of the bodies may be badly mangled or incinerated.

There are many different means of identification; and the golden rule is firstly to use all the means of identification that are available, so that one cross-checks another, and secondly not to release any of the bodies until they have all been identified. It is all too easy to release some bodies, and later further evidence is found which shows that an error has been made; then there is a very difficult situation which cannot be dealt with without exhumations, causing great distress to relatives. Effectively, there are two classes of identification methods. Firstly, identification by comparing parts of the body, such as warts, or deformed toes, or teeth with ante-mortem records, which may give positive proof of identification. Secondly, comparison of possessions found on the body, such as clothing or papers or jewellery, may provide a helpful starting point but not positive proof, because people may exchange possessions for all sorts of romantic or criminal reasons. Nevertheless, a wallet firmly buttoned into a hip pocket is likely to belong to that person, unless he has stolen it from someone, and possessions may well be the easiest way to start the identification process; but other and more reliable methods must be used to confirm or refute the working hypothesis. Dental identification has proved to be the most

reliable and successful single means of identification, and is considered in detail in Chapter 55. Even if a body has no teeth, it may well be that the dentures have been retained in the mouth and protected from fire by the moist cheeks and tongue; they may indicate the identity, especially if they have a name or a number on them.

The pathology team

The size of the team taken to the site will depend upon the size of the accident; IPTM normally send a pathologist, a laboratory scientific officer, and an odontologist with forensic experience if there is any difficulty with the identifications, and are prepared to send further experts and photographers as required. Suitable forms for recording the findings are only a small part of the equipment which the Aviation Pathology team must bring with them to the accident; ideally they should also have a portable computer and modem so that the findings can be rapidly transferred to the large computer at their home base, where other workers can gather and transmit to the team information that may assist with identification, or the clarification of the autopsy findings in the light of the past medical history of the casualty. The team will also have to carry post-mortem kit, and containers for specimens sufficient for the estimated number of casualties; IPTM have cases with equipment for 200 casualties standing by permanently, with arrangements to provide others rapidly if needed; the cases are of watertight metal alloy suitable for air transport.

After the autopsies and all the special investigations have been completed, all the information available has to be collated and arranged logically to see what deductions can be made from it. This appraisal has to be a joint function of all the investigators because both medical and technical evidence is important, as in the Rhodes Comet accident (Mason and Tarlton, 1969). There may be evidence of a probable or possible medical cause for the accident, but this is unusual, as one would expect when all aircrew have regular medical examinations. Nevertheless, the previous medical history of the aircrew, if not of everybody on board the aircraft, must be scrutinized and any medical factors that might have caused or contributed to the accident examined in detail. The question of pilot incapacitation by alcohol or other self-administered drugs must always be considered, but the toxicological examination will usually provide the answer here if suitable specimens for analysis were available; but in some cases the material available for examination is such that a reliable result cannot be obtained. Histology may indicate previous disease, or one may be in the unsatisfactory position of having to say that while there was no evidence of incapacitation one could not disprove it either. There are other human factors to be considered besides pathological changes, and as well as the previous medical history attempts should be made to assess the psychological state of the aircrew before the accident. This may be relatively straightforward when there is a history of mental disturbance or a suicide note has been left, but very often it is a matter of questioning the family and friends; this is outside the scope of pathology, but has to be considered as part of the medical investigation process. The position is often easier with a service accident, where the flight medical officer on a flying station may know the pilot and his aircraft and its task well, so that he is in a position to answer many of these questions himself.

The safety equipment associated with the aircrew must be examined in detail, by experts with experience in finding any traces of malfunction, and who can also recognize damage that may have been caused during the accident sequence. Ejection seats are a good example, as expert examination may reveal some fault in the escape sequence or damage which can be shown to have been caused before the accident rather than at ground impact. Recent changes in legislation and product liability claims may or may not concern the pathologist directly, but they have certainly led to more searching enquiries in court and the need for a higher standard of technical evidence and of preparation before court appearances.

Pathologists can never tell beforehand which accidents are the ones in which the medical evidence will be of great value, as against those in which it makes little or no contribution; so the aviation pathologist must try to attend every fatal aircraft accident within his field of action. This may not be possible to achieve, and unless the bodies have been recovered there is nothing useful that the pathologist can do to help. No discoveries are made except by looking for them, and if one does look carefully and finds nothing unusual it may be possible to say it was because there was nothing to be found—and this is, of itself, a valuable result for the accident investigators. Tench (1985) records many accidents where successful technical or medical investigations have led to notable improvements in flight safety, which have reduced the loss of lives in aviation accidents.

References

Accidents Investigation Branch, Department of Transport (1984) *Memorandum on the Investigation of Civil Air Accidents*. London: HMSO

ARMSTRONG, J.A., FRYER, D.I., STEWART, W.K. and WHITTINGHAM, H.E. (1955) Interpretation of injuries in the Comet aircraft disasters. *Lancet*, **i**, 1135–1144

International Civil Aviation Organisation (1981) *Aircraft Accident Investigation: Annex 13 to the Convention on Civil Aviation*, 6th edn. Montreal: ICAO

MASON, J.K. and REALS, W.J. (eds) (1973) *Aerospace Pathology*. Chicago: College of American Pathologists Foundation

MASON, J.K. and TARLTON, S.W. (1969) Medical investigation of the loss of the Comet 4B aircraft, 1967. *Lancet*, **i**, 431–434

STAMM, W.P. (1968) Aviation accident pathology. *Proceedings of the Royal Society of Medicine*, **61**, 1705–1706

TEARE, D. (1951) Post mortem examinations on aircraft victims. *British Medical Journal*, **ii**, 707–708

TENCH, W.H. (1985) *Safety is No Accident*, 1st edn. London: Collins.

54

Aviation pathology

A.J.C. Balfour

'Aviation in itself is not inherently dangerous. But to an even greater degree than the sea, it is terribly unforgiving of any carelessness, incapacity or neglect.'

(Lamplugh, 1932)

Aviation pathology is the application of the disciplines of traumatic pathology in the service of flight safety; it has been defined (Mason, 1962) as the comprehensive study of aviation fatalities whereby the medical history of the casualty and the findings at autopsy can be correlated with the environmental factors, the structural or other damage to the aircraft and the use or abuse of equipment so that a complete picture of the accident may be formed. The object of investigating fatal aircraft accidents is to find their causes and prevent similar accidents occurring in the future, and if this is to be achieved the investigation must be as thorough and complete as circumstances permit; this demands a multi-disciplined team approach, and the areas of interest covered are very wide.

The pathologist is primarily concerned with the human factors in the accident, and he may often be able to implicate a contributory or even a main cause of the accident, and be of assistance to the accident investigators in seven main fields:

1. Demonstration of disease in the pilot which may be causative, contributory or coincidental to the accident.
2. Circumstantial medical evidence, such as a history of psychiatric illness.
3. Toxicological evidence: alcohol, carbon monoxide or drugs.
4. Mechanical defects manifesting as toxicological findings, e.g. fumes in cockpit.
5. Sequence of events in the accident.

6. Whether emergency was anticipated, or occurred without warning.
7. Questions relating to survivability.

The pathologist's investigation is undertaken to find medical evidence which might reveal natural disease, or some abnormality that could have caused incapacitation, or led to impaired function. Circumstantial evidence can be an important factor in the interpretation of pre-existing disease in aircrew, but the main source of medical evidence is from detailed autopsies on the bodies of all those who have been killed.

These findings have to be correlated with the medical histories of the aircrew, and the laboratory examinations of the specimens taken at autopsy, the evidence from the victims' clothing and equipment, and the evidence at the scene of the accident. It is important that the pathological evidence should be interpreted together with the evidence found by the non-medical investigators, and that all the evidence available should be correlated. It is essential that the pathologist should visit the scene of the accident whenever it is possible to do so, in order to appreciate the circumstances and discover the significance of the injuries; and it will often be important to examine an intact aircraft similar to the one in the accident.

Pre-existing disease

Aircrew have regular medical examinations with ECGs and chest X-rays as appropriate, so it is likely that any evidence of disease found at autopsy following a fatal aircraft accident will be covert; and any pilot known to be suffering from a condition liable to cause sudden incapacitation would only be licensed to fly with a safety pilot, if at all. Coronary artery disease is a good example, because it is common both in aircrew and in the general population and because it is all too likely that a pilot who has a heart attack in the air will also have an accident. The prevalence of significant coronary artery disease in one series of 288 aircrew killed in 210 aircraft accidents (Underwood Ground, 1981) was found to be 17% in 135 military aircrew with a mean age of 29, 22% in 100 private pilots with a mean age of 37, and 25% in 53 commercial pilots with a mean age of 40. The prevalence in 132 apparently healthy men between the ages of 18 and 62 who had been killed accidentally was 18%, with a mean age of 30; by contrast, 11 glider pilots with a mean age of 49 had a 36% prevalence. There appeared to be no significant difference in the prevalence in the four main groups, although the older glider pilots did have a higher prevalence. An earlier series (Mason, 1963) found a prevalence of 25% in 180 aircrew with a mean age of 28, suggesting no significant change over two decades. As the disease is common, it is not unusual to find some degree of arteriosclerosis in solo pilots who have been killed in accidents; the important question for the aviation pathologist is then whether the disease caused or contributed to the accident, or whether it is a purely coincidental finding. If a man has a heart attack on land and collapses there is often no medical evidence of the acute attack, but the fact that he has collapsed is known; with a pilot flying an aircraft, as with a driver in a car, it is possible that he may collapse at the controls or perhaps suffer symptoms which distract him so that he crashes, and unless he has had time to give a distress signal there may be no evidence of his incapacitation. At autopsy and on histology there may well be evidence of previous heart attacks, but evidence of the terminal attack is likely to be lacking; so that it becomes necessary to examine every piece of circumstantial evidence in detail to try to determine the true course of events.

A rather similar problem is posed by focal myocarditis, which is found from time to time (Stevens and Underwood Ground, 1970), and may or may not have contributed to the accident and the death. In one airline accident focal myocarditis was found in the captain of an airliner taking off at night, but the presence of pulmonary fat and bone marrow emboli indicated that his circulatory system had been intact at impact, which suggested that the myocarditis had not caused cardiac symptoms before the accident although it did not prove it conclusively.

Sarcoidosis is another disease which may cause sudden collapse, and the prevalence of 'sarcoid-like-granulomata' at autopsy was found to be 3% in 294 military aircrew, but only 1% in 268 civil pilots and in 290 passengers or glider pilots (Balfour, 1982); this raised the questions of whether there might be an association between these lesions and accidents, or whether some environmental factor led to their occurrence in aircrew more often than in passengers; both speculations are fascinating, but there is no other evidence to support either idea and it is possible that the findings are due to chance because the numbers are small.

Professional pilots not only have regular medical examinations but also have constant contact with their colleagues and managers, so that any developing problem which might later lead to an accident may well be recognized and dealt with before the accident occurs; but private pilots are unsupervised, and from time to time irregularities occur. After a fatal accident a glider pilot who was believed to be fit was found to have been suffering from severe epilepsy since childhood (Stevens, 1970), and the supply that he had left suggested that he had not been taking his treatment as he should have been. The evidence was circumstantial, but there was reason to believe that the accident was caused by the instructor having a fit, presumably because he had not taken his treatment as prescribed; the problem remained as to why a very competent instructor should have failed to take his medicine. No explanation was found for this, and the only suggestion was that it was so important to him to fly that he suppressed the realization of his illness even in his own mind.

The interpretation of the autopsy findings may be made more difficult by the severe or fatal injuries caused at impact, and it is obviously more difficult to form an opinion on the previous state of an organ when it has been severely traumatized. However, the history of the accident, the previous medical history of the individual, and the findings at autopsy and on histology may add up to a convincing hypothesis when they are all considered together.

Pilots in multi-pilot aircraft occasionally suffer cardiovascular or other symptoms; and the fact that there have been very few civil air transport accidents attributed to coronary artery disease is a tribute not to the medical profession for ensuring that pilots are fit, but to the co-pilots who have taken over the controls very promptly when their colleagues have become incapacitated.

Intoxication

Intoxication crops up as a factor in aircraft accidents as well as in road traffic accidents, and is an equally controversial subject. Alcohol determinations on the tissue of 102 pilots killed in 86 fatal light-aircraft accidents in the UK (Underwood Ground, 1975) were positive in 34 cases varying from small amounts to 313 mg/100 ml; the difficulties of interpreting post-mortem tissue alcohol levels were recognized, but 12 pilots involved in 10 of the accidents were considered to have ingested alcohol before flying, giving an incidence of 11.6% fatal light-aircraft accidents in which alcohol played a part. Drinking undoubtedly played a significant part in the fatal accidents of pilots with a high level of alcohol in their blood; but, as with road traffic accidents, there has been considerable argument as to the likely effects of lower levels. There can be no disagreement with the view that alcohol does impair performance, and that any pilot who places himself under its influence is subjecting himself to an avoidable hazard.

The classic study (Billings *et al.*, 1973) showed that blood alcohol concentrations of 40 mg/100 ml and over were associated with an increase in serious errors both in inexperienced and in experienced pilots; and at a level of 120 mg/100 ml pilots flew in a grossly unsafe manner on 16 out of 30 flights. More recently (Flanagan *et al.*, 1983) a study on road vehicle drivers confirmed yet again the wide individual variation in response to low blood alcohol levels; some people show marked impairment at very low levels, together with mild euphoria, so that the drivers were surprised that their performance had deteriorated. Alcohol levels of 50 mg/100 ml or over clearly induce significant deterioration of performance in aircraft pilots; levels of 20 mg/100 ml or even less probably also increase the risk of an accident, although this has not been proved. A study of fatal accidents in the USA (Ryan and Mohler, 1972) found that the proportion of accidents with alcohol levels of 50 mg/100 ml or more was fairly stable, but that the proportion of accidents with levels of 150 mg/100 ml or more was higher since the introduction of an 8 hour abstinence period before flying in 1970. The comment was made (Mason, 1983) that, since the proportion of fatal accidents associated with a very high blood alcohol level had risen since the Federal Aviation Authority introduced a regulation forbidding private flying within 8 hours of alcohol intake, the conclusion must be that at one end of the scale were the social drinkers who were amenable to reason and regulation, and at the other end the hardened alcoholics who were indifferent to moral or punitive measures. It is an offence to fly in UK airspace while under the influence of drink or drugs so as to impair the capacity of the crew member, but at present there is no authority to test the biological fluids of living pilots for alcohol content as there is with drivers of automobiles.

Alcohol is a difficult subject to discuss, firstly because most people have strong feelings on the subject one way or the other, and secondly because there are so many variables that it is difficult to predict the effects of an alcoholic drink with any certainty. It may not be easy to discover how many drinks a subject has had, as after he has had a few his memory is likely to be uncertain; and often it is

uncertain how much alcohol there is in the drink, although a useful generalization is that there is likely to be about 20 g of alcohol in a pint of beer or a double measure of spirits. The amount of alcohol absorbed and the time taken for this varies greatly according to the nature of the drink and the amount of food in the stomach, but commonly 85–90% of the alcohol is absorbed within an hour. The concentration of alcohol in the tissues will vary with the volume of the total body water into which it is diluted; this will vary not only with the size and weight of the drinker but with the percentage of his total weight which is body water, 55–60% being usual. The range extends from 42% to 70% according to age and sex (Documenta Geigy, 1956), and the state of health and hydration would also be relevant. Most of the alcohol in the body is detoxicated by the liver, often at a steady rate which has the effect of lowering the blood alcohol level by 15 mg/100 ml each hour, but according to the state of liver function this figure may vary from 8 to 25 mg/100 ml. There may also be doubts about the time available for absorption and for detoxication, so that there are difficulties about extrapolating back to previous blood alcohol levels from a single measurement, although a recent study (Lewis, 1986) proposes an improved procedure for retrospective estimations.

All these variable factors mean that the only two reliable deductions one can make about an individual are the highest peak level his blood alcohol might reach after ingesting a certain quantity of alcohol, and also the lowest amount of alcohol he must ingest to reach a particular blood level; other speculations may be helpful as a working hypothesis, but estimates as to previous blood level and the amount of alcohol consumed must be made with considerable caution even in the living.

The position is more difficult with autopsy specimens, as although the amount of alcohol in the specimen bottle can be measured accurately on the gas chromatograph the level may or may not reflect the amount of alcohol present in the body at death. Under the circumstances of a fatal aircraft accident organisms from the gut and elsewhere are likely to get into the bloodstream, and many of them will ferment glucose and other substances to produce alcohol (Corry, 1978); so that, unless the autopsy is carried out very soon after death, alcohol from early putrefactive changes may be present. Ideally one should obtain clean limb blood at autopsy for alcohol estimations in a fluoride container and refrigerate them until the analysis can be completed, but if the body is badly injured the only material available may well be contaminated already. If only ethyl alcohol is present, it is likely to be due to drinking; but if a mixture of alcohols including methyl, propyl, etc. are present then that suggests the presence of putrefaction. Bacteriological studies should also be carried out routinely to see whether alcohol-producing organisms are present, but there is always the risk of failing to detect them because they have died or because they are reluctant to grow on culture. The remedy is to examine other specimens as well as blood, urine being less likely to be contaminated; but the best specimen is normally vitreous humour, which is likely to remain uncontaminated unless the eye has been injured directly. Bile and CSF may also be tested.

If there are consistent raised levels in all the fluids tested, then it is highly likely that the subject was drinking before death; but if there is a raised level in the blood and not in the other fluids, then the raised blood level should be attributed to contamination. The interpretation may be straightforward, or may be so difficult as to be virtually impossible; it is important to get all the information available both from the toxicology and from the known history of the subject before giving an opinion, and to be prepared to say that one does not know when the facts do not lend themselves to a clear opinion.

It is impossible to be certain what level of blood alcohol will be produced in a given individual by drinking a certain quantity of alcohol, but it is a useful rule of thumb that drinking a pint of beer or a double measure of spirits (either containing about 20 g of alcohol) will raise the blood alcohol level by about 30 mg/100 ml and that the liver will lower this level by about 15 mg/100 ml per hour. This allows one to make a reasonable estimate of the amount of alcohol likely to have been consumed which may be helpful in directing further enquiries in the right direction. One can also deduce that the subject is in the post-absorptive phase if the urine alcohol level is much above the blood level, and conversely that he had been drinking recently if the blood level is higher than the urine level. But, once again, it is essential to take into consideration both the analysis and the eye-witness accounts of the subject's previous conduct before giving an opinion.

The effects of a given blood alcohol level upon the conduct and ability of a pilot are difficult enough to predict; but the effects of a hangover are even more difficult to assess. Intoxicating doses of ethanol disturb the brain's metabolism for a period which outlasts the measurable concentration of alcohol in the blood (O'Hanlon, 1983); and although contaminants in beverages or sleep disturbance may contribute to the effects, there seems little question but that alcohol alone is sufficient to produce this condition although the mechanism is unknown. Tests on subjects with hangovers have produced very variable results, but a recent study (Laurell and Tornros, 1982) found that on the day after ingesting enough alcohol to raise the blood concentration to around 150 mg/100 ml all 22 subjects showed impairment of performance in a staged 'avoidance manoeuvre' test.

Alcohol also has an effect on the inner ear, which may lead to loss of balance and liability to disorientation for many hours after drinking (Money and Landlot, 1983). The findings of the study by Money and Landlot included the following:

1. Alcohol in the blood at concentration of 20 mg/100 ml or above caused measurable performance deficits and was associated with a large fraction of fatal aircraft accidents in general aviation.
2. Alcohol in the blood at higher levels, around 50 mg/100 ml, impaired the ability to fixate visually and perform tracking tasks while receiving vestibular stimulation.
3. The performance deficits caused by alcohol were potentiated by low partial pressures of oxygen in the inspired air.
4. Alcohol can cause hypoglycaemia with severe performance deficits, usually between 6 and 36 hours after ingestion when the alcohol is no longer detectable in the blood.
5. Alcohol can predispose to visual problems; disorientation can persist for at least 6 hours after the blood alcohol concentration has reached zero.
6. Since a person with blood alcohol concentration of 150 mg/100 ml is likely to take more than 10 hours to reduce his blood level to zero, and since the vestibular problems can persist for a further 6 or 7 hours or possibly longer, it would be prudent for pilots to abstain from alcohol for at least 24 hours before flying.

Carbon monoxide and other products of combustion may be present in the exhaust fumes of piston engines, and may affect the aircrew if they get into the cockpit; this problem does not arise with jet engines. The effects of low concentrations of carbon monoxide are usually insidious over a period, so that the subject may not realize that he has been affected until his symptoms are severe; this situation occurs occasionally with road traffic accidents. The position is quite different in fires, especially aircraft fires which are particularly intense; then there may be high levels of carbon monoxide in the atmosphere which is rapidly absorbed, and incapacitating symptoms often occur very rapidly. Where fire breaks out after an impact, escape may be difficult or impossible once the fire has taken hold and filled the cabin with toxic fumes. The heat effects from fires may kill people rapidly from peripheral circulatory effects at temperatures around 200°C; but at high temperatures, particularly those of the order of 1000°C, death may occur within seconds from central effects. Inhalation of hot gases is often considered a cause of death (Hill, 1986) but there are also many toxic substances in a fire besides carbon monoxide—cyanide and other highly toxic substances being produced by burning plastics and other materials.

Routine toxicology following an aviation autopsy includes estimates of alcohol levels in vitreous humour, urine, bile and blood, together with analysis for carboxyhaemoglobin and volatiles, and a drug screen on the urine and liver tissue. This may reveal the presence of medicinal drugs which may have had an effect upon the aircrew, or the condition for which they were being taken may be significant; nicotine and caffeine are common findings, and occasionally quinine from drinking tonic water which may contribute to disorientation (Stockwell, 1982; Balfour, 1986). Drugs of abuse have not been found in pilots in UK, but if drug abuse becomes commoner in the general population the situation may change.

Accident reconstruction

The pattern of injuries sustained at impact may give an indication of what the subject was doing at the time. In light aircraft it is common for the floor to break up in a severe impact so that leg injuries are not unusual, and also for arms to flail around so that injury on the back of the hand is common. Injuries to the palms of the hands, especially between thumb and forefinger, suggest that at impact the individual was holding something—possibly the controls, and therefore that he was perhaps the pilot in control; and injuries to the foot may indicate he had his feet on the rudder pedals at impact. X-rays are particularly helpful here.

Patterns of injury may recur in different situations; after the Aer Lingus Viscount crashed into the sea near the Tusker Rock, the bodies of the casualties all showed head, limb and trunk injuries consistent with being tightly strapped into a forward facing seat. This made sense, as the aircraft had been sending out distress calls, so that the emergency was anticipated and the passengers would have been told to strap in. A subsequent accident on land showed a similar pattern of injury, which suggested that again all the passengers had been strapped in, so that perhaps this emergency also had been anticipated; but this would not be a safe deduction to make nowadays, as many airlines advise that passengers should remain strapped in throughout the flight. Having all the bodies in one mortuary makes it easier to spot variations from the usual pattern, and the odd man out is always important. In the Rhodes Comet accident (Mason and Tarlton, 1969), one passenger showed a pattern of shrapnel injuries, which confirmed the suggestion that an explosive device had gone off in the cabin; the injuries to other passengers were consistent with those in the back cabin being thrown around and severely injured on parts of the aircraft, while many of the people in the front cabin had lesser injuries, consistent with falling out into the sea after the aircraft broke up at altitude.

Safety equipment

The question of safety equipment is important; if the impact is severe enough to crush the cockpit then it is unlikely that the safety equipment can help the crew, but if the seats and harness attachments have held firm in an intact cockpit then the crew should not be killed by hitting their heads on the instrument panel unless their harness has been undone. An efficient restraining harness is a lifesaver, but it has to be properly fitted to secure parts of the aircraft and the aircrew must use it.

People occasionally survive in apparently non-survivable accidents by sheer good fortune; of greater concern are the survivable accidents in which people are killed. A survivable accident is not one in which people do or do not survive, but rather one in which they should be expected to survive considering firstly that the accident forces do not exceed human tolerance under the conditions prevailing, and secondly that there is enough room inside the aircraft for the occupants. In one such accident the pilot died from fractured ribs and ruptured heart inflicted by the controls because he had no effective shoulder restraint, although it was mandatory by law at that time. In another, the seat attachments failed and allowed pilot and seat to rotate forwards, and in yet others excellent and well-mounted harnesses were not used owing to haste or human error. No equipment will save life in high-speed impacts, but the major worry is unnecessary deaths in relatively gentle impacts where slight incapacitation has led to people failing to escape from the aircraft before fire breaks out. In the Stockport accident an airliner crashed on the approach with fuel problems, and the police were able to rescue about a dozen people before fire broke out; the remaining occupants all perished rapidly from the fumes in the fire, many being unable to escape because of leg injuries due to bars at the back of the old-type seats and failure of the mountings. By contrast, at about the same time an RAF Hastings crashed in Africa under very similar circumstances; all of the passengers were in strongly mounted backward facing seats, and survived the impact without incapacitation, so that they escaped successfully before fire broke out and destroyed the aircraft.

The severe impacts of high-speed accidents are non-survivable, and often the only comment that can be made is that death was due to multiple injuries; but in less severe impacts death may have been due to particular localized injuries. The safety equipment provided and the way it was used may be very relevant, as in the low-speed accidents with an intact cockpit and no fire—where death is too often due to fatal head or chest injury because the shoulder harness was not effective and no protective helmet was worn. Death after a period of survival on land or in the sea must cause one to question whether the survival equipment was adequate, and how the rescue services could have got there more quickly; one must always ask how the death could have been prevented, and even if death has been prevented one must constantly ask how things could be done better next time.

Medico-legal considerations

The pathologist is concerned to assist the accident investigators with any evidence of a medical cause for the accident, due either to previous disease in the aircrew or to some partial incapacitation to alcohol, drugs, or toxic fumes from an engine malfunction or fire; but there is also an obligation to provide the coroner with the precise cause of death, for legal and registration purposes, and any form of intoxication may carry an implication of negligence either by the aircrew if the substance was self-administered, or by some other person if it was due to an avoidable malfunction of the aircraft. To the investigators, length of survival is important as an indication of the sequence of events in the accident and the effectiveness of the safety equipment; while to the lawyers survival is important because of the implications for inheritance and tax purposes. In the UK the law of Commorientes assumes that the older person has died first, if there is no evidence to show otherwise; in other countries the law is often different, and in the USA is said to be 'as if each had survived the other' which may be difficult for a layman to comprehend. Identification is of obvious legal importance, quite apart from its significance to the accident investigator and to the family of the deceased.

Conclusions

1985 was a bad year for aircraft accidents, and worldwide over 2000 people were killed in them; but it puts these grim figures in better perspective to realize that within the UK alone over 7000 were killed on the roads in the same time. Fatal accidents to large passenger carrying aircraft are relatively uncommon, for instance six in the UK in the 10 years 1970–79 as against over 160 in general aviation; and the rate for fatal accidents per 100 000 hours was 0.02 for public transport aircraft as against 2.76 for general aviation.

Aviation pathology is a relatively small corner of forensic medicine; simple procedures scrupulously carried out often provide the evidence on which important conclusions can be drawn later, and from these ways of saving lives in the future may be deduced. Aviation pathology is a small but worthwhile part of flight safety, important because it may provide evidence that cannot be found by any other means; but it is only part of the story, and in order to discover the truth and save lives it is essential that all

the workers in accident investigation should record their evidence in detail, and then correlate it with all the other evidence available until the truth emerges.

References

BALFOUR, A.J.C. (1982) Sarcoidosis in aircrew. *Aviation Space and Environmental Medicine*, **53**, 269–272

BALFOUR, A.J.C. (1986) The Bite of Jesuit's Bark. Presented at the *Biennial Scientific Session of Joint Committee on Aviation Pathology* (in press)

BILLINGS, C.E., WICK, R.L., GERKE, R.J. and CHASE, R.C. (1973) Effects of ethyl alcohol on pilot performance. *Aerospace*, **44**, 379–382

CORRY, J.E.L. (1978) Possible sources of ethanol ante- and post-mortem: its relationship to the biochemistry and microbiology of decomposition. *Journal of Applied Bacteriology*, **44**, 1–56

Documenta Geigy (1956) *Scientific Tables*, p. 295. Geigy: Basle

FLANAGAN, N.G., STRIKE, P.W., RIGBY, C.J. and LOCHRIDGE, G.K. (1983) The effects of low doses of alcohol on driving performance. *Medicine, Science and the Law*, **23**, 203–208

HILL, I.R. (1986) The immediate problems of aircraft fires. *The American Journal of Forensic Medicine and Pathology*, **7**, 271–277

LAMPLUGH, A.G. (1932) Accidents in civil aviation. *Proceedings of the Royal Aeronautical Society*, **36**, 93–110

LAURELL, H. and TORNROS, J. (1982) *Hang-over effects of alcohol on driver performance*. Report No. 222A. Linkoping, Sweden: National Road and Traffic Research Institute

LEWIS, M.J. (1986) Blood alcohol: the concentration–time curve and retrospective estimation of level. *Journal of the Forensic Science Society*, **26**, 95–113

MASON, J.K. (1962) *Aviation Accident Pathology*. London: Butterworths

MASON, J.K. (1963) Asymptomatic disease of coronary arteries in young men. *British Medical Journal*, ii, 1234–1237

MASON, J.K. (1983) *Forensic Medicine for Lawyers*, 2nd edn. London: Butterworths

MASON, J.K. and TARLTON, S.W. (1969) Medical investigation into the loss of the Comet 48 aircraft, 1967. *Lancet*, i, 431–434

MONEY, K.E. and LANDOLT, J.P. (1983) *An Unusual Toxicological Property of Alcohol. The Density Effect on the Organ of Balance*. DCIEM Publication No 83-P-44. Downsview, Ontario: Defence and Civil Institute of Environmental Medicine

O'HANLON, J.F. (1983) Alcohol and hypnotic hangovers as an influence on driving performance. *Travel and Traffic Medicine International*, **1**, 147–152

RYAN, L.C. and MOHLER, S.R. (1972) Intoxicating liquor and the general aviation pilot in 1971. *Aerospace Medicine*, **43**, 1024–1026

STEVENS, P.J. and UNDERWOOD GROUND, K.E. (1970) Occurrence and significance of myocarditis in trauma. *Aerospace Medicine*, **41**, 776–780

STEVENS, P.J. (1970) *Fatal Civil Aircraft Accidents*. Bristol: John Wright

STOCKWELL, J.R. (1982) Aeromedical considerations of malaria prophylaxis with mefloquine hydrochloride. *Aviation Space and Environmental Medicine*, **53**, 1011–1101

UNDERWOOD GROUND, K.E. (1975) Alcohol associated with fatal light aircraft accidents, United Kingdom, 1964–1973. *Aviation, Space and Environmental Medicine*, **46**, 1275–1279

UNDERWOOD GROUND, K.E. (1981) Prevalence of coronary atherosclerosis in healthy United Kingdom aviators. *Aviation, Space and Environmental Medicine*, **52**, 696–701

55

Dental identification

I.R. Hill

Introduction

Odontological evidence has been used to identify individuals for thousands of years. The techniques are well known and essentially straightforward; however, success depends upon accurate observation and painstaking attention to detail. Genetic variations, disease patterns and a variety of other factors such as thumb-sucking, orthodontic and other treatment all combine to make an individual's dentition unique, so that they can be distinguished from other people. As teeth are the hardest-known biological tissues and as the mouth is often preserved, either whole or in part, in accidents, dental identification has proved to be the most useful method available (Hill, 1980, 1984).

Method

Ideally the odontologist and the pathologist should examine the body together, but in a mass disaster they may have to work separately. The odontologist must carry out a comprehensive post-mortem examination of the human remains to see if any of the oral tissues have been dislodged. Teeth and dentures may be found in the oesophagus for example, or if the body is fragmented they may be mixed with other tissues. Once all of the available material for that victim is found it must be comprehensively examined and a detailed record must be made of the findings. This should include radiography of the jaws. The following information should be collected:

1. Body number.
2. Sex.

3. Type of occlusion.
4. The decayed, missing, filled teeth.
5. The number of teeth present.
6. The number of teeth missing or fractured due to the accident.
7. Types and nature of restorations.
8. Type and nature of prostheses.
9. Racial characteristics.
10. An estimation of age.
11. Radiological appearances.
12. Pathological lesions.
13. Soft-tissue injuries to the head and face.
14. Skeletal injuries to the head and face.

Access to the jaws may be difficult, especially in incinerated bodies. When this occurs the jaws may have to be removed. The two techniques commonly used are shown in *Figures 55.1* and *55.2*.

Ideally one dentist will examine the body, whilst a second records the findings. In most instances though this may not be practical and either the operator will have to make the record himself, or instruct a lay person such as a policeman how to do it, checking that each recording is correct. In these circumstances it may be preferable to ask the person making the record to write down exactly what is said, e.g. 17 MOD amalgam, rather than drawing the filling on a chart. If necessary an accurate pictorial representation can be drawn at a later date. This may be needed in cases where there is doubt.

Completed post-mortem records, radiographs and photographs must all be carefully labelled with the body number and stored until the identification process can be carried out. They should be put in a safe, secure place, preferably separate from the post-mortem room, where there is a danger of contamination by body fluids.

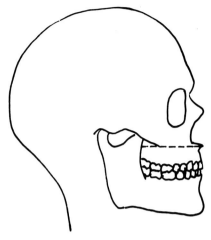

Figure 55.1 Removal of jaws. The face is dissected first and the skin flap raised, exposing the jaws. The lower jaw is dissected out and then a cut is made across the maxilla, freeing it in the direction of the dotted line.

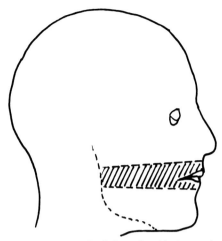

Figure 55.2 In badly disfigured and incinerated cases this technique may be used to expose the teeth, the soft tissues being cut away. It must never be used in cases in which there is no disfigurement.

Equipment

The amount and type of equipment needed is the subject of much argument amongst experts. This ought to be resolved by saying that it is largely a matter of personal preference. Apart from protective clothing, many of the instruments can be shared with the pathologist. When this is not possible a separate supply of dissecting instruments, including a saw, should be carried. In addition mirrors, probes, scalers, toothbrushes and impression materials are all that need be carried routinely. A subsidiary light source can be useful. The Royal Air Force team keeps its kit in a sturdy box (*Figure 55.3*) which is kept packed and routinely checked at regular intervals.

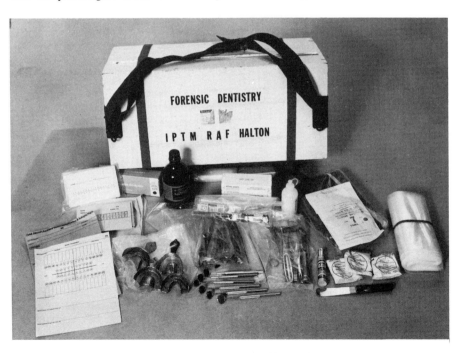

Figure 55.3 Forensic odontological equipment taken to accidents. The forms are colour coded, blue for males and pink for females.

Special procedures

Apart from dissection of the jaws there are just two other procedures which may be routinely useful in dental identifications. Antero-posterior radiographs of the skull may be matched to either photographs or pre-existing radiographs. This is discussed below. The other technique concerns the hardening of viable dental material. Heat may make the teeth brittle, so that they break easily. If they are to be examined, then the soot and debris may be removed. This can be done by a mixture of very gentle scaling and brushing in soapy water preferably over a fine-mesh wire basket, so that any pieces which break off can be collected and matched up to the specimens. Some workers spray the jaws with bioplastic materials which set hard, so that the jaws can be removed safely and then radiographed. This does not inhibit scaling and cleaning, but it makes it more difficult.

Collecting ante-mortem information

Ascertaining the name of the victim's dentist and getting the dental records can be difficult, especially if the accident involves people of many different nationalities. The best results are obtained when relatives have a central reference point to whom they can refer, the telephone number of which is widely advertised by the media. Those manning such a centre can be given a standard set of questions which they must ask. After recording the details these can then be transmitted to the mortuary; where on receipt, the dentist can contact the victim's practitioner. Alternatively, if there is a dentist on call at the relevant centre, he can obtain a telephone charting and request the records, including models, X-rays, photographs and other relevant material. Unless the circumstances are unusual, such as the Mt Erebus accident, all records probably have to be telephoned in the first instance and the definitive material sent later. At Mt Erebus, because the bodies were deep frozen it was practical to travel with the transcribed documents. If this is done a spare set should be kept; otherwise if there is another accident, some may be destroyed, as happened in the USAF crash at Gander (Hartman, 1986).

Methods of data transmission have been widely studied (Vermylen, 1980; de Valck, 1984). In practice two systems operate. If distance permits records can be placed in sealed envelopes marked 'Medical-in-Confidence' and carried by the police to the mortuary. They may also be sent via the airlines. Immediate transmission of data is usually done by telex. Methods of computer transmission are being studied.

Making an identification

Making an identification involves matching ante-mortem records of an individual with post-mortem findings. In a large accident this can be a lengthy procedure. Usually the medical team sets up an identification commission, comprising the pathologists and dentists, who review all of the available material. The victims are divided into males and females, adults and children. Whilst the two groups may work separately, their efforts are co-ordinated, so that when a body is provisionally identified either dentally or by fingerprints, for example, that victim's records are placed separately.

Matching the records is a laborious task, which can be achieved only by carefully examining each one to see if it matches another. This is done until a small number of cases are left in which there is some difficulty. The major problems are usually a result of mis-chartings either of premolars or molars, especially when there have been extractions followed by mesial drift. This usually occurs in heavily filled teeth where the morphology may not be clear. It may result in incompatibilities, of which two types are recognized. Compatible incompatibilities are those in which a filling or extraction has occurred after the last known charting. One that is wholly incompatible is one in which, for example, a filling is found in a tooth known to have been extracted. In the former case, if evidence can be adduced that this has happened and there is other evidence of identification, together with evidence that that person actually boarded the aeroplane, then it may be reasonable to accept the identification—but considerable care is needed.

Victims who have been dentally identified must be examined for corroborative evidence, such as documents and clothing. Ideally everything about the victim should match with what is known about them. The dentist and other members of the team must discuss their mutual findings; after they have agreed, then that victim can be declared to have been identified. This process can then be presented to the locally appointed legal authority in charge of the investigation.

Discussion

The identification of the victims of mass disasters is carried out for medico-legal reasons, such as the proving of wills; for sociological reasons; so that the relatives can be satisfied and the appropriate rights given; and so that the accident can be reconstructed. It is not an easy task and it has to be completed expeditiously, without bowing to the many extraneous pressures that may be put upon the team. Because it is laborious and because much depends upon it, it is essential that there is a team leader who accepts responsibility for the diagnoses and that the team work harmoniously.

Ultimately responsibility is vested in the coroner or his counterpart in other jurisdictions, which may be deputed to a policeman. The important task is to make the identifications and to get them right. The dental evidence should be presented formally, with copies of the ante- and post-mortem charts juxtaposed, so that the similarities can be seen. The findings should be explained and the conclusions given.

Because aircraft accidents are often very destructive, identifications may depend upon small pieces of evidence. Therefore, it is essential that minute detail has to be recorded, in every case. Gross findings are easily recognizable, but it may be necessary to match fillings by shape and to use the pattern of bone trabeculation in the jaws to identify victims. Occasionally, frontal sinus patterns on pre- and post-mortem radiographs may be used. Sometimes, photographs may be matched to post-mortem radiographs, after they have been lined up using various landmarks such as the teeth (McKenna, 1984).

If all else fails then the victims may have to be differentiated by age. Radiographs of children's jaws may be compared with standardized charts; and although variations do occur, it ought to be possible to achieve an accuracy of within 1 year. Between 20 and 28 weeks *in utero*, the deciduous dentition begins to calcify. Prior to birth, the permanent dentition starts to mineralize. Between 6 and 25 years of age, there is a progressive replacement of the deciduous dentition by permanent teeth. Whereas in children the start of mineralization, the completion of the crown, the completion of eruption and finally root formation confer accuracy, in adults attrition, secondary dentine formation and obliteration of the pulp cavity are inaccurate. Thus in adults age estimation may only achieve an accuracy of within 10 years.

Dentures are rarely marked and so much of their value in identification is lost. However, they can occasionally be matched to models, on the rugal pattern identified from pre-existing models of the patient's mouth and this may be used to differentiate otherwise unidentifiable people. Partial dentures, especially if of a distinctive construction, may also be helpful. Racial characteristics, such as melanin pigment in the gingivae and shovel-shaped incisors in Mongoloid people, and the type of restoration may also assist in otherwise doubtful cases.

Conclusions

Whilst dental identification is the method of choice, it is difficult to say what amount of evidence is needed. Ideally a perfect match in all 32 teeth is needed, but circumstances may dictate that less evidence is accepted. All workers can recall an example of a single tooth being used, but this would have to have some very special features, such as a perfect radiographic match of a complex restoration. Because aircraft accidents are closed disasters the amount of evidence acceptable can be less than that demanded in other circumstances, but the standard of proof does not vary. Dental evidence must match other information and there must be no doubt.

References

de VALCK, E. (1984) A new type of telecopier in the long distance transmission of information. *Journal of the Forensic Science Society*, **24**, 375

HARTMAN, K.S. (1986) *Problems Encountered During Dental Identification of Arrow Air Crash Gander Newfoundland*. RAF Halton: Joint Committee on Aviation Pathology

HILL, I.R. (1980) Dental identification in fatal aircraft accidents. *Aviation, Space and Enviromental Medicine*, **51**, 1021–1025

HILL, I.R., KEISER-NIELSEN, S., VERMYLEN, Y., FREE, E., DE-VALCK, E. and TORMENS, E. (eds) (1984) *Forensic Odontology—Its Scope and History*. Leuven, Belgium: International Organization for Forensic Odontostomatology Publications

MCKENNA, J.J.I. (1984) Further studies in the method of matching skulls with photographic portraits using landmarks and measurements of the dentition. *Journal of the Forensic Science Society*, **4**, 326

VERMYLEN, Y. (1980) The use of the telecopier in the long distance transmission of dental data in mass disasters. *Medicine, Science and The Law*, **20**, 89–92

Appendix: Units of Measurement

Table A1 — General physical units and useful equivalents
Table A2 — Derivation of SI units
Table A3 — Conversion table for units of pressure
Table A4 — Conversion table for units of energy
Table A5 — Respiratory symbology
Table A6 — Thermal symbology
Table A7 — Vibration/biodynamics symbology

Table A1 General physical units and useful equivalents

Quantity	Symbol	SI unit	Other units	Abbreviation	Useful equivalents	Notes
Acceleration:						
Linear	a	metre per second squared		m/s^2	$3.281\ ft/s^2$	1
			foot per second squared	ft/s^2	$0.305\ m/s^2$	
			inch per second squared	in/s^2	$0.025\ m/s^2$	
Angular	α	radian per second squared		rad/s^2	$57.296°/s^2$	
			Degree per second squared	$°/s^2$	$0.017\ rad/s^2$	
Angle:						
Plane	$\alpha,\ \beta,\ \gamma$ etc	radian		rad	$0.001\ rad$	2,3
			milliradian	mrad	$1.745 \times 10^{-2}\ rad$	
			degree	°	$2.909 \times 10^{-4}\ rad$	
			minute of arc	′	$4.898 \times 10^{-6}\ rad$	
			second of arc	″		
Solid	Ω	steradian		sr		2
Area	A or S	square metre		m^2	$10.76\ ft^2$	
			square kilometre	km^2	$1.0 \times 10^6\ m^2$	
			square centimetre	cm^2	$1.0 \times 10^{-4}\ m^2$	
			square millimetre	mm^2	$1.0 \times 10^{-6}\ m^2$	
			square inch	in^2	$6.452\ cm^2$	
			square foot	ft^2	$0.093\ m^2,\ 929.03\ cm^2$	
			square yard	yd^2	$0.836\ m^2$	
			square mile	$mile^2$	$2.59\ km^2$	
Density	ρ	kilogram per cubic metre		kg/m^3	$1.0 \times 10^{-3}\ kg/m^3$	
			gram per cubic centimetre	g/cm^3	$2.768 \times 10^4\ kg/m^3$	
			pound mass per cubic inch	$lb\ m/in^3$	$16.018\ kg/m^3$	
			pound mass per cubic foot	$lb\ m/ft^3$		
Electric current intensity	I	ampere		A		
Energy, work, amount of heat	J	joule (J) (newton metre)		$J = N.m$	$0.738\ ft\ lb\ f,\ 9.478 \times 10^{-4}\ BTU,$	4
					$0.239\ cal$	
			foot pound force	ft lb f	$1.356\ J$	
			British Thermal Unit	BTU	$1055.06\ J$	
			kilowatt hour	kWh	$3.6 \times 10^6\ J$	
			kilocalorie	kcal	$4185.5\ J$	
			calorie	cal	$4.185\ J$	
			horsepower hour	hph	$2.684 \times 10^6\ J$	
			foot poundal	ft pdl	$0.042\ J$	
			erg	erg	$1.0 \times 10^{-7}\ J$	

Quantity	Symbol	SI unit	Unit symbol	Conversion	Notes
Force	F	newton (N)	$N = kg/m/s^2$	0.245 lbf	5
		kilogram force (kilopond)	kgf (kp)	9.807 N	
		pound force	lbf (Lb)	4.448 N	
		ounce force	ozf	0.278 N	
		poundal	pdl	0.138 N	
		dyne	dyn	1.0×10^{-5} N	
		pond	p	9.807×10^{-3} N	
Frequency	f	Hertz (Hz) (events per second)	$Hz = .s^{-1}$		
		cycles per second	cps		
Heat, production	H	watt	W = J/s		
Heat, transfer: Convective	C				
Conductive	K	watt (W)	W = J/s		
Evaporative	E				
Radiant	R				
Illumination		lumen per square metre (lux (lx))	$lx = lm/m^2 =$		6
			$cd/sr/m^2$		
		lumen per square foot	lm/ft^2	10.764 lx	
		foot-candle	ft-candle	10.764 lx	
Length	L	metre	m	3.281 ft	7
		kilometre	km	1.0×10^3 m, 0.621 mile	
		centimetre	cm	1.0×10^{-2} m, 0.594 in	
		millimetre	mm	1.0×10^{-3} m	
		micrometre	μm	1.0×10^{-6} m	
		inch	in	2.54 cm	
		foot	ft	0.305 m	
		yard	yd	0.914 m	
		mile: statute	mile	1.609 km	
		nautical (UK)	nm (UK)	1.853 km, 1.152 mile	
		nautical (Int)	nm (Int)	1.852 km	
Luminance (surface brightness)		candelas per square metre	cd/m^2	10.764 cd/m^2	8
		candelas per square foot	cd/ft^2		
		foot-Lambert	ft L	3.426 cd/m^2	
Luminous flux		lumen	cd/sr		7
Luminous intensity		candela	cd		7
Mass	m	kilogram	kg	2.205 lb	
		gram	g	1.0×10^{-3} kg	
		ounce	oz	28.35 g	
		pound	lb	0.454 kg	
		ton (imperial)	ton	1016.05 kg	
		tonne (metric ton)	t	1.0×10^3 kg	
Matter	n	mole	mol		7, 9

Quantity	Symbol	SI unit	Other units	Abbreviation	Useful equivalents	Notes
Pressure	p	pascal (Pa) (newton per square metre)		Pa = N/m²	0.021 lbf/ft²	
			kilopascal	kPa	1000 Pa, 7.501 mm Hg (Torr)	
			micropascal	µPa	1.0×10^{-6} Pa	
			bar	b	1.0×10^{5} Pa, 14.504 lbf/in²	
			millibar	mbar	1.0×10^{2} Pa, 1.0×10^{-3} b	
			millimetre of water	mm H₂O	9.807 Pa	
			centimetre of water	cm H₂O	98.067 Pa	
			inch of water	in H₂O	249.081 Pa, 1.868 mm Hg (Torr)	
			millimetre of mercury (Torr)	mm Hg (Torr)	133.322 Pa, 0.133 kPa, 0.019 lbf/in²	
			pound force per square foot	lbf/ft²	47.88 Pa, 0.359 mm Hg (Torr)	
			pound force per square inch	lbf/in² (psi)	6894.74 Pa, 68.948 mbar, 51.715 mm Hg (Torr)	
			atmosphere (standard)	atm	101.325 kPa, 1013.25 mbar, 760.00 mm Hg (Torr), 14.696 lbf/in² (psi)	10
Power (work rate)	P	watt (W)		W = J/s	0.738 ft lbf/s, 0.102 kgf m/s	
			kilogram force metre per second	kgf m/s	9.807 W	
			foot pound force per second	ft lbf/s	1.356 W	
			horsepower	hp	745.7 W, 550.0 ft lbf/s	
			kilocalorie per hour	kcal/h	1.16 W	
Radiation:						
Quantity	D	Gray (Gy)	radiation absorbed dose	Gy = J/kg	100.0 rad	
				rad	0.01 Gy	
Dose equivalent		Sievert (Sv)	Roentgen equivalent, man	Sv = J/kg	100.0 rem	
				rem	0.01 Sv	
Relative humidity	rh			%		
Revolution (frequency of rotation)	n(r)	units per minute		n/min = (rpm)		
Skin wettedness	w			%		
Sound:						
Pressure	p	pascal (Pa) (newton per square metre)		Pa = N/m²		
			dynes per square centimetre (microbar)	dyn/cm (µbar)		
Pressure level	Lp		decibel	dB		11
Specific heat	c	joule per kilogram per degree celsius		J/kg/°C		
Temperature	T	Kelvin		K	°C + 273.15, (5/9) (°F + 459.67)	7
			degree Celsius	°C	K − 273.15, (5/9) (°F − 32)	
			degree Fahrenheit	°F	(9/5)°C + 32, (9/5)K − 459.67	
Thermal:						
Conductance	C			W/m²/°C		

Quantity	Symbol	SI unit	Unit symbol	Conversions	Note
Conductivity	k or λ	watt per metre per Kelvin	W/m/K		
Insulation	I		°C·m²/W		7
		tog		0.1°C·m²/W, 0.645 clo	
		clo		1.55 tog	
Resistance	R		°C·m²/W		
Storage	S	watt (W)	W = J/s		
Time	t	second	s		
		minute	min		
		hour	h		
		day	d		
Velocity: Linear	v	metre per second	m/s	3.281 ft/s	
		kilometre per hour	km/h	0.278 m/s, 0.621 mph	
		feet per minute	ft/min	0.005 m/s	
		feet per second	ft/sec	0.305 m/s	
		mile per hour	mph	0.447 m/s, 1.609 km/h, 1.46 ft/s	
		nautical mile (UK) per hour (knot)	kn/h	0.515 m/s, 1.853 km/h	
Angular	ω	radian per second	rad/s	57.296°/s	
		degree per second	°/s	0.017 rad/s	
Volume	V	cubic metre	m³	2.832×10^{-2} ft³	
		cubic centimetre	cm³ (cc)	1.0×10^{-6} m³	
		cubic decimetre	dm³	1.0×10^{-3} m³, 1000 cm³ = 1000 ml	
		litre	L (dm³)	0.035 ft³, 1000 cm³, 61.025 in³	
		millilitre	ml (cm³)	1.0×10^{-6} m³	
		cubic inch	in³	16.387 cm³, 0.016 L	
		cubic foot	ft³	28.317 L	
		pint	pint	0.568 L	
		gallon (UK)	gal (UK)	4.546 L	
		gallon (US)	gal (US)	3.785 L	
Volume flow	V̇	cubic metre per second	m³/s		12
		litres per second	L/s	1.0×10^{-3} m³/s	
		litres per minute	L/min	1.667×10^{-5} m³/s, 0.035 ft³/min	
		cubic foot per minute	ft³/min	28.317 L/min	
		gallon per hour	gal/h	4.546 L/h	

1. Gravitational acceleration (g) = 9.80665 m/s² = 32.174 ft/s².
2. Supplementary base unit of the SI.
3. A complete circle subtends an angle of 2π rad.
4. The joule is the energy expended in the application of a force of 1 newton through a distance of 1 metre.
5. The newton is the force required to accelerate a mass of 1 kilogram at 1 metre per second per second.
6. The lux is the illumination of a surface at an intensity of 1 lumen per square metre.
7. Base unit of the SI.
8. The lumen is the luminous flux emitted within a solid angle of 1 steradian by a point source having a luminous intensity of 1 candela.
9. One mole of an atomic, molecular or ionic substance is the amount of the substance that contains 6.023×10^{23} atoms, molecules or ions.
10. The watt is the power which in 1 second gives rise to an energy of 1 joule.
11. The decibel (dB) is a logarithmic measure of relative intensity, and dB = $20.\log_{10}$ (P measured/P reference). In the measurement of sound, P reference is a sound pressure of 2.0×10^{-5} Pa = 2.0×10^{-4} μbar = 20 μPa.
12. 1 lb air at 760 mm Hg (Torr) and 20°C occupies 13.3 ft³ or 376.6 L; 1 ft³ air at 760 mm Hg (Torr) and 20°C weighs 0.075 lbf or 34.0 g.

Table A2 Derivation of SI units

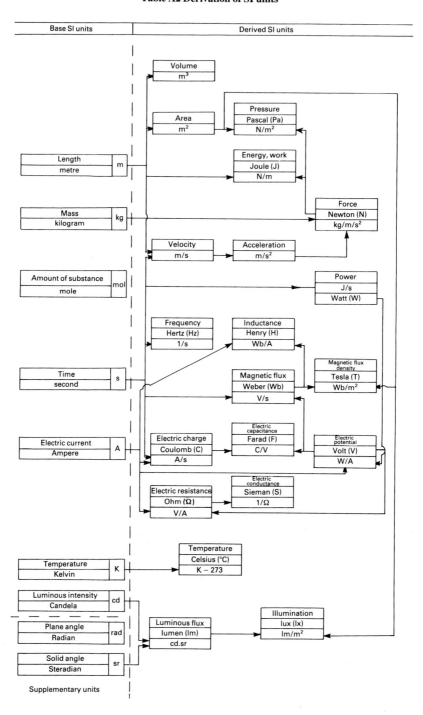

Table A3 Conversion table for units of pressure

From \ To	kPa	$Pa\ (N/m^2)$	b	$mbar$	atm	$mm\ Hg$ $(Torr)$	$in\ Hg$	$cm\ H_2O$	$in\ H_2O$	lbf/ft^2	lbf/in^2
kPa	1	1000	0.01	10	9.872×10^{-3}	7.501	0.295	10.197	4.014	20.885	0.145
Pa (N/m²)	0.001	1	1×10^{-5}	0.01	9.872×10^{-6}	7.501×10^{-3}	2.953×10^{-4}	0.01	4.014×10^{-3}	0.021	1.45×10^{-4}
b	100	1×10^5	1	1000	0.987	750.062	29.53	1019.71	401.436	2088.543	14.504
mbar	0.1	100	0.001	1	9.87×10^{-4}	0.75	0.029	1.02	0.401	2.088	0.014
atm	101.325	1.013×10^5	1.013	1013.25	1	760	29.92	1033.26	406.78	2116.216	14.696
mm Hg (Torr)	0.133	133.322	1.333×10^{-3}	1.333	1.316×10^{-3}	1	0.039	1.359	0.535	2.784	0.019
in Hg	3.386	3386.4	0.034	33.864	0.033	25.4	1	34.531	13.595	70.726	0.491
cm H₂O	0.098	98.067	9.806×10^{-4}	0.981	9.679×10^{-4}	0.735	0.029	1	0.394	2.048	0.014
in H₂O	0.249	249.081	2.491×10^{-3}	2.491	2.458×10^{-3}	1.868	0.074	2.54	1	5.202	0.036
lbf/ft²	0.048	47.88	4.788×10^{-4}	0.479	4.725×10^{-4}	0.359	0.014	0.488	0.192	1	6.94×10^{-3}
lbf/in²	6.895	6894.74	0.069	68.948	0.068	51.715	2.036	70.376	27.707	144	1

Table A4 Conversion table for units of energy

From \ To	J (N.m)	ftlbf	BTU	kWh	kilocal	cal	hph
J (N.m)	1	0.738	9.471×10^{-4}	2.778×10^{-7}	2.387×10^{-4}	0.239	3.777×10^{-7}
ftlbf	1.356	1	1.284×10^{-3}	3.766×10^{-7}	3.236×10^{-4}	0.324	5.12×10^{-7}
BTU	1055.06	778.768	1	2.933×10^{-4}	0.252	251.2	3.987×10^{-4}
kWh	3.6×10^6	2.655×10^{-6}	3409.52	1	859.184	8.592×10^5	1.36
kilocal	4185.5	3090.4	3.968	1.164×10^{-3}	1	1000	1.581×10^{-3}
cal	4.185	3.09	3.968×10^{-3}	1.164×10^{-6}	0.001	1	1.581×10^{-6}
hph	2.684×10^6	1.952×10^6	2507.9	0.735	632.61	6.326×10^5	1

Table A5 Respiratory symbology

	Symbol	Definition
Quantitative variables	F	Fractional concentration of gas
	f	Respiratory frequency
	P	Pressure in general
	Q	Blood volume in general
	$\dot{Q}$	Blood volume per unit time (flow)
	R	Respiratory exchange ratio
	S	Saturation
	t	Temperature
	V	Gas volume in general
	$\dot{V}$	Gas volume per unit time (flow)
	$\dot{v}$	Instantaneous gas flow per unit time
Qualifying terms (subscripts):		
Gas phase	A	Alveolar
	B	Barometric
	D	Dead space
	E	Expired
	$\overline{E}$	Mixed expired*
	ET	End-tidal
	I	Inspired
	T	Tidal
Blood phase	a	Arterial
	c	Capillary
	v	Venous
General	ATPD	Ambient temperature and pressure, dry
	ATPS	Ambient temperature and pressure, saturated with water
	BTPS	Body temperature (37°C) and ambient temperature, saturated with water
	STPD	Standard temperature (0°C) and pressure (760 mm Hg), dry
	NTP	Normal temperature (15°C) and pressure (760 mm Hg)

*NB. A bar over any symbol indicates a mean value.

Table A6 Thermal symbology

	Symbol	Definition
Quantitative variables:	A	Area
	I	Thermal insulation
	P	Pressure in general
	T	Temperature
Qualifying terms (subscripts):		
Physical	a	Air
	b	Body
	c	Convective
	cl	Clothing
	db	Dry bulb
	dp	Dew point
	e	Evaporative
	eff	Effective
	g	Globe
	k	Conductive
	n	Natural (vs ventilated)
	o	Operative
	r	Radiant
	v	Ventilated
	w	Water (vapour)
	wb	Wet bulb
Physiological	a	Arterial
	ac	Auditory canal
	b	Body
	bl	Blood
	bs	Body surface
	co	Core
	gi	Gastrointestinal
	lb	Lean body
	oe	Oesophageal
	re	Rectal
	sk	Skin
	tr	Tracheal
	ty	Tympanic

Table A7 Vibration/biodynamics symbology

	Symbol	Definition
Quantitative variables:	g	Gravitational constant
	G	Gravitoinertial force
	S	Displacement
	v	Velocity
	a	Acceleration
	c	Coefficient of damping
	c_c	Coefficient for initial damping
		Damping factor (c/c_c)
	m	Mass
	k	Stiffness
	f	Frequency
	f_n	Undamped natural frequency
	ς	Angular frequency
Qualifying terms:	x	Antero-posterior
(directional subscripts with	y	Lateral
respect to body)	z	Cranio-caudal
	α	Rotation about x axis (roll)
	β	Rotation about y axis (pitch)
	γ	Rotation about z axis (yaw)

Index

Abdominal pain from pressure
    change, 17
Acceleration,
    angular, 293
    backward, 157
    blackouts and greyouts, 145
    body build and, 611
    causing head injury, 177
    centrifugal forces, 142
    classification of, 139
    contact lenses and, 672
    effects on prone man, 158
    effect on seated man, 157
    in ejection, 210
    forward, 155
        general effects, 155
        pulmonary effects, 156
        tolerance to, 156
    haematuria and, 605
    hyperventilation and, 153
    intermediate duration, 139
    jolt, 140
    lateral, 157
    linear, 141
    long duration, 139
        effects of, 139–158
        positive, 144
        protection against, 159–165
        negative, 153
        transverse, 154
    maximum tolerance, 164
    negative, 153
        cardiovascular effects, 153
        cerebral effects, 154
        general effects, 154
        hydrostatic effect, 154
        pulmonary effects, 154
        tolerance to, 155
    physical considerations, 139
    positive,
        cardiovascular effects, 145
        cerebral effects, 147
        circulatory effects, 146

Acceleration (cont.)
    positive (cont.)
        gas exchange affected by, 150
        general effects, 144
        hormonal effects, 151
        hydrostatic effects, 145
        hypoglycaemia and, 153
        loss of consciousness in, 145
        mobility affected by, 144
        pulmonary effects, 148, 149
        tolerance to, 151
        visual effects, 144, 147
    prolonged, 141
    protection against, 159–165
        abdominal counter-pressure, 162
        anti-G suits, 162, 163
        arterial occlusion, 162
        centrifuge training, 161
        drug therapy, 162
        L-1 procedure, 160
        M-1 procedure, 160
        muscle tensing, 159
        physical training, 161
        positive pressure breathing, 160
        posture for, 161
        Valsalva manoeuvre, 159
        voluntary actions, 159
        water immersion, 162
    radial, 141
    renal response to, 604
    rotational, 180, 182
    short duration, 139
    in spacecraft, 482, 484
    speed, velocity and, 139
    terminology, 143
    vestibular apparatus and, 283, 284,
        287
    weight factor, 140
Acceleration atelectasis, 160
Accelerometers, 190
Accidents,
    alcohol and, 704
    carbon monoxide causing, 706

Accidents (cont.)
    dental identification of victims, see
        Dental identification
    disorientation error, 279
    escape from aircraft, see Escape
        from aircraft
    fire following, 706
    high-speed, 707
    human error causing, 621
    identification of victims, 701
    investigation, 697–702, 703
        approach to, 697
        international agreements, 698
        medico-legal considerations, 708
        pathology of, 700
        personnel for, 698
    involving helicopters, 472, 475
        survivability of, 472
    life stress causing, 436
    memory of, 405
    military, 699
    mortuary organization, 700
    orientation error causing, 278
    passenger behaviour in, 464
    reconstruction of, 707
    see also Crash(es), etc.
Accident-prone personality, 418
Acclimatization, 244
Accommodation of eye, 682
Acetaldehyde, 130
Achievement tests, 420
Acoustic neuroma, 659
Acoustic reflex, 358
Acquired immunodeficiency
    syndrome (AIDS), 526
Acrolein, 130
Active noise reduction, 374
Aeroembolism, 19
Aeropathy, 19
Aerosinusitis see Sinus barotrauma
Aerotitis media, see Otic barotrauma
Affective disorders, 632
    major, 634

Agricultural chemicals, toxicity of, 133
Airbags, 172
Aircraft,
    animal carriage in, 548
        cleaning after, 561
    communication systems, 371
    controls, *see* Controls
    design
        concepts, 497
        fire precautions, 499
        health and safety aspects, 497–500
        noise requirements, 498
        oxygen systems, 499
        pollution aspects, 498
        requirements of, 498
        with accidents in mind, 465
    disinfection of, 540
    disinsection of, 524, 525
        methods, 538
    door opening in emergency, 465
    drinking water on, 535
    escape from, *see* Escape from aircraft
    evacuation from, 463
    exits, 464
    fire precautions, 499
    food on, 534
    fumigation of, 540
    general declaration of health, 530
    health documentation, 524
    jet,
        noise levels, 357, 362
    noise from, 362
        effect on environment, 379
    on fire, fear and, 465
    passenger,
        noise levels, 366, 371
    pest control, 538
    piston-engined,
        noise levels, 365
    protective paints, 500
    skin temperatures, 250
    stretchers in, 553
    supersonic,
        kinetic heating, 479
        medical aspects of, 477
        noise levels, 367, 379
    toilets, 537
    turbo-prop,
        noise levels, 365
    V/STOL,
        battle operations, 477
        escape from, 476
        medical aspects, 475
        noise and communication in, 477
        noise levels in, 366
        visual problems of, 476
    water and waste systems, 499
Aircraft shelters, 247
Aircrew,
    advice on disorientation, 316
    alcoholism in, 509, 637
    anxiety in, 628

Aircrew (*cont.*)
    as flight deck group, 458
    cabin group, 462
    cardiovascular disease in, 585–596
        see also under specific conditions
    civilian,
        authorized examiners, 502
        cardiovascular standards, 504
        medical assessment standards, 502
        medical standards for, 500–514
        personality, 620
        physical standards, 504
        respiratory system standards, 505
    combat-stress reactions, 632
    compliance and conformity, 459
    contact lenses for, 672
    co-ordination of, 425
    cultural effects of group, 466
    deafness in, 654, 657
    diseases of, *see under* specific conditions
    during crashes, 167
    ear, nose and throat examination, 510
    group decision-making, 460
    group formation among, 458
    health documentation, 524
    hearing requirements, 509
    leadership styles, 460, 461
    loss of sleep, 437
    mental and behavioural disorders in, 507
    military, personality, 619
    obedience to authority, 459
    perception, 391
    personality characteristics, 619
    quality of, 494
    responsibility for fitness, 501
    seating, 455
        in helicopters, 472
    selection, *see* Selection of aircrew
    sleep of, *see under* Sleep
    standard of fitness, 609
    stress in, 623
    training of, *see* Training of aircrew
    visual acuity, 666
    visual standards, 511
Airline(s)
    ground staff
        see Ground staff
    hygiene
        see under Aircraft and specific subjects
    medical department, 494
        research and development by, 496
    preservice planning, 500
Air movement, measurement, 224
Airport(s)
    accommodation of animals at, 559
    buildings,
        health aspects of, 549
    control of working environment, 544

Airport(s) (*cont.*)
    emergency facilities, 544
    health organization at, 520
    offices,
        health factors, 548
    'sanitary', 521
    treatment services, 542
    veterinary facilities at, 559
Air temperature, 220
Air traffic controllers,
    hearing in, 659
    migraine in, 648
    standard of fitness, 609
    stress in, 623
Airways,
    chronic obstruction, 600
Alcohol,
    acceleration and, 152
    accidents and, 704
    disorientation and, 315
    measurement of levels of, 705
    nystagmus and, 292, 315, 326
Alcoholism, 631, 637–639
    among aircrew, 509
    management of, 638
Alimentary canal,
    pressure changes in, 17
Altimeters, 445
Altitude,
    decompression sickness and, 22
    perception of, 290
    physiologically equivalent, 49
    pressure and temperature variations, 7
Alveolar–arterial gas tensions, 39
Alveolar ventilation, 36
Alveoli, 34
    capillary membrane, 35
    gases in, 47, 48, 49
Amaurosis fugax, 684
Ambient temperature and pressure, 11
Amnesia, 404, 646
Amphetamine abuse, 637, 640
Anaemia, 616
    in aircrew, 507
Angular motion, perception of, 303
Animals, transport of, 548, 558–561
    airport arrangements, 559
    aircraft cleaning after, 561
    collection of, 558
    disinfection following, 559
    during flight, 560
    factors affecting animal, 558
    hygiene problems, 560
    packaging, 559
Ankle, 688
Anti-depressants, 636
Anti-detonant compounds, toxicity of, 131
Anti-G suits, 151, 162
    evaporation and, 229
    heat stress and, 220
    mode of action, 164
Anti-icing compounds, toxicity of, 131

Anxiety, 280, 626
  management of, 621, 627
  metabolic causes, 631
  motion sickness and, 332
  somatic, 629
Anxiety neurosis, 626, 628
Aorta, coarctation of, 596
Aortic valve disease, 593
Aphakia in aircrew, 512
Aptitudes, 420
Arousal, performance and, 436, 439
Arterial occlusion during
    acceleration, 162
Arteriosclerosis, 704
Asthenia, 624
Asthma, 597
  aeromedical problems, 598
  in aircrew, 506
Astigmatism, 670, 686
Atelectasis, acceleration, 62, 150,
    154, 156, 160
Atmosphere, 3
  composition of, 5
  influencing sound, 356
  physics of, 3
  standard, 7
  structure of, 6
Atmospheric pressure, 3, 10
Atrial septal defect, 595
Atrial fibrillation and flutter, 594
Attention, 406
  divided, 409
  failure of, 411
  selective, 406
Attitude,
  errors in perception of, 297
Attitude indicators, 448
Audiometry, 654, 664
Autokinesis, 348
Avalanche phenomenon in motion
    sickness, 319
Aviation fuels, 130

BCG, 532
Back,
  injury of, 689
    during ejection, 212
Backache, 690
Barbiturate abuse, 637, 640
Barotrauma,
  external auditory meatus, 651
  otic, 15, 649
  sinus, 15, 652
Behaviour, 414
Behaviourism, 386
Behaviour therapy, 628
Bends, 19, 20
Bereavement causing depression, 633
Biliary tract disease, 615
Biological hazards, 548
Biosphere, 3
Birdstrike, 182, 348, 671
Black-outs, 145
Bladder,
  carcinoma of, 605

Blood,
  carbon dioxide content, 34
  carbon dioxide dissociation curve,
    33
  carbon dioxide transport in, 33
  gas transport in, 31
  oxygen dissociation curve, 32
  oxygen tension, 37, 39, 43
  oxygen transport, 31
  oxygen uptake, 37
  pooling,
    during pressure breathing, 67
    from acceleration, 147
  pulmonary flow, 38
Blood disorders, 555
Blood flow
  during hypobaric hypoxia, 51, 53
Blood gases in hypoxia, 50
Blood pressure
  during hypoxia, 51
  pressure breathing affecting, 69
  vibration affecting, 194
Blood–tissue exchange, 30
Blood volume during pressure
    breathing, 68
Body,
  core temperature, 241
  heat conservation, 237
  heat loss to environment, 239
  heat production, 239
  homeostasis and homeothermy, 235
  in free fall, 201
Body build and acceleration, 611
Body cavities,
  closed
    pressure changes affecting, 17
    gas filled, 13, 22
  semi-closed,
    pressure changes affecting, 14
Bone lesions in decompression
    sickness, 25
Boyle's law, 8, 9
Brachalgia, 691
Bradycardia, 594
  from pressure breathing, 70
Brain,
  circulation
    acceleration affecting, 147
    hypobaric hypoxia affecting, 52
  contre-coup injury, 175
  disease, 631
  effect of acceleration, 154
  effect of hypoxia, 52, 53, 54, 57
  effect of decompression, 123
  function,
    disorientation and, 293, 294
  injury to, 174
  tumours, 639, 644
    mental disorder in, 631
Break-off phenomenon, 310, 313
British Helicopter Experimental
    Blade Program, 474
Broadbent's dichotic listening tank,
    407, 409
Bromochlorodifluoromethane, 133

Bronchus,
  anatomy, 34
  cancer, 602
Bronchitis, 600
Butyl cellosolve, 131

Cabins,
  see also Cockpits; Pressure cabins;
      Flight deck etc.
  aircrew group, 462
  cleanliness, 541
  contamination of, 134
  design of workspace, 455
  differential pressure, 112
  disinsection, 539
  environmental control systems, 247
    design limitations, 250
    distribution ductwork, 249
    ground equipment, 251
    insulation, 250
    principles, 248
    specification, 248
  heating, 219
  noise level in, 250, 362, 371
    reduction of, 367
  seating, 455
  in supersonic aircraft, 477
  water condensation, 250
Caisson disease, 19
Cancer, 617
Canopy, fragmentation, 350
Carbamates, toxicity of, 134
Carbon dioxide, 33
  disposal in oxygen equipment, 74
  toxicity of, 132
  ventilation response to, 40
Carbon dioxide dissociation curve of
    blood, 33
Carbon dioxide tension,
  during ascent, 47
  during decompression, 50
  gradients, 41
  in hyperventilation, 58
  in lung, 39
  in ventilation, 128
Carbon monoxide,
  blood concentrations, 129
  causing accidents, 706
Carbon tetrachloride, toxicity of, 132
Carboxyhaemoglobin, 128
Cardiac arrhythmias
  from acceleration, 148
Cardiac output,
  acceleration affecting, 147, 154
  hypobaric hypoxia and, 51, 52
  pressure breathing reducing, 69
Cardiomyopathies, 592
Cardiovascular disease
  among aircrew, 585–596
  see also specific conditions
Cargo,
  health regulations, 522
Carotid bodies, 40
Carotid sinus, 153
Cataplexy, 571

Cataract, 683
Cellular metabolism, 27
Central serous retinopathy, 684
Centrifugal forces in flight, 142
Centrifuge training, 161
Cerebral competence, diminution of,
    295
Cervical disc prolapse, 691
Cervical spine,
    ejection injury, 691
Charles's law, 8, 9
Chemical hazards for ground staff,
    546
Chemoreceptors, 40
Cherry's shadowing task, 407, 409
Chest during pressure breathing, 66
Chlorinated cyclic hydrocarbons,
    toxicity of, 134
Chlorobromomethane,
    toxicity of, 132
Chokes, 19, 20
Cholera, 518, 548
    immunization, 529, 530
    regulations, 523
Ciliary muscles, 340
Circulation,
    acceleration affecting, 146, 157
Clothing,
    air-ventilated suits, 255
    contributing to heat stress, 220
    electrical heating, 253
    evaporation and, 229
    exercise and, 227
    for cold conditions, 251
    for heat protection, 255
    heated, 253
    immersion suits, 228, 252, 268
        protocol for use, 269
        testing, 269
    insulation from, 228, 251
    liquid cooled, 256
    permeability of, 230
    radiation and, 229
    survival suits, 228
    thermal effects of, 227
    wind and waterproofing, 251
Coarctation of aorta, 596
Cocaine, 641
Cochlea, 358
Cockpit,
    design of workspace, 455
    ergonomics,
        disorientation and, 313
        in V/STOL aircraft, 477
    heating, 219
    instrumental display, *see*
        Instrumental displays
    seating, 455
Cockroaches, 539
Cognitive processes, 402–413
Cognitive therapy in depression, 635
Cold,
    acclimatization, 245
    protection from, 270
        clothing, 251, 255

Cold (*cont.*)
    protection from (*cont.*)
        head, hands and feet, 252
        in water, 268
        liquid cooled suits, 256
        on land, 270
        vascular response to, 237
Cold receptors, 236
Cold stress, 219, 244
    clothing causing, 220
Collison, mid-air, 399
    see also Accidents, etc.
Colour vision, 513, 676
Combat stress reactions, 626, 632
Combustion, products of, 128
Communicable disease, 517
Communication, 368–375
    signal to noise ratio, 369
    systems, 369, 372
    in V/STOL aircraft, 477
Compression therapy, 25
Concorde,
    heating in, 479
    medical problems, 477
    noise levels, 479
    see also under Supersonic aircraft
Concussion, 175
    memory loss from, 405
Congenital heart disease, 595
Contact lenses, 511, 672
Controls, 452
    coding and confusability, 453
    compatibility, 453
    current trends in design, 454
    dynamic control, 454
    locations of, 456
    types of, 452
Convergence, 674
Convulsions, hypoxic, 57
Coolant fluids,
    toxicity of, 131
Cornea, 340
Coronary angiography, 587
Coronary artery disease, 589, 704
    by-pass grafting for, 592
    diagnosis, 590
    investigation of, 505
    management of, 591
    presymptomatic stage, 591
    stress and, 622
Coronary circulation during hypoxia,
    52
Cosmic radiation, 4, 478
Cranial nerve disorders, 645
Crash(es)
    dynamics, 166
    forces acting on occupants, 167
    from disorientation, 279
    prevention of injury,
        airbags, 172
        backward facing seats, 172
        harnesses, 170
    structural damage causing injury,
        168
    see also Accidents etc.

Creeps, 19, 21
Crohn's disease, 507, 615
Cyanosis in hypoxia, 54

Dalton's law, 8, 9
Deafness, 375
    in aircrew, 510
    conductive, 654
    established, 665
    from barotrauma, 650
    management of, 664
    otosclerotic, 656
    sensorineural, 657
Deceleration,
    definition of, 167
    human tolerance to, 168
    in crashing aircraft, 166
    profile of forces, 167
Decibels, 354, 715
Decompression,
    alveolar gases during, 49
    at altitude of 63 000 feet, 124
    carbon dioxide tension during, 50
    contact lenses and, 673
    effect of gas in body cavities, 122
    effect on mental performance, 124
    loss of consciousness from, 123
    oxygen tension during, 50
    pulmonary damage from, 16
    rapid, 55
    'safe', 17
    see also Decompression sickness;
        Pressure cabins, etc.
Decompression rate of lungs, 15
Decompression sickness, 19–26, 106,
    556
    altitude and, 22
    body build and, 611
    bubble formation, 19
    cause of, 19
    clinical features, 20
    collapse in, 21
    compression therapy, 25
    differential diagnosis, 24
    exercise and, 23
    factors involved, 22
    from failure of pressure cabin, 124
    identification of, 19
    incidence of, 22
    management of, 24
    mortality from, 22
    personal factors in, 23
    post-decompression collapse, 22
    presentation of, 20
    prevention of, 25
        by pressure suits, 107
        in oxygen equipment, 74
    rate of ascent and, 22
    sequelae of, 25
    in space, 480
    supportive treatment, 24
    terminology, 19
Dehydration,
    in motion sickness, 320

Dehydration (*cont.*)
  survival and, 270
  sweating causing, 240
  symptoms of, 271
Denitrogenation, 26
Density and pressure, 3
Dental identification, 700, 710–713
  collecting ante-mortem
      information, 712
  conclusions, 712
  equipment, 711
  methods, 710
  special procedures, 712
Depression, 630, 632, 633, 634
  in aircrew, 508
  alcoholism and, 639
  choice of treatment, 635
  management of, 634
  non-compliance with treatment,
    636
Diabetes mellitus, 611, 612–614
  in aircrew, 507
  air travel and, 556
  retinopathy, 685
Dialysis for renal failure, 607
Dichotic listening, 407
Diphteria, 531
Disabled passengers,
  carriage of, 495
  see also under Invalids
Disinfection of aircraft, 540
Disinsection, 524, 525, 538
  against cockroaches, 539
Disorientation, 391
  during approach and landing, 311
  see also Orientation; Spatial
    disorientation
Disorientation stress, 280
Ditching, 473
  see also Survival
Documentation, health, 524
Drowning, 264, 267
Drowsiness, 571
  in motion sickness, 319
Drug abuse, 509, 637
Duodenal ulcer, 615
Dupuytren's contracture, 689
Dysbarism, *see* Decompression
  sickness

Ear,
  anatomy of, 257
  discomfort from pressure
    breathing, 65
  diseases of, 555
  effect of decompression on, 122
  examination in aircrew, 510
  inner, 358
  middle, 357
  in orientation, 282
  outer, 357
  pressure changes affecting, 14
  protection of, 377
  reversed, 651

Ear (*cont.*)
  see also Hearing; Vestibular
    system, etc.
Ear muffs and plugs, 373, 662, 663
Ebola virus disease, 528
Echocardiography, 587
Ejection, 262
  acceleration in, 210
  at high altitude, 213
  back injury during, 212, 619, 692,
    693
  canopy jettison, 206, 209
  canopy materials and, 208
  clearance of path, 208
  forces of, 210
  from helicopters, 214
  high speed, 213
  initiation of, 209
  injury from, 691
  protection of face during, 349
  psychiatric consequences, 620
  seat anatomy and, 205
  seat stabilization, 210
  sequence of operations, 206
  under extreme conditions, 21
  from VTOL aircraft, 214, 476
  windblast protection, 180
Elevator illusions, 301
Emergencies,
  passenger behaviour, 463
Emmetropia, 668
Emphysema, 600
Encephalitis, 532
Endocrine disorders, 506
Engine exhaust gases, 128
Environment,
  aircraft noise in, 379
  causing stress, 438
Epidemiological problems, 527–533
Epilepsy, 644, 645, 657–648
  accidents and, 704
  air travel and, 555
  in aircrew, 509
  personality and, 631
  traumatic, 646
Ergonomics of aircraft cockpits, 445–
    457
  ground personnel, 548
  of V/STOL aircraft, 477
Escape from aircraft, 200–215
  after crashing, 464
  assisted, 205–215
    acceleration forces, 210
    back injury during, 212
    canopy factors, 206, 208, 209, 350
    clearance of ejection path, 208
    ejection forces, 210
    requirement of system, 205
    seat stabilization, 210
    sequence of operations, 206
    see also Ejection
  canopy fragmentation, 209, 350
  descent, 201
    speed of, 202
  design factors, 499

Escape from aircraft (*cont.*)
  evacuation, 463
  face protection, 349
  free fall, 201
  helicopters, 214
  high altitude, 213
  high speed, 213
  initiation of ejection, 209
  terminal velocity, 201
  unassisted, 200
    descent, 201
    exit, 200
    landing and recovery, 203
    technique, 200
  see also Parachutes
  under extreme conditions, 213
  under water, 263
  V/STOL aircraft, 214, 476
Esophoria, 679
Ethics, 610
Ethylene glycol, 131
Eustachian tubes,
  during pressure breathing, 65
  patency, 510
  pressure changes, 14
  vibration affecting, 196
Evaporation, 226
  clothing and, 229
Exercise,
  affecting ventilation, 41
  blood gases and, 51
  clothing and, 227
  hyperthermia, 241
  in heat, 245
Exophoria, 679
Exosphere, 4, 6, 7
Extraversion, 415, 418
Eye,
  accommodation, 667, 682
  adjustment to light, 343
  anatomy of, 339
  contamination of, 547
  convergence, 682
  counter-folling, 290
  diseases of, 668
    see also specific conditions
  dry, 683
  examination of, 676
  extra-ocular muscles, 340
  fundi, 683, 686
  hypoxia affecting, 55
  lens, 341
  movements, 287
  stereopsis, 674
  vibration affecting, 194
  see also Vision
Eyelids,
  in pressure breathing
Eysenck personality questionnaire, 41

Face,
  protection,
    during ejection, 349
    from windblast, 180
Fear, 465

Fear of flying syndrome, 310, 620, 627, 690
Fever, thermoregulatory response, 241
Fick's law, 10, 30, 33, 37
Fire extinguishing agents, 132
Fire precautions, 499
Flicker vertigo, 309, 348
Flight deck,
    aircrew as group, 458
        authority, 459
    design of workspace, 455
    instrumental display, 445
        see also Instrumental displays
    seating, 455
    simplification, 450
Flight simulators, 432
Flight simulator sickness, 324
Food,
    bacteriological examination of, 535
    examination of handlers, 543
    for survival, 271
Food hygiene, 496
Food poisoning, 534, 535
    prevention of, 496
Free fall, 201
Frenzel manoeuvre, 15
Frostbite, 244
    prediction of, 232
    protection from, 270
Frostnip, 244
Fumigation of aircraft, 540
Fundi, examination of, 682, 686

G *see under* Acceleration
G excess illusion, 299, 308, 313
Galactic cosmic radiation, 4
Gall stones, 615
Gases
    absolute pressure, 10
    expansion of, 13
Gas exchange in lung, 34
Gas flow patterns, 62
Gas laws, 8–10
Gastric ulcer, 615
Gastrointestinal disease, 614
    in aircrew, 507
Gastro-intestinal tract
    effect of decompression on, 122
    expansion of gases at altitude, 113
Gauge pressure, 10
Gay-Lussac's law, 8, 9
Geographic disorientation, 277
Glaucoma, 512, 684
Glomerular nephritis, 605
Glucose tolerance, 613
Glycosuria, 613
Gout, 616
Graham's law, 10
Gravity,
    see also Anti-G suits
    muscles and, 486
Greenhouse effect, 4, 221
Grey-out, 145, 684

Ground staff,
    biological hazards, 548
    chemical hazards, 546
    clinical services, 542
    consultation and advisory services, 543
    effects of ageing on, 544
    ergonomics, 548
    exposure to pressure, 546
    exposure to radiation, 544
    health of, 495, 542–560
    hearing conservation in, 661
    medical hazards, 544
    medical records, 547
    noise exposure, 545, 549
    occupational stress, 549
    periodic medical examination, 543
    physical hazards, 544
    safety and control procedures, 547
    sickness absence, 543
    treatment services, 542
    vibration exposure, 546
Groups, 458
    decision making, 460
    motivation, 465

Haematuria, 605
Haemoglobin, 31
    reduced, 33
    in hypoxia, 54
Hallucinogens, 640
Harnesses for restraint, 170, 707
Harrier, problems of, 476
    see also V/STOL aircraft
Head,
    conduction, 225
    effect of vibration on, 192, 193
    injury, 174
    protection, 174
        absorbant materials, 179
        ALPHA helmet, 179
        assessment of, 181
        from cold, 252
        from heat, 258
        helmets, 178, 181
        provision of finite stopping distance, 179
        shock absorption, 181
        treatment of cockpit surfaces, 178
    injury,
        acceleration forces, 117
        in aircrew, 109, 508
        bone and soft-tissue, 177
        epilepsy following, 646
        mechanisms of, 174
        prevention of, 177
        psychiatric sequelae, 631, 646
        tolerance to, 176, 177
    movements, 299
        in disorientation, 308
        semicircular canals in, 288
Health regulations, international, *see* International Health Regulations

Hearing, 391
    air traffic controllers, 659
    checking, 664
    conservation in ground staff, 661
    hypoxia affecting, 55
    measurement of, 654
    mechanism of, 353, 357
    protection of, 377, 662
        advice on, 664
    requirements for aircrew, 509
Hearing loss, *see* Deafness
Heart
    acceleration affecting, 147, 148, 156
    disturbance of conduction, 595
    ectopic beats, 594
    imaging, 587
    radionuclide scanning, 591
    rate and rhythm, 586
        disturbances of, 594
        during hypoxia, 51
    valve replacement, 593
    valvuloplasty, 593
Heart block, 595
Heart disease,
    air travel and, 555
    congenital, 595
    ischaemic, 589–592
        diagnosis, 590
        management of, 591
        risk factors, 589
    valvular, 592
Heat,
    acclimatization to, 245
    conservation of, 237
    convection, 225
    loss of environment, 239
    production, 239
    protection from, 270
        clothing, 255
        personal cooling system, 255
Heat exchange, 225, 227
Heat stress, 152, 243, 438
    aircraft factors, 219
    aircrew factors, 220
    clothing causing, 220
    corrected effective temperature, 230, 231
    fighter index of (FITS), 232
    from solar radiation, 219
    in helicopters, 472
    indices of, 230
    origins of, 219
    physiological responses, 220
    solar radiation causing, 219
    wet bulb globe temperature, 232
Helicopters,
    accidents from disorientation, 279
    accident rate, 475
    aircrew comfort, 472
    blade flicker, 475
    break-off phenomenon, 310
    British Experimental Blade Program, 474
    comfort and fatigue in, 471
    crashing, 168

Helicopters (*cont.*)
  crashworthiness, 472
  crew fatigue, 472
  disorientation of crew, 475
  ditching, 473
  escape from, 214
    under water, 263
  evacuation of casualties, 198
  exits, 473
  fires in, 473
  heat stress in, 472
  medical aspects of, 471
  noise levels, 364, 438, 474
    communication and, 372
  passenger seats in, 472
  safety designs, 473
  seating in, 472
  spatial disorientation and, 277, 278
  vibration in, 188, 189, 194, 474
    effect on pilots, 198
    effect on vision, 194
    protection against, 197
Helicopter pilots,
  backache in, 690
  disorientation in, 277, 279, 291, 475
  flicker vertigo in, 309
  heat stress, 438
  selection of, 427
Helmets,
  ALPHA, 179
  assessment of, 181
  colour of, 229
  comfort and fit, 183
  communication and noise exclusion
    by, 182, 373
  facemask fitted to, 182
  protective, 178
    hearing, 663
  non-protective functions, 182
  retention, 180, 181
  vibration and, 192
  weight, size and shape, 183
Helmet-mounted displays, 183
  effect of vibration on, 194
Henry's law, 8, 9
Hepatitis, 532
Herbicides,
  toxicity of, 133
Heroin abuse, 641
Heterophoria, 673
Hijacks, 466
Hodgkin's disease, 617
Homeostasis, 235
Homeothermy, 235
  control of, 241
  physiological mechanism, 243
Hormones,
  acceleration affecting, 151
  sleep and, 569
Humidity, 223
Hydraulic fluids,
  toxicity of, 131
Hyperaciduricaemia, 616
Hypercapnia, 64
Hyperglycaemia, 613

Hyperlipidaemia, 616
Hypermetria, 686
Hypermetropia, 668, 678
  treatment, 670
Hypersomnia, 571
Hypertension, 587–589
  assessment of, 588
  follow-up, 589
  in aircrew, 505
  management of, 588
  in renal failure, 607
  retinopathy, 685
Hyperthermia, 241
Hyperthyroidism, 614
Hypertrophic cardiomyopathy, 592
Hyperventilation, 58–59
  acceleration and, 152
  aetiology, 58
  causes of, 41
  clinical features, 59
  definition, 46
  effect on oxygen tension, 53
  from pressure breathing, 70
  in motion sickness, 319
  physiological features, 58
  vibration and, 194
Hypnagogic hallucinations, 571
Hypnotics, 572
Hypocapnia, 46
  induced by vibration, 194
  of hyperventilation, 58
Hypoglycaemia
  acceleration and, 152
Hypotension
  pressure breathing and, 70
Hypothalamus,
  in homeothermy, 236
  in motion sickness, 328
  thermoreceptors, 237
Hypothermia, 244
  in immersion, 268
Hypothyroidism, 614
Hypoxia, 45–58
  acceptable degree of, 70
  anaemic, 45
  convulsions in, 57
  decompression sickness and, 23
  definition, 45
  effect on tolerance of acceleration,
    153
  following pressure cabin
    decompression, 122, 125
  histotoxic, 45
  hypobaric, 45, 46
    aetiology, 46
    blood flow in, 51, 53
    cardiac output during, 51, 52
    cardiovascular response, 51
    cerebral circulation in, 52, 53
    cerebral features, 57
    clinical features, 56
    cyanosis in, 54
    effect on special senses, 55
    factors modifying, 56
    mental performance in, 54

Hypoxia (*cont.*)
  hypobaric (*cont.*)
    neurological effects, 54
    pulmonary circulation in, 52
    regional cardiovascular changes
      in, 52
    respiratory response to, 46
    syncope in, 52
    time of useful consciousness, 57
    tissue oxygen tension in, 52
  hypoxic, 45
  invalid passengers and, 551, 552,
    554
  ischaemic, 45
  oxygen paradox and, 57
  pressure cabins and, 113
  prevention of, 60–71
  recovery from, 57
  susceptibility to, 56
  types of, 45

Illusions, 392
  see also Spatial disorientation
Immersion suits, 228, 252, 268
  heat stress and, 472
  protocol for use, 269
  testing and maintenance, 269
Immunization, 530
Immunological problems, 527
Infectious disease
  among passengers, 554
  exclusion from aircraft, 529
Inflammatory bowel disease, 615
Infra-red radiation, 4
Infrasonic vibration, 195
Insecticides,
  toxicity of, 133
Insomnia,
  in aircrew, 583
  EEG recording, 570
  hypnotics in, 574
  short term, 570
Instrument displays, 445
  aircraft status, 449
  altimeters, 445
  attitude, 448
  compatibility with controls, 453
  current trends in design, 450
  location of, 456
  location flexibility, 451
  perceptual distance, 451
  principles of, 451
  use of colour, 450
Intelligence, 418, 419
  tests, 420
International Air Transport
    Association,
  transport of animals regulations,
    559, 560
International Civil Aviation
    Organization,
  medical standards, 500
  standard atmosphere, 7
International health regulations, 496,
  517–526

International health regulations (*cont.*)
  application of, 519
  at and between airports, 521
  disease control in future, 525
  disease subject to, 518
  documentation, 524
  for communicable diseases, 528
  goods and cargo, 522
  liberties of individuals, 529
  notification and epidemiological
      information, 520
  provisions relating to disease, 523
  see also under Epidemiology;
      Immunological problems, etc.
Intervertebral disc, 690, 691
Intestines,
  pressure changes affecting, 17
Intracranial haemorrhage, 174
Intra-ocular tension,
  management of, 683
Intra-pleural pressure, 67
Invalids,
  carriage of, 495, 551–557
    accommodation problems, 552
    clinical aspects, 553
    conditions susceptable to
        hypoxia, 554
    contraindications, 553
    gastrointestinal conditions, 556
    hypoxia and, 551, 552, 554
    on stretchers, 553
    physiological and physical
        factors, 551
    psychiatric illness, 557
    susceptible to pressure changes,
        555
Ionizing radiation, 4
  effects of, 483
  exposure to, 544
Ionosphere, 4, 7
Iron deficiency anaemia, 616
Isopropyl nitrate, 130

Japanese encephalitis, 532
Jaws, wiring of, 556
Jerkins for sound protection, 663
Jolt, 140
Jungles, survival in, 271

Kidney,
  anomalies of, 607
  chronic failure, 607
  diseases of, 604
  polycystic, 607
  response to flying, 604
  stones, 606
  transplantation, 607
Kreb's cycle, 28

Labyrinthitis, 511
Landing,
  accidents during, 697
  disorientation during, 311
  of spacecraft, 482
  visual approach to, 397

Landing (*cont.*)
  visual cues used in, 311
  V/STOL aircraft, 476
Lap belts, 170
Lasers, 350
Lassa fever, 528
Leadership, 460, 461
Leans, 278, 302, 313
Learning, 427, 429, 430
Life-preservers, 264
  inflation systems, 267
Liferafts, 267
  motion sickness in, 336
Life support systems, 481
Lighting, 549
Listening, dichotic, 407
Lithium treatment, 636
Loudness,
  measurement of, 360
  sensation of, 359
Lown–Ganong–Kevine patterns, 595
LSD, 640
Lubricating oils,
  toxicity of, 131
Lung,
  acceleration affecting, 148, 154, 155
  blood flow in, 38
    in capillaries, 38
  bullae, 602
  cancer of, 602
  collapse from acceleration, 150,
      156, 160
  decompression damage, 16, 122
  decompression rate, 15
  distension of from pressure
      breathing, 66
  effect of ozone on, 6
  expansion of, 16
  functional anatomy, 34
  functional residual capacity, 35
  gas diffusion in, 36, 37
  gas distribution in, 36, 37
  gases in, physics of, 11
  gas exchange, 34
    acceleration affecting, 150, 156
    pressure changes affecting, 15
  pressure in,
    relation to cabin pressure, 16
  residual capacity, 151
  residual volume, 35
  structure of, 34
  tidal volume, 35, 36
  total capacity, 35
  ventilation, 35
  vital capacity, 35
  volumes, 35
    acceleration affecting, 148, 149,
        151

Maddox rod and wing tests, 681
Malaria, 517, 518, 519, 526, 532, 548
Mal de debarquement, 320, 322
Malignant disease, 617
  in aircrew, 507
Manic depressive psychosis, 633

Man-machine interaction, 445
Marburg fever, 528
Marijuana, 641
Medical ethics, 610
Medical examination, 587
  biochemical, 613
  cardiac imaging, 587, 591
  colour vision, 676
  electrocardiography, 586
  eyes, 676, 685
  for cardiovascular disease, 585
  for groundstaff, 543
  pre-employment, 543
  urine testing, 604
Medical standards,
  for civilian aircrew, 500–514
    national, 501
Medication, inappropriate, 641
Memory, 402
  episodic, 404
  long-term, 404
  loss of, 404
  short-term, 403
  working, 404
Meniere's disease, 510, 660
Meningitis, 532
Mental disorders,
  classification, 620
  grounding and, 621
  in aircrew, 507
Mental performance
  acceleration affecting, 145
  hypoxia affecting, 54, 56
  pressure breathing and, 70
Mesosphere, 6, 7
Metabolic disorders,
  emotional symptoms, 631
Methyl bromide,
  toxicity of, 132
Microgravity, 485
Micrometeorites, 484
Microphones, 372
Micropsia, 684
Migraine, 509, 648
Minnesota multiphasic personality
    inventory, 417
Minute volume, 36
Mitral regurgitation, 593
Mitral valve disease, 592
Molecular sieve oxygen concentration
    systems, 81, 102
Molecular Sieve Oxygen
    Concentrator, 75
Morphine abuse, 637, 641
Motion maladaptation syndrome, 318
Motion platforms, 433
Motion sickness, 318–338
  aetiology of, 320
  age factors, 331
  among aircrew, 319
  among passengers, 320
  anxiety and, 332
  associated symptoms and signs, 319
  avalanche phenomenon, 319
  canal–otolith mismatch in, 323, 324

Motion sickness (*cont.*)
definitions, 318
environmental factors, 335
factors influencing susceptibility, 330
incidence of, 328
factors involved, 328
prediction of, 330
mental activity and, 332
nature of stimulus, 322
neural mismatch theory, 321, 333
neural pathways in, 327
neurotic reactions and, 332
operational significance of, 319
prevention and treatment, 333
adaptation, 333
aircraft factors, 334
behavioural measures, 333
desensitization, 333
drugs, 335
vomiting, 336
sex differences, 331
in space, 486
symptoms and signs, 318
slow development of, 322, 328
vibration and, 195
visual–vestibular mismatch in, 323
Multiple sclerosis, 644
Muscles,
effect of vibration on, 195
hypoxia affecting, 54
Muscle spasms in hyperventilation, 59
Myocardial abnormalities, 586
Myocardial sarcoidosis, 599
Myopia, 669
assessment of, 686
treatment, 670

Narcolepsy, 570
Neck injury from ejection, 691
Nephritis, 605
Nervous system,
diseases of, 644
air travel and, 555
in aircrew, 508
progressive disorders, 645
static disorders, 644
in decompression sickness, 21
transient disability, 647
Neuralgia, 647
Neuroendocrinology, sleep and, 569
Neuroses, 620, 621, 623, 625–631
affective and depressive, 632
anxiety, 626
motion sickness and, 332
post-traumatic, 631
Neuroticism, 415, 418
Newton's law of motion, 140
Night blindness, 686
Nitrogen,
supersaturation of tissue with, 19
Nitrogen oxides, 130
Nitrophenols,
toxicity of, 134

Noise, 353–368
acceptable levels of, 377
active reduction of, 374
in aircraft design, 498
annoyance and, 361, 380
assessment of risk of damage from, 661
atmospheric influences on, 356
definition of, 353
duration of exposure, 379
from aircraft, 362
sources, 362
ground staff exposure to, 545, 549
helicopters, 364, 474
jet aircraft, 357
line source, 356
measurement of, 361, 375, 661
passenger aircraft, 366
perceived level of, 361, 379
point source, 356
propagation of, 356
protection from, 661
psychological effects of, 377
reducing levels of, 381
sensation of, 359
sources of, 356
stress factors interacting with, 378
stress from, 438
from supersonic aircraft, 367, 479
V/STOL aircraft, 366, 477
Noise and number index, 380
Noise induced temporary threshold shift, 376
Nominal Ocular Hazard Distance for laser irradiation, 351
Nose
examination of, 510
Noy (unit of noisiness), 361
Nuclear flash,
protection from, 183, 351
Nystagmus, 292
alcohol, 315, 326
examination, 677
from roll, 304
from vibration, 196
positional, 661
types of, 678
vestibular, 288

Obesity, 611, 612
hazards of, 612
sleep apnoea syndrome and, 572
Obsessional disorder, 629
Occupational stress, 549
Ocular counter-rolling, 290
Ocular movements, 677
Ocular muscle balance, 673
assessment of, 686
examination of, 679
in aircrew, 512
Organophosphates, 134
Orientation,
ear in, 282
external visual cues, 290
eyes and, 282

Orientation (*cont.*)
kinaesthesis, 283
mechanisms of, 281
otolith organ in, 287
semicircular canals in, 283
vestibular apparatus in, 283
visual cues from instruments, 291
Orientation error accident, 278
Oronasal masks, 65
Orthopaedics, 688–693
Orthophoria, 673, 679
Otic baratrauma, 15, 114, 649
chronic, 650
delayed, 62, 651
prognosis, 651
treatment, 651
Otitis media, 656
Otolith organs
in motion sickness, 323
in orientation, 287
Otosclerosis, 656
in aircrew, 510
Oxygen,
breathing, 61, 62
consumption of, 29
maximum acceptable concentration, 61
minimum acceptable concentration, 60
production of, 81
supply to tissue, 29, 31
therapeutic, provision of, 499
transport by blood, 31
uptake, 37, 51
ventilatory response to, 41
Oxygen dissociation curve, 32
Oxygen equipment, 72–106
adequate supply, 73
air dilution, 88
in aircraft design, 499
body-mounted regulator systems, 100
breathing gas on demand, 87
carbon dioxide disposal in, 74
classes of, 72
closed circuit systems, 72
combat aircraft, 98
components of, 75
continuous flow delivery systems, 83
convenience of, 74
delivery, 79
demand flow delivery systems, 86
demand regulators, 86
direct flow sytems, 84
duplication in, 74
for bail-out, 84
for underwater breathing, 75
gaseous oxygen storage, 76
hoses and personal connectors, 91
indication of failure, 74
indication of flow, 90
liquid oxygen storage, 77
disadvantages of, 80
masks, 93–98, 109
for aircrew, 93

Oxygen equipment (*cont.*)
  masks (*cont.*)
    for passengers, 96
  maximum acceptable concentration
    of oxygen, 61
  minimum acceptable concentration
    of oxygen, 60
  molecular sieve concentration
    systems, 81, 102
  nitrogen supply, 73
  non-rebreathing reservoir systems,
    85
  onboard oxygen production, 81
  open-circuit systems, 73
  oxygen sources, 75
  panel-mounted regulator systems,
    98
  passenger aircraft installation, 103
  physiological requirements, 60, 73
  pressure breathing in, 90
  protection against toxic fumes, 74
  protection during high-altitude
    escape, 75
  pulmonary ventilation and, 62
  purpose of, 60, 72
  RAF economizer system, 85
  rebreathing reservoir systems, 84
  resistance to breathing in, 64
  respiratory gas flow patterns and,
    62
  safety pressure, 74, 89
  seat-mounted regulator systems,
    101
  servo-controlled demand
    regulators, 87
  sodium chlorate candles, 80
  solid chemical oxygen storage, 80
  in supersonic aircraft, 477
  temperature of inspired gas, 74
  therapeutic sets, 106
  typical systems, 98
Oxygen masks, 93–98, 109
  aircrew, 93
  anti-suffocation facility, 96
  demand, 94
  fitted to helmet, 192
  for ejection, 94
  for passengers, 96
  regulator systems on, 101
  requirements of, 94
  valves, 95, 96
  with trunk and lower limb
    counterpressure, 110
Oxygen paradox, 57
Oxygen tension, 28, 43
  alveolar, 39
  in blood, 37, 39, 43
  during ascent, 47
  during decompression, 50
  during oxygen breathing, 48
  gradients, 42
  hyperventilation affecting, 53
  variations in, 43
  ventilation and, 40
Oxyhaemoglobin, 31

Ozone, 5–6
  effects of, 478
  toxicity of, 133
Ozonosphere, 4

Pain causing hyperventilation, 58
Paints, protective, 500
Pancreatitis, 507, 616
Parachutes, 203–205
  automatic operation, 202
  canopy, 204
  harness, 203
  opening, 201, 202
  packs, 204
Paranasal sinuses,
  see also Sinus barotrauma
  air travel and, 555
  examination of, 510
  pressure changes affecting, 15
Paratroops,
  motion sickness among, 329, 336
Parawings, 205
Paroxysmal tachycardia, 594
Pascals, 354, 715
Passengers,
  as group, 463
  behaviour in emergency, 463
  comfort of, 494
  health documentation, 524
  infectious disease among, 554
  invalid *see under* Invalids
  opening doors in emergency, 465,
    466
  panic among, 464
  pregnant, 554
Pelvic-ureteric junction obstructing,
  607
Peptic ulcer, 507, 615
Perception, 391–401
Performance,
  aptitude, 420
  arousal and, 436, 439
  control design and, 455
  motivation, 420
  noise affecting, 438
  of several tasks, 410
  workload and, 441
  see also specific conditions
Performance operating characteristic,
  410
Peripheral nerve injuries, 689
Peripheral vascular disease, 595
Persistent ductus arteriosus, 596
Personality, 414
  accident-prone, 418
  in aircrew, 619
  assessment of, 416
  classification of, 414
  epilepsy and, 631
  factors, 415
  head injury affecting, 631
  measurement of, 623
  obsessional, 630
  stress and, 439, 621
  type A, 622

Pest control, 538
Phobic anxiety states, 627
Phons, 360, 715
Physiologically equivalent altitudes,
  49
Pilgrims and international health
  regulations, 522
Pilots,
  as leaders, 462
  effectof thermal stress, 248
  errors causing accidents, 621
  eye examination, 685
  incapacitation of, 500
  motion sickness among, 329
  perception in visual approach, 397
  personality of, 417
  seating, 455
  selection of, 425
    for helicopters, 427
    military, 425
    RAF procedure, 426
  stress among, 466
  training, 387
  visual searching by, 401
Plague, 518, 532, 533
Pneumothorax in passengers, 556
  in aircrew, 506
  spontaneous, 600
  traumatic, 600
Poliomyelitis, 518, 531
Pollution by aircraft, 498
Polycystic kidney, 607
Positional nystagmus, 661
Prebyacusis, 378
Pregnancy, 554
Pre-oxygenation, 26
Presbyopia, 670
Pressure, 3
  ambient, 11
  atmospheric, 3, 10
  changes,
    effects of, 13–18
    gas expansion, 13
    on closed cavities, 17
    on semi-closed cavities, 14
    paranasal sinuses affected by, 15
    pulmonary effects of, 15
  differential, 112
  exposure to
    by ground staff, 546
  gauge, 10
  measurement of, 10
  spacecraft problems, 480
  transthoracic, 16
  variation with altitude, 7
Pressure breathing, 58, 109
  affecting intra-ocular pressure, 684
  blood pooling during, 67
  breathing effort in, 66
  circulatory effects, 67
  during acceleration, 160
  effects of, 65
    blood pressure, 69
    cardiac output, 69
    circulatory, 69

Pressure breathing (*cont.*)
  effects of (*cont.*)
    head and neck, 65
    hyperventilation, 70
    mental performance, 70
    respiratory, 66
  in oxygen equipment, 90
  reduction of blood volume by, 68
  residual capacity affecting, 151
  respiratory counterpressure and, 67
  syncope from, 69
  ventilation in, 67
  with oronasal mask, 65
  with pressure helmet, 66
Pressure cabins, 60, 112–126
  accidental decompression,
    aerodynamic suction, 121
    above 63 000 feet, 124
    airblast, 122
    cabin altitude profiles, 121
    causes of, 119
    cold following, 124
    effect of inflow of air, 120
    effect on mental performance,
      124
    effect on occupants, 122
    hypoxia and, 122, 125
    incidence of, 119
  causes of failure, 118
  decompression of, 114
    rapid, 118
  decompression sickness and, 113,
    124
  design of, 112
  differential control, 115
  differential pressure, 10, 115
  discharge valves, 117
  failure, 49, 106
  gastro-intestinal gas expansion and,
    113
  high-differential,
    combat, 115
    decompression, 125
    oxygen equipment, 104
    passenger, 115, 125
  hypoxia and, 113, 122, 125
  indicators and warning systems, 118
  low differential,
    combat, 116, 125
    decompression, 125
    oxygen systems in, 98
  maximum cabin altitude, 113
  maintaining pressure in, 112
  passenger comfort in, 494
  physiological requirements for, 113
  pressure controllers, 117
  presurization schedules, 114
  principles of, 117
  rapid decompression, 118
    physics of, 119
  rate of change, 114, 115
  reduced air inflow, 118
  relation between cabin altitude and
    aircraft altitude, 114
  safety and inward vent valves, 117

Pressure cabins (*cont.*)
  sealed, 112
  source of air, 117
  structural failure, 118
  in supersonic aircraft, 477
  time of decompression, 16, 120
  toxic contamination of, 134
  see also Cabins, etc.
Pressure clothing, 106–111
  air control systems, 108
  full pressure suits, 107
  oxygen pressure control system,
    108
  partial pressure suits, and
    asemblies, 108
  physiological and general
    requirements, 107
  trunk and lower limb counter
    pressure, 110
Pressure helmets,
  pressure breathing with, 66
  with trunk and limb counter
    pressure, 110
Pressure vertigo, 292, 308, 326
Protective equipment design, 49
Proteinuria, 605
  acceleration and, 604
Psychiatric disorders,
  air travel and, 557
  grounding and, 621
Psychiatry, 619–643
Psychology, 385–390
  aviation, 387
  scientific factors, 385
  social, 458
  terminology, 388
Psychosomatic disorders, 621
Psychoticism, 415
Psychrometers, 224
Ptosis, 685
Pulfrich effect, 348
Pulmonary arteries, 35
Pulmonary blood flow, 38
  acceleration affecting, 149
  relationship to ventilation, 38
  hypobaric hypoxia affecting, 52
Pulmonary oedema, 6, 130, 133, 592
Pulmonary stenosis, 596
Pulmonary ventilation, 35
  acceleration affecting, 148, 156
  control of, 40, 41
  during pressure breathing, 67
  effect of altitude, 47
  exercise affecting, 41
  in flight, 62

Quarantine, 517, 560

Rabies, 526, 531, 560
Radiant heat, 221
Radiation,
  clothing and, 229
  effects of, 478
  electromagnetic, 545
  exposure to by ground staff, 544

Radiation (*cont.*)
  heat exchange by, 226
  infra-red, 4
  ionizing, 4, 483
  solar, 4
  spacecraft and, 482, 483
  ultra-violet, 4, 5
Raynaud's disease, 198
Raynaud's phenomenon, 244
Refractive conditions, 668
Refrigerants, toxicity of, 133
Relapsing fever, 518
Renal calculi, 606
Renal colic, 606
Renal dialysis, 607
Renal disease, 604–608
Renal failure, 607
Resonance,
  concept of, 187
  in body, 192
Respiration,
  cellular metabolism in, 27
  in decompression sickness, 21
  effect of 100% oxygen on, 62
  external, 27
  internal, 27
  neural control of, 40
  physiology, 27–43
  pressure *see* Pressure breathing
  tissue, 27
  vibration affecting, 194
Respiratory diseases, 597–603
  air travel and, 555
  see also specific conditions
Respiratory muscles, 40
Respiratory system
  in aircrew standards, 505
  infection, 15, 309
Restless legs syndrome, 572
Restraint, 170–173
  airbags, 172
  avoiding head injury, 177
  harnesses, 170
    motion sickness and, 335
Retina, 341, 394, 395
  circulation, 147
  size and actual size, 394, 395
  mid air collisions and, 400
Retinopathy,
  central serous, 684
  diabetic, 685
  hypertensive, 685
Reversed fuel cells, 81
Rorschach test, 417

Safety equipment, 707
Salt, survival and, 273
Salt loss in sweating, 240
Sarcoidosis, 506, 598, 704
Sea sickness, 320, 329
Seating,
  backward facing, 172
  energy attenuating, 172
Selection of aircrew, 423–427
  civilian, 426

Selection of aircrew (*cont.*)
  health factors, 314
  military, 426
  motion sickness, 334
  practical aspects, 424
  principles of, 423
  reliability of tests, 423
  susceptibility to disorientation and, 314
  testing, 420
  validity of tests used, 423
Semicircular canals,
  cross-coupled (Coriolis) stimulation, 305, 325, 330, 334
  in disorientation, 292
  in orientation, 274, 283–287
Semicircular canal–otolith mismatch, 323
Sexual problems, 630, 642
Sinus barotrauma, 15, 114, 652
Sinus tachycardia, 594
Skin,
  contamination of, 547
  vasoconstriction and vasodilatation, 239
Skin capillaries,
  acceleration affecting, 148
Skin lesions in decompression sickness, 21
Skull,
  injury to, 174
  prevention of deformities, 178
Sleep,
  age affecting, 568
  aircrew, 496, 565, 576–584
    clinical considerations, 582
    flight-time limitations and, 580
    irregularity of work affecting, 578
    persistent disturbance, 583
    rate of working and, 581
    transmeridian flights and, 576
    unusual hours affecting, 576
  anticipatory, 580
  circadian rhythms, 569
  clinical considerations, 565
  daytime, 583
  daytime latencies, 568
  disorders of, 570
    aetiology, 570
    among aircrew, 576
    circadian rhythm and, 569
    use of hypnotics, 583
  excessive daytime, 570
  hormones and, 568
  loss of, 437
  multiple latency test, 568
  neuroendocrinology and, 569
  onset of, 565
  paralysis, 571
  REM, 565, 569, 571
  total time, 568
  use of hypnotics, 572
Sleep apnoea syndrome, 572
Sleep-wakefulness continuum, 565, 570

Smallpox, 518, 527
Smoke hoods, 97, 464
Snow, protection from, 270
Social psychology, 458–467
  aircrew groups, 458
  cabin crew group, 462
  flight deck group, 458
  passenger group, 463
Sodium chlorate candles, 80
Sodium loss in sweating, 240
Solar flares, 483
Solar glare, 182, 348
Solar radiation, 219, 478
Somatic anxiety, 629
Sones, 360
Sonic boom, 367
Sound,
  atmospheric influences on, 356
  complex, 355
  frequency analysis, 355
  physical characteristics, 353
  pressure, 353, 354
  production of, 353
  subjective sensation, 359
Space,
  motion sickness in, 320, 326, 330
Space craft, 479–488
  acceleration, 482, 485
  environmental control in, 480
  food in, 484
  long-term problems, 485
  medical problems of, 486
  microgravity in, 485
  micrometeoroids hitting, 484
  motion sickness in, 486
  personal hygiene in, 485
  problems of, 479
  radiation affecting, 483
  waste management in, 484
  water management in, 484
Space flight,
  acceleration in, 155
  behavioural aspects, 488
  renal response to, 604
Space suits, 481
  life support systems, 481
Space walking, 481
Spatial disorientation, 277–296, 297–317
  advice to aircrew, 316
  aetiology of, 290
  aircraft factors, 312
  aircrew factors, 314
  among helicopter crews, 475
  angular motion, 303
  anxiety reactions, 280
  break-off phenomenon, 310, 313
  in civil aviation pilots, 278
  cockpit ergonomics and, 313
  common illusions, 297–317
  coning of attention, 294
  cross-coupled stimulation causing, 305
  definitions, 277
  dissociative sensations, 310

Spatial disorientation (*cont.*)
  drugs and, 315
  environmental factors, 313
  errors of attitude, 297, 298
  in fixed wing aircraft pilots, 278
  G excess illusion, 299, 306, 313
  general aspects, 277–296
  in helicopter pilots, 277, 278, 475
  illusions, 392
  impairment of vision in, 291
  imput error, 290
  inadequate cues, 292
  incidence of, 277
  instruments and, 312
  oculogravic illusions, 297, 300, 301
  oculogyral illusion, 304
  operational factors, 314
  operational significance, 278
  prophylaxis, 312
  somatogravic illusion, 297
  somatogyral illusion, 303
  the leans, 302, 313
  training and, 315
  visual cues and, 290, 291
Spectacles, 671
Speech,
  intelligibility of, 368
    noise levels and, 377
  physical nature of, 368
Spine, 689
  ejection injury, 212, 691, 693
  vibration affecting, 198
Squint, 680, 685
  in aircrew, 512
Staggers, 19, 21
Standard atmosphere, 7
Stapedectomy, 665
Stereopsis, 347, 394
  effective, 674
  measurement of, 682
Stomach,
  distension, 153
  effect of vibration on, 199
  pressure changes affecting, 17
Strabismus, 680
Stratosphere, 6
Stress, 620, 626
  cognitive, 435
  cultural, 466
  environmental, 435, 436, 438
  from hijacks, 466
  life, 435, 436
  noise causing, 438
  personality and, 439, 622
  psychological, 435
  workload and, 435
  measurement of, 440
  Yerkes–Dodson law, 439
Suicide, 639
Sun shades, 247
Supersonic aircraft,
  cabins, 477
  kinetic heating, 479
  medical aspects, 367, 479
  noise levels, 367, 479

Supersonic aircraft (*cont.*)
  oxygen equipment, 477
Survival, 262–281
  cold protection,
    on land, 270
    in water, 268
  dehydration and, 270
  energy requirements, 272
  in jungle, 271
  location, 271
  packs, 271, 273
  protection, 262
  salt requirements, 273
  search and rescue, 269
  sources of drinking water, 272
  training in, 273
  in water,
    cold protection, 268
    life preservers, 264
  water and food needed, 271
  water rationing, 272
Survival suits, 228
Sweat glands, 245
Sweating, 240, 245
  causing dehydration, 240
  control of, 241
  in motion sickness, 318
Syncope,
  from pressure breathing, 69
  in decompression sickness, 21
  in hypobaric hypoxia, 52, 55

Tachycardia, paroxysmal, 594
Take-off,
  illusions during, 299
Task analysis, 440
Teeth,
  pressure changes affecting, 18
Temperature, 4
  ambient, 11
  core, 241
  decompression sickness and, 23
  equivalent chill, 233
  hypoxia and, 56
  operative, 226
  oxygen equipment and, 74, 80
  relation to altitude, 7
Temperature stratification, 80
Tetanus, 531
Tetany, 59
Thematic apperception test, 417
Thermal blankets, 247
Thermal environment, 219
  air movement, 224
  air temperature, 220
  components of, 220
  conduction and convection, 225, 226
  evaporation, 226
  heat radiation, 226
  human heat exchange in, 225
  humidity, 223
  operative temperature, 226
  radiant heat, 221
Thermal physiology, 235–246

Thermal protection, 247–260
Thermal stress, 438
  aircrew factors, 220
  clothing causing, 220
  effective temperature, 230, 231
  effect on pilot performance, 248
  electrical, 219
  fighter index, 232
  in helicopters, 472
  indices of, 230
  origins of, 219
  physiological responses, 220
  protection from, 247
  solar, 219
Thermoreceptors, 236, 237
Thermoregulation, 225
  control of, 241
  problems, 243
  stimulation of, 245
Thermosphere, 6, 7
Thoraco-lumbar injury from ejection, 691
Thoraco-lumbar spine, 689
Throat,
  examination of, 510
Thromboembolism, 595
Thyroid gland,
  disease of, 506, 614
Tick borne encephalitis, 532
Tinnitus, 377, 650
  control of, 665
  in Meniere's disease, 660
Tissue,
  carbon dioxide tension in, 41
  elasticity, 187
  freezing damage to, 244
  hypoxia, 45
  mechanical properties of, 187
  oxygen consumption, 30, 41
  oxygen requirements, 29
  oxygen supply, 31
  oxygen tension, 42, 52
  respiration in, 27
  supersaturation with nitrogen, 19
Toilets in aircraft, 537
Toxic gases and vapours, 127–135
  escape and, 263
  exposure limits, 127
  sources of, 127
  threshold limit valve, 127
  see also under specific compounds
Toxicology, 547
Toynbee manoeuvre, 15
Tracheostomy,
  air travel and, 557
Training of aircrew, 427–434
  instrumental conditioning, 428
  learning process, 427
  motion platforms in, 433
  psychomotor skills, 431
  simulation, 432
  transfer, 431
Transthoracic pressure, 16
Tropical medicine, 495
Troposphere, 6

Tuberculosis, 506, 601
Turbulence, 189
Tympanic membrane,
  during pressure breathing, 65
  perforation of, 656
  pressure changes, 14
  rupture of, 650
  vibration affecting, 196
Typhoid, 530
Typhus, 518

Ulcerative colitis, 615
Ultra-violet radiation, 4
  absorption of, 6
Urinary calculi, 507
Urine, abnormal findings in, 604
Uveal tract, 340
Uveitis, 686

Valsalva manoeuvre, 15, 159
Vasodilatation, 238
Vection stimuli, 291
Venous thrombosis, 595
Ventilation
  acceleration affecting, 148, 154, 156
  alveolar, 36
  blood flow relationship, 38
  control of, 39, 41
  during pressure breathing, 67
  effect of altitude, 47
  exercise affecting, 41
  in flight, 62
  pulmonary, 35
  response to carbon dioxide, 40
  response to oxygen tension, 41
Ventricular septal defect, 596
Vertigo, 659–661
  in aircrew, 510
  alternobaric *see* Pressure vertigo
  aviator's, 277
  benign paroxysmal, 326
  flicker, 309, 348
  from barotrauma, 650
  in Meniere's disease, 660
  paroxysmal, 647
  positional, 326
  pressure, 308, 326
  traumatic, 659
Vestibular neuronitis, 660
Vestibular nystagmus, 288
Vestibular system, 391
  acceleration and, 283, 284, 287
  disease, 659
  erroneous cues from, 293
  form and function, 283
  inadequate cues from, 293
  in motion sickness, 320, 327
  pressure changes in, 309
  spatial disorientation and, 292
Vestibular threshold mechanisms, 303
Vibration, 185–199
  accelerations, 190
  assessment of severity, 196
  biomechanical effects of, 191
  cardiovascular effects, 194

Vibration (*cont.*)
  damping, 186, 188
  definition, 185
  effect on vision, 192, 193
  in fixed wing aircraft, 189
  forced, 186
  ground staff exposure to, 546
  in helicopters, 188, 189, 194, 474
    effect on pilots, 198
    protection from, 197
  infrasonic, 195
  measurement of, 189
  motion sickness and, 195
  neurological effects, 195
  occupational hazard, 198
  protection from, 197
  respiratory effects of, 194
  sources of, 188
  theoretical principles, 185
  tolerance to, 196
Viral haemorrhagic fever, 525, 528
Vision,
  acceleration affecting, 144, 147
  accommodation, 394, 667
  anatomy and physiology of, 339
  autokinesis, 348
  colour sense, 345
  convergence, 394
  in decompression sickness, 21
  depth perception, 347, 394
  effect of intravascular pressure, 65
  errors during approach and
    landing, 311
  in flight, 339–351
  form sense, 344
  in high speed flight, 346
  hypoxia affecting, 55, 57
  illusions, 348, 392
  importance of, 666
  light sense, 342

Vision (*cont.*)
  monocular cues, 347
  orientation and, 282, 291
  perception, 391
  problems in VTOL aircraft, 476
  protective devices, 348
  recognition of targets, 344
  refractive conditions, 668
  retinal and actual size, 394, 395
  shape constancy, 396
  size and colour constancy, 396
  standards, 511
  stereopsis, 347, 394
  testing, 346
  uniocular, 685
  vibration and, 192, 193
Visors, 348, 349, 350, 351
Visual acuity, 344, 666
  assessment of, 686
  dynamic, 347
  examination of, 677
  in aircrew, 511
Visual cues
  during approach and landing, 311,
    397
  for orientation, 290
  from instruments, 291
Visual fields, 674
  in aircrew, 512
  examination of, 682, 686
Visual illusions, 300, 301
Visual-vestibular mismatch, 323
Vitreous humour, alcohol level in,
  706
von Karman line, 3
V/STOL aircraft,
  battle operations, 477
  cockpit in, 477
  communication in, 477
  ergonomics of, 477

V/STOL aircraft (*cont.*)
  escape from, 214, 476
  landing, 476
  medical aspects of, 475
  noise levels, 477
  visual problems, 476

Warm receptors, 236
Water,
  drinking, 535
  escape from, 263
  for survival, 271
  protection from cold in, 268
  protection from drowning, 264
  sources of, 272
Water immersion,
  clothing for, 251
  during acceleration, 162
Water vapour,
  saturation, 11
Wet bulb globe temperature index,
  232
Windblast protection, 180
Windchill index, 232
Wolff–Parkinson–White pattern, 595
Woodcock's permeability index, 230
Work efficiency, 445
Workload,
  assessment of, 440, 442
  reducing, 443
Workspace,
  design of, 455

Yellow fever, 518, 522
  immunization, 529, 530
  regulations, 523
Yerkes–Dodson law, 436, 437, 439
  stress and, 439